MEDICAL LANGUAGE

Susan M. Turley

Fourth Edition

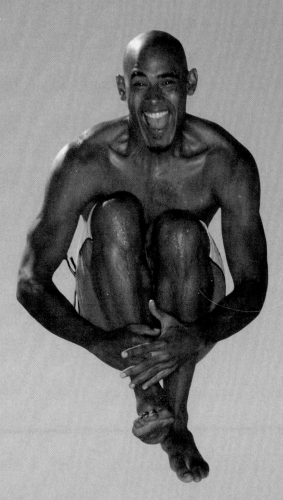

IMMERSE YOURSELF

PEARSON

Boston   Columbus   Indianapolis   New York   San Francisco
Amsterdam   Cape Town   Dubai   London   Madrid   Milan   Munich   Paris   Montreal   Toronto
Delhi   Mexico City   Sao Paulo   Sydney   Hong Kong   Seoul   Singapore   Taipei   Tokyo

Publisher: Julie Levin Alexander
Publisher's Assistant: Sarah Henrich
Executive Editor: John Goucher
Program Manager: Nicole Ragonese
Editorial Assistant: Amanda Losonsky
Development Editor: Cathy Wein
Director of Marketing: David Gesell
Marketing Manager: Brittany Hammond
Marketing Specialist: Michael Sirinides
Project Management Lead: Cynthia Zonneveld
Project Manager: Patricia Gutierrez
Operations Specialist: Mary Ann Gloriande

Art Director: Andrea Nix
Creative Director: Maria Guglielmo-Walsh
Cover/Interior Designer: Wee Group Design
Cover Art: Radius Images/Getty Images
Media Director: Amy Peltier
Lead Media Project Manager: Lorena Cerisano
Full-Service Project Management: Patty Donovan
Composition: SpiGlobal
Printer/Binder: Manufactured in the United States by RR Donnell
Cover Printer: Phoenix Color/Hagerstown
Text Font: Palatino LT Pro 9.5/13

Credits and acknowledgments for content borrowed from other sources and reproduced, with permission, in this textbook appear on appropriate pages within the text.

Library of Congress Cataloging-in-Publication Data

Names: Turley, Susan M., author.
Title: Medical Language : Immerse Yourself / Susan M. Turley.
Description: Fourth edition. | Upper Saddle River, NJ : Pearson, 2017. |
  Includes index.
Identifiers: LCCN 2015045277| ISBN 9780134318127 | ISBN 0134318129
Subjects: | MESH: Terminology as Topic--Problems and Exercises.
Classification: LCC R123 | NLM W 18.2 | DDC 610.1/4--dc23 LC record available at http://lccn.loc.gov/2015045277

V011

10 9 8 7 6 5 4 3 2 1
ISBN-13: 978-0-13-431812-7
ISBN-10: 0-13-431812-9

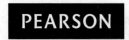

www.pearsonhighered.com

DEDICATION

To my husband Al

To my family
Daniel, Minh, Adam, Lien, and Latrise

Two Journeys

In August 2000, I began two journeys—the adoption of children into our family and the writing of this textbook. Although very different, these two journeys shared a common thread of language and communication.

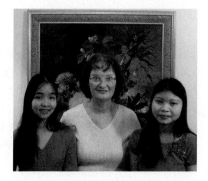

The first journey was the adoption of two beautiful children, Minh and Lien (ages 8 and 9), who joined our family from an orphanage in Vietnam in 2001. This journey of adoption involved completing much paperwork and research, learning a new language and culture, and traveling to an exotic land.

For many months prior to the adoption, nearly everything I did on a day-to-day basis was, in some way, affected by the decision to adopt. I purchased Vietnamese language study aids and began to spend an hour each day studying. A Vietnamese-American friend tutored me, teaching me Vietnamese phrases and laughed with me when I unknowingly said something I didn't intend to say. My studies were rewarded, however, when I was able to communicate with my new daughters, even as they quickly learned to speak English.

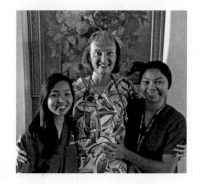

The second journey was the process of writing this textbook. This journey also involved paperwork and research, but I did not need to learn a new language or culture. Because of my many years of experience in the healthcare field, I already understood medical language and culture.

I did, however, need to determine the best way to convey that knowledge to each student who studies this textbook. And so, as I wrote, I drew on my own efforts and struggles to learn a new language during the adoption process. Those insights helped me identify with students who are learning medical language for the first time and enabled me to include textbook features that would support and strengthen students' efforts as they learned.

As I write this page in late 2015, I am ever-mindful of the many children in this country and overseas who are in need of help, food, and homes.

DID YOU KNOW?

The royalties from this textbook are given to provide ongoing financial support to orphanages and feed-and-read school programs for destitute children in several countries, as well as help poor and homeless children in the United States.

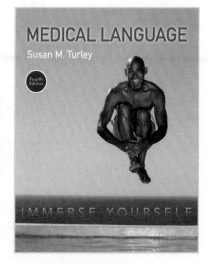

Immerse Yourself in Something Different

No new medical terminology book has touched the lives of so many people as profoundly as *Medical Language*. We credit the astounding success of the award-winning first edition and all subsequent editions to their special ability to meet the needs of students and instructors. This new fourth edition builds on our commitment to excellence, and so we have once again challenged the author and our development team (see page xvii) to critique every feature, every page, every word—all to help enhance the learning and teaching process. The result has been an integration of features that "you," our customer, have asked for and will not find in other books.

CHAPTER FORMAT

Each chapter follows a consistent organization designed for student success.

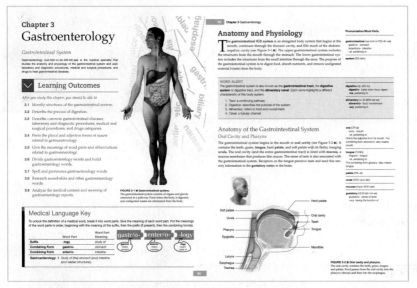

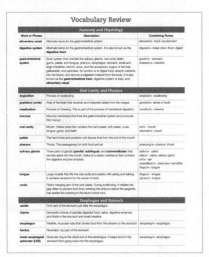

1 **Learning Outcomes/Medical Language Key**—This page focuses students on the learning outcomes for the chapter and provides a word analysis of the chapter title.

2 **Anatomy and Physiology**—This section presents the anatomy and physiology of a body system in a way that reflects the level of detail that the majority of instructors told us they need. To prepare students for the real world of health care, this section provides detailed illustrations, see-and-say pronunciations, and word parts and their meanings for each bolded word in the text.

3 **Vocabulary Review**—This section reinforces anatomy and physiology understanding with an at-a-glance review of each bolded word or phrase, its description, and related combining forms. A self-study quiz section follows with an emphasis on anatomy labeling, word parts and their meanings, and building medical words.

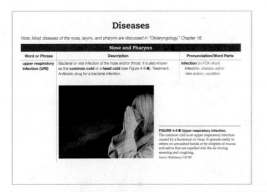

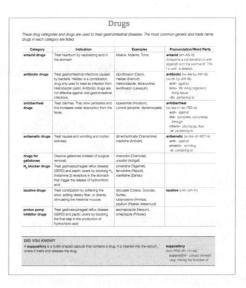

4 **Diseases and Procedures**—These sections provide descriptions, rich visuals, and treatments for diseases. Subsequent sections provide the same for laboratory, medical, and surgical procedures.

5 **Drugs**—This section describes the most common generic and trade name drugs used to treat the diseases presented in the chapter.

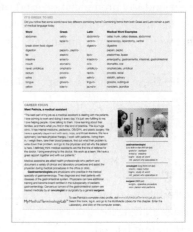

6 **Abbreviations**—This section provides a quick-reference listing of the abbreviations presented in the chapter with a caution about sound-alike abbreviations.

7 **Career Focus**—This section orients students to a different career in each chapter. A full-length, in-depth career video of a real person is online at www.MyMedicalTerminologyLab.com.

8 **Chapter Review Exercises**—This section fortifies students with a fun and extensive variety of exercises linked to each chapter learning outcome and designed for a range of learning styles.

9 **MyMedicalTerminologyLab Preview**—This end-of-chapter reminder encourages students to use the online interactive activities and games at www.MyMedicalTerminologyLab.com.

SPECIAL FEATURES

"How would you describe the ideal medical terminology textbook?" That is the question we asked our development team of students and instructors. Their responses helped us craft an array of special features that make this book unique.

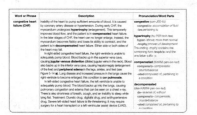

Pronunciation/Word Parts—This section is in the page margins and within various tables throughout, whenever a bolded word is introduced. It gives students the tools to understand unfamiliar words on their own—a see-and-say pronunciation guide and the word parts and meanings of each bolded word—reinforcing that word building is an ongoing process.

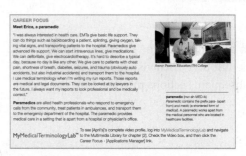

Vibrant Medical Illustrations and Photographs—These bring medical language to life and facilitate understanding, especially for visual learners.

Special Boxes—These feature boxes spark student interest with key details relating the material to the real world of medicine.

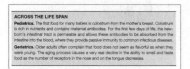

Across the Life Span—This feature box brings an infusion of relevant information related to pediatrics and geriatrics.

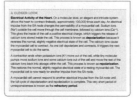

A Closer Look—This feature box presents a quick, focused glance at pertinent details related to material being covered.

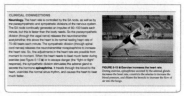

Clinical Connections—This feature box highlights the relationships between medical specialties.

Word Alert—This feature box presents important notes about the nuances, meanings, variations, and peculiarities of selected bolded words in the chapter.

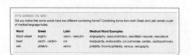

Did You Know?—This feature box showcases fun, interesting information designed to stimulate student curiosity.

Technology in Medicine—This feature box presents snapshots of the ways technology is changing health care.

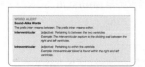

It's Greek to Me!—This feature box gives useful reminders about how Greek and Latin combining forms remain part of medical language today.

MyMedicalTerminologyLab™

www.MyMedicalTerminologyLab.com

What is MyMedicalTerminologyLab?

MyMedicalTerminologyLab is a comprehensive online program that gives you, the student, the opportunity to test your understanding of information, concepts and medical language to see how well you know the material. From the test results, MyMedicalTerminologyLab builds a self-paced, personalized study plan unique to your needs. Remediation in the form of etext pages, illustrations, exercises, audio segments, and video clips is provided for those areas in which you may need additional instruction, review, or reinforcement. You can then work through the program until your study plan is complete and you have mastered the content. MyMedicalTerminologyLab is available as a standalone program or with an embedded etext.

MyMedicalTerminologyLab is organized to follow the chapters and learning outcomes in *Medical Language*, fourth edition. With MyMedicalTerminologyLab, you can track your own progress through your entire med term course.

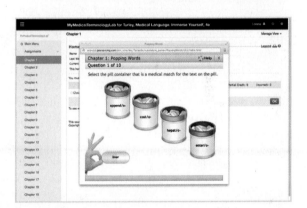

How do Students Benefit?

Here's how MyMedicalTerminologyLab helps you.

- Keep up with information presented in the text and lectures.
- Save time by focusing study and review just the content you need.
- Increase understanding of difficult concepts with study material for different learning styles.
- Remediate in areas in which you need additional review.

Key Features of MyMedicalTerminologyLab

Pre-Tests and Post-Tests. Using questions aligned to the learning outcomes in *Medical Language*, multiple tests measure your understanding of topics.

Personalized Study Material. Based on the topic pre-test results, you receive a personalized study plan, highlighting areas where you may need improvement. It includes these study tools

- Links to specific pages in the etext
- Images for review
- Interactive exercises
- Animations and video clips
- Audio glossary
- Access to full Personalized Study Material.

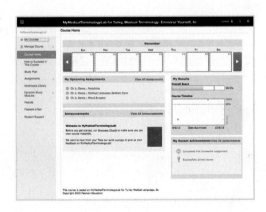

How do Instructors Benefit?

- Save time by providing students with a comprehensive, media-rich study program.
- Track student understanding of course content in the program gradebook.
- Monitor student activity with viewable student assignments.

Preface

Something Different

You may have already noticed that there is something different about this book. Perhaps by examining the cover and thumbing through the pages, you have taken note of the abundance of real-world healthcare images. Maybe you have discovered some of the practice exercises that abound within these pages, many of which place you in your soon-to-be-realized role of a healthcare professional. Or perhaps you have already begun exploring the revolutionary student media materials that are rich with highly engaging and interactive activities that add a unique dimension to your learning. As you begin this exciting and important journey into the world of medical language and health care, we offer you a single promise— that you will soon be immersed in a new, exciting learning experience.

As a soon-to-be healthcare professional, your knowledge, hard work, and interpersonal skills will have a direct impact on health care throughout your career. Therefore, we do everything we can to help you learn and to empower you so you can use what you learn to positively impact the lives of others. And so, we encourage you to immerse yourself in this book and the rich variety of resources it offers to help you learn medical language, the language of your chosen career!

The Title of This Book

Let's start at the beginning and take a close look at the title of this book: *Medical Language.*

Medical

Medicine is the drama of life and death, and few subjects are as compelling, profound, or worthy of study. This book is about real medicine that affects real patients—their lives, their families, and their futures. As a healthcare professional, no matter which aspect of health care you choose, you will have important responsibilities. Therefore, we feel it is our responsibility to provide you with as realistic a view as possible of health care today. Here are some examples of how we have done this:

- The majority of the images in this book incorporate medical illustrations and photographs that include a diverse array of real people, instead of cartoon-like illustrations. The photographs are of real patients and real healthcare professionals in real healthcare settings.

- The chapter review exercises present real medical reports with related critical-thinking questions. There are also exercises where you play the role of the healthcare professional in interpreting a patient's condition and rephrasing it as medical language.

- The student media will immerse you in the virtual world of MyMedicalTerminologyLab, where you will explore a variety of fun study opportunities. In one of them, you will listen to real doctors dictating real medical sentences for you to interpret.

- Within MyMedicalTerminologyLab, you will find the video library *Real People, Real Medicine,* which was filmed in association with this book to profile a variety of healthcare professionals on the job.

Language

A language is a method of communicating and an expression of the people, events, and culture it represents. This book is about medical language. As opposed to simply memorizing vocabulary words, this book offers a complete experience—the opportunity to embrace the world of health care, just as if you were learning a foreign language. Like traveling to Tokyo for a year to learn Japanese, the goal here is for you to become immersed in the sights and sounds of your new culture of health care. This book surrounds you with context that brings the medical words to life.

A Living Language

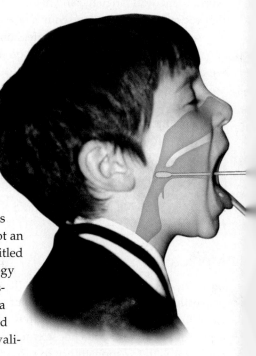

You will not be a passive reader of this book. Instead, you will be challenged to listen, speak, write, watch, respond, examine, think, and make connections. You should consume this book by writing notes in it and filling in your answers. By being an active participant in your own learning process, the concepts presented here will come alive in vibrant color and full texture. This book is a *living* document about a *living* language. Through the features of this book and the accompanying multimedia resources, you will get a true taste of the world of health care in *living* color.

You will notice that, unlike other medical terminology books, the chapters in this book are titled by medical specialties, as well as by body systems. This reflects the real world. For example, people with skin conditions visit a dermatologist, not an "integumentary system specialist." That's why the related chapter in our book is titled "Dermatology." A patient with heart problems is treated in a hospital's cardiology department and not in a "cardiovascular system department." The decision to present the chapters in this way is an example of our commitment to make this book a realistic reflection of health care as it is in the real world. This distinction was tested extensively, and instructors and students alike overwhelmingly supported and validated this way to learn.

Immerse Yourself!

You are about to begin an interactive learning experience between you, this book, and your instructor—one that will equip you and inspire you to become an expert in medical language. The goal of this book is to connect with you, to engage your visual, auditory, and kinesthetic senses, to stimulate you, and to fuel your complete understanding of medical language. As you engage in the multisensory experience within these pages, remember to *discover, learn, know,* and *understand* the information. But—even more—experience it and ***live it!*** So dive in and immerse yourself!

New to This Edition

This new fourth edition maintains the best aspects of previous editions while continuing to facilitate the learner's mastery of medical language. We have revised this edition so that it provides an even more valuable teaching and learning experience. Here are the enhancements that we have made:

- Learning outcomes whose numbers are correlated to all parts of the text and to all review exercises.
- Many **new, updated medical photos** and medically realistic, and newly enhanced medical illustrations.
- Updated word part meanings that are now alphabetized for easier memorization.
- Updated abbreviations and drug names related to the chapter.
- Additional medical reports and questions at the end of the chapter.
- A new format that is compatible with any device that a student might use to view the e-text.
- **Updated review exercises** to give you more practice with dividing and building medical words. Also new exercises for forming the plurals and adjectives of medical nouns. And new exercises for researching the meanings of what can be confusing sound-alike medical words.
- A new Answer Key that only includes every other answer. This encourages students to think for themselves about the answers, rather than just copying them from the Answer Key. A full Answer Key is provided to the instructor. This format now allows the instructor to use any exercise as a homework assignment that contributes to the student's overall grade.

What Makes This Book Different

We Listened

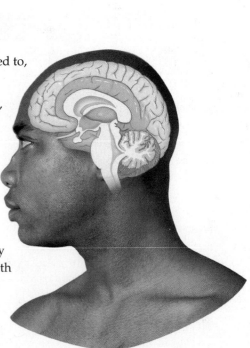

In developing this book over four editions, we have immersed ourselves in the perspective of you, our readers. We have strived to make *Medical Language* a customer-driven text by aggressively and comprehensively researching the needs and desires of current medical terminology students and instructors. We aimed to guarantee that we were "speaking the same language" as those who would ultimately be using this book. To do this, we gathered a highly qualified development team of over 160 reviewers, with over 2,250 years of teaching experience, four physician specialists, as well as 11 students from across the United States to help steer us toward success.

Over the past 14 years we sat in classrooms, hosted focus groups, and conducted thorough manuscript reviews. We asked for blunt and uncompromising opinions and insights. We also commissioned dozens of detailed reviews from instructors, asking them to analyze and evaluate each chapter of the textbook. They not only told us what they did and didn't like, but they identified, page by page, numerous ways in which we could refine and enhance our key features. Their invaluable feedback was compiled, analyzed, and incorporated throughout *Medical Language*, 4th edition.

We asked our team to imagine their ideal medical terminology book—what it should include, how it should look. We had the author meet personally with several instructors to discuss the specifics of the book's organization, layout, format, and features. We asked question after question. This book is truly the product of a successful partnership between the author, the publisher, and our development team of students and instructors. We listened.

And We Learned

Here are some of the recommendations that we heard from our team, responded to, and included in all four editions:

- **Design**. Students and instructors alike told us they wanted an appealing, uncluttered design with lots of rich images and enough white space to allow for notetaking.

- **Exercises**. Both students and instructors suggested that we provide a greater quantity and variety of exercises than any other book, thus providing maximum opportunities to reinforce learning. Instructors asked that we only provide the answers to some of the exercises so that the exercises could become graded homework assignments.

- **Illustrations**. Students and instructors alike suggested that we display colorful and interesting illustrations as large as possible on the page, with opportunities to label those images as practice opportunities.

- **Special Feature Boxes**. Students asked for highlighted boxes that would help break up the reading and also provide them with opportunities to learn something new or interesting, thereby providing additional context.

- **Medical Specialties Approach**. A substantial majority (75%) of instructors told us that they wanted a medical specialties approach, rather than an approach based only on body systems.

- **Focus on Word Building**. Another substantial majority of instructors (over 70%) told us that they wanted a focus on word building with analysis of combining forms, suffixes, and prefixes right within the text and not just at the end of each chapter or in isolated boxes.

- **Medical Report Activities**. Instructors wanted an activity in each chapter that challenged students to analyze actual medical reports.

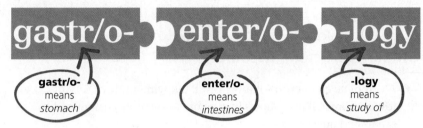

- **Lecture Support Materials**. Instructors told us about the increased challenge of creating interesting lectures and suggested that we create a fully loaded PowerPoint presentation system complete with a multitude of illustrations and photographs, plus animations and embedded, real-life medical videos. In addition, we created Guided Lectures, a comprehensive auditory and visual learning experience, narrated by the author. It includes the PowerPoint presentation coordinated with a full lecture, including the author's many personal experiences in various healthcare fields. This is an especially helpful feature for students enrolled in online courses or for students who miss a lecture.

- **Tools for Testing**. Instructors asked for a complete testing package that is customizable to fit their needs. Additionally, they asked for these test items to be available in online course formats.

A Commitment to Accuracy

As part of our respect for real medicine, and the importance of getting it right the first time, we made a commitment to accuracy. It was important to us to attain the highest level of accuracy possible throughout this educational package in order to match the precision required in today's healthcare environment. The author drew on her 30 years of experience in nursing, health information management, medical transcription, medical publications, and as a college instructor to provide accurate and complete information. Our development team read every page, every test question, and every vocabulary word. No less than 12 content experts read each chapter for accuracy and analyzed every bit of content in the ancillary resources. We also engaged the technical editing services of four physician specialists who carefully reviewed the chapters that correspond to their respective practices.

We welcome any and all feedback you may have to help us enhance the accuracy of this book. If you identify any errors that need to be corrected in a subsequent printing, please send them to: Pearson Health Science Editorial, Medical Terminology Corrections.

COMPREHENSIVE TEACHING PACKAGE

Perhaps the most gratifying part of an instructor's work is the "aha" learning moment when the light bulb goes on and a student truly understands a concept—when that connection is made. Along these lines, Pearson is pleased to help instructors foster more of these educational connections by providing a complete suite of resources to support teaching and learning. Qualified adopters are eligible to receive a wealth of tools designed to help instructors prepare, present, and assess. For more information, please contact your Pearson sales representative or visit www.pearsonhighered.com/educator.

Online Instructor's Resources

- A complete chapter-by-chapter Test Bank with a full variety of test questions. It also allows instructors to generate customized exams and quizzes.

- A comprehensive, turn-key lecture package with fully narrated chapter-by-chapter lectures by the author ("Guided Lectures") in an audio format, as well as an accompanying PowerPoint presentation containing discussion points and images, animations, and videos.

- A sample course syllabus.

- PowerPoint content to support instructors who are using Personal Response Systems ("clickers").

- A complete image library that includes every photograph and illustration from the book.

- Articles with useful ideas, such as classroom management tips, how to construct test questions, and how to put students at ease on the first day of class.

- Nearly 100 ready-made worksheets that can be used for quizzes or homework assignments.

- An array of teaching pearls and tips.

- Interesting facts and anecdotes.

- Extra content, such as word origins and the stories behind anatomical structures and diseases named for someone (eponymns)—things not covered in the book.

- A complete Answer Key that includes the answers to each of the student questions in each chapter.

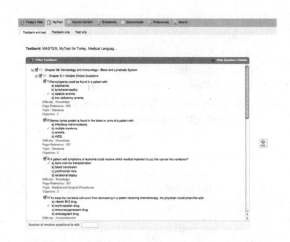

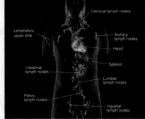

Click on the screenshot to view an animation on the topic of the lymphatic system.

Our Development Team

We can truly say that each individual on our development team has infused this book with ideas, vision, and passion for medical language. Our team crafted the blueprints for this book and contributed to this landmark educational tool. Their influence will continue to have an impact for decades to come. We are pleased to introduce the members of our team.

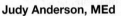

Physician Specialist Consultants

Stephen Caldwell, MD
Director of Hepatology
Digestive Health Center of Excellence
Charlottesville, Virginia

John H. Dirckx, MD
Former Medical Director
University of Dayton
Student Health Center
Dayton, Ohio

Joseph Gibbons, MD
Internal Medicine Physician
Centennial Medical Group
Elkridge, Maryland

James Michelson, MD
Professor of Orthopedic Surgery
George Washington University
School of Medicine
Washington, D.C.

Quality Assurance Editor

Garnet Tomich, BA
San Diego, California

Ancillary Content Providers

James F. Allen, Jr., RN, BSN, MBA/HCM, JD
Lansing Community College
Lansing, Michigan

Michael Battaglia, MS, Ed
Greenville Technical College
Greenville, South Carolina

Dale Brewer, BS, MEd, CMA, (AAMA)
Pensacola Junior College
Pensacola, Florida

Dean Chiarelli, MA, RD, HFS, CHES
Arizona State University
Phoenix, Arizona

Dianne Davis, BS, MS, ABD EdD
West Virginia University at Parkersburg
Parkersburg, West Virginia

Sarah E.W. Finch, PhD
Florida State College at Jacksonville
Jacksonville, Florida

Jean M. Krueger-Watson, PhD
Clark College
Vancouver, Washington

Angela Moderow, PT, MPT
Carolinas Rehabilitation
Charlotte, North Carolina

Janet Pandzik, MS, CMT, RMA
Good Careers Academy
San Antonio, Texas

Garnet Tomich, BA
San Diego, California

Katherine Twomey, MLS
Greenville Technical College
Greenville, South Carolina

Manuscript Reviewers
(*Reviewer conference attendee)

Denise M. Abrams, PT, MASS
SUNY Broome Community College
Appalachian, New York

Betsy Adams, AAS, BS, MSBE
Alamance Community College
Graham, North Carolina

Mercedes Alafriz-Gordon, BS
High Tech Institute
Phoenix, Arizona

Diana Alagna, RN, AHI, CPT
Branford Hall Career Institute
Southington, Connecticut

Jana Allen, BS, MT*
Volunteer State Community College
Gallatin, Tennessee

Pam Anania, RN, APRN, MSN
Brookdale Community College
Lincroft, New Jersey

Ellen Anderson, RHIA
College of Lake County
Northfield, Illinois

Judy Anderson, MEd
Coastal Carolina Community College
Jacksonville, North Carolina

Wendy Anderson
MTI College
Sacramento, California

Lori Andreucci, MEd, CMT, CMA
Gateway Technical College
Racine, Wisconsin

Leah Beall, CST, BS
Fortis College
Westerville, Ohio

Debbie Bedford, CMA, AAS
North Seattle Community College
Seattle, Washington

Tricia Berry, OTR/L
Hamilton College
Urbandale, Iowa

Sue Biederman, MSHP, RHIA
Texas State University
San Marcos, Texas

Richard Boan, BS, MS, PhD
Midlands Technical College
Columbia, South Carolina

Jennifer Boles, MSN, RN, NCSN
Cincinnati State Technical and
Community College
Cincinnati, Ohio

Julie E. Boles, MS, RHIA
Ithaca College
Ithaca, New York

Annie M. Boster, PT
Bishop State Community College
Mobile, Alabama

Susan A. Boulden, RN
Mt. Hood Community College
Aloha, Oregon

Beth Braun, MA, PhD
Truman College
Chicago, Illinois

Shannon Bruley, BAS, AEMT-IC
Henry Ford Community College
Dearborn, Michigan

Juanita R. Bryant, CMA-A/C
Sierra College
Penn Valley, California

Thomas Bubar, BA, MS
Erie Community College
Williamsville, New York

Susan Buboltz, RN, MS, CMA
Madison Area Technical College
Madison, Wisconsin

Patricia Bufalino, MA, MN, RN, FNP
Riverside Community College
Moreno Valley, California

Ginger Bushway
Mendocino College
Ukiah, California

Mary Butler, BS
Collin County Community College
McKinney, Texas

Toni Cade, MBA, RHIA, CCS, FAHIMA
University of Louisiana at Lafayette
Lafayette, Louisiana

Cara L. Carreon, BS, RRT, CMA, CPC
Ivy Tech Community College
Lafayette, Indiana

Rafael Castilla, MD
Ho Ho Kus School
Ramsey, New Jersey

Julia I. Chapman, BS
Stark State College of Technology
North Canton, Ohio

Dean Chiarelli, MA, RD, HFS, CHES
Arizona State University
Phoenix, Arizona

Kim Christmon, BS, RRT
Volunteer State Community College
Gallatin, Tennessee

Paula-Beth Ciolek
National College of Business and
Technology
Richmond, Kentucky

Deresa Claybrook, MS, RHIT
Oklahoma City Community College
Oklahoma City, Oklahoma

Mike Cochran, BA, RT(R)(CT), ARRT, VSRT, SWDSRT
Southwest Virginia Community
College
Richlands, Virginia

Christine Cole, CCA
Williston State College
Williston, North Dakota

Ronald Coleman, EdD
Volunteer State Community College
Gallatin, Tennessee

Bonnie Crist
Harrison College
Indianapolis, Indiana

Cathleen Currie, RN, BS
College of Southern Idaho
Twin Falls, Idaho

Dianne Davis, BS, MS, ABD EdD
West Virginia University at Parkersburg
Parkersburg, West Virginia

Denise J. DeDeaux, AAS, BS, MBA*
Fayetteville Technical Community
College
Fayetteville, North Carolina

Anita Denson, BS, CMA
National College of Business and
Technology
Danville, Kentucky

Susan D. Dooley, CMT*
Seminole Community College
Sorrento, Florida

Robert Fanger, MSEd
Del Mar College
Corpus Christi, Texas

Sarah E.W. Finch, PhD
Florida State College at Jacksonville
Jacksonville, Florida

Vickie Findley, MPA, RHIA
Fairmont State College
Fairmont, West Virginia

Kathie Folsom, MS, BSN, RN
Skagit Valley College—Whidbley Island
Campus
Oak Harbor, Washington

Joyce Foster
State Fair Community College
Sedalia, Missouri

Elaine Garcia, RHIT
Spokane Community College
Spokane, Washington

Suzanne B. Garrett, MSA, RHIA
Central Florida Community College
Ocala, Florida

Cheryl Gates, RN, MSN, PHN
Cerro Coso Community College
Ridgecrest, California

Barbara E. Geary, RN, MA
North Seattle Community College
Seattle, Washington

Paige Gebhardt, RMT
Sussex County Community College
Newton, New Jersey

Laura Ristrom Goodman, MSSW
Pima Medical Institute
Tucson, Arizona

Patricia Goshorn, MA, RN, CMA-AC
Cosumnes River College
Sacramento, California

Debra Griffin, RN, BSN
Tidewater Community College
Virginia Beach, Virginia

Dawn Guzicki, RN
Detroit Business Institute—Downriver
Riverview, Michigan

Paula Hagstrom, MM, RHIA
Ferris State University
Big Rapids, Michigan

Dotty Hall, RN, MSN, CST
Ivy Tech Community College
Lafayette, Indiana

Karen Hardney, MSEd, RT
Chicago State University
Chicago, Illinois

Marie Hattabaugh, RT(R)(M)
Pensacola Junior College
Pensacola, Florida

Tiffany Heath, CMA, CMAS, AHI, CS
Porter and Chester Institute
Chicopee, Massachusetts

Barbara L. Henry, RN, BSN
Gateway Technical College
Racine, Wisconsin

Forrest Heredia
Pima Medical Institute
Tucson, Arizona

Cathy Hess, RHIA
Texas State University
San Marcos, Texas

Dori L. Hess, MS, LMT, BS
Stark State College of Technology
Canton, Ohio

Jan C. Hess, MA
Metropolitan Community College
Omaha, Nebraska

Denise M. Hightower, RHIA
Cape Fear Community College
Wilmington, North Carolina

Beulah A. Hofmann, RN, MSN, CMA
Ivy Tech Community College
Greencastle, Indiana

Valentina Holder, MA.Ed, RHIA
Pitt Community College
Winterville, North Carolina

Joe Horan
Seacoast Career School
Manchester, New Hampshire

Pamela S. Huber, MS, MT(ASCP)
Erie Community College
Williamsville, New York

James E. Hudacek, MSEd*
Loraine County Community College
Amherst, Ohio

Bud W. Hunton, MA, RT (R) (QM)
Sinclair Community College
Dayton, Ohio

Karen Jackson, NR-CMA
Remington College
Garland, Texas

Donna Jimison RN, MSN
Cuyahoga Community College
Parma, Ohio

Timothy J. Jones, MA
Oklahoma City Community College
Oklahoma City, Oklahoma

Kathleen Kearney, BS, MEd, EMT-P
Kent State University
Kent, Ohio

**Cathy Kelley-Arney,
CMA, MLTC, BSHS, AS**
National College of Business
and Technology
Bluefield, Virginia

Winifred Khalil, RN, MS
San Diego Mesa College
San Diego, California

Heather Kies, MHA
Goodwin College
East Hartford, Connecticut

Jan Klawitter, CMA (AAMA), CPC
San Joaquin Valley College
Bakersfield, California

Marsha Lalley, BSM, MSM
Minneapolis Community and Technical
College
Minneapolis, Minnesota

Joyce Lammers, PT, MHS, PCS
University of Findlay
Findlay, Ohio

Carol A. Lehman, ART
Hocking College
Nelsonville, Ohio

Sandra Lehrke, MS, RN
Anoka Technical Community College
Anoka, Minnesota

Randall M. Levin, FACEP
Sanford Brown College
Milwaukee, Wisconsin

Maria Teresa Lopez-Hill, MS
Laredo Community College
Laredo, Texas
Bow Valley College
Calgary, Alberta
Collin County Community College
McKinney, Texas

Michelle Lovings, BA
Missouri College
Brentwood, Missouri

Carol Loyd, MSN, RN
University of Arkansas
Community College
Morrilton, Arkansas

Patricia McLane, RHIA, MA
Henry Ford Community College
Dearborn, Michigan

Michael C. McMinn, MA, RRT
Mott Community College
Flint, Michigan

Aimee Michaelis
Pima Medical Institute
Denver, Colorado

Michelle G. Miller, M, CMA, COMT
Lakeland Community College
Kirtland, Ohio

Ann Minks, FAAMT
Lake Washington Technical College
Kirkland, Washington

Suzanne Moe, RN
Northwest Technical College
Bemidji, Minnesota

Barbara S. Moffet, PhD, RN
Southeastern Louisiana University
Hammond, Louisiana

**Debby Montone, BS, RN,
CCS-P, RCVT**
Eastwick College/Ho Ho Kus Schools
Ramsey, New Jersey

Karen Myers, CPC
Pierce College Puyallup
Puyallup, Washington

Gloria Newton, MA-ED
Shasta College
Redding, California

Amanda Niebur, BA
Minneapolis Business College
Roseville, Minnesota

Erin Nixon, RN
Bakersfield College
Bakersfield, California

**Alice M. Noblin, MBA, RHIA,
CCS, LHRM**
University of Central Florida
Orlando, Florida

Wendy Oguz, AS, BA
National College
Indianapolis, Indiana

Evie O'Nan, RMA
National College
Florence, Kentucky

Kerry Openshaw, PhD
Bemidji State University
Bemidji, Minnesotta

Bob Osborn
Lansing Community College
Lansing, Michigan

Janet Pandzik, MS, CMT, RMA
Good Careers Academy
San Antonio, Texas

Mirella G. Pardee, MSN, RN
University of Toledo
Toledo, Ohio

Sherry Pearsall, MSN
Bryant & Stratton College
Liverpool, New York

Tina Peer, MS, RN
The College of Southern Idaho
Twin Falls, Idaho

Tammie C. Petersen, RNC-OB, BSN
Austin Community College
Austin, Texas

Susan Prion, EdD, RN
University of San Francisco
San Francisco, California

Mary Rahr, MS, RN, CMA
Northeast Wisconsin Technical College
Madison, Wisconsin

Edilberto A. Raynes, MD
Tennessee State University
Nashville, Tennessee

Deward Reece, DC
Sanford Brown College
Milwaukee, Wisconsin

**Joy Renfro, EdD, RHIA, CMA,
CCS-P, CPC**
Eastern Kentucky University
Richmond, Kentucky

**Sheila G. Rockoff, EdD, MSN,
BSN, AS, RN**
Santa Ana College
Santa Ana, California

Mary Sayles, RN, MSN
Sierra College—Nevada County Campus
Rocklin, California

Jody E. Scheller, MS, RHIA
Schoolcraft College
Garden City, Michigan

Patricia Schrull, MSN, MBA, MEd, RN
Lorain County Community College
Elyria, Ohio

**Theresa R. Schuldt, MEd, HT/HTL
(ASCP)** Rose State College
Midwest City, Oklahoma

Jan Sesser, BS, RMA (AMT), CMA
High Tech Institute
Phoenix, Arizona

Julie A. Shellenbarger, MBA, RHIA
University of Northwestern Ohio
Lima, Ohio

Donna Sue Shellman, MA, CPC
Gaston College
Dallas, North Carolina

Karin Sherrill, BSN
Mesa Community College
Gilbert, Arizona

Vicki Simpson, PhD, RN, CHES
Purdue University West Lafayette
West Lafayette, Indiana

Paula Silver, PharmD
ECPI University
Newport News, Virginia

Erin Sitterley
North Seattle Community College
Seattle, Washington

Tim J. Skaife, RT(R), MA
National Park Community College
Hot Springs, Arizona

Lynn G. Slack, CMA
ICM School of Business and
Medical Careers
Pittsburgh, Pennsylvania

Ellie Smith, RN, MSN
Cuesta College
San Luis Obispo, California

Sherman K. Sowby, PhD, CHES
California State University—Fresno
Fresno, California

Darla K. Sparacino, MEd, RHIA
Arkansas Tech University
Russelville, Arkansas

Carolyn Stariha, BS, RHIA
Houston Community College—
Coleman Campus
Houston, Texas

Kathy Stau, CPhT
Medix School
Smyrna, Georgia

Twila Sterling-Guillory, RN, MSN
McNeese State University
Lake Charles, Louisiana

Deb Stockberger, MSN, RN
North Iowa Community College
Mason City, Iowa

Paula L. Stoltz, CMT-F
Medical Transcription Education Center
Fairlawn, Ohio

Diane Swift
State Fair Community College
Sedalia, Missouri

J. David Taylor, PhD, PT, CSCS
University of Central Arkansas
Conway, Arkansas

Sylvia Taylor, CMA, CPCA
Cleveland State Community College
Cleveland, Tennessee

Jean Ternus, RN, MS
Kansas City Community College
Kansas City, Kansas

Cindy B. Thompson, BSRT, MA*
Alamance Community College
Graham, North Carolina

Lenette Thompson, CST
Piedmont Technical College
Greenwood, South Carolina

Margaret A. Tiemann, RN, BS
St. Charles Community College
Cottleville, Missouri

Mary Jane Tremethick, PhD, RN, CHES
Northern Michigan University
Marquette, Michican

Valeria D. Truitt, BS, MAEd
Craven Community College
New Bern, North Carolina

Christine Tufts-Maher, MS, RHIA
Seminole Community College
Altamonte Springs, Florida

**Pam Ventgen, CMA (AAMA),
CCS-P, CPC, CPC-I**
University of Alaska Anchorage
Anchorage, Alaska

Patricia Von Knorring
Tacoma Community College
Gig Harbor, Washington

**Jane C. Walker, BBA, PhD, RN,
ASLNC-C, CPN, CNE**
Walters State Community College
Morristown, Tennessee

Mary Warren-Oliver, BA
Gibbs College
Vienna, Virginia

Kristen Waterstram-Rich, MS, CNMT
Rochester Institute of Technology
Rochester, New York

Kim Webb, RN, MN
Northern Oklahoma College
Tonkawa, Oklahoma

Richard Weidman, RHIA, CCS-P
Tacoma Community College
Tacoma, Washington

Bonnie Welniak, RN, MSN
Monroe County Community College
Monroe, Michigan

Connie Werner, MS, RHIA
York College of Pennsylvania
York, Pennsylvania

Victoria Lee Wetle, RN, EdD
Chemeketa Community College
Salem, Oregon

David J. White, MA, MLIS
Baylor University
Waco, Texas

Jay W. Wilborn, MEd, MT(ASCP)
National Park Community College
Hot Springs, Arkansas

Tammy L. Wilder, RN, MSN, CMSRN
Ivy Tech Community College
Evansville, Indiana

Antionette Woodall
Remington College-Cleveland
North Olmsted, Ohio

Scott Zimmer, MS
Metropolitan Community College
Omaha, Nebraska

Focus Group Participants

Kim Anthony Aaronson, BS, DC
Harry S. Truman College
Chicago, Illinois
Harold Washington College
Chicago, Illinois

Kendra J. Allen, LPN
Ohio Institute of Health Careers
Columbus, Ohio

Delena Kay Austin, BTIS, CMA
Macomb Community College
Clinton Township, Michigan

Molly Baxter
Baker College—Port Huron
Port Huron, Michigan

Joan Berry, RN, MSN, CNS
Lansing Community College
Lansing, Michigan

Kenneth Bretl, MA, RRT
College of DuPage
Glen Ellyn, Illinois

Carole Bretscher
Southwestern College
Bellrook, Ohio

Adrienne L. Carter, MEd, NRMA
Riverside Community College
Moreno Valley, California

Mary Dudash-White, MA, RHIA, CCS
Sinclair Community College
Dayton, Ohio

Cathy Flite, MEd, RHIA
Temple University
Philadelphia, Pennsylvania

Sherry Gamble, RN, CNS, MSN, CNOR
University of Akron
Akron, Ohio

Mary Garcia, BA, AD, RN
Northwestern Business College
Northeastern Illinois University
Truman College
Chicago, Illinois

Joyce Garozzo, MS, RHIA, CCS
Community College of Philadelphia
Philadelphia, Pennsylvania

Patsy Gehring, PhD, RN, CS
Lakeland Community College
Kirkland, Ohio

Michelle Heller, CMA, RMA
Ohio Institute of Health Careers
Columbus, Ohio

Janet Hossli
Northwestern Business College
Chicago, Illinois

Trudi James-Parks, RT, BS,
Lorain County Community College
Elyria, Ohio

Sherry L. Jones, RN, ASN
Western School of Health and Business
Community College of Allegheny County
Pittsburgh, Pennsylvania

Esther H. Kim
Chicago State University
Chicago, Illinois

Richelle S. Laipply, PhD, CMA
University of Akron
Akron, Ohio

Andrea M. Lane, CMA-C, BAS RN, MS
Brookdale Community College
Lincroft, New Jersey

Mary Lou Liebal, BS, RTR, MA
Cuyahoga Community College
Cleveland, Ohio

Stacey Long, BS
Miami Jacobs Career College
Dayton, Ohio

Anne Loochtan, MEd
Columbus State Community College
Cincinnati, Ohio

Anne M. Lunde, BS, CMT
Waubonsee Community College
Sugar Grove, Illinois

Janice Manning, MA, PCP
Baker College
Jackson, Michigan

Sandy Marks, RN, MS(HCA)
Cerritos College
Norwalk, California

Kathleen Masters, MS, RN
Monroe County Community College
Monroe, Michigan

Mary Morgan, MS, CNMT
Columbus State Community College
Columbus, Ohio

Andrew Muniz, OT, BBA, MBA
Baker College
Auburn Hills, Michigan

Michael Murphy, AAS, CMA, CLP
Berdan Institute
Union, New Jersey

Stephen Nardozzi, BA
SUNY-Westchester Community College
Valhalla, New York

Ruth Ann O'Brien, MHA, RRT
Miami Jacobs Career College
Dayton, Ohio

Donna Schnepp, MHA, RHIA
Moraine Valley Community College
Palos Hills, Illinois

Ann M. Smith, MS
Joliet Junior College
Joliet, Illinois

Mark Velderrain
Cerritos College
Norwalk, California

**Jane C. Walker, BBA, RN,
ASLNC-C, CPN, CNE**
Walters State Community College
Morristown, Tennessee

Barbara Wiggins, MT(ASCP)
Delaware Technical & Community
College
Georgetown, Delaware

**Gail S. Williams, Ph.D., MT(ASCP)SBB,
CLS(NCA)**
Northern Illinois University
DeKalb, Illinois

Karen Wright, RHIA, MHA
Hocking College
Nelsonville, Ohio

Student Advisors

Tobi Burch
Community College of Philadelphia
Philadelphia, Pennsylvania

Calvin Byrd
Temple University
Philadelphia, Pennsylvania

Kimberly Clark
Community College of Philadelphia
Philadelphia, Pennsylvania

Susan DiMaria
Brookdale Community College
Lincroft, New Jersey

Avelina Elam
Thomas Jefferson University
Philadelphia, Pennsylvania

Michael Flores
Berdan Institute
Union, New Jersey

Frederick Herbert
Temple University
Philadelphia, Pennsylvania

Brenda Merlino
Thomas Jefferson University
Philadelphia, Pennsylvania

Megan Milos
Ocean County College
Toms River, New Jersey

Payam Mohadjeri
Temple University
Philadelphia, Pennsylvania

Monica Narang
Westchester Community College
Valhalla, New York

Medical Terminology Advisory Board

Jeff Anderson, MA, RRT
Boise State University
Boise, ID

Beverly Bartholomew, M.Ed, CPC
Wake Tech Community College
Raleigh, NC

Amy Bolinger Snow, MS
Greenville Technical College
Greenville, SC

Richard Brown, MS, CPhT /RPT
Program Chair, MAA/MOBS
Ultimate Medical Academy
Clearwater, FL

Kerry Cirillo, MS, BS
Mildred Elley
New York, NY

Rosana Darang, MD, Dept. Chair
Bay State College
Boston, MA

Robert Fanger, MSEd
Del Mar College
Corpus Christi, TX

Gerry Gordon, BA CPC, CPB
Daytona College
Ormond Beach, FL

Timothy J. Jones, BA, MA (English),
MA (Classics)
Oklahoma City Community College
Oklahoma City, Oklahoma
The University of Oklahoma
Norman, Oklahoma

Tammie Petersen, RNC, BSN
Austin Community College
Austin, TX

About the Author

Susan M. Turley, MA (Educ), BSN, RN, RHIT, CMT, is a full-time author and editor. In the recent past, she was an adjunct professor in the School of Health, Wellness, and Physical Education at Anne Arundel Community College in Arnold, Maryland, where she taught courses in medical terminology and pharmacology. She was instrumental in gaining initial accreditation for the college's medical assisting program.

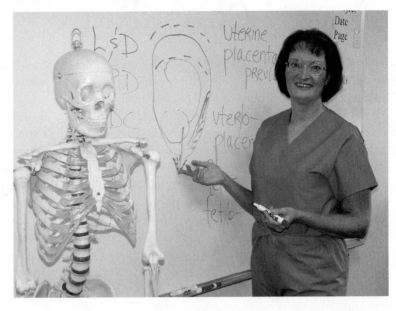

As a healthcare professional, Susan has worked in a variety of healthcare settings: acute care/ICU, long-term care, physicians' offices, and managed care. She has held positions as an intensive care nurse, plasmapheresis nurse, infection control officer, physician office auditor, medical transcriptionist, medical writer/editor for physician publications, director of education, and director of quality management and corporate compliance for an HMO.

Susan is also the author of *Understanding Pharmacology for Health Professionals, 5th edition* (Pearson, 2016) and more than 40 articles published in medical transcription and health information management journals. She is a codeveloper of *The SUM Program for Medical Transcription Training* and reference books for Health Professions Institute. With physician coauthors, she has written three nationally funded grants, two chapters in physicians' anesthesiology and ENT textbooks, and numerous abstracts and articles published in nationally known medical journals.

She has been a guest speaker at national seminars for accreditation of utilization management programs, medical transcription teacher training, and health information management certification exam review.

Susan holds a Master of Arts degree in adult education from Norwich University in Vermont, a Bachelor of Science degree in nursing from the Pennsylvania State University, and has state licensure as an RN. She is a member and has national certification in medical transcription from the Association for Healthcare Documentation Integrity (AHDI) and is a member and has national certification from the American Health Information Management Association (AHIMA).

About the Illustrator

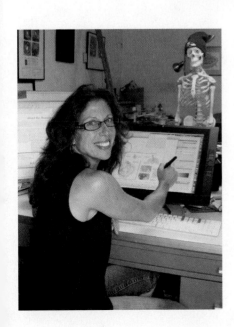

The illustrations throughout this book were carefully coordinated through a close collaborative effort between the author and artist. Every figure was custom developed specifically for this book, and refined to be medically accurate, precise, unique, and fresh. From a pedagogical point of view, it was important that all of the art be consistent throughout, rather than presenting a conglomeration of styles and levels of detail.

Anita Impagliazzo is a medical illustrator and designer in Charlottesville, Virginia. A graduate of the University of Virginia, she went on to complete the Biomedical Illustration Graduate Program at the University of Texas Southwestern Medical Center at Dallas and spent several years specializing in illustrating for medical malpractice litigation. She has been self-employed since 2001, planning, creating, and collaborating on artwork for the University of Virginia Health System, for medical malpractice defense attorneys nationwide, and for multiple journals and textbooks (including the popular *Martini Human Anatomy and Physiology* series, and the revered *Netter Collection of Medical Illustrations*). She is a member of the Association of Medical Illustrators and has received several awards in its annual juried salons. She never tires of using medical language to learn new things about the human body: how it works, how it fails, how it is fixed, and how the fixing fails.

About the Educational Consultant

James F. Allen, Jr., RN, BSN, MBA/HCM, JD, is an Adjunct Associate Professor at Lansing Community College in Lansing, Michigan. He earned both his bachelor's degree in nursing (BSN) and a master's of business administration in healthcare management (MBA/HCM) from the University of Phoenix. He also earned his Juris Doctorate (JD) from Thomas M. Cooley School of Law. Jim has taught courses in medical terminology, pathophysiology, pharmacology, and medical law and ethics. Since his college adopted the first edition of *Medical Language*, Jim has been an invaluable source of information and suggestions for the improvement of *Medical Language*. Jim is the co-author of *Medical Language Stat!* (Pearson, 2009, out of print) and the author of *Health Law and Medical Ethics for Healthcare Professionals* (Pearson, 2013).

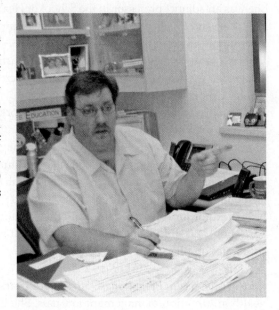

To the Pearson Development Team

My utmost thanks go to John Goucher, Executive Acquisitions Editor for *Medical Language*, for the very successful 3rd and 4th editions of this textbook.

My sincere thanks go to Mark Cohen, former Pearson Health Science Editor-in-Chief for the 1st and 2nd editions. (He is now the Head of Concept Development for Pearson Higher Learning.) His initial vision of this book was one with mine, but he also envisioned the next level of excellence and expertly guided this book from idea to reality.

My gratitude and thanks go to Anita Impagliazzo, my medical illustrator. She embraced much more than her original role and quickly became a creative collaborator and advisor for all four editions. She is a wonderfully talented medical illustrator whose efforts made this book medically accurate, artistically unique, and without equal. By combining real-life people with superimposed medical illustrations, she created a never-before-seen level of medical realism, to the delight of the author and the awe of students and instructors alike.

My sincere thanks go to Cathy Wein, my development editor. She coordinated communication, manuscript copyediting review, art spec sheets, and deadlines for everyone involved. Her professional expertise was a constant through all four editions, and they would have been difficult to complete without her all-encompassing and timely editorial assistance and personal support.

My thanks go to Pearson design directors for creating a new design and format that is now accessible to all devices and across all platforms.

My thanks go to all of members of the Pearson team from editorial assistants to program managers to marketing managers and sales representatives to the executive editors and the publisher!

My thanks go to the talented team at SPi Global, led by Patty Donovan, Senior Production Editor, who oversaw the extensive editing, layout, typesetting and indexing of the fourth edition. In light of the complexity of the book, I especially appreciated her professionalism, flexibility, creative insights, and can-do approach.

My thanks go to the Pearson media team that designed and produced a spectacular array of learning applications to support my textbook.

My thanks go to Sally Pitman of Health Professions Institute for granting permission for using authentic medical dictation from *The SUM Program for Medical Transcription Training* as exercises in online activities in MyMedicalTerminologyLab.

To Students and Instructors

As the author, my thanks go to the many classes of students who motivated me to continually research and present medical language clearly and thoroughly. It was their warm response to my teaching methods and materials that encouraged me to keep improving in the classroom and throughout all four editions of the textbook.

My thanks go to the many instructors and practitioners—my colleagues—who have overwhelmingly validated my efforts to write about medical language with a uniquely interesting, lively, and fresh approach. Each and every person listed played an important role in the development of this book, and I hope they share my sense of pride and accomplishment in this fourth edition.

Contents

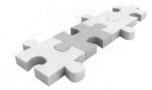
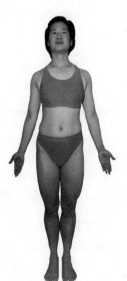
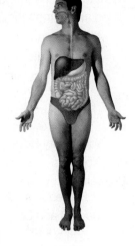
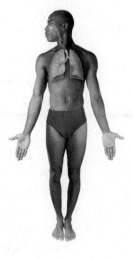

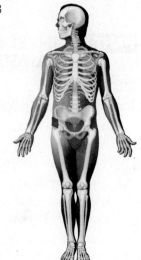
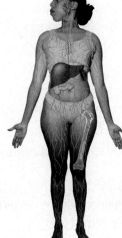
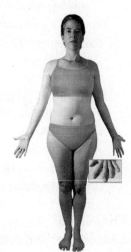

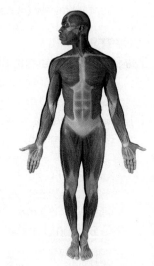
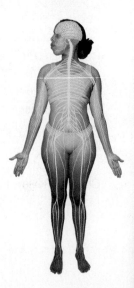

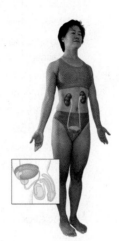

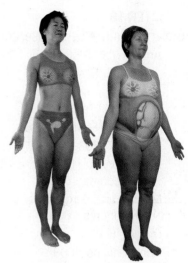

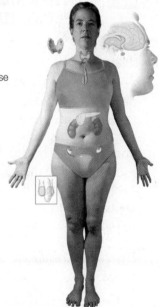

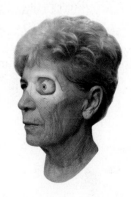

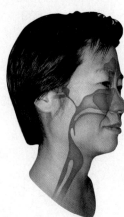

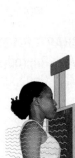

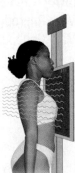

Chapter 1

The Structure of Medical Language

Medical language is the framework on which the practice of medicine is built. Healthcare professionals use medical language every day to communicate with each other.

 ## Learning Outcomes

After you study this chapter, you should be able to

1.1 Identify the five skills of medical language communication.

1.2 Describe the origins of medical language.

1.3 Recognize common Latin and Greek singular nouns and form their plurals.

1.4 Identify and describe the characteristics of a combining form, a suffix, and a prefix.

1.5 Give the meanings of common word parts.

1.6 Divide medical words into word parts and build medical words from word parts.

1.7 Spell and pronounce common medical words.

1.8 Describe the format and contents of the medical record.

1.9 Define abbreviations related to the medical record.

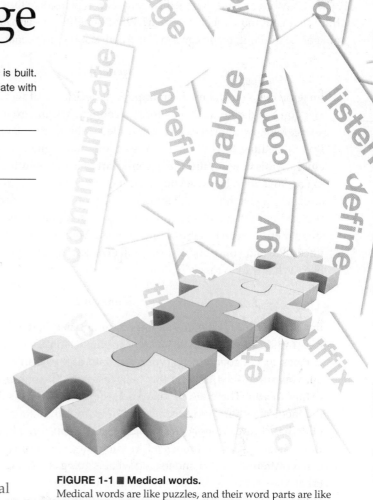

FIGURE 1-1 ■ Medical words.
Medical words are like puzzles, and their word parts are like the pieces. If you put the pieces together correctly, you can understand the definition of the medical word.
Source: VERSUSstudio/Shutterstock

Welcome to Medical Language

You are about to begin the study of medical language! Right now, medical words may seem like puzzles (see Figure 1-1 ■), but, as you study, you will learn their meanings. Studying medical language will involve time and effort on your part. But what can you expect in return? What benefits come from learning medical language? To find out, read Scenario 1 and contrast it with Scenario 2.

Scenario 1

Imagine that you just made an important decision that will affect the rest of your life: You decided to move to a foreign country. You are excited and anxious to get going! When you arrive, you are thrilled to be in this new, exotic environment. It is fascinating to you! There are so many new sights and sounds. You want to embrace this new culture and become part of it, but your first attempts at interacting are awkward because you do not know the language. You can't seem to make anyone understand you. All around you, people are engaged in interesting activities and important conversations, but you can't join in because you can't understand them. You feel confused and helpless. Your future in this country now seems uncertain, and you wonder if you will ever be anything more than just a spectator here. What went wrong?

Scenario 2

Imagine that you just made an important decision that will affect the rest of your life: You decided to pursue a career in the healthcare field. You are excited and anxious to get going! When you walk into a physician's office, clinic, or hospital, you are thrilled to be in this new, fast-paced, exotic environment. It is fascinating to you! There are so many new sights and sounds. You want to embrace the medical culture and become part of it. Your first attempts at interacting with other healthcare professionals are successful because you know medical language. Immediately, you are immersed in interesting medical activities and important conversations, and you understand what is going on. You feel excited and empowered! Your future in the healthcare field is certain because you took the time to study medical language.

CLINICAL CONNECTIONS

Healthcare professionals know that there is no substitute for a thorough, working knowledge of medical language (see Figure 1-2 ■). If you want to "walk the walk," you have to "talk the talk." Medical language is the language of the healthcare profession, and medical words are the tools of the trade! Learning medical language is your key to a successful career in the healthcare field.

DID YOU KNOW?

There is more than one way to learn medical language. Which one do you prefer?

1. Memorize a medical dictionary.

2. Take courses in Latin, Greek, and other languages.

3. Learn medical language by studying this textbook!

The third option is the easiest. Of course, there is still effort involved; but, with practice, you will learn medical language!

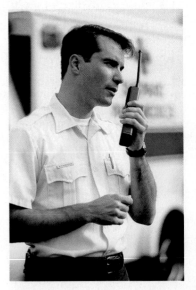

FIGURE 1-2 ■ Medical language.
This paramedic is using medical language to communicate with healthcare professionals in the emergency department to describe the condition of a patient in the ambulance. How important do you think it is for this paramedic to have a thorough, working knowledge of medical language?
Source: Keith Brofsky/Photodisc/Getty Images

Pronunciation/Word Parts

DID YOU KNOW?

Medical Language versus Medical Terminology

There are many medical **terminology** books on the market. These books teach medical terms, but not medical language. It is medical language that doctors, nurses, therapists, and other healthcare workers use. Medical language is the language of medicine. Also, the practice of medicine is always divided into medical specialties, not body systems, as taught in medical terminology books. Only medical language, as taught in this textbook, reflects the way communication really happens in medicine and health care today!

terminology (TER-mih-NAW-loh-jee)
  termin/o- *boundary; end; word*
  -logy *study of*

Medical Language and Communication

Communication in any language consists of five language skills. These same skills apply to **medical language**. You need to master all five skills in order to communicate on the job with other healthcare professionals (see Figure 1-3 ■).

communication (koh-MYOO-nih-KAY-shun)
  communicat/o- *impart; transmit*
  -ion *action; condition*

medical (MED-ih-kal)
  medic/o- *medicine; physician*
  -al *pertaining to*

language (LANG-gwij)

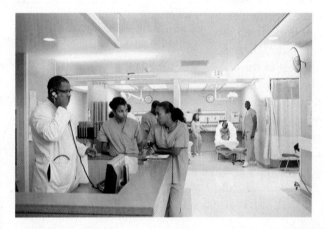

FIGURE 1-3 ■ Medical language communication.
These healthcare professionals are using all five medical language skills in order to communicate successfully.
Source: Blend Images/ERproductions Ltd/Getty Images

1. **Reading**

2. **Listening**

   These two skills involve receiving medical language. This is similar to input coming into a computer.

   - You read medical words. Each chapter in this book contains many medical words.

   - You read actual medical reports in the Chapter Review Exercises.

   - You listen to your course instructor speak medical language.

   - You listen to exercises with actual physicians speaking medical language from medical reports on the website at www.MyMedicalTerminologyLab.com.

3. **Thinking, analyzing, and understanding**

   This three-part skill involves processing medical language. This is similar to the processing function of a computer.

   - You divide medical words into their word parts.

   - You recall the meanings of word parts.

   - You build medical words from word parts.

   - You answer questions after reading electronic patient records.

   - You relate common English words to their medical word equivalents.

   - You research the definitions of new medical words.

4. **Writing (or typing) and spelling**

5. **Speaking and pronouncing**

These two skills involve relaying medical language. This is similar to output coming from a computer.

- You write or type a medical word and spell it correctly.
- You spell the plural and adjective forms of medical words.
- You identify misspelled medical words.
- You identify the primary accented syllable in a medical word.
- You pronounce medical words correctly, using "see-and-say" pronunciation guides.

All of these skills are critical to the communication of medical language. This textbook, *Medical Language*, helps you develop all of these skills by giving you many opportunities to practice until you have mastered all of them.

The Beginning of Medical Language

Let's begin the study of medical language by looking at how medical language began. **Etymology** is the study of word origins. In medical language, many words come from other languages, particularly from Latin and Greek. Why? The Greek physician Hippocrates is known as the "father of medicine." He founded what is thought to be the first school of medicine. He spoke Greek but, during his time, the rest of the civilized world, centered in Rome, spoke Latin. In ancient times, both the Greeks and the Romans advanced the study and practice of medicine. They named anatomical structures, diseases, and treatments in their own languages, and these Latin and Greek words remain a part of medical language today. You'll be surprised to see how many of these words are familiar to you.

etymology (ET-ih-MAW-loh-jee)
 etym/o- *word origin*
 -logy *study of*

WORD ALERT

Some medical words are identical to the original Latin and Greek words used centuries ago.

Medical Word	Language of Origin
nucleus	Latin *nucleus*
pelvis	Latin *pelvis*
sinus	Latin *sinus*
paranoia	Greek *paranoia*
thorax	Greek *thorax*

Some medical words are similar (but not identical) to Latin and Greek words.

Medical Word	Language of Origin
artery	Latin *arteria*
muscle	Latin *musculus*
patient	Latin *patiente*
vein	Latin *vena*
phobia	Greek *phobos*
sperm	Greek *sperma*
urine	Latin *urina*

Some medical words are similar to words from Old English, Dutch, or French.

Medical Word	Language of Origin
bladder	English *blaedre*
heart	English *heorte*
drug	Dutch *droog*
physician	French *physicien*

This *It's Greek to Me!* feature appears in each chapter. It lists common combining forms, their language of origin, and the medical words in which they were used in that chapter. You will learn about combining forms later in this chapter.

IT'S GREEK TO ME!

Did you notice that some words have two different combining forms? Combining forms from both Greek and Latin remain a part of medical language today.

Medical Singular and Plural Nouns

The Latin and Greek languages are the main sources of medical words. These languages had rules that told how to form plural nouns and how to pronounce singular and plural nouns; those rules still apply today. *Note*: When a Latin or Greek word is used in a chapter, there will be a note there to remind you of those rules. Here are some common Latin and Greek singular and plural nouns and their pronunciations.

Latin Singular and Plural Nouns and Pronunciations

1. When a Latin singular noun ends in *-a*, form the plural by changing *-a* to *-ae*.

Singular	Pronunciation	Plural	Pronunciation
areola	(ah-REE-oh-lah)	areolae	(ah-REE-oh-lee)
conjunctiva	(CON-junk-TY-vah)	conjunctivae	(CON-junk-TY-vee)
patella	(pah-TEL-ah)	patellae	(pah-TEL-ee)
scapula	(SKAP-yoo-lah)	scapulae	(SKAP-yoo-lee)
sclera	(SKLEER-ah)	sclerae	(SKLEER-ee)
vertebra	(VER-teh-brah)	vertebrae	(VER-teh-bree)

2. When a Latin singular noun ends in *-us*, form the plural by changing *-us* to *-i*.
   (*Note*: Exceptions to this rule are the Latin words *fetus*, *virus*, and *sinus*, whose plural forms are the English-type plurals *fetuses*, *viruses*, and *sinuses*.)

alveolus	(al-VEE-oh-lus)	alveoli	(al-VEE-oh-lie)
bronchus	(BRONG-kus)	bronchi	(BRONG-ki)
glomerulus	(gloh-MAIR-yoo-lus)	glomeruli	(gloh-MAIR-yoo-lie)
nucleus	(NOO-klee-us)	nuclei	(NOO-klee-eye)
thrombus	(THRAWM-bus)	thrombi	(THRAWM-by)

3. When a Latin singular noun ends in *-um*, form the plural by changing *-um* to *-a*.

atrium	(AA-tree-um)	atria	(AA-tree-ah)
bacterium	(bak-TEER-ee-um)	bacteria	(bak-TEER-ee-ah)
diverticulum	(DY-ver-TIH-kyoo-lum)	diverticula	(DY-ver-TIH-kyoo-lah)
labium	(LAY-bee-um)	labia	(LAY-bee-ah)
ovum	(OH-vum)	ova	(OH-vah)

4. When a Latin singular noun ends in *-is*, form the plural by changing *-is* to *-es*.

diagnosis	(DY-ag-NOH-sis)	diagnoses	(DY-ag-NOH-seez)
testis	(TES-tis)	testes	(TES-teez)

5. When a Latin singular noun ends in *-ex*, form the plural by changing *-ex* to *-ices*.

apex	(AA-peks)	apices	(AA-pih-seez)
cortex	(KOR-teks)	cortices	(KOR-tih-seez)
index	(IN-deks)	indices	(IN-dih-seez)

Greek Singular and Plural Nouns and Pronunciations

1. When a Greek singular noun ends in *-is*, form the plural by changing *-is* to *-ides*.

| epididymis | (EP-ih-DID-ih-mis) | epididymides | (EP-ih-dih-DIM-ih-deez) |
| iris | (EYE-ris) | irides | (IH-rih-deez) |

2. When a Greek singular noun ends in *-nx*, form the plural by changing *-nx* to *-nges*.

| phalanx | (FAY-langks) | phalanges | (fah-LAN-jeez) |

3. When a Greek singular noun ends in *-oma*, form the plural by changing *-oma* to *-omata*.

| carcinoma | (KAR-sih-NOH-mah) | carcinomata | (KAR-sih-NOH-mah-tah) |
| fibroma | (fy-BROH-mah) | fibromata | (FY-broh-MAH-tah) |

4. When a Greek singular noun ends in *-on*, form the plural by changing *-on* to *-a*.

| ganglion | (GANG-glee-on) | ganglia | (GANG-glee-ah) |
| mitochondrion | (MY-toh-CON-dree-on) | mitochondria | (MY-toh-CON-dree-ah) |

WORD ALERT

Carcinomata and *fibromata* are the plural forms of the Greek words. However, English-type plural forms are also acceptable, according to medical dictionaries, and these plural forms are commonly used by healthcare professionals: *carcinomas, fibromas*.
Note that both Latin and Greek nouns can end in *-is*, but their plurals are formed differently.

Medical Word Parts

Medical language contains medical words, and most medical words contain word parts. The smallest components of a word are its word parts. Even the longest medical word only has three types of word parts: combining forms, suffixes, and prefixes. Medical words can be broken down into their word parts. Word parts are like puzzle pieces that, when fit together, build a medical word.

There are three different types of word parts.

Word Part	Meaning
prefix	an optional word beginning
combining form	the foundation of a medical word
suffix	the word ending

DID YOU KNOW?

When you learn something new, it is always best to learn it the right way the very first time! That is why the spelling and punctuation of combining forms, suffixes, and prefixes used in this book agree with those used in medical dictionaries, the recognized authorities on medical language origin and use.

Combining Forms

Because the combining form is the foundation of a medical word, we begin our study of word parts by looking at combining forms.

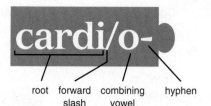

Characteristics of a Combining Form

Combining forms have the following characteristics.

- A combining form is a word part that is the foundation of a word.
- A combining form gives the word its main medical meaning.
- A combining form has a root, a forward slash, a combining vowel (usually an *o*, but occasionally an *a, e, i,* or *y*), and a final hyphen (see Figure 1-4 ■).
- Most medical words contain a combining form. (*Note:* Some medical words, such as *blood, health, heart,* or *nurse,* do not contain any word parts.)
- Sometimes a medical word contains two or more combining forms, one right after the other. Example: *gastrointestinal.*

FIGURE 1-4 ■ Combining form.
A combining form contains a root, forward slash, combining vowel, and hyphen. The hyphen shows that the combining form is a word part, not a complete word. The combining form *cardi/o-* means *heart.*

Source: Pearson Education

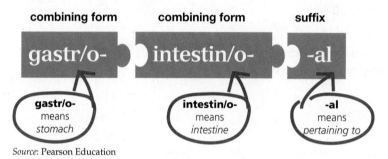

Source: Pearson Education

WORD ALERT

Two combining forms can have the same medical meaning. For example, the combining forms *enter/o-* and *intestin/o-* both mean *intestine.* When this occurs in a chapter, there will be a note to remind you.

A CLOSER LOOK

Learning medical language requires some memorization of combining forms and their meanings. Knowing the meaning of the combining form allows you to look at a medical word and already have an idea about its definition; and that same combining form appears in many different medical words. If you know the meanings of combining forms, you don't have to use a medical dictionary to look up the definition of each new medical word you encounter!

Here are some tips on how to manage your time and the amount of memorization you need to do as you study medical language.

Tip #1: Some combining forms are nearly identical to their medical meanings. When you see combining forms such as these, you already know their medical meanings.

Combining Form	Meaning
abdomin/o-	abdomen
append/o-	appendix; small structure hanging from a larger structure
arteri/o-	artery

Combining Form	Meaning
intestin/o-	intestine
laryng/o-	larynx; voice box
muscul/o-	muscle
thyroid/o-	thyroid gland
tonsill/o-	tonsil
ven/o-	vein

Tip #2: Some combining forms bring to mind a word you already know. That helps you to remember the medical meaning of combining forms such as these.

Combining Form	Meaning	Related Word
arthr/o-	joint	arthritis
cardi/o-	heart	cardiac
dermat/o-	skin	dermatologist
gastr/o-	stomach	gastric
mamm/o-	breast	mammogram
nas/o-	nose	nasal
psych/o-	mind	psychiatrist

Tip #3: Other combining forms are very different from their medical meanings. Combining forms such as these and their medical meanings need to be memorized.

Combining Form	Meaning
cholecyst/o-	gallbladder
cost/o-	rib
enter/o-	intestine
hepat/o-	liver
hyster/o-	uterus; womb
lapar/o-	abdomen

Tip #4: Combining forms can have the meaning of a color.

Combining Form	Meaning
chrom/o-	color
erythr/o-; rub/o-	red
jaund/o-	yellow
verd/o-	green
cyan/o-	blue
melan/o-	black
albin/o-; leuk/o-	white

Suffixes

Now let's turn our attention to another type of word part: suffixes.

Characteristics of a Suffix

Suffixes have the following characteristics.

- A suffix is a word part that is at the end of a word.
- A suffix modifies or clarifies the medical meaning of the combining form.
- A suffix is a single letter or group of letters that begins with a hyphen (see Figure 1-5 ■).
- Most medical words contain a suffix (see *Note* with *Combining Forms*).
- Occasionally, a medical word has two suffixes, one right after the other. Example: *nutritional*.

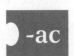

FIGURE 1-5 ■ Suffix.
A suffix begins with a hyphen to show that it is a word part, not a complete word. The suffix -ac means *pertaining to.*
Source: Pearson Education

Here are some common suffixes. Take a moment to review them and learn their meanings so that you will be ready to use them in medical words.

Suffixes for an Adjective			
Suffix	**Meaning**	**Medical Word Example**	**Definition**
-ac	pertaining to	cardiac (KAR-dee-ak) (*cardi/o-* means *heart*)	<u>pertaining to</u> the heart
-al	pertaining to	intestinal (in-TES-tih-nal) (*intestin/o-* means *intestine*)	<u>pertaining to</u> the intestine
-ar	pertaining to	muscular (MUS-kyoo-lar) (*muscul/o-* means *muscle*)	<u>pertaining to</u> the muscle
-ary	pertaining to	urinary (YOOR-ih-NAIR-ee) (*urin/o-* means *urinary system; urine*)	<u>pertaining to</u> the urine
-ic	pertaining to	pelvic (PEL-vik) (*pelv/o-* means *hip bone; pelvis; renal pelvis*)	<u>pertaining to</u> the pelvis
-ine	pertaining to	uterine (YOO-ter-in) (*uter/o-* means *uterus; womb*)	<u>pertaining to</u> the uterus
-ive	pertaining to	digestive (dy-JES-tiv) (*digest/o-* means *break down food; digest*)	<u>pertaining to</u> break(ing) down food
-ous	pertaining to	venous (VEE-nus) (*ven/o-* means *vein*)	<u>pertaining to</u> a vein

Suffixes for a Process			
-ation	being; having; process	urination (YOOR-ih-NAY-shun) (*urin/o-* means *urine; urinary system*)	<u>process</u> (of making) urine
-ion	action; condition	digestion (dy-JES-chun) (*digest/o-* means *break down food; digest*)	<u>action</u> of break(ing) down food

Suffixes for a Disease			
-ia	condition; state; thing	pneumonia (noo-MOHN-yah) (*pneumon/o-* means *air; lung*)	<u>condition</u> of the lung
-ism	disease from a specific cause; process	hypothyroidism (HY-poh-THY-royd-izm) (*thyroid/o-* means *thyroid gland*)	<u>disease from a specific cause</u> of deficient thyroid gland (hormone)
-itis	infection of; inflammation of	tonsillitis (TAWN-sil-EYE-tis) (*tonsill/o-* means *tonsil*)	<u>infection of</u> the tonsil
-megaly	enlargement	cardiomegaly (KAR-dee-oh-MEG-ah-lee) (*cardi/o-* means *heart*)	<u>enlargement</u> of the heart
-oma	mass; tumor	neuroma (nyoor-OH-mah) (*neur/o-* means *nerve*)	<u>tumor</u> of a nerve
-osis	condition; process	psychosis (sy-KOH-sis) (*psych/o-* means *mind*)	<u>condition</u> of the mind
-pathy	disease	arthropathy (ar-THRAW-pah-thee) (*arthr/o-* means *joint*)	<u>disease</u> of a joint

Suffixes for a Diagnostic, Medical, or Surgical Procedure

Suffix	Meaning	Medical Word Example	Definition
-ectomy	surgical removal	appendectomy (AP-en-DEK-toh-mee) (*append/o-* means *appendix; small structure hanging from a larger structure*)	surgical removal of the appendix
-gram	picture; record	mammogram (MAM-oh-gram) (*mamm/o-* means *breast*)	picture of the breast
-graphy	process of recording	mammography (mam-AW-grah-fee) (*mamm/o-* means *breast*)	process of recording the breast
-metry	process of measuring	spirometry (spih-RAW-meh-tree) (*spir/o-* means *breathe; coil*)	process of measuring the breathing
-scope	instrument used to examine	colonoscope (koh-LAW-noh-skohp) (*colon/o-* means *colon*)	instrument used to examine the colon
-scopy	process of using an instrument to examine	gastroscopy (gas-TRAW-skoh-pee) (*gastr/o-* means *stomach*)	process of using an instrument to examine the stomach
-stomy	surgically created opening	colostomy (koh-LAW-stoh-mee) (*col/o-* means *colon*)	surgically created opening in the colon
-therapy	treatment	psychotherapy (SY-koh-THAIR-ah-pee) (*psych/o-* means *mind*)	treatment of the mind
-tomy	process of cutting; process of making an incision	laparotomy (LAP-ar-AW-toh-mee) (*lapar/o-* means *abdomen*)	process of making an incision in the abdomen

Suffixes for a Medical Specialty or Specialist

Suffix	Meaning	Medical Word Example	Definition
-iatry	medical treatment	psychiatry (sy-KY-ah-tree) (*psych/o-* means *mind*)	medical treatment for the mind
-ics	knowledge; practice	dietetics (DY-eh-TEH-tiks) (*dietet/o-* means *diet; foods*)	knowledge and practice of diet and foods
-ist	person who specializes in; thing that specializes in	therapist (THAIR-ah-pist) (*therap/o-* means *treatment*)	person who specializes in treatment
-logy	study of	cardiology (KAR-dee-AW-loh-jee) (*cardi/o-* means *heart*)	study of the heart

Prefixes

Finally, let's look at the third type of word part: prefixes.

Characteristics of a Prefix

Prefixes have the following characteristics.

- A prefix is a word part that is at the beginning of a word. A prefix is an optional word part, and not every medical word contains a prefix.
- A prefix modifies or clarifies the medical meaning of the combining form.
- A prefix is a single letter or group of letters that ends with a hyphen (see Figure 1-6 ■).
- Occasionally, a medical word has two prefixes, one right after the other.

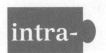

FIGURE 1-6 ■ Prefix.
A prefix ends with a hyphen to show that it is a word part, not a complete word. The prefix *intra-* means *within*.
Source: Pearson Education

Here are some common prefixes. Take a moment to review them and learn their meanings so that you will be ready to use them in medical words.

Prefixes for Location or Direction			
Prefix	**Meaning**	**Medical Word Example**	**Definition**
endo-	innermost; within	endotracheal (EN-doh-TRAY-kee-al) (*trache/o-* means *trachea; windpipe*)	pertaining to <u>within</u> the trachea
epi-	above; upon	epidermal (EP-ih-DER-mal) (*derm/o-* means *skin*)	pertaining to <u>upon</u> the skin
inter-	between	intercostal (IN-ter-KAW-stal) (*cost/o-* means *rib*)	pertaining to <u>between</u> the ribs
intra-	within	intravenous (IN-trah-VEE-nus) (*ven/o-* means *vein*)	pertaining to <u>within</u> a vein
peri-	around	pericardial (PAIR-ih-KAR-dee-al) (*cardi/o-* means *heart*)	pertaining to <u>around</u> the heart
post-	after; behind	postnasal (post-NAY-zal) (*nas/o-* means *nose*)	pertaining to <u>behind</u> the nose
pre-	before; in front of	premenstrual (pree-MEN-stroo-al) (*menstru/o-* means *monthly discharge of blood*)	pertaining to <u>before</u> the monthly discharge of blood
sub-	below; underneath	subcutaneous (SUB-kyoo-TAY-nee-us) (*cutane/o-* means *skin*)	pertaining to <u>underneath</u> the skin
trans-	across; through	transvaginal (trans-VAJ-ih-nal) (*vagin/o-* means *vagina*)	pertaining to <u>through</u> the vagina

Prefixes for Amount, Number, or Speed			
bi-	two	bilateral (bi-LAT-er-al) (*later/o-* means *side*)	pertaining to <u>two</u> sides
brady-	slow	bradycardia (BRAD-ee-KAR-dee-ah) (*card/i-* means *heart*)	condition of a <u>slow</u> heart
hemi-	one half	hemiplegia (HEM-ee-PLEE-jah) (*pleg/o-* means *paralysis*)	condition of <u>one half</u> (of the body with) paralysis
hyper-	above; more than normal	hypertension (HY-per-TEN-shun) (*tens/o-* means *pressure; tension*)	condition of <u>more than normal</u> pressure
hypo-	below; deficient	hypothyroidism (HY-poh-THY-royd-izm) (*thyroid/o-* means *thyroid gland*)	disease from a specific cause of <u>deficient</u> thyroid gland (hormone)
poly-	many; much	polyneuritis (PAW-lee-nyoor-EYE-tis) (*neur/o-* means *nerve*)	inflammation of <u>many</u> nerves
quadri-	four	quadriplegia (KWAH-drih-PLEE-jah) (*pleg/o-* means *paralysis*)	condition of <u>four</u> (limbs with) paralysis
tachy-	fast	tachycardia (TAK-ih-KAR-dee-ah) (*card/i-* means *heart*)	condition of a <u>fast</u> heart
tri-	three	trigeminal (try-JEM-ih-nal) (*gemin/o-* means *group; set*)	pertaining to <u>three</u> (nerve branches in a) group

Prefixes for Degree or Quality

Prefix	Meaning	Medical Word Example	Definition
a-	away from; without	aspermia (aa-SPER-mee-ah) (*sperm/o-* means *sperm*)	condition (of being) <u>without</u> sperm
an-	not; without	anesthesia (AN-es-THEE-zha) (*esthes/o-* means *feeling; sensation*)	condition (of being) <u>without</u> sensation
anti-	against	antibiotic (AN-tee-by-AW-tik) (*bi/o-* means *life; living organism; living tissue*)	pertaining to (a drug that is) <u>against</u> living organisms (such as bacteria)
de-	reversal of; without	dementia (deh-MEN-sha) (*ment/o-* means *chin; mind*)	condition (of being) <u>without</u> a mind
dys-	abnormal; difficult; painful	dysphagia (dis-FAY-jee-ah) (*phag/o-* means *eating; swallowing*)	condition of <u>difficult or painful</u> eating and swallowing
eu-	good; normal	euthyroidism (yoo-THY-royd-izm) (*thyroid/o-* means *thyroid gland*)	process of <u>normal</u> thyroid gland (function)
mal-	bad; inadequate	malnutrition (MAL-noo-TRIH-shun) (*nutrit/o-* means *nourishment*)	condition of <u>inadequate</u> nourishment
re-	again and again; backward; unable to	respiration (RES-pih-RAY-shun) (*spir/o-* means *breathe; coil*)	process of <u>again and again</u> breathing

Vocabulary Review

Here are the word parts presented in this chapter. (You will see these word parts in other chapters in the book.) Take time to review them and learn their meanings so that you will be ready to use them in medical words.

Combining Forms

Combining Form	Meaning	Combining Form	Meaning
abdomin/o-	abdomen	later/o-	side
append/o-	appendix; small structure hanging from a larger structure	mamm/o-	breast
arteri/o-	artery	medic/o-	medicine; physician
arthr/o-	joint	menstru/o-	monthly discharge of blood
bi/o-	life; living organism; living tissue	ment/o-	chin; mind
card/i-	heart	muscul/o-	muscle
cardi/o-	heart	nas/o-	nose
cholecyst/o-	gallbladder	neur/o-	nerve
col/o-	colon	nutrit/o-	nourishment
colon/o-	colon	pelv/o-	hip bone; pelvis; renal pelvis
communicat/o-	impart; transmit	phag/o-	eating; swallowing
cost/o-	rib	pleg/o-	paralysis
cutane/o-	skin	pneumon/o-	air; lung
derm/o-	skin	psych/o-	mind
dietet/o-	diet; foods	sperm/o-	sperm; spermatozoon
digest/o-	break down food; digest	spir/o-	breathe; coil
enter/o-	intestine	tens/o-	pressure; tension
esthes/o-	feeling; sensation	therap/o-	treatment
etym/o-	word origin	thyroid/o-	thyroid gland
gastr/o-	stomach	tonsill/o-	tonsil
gemin/o-	group; set	trache/o-	trachea; windpipe
hepat/o-	liver	urin/o-	urinary system; urine
hyster/o-	uterus; womb	uter/o-	uterus; womb
intestin/o-	intestine	vagin/o-	vagina
lapar/o-	abdomen	ven/o-	vein
laryng/o-	larynx; voice box		

Suffixes

Suffix	Meaning	Suffix	Meaning
-ac	pertaining to	-gram	picture; record
-al	pertaining to	-graphy	process of recording
-ar	pertaining to	-ia	condition; state; thing
-ary	pertaining to	-iatry	medical treatment
-ation	being; having; process	-ic	pertaining to
-ectomy	surgical removal	-ics	knowledge; practice

Suffix	Meaning	Suffix	Meaning
-ine	pertaining to; thing pertaining to	-oma	mass; tumor
-ion	action; condition	-osis	condition; process
-ism	disease from a specific cause; process	-ous	pertaining to
-ist	person who specializes in; thing that specializes in	-pathy	disease
-itis	infection of; inflammation of	-scope	instrument used to examine
-ive	pertaining to	-scopy	process of using an instrument to examine
-logy	study of	-stomy	surgically created opening
-megaly	enlargement	-therapy	treatment
-metry	process of measuring	-tomy	process of cutting; process of making an incision

Prefixes			
Prefix	**Meaning**	**Prefix**	**Meaning**
a-	away from; without	inter-	between
an-	not; without	intra-	within
anti-	against	mal-	bad; inadequate
bi-	two	peri-	around
brady-	slow	poly-	many; much
de-	reversal of; without	post-	after; behind
dys-	abnormal; difficult; painful	pre-	before; in front of
endo-	innermost; within	quadri-	four
epi-	above; upon	re-	again and again; backward; unable to
eu-	good; normal	sub-	below; underneath
hemi-	one half	tachy-	fast
hyper-	above; more than normal	trans-	across; through
hypo-	below; deficient	tri-	three

Divide Medical Words

The third skill of medical language involves thinking, analyzing, and understanding. When you analyze something, you divide it into smaller pieces that are easier to understand. To analyze a medical word, divide it into its word parts. Then you combine the meanings of the word parts to give you the definition of the medical word. Here are the steps for dividing and defining a medical word.

● Medical Word with a Combining Form and Suffix

Let's say you read or hear this word and want to know its definition.

cardiology

Step 1. Divide the medical word into its combining form and suffix.

   (*Note*: At this point in your study, you may not be able to look at a medical word and know that it contains a combining form and a suffix. However, as you memorize various word parts and their meanings, you will be able to do this.)

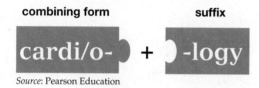

Source: Pearson Education

Step 2. Give the meaning of each word part.

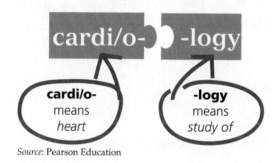

Source: Pearson Education

Step 3. Put the meanings of the word parts in order, beginning with the meaning of the suffix, then the meaning of the combining form. Then, add small connecting words to make the definition.

suffix	combining form
study of	*heart*

Cardiology: *Study of (the) heart (and related structures)*

● Medical Word with a Prefix, Combining Form, and Suffix

Let's say you read or hear this word and want to know its definition.

pericardial

Step 1. Divide the medical word into its prefix, combining form, and suffix.

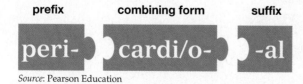

Source: Pearson Education

Step 2. Give the meaning of each word part.

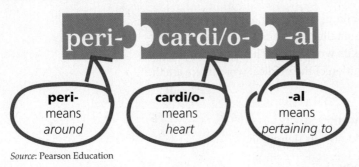

Source: Pearson Education

Step 3. Put the word part meanings in order, beginning with the meaning of the suffix, then the meaning of the prefix, then the meaning of the combining form. Then, add small connecting words to make the definition.

suffix	prefix	combining form
pertaining to	*around*	*heart*

Pericardial: *Pertaining to around (the) heart*

Build Medical Words

Medical words are like puzzles, and their word parts are the pieces of the puzzle. To build a medical word, begin with its definition. Select word parts that match that definition, and put the word part puzzle pieces together in the correct way. Here are the steps for building a medical word.

● Suffix that Begins with a Consonant

Let's say you want to build a medical word with this definition.

Study of the heart

Step 1. Select the suffix and combining form whose meanings match the definition of the medical word.

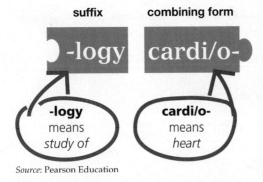

Source: Pearson Education

Step 2. Change the order of the word parts to put the suffix last.

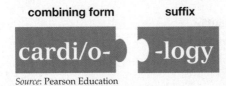

Source: Pearson Education

Step 3. Because the suffix begins with a consonant, you will need to keep the combining form's vowel.

Delete the forward slash and hyphen from the combining form. Delete the hyphen from the suffix. Then, join the two word parts.

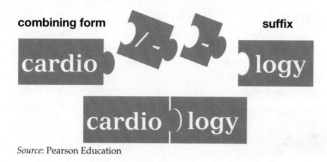

Source: Pearson Education

● Suffix that Begins with a Vowel

Let's say you want to build a medical word with this definition.

Pertaining to the heart

Step 1. Select the suffix and combining form whose meanings match the definition of the medical word.

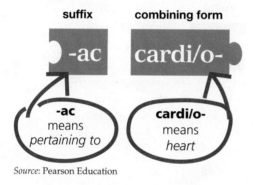

Source: Pearson Education

Step 2. Change the order of the word parts to put the suffix last.

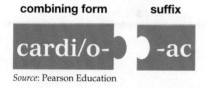

Source: Pearson Education

Step 3. Because the suffix begins with a vowel, you will need to delete the combining form's vowel.

Delete the forward slash, combining vowel, and hyphen from the combining form. Delete the hyphen from the suffix. Then, join the two word parts.

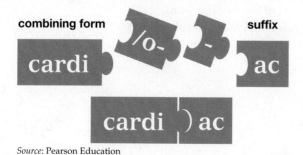

Source: Pearson Education

• Contains a Prefix

Let's say you want to build a medical word with this definition.

Pertaining to within the heart

Step 1. Select the suffix, prefix, and combining form whose meanings match the definition of the medical word.

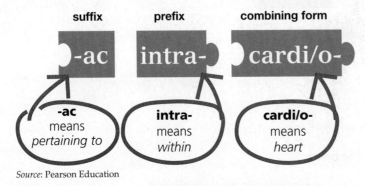

Source: Pearson Education

Step 2. Change the order of the word parts to put the suffix last.

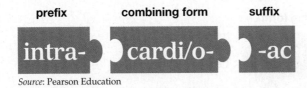

Source: Pearson Education

Step 3. Delete the hyphen from the prefix. Delete the forward slash, combining vowel, and hyphen from the combining form. Delete the hyphen from the suffix. Then, join the three word parts.

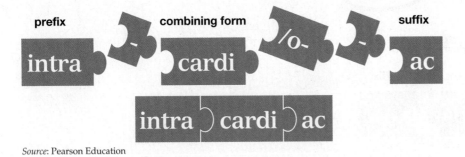

Source: Pearson Education

Spell Medical Words

One of the five medical language skills is the spelling of medical words. Remembering the spelling of combining forms and other word parts and how to correctly build a medical word will also help you achieve the correct spelling of the medical word. Spelling of medical words is emphasized in the Chapter Review Exercises in subsequent chapters, in exercises such as "Plural Noun and Adjective Exercise," "Proofreading and Spelling Exercise," and "You Write the Medical Report."

Pronounce Medical Words

Knowing the definition of a medical word is important, but being able to pronounce the word correctly is equally important. One of the five medical language skills is the pronunciation of medical words. In each chapter, as you read a medical word (in bold in the text), there is an accompanying "see-and-say" pronunciation guide, so you can immediately pronounce the word you are learning. These pronunciation guides are straight-forward and easy to use. The syllables in the medical word are separated by hyphens. The primary (main) accented syllable is in all capital letters. The secondary accented syllable is in smaller capital letters. Just say each syllable by following the "see-and-say" pronunciation guide. When you read a medical word and then speak and pronounce it correctly, you are forming an accurate word memory for that medical word.

Now use the "see-and-say" pronunciation guides to practice pronouncing common medical words, many of which are presented in this chapter.

PRONOUNCING MEDICAL WORDS   Look at each medical word and its "see-and-say" pronunciation guide. Practice pronouncing the word several times.

Medical Word	**Pronunciation**
1. abdominal	(ab-DAW-mih-nal)
2. appendectomy	(AP-en-DEK-toh-mee)
3. arthritis	(ar-THRY-tis)
4. cardiac	(KAR-dee-ak)
5. cardiology	(KAR-dee-AW-loh-jee)
6. digestion	(dy-JES-chun)
7. gastric	(GAS-trik)
8. intestinal	(in-TES-tih-nal)
9. intravenous	(IN-trah-VEE-nus)
10. laryngitis	(LAIR-in-JY-tis)
11. mammography	(mam-AW-grah-fee)
12. muscular	(MUS-kyoo-lar)
13. pneumonia	(noo-MOHN-yah)
14. psychiatry	(sy-KY-ah-tree)
15. therapist	(THAIR-ah-pist)
16. tonsillectomy	(TAWN-sil-EK-toh-mee)
17. urinary	(YOOR-ih-NAIR-ee)

The Medical Record

Many of the medical language skills discussed at the beginning of the chapter are used when dealing with medical records. Let's briefly look at some of the more common types of medical records.

The **medical record** is where healthcare professionals document all care provided to a patient. In the past, the medical record was mainly used to document diseases, treatments, surgeries, etc. Now, the medical record reflects an emphasis on keeping the patient in good health and preventing disease. Most physicians' office medical records include a checklist that documents preventive care given to the patient (immunizations, routine physical exams, etc.), as well as things the patient should do (limit sun exposure and apply sunscreen, have smoke detectors in the home, use seat belts, do monthly self-examination of the breasts or testicles, secure firearms kept in the home, etc.).

The paper medical record has been the traditional form of medical record. Its disadvantages are that only one healthcare professional can access it at a time, it can be lost or damaged, and it can take hours or even days to retrieve a patient's past medical records that are stored off-site. This delay can compromise the delivery of quality care.

Most physicians' offices, hospitals, and other healthcare facilities have converted some or all of their paper medical records to **electronic patient records (EPRs)** (see Figure 1-7 ■). In those facilities, several healthcare professionals can access the same record at the same time, the record cannot be lost or damaged (because there is always a back-up electronic copy), and it takes only seconds to retrieve a patient's past medical records (because the record is stored in a computer that is on-site or can be accessed electronically in a remote location).

Pronunciation/Word Parts

medical (MED-ih-kal)
  medic/o- *medicine; physician*
  -al *pertaining to*

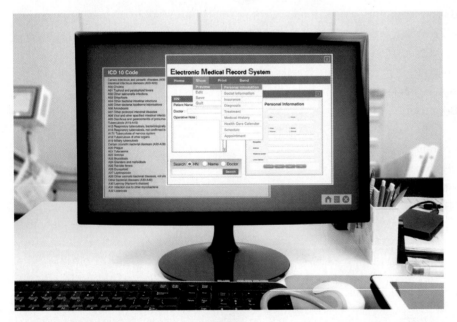

FIGURE 1-7 ■ Electronic patient record (EPR).
The electronic patient record can provide immediate access to a patient's current and previous medical records in one medical facility or between related facilities.
Source: pandpstock001/Shutterstock

TECHNOLOGY IN MEDICINE

The **electronic medical record (EMR)**, **electronic patient record (EPR)**, or **electronic health record (EHR)** provides seamless, immediate, and simultaneous access for several healthcare professionals to all parts of a patient's record regardless of where those parts were created or stored. The federal government set a goal to have the electronic medical record and electronic prescribing of drugs (e-prescribing) available everywhere in health care. Now these electronic records go beyond storing a patient's medical information. They alert physicians to potential errors, suggest additional tests, spot trends in the patient's condition, and warn about prescribing the wrong drug.

Types of Documents in the Medical Record

The medical record varies in format and content from one facility to the next. Short narrative notes and checklists are used in many physicians' offices and clinics. These notes usually contain a brief history of the present illness, pertinent past medical or surgical history, a physical examination, a diagnosis, treatments given, and a follow-up plan.

Hospitals have more extensive documentation than physicians' offices. Common documents for a hospitalized patient include the Admission History and Physical Examination (H&P), Operative Report, and Discharge Summary (DS). These documents include standard headings, as described below.

Standard Headings in Healthcare Documents

- Chief Complaint (CC)
- History of Present Illness (HPI)
- Past Medical (and Surgical) History (PMH)
- Social History (SH) and Family History (FH)
- Review of Systems (ROS)
- Physical Examination (PE)
- Laboratory and X-ray Data
- Diagnosis (Dx)
- Disposition

In addition, physicians write orders and progress notes, nurses write nurses' notes, and other departments contribute to these notes or use preprinted forms to record information in the hospital medical record.

A CLOSER LOOK

The medical record is a medicolegal record. This means that it not only contains medical documents but that those are also legal documents that can be used in a court of law.

Before patients can be treated at any type of healthcare facility, they must sign a **consent to treatment** form that gives physicians and other healthcare professionals the right to treat them. Treatment without consent is against the law and could constitute battery (touching another person without his or her consent or causing harm). For a patient who is a minor, the parent or legal guardian signs the consent to treatment form. In an emergency situation, implied consent allows care to be provided until the patient is awake and able to consent or until a legally appropriate person is able to consent for the patient. Prior to a surgery, the physician describes the purpose of the surgery and informs the patient of alternatives, risks, and possible outcomes or complications. Then the patient signs a consent to surgery form.

A patient must also sign a form that allows the facility to contact the insurance company to obtain payment for any health care that is provided. Under the federal regulations of **HIPAA** (**Health Insurance Portability and Accountability Act** of 1996), all healthcare settings must provide patients with a statement verifying that their medical record information is secure and is released only to authorized healthcare providers, insurance companies, or healthcare quality monitoring organizations.

Abbreviations

Abbreviations are commonly used in medical language and understanding their meanings is a part of learning medical language. Each chapter in this book includes a list of commonly used abbreviations.

CC	chief complaint	**H&P**	history and physical (examination)
D/C*■	discharge; discontinue	**HIPAA**	Health Insurance Portability and
DS	discharge summary		Accountability Act (pronounced "HIP-ah")
DX, Dx	diagnosis	**HPI**	history of present illness
EHR	electronic health record	**ISMP**	Institute for Safe Medication Practices
EMR	electronic medical record	**PE**	physical examination
EPR	electronic patient record	**PMH**	past medical (and surgical) history
FH	family history	**ROS**	review of systems
		SH	social history

*According to The Joint Commission and ■ the Institute for Safe Medication Practices (ISMP), this abbreviation should not be used. Because it is still used by some healthcare professionals, it is included here.

WORD ALERT

Abbreviations

Abbreviations are commonly used in all types of medical documents; however, they can mean different things to different people and their meanings can be misinterpreted. Always verify the meaning of an abbreviation.

CC means *chief complaint,* but it also means *cubic centimeter* (a measure of volume).

H&P means *history and physical* (*examination*), but the sound-alike abbreviation *HNP* stands for *herniated nucleus pulposus.*

PE means *physical examination,* but it also means *pressure-equalizing tube* and *pulmonary embolus.*

DID YOU KNOW?

Each healthcare facility develops its own list of acceptable abbreviations (that can be used in medical records produced in that facility) and a list of unacceptable or "do not use" abbreviations. In addition to that, The Joint Commission, an accrediting body for hospitals, has a list of abbreviations that should not be used because they cause errors. Their National Safety Goal states that these abbreviations should appear on a facility's "Do Not Use" list. The Joint Commission's list is a short list because it is the minimum required for a facility to be accredited. Some of these "do not use" abbreviations are included in this book because they are still in common use by some healthcare professionals. These abbreviations are marked with an asterisk (*). Other "do not use" abbreviations, compiled by the Institute for Safe Medication Practices (ISMP), are also marked (■). Finally, some abbreviations (such as the abbreviation *SOB,* meaning *shortness of breath*) have an alternate undesirable meaning and should not be used. However, these questionable abbreviations still continue to be used in medical records and are noted whenever they occur in a chapter.

Chapter 2
The Body in Health and Disease

The human body is a marvelous, intricate creation that can be organized and studied in different ways. When functioning properly, the body operates in a state of health; when it fails, it experiences disease.

 ## Learning Outcomes

After you study this chapter, you should be able to

2.1 Define health and describe approaches used to organize information about the human body.

2.2 Identify body planes, body directions, body cavities, abdominal quadrants and regions, body systems, medical specialties, and structures of the cell.

2.3 Describe categories of diseases.

2.4 Describe techniques used to perform a physical examination.

2.5 Describe categories of healthcare professionals and settings in which health care is provided.

2.6 Give the meanings of word parts and abbreviations related to the body, health, and disease.

2.7 Divide words and build words about the body, health, and disease.

2.8 Spell and pronounce words about the body, health, and disease.

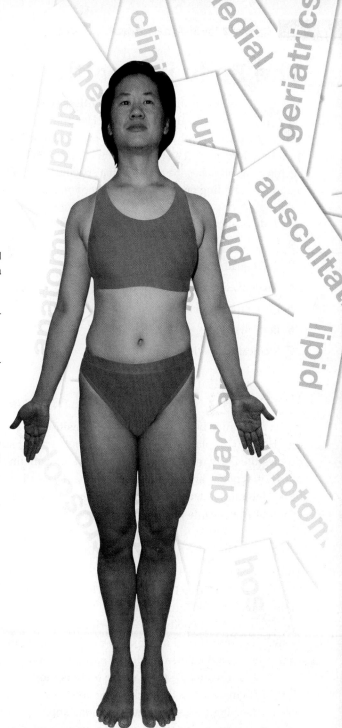

FIGURE 2-1 ■ Human body in anatomical position.
Anatomical position is a standard position in which the body is standing erect, the head is up with the eyes looking forward, the arms are by the sides with the palms facing forward, and the legs are straight with the toes pointing forward.

Source: Pearson Education

The Body in Health

When the human body's countless parts function correctly, the body is in a state of **health**. The World Health Organization defines health as a state of complete physical, mental, and social well-being (and not just the absence of disease or infirmity). The healthy human body can be studied in several different ways. Each way approaches the body from a specific point of view and provides unique information by dividing or organizing the body in a logical way. These ways include:

1. Body planes and body directions
2. Body cavities
3. Body quadrants and regions
4. Anatomy and physiology
5. Microscopic to macroscopic
6. Body systems
7. Medical specialties.

Body Planes and Body Directions

When the human body is in **anatomical position** (see Figure 2-1 ■), it can be studied by dividing it with planes. A **plane** is an imaginary flat surface (like a plate of glass) that divides the body into two parts. There are three main body planes: the coronal plane, the sagittal plane, and the transverse plane. These planes divide the body into front and back, right and left, and upper and lower sections, respectively. Body directions represent movement away from or toward these planes.

Coronal Plane and Body Directions

The **coronal plane** or **frontal plane** is a vertical plane that divides the body into front and back sections (see Figure 2-2 ■). The coronal plane is named for the coronal suture in the cranium (see Figure 2-3 ■).

The front of the body is the **anterior** or **ventral** section. The back of the body is the **posterior** or **dorsal** section. Lying face down is being in the **prone** position. Lying on the back is being in the **dorsal** or **dorsal supine** position.

Moving toward the front of the body is moving in an anterior direction, or anteriorly. Moving toward the back of the body is moving in a posterior direction, or posteriorly (see Figure 2-4 ■). The directions anterior and posterior can be combined as anteroposterior or posteroanterior. An **anteroposterior (AP)** direction moves from outside the body through the anterior section and then through the posterior section. A **posteroanterior (PA)** direction moves from outside the body through the posterior section and then through the anterior section (see Figure 2-5 ■).

Pronunciation/Word Parts

health (HELTH)

anatomical (AN-ah-TAW-mih-kal)
  ana- *apart; excessive*
  tom/o- *cut; layer; slice*
  -ical *pertaining to*

plane (PLAYN)

coronal (kor-OH-nal)
  coron/o- *structure that encircles like a crown*
  -al *pertaining to*

frontal (FRUN-tal)
  front/o- *front*
  -al *pertaining to*

anterior (an-TEER-ee-or)
  anter/o- *before; front part*
  -ior *pertaining to*

ventral (VEN-tral)
  ventr/o- *abdomen; front*
  -al *pertaining to*

posterior (pohs-TEER-ee-or)
  poster/o- *back part*
  -ior *pertaining to*

dorsal (DOR-sal)
  dors/o- *back; dorsum*
  -al *pertaining to*

prone (PROHN)

supine (soo-PINE) (SOO-pine)

anteroposterior
(AN-ter-OH-pohs-TEER-ee-or)
  anter/o- *before; front part*
  poster/o- *back part*
  -ior *pertaining to*

posteroanterior
(POHS-ter-OH-an-TEER-ee-or)
  poster/o- *back part*
  anter/o- *before; front part*
  -ior *pertaining to*

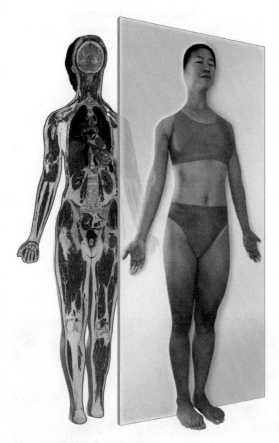

FIGURE 2-2 ■ Coronal plane.
The coronal or frontal plane divides the body into anterior (front) and posterior (back) sections.
Source: Pearson Education

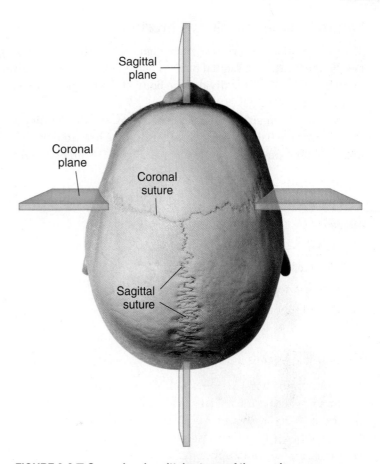

FIGURE 2-3 ■ Coronal and sagittal sutures of the cranium.
The coronal and sagittal planes are named for the coronal and sagittal sutures that join together the bones of the cranium. Each plane is oriented in the same direction as the suture for which it is named.
Source: Pearson Education

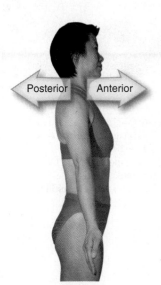

FIGURE 2-4 ■ Anterior and posterior directions.
Moving in an anterior direction is moving toward the front of the body. Moving in a posterior direction is moving toward the back of the body. Anterior and posterior are opposite directions.
Source: Pearson Education

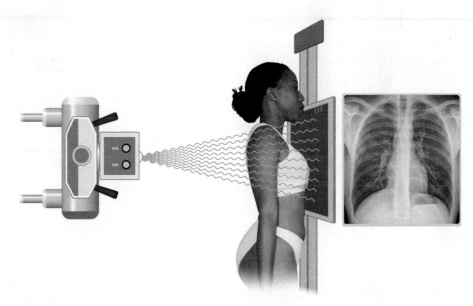

FIGURE 2-5 ■ Posteroanterior direction.
Anteroposterior and *posteroanterior* are commonly used in radiology to indicate the path of an x-ray beam. For a posteroanterior (PA) chest x-ray, the x-ray beam enters the posterior chest, goes through the anterior chest, and enters the x-ray plate to produce an image.
Source: Pearson Education

Sagittal Plane and Body Directions

The **sagittal plane** is a vertical plane that divides the body into right and left sections (see Figure 2-6 ■). The sagittal plane is named for the sagittal suture in the cranium (see Figure 2-3). If this plane divides the body at the midline into equal right and left sections, it is a midsagittal plane (see Figure 2-7 ■).

Moving from either side of the body toward the midline is moving in a **medial** direction, or medially. Moving from the midline toward either side of the body is moving in a lateral direction, or laterally (see Figure 2-8 ■). **Bilateral** indicates both sides.

Pronunciation/Word Parts

sagittal (SAJ-ih-tal)
  sagitt/o- *front to back*
  -al *pertaining to*

medial (MEE-dee-al)
  medi/o- *middle*
  -al *pertaining to*

lateral (LAT-er-al)
  later/o- *side*
  -al *pertaining to*

bilateral (by-LAT-er-al)
  bi- *two*
  later/o- *side*
  -al *pertaining to*

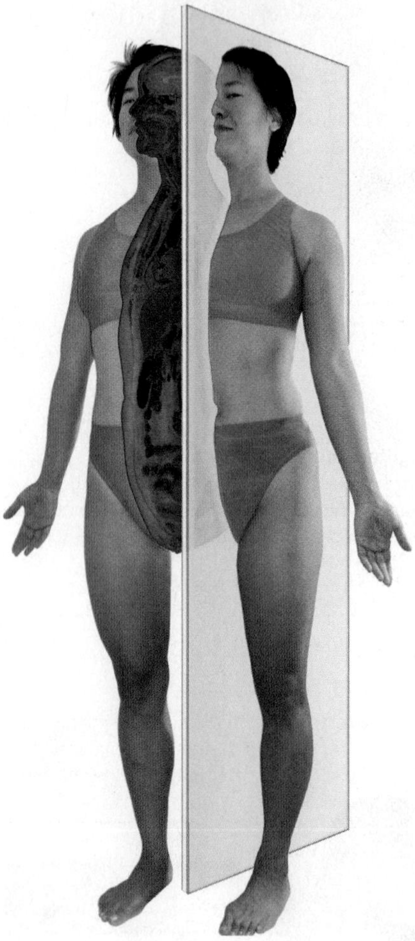

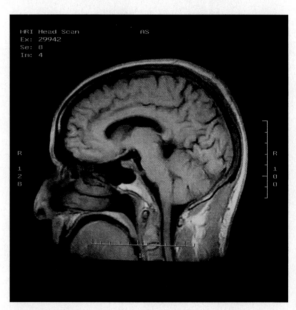

FIGURE 2-6 ■ Sagittal plane.
The sagittal plane divides the body into right and left sections.
Source: Pearson Education

FIGURE 2-7 ■ Midsagittal image of the head on an MRI scan.
A magnetic resonance imaging (MRI) scan uses a magnetic field to create many individual images of the body in "slices." This is an image of the head, taken in the midsagittal plane. The prefix *mid-* means *middle*. Other images taken during this scan would show "slices" along many parasagittal planes on either side of the midline. One of the meanings of the prefix *para-* is *beside*.
Source: CGinspiration/Shutterstock

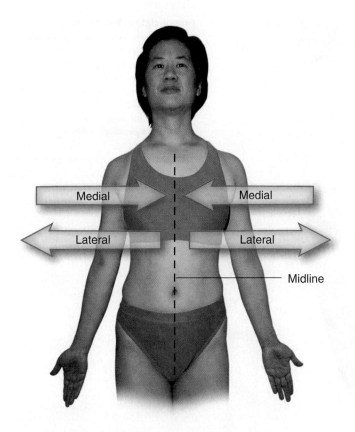

FIGURE 2-8 ■ Medial and lateral directions.
Moving in a medial direction is moving toward the midline of the body.
Moving in a lateral direction is moving away from the midline. Medial
and lateral are opposite directions.
Source: Pearson Education

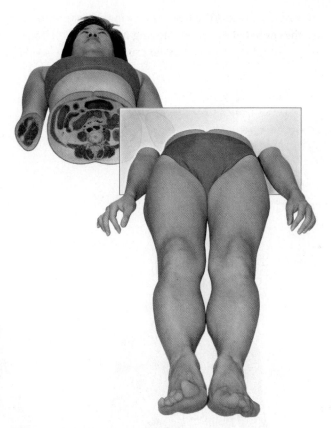

FIGURE 2-9 ■ Transverse plane.
The transverse plane divides the body into superior (upper) and
inferior (lower) sections.
Source: Pearson Education

Transverse Plane and Body Directions

The **transverse plane** is a horizontal plane that divides the body into upper and lower
sections (see Figure 2-9 ■). The upper half of the body is the **superior** section, and the
lower half is the **inferior** section. Some anatomical structures have superior and inferior
parts (see Figure 2-10 ■).

Pronunciation/Word Parts

transverse (trans-VERS)
  trans- *across; through*
  -verse *travel; turn*
Most medical words contain a combining
form. The ending *-verse* contains the
combining form **vers/o-** and the one-letter
suffix *-e*.

superior (soo-PEER-ee-or)
  super/o- *above*
  -ior *pertaining to*

inferior (in-FEER-ee-or)
  infer/o- *below*
  -ior *pertaining to*

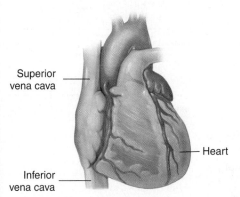

FIGURE 2-10 ■ Superior and inferior parts.
The superior vena cava brings blood from the head
to the heart. The inferior vena cava brings blood
from the lower body to the heart.
Source: Pearson Education

Moving toward the head is moving in a superior direction, or superiorly. This is also the **cephalad** direction. Moving toward the tail bone is moving in an inferior direction, or inferiorly. This is also the **caudad** direction (see Figure 2-11 ■).

Pronunciation/Word Parts

cephalad (SEF-ah-lad)
  cephal/o- *head*
  -ad *in the direction of; toward*

caudad (KAW-dad)
  caud/o- *tail bone*
  -ad *in the direction of; toward*

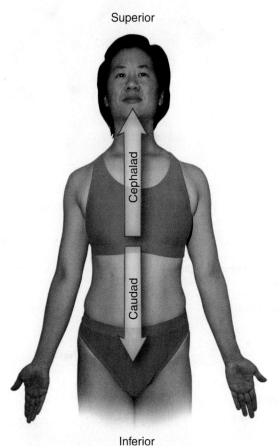

Superior

Cephalad

Caudad

Inferior

FIGURE 2-11 ■ Cephalad and caudad directions.
Moving in a cephalad direction is moving toward the head. Moving in a caudad direction is moving toward the tail bone. Cephalad and caudad are opposite directions.
Source: Pearson Education

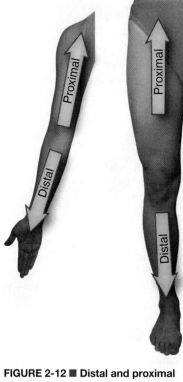

Proximal

Distal

Proximal

Distal

FIGURE 2-12 ■ Distal and proximal directions.
Moving in a distal direction is moving away from the trunk of the body (where the limb is attached) toward the fingers or toes. Moving in a proximal direction is moving away from the fingers or toes toward the trunk of the body. Distal and proximal are opposite directions.
Source: Pearson Education

distal (DIS-tal)
  dist/o- *away from the center; away from the point of origin*
  -al *pertaining to*

proximal (PRAWK-sih-mal)
  proxim/o- *near the center; near the point of origin*
  -al *pertaining to*

external (eks-TER-nal)
  extern/o- *outside*
  -al *pertaining to*

internal (in-TER-nal)
  intern/o- *inside*
  -al *pertaining to*

Other Body Directions and Locations

Moving from the trunk of the body toward the end of a limb (arm or leg) is moving in a **distal** direction, or distally. Moving from the end of a limb toward the trunk of the body is moving in a **proximal** direction, or proximally (see Figure 2-12 ■).

Structures on the surface of the body are superficial or **external**. Structures below the surface and inside the body are deep or **internal** (see Figure 2-13 ■).

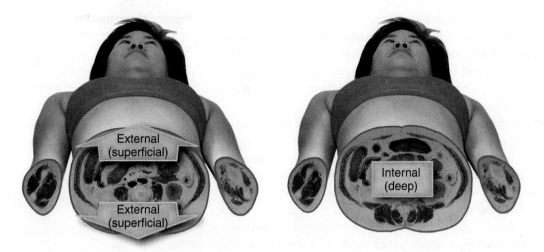

FIGURE 2-13 ■ External and internal locations.
External refers to the superficial or outer part of the body or an organ. *Internal* refers to deep inside the body or an organ. Internal and external are opposite locations.
Source: Pearson Education

Body Cavities

The human body can be studied according to its body cavities and their internal organs (see Figure 2-14 ■). A **cavity** is a hollow space. It is surrounded by bones or muscles that support and protect the organs and structures within the cavity. There are five body cavities.

The **cranial cavity** is within the bony cranium of the head. The cranial cavity contains the brain, cranial nerves, and related structures.

The **spinal cavity** or spinal canal is a continuation of the cranial cavity as it travels down the midline of the back. The spinal cavity is within the bones of the spine. The spinal cavity contains the spinal cord, spinal nerves, and related structures.

Pronunciation/Word Parts

cavity (KAV-ih-tee)
  cav/o- *hollow space*
  -ity *condition; state*

cranial (KRAY-nee-al)
  crani/o- *cranium; skull*
  -al *pertaining to*

spinal (SPY-nal)
  spin/o- *backbone; spine*
  -al *pertaining to*

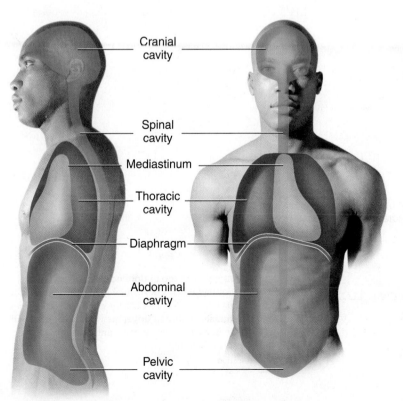

Cranial cavity

Spinal cavity

Mediastinum

Thoracic cavity

Diaphragm

Abdominal cavity

Pelvic cavity

FIGURE 2-14 ■ Body cavities.
The cranial cavity becomes the spinal cavity along the back. The thoracic cavity is separated from the abdominal cavity by the diaphragm. The abdominal cavity is continuous with the pelvic cavity and is often called the *abdominopelvic cavity.*
Source: Pearson Education

The **thoracic cavity** is within the chest and is surrounded by the breast bone (sternum) anteriorly, the ribs bilaterally, and the bones of the spine posteriorly. The thoracic cavity contains the lungs. The mediastinum—a smaller, central area within the thoracic cavity—contains the trachea, esophagus, heart, and related structures. The inferior border of the thoracic cavity is the large, muscular diaphragm that functions during respiration. The diaphragm separates the thoracic cavity from the abdominal cavity.

The **abdominal cavity** is within the abdomen. It is surrounded by the diaphragm superiorly, the abdominal wall anteriorly, and the bones of the spine posteriorly. The **pelvic cavity** is a continuation of the abdominal cavity. The pelvic cavity is surrounded by the pelvic (hip) bones anteriorly and bilaterally and the bones of the spine posteriorly. These two cavities are often called the **abdominopelvic cavity** because it is one continuous cavity with no dividing structure. The abdominopelvic cavity contains many organs of the gastrointestinal, endocrine, reproductive, and urinary systems, such as the stomach, intestines, liver, gallbladder, pancreas, ovaries, uterus, and bladder. These large internal organs are the **viscera**.

Body Quadrants and Regions

The human body can be studied according to its quadrants and regions. The anterior surface of the abdominopelvic area can be divided into four quadrants or nine regions, both of which are helpful as references during a physical examination of the internal organs.

The four **quadrants** include the right upper quadrant (RUQ), left upper quadrant (LUQ), right lower quadrant (RLQ), and left lower quadrant (LLQ) (see Figure 2-15 ■).

Pronunciation/Word Parts

thoracic (thor-AS-ik)
  thorac/o- *chest; thorax*
  -ic *pertaining to*

abdominal (ab-DAW-mih-nal)
  abdomin/o- *abdomen*
  -al *pertaining to*

pelvic (PEL-vik)
  pelv/o- *hip bone; pelvis; renal pelvis*
  -ic *pertaining to*

abdominopelvic (ab-DAW-mih-noh-PEL-vik)
  abdomin/o- *abdomen*
  pelv/o- *hip bone; pelvis; renal pelvis*
  -ic *pertaining to*

viscera (VIS-er-ah)

visceral (VIS-er-al)
  viscer/o- *large internal organs*
  -al *pertaining to*

quadrant (KWAH-drant)
  quadr/o- *four*
  -ant *pertaining to*

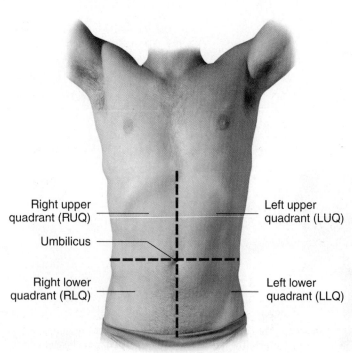

Right upper quadrant (RUQ)

Left upper quadrant (LUQ)

Umbilicus

Right lower quadrant (RLQ)

Left lower quadrant (LLQ)

FIGURE 2-15 ■ Quadrants of the abdominopelvic area.
Four quadrants are formed when a horizontal line and a vertical line cross at the umbilicus (navel). The liver can be felt in the right upper quadrant, and the stomach in the left upper quadrant. A patient with appendicitis has pain in the right lower quadrant, and the rectum can be felt in the left lower quadrant.
Source: Pearson Education

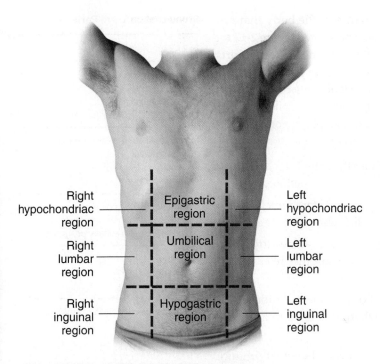

Right hypochondriac region

Epigastric region

Left hypochondriac region

Right lumbar region

Umbilical region

Left lumbar region

Right inguinal region

Hypogastric region

Left inguinal region

FIGURE 2-16 ■ Regions of the abdominopelvic area.
Nine regions are formed when two horizontal lines and two vertical lines form a square around the umbilicus.
Source: Pearson Education

The nine regions include the right and left **hypochondriac** regions, the **epigastric** region, the right and left **lumbar** regions, the **umbilical** region (centered around the umbilicus or navel), the right and left **inguinal** regions, and the **hypogastric** region (see Figure 2-16 ■).

CLINICAL CONNECTIONS

The lumbar regions of the abdominal area are so named because they are on the same level as the lumbar area of the lower back. Remember, when you are facing the patient (as in this illustration), your right side corresponds to the patient's left side. Correctly identifying right and left is an important patient safety issue.

DID YOU KNOW?

The Greeks considered the hypochondriac regions to be the seat of melancholy (sad feelings) because they contained the liver and spleen, organs that were thought to release substances that caused different moods. Today, a hypochondriac is a person who is constantly concerned about real or imagined symptoms, many of which are in these regions.

The anatomy of the human body was first studied by physicians who secretly carried away and dissected the unclaimed dead bodies of criminals.

Cells, Tissues, and Organs

The human body can be studied according to its structures and functions. **Anatomy** is the study of the structures of the human body. **Physiology** is the study of the functions of those structures.

The human body can be studied according to its smallest parts and how they combine to make larger and more complex structures and systems.

---

hypochondriac (HY-poh-CON-dree-ak)
  hypo- *below; deficient*
  chondr/o- *cartilage*
  -iac *pertaining to*
Add words to make a complete definition of *hypochondriac: pertaining to below (the) cartilage (of the ribs).*

---

epigastric (EP-ih-GAS-trik)
  epi- *above; upon*
  gastr/o- *stomach*
  -ic *pertaining to*

---

lumbar (LUM-bar)
  lumb/o- *area between the ribs and pelvis; lower back*
  -ar *pertaining to*

---

umbilical (um-BIL-ih-kal)
  umbilic/o- *navel; umbilicus*
  -al *pertaining to*

---

inguinal (ING-gwih-nal)
  inguin/o- *groin*
  -al *pertaining to*

---

hypogastric (HY-poh-GAS-trik)
  hypo- *below; deficient*
  gastr/o- *stomach*
  -ic *pertaining to*

---

anatomy (ah-NAT-oh-mee)
  ana- *apart; excessive*
  -tomy *process of cutting; process of making an incision*
The ending *-tomy* contains the combining form *tom/o-* and the one-letter suffix *-y*.

---

physiology (FIZ-ee-AW-loh-jee)
  physi/o- *physical function*
  -logy *study of*

A **cell** is the smallest independently functioning structure in the body that can reproduce itself by division. All cells contain certain basic structures (see Figure 2-17 ■). The **cell membrane** around the cell is a permeable barrier that protects and supports the **intracellular contents**. It allows water and nutrients to enter the cell and cellular waste products to leave the cell. It also contains ion pumps that actively bring electrolytes (sodium, potassium, and so forth) in and out of the cell.

The **cytoplasm** is a gel-like substance that fills the cell. The cytoplasm contains several different types of structures known as **organelles**.

- **Endoplasmic reticulum**. Network of channels throughout the cytoplasm that transports materials. It is also the site of protein, fat, and glycogen production.

- **Golgi apparatus**. Curved, stacked membranes that process and store proteins (such as hormones or enzymes) until they are released by the cell. It also makes lysosomes.

- **Lysosomes**. Small sacs that contain powerful digestive enzymes to destroy a bacterium or virus that invades the cell. When a cell dies, the lysosomes release their enzymes into the cytoplasm, and the cell is slowly dissolved.

- **Messenger RNA**. Messenger RNA (**ribonucleic acid**) duplicates the information contained in a gene and carries it to the ribosome where it is used to assemble amino acids to make a protein molecule.

- **Mitochondria**. Capsule-shaped structures with sectioned chambers that produce and store ATP, a high-energy molecule obtained from the metabolism of glucose. As needed, the mitochondria convert ATP to ADP to release energy for cellular activities.

- **Nucleus**. Large, round, centralized structure that is surrounded by a membrane. The nucleus controls all of the activities that take place within the cell. The **nucleolus** is a round, central region within the nucleus. It produces RNA and ribosomes. **Chromosomes** are paired structures within the nucleus. Each cell nucleus contains 23 pairs of chromosomes for a total of 46 chromosomes. In each of the 23 pairs, one of the chromosomes was inherited from the mother and the other from the father. A single chromosome is made of one long DNA (**deoxyribonucleic acid**) molecule. A DNA molecule consists of repeating pairs of amino acids sequenced along two strands that form a double helix.

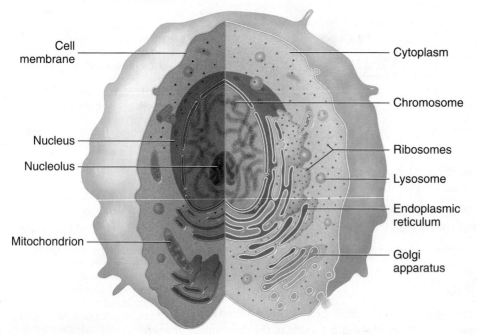

FIGURE 2-17 ■ Structures of a cell.
A cell consists of many different structures, each of which plays a unique role in securing nutrients, producing energy, building proteins, and fighting invading pathogens. All of these functions are essential to the continuing health of the body.
Source: Pearson Education

Pronunciation/Word Parts

cell (SEL)

cellular (SEL-yoo-lar)
  cellul/o- *cell*
  -ar *pertaining to*
The combining form **cyt/o-** also means *cell*.

intracellular (IN-trah-SEL-yoo-lar)
  intra- *within*
  cellul/o- *cell*
  -ar *pertaining to*

cytoplasm (SY-toh-plazm)
  cyt/o- *cell*
  -plasm *formed substance; growth*

organelle (OR-gah-NEL)
  organ/o- *organ*
  -elle *small thing*

endoplasmic (EN-doh-PLAS-mik)
  endo- *innermost; within*
  plasm/o- *plasma*
  -ic *pertaining to*

reticulum (reh-TIH-kyoo-lum)

Golgi (GOL-jee)

lysosome (LY-soh-sohm)
  lys/o- *break down; destroy*
  -some *body*
Add words to make a complete definition of *lysosome*: body (that contains enzymes that) break down or destroy.

ribonucleic acid
(RY-boh-noo-KLEE-ik AS-id)

mitochondrion (MY-toh-CON-dree-on)

mitochondria (MY-toh-CON-dree-ah)
Mitochondrion is a Greek singular noun. Form the plural by changing -on to -a.

nucleus (NOO-klee-us)

nuclei (NOO-klee-eye)
Nucleus is a Latin singular noun. Form the plural by changing -us to -i. The combining form **kary/o-** means *nucleus of a cell*.

nuclear (NOO-klee-ar)
  nucle/o- *nucleus of an atom; nucleus of a cell*
  -ar *pertaining to*

nucleolus (noo-KLEE-oh-lus)

nucleoli (noo-KLEE-oh-lie)
Nucleolus is a Latin singular noun. Form the plural by changing -us to -i.

chromosome (KROH-moh-sohm)
  chrom/o- *color*
  -some *body*
Add words to make a complete definition of *chromosome*: (microscopic) body (that takes on) color (when stained).

A **gene** is one segment of a DNA molecule that contains enough amino acid pairs to provide the information needed to produce one protein molecule. In a cell that is not dividing, each long DNA molecule is loosely coiled, giving the nucleus a woven, grainy appearance under the microscope. As the cell prepares to divide, each DNA molecule coils tightly, making the chromosomes visible as rodlike structures in the nucleus.

- **Ribosomes**. Granular structures in the cytoplasm and on the endoplasmic reticulum. Ribosomes contain RNA and proteins and are the site where proteins are produced.

DID YOU KNOW?

Most body cells contain one nucleus. However, a mature erythrocyte (red blood cell) does not contain any nucleus, and a skeletal muscle cell contains many nuclei.

Mitosis is the process by which a cell divides. Mitosis begins in the cell's nucleus as each chromosome makes an exact copy of itself. (The double helix of its DNA molecule splits down its length and rebuilds to form another double helix.) All of the chromosomes and their identical copies align themselves along thread-like strands in the nucleus and then separate to opposite sides of the nucleus. Then the entire nucleus and cytoplasm split, forming two cells that are identical to the original cell.

Most cells and cellular structures are **microscopic** in size and can be seen only through a **microscope** (see Figure 2-18 ■), although some cells—a female ovum, for example—can be seen with the naked eye. Cells combine to form **tissues**, and tissues combine to form **organs**. (Different kinds of tissues and organs are discussed in specific chapters.) Tissues and organs are **macroscopic** and can be seen with the naked eye. Organs combine to form a body system. The human body contains many different body systems, as discussed in the next section.

MACROSCOPIC

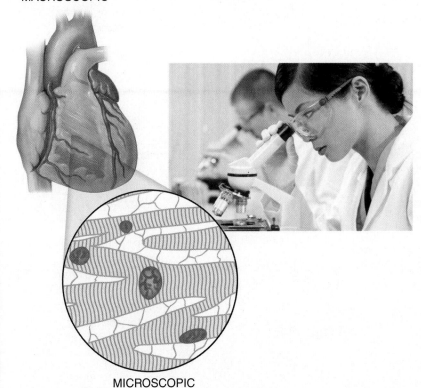

MICROSCOPIC

FIGURE 2-18 ■ Using a microscope to study the human body.
A microscope enhances our understanding of the human body because it allows us to see anatomical structures not visible to the naked eye. With its magnification, we can see cells and even tiny structures within cells.

Source: Pearson Education; Darren Baker/Fotolia

Pronunciation/Word Parts

deoxyribonucleic acid
(dee-AWK-see-RY-boh-noo-KLEE-ik AS-id)

gene (JEEN)

genetic (jeh-NET-ik)
  gene/o- *gene*
  -tic *pertaining to*

ribosome (RY-boh-sohm)
  rib/o- *ribonucleic acid*
  -some *body*

mitosis (my-TOH-sis)
  mit/o- *thread-like structure*
  -osis *condition; process*
Add words to make a complete definition of *mitosis*: *process (of cell division during which the chromosomes align along) thread-like structures (in the nucleus).*

microscopic (MY-kroh-SKAW-pik)
  micr/o- *one millionth; small*
  scop/o- *examine with an instrument*
  -ic *pertaining to*

microscope (MY-kroh-skohp)
  micr/o- *one millionth; small*
  -scope *instrument used to examine*
A microscope is an *instrument used to examine small (things). Note:* To define this word correctly, you must start with the meaning of the suffix followed by the meaning of the combining form. If not, you will get the incorrect definition of *small instrument used to examine (things).*

tissue (TIH-shoo)

organ (OR-gan)

macroscopic (MAK-roh-SKAW-pik)
  macr/o- *large*
  scop/o- *examine with an instrument*
  -ic *pertaining to*

Body Systems

The human body can be studied according to its structures and how they function together as a **body system**. Studying the body systems is the standard approach used in anatomy and physiology textbooks. However, in medicine, body systems are studied within the context of medical specialties. Because this textbook is about medical language, we will study by medical specialties, just as in the real world of medicine!

Medical Specialties

The human body can be studied according to the **medical specialties** that make up the practice of medicine. Each medical specialty includes the anatomy (structures), physiology (functions), diseases, laboratory and diagnostic procedures, medical and surgical procedures, and drugs for a particular body system. Medical specialties (not body systems) are used to name departments in the hospital and other medical facilities (example: the Department of Cardiology).

Pronunciation/Word Parts

system (SIS-tem)

medical (MED-ih-kal)
  medic/o- *medicine; physician*
  -al *pertaining to*

Medical Specialty and Body System	Structures	Functions	Pronunciation/Word Parts
Gastroenterology **Gastrointestinal** **System** (Chapter 3) Gastroenterology is the study of the stomach and intestines (and related structures). A gastroentero-logist is a physician who specializes in gastroenterology. *Source*: Pearson Education	• mouth (teeth and tongue) • salivary glands • pharynx (throat) • esophagus • stomach • small intestine • large intestine • liver • gallbladder • pancreas	• receive sensory information (taste) • digest food • absorb nutrients into the blood • excrete undigested wastes	**gastroenterology** (GAS-troh-EN-ter-AW-loh-jee) **gastr/o-** *stomach* **enter/o-** *intestine* **-logy** *study of* **gastrointestinal** (GAS-troh-in-TES-tih-nal) **gastr/o-** *stomach* **intestin/o-** *intestine* **-al** *pertaining to*
Pulmonology **Respiratory** **System** (Chapter 4) Pulmonology is the study of the lungs (and related structures). A pulmonologist is a physician who specializes in pulmonology. *Source*: Pearson Education	• nose • pharynx (throat) • larynx (voice box) • trachea • bronchi • bronchioles • alveoli (in the lungs)	• inhale oxygen • exhale carbon dioxide • exchange gases in the alveoli	**pulmonology** (PUL-moh-NAW-loh-jee) **pulmon/o-** *lung* **-logy** *study of* **respiratory** (RES-pih-rah-TOR-ee) (reh-SPY-rah-TOR-ee) **re-** *again and again; backward; unable to* **spir/o-** *breathe; coil* **-atory** *pertaining to*

Medical Specialty and Body System	Structures	Functions	Pronunciation/Word Parts
Cardiology **Cardiovascular System** (Chapter 5) Cardiology is the study of the heart (and related structures). A cardiologist is a physician who specializes in cardiology. *Source*: Pearson Education	• heart • arteries • veins • capillaries	• circulate blood throughout the body	**cardiology** (KAR-dee-AW-loh-jee) **cardi/o-** *heart* **-logy** *study of* **cardiovascular** (KAR-dee-oh-VAS-kyoo-lar) **cardi/o-** *heart* **vascul/o-** *blood vessel* **-ar** *pertaining to*
Hematology **Blood** (Chapter 6) Hematology is the study of the blood. A hematologist is a physician who specializes in hematology.	• blood (blood cells and plasma)	• transport oxygen and nutrients to the cells • transport carbon dioxide to the lungs and wastes to the kidneys	**hematology** (HEE-mah-TAW-loh-jee) **hemat/o-** *blood* **-logy** *study of* **blood** (BLUD)
Immunology **Blood, Lymphatic System** (Chapter 6) Immunology is the study of the immune response. An immunologist is a physician who specializes in immunology. *Source*: Pearson Education	• lymphatic vessels, lymph nodes, and lymph fluid • spleen • thymus • white blood cells	• recognize and destroy disease-causing organisms and abnormal cells	**immunology** (IH-myoo-NAW-loh-jee) **immun/o-** *immune response* **-logy** *study of* **lymphatic** (lim-FAT-ik) **lymph/o-** *lymph; lymphatic system* **-atic** *pertaining to*
Dermatology **Integumentary System** (Chapter 7) Dermatology is the study of the skin (and related structures). A dermatologist is a physician who specializes in dermatology. *Source*: Pearson Education	• skin • hair • nails • sweat glands • oil glands	• receive sensory information (pain, touch, temperature) • protect internal organs • regulate body temperature by sweating	**dermatology** (DER-mah-TAW-loh-jee) **dermat/o-** *skin* **-logy** *study of* **integumentary** (in-TEH-gyoo-MEN-tair-ee) **integument/o-** *skin* **-ary** *pertaining to*

Medical Specialty and Body System	Structures	Functions	Pronunciation/Word Parts
Orthopedics **Skeletal System** (Chapter 8) Orthopedics is the knowledge and practice of producing straightness of the bones and muscles in a child or adult. An orthopedist is a physician who specializes in orthopedics. *Source*: Pearson Education	• bones • cartilage • ligaments • joints	• support the body	**orthopedics** (OR-thoh-PEE-diks) **orth/o-** *straight* **ped/o-** *child* **-ics** *knowledge; practice* Add words to make a complete definition of *orthopedics: knowledge and practice (of producing) straight(ness of the bones and muscles in a) child (or adult).* **skeletal** (SKEL-eh-tal) **skelet/o-** *skeleton* **-al** *pertaining to*
Orthopedics **Muscular System** (Chapter 9) *Source*: Pearson Education	• muscles • tendons	• produce movement of the body	**muscular** (MUS-kyoo-lar) **muscul/o-** *muscle* **-ar** *pertaining to*
Neurology **Nervous System** (Chapter 10) Neurology is the study of the nerves (and related structures). A neurologist is a physician who specializes in neurology *Source*: Pearson Education	• brain • cranial nerves • spinal cord • spinal nerves • cerebrospinal fluid • neurons	• receive, relay, and interpret sensory information (vision, hearing, smell, taste) and sensations (pain, touch, temperature, body position, balance) • coordinate movement • store and interpret memory and emotion	**neurology** (nyoor-AW-loh-jee) **neur/o-** *nerve* **-logy** *study of* **nervous** (NER-vus) **nerv/o-** *nerve* **-ous** *pertaining to*

Medical Specialty and Body System	Structures	Functions	Pronunciation/Word Parts
Urology **Urinary System** (Chapter 11) Urology is the study of the urine and the urinary system. A urologist is a physician who specializes in urology. *Source*: Pearson Education	• kidneys • ureters • bladder • urethra • nephrons	• filter out waste products from the blood and excrete them in the urine	**urology** (yoor-AW-loh-jee) 　**ur/o-** *urinary system; urine* 　**-logy** *study of* **urinary** (YOOR-ih-NAIR-ee) 　**urin/o-** *urinary system; urine* 　**-ary** *pertaining to*
Male Reproductive Medicine **Male Genital and Reproductive System** (Chapter 12) Reproductive medicine studies the structures that produce children. A reproductive specialist is a physician who specializes in reproductive medicine. *Source*: Pearson Education	• scrotum • testes • epididymides • vas deferens • seminal vesicles • prostate gland • urethra • penis	• secrete male hormones • develop male secondary sexual characteristics • produce and release sperm	**reproductive** (REE-proh-DUK-tiv) 　**re-** *again and again; backward; unable to* 　**product/o-** *produce* 　**-ive** *pertaining to* **genital** (JEN-ih-tal) 　**genit/o-** *genitalia* 　**-al** *pertaining to*
Gynecology and Obstetrics **Female Genital and Reproductive System** (Chapter 13) Gynecology is the study of females. A gynecologist is a physician who specializes in gynecology. Obstetrics is the knowledge and practice of treating women during pregnancy and childbirth. An obstetrician is a physician who specializes in obstetrics. *Source*: Pearson Education	• breasts • ovaries • uterine tubes • uterus • vagina • external genitalia	• secrete female hormones • develop female secondary sexual characteristics • produce ova • menstruate • conceive and bear children • produce milk to nourish children	**gynecology** (GY-neh-KAW-loh-jee) 　**gynec/o-** *female; woman* 　**-logy** *study of* **obstetrics** (awb-STEH-triks) 　**obstetr/o-** *pregnancy and childbirth* 　**-ics** *knowledge; practice* Add words to make a complete definition of *obstetrics*: *knowledge and practice (of treating women during) pregnancy and childbirth.* **genital** (JEN-ih-tal) 　**genit/o-** *genitalia* 　**-al** *pertaining to*

Medical Specialty and Body System	Structures	Functions	Pronunciation/Word Parts
Endocrinology Endocrine System (Chapter 14) *Source*: Pearson Education Endocrinology is the study of glands within the body that secrete hormones into the blood. An endocrinologist is a physician who specializes in endocrinology.	• pituitary gland • pineal gland • thyroid gland • parathyroid glands • thymus • pancreas • adrenal glands • ovaries • testes	• secrete hormones into the blood • direct the activities of the body	**endocrinology** (EN-doh-krih-NAW-loh-jee) **endo-** *innermost; within* **crin/o-** *secrete* **-logy** *study of* Add words to make a complete definition of *endocrinology*: *study of (glands) within (the body that) secrete (hormones into the blood)*. **endocrine** (EN-doh-krin) (EN-doh-krine) **endo-** *innermost; within* **crin/o-** *secrete* **-ine** *pertaining to; thing pertaining to* *Note*: The duplicated letters "in" are deleted when the word is formed.
Ophthalmology Eyes (Chapter 15) Ophthalmology is the study of the eye (and related structures). An ophthalmologist is a physician who specializes in ophthalmology. *Source*: Pearson Education	• eyes	• receive sensory information (vision)	**ophthalmology** (OFF-thal-MAW-loh-jee) **ophthalm/o-** *eye* **-logy** *study of*
Otolaryngology Ears, Nose, and Throat (ENT) System (Chapter 16) Otolaryngology is the study of the ears, nose, pharynx (throat), larynx (voice box), and related structures. An otolaryngologist is a physician who specializes in otolaryngology. *Source*: Pearson Education	• ears • nose • sinuses • pharynx (throat) • larynx (voice box)	• receive sensory information (hearing, balance, smell) • produce speech	**otolaryngology** (OH-toh-LAIR-ing-GAW-loh-jee) **ot/o-** *ear* **laryng/o-** *larynx; voice box* **-logy** *study of*

Other Medical Specialties

These medical specialties are not directly related to body systems.

Medical Specialty	Chapter	Description	Pronunciation/Word Parts
Psychiatry	17	Psychiatry is the medical treatment of the mind. A psychiatrist is a physician who specializes in psychiatry.	**psychiatry** (sy-KY-ah-tree) **psych/o-** *mind* **-iatry** *medical treatment*
Oncology	18	Oncology is the study of a (cancerous) mass or tumor. An oncologist is a physician who specializes in oncology.	**oncology** (ong-KAW-loh-jee) **onc/o-** *mass; tumor* **-logy** *study of*
Radiology and Nuclear Medicine	19	Radiology is the study and use of x-rays, sound waves, and other forms of radiation and energy to diagnose diseases. Nuclear medicine uses radioactive substances to diagnose and treat diseases. A radiologist is a physician who specializes in radiology and nuclear medicine.	**radiology** (RAY-dee-AW-loh-jee) **radi/o-** *forearm bone; radiation; x-rays* **-logy** *study of* Select the correct combining form meaning to get the correct definition of *radiology*: *study of x-rays.* **nuclear** (NOO-klee-ar) **nucle/o-** *nucleus of an atom; nucleus of a cell* **-ar** *pertaining to* **medicine** (MED-ih-sin) **medic/o-** *medicine; physician* **-ine** *pertaining to; thing pertaining to*
Dentistry		Dentistry is a process related to the specialty of the teeth. A dentist is a doctor of dentistry who specializes in the teeth.	**dentistry** (DEN-tis-tree) **dent/o-** *tooth* **-istry** *process related to a specialty*
Dietetics	*	Dietetics is the knowledge and practice of diet and foods. A dietitian is a healthcare professional who specializes in dietetics.	**dietetics** (DY-eh-TEH-tiks) **dietet/o-** *diet; foods* **-ics** *knowledge; practice*
Pharmacology	*	Pharmacology is the study of medicines and drugs. A pharmacist has a doctoral degree in pharmacy and specializes in medicines and drugs.	**pharmacology** (FAR-mah-KAW-loh-jee) **pharmac/o-** *drug; medicine* **-logy** *study of*
Neonatology	*	Neonatology is the study of newborn babies with medical problems. A neonatologist is a physician who specializes in neonatology.	**neonatology** (NEE-oh-nay-TAW-loh-jee) **ne/o-** *new* **nat/o-** *birth* **-logy** *study of*
Pediatrics	*	Pediatrics is the knowledge and practice of children and their medical treatment. A pediatrician is a physician who specializes in pediatrics.	**pediatrics** (PEE-dee-AT-riks) **ped/o-** *child* **iatr/o-** *medical treatment; physician* **-ics** *knowledge; practice*
Geriatrics	*	Geriatrics is the knowledge and practice of persons of old age and their medical treatment. A gerontologist is a physician who specializes in geriatrics.	**geriatrics** (JAIR-ee-AT-riks) **ger/o-** *old age* **iatr/o-** *medical treatment; physician* **-ics** *knowledge; practice*

*These medical specialties are mentioned in feature boxes throughout the book.

Vocabulary Review

The Body in Health		
Word or Phrase	**Description**	**Combining Forms**
abdominal cavity	Cavity that is surrounded by the diaphragm superiorly, the abdominal wall anteriorly, and the bones of the spine posteriorly	**abdomin/o-** *abdomen*
abdominopelvic cavity	Continuous cavity formed by the abdominal and pelvic cavities	**abdomin/o-** *abdomen* **pelv/o-** *hip bone; pelvis; renal pelvis*
anatomical position	Standard position of the body for the purpose of study. The body is erect, head up, hands by the side with palms facing forward, and the legs are straight with the toes pointing forward.	**tom/o-** *cut; layer; slice*
anatomy	Study of the structures of the human body	**tom/o-** *cut; layer; slice*
anterior	Pertaining to the front of the body, an organ, or a structure	**anter/o-** *before; front part*
anteroposterior	Pertaining to the anterior section and then the posterior section of the body	**anter/o-** *before; front part* **poster/o-** *back part*
blood	Body system of blood cells and plasma. It transports oxygen and nutrients to the cells, carbon dioxide to the lungs, and wastes to the kidneys.	**hemat/o-** *blood*
body system	A way to study the body according to its structures and how they function	
cardiology	Medical specialty that deals with the cardiovascular system	**cardi/o-** *heart*
cardiovascular system	Body system that includes the heart, arteries, veins, and capillaries. It circulates the blood throughout the body.	**cardi/o-** *heart* **vascul/o-** *blood vessel*
caudad	Toward the tail bone	**caud/o-** *tail bone*
cavity	Hollow space surrounded by bones or muscles, It contains organs and related structures	**cav/o-** *hollow space*
cell	Smallest, independently functioning structure in the body that can reproduce itself by division	**cellul/o-** *cell* **cyt/o-** *cell*
cell membrane	Permeable barrier that surrounds a cell and holds in the cytoplasm. It allows water and nutrients to enter and waste products to leave the cell.	
cephalad	Toward the head	**cephal/o-** *head*
chromosome	Paired, rodlike structures within the nucleus. Each cell contains 46 chromosomes (23 pairs).	**chrom/o-** *color*
coronal plane	Plane that divides the body into front and back sections, anterior and posterior. It is also known as the **frontal plane**.	**coron/o-** *structure that encircles like a crown* **front/o-** *front*
cranial cavity	Cavity in the head that is surrounded by the bony cranium and contains the brain, cranial nerves, and related structures	**crani/o-** *cranium; skull*
cytoplasm	Gel-like intracellular substance. Organelles are embedded in it.	**cyt/o-** *cell*
dentistry	Medical specialty that deals with the teeth	**dent/o-** *tooth*

Word or Phrase	Description	Combining Forms
dermatology	Medical specialty that deals with the integumentary system	**dermat/o-** *skin*
dietetics	Medical specialty that deals with nutrition, nutrients, foods, and diet	**dietet/o-** *diet; foods*
distal	Pertaining to away from the point of origin, such as on an arm or leg	**dist/o-** *away from the center; away from the point of origin*
DNA	Deoxyribonucleic acid. Sequenced pairs of amino acids that form a double helix chain within a chromosome. One segment of DNA makes up a gene.	
dorsal	Pertaining to the posterior of the body. Lying on the back is being in the dorsal or dorsal supine position.	**dors/o-** *back; dorsum*
endocrine system	Body system that includes the pituitary gland, pineal gland, thyroid gland, parathyroid glands, thymus, pancreas, adrenal glands, ovaries, and testes. It secretes hormones into the blood that direct the activities of the body.	**crin/o-** *secrete*
endocrinology	Medical specialty that deals with the endocrine system	**crin/o-** *secrete*
endoplasmic reticulum	Organelle that is a network of channels that transport materials within the cell. It is also the site of protein, fat, and glycogen production.	**plasm/o-** *plasma*
epigastric region	Region on the surface of the abdominopelvic area. It is superior to the umbilical region and medial to the hypochondriac regions.	**gastr/o-** *stomach*
external	Pertaining to the outer, superficial surface of the body, an organ, or other structure	**extern/o-** *outside*
gastroenterology	Medical specialty that deals with the gastrointestinal system	**gastr/o-** *stomach* **enter/o-** *intestine*
gastrointestinal system	Body system that includes the mouth, teeth, tongue, salivary glands, pharynx (throat), esophagus, stomach, small intestine, large intestine, liver, gallbladder, and pancreas. It receives sensory information for the sense of taste. It digests food, absorbs nutrients into the blood, and excretes undigested wastes.	**gastr/o-** *stomach* **intestin/o-** *intestine*
gene	An area on a chromosome that contains all the DNA information needed to produce one type of protein molecule	**gene/o-** *gene*
genital	Pertaining to the male or female genitalia	**genit/o-** *genitalia*
geriatrics	Medical specialty that deals with older adults	**ger/o-** *old age* **iatr/o-** *medical treatment; physician*
Golgi apparatus	Organelle that consists of curved, stacked membranes that process and store hormones and enzymes. It also makes lysosomes.	
gynecology	Medical specialty that deals with the female genital system	**gynec/o-** *female; woman*
health	State of complete physical, mental, and social well-being	
hematology	Medical specialty that deals with the blood	**hemat/o-** *blood*
hypochondriac regions	Right and left regions on the surface of the abdominopelvic area. They are lateral to the epigastric region and inferior to the ribs.	**chondr/o-** *cartilage*

Word or Phrase	Description	Combining Forms
hypogastric region	Region on the surface of the abdominopelvic area. It is inferior to the umbilical region and medial to the inguinal regions.	**gastr/o-** *stomach*
immunology	Medical specialty that deals with the lymphatic system and the immune response	**immun/o-** *immune response*
inferior	Pertaining to the lower part of the body, an organ, or a structure	**infer/o-** *below*
inguinal regions	Right and left regions on the surface of the abdominopelvic area. They are lateral to the hypogastric region.	**inguin/o-** *groin*
integumentary system	Body system that includes the skin, hair, nails, sweat glands, and oil glands. It receives sensory information for sensations of pain, touch, and temperature. It protects the internal organs from infection and trauma. It regulates the body temperature by sweating.	**integument/o-** *skin*
internal	Pertaining to the inside of the body, an organ, or a structure	**intern/o-** *inside*
intracellular	Within a cell	**cellul/o-** *cell*
lateral	Pertaining to the side of the body, an organ, or a structure	**later/o-** *side*
lumbar regions	Right and left regions on the surface of the abdominopelvic area. They are lateral to the umbilical region.	**lumb/o-** *area between the ribs and pelvis; lower back*
lymphatic system	Body system that includes the lymphatic vessels, lymph nodes, lymph fluid, spleen, thymus, and white blood cells. It recognizes and destroys disease-causing organisms and abnormal cells.	**lymph/o-** *lymph; lymphatic system*
lysosome	Organelle that consists of a small sac with digestive enzymes in it. It destroys pathogens that invade the cell.	**lys/o-** *break down; destroy*
macroscopic	Pertaining to large structures that can be seen with the naked eye	**macr/o-** *large* **scop/o-** *examine with an instrument*
medial	Pertaining to the middle of the body, an organ, or a structure	**medi/o-** *middle*
medical specialty	Basis of the practice of medicine. Each medical specialty includes the structures, functions, and diseases for a body system plus related laboratory and diagnostic procedures, medical and surgical procedures, and drugs.	**medic/o-** *medicine; physician*
microscope	Instrument used to examine very small structures	**micr/o-** *one millionth; small*
microscopic	Pertaining to small structures that cannot be seen with the naked eye	**micr/o-** *one millionth; small* **scop/o-** *examine with an instrument*
mitochondria	Organelles that are capsule shaped and produce and store ATP and then convert it to ADP to release energy for cellular activities	
mitosis	Process of cellular division. The chromosomes duplicate, align along thread-like strands, and then migrate to either end of the nucleus as the cell divides.	**mit/o-** *thread-like structure*
muscular system	Body system that includes the muscles and tendons. It produces body movement.	**muscul/o-** *muscle*
neonatology	Medical specialty that deals with newborn babies with medical problems	**ne/o-** *new* **nat/o-** *birth*

Word or Phrase	Description	Combining Forms
nervous system	Body system that includes the brain, cranial nerves, spinal cord, spinal nerves, cerebrospinal fluid, and neurons. It receives, relays, and interprets sensory information for the senses of vision, hearing, smell, and taste and sensations of pain, touch, temperature, body position, and balance. It coordinates body movement and stores and interprets memory and emotion.	**nerv/o-** *nerve*
neurology	Medical specialty that deals with the nervous system	**neur/o-** *nerve*
nucleolus	Round, central region within the nucleus. It makes RNA and ribosomes.	
nucleus	Large, round, centralized intracellular structure that contains chromosomes and their DNA. It controls all of the cell's activities. It is surrounded by a membrane.	**nucle/o-** *nucleus of an atom; nucleus of a cell* **kary/o-** *nucleus of a cell*
obstetrics	Medical specialty that deals with the female reproductive system during pregnancy and childbirth	**obstetr/o-** *pregnancy and childbirth*
oncology	Medical specialty that deals with cancer	**onc/o-** *mass; tumor*
ophthalmology	Medical specialty that deals with the eyes. The eyes receive sensory information for the sense of vision.	**ophthalm/o-** *eye*
organ	Body structure composed of tissues	
organelles	Small structures in the cytoplasm that have specialized functions. They include mitochondria, ribosomes, the endoplasmic reticulum, the Golgi apparatus, and lysosomes.	**organ/o-** *organ*
orthopedics	Medical specialty that deals with the skeletal system and muscular system	**orth/o-** *straight* **ped/o-** *child*
otolaryngology	Medical specialty that deals with the ears, nose, sinuses, throat, and voice box. The ears receive sensory information for the sense of hearing and the sensation of balance. The nose receives sensory information for the sense of smell. The pharynx (throat) and the larynx (voice box) help produce speech.	**ot/o-** *ear* **laryng/o-** *larynx; voice box*
pediatrics	Medical specialty that deals with infants and children	**ped/o-** *child* **iatr/o-** *medical treatment; physician*
pelvic cavity	Cavity that is continuous with and inferior to the abdominal cavity. It is surrounded by the pelvic bones anteriorly and bilaterally and bones of the spine posteriorly.	**pelv/o-** *hip bone; pelvis; renal pelvis*
pharmacology	Medical specialty that deals with the study of drugs and medicines	**pharmac/o-** *drug; medicine*
physiology	Study of the functions of the human body	**physi/o-** *physical function*
plane	An imaginary flat surface that divides the body into sections. There are three planes: the coronal plane (frontal plane), sagittal plane, and transverse plane.	
posterior	Pertaining to the back of the body, an organ, or a structure	**poster/o-** *back part*
posteroanterior	Pertaining to the posterior section and then the anterior section of the body	**poster/o-** *back part* **anter/o-** *before; front part*
prone	Position of lying on the anterior surface of the body	

Word or Phrase	Description	Combining Forms
proximal	Pertaining to near the point of origin, such as on an arm or leg	**proxim/o-** *near the center; near the point of origin*
psychiatry	Medical specialty that deals with the mind	**psych/o-** *mind*
pulmonology	Medical specialty that deals with the respiratory system	**pulmon/o-** *lung*
quadrant	Each of four equal divisions on the surface of the abdominopelvic area: the left upper quadrant (LUQ), right upper quadrant (RUQ), left lower quadrant (LLQ), and right lower quadrant (RLQ)	**quadr/o-** *four*
radiology and nuclear medicine	Medical specialty that deals with the use of x-rays, sound waves, and other forms of radiation and energy to create images and diagnose disease. Nuclear medicine uses radioactive substances to treat disease.	**radi/o-** *forearm bone; radiation; x-rays* **nucle/o-** *nucleus of an atom; nucleus of a cell*
reproductive medicine	Medical specialty that deals with the reproductive system	**product/o-** *produce*
reproductive system	Body system that, in the female, includes the breasts, ovaries, uterine tubes, uterus, vagina, and external genitalia. It secretes hormones, produces ova, and regulates menstruation, pregnancy, and milk production from the breasts. In the male, it includes the scrotum, testes, epididymides, vas deferens, seminal vesicles, prostate gland, urethra, and penis. It secretes hormones and produces and releases sperm.	**product/o-** *produce*
respiratory system	Body system that includes the nose, pharynx (throat), larynx (voice box), trachea, bronchi, bronchioles, and alveoli (in the lungs). It inhales oxygen, exhales carbon dioxide, and exchanges gases in the alveoli.	**spir/o-** *breathe; coil*
ribosomes	Granular organelles in the cytoplasm and on the endoplasmic reticulum. Ribosomes contain RNA and proteins and are the site where proteins are produced.	**rib/o-** *ribonucleic acid*
RNA	**Ribonucleic acid.** It is created in the nucleolus and stored in ribosomes. Messenger RNA duplicates DNA information in the nucleus and carries it to the ribosome.	
sagittal plane	Plane that divides the body into right and left sections	**sagitt/o-** *front to back*
skeletal system	Body system that includes the bones, cartilage, ligaments, and joints. It supports the body.	**skelet/o-** *skeleton*
spinal cavity	Cavity that is within the bones of the spine and contains the spinal cord, spinal nerves, and related structures	**spin/o-** *backbone; spine*
superior	Pertaining to the upper part of the body, an organ, or a structure	**super/o-** *above*
thoracic cavity	Cavity that is surrounded by the breast bone (sternum), ribs, and bones of the spine. The diaphragm is the inferior border. The thoracic cavity contains the lungs and the mediastinum (and the structures within it).	**thorac/o-** *chest; thorax*
tissue	Body structure formed of cells	
transverse plane	Plane that divides the body into upper (superior) and lower (inferior) parts	**vers/o-** *travel; turn*
umbilical region	Region on the surface of the abdominopelvic area. It is centered around the umbilicus.	**umbilic/o-** *navel; umbilicus*

Give Word Part Meanings

Use the Answer Key at the end of the book to check your answers.

Combining Forms Exercise

Next to each combining form, write its meaning. The first one has been done for you.

Combining Form	Meaning	Combining Form	Meaning
1. **dors/o-**	back; dorsum	36. later/o-	
2. abdomin/o-		37. lumb/o-	
3. anter/o-		38. lymph/o-	
4. cardi/o-		39. lys/o-	
5. caud/o-		40. macr/o-	
6. cav/o-		41. medic/o-	
7. cellul/o-		42. medi/o-	
8. cephal/o-		43. micr/o-	
9. chondr/o-		44. muscul/o-	
10. coron/o-		45. nat/o-	
11. crani/o-		46. ne/o-	
12. crin/o-		47. nerv/o-	
13. cyt/o-		48. neur/o-	
14. dent/o-		49. nucle/o-	
15. dermat/o-		50. obstetr/o-	
16. dietet/o-		51. onc/o-	
17. dist/o-		52. ophthalm/o-	
18. dors/o-		53. organ/o-	
19. enter/o-		54. orth/o-	
20. extern/o-		55. ot/o-	
21. front/o-		56. ped/o-	
22. gastr/o-		57. pelv/o-	
23. genit/o-		58. pharmac/o-	
24. ger/o-		59. physi/o-	
25. gynec/o-		60. poster/o-	
26. hemat/o-		61. product/o-	
27. iatr/o-		62. proxim/o-	
28. immun/o-		63. psych/o-	
29. infer/o-		64. pulmon/o-	
30. inguin/o-		65. quadr/o-	
31. integument/o-		66. radi/o-	
32. intern/o-		67. rib/o-	
33. intestin/o-		68. sagitt/o-	
34. kary/o-		69. scop/o-	
35. laryng/o-		70. skelet/o-	

Combining Form	Meaning	Combining Form	Meaning
71. spin/o-	________	77. urin/o-	________
72. spir/o-	________	78. ur/o-	________
73. super/o-	________	79. vascul/o-	________
74. thorac/o-	________	80. ventr/o-	________
75. tom/o-	________	81. vers/o-	________
76. umbilic/o-	________	82. viscer/o-	________

Build Medical Words

Combining Form and Suffix Exercise

Read the definition of the medical word. Look at the combining form that is given. Select the correct suffix from the Suffix List and write it on the blank line. Then build the medical word and write it on the line. (Remember: You may need to remove the combining vowel. Always remove the hyphens and slash.) Be sure to check your spelling. The first one has been done for you.

SUFFIX LIST

-ad (in the direction of; toward)	-ary (pertaining to)	-ics (knowledge; practice)	-ity (condition; state)
-al (pertaining to)	-atic (pertaining to)	-ior (pertaining to)	-logy (study of)
-ar (pertaining to)	-iatry (medical treatment)	-istry (process related to a specialty)	-ous (pertaining to)
	-ic (pertaining to)		

Definition of the Medical Word	Combining Form	Suffix	Build the Medical Word
1. Pertaining to the abdomen	abdomin/o-	-al	abdominal
(You think *pertaining to* (-al) + *(the) abdomen* (abdomin/o-). You change the order of the word parts to put the suffix last. You write *abdominal*.)			
2. Study of (the) physical function (of the body)	physi/o-	________	________
3. Pertaining to (the) lower back	lumb/o-	________	________
4. In the direction of (the) head	cephal/o-	________	________
5. Pertaining to away from the point of origin	dist/o-	________	________
6. Pertaining to (the) chest	thorac/o-	________	________
7. Pertaining to (the) skull	crani/o-	________	________
8. Pertaining to (the) back part	poster/o-	________	________
9. Study of (the) skin	dermat/o-	________	________
10. Pertaining to (the) lymph	lymph/o-	________	________
11. Pertaining to (the) side	later/o-	________	________
12. Pertaining to inside	intern/o-	________	________
13. Study of (the) heart	cardi/o-	________	________
14. Knowledge and practice (of treating women during) pregnancy and childbirth	obstetr/o-	________	________
15. Study of (the) urinary system	ur/o-	________	________
16. Study of (the) lungs	pulmon/o-	________	________
17. Study of (the) eye	ophthalm/o-	________	________
18. Pertaining to (the) skin	integument/o-	________	________

Definition of the Medical Word	Combining Form	Suffix	Build the Medical Word
19. Study of females	gynec/o-	_____	_____
20. Medical treatment (of the) mind	psych/o-	_____	_____
21. Pertaining to (the) nerves	nerv/o-	_____	_____
22. Pertaining to (the) urine (and its system)	urin/o-	_____	_____
23. Study of (cancerous) tumors	onc/o-	_____	_____
24. Pertaining to (the) front part	anter/o	_____	_____
25. Pertaining to (the) groin	inguin/o-	_____	_____
26. State (of having a) hollow space	cav/o-	_____	_____
27. Study of (the) blood	hemat/o-	_____	_____
28. Process related to a specialty (of the) tooth	dent/o-	_____	_____
29. Study of (the) nerves	neur/o-	_____	_____
30. Pertaining to (the) muscles	muscul/o-	_____	_____
31. Pertaining to (the) middle	medi/o-	_____	_____
32. Pertaining to (being) above	super/o-	_____	_____
33. Study of (the) heart	cardi/o-	_____	_____
34. Study of drugs and medicines	pharmac/o-	_____	_____
35. Knowledge and practice (of) diet and foods	dietet/o-	_____	_____
36. Study of x-rays	radi/o-	_____	_____
37. Pertaining to (the) large internal organs	viscer/o-	_____	_____

Prefix Exercise

Read the definition of the medical word. Look at the medical word or partial word that is given (it already contains a combining form and a suffix). Select the correct prefix from the Prefix List and write it on the blank line. Then build the medical word and write it on the line. Be sure to check your spelling. The first one has been done for you.

PREFIX LIST			
ana- (apart; excessive)	epi- (above; upon)	intra- (within)	re- (again and again)
endo- (innermost; within)	hypo- (below; deficient)	mid- (middle)	

Definition of the Medical Word	Prefix	Word or Partial Word	Build the Medical Word
1. Thing (gland) that secretes within (the body)	endo-	-crine	*endocrine*
2. Pertaining to (taking the body) apart (as a) cut, layer, or slice	_____	tomical	_____
3. Pertaining to (in the) middle (of the body with a plane going) front to back	_____	sagittal	_____
4. Pertaining to (a region) below (the) cartilage (of the ribs)	_____	chondriac	_____
5. Pertaining to again and again breath(ing)	_____	spiratory	_____
6. Pertaining to (a region) above (the) stomach	_____	gastric	_____
7. Pertaining to again and again produc(ing) (children)	_____	productive	_____
8. Pertaining to within the cell	_____	cellular	_____

The Body in Disease

Preventive medicine is the healthcare specialty that focuses on keeping a person healthy and preventing disease. But despite the best efforts of modern medicine, the human body does not always remain in a state of health. Much of medical language deals with diseases and conditions and how they are diagnosed and treated. **Disease** is any change in the normal structure or function of the body. This change might be slight and short lived or severe and life threatening. The **etiology** is the cause or origin of a disease. In most cases, the cause of a disease is known or can be discovered through a physical examination and laboratory and diagnostic procedures. In some cases, however, the exact cause of a disease is never completely understood.

Pronunciation/Word Parts

preventive (pree-VEN-tiv)
  prevent/o- *prevent*
  -ive *pertaining to*

medicine (MED-ih-sin)
  medic/o- *medicine; physician*
  -ine *pertaining to; thing pertaining to*

disease (dih-ZEEZ)

etiology (EE-tee-AW-loh-jee)
  eti/o- *cause of disease*
  -logy *study of*

Disease Categories

Diseases can be divided into different categories based on their etiology (cause or origin) (see Table 2-1 ■).

Table 2-1 Disease Categories

Disease Type	Etiology	Pronunciation/Word Parts
congenital	Caused by an abnormality in the fetus as it develops or caused by an abnormal process that occurs during gestation or birth Examples: Cleft lip and palate, cerebral palsy	**congenital** (con-JEN-ih-tal) **congenit/o-** *present at birth* **-al** *pertaining to*
degenerative	Caused by the progressive destruction of cells due to disease or the aging process Examples: Multiple sclerosis, loss of hearing, arthritis	**degenerative** (dee-JEN-er-ah-TIV) **de-** *reversal of; without* **gener/o-** *creation; production* **-ative** *pertaining to*
environmental	Caused by exposure to external substances in the environment Examples: Smoke, allergies to pollen, skin cancer from the sun	**environmental** (en-VY-rawn-MEN-tal)
genetic	Spontaneous mutation in a person's own gene and chromosome during fetal development Example: Down syndrome	
hereditary	An inherited recessive defective gene, passed to the child from a parent who carries the defective gene but does not have the disease Examples: Cystic fibrosis, hemophilia, sickle cell disease	**hereditary** (heh-RED-ih-TAIR-ee) **heredit/o-** *genetic inheritance* **-ary** *pertaining to*
iatrogenic	Caused by medicine or treatment that was given to the patient Examples: Wrong drug given to a patient, surgery performed on the wrong leg, an incompatible blood type given as a blood transfusion	**iatrogenic** (eye-AT-roh-JEN-ik) **iatr/o-** *medical treatment; physician* **gen/o-** *arising from; produced by* **-ic** *pertaining to*
idiopathic	Having no identifiable or confirmed cause Example: Sudden infant death syndrome (SIDS)	**idiopathic** (ID-ee-oh-PATH-ik) **idi/o-** *individual; unknown* **path/o-** *disease* **-ic** *pertaining to*

Table 2-1 Disease Categories (*continued*)

Disease Type	Etiology	Pronunciation/Word Parts

infectious	Caused by a **pathogen** (a disease-causing microorganism such as a bacterium, virus, fungus, etc.). A **communicable** disease is an infectious disease that is transmitted by direct or indirect contact with an infected person, animal, or insect. Examples: Gonorrhea (a sexually transmitted disease), rabies (from an animal bite), tuberculosis (from being in close proximity to a person with tuberculosis)	**infectious** (in-FEK-shus)
		  infect/o- *disease within*
		  -ious *pertaining to*
		Add words to make a complete definition of *infectious*: *pertaining to disease (causing organisms) within (the body).*
		
		pathogen (PATH-oh-jen)
		  path/o- *disease*
		  -gen *that which produces*
		
		communicable
		(koh-MYOO-nih-kah-BL)
		  communic/o- *impart; transmit*
		  -able *able to be*

neoplastic	Caused by the new growth of either a benign (not cancerous) or malignant (cancerous) mass or tumor
	Examples: Benign cyst, cancerous tumor of the skin
		neoplastic (NEE-oh-PLAS-tik)
		  ne/o- *new*
		  plast/o- *formation; growth*
		  -ic *pertaining to*

nosocomial	Caused by exposure to a disease-causing agent while in the hospital environment
	Example: Surgical wound infection
		nosocomial (NOH-soh-KOH-mee-al)
		  nosocomi/o- *hospital*
		  -al *pertaining to*

nutritional	Caused by a lack of nutritious food, insufficient amounts of food, or an inability to utilize the nutrients in food
	Examples: Malnutrition, pernicious anemia (caused by a lack of intrinsic factor in the stomach and inability to absorb vitamin B_{12})
		nutritional (noo-TRIH-shun-al)
		  nutrit/o- *nourishment*
		  -ion *action; condition*
		  -al *pertaining to*

Onset, Course, and Outcome of Disease

Onset of a Disease

The beginning or onset of disease is often noticed because of symptoms and/or signs. A **symptom** is any deviation from health that is experienced or felt by the patient. When a symptom can be seen or detected by others, it is known as a **sign**. An elevated temperature, coughing, tremors, paleness, vomiting, or a lump that can be seen or felt would all be signs of disease. **Symptomatology** is the clinical picture of all of the patient's symptoms and signs. A **syndrome** is a set of symptoms and signs associated with, and characteristic of, one particular disease. Patients who are **asymptomatic** (showing no symptoms or signs) can still have a disease, but one that can only be detected by laboratory and diagnostic procedures.

Course and Outcome of a Disease

The course of a disease includes all events from the onset of the disease until its final outcome. During the course of a disease, the symptoms and signs may be **acute** (sudden in nature and severe in intensity), **subacute** (less severe in intensity), or **chronic** (continuing for 3 months or more). An **exacerbation** is a sudden worsening in the severity of the symptoms or signs. A **remission** is a temporary improvement in the symptoms and

Pronunciation/Word Parts

symptom (SIMP-tom)

symptomatology
(SIMP-toh-mah-TAW-loh-jee)
  symptomat/o- *collection of symptoms*
  -logy *study of*

syndrome (SIN-drohm)
  syn- *together*
  -drome *running*
Most medical words contain a combining form. The ending *-drome* contains the combining form *drom/o-* and the one-letter suffix *-e.*

asymptomatic (AA-simp-toh-MAT-ik)
  a- *away from; without*
  symptomat/o- *collection of symptoms*
  -ic *pertaining to*

acute (ah-KYOOT)

subacute (SUB-ah-KYOOT)

signs of a disease without the underlying disease being cured. A relapse or recurrence is a return of the original symptoms and signs of the disease. A **sequela** is an abnormal condition or complication that arises because of the original disease and remains after the original disease has resolved.

The course and outcome of a disease can be affected by treatment: the physician prescribes drugs or orders therapy for the patient. If the treatment is **therapeutic**, the symptoms or signs of the disease disappear. A disease that is **refractory** (resistant) is one that does not respond to treatment. Certain diseases that cannot be treated with drugs or therapy may require **surgery**.

The **prognosis** is the predicted outcome of a disease. The natures of many diseases are so well known that the physician can predict with a great deal of accuracy what the patient's prognosis will be.

The course of a disease ends in one of the following outcomes. **Recuperation** or recovery is a return to a normal state of health. When recuperation is not complete, residual chronic disease or disability remains. A **disability** is a permanent loss of the ability to perform certain activities or to function in a given way. A **terminal illness** is one from which the patient cannot recover, and one that eventually results in death.

Physical Examination

To fully understand the patient's symptoms and signs, the physician takes a history and performs a physical examination. For the history of the present illness, the physician asks the patient in detail about the location, onset, duration, and severity of the symptoms. The physician also asks about the patient's past medical history, past surgical history, family history, social history, and history of allergies to drugs. Then the physician performs a physical examination to look for signs of disease. The physician uses the following techniques (as needed) during the physical examination: **inspection**, **palpation**, **auscultation**, and **percussion** (see Figures 2-19 ■ through 2-22 ■).

Based on the patient's history and the results of the physical examination, the physician can rule out (R/O) most diseases and make a **diagnosis** that identifies the nature and cause of the disease or condition. If it is not possible to make a diagnosis, the physician makes a tentative or working diagnosis and orders further diagnostic procedures or refers the patient to a specialist for a more detailed evaluation.

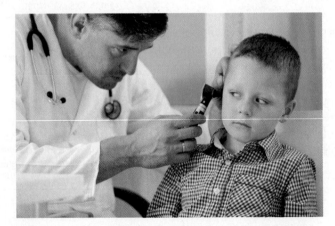

FIGURE 2-19 ■ Inspection.
Inspection is using the eyes or an instrument to examine the external surfaces or internal cavities of the body. This physician is using his eyes and a lighted instrument (an otoscope) to examine the patient's internal ear canal.
Source: Photographee.eu/Fotolia

Pronunciation/Word Parts

chronic (KRAW-nik)
  chron/o- *time*
  -ic *pertaining to*

exacerbation (eg-ZAS-er-BAY-shun)
  exacerb/o- *increase; provoke*
  -ation *being; having; process*

remission (ree-MIH-shun)
  remiss/o- *send back*
  -ion *action; condition*

sequela (see-KWEL-ah)
Sequela is a Latin singular noun. Form the plural by changing -a to -ae.

therapeutic (THAIR-ah-PYOO-tik)
  therapeut/o- *therapy; treatment*
  -ic *pertaining to*

refractory (ree-FRAK-tor-ee)
  re- *again and again; backward; unable to*
  fract/o- *bend; break up*
  -ory *having the function of*
Add words to make a complete definition of *refractory: having the function of (a disease that treatment is) unable to break up (or cure).*

surgery (SER-jer-ee)
  surg/o- *operative procedure*
  -ery *process*

prognosis (prawg-NOH-sis)
  pro- *before*
  gnos/o- *knowledge*
  -osis *condition; process*

recuperation (ree-KOO-per-AA-shun)
  recuper/o- *recover*
  -ation *being; having; process*

disability (DIS-ah-BIL-ah-tee)

terminal (TER-mih-nal)
  termin/o- *boundary; end; word*
  -al *pertaining to*

inspection (in-SPEK-shun)
  inspect/o- *looking at*
  -ion *action; condition*

palpation (pal-PAY-shun)
  palpat/o- *feeling; touching*
  -ion *action; condition*

auscultation (AWS-kul-TAY-shun)
  auscult/o- *listening*
  -ation *being; having; process*

percussion (per-KUH-shun)
  percuss/o- *tapping*
  -ion *action; condition*

diagnosis (DY-ag-NOH-sis)
  dia- *complete; completely through*
  gnos/o- *knowledge*
  -osis *condition; process*
Diagnosis is a Greek singular noun. Form the plural by changing -is to -es.

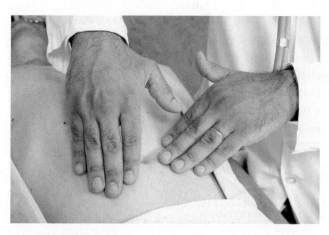

FIGURE 2-20 ■ Palpation.
Palpation is using the fingers to feel masses or enlarged organs or to detect tenderness or pain. This physician is palpating the patient's abdomen.
Source: Pearson Education/PH College Michael Heron

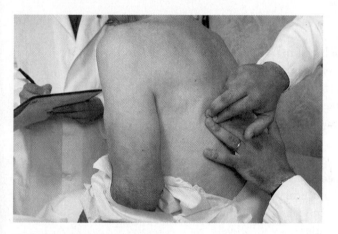

FIGURE 2-22 ■ Percussion.
Percussion is using the finger of one hand to tap on the finger of the other hand that is spread over a body cavity. After a few taps, the hand is moved to another location. This physician is using percussion over the thoracic cavity and left lung and listening to the sound that is produced.
Source: Pearson Education/PH College Michael Heron

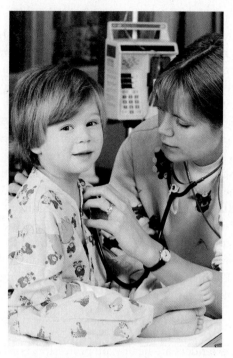

FIGURE 2-21 ■ Auscultation.
Auscultation is using a stethoscope to listen to the sounds of the heart, lungs, or intestines. This nurse is using a stethoscope to listen to this child's lungs and breath sounds.
Source: Corbis Real Life Medicine Royalty Free CD

TECHNOLOGY IN MEDICINE

In the past, physician–patient contact was always face to face. Now, telecommunication advances allow patients to receive care via telemedicine—also known as *televisiting*— through life-sized videoconferencing screens, remote monitoring of vital signs, etc. Physicians use videoconferencing to consult with specialists (eConsulting). Surgeons in one part of the world do telesurgery with on-site and remote robots and 3-D visualization to operate on a patient thousands of miles away.

Healthcare Professionals and Healthcare Settings

Healthcare Professionals

Physicians

A **physician** or **doctor** leads the members of the healthcare team and directs their activities. The physician examines the patient, orders tests (if necessary), diagnoses diseases, and treats diseases by prescribing medicines or therapy. Physicians who graduate from

Pronunciation/Word Parts

physician (fih-ZIH-shun)
 physic/o- *body*
 -ician *skilled expert; skilled professional*
 Note: The duplicated letters "ic" are deleted when the word is formed.

doctor (DAWK-ter)

medical school receive a Doctor of Medicine (M.D.) degree. Physicians who graduate from a school of osteopathy receive a Doctor of Osteopathy or Osteopathic Medicine (D.O.) degree. After medical school, physicians complete residency training and select a specialized area for their medical practice (e.g., family practice, pediatrics, psychiatry, etc.). **Surgeons** are physicians who complete additional training in surgical techniques.

Primary care physicians (PCPs) are physicians who specialize in family practice or pediatrics. They see the majority of patients on a day-to-day basis in their offices. A physician or doctor who is on the medical staff of a hospital and admits a patient to the hospital is known as the **attending physician.**

Other doctors graduate from schools that focus their training on just one part of the body or one aspect of medicine. Chiropractors have a Doctor of Chiropracty or Chiropractic Medicine (D.C.) degree and only treat the alignment of the bones, muscles, and nerves. Optometrists have a Doctor of Optometry (O.D.) degree and only treat the eyes. Podiatrists have a Doctor of Podiatric Medicine (D.P.M.) degree and only treat the feet. Dentists have a Doctor of Dental Surgery (D.D.S.) degree and only treat the teeth. Pharmacists have a Doctor of Pharmacy (Pharm. D.) degree. They fill prescriptions for medicines as well as consult with physicians and patients.

Physician Extenders

Physician extenders are healthcare professionals who perform some of the duties of a physician. They examine, diagnose, and treat patients and some of them can prescribe medicines. They work under the supervision of a physician or doctor (M.D. or D.O.).

Physician extenders include physician's assistants (PAs), nurse practitioners (NPs), certified nurse midwives (CNMs), and certified registered nurse anesthetists (CRNAs).

Allied Health Professionals

Allied health professionals support the physician and perform specific services ordered by the physician. **Nurses**, such as a registered nurse (RN), licensed practical nurse (LPN), or licensed vocational nurse (LVN), are allied health professionals who examine patients, make nursing diagnoses, and administer treatments or medicines ordered by the physician. Nurses give hands-on care and focus on the physical and emotional needs of the patient and the family.

Other allied health professionals include **technologists**, **technicians**, and **therapists**, as well as dietitians, medical assistants, phlebotomists, dental hygienists, and audiologists.

Healthcare Settings

Health care is provided in many different settings, depending on the healthcare needs of the patient and which setting can medically and cost effectively meet those needs.

Hospital

A **hospital** is a healthcare facility that is the traditional setting for providing care for patients who are acutely ill and require medical or surgical care for longer than 24 hours. Each hospital stay begins with admission and ends with **discharge** from the hospital. The attending physician must write an order in the patient's medical record to admit or discharge the patient. The attending physician also monitors the patient's care and orders diagnostic tests, treatments, therapies, medicines, and surgeries, as needed. A patient in the hospital is an **inpatient**.

A hospital is divided into floors or nursing units that provide care for specific types of patients. There are also specialty care units such as the intensive care unit (ICU). **Ancillary** departments in the hospital provide additional types of services and include the radiology department, physical therapy (PT) department, dietary department, emergency department (ED) or emergency room (ER), clinical laboratory, and

---

Pronunciation/Word Parts

surgeon (SER-jun)
  surg/o- *operative procedure*
  -eon *person who performs*

nurse (NERS)

technologist (tek-NAW-loh-jist)
  techn/o- *technical skill*
  log/o- *study of; word*
  -ist *person who specializes in; thing that specializes in*

technician (tek-NIH-shun)
  techn/o- *technical skill*
  -ician *skilled expert; skilled professional*

therapist (THAIR-ah-pist)
  therap/o- *treatment*
  -ist *person who specializes in; thing that specializes in*

hospital (HAWS-pih-tal)

discharge (DIS-charj)

inpatient (IN-pay-shent)

ancillary (AN-sih-LAIR-ee)
  ancill/o- *accessory; servant*
  -ary *pertaining to*

pharmacy. Nonmedical departments provide other services such as health information management (medical records), finances and billing, housekeeping, etc.

Physician's Office

The physician's office is one of the most frequently used healthcare settings. A single physician (or group of physicians in a group practice) maintains an office where patients are seen, diagnosed, treated, and counseled. Some offices have their own laboratory and x-ray equipment for performing diagnostic tests. Seriously ill patients who cannot be quickly diagnosed or adequately treated in the office are sent to a hospital.

Clinic

A **clinic** provides healthcare services similar to that of a physician's office but for just one type of patient or one type of disease. For example, a well-baby clinic provides care to newborn infants, and a methadone clinic treats recovering drug addicts. Outpatient clinics are located in a hospital or in their own separate facility. Their patients are known as **outpatients** because they are not admitted to the clinic and do not stay overnight.

Ambulatory Surgery Center

An **ambulatory surgery center (ASC)** is a facility where minor surgery is performed and the patient does not stay overnight.

Long-Term Care Facility

A **long-term care facility,** previously known as a *nursing home,* is primarily a residential facility for older adults or those with disabilities who are unable to care for themselves. Long-term care facilities provide 24-hour nursing care. Persons in long-term care facilities are referred to as **residents** rather than *patients* because the facility is considered their home or residence. **Skilled nursing facilities (SNFs)** are long-term care facilities with a special nursing unit that provides a higher level of medical and nursing care that is needed for patients who have recently been discharged from the hospital. Many long-term care facilities also provide **rehabilitation** services to prepare a patient to live independently at home.

Home Health Agency

A **home health agency** provides a range of healthcare services to persons (who are known as **clients**) in their homes. These services are particularly useful for those who are unable to come to a physician's office or clinic and do not want to live in a long-term care facility (see Figure 2-23 ■).

Pronunciation/Word Parts

clinic (KLIN-ik)

outpatient (OUT-pay-shent)

ambulatory (AM-byoo-lah-TOR-ee)
  ambulat/o- *walking*
  -ory *having the function of*

rehabilitation (REE-hah-BIL-ih-TAY-shun)
  re- *again and again; backward; unable to*
  habilitat/o- *give ability*
  -ion *action; condition*
Select the correct prefix meaning to get the correct definition of *rehabilitation*: action (of to) again and again give ability.

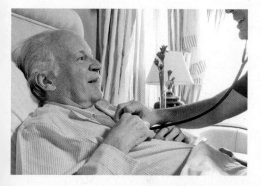

FIGURE 2-23 ■ Home health nurse.
This home health nurse is making one of his regularly scheduled visits to an elderly client in his home. He will assess the client's physical status, emotional needs, and medications. He will also offer emotional support to other family members. The home health nurse supervises the home health aide who see the client several times a week to help him with his physical care.
Source: iceteastock/Fotolia

Hospice

A **hospice** is an inpatient facility for patients who are dying from a terminal illness, and their physicians have certified that they have less than 6 months to live. Hospice services include **palliative** care (supportive medical and nursing care to keep the patient comfortable), pain management, counseling, and emotional support for the patient and family. Hospice care can also be provided in the patient's home.

Pronunciation/Word Parts

hospice (HAWS-pis)

palliative (PAL-ee-ah-TIV)
 palliat/o- *reduce the severity*
 -ive *pertaining to*

ACROSS THE LIFE SPAN

Most people think of the healthcare settings of a long-term care facility and hospice as only pertaining to older adults. In fact, some chronically ill or severely handicapped children and young adults are cared for in long-term care facilities. All ages of patients who are terminally ill can receive hospice care in a hospice facility or at home.

Vocabulary Review

The Body in Disease		
Word or Phrase	**Description**	**Combining Forms**
acute	Symptoms and signs that occur suddenly and are severe in nature	
allied health professionals	Healthcare professionals who support the work of physicians and perform specific services ordered by the physician. Allied health professionals include nurses, technologists, technicians, therapists, and others.	
ambulatory surgery center (ASC)	Facility where minor surgical procedures are performed. The patient is an **outpatient** who arrives in time for the surgery and does not stay overnight.	**ambulat/o-** *walking* **surg/o-** *operative procedure*
ancillary department	Department that provides services to support the medical and surgical care given in a hospital. Examples: Radiology department, physical therapy department, dietary department, emergency department, clinical laboratory, and pharmacy.	**ancill/o-** *accessory; servant*
asymptomatic	Showing no symptoms or signs of disease	**symptomat/o-** *collection of symptoms*
attending physician	Physician on the medical staff of a hospital who admits patients, directs their care, and discharges them	**physic/o-** *body*
auscultation	Using a stethoscope to listen to the heart, lungs, or intestines	**auscult/o-** *listening*
chronic	Symptoms or signs that continue for 3 months or longer	**chron/o-** *time*
clinic	An ambulatory facility that provides healthcare services, often for just one type of patient or one type of disease. Example: Well-baby clinic for newborns. Clinic patients are known as **outpatients** and the facility is an outpatient clinic.	
congenital	Disease caused by an abnormality in fetal development or an abnormal process that occurs during gestation or birth. Examples: Cleft lip, cerebral palsy	**congenit/o-** *present at birth*
degenerative	Disease caused by progressive destruction of cells due to disease or the aging process. Examples: Multiple sclerosis, hearing loss, arthritis	**gener/o-** *creation; production*
diagnosis	A determination based on knowledge about the cause of the patient's symptoms and signs	**gnos/o-** *knowledge*
disability	Permanent inability to perform certain activities or function in a given way	
discharge	Release from the hospital of a patient who no longer needs hospital-level care. The patient can be discharged to home or transferred to another healthcare facility. (*Note: Discharge* also refers to a fluid or semisolid substance produced by a disease process or condition.)	
disease	Any change in the normal structure or function of the body	
environmental	Disease caused by exposure to substances in the environment. Examples: Smoke, pollen, sun rays, etc.	
etiology	The cause or origin of a disease	**eti/o-** *cause of disease*
exacerbation	Sudden worsening in the severity of symptoms or signs	**exacerb/o-** *increase; provoke*
genetic	Disease caused by a spontaneous mutation in a person's own gene or chromosome during fetal development. Example: Down syndrome	**gene/o-** *gene*

Word or Phrase	Description	Combining Forms
hereditary	An inherited recessive defective gene, passed to the child from a parent who carries the defective gene but does not have the disease. Examples: Cystic fibrosis, sickle cell disease	**heredit/o-** *genetic inheritance*
home health agency	Agency that provides nursing and non-nursing services to patients in their homes. These patients are known as **clients**.	
hospice	Facility for patients who have a terminal illness and require **palliative** supportive care, counseling, and emotional support for themselves and their families. Hospice care can also be provided in the patient's home.	**palliat/o-** *reduce the severity*
hospital	Healthcare facility that provides care for acutely ill medical and surgical patients for longer than 24 hours. The patient being treated is an **inpatient**. The patient is admitted, occupies a bed in the hospital, and is discharged.	
iatrogenic	Disease caused by medicine or treatment given to the patient. Examples: Wrong drug given to a patient; surgery on the wrong part	**iatr/o-** *medical treatment; physician* **gen/o-** *arising from; produced by*
idiopathic	Disease having no identifiable or confirmed cause. Example: Sudden infant death syndrome	**idi/o-** *individual; unknown* **path/o-** *disease*
infectious	Disease caused by a pathogen. A **communicable** disease is an infectious disease that is transmitted by direct or indirect contact with an infected person, animal, or insect. Examples: Gonorrhea, rabies, tuberculosis	**infect/o-** *disease within* **communic/o-** *impart; transmit*
inpatient	A patient in a hospital	
inspection	Using the eyes or an instrument to examine the body	**inspect/o-** *looking at*
long-term care facility	Residential facility for persons who are unable to care for themselves. A long-term care facility, also known as a *nursing home,* provides 24-hour nursing care and **rehabilitation** services. Persons in this facility are known as **residents**.	**habilitat/o-** *give ability*
neoplastic	Disease caused by the growth of a benign (not cancerous) or a malignant (cancerous) tumor or mass	**ne/o-** *new* **plast/o-** *formation; growth*
nosocomial	Disease caused by exposure to a disease-causing agent while the patient is in the hospital. Example: Surgical wound infection	**nosocomi/o-** *hospital*
nurse	Allied health professional who examines patients, makes nursing diagnoses, and gives medicines and treatment ordered by a physician	
nutritional disease	Disease caused by lack of nutritious food, too little food, or an inability to utilize the food that is eaten. Example: Malnutrition	**nutrit/o-** *nourishment*
palliative care	Supportive medical and nursing care that keeps the patient comfortable but does not cure the disease	**palliat/o-** *reduce the severity*
palpation	Using the fingers to press on a body part to detect a mass, an enlarged organ, tenderness, or pain	**palpat/o-** *feeling; touching*
pathogen	Disease-causing microorganism, such as a bacterium, virus, fungus, etc.	**path/o-** *disease*
percussion	Tapping one finger on another finger of a hand that is spread across the chest or abdomen to listen for differences in sound in a body cavity	**percuss/o-** *tapping*
physician	Healthcare professional who directs the activities of the healthcare team. The physician orders tests, diagnoses, and treats patients. Other healthcare professionals who graduate from schools that focus their training on just one part of the body or one aspect of medicine are known as **doctors**. A primary care physician (PCP) is a general practitioner who specializes in family practice or pediatrics.	**physic/o-** *body*

Word or Phrase	Description	Combining Forms
physician extender	Healthcare professionals who perform some of the duties of physicians or doctors (M.D. or D.O.) and work under their supervision. They examine, diagnose, and treat patients. Some can prescribe medicines. Physician extenders include physician's assistants, nurse practitioners, certified nurse midwives, and certified registered nurse anesthetists.	
physician's office	Facility where a physician (or a group of physicians in a group practice) maintains an office. The ambulatory patients here are outpatients and are seen for a short period of time to diagnose and prescribe treatment for diseases that do not require hospitalization.	
preventive medicine	Medicine that keeps a person in a state of health and prevents the occurrence of disease	**prevent/o-** *prevent* **medic/o-** *medicine; physician*
prognosis	Predicted course and outcome of a disease	**gnos/o-** *knowledge*
recuperation	Process of return to a normal state of health	**recuper/o-** *recover*
refractory	Pertaining to a disease that does not respond well to treatment	**fract/o-** *bend; break up*
remission	Temporary improvement in the symptoms and signs of a disease without the underlying disease being cured	**remiss/o-** *send back*
sequela	Abnormal condition or complication that is caused by the original disease and remains after the original disease has resolved	
skilled nursing facility (SNF)	Long-term care facility with a special nursing unit that admits patients from the hospital and provides a higher level of medical and nursing care. Persons in this facility are known as **residents**.	
symptom	A deviation from health that is only experienced and felt by the patient	
symptomatology	The clinical picture of all the patient's symptoms and signs	**symptomat/o-** *collection of symptoms*
syndrome	Set of symptoms and signs associated with a specific disease	
subacute	Symptoms and signs that are less severe in intensity than acute symptoms	
surgeon	Physician or doctor who performs surgery	**surg/o-** *operative procedure*
surgery	A treatment that involves invading the patient's body, often by cutting	**surg/o-** *operative procedure*
technician	Allied health professional who has technical skill in a particular field of medicine	**techn/o-** *technical skill*
technologist	Allied health professional who specializes in a technical area of a field of medicine and performs technical tests	**techn/o-** *technical skill* **log/o-** *study of; word*
terminal illness	A disease from which there is no hope of recovery and one that will eventually result in the patient's death	**termin/o-** *boundary; end; word*
therapeutic	Pertaining to an action (from therapy or medicines) that results in improvement in the symptoms or signs of a disease	**therapeut/o-** *therapy; treatment*
therapist	Allied health professional who performs therapy on patients to treat a specific disease or condition	**therap/o-** *treatment*

Give Word Part Meanings

Use the Answer Key at the end of the book to check your answers.

Combining Forms Exercise

Next to each combining form, write its meaning. The first one has been done for you.

Combining Form	Meaning	Combining Form	Meaning
1. **termin/o-**	boundary; end; word	21. log/o-	
2. ambulat/o-		22. medic/o-	
3. ancill/o-		23. ne/o-	
4. auscult/o-		24. nosocomi/o-	
5. chron/o-		25. nutrit/o-	
6. communic/o-		26. palliat/o-	
7. congenit/o-		27. palpat/o-	
8. eti/o-		28. path/o-	
9. exacerb/o-		29. percuss/o-	
10. fract/o-		30. physic/o-	
11. gener/o-		31. plast/o-	
12. gen/o-		32. prevent/o-	
13. genit/o-		33. recuper/o-	
14. gnos/o-		34. remiss/o-	
15. habilitat/o-		35. surg/o-	
16. heredit/o-		36. symptomat/o-	
17. iatr/o-		37. techn/o-	
18. idi/o-		38. therapeut/o-	
19. infect/o-		39. therap/o-	
20. inspect/o-			

Build Medical Words

Combining Form and Suffix Exercise

Read the definition of the medical word. Look at the combining form that is given. Select the correct suffix from the Suffix List and write it on the blank line. Then build the medical word and write it on the line. (Remember: You may need to remove the combining vowel. Always remove the hyphens and slash.) Be sure to check your spelling. The first one has been done for you.

SUFFIX LIST

-al (pertaining to)
-ary (pertaining to)
-ation (being; having; process)

-eon (person who performs)
-ery (process)
-gen (that which produces)
-ic (pertaining to)

-ician (skilled expert; skilled professional)
-ion (action; condition)
-ious (pertaining to)

-ist (person who specializes in)
-ive (pertaining to)
-logy (study of)

Definition of the Medical Word	Combining Form	Suffix	Build the Medical Word
1. Action (of) looking at (the body)	inspect/o-	-ion	inspection
(You think *action* (-ion) + *looking at* (inspect/o-). You change the order of the word parts to put the suffix last. You write *inspection*.)			
2. Pertaining to (the) end (of life)	termin/o-	_____	_____
3. Person who specializes in treatment	therap/o-	_____	_____
4. Person who performs operative procedures	surg/o-	_____	_____
5. Pertaining to reducing the severity	palliat/o-	_____	_____
6. Skilled professional (with) technical skill	techn/o-	_____	_____
7. Pertaining to genetic inheritance	heredit/o-	_____	_____
8. That which produces disease	path/o	_____	_____
9. Study of (a) collection of symptoms	symptomat/o-	_____	_____
10. Action (of) feeling or touching	palpat/o-	_____	_____
11. Process (of) listening	auscult/o-	_____	_____
12. Pertaining to disease (-causing organisms) within (the body)	infect/o-	_____	_____
13. Pertaining to therapy or treatment	therapeut/o-	_____	_____
14. Process (of an) operative procedure	surg/o-	_____	_____
15. Action (of) tapping	percuss/o-	_____	_____
16. Pertaining to (continuing over) time	chron/o-	_____	_____
17. Pertaining to (being) present at birth	congenit/o-	_____	_____
18. Study of (the) cause of disease	eti/o-	_____	_____

Prefix Exercise

Read the definition of the medical word. Look at the medical word or partial word that is given (it already contains a combining form and a suffix). Select the correct prefix from the Prefix List and write it on the blank line. Then build the medical word and write it on the line. Be sure to check your spelling. The first one has been done for you.

PREFIX LIST

a- (away from; without)	dia- (complete; completely through)	re- (again and again; backward; unable to)
de- (reversal of; without)	pro- (before)	

Definition of the Medical Word	Prefix	Word or Partial Word	Build the Medical Word
	dia-	**gnosis**	
1. Condition (of) complete knowledge			*diagnosis*
2. Pertaining to (the) reversal of (the) production (of tissues)	_____	generative	_____
3. Pertaining to (being) without symptoms	_____	symptomatic	_____
4. Condition (of having) before knowledge (foreknowledge about the course of a disease)	_____	gnosis	_____
5. Having the function of (being) unable to break up	_____	fractory	_____

Abbreviations

A&P	anatomy and physiology		**LPN**	licensed practical nurse
AP	anteroposterior		**LUQ**	left upper quadrant (of the abdomen)
ASC	ambulatory surgery center		**LVN**	licensed vocational nurse
CNM	certified nurse midwife		**M.D.**	Doctor of Medicine
CRNA	certified registered nurse anesthetist		**NP**	nurse practitioner
CV	cardiovascular		**OB**	obstetrics
D.C.	Doctor of Chiropracty or Chiropractic Medicine		**OB/GYN**	obstetrics and gynecology
D.D.S.	Doctor of Dental Surgery		**O.D.**	Doctor of Optometry
D.O.	Doctor of Osteopathy or Osteopathic Medicine		**PA**	physician's assistant; posteroanterior
D.P.M.	Doctor of Podiatry or Podiatric Medicine		**PCP**	primary care physician
Dr.	doctor		**PE**	physical examination
DX, Dx	diagnosis		**Pharm.D.**	Doctor of Pharmacy
ED	emergency department		**PT**	physical therapist; physical therapy
ENT	ears, nose, and throat		**RLQ**	right lower quadrant (of the abdomen)
ER	emergency room		**RN**	registered nurse
GI	gastrointestinal		**R/O, r/o**	rule out
GYN	gynecology		**RUQ**	right upper quadrant (of the abdomen)
H&P	history and physical (examination)		**SNF**	skilled nursing facility (pronounced "sniff")
HX, Hx	history		**SX, Sx**	symptoms
ICU	intensive care unit		**TX, Tx**	treatment
LLQ	left lower quadrant (of the abdomen)			

Chapter 3
Gastroenterology

Gastrointestinal System

Gastroenterology (GAS-troh-EN-ter-AW-loh-jee) is the medical specialty that studies the anatomy and physiology of the gastrointestinal system and uses laboratory and diagnostic procedures, medical and surgical procedures, and drugs to treat gastrointestinal diseases.

 ## Learning Outcomes

After you study this chapter, you should be able to

3.1 Identify structures of the gastrointestinal system.

3.2 Describe the process of digestion.

3.3 Describe common gastrointestinal diseases, laboratory and diagnostic procedures, medical and surgical procedures, and drugs.

3.4 Form the plural and adjective forms of nouns related to gastroenterology.

3.5 Give the meanings of word parts and abbreviations related to gastroenterology.

3.6 Divide gastroenterology words and build gastroenterology words.

3.7 Spell and pronounce gastroenterology words.

3.8 Research sound-alike and other gastroenterology words.

3.9 Analyze the medical content and meaning of gastroenterology reports.

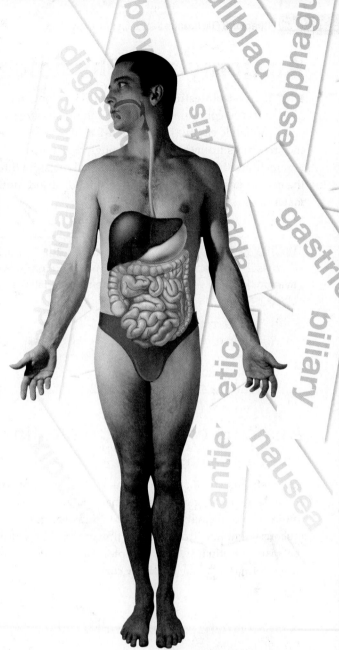

FIGURE 3-1 ■ Gastrointestinal system.
The gastrointestinal system consists of organs and glands connected in a pathway. Food enters the body, is digested, and undigested wastes are eliminated from the body.
Source: Pearson Education

Medical Language Key

To unlock the definition of a medical word, break it into word parts. Give the meaning of each word part. Put the meanings of the word parts in order, beginning with the meaning of the suffix, then the prefix (if present), then the combining form(s).

	Word Part	Word Part Meaning
Suffix	**-logy**	*study of*
Combining Form	**gastr/o-**	*stomach*
Combining Form	**enter/o-**	*intestine*

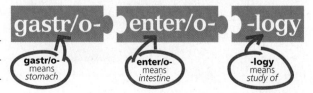

Gastroenterology: ▶ *Study of (the) stomach (and) intestine (and related structures).*

Anatomy and Physiology

The **gastrointestinal (GI) system** is an elongated body system that begins at the mouth, continues through the thoracic cavity, and fills much of the abdominopelvic cavity (see Figure 3-1 ■). The upper gastrointestinal system includes the structures from the mouth through the stomach. The lower gastrointestinal system includes the structures from the small intestine through the anus. The purpose of the gastrointestinal system is to digest food, absorb nutrients, and remove undigested material (waste) from the body.

Pronunciation/Word Parts

gastrointestinal (GAS-troh-in-TES-tih-nal)
  gastr/o- *stomach*
  intestin/o- *intestine*
  -al *pertaining to*

system (SIS-tem)

> **WORD ALERT**
>
> The gastrointestinal system is also known as the **gastrointestinal tract,** the **digestive system** or digestive tract, and the **alimentary canal**. Each name highlights a different characteristic of this body system.
>
> 1. Tract: a continuing pathway
> 2. Digestive: describes the purpose of the system
> 3. Alimentary: refers to food and nourishment
> 4. Canal: a tubular channel

digestive (dy-JES-tiv)
  digest/o- *break down food; digest*
  -ive *pertaining to*

alimentary (AL-ih-MEN-tair-ee)
  aliment/o- *food; nourishment*
  -ary *pertaining to*

Anatomy of the Gastrointestinal System

Oral Cavity and Pharynx

The gastrointestinal system begins in the mouth or **oral cavity** (see Figure 3-2 ■). It contains the teeth, gums, **tongue**, hard **palate**, and soft palate with its fleshy, hanging **uvula**. The oral cavity (and the entire gastrointestinal tract) is lined with **mucosa**, a mucous membrane that produces thin mucus. The sense of taste is also associated with the gastrointestinal system. Receptors on the tongue perceive taste and send this sensory information to the **gustatory cortex** in the brain.

oral (OR-al)
  or/o- *mouth*
  -al *pertaining to*
Oral is the adjective form for *mouth*. The combining form **stomat/o-** also means *mouth*.

tongue (TUNG)
  lingu/o- *tongue*
  -al *pertaining to*
The combining form **gloss/o-** also means *tongue*.

palate (PAL-at)

uvula (YOO-vyoo-lah)

mucosa (myoo-KOH-sah)

gustatory (GUS-tah-TOR-ee)
  gustat/o- *sense of taste*
  -ory *having the function of*

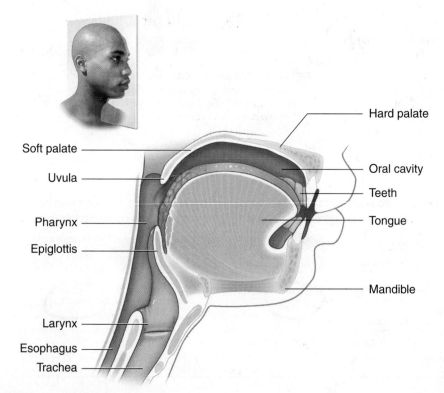

Soft palate —
Uvula —
Pharynx —
Epiglottis —
Larynx —
Esophagus —
Trachea —

— Hard palate
— Oral cavity
— Teeth
— Tongue
— Mandible

FIGURE 3-2 ■ Oral cavity and pharynx.
The oral cavity contains the teeth, gums, tongue, and palate. Food passes from the oral cavity into the pharynx (throat) and then into the esophagus.
Source: Pearson Education

The sight, smell, and taste of food cause the salivary glands to release saliva into the mouth. **Saliva** is a lubricant that moistens food as it is chewed and swallowed. Saliva also contains the enzyme amylase that begins the process of digestion. There are three pairs of **salivary glands:** the **parotid glands**, **sublingual glands**, and **submandibular glands** (see Figure 3-3 ■).

The teeth tear, chew, and grind food during the process of **mastication**. The tongue moves food toward the teeth and mixes food with saliva. Swallowing or **deglutition** moves food into the **pharynx** (throat), and then into the esophagus.

It is important to remember that the pharynx is a passageway for food as well as for inhaled and exhaled air. When food is swallowed, muscles in the neck pull the larynx (voice box) upward against the epiglottis, and that seals off the opening to the larynx, so that food in the pharynx does not enter the larynx, trachea, and lungs. If the larynx is not closed, food in the back of the pharynx presses on the uvula and initiates the gag reflex.

ACROSS THE LIFE SPAN

Pediatrics. The first food for many babies is colostrum from the mother's breast. Colostrum is rich in nutrients and contains maternal antibodies. For the first few days of life, the newborn's intestinal tract is permeable and allows these antibodies to be absorbed from the intestine into the blood, where they provide passive immunity to common infectious diseases.

Geriatrics. Older adults often complain that food does not seem as flavorful as when they were young. The aging process causes a very real decline in the ability to smell and taste food as the number of receptors in the nose and on the tongue decreases.

Pronunciation/Word Parts

saliva (sah-LY-vah)

salivary (SAL-ih-VAIR-ee)
  saliv/o- *saliva*
  -ary *pertaining to*
The combining form **sial/o-** means *saliva; salivary gland.*

parotid (pah-RAW-tid)
  par- *beside*
  ot/o- *ear*
  -id *origin; resembling; source*

sublingual (sub-LING-gwal)
  sub- *below; underneath*
  lingu/o- *tongue*
  -al *pertaining to*

submandibular (SUB-man-DIH-byoo-lar)
  sub- *below; underneath*
  mandibul/o- *lower jaw; mandible*
  -ar *pertaining to*

mastication (MAS-tih-KAY-shun)
  mastic/o- *chewing*
  -ation *being; having; process*

deglutition (DEE-gloo-TIH-shun)
  degluti/o- *swallowing*
  -tion *being; having; process*

pharynx (FAIR-ingks)
Pharynx is a Greek word that means *throat.*

pharyngeal (fah-RIN-jee-al)
  pharyng/o- *pharynx; throat*
  -eal *pertaining to*

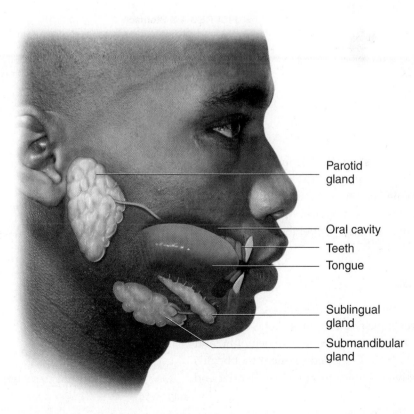

Parotid gland

Oral cavity

Teeth

Tongue

Sublingual gland

Submandibular gland

FIGURE 3-3 ■ Salivary glands.
The large, flat parotid glands are on either side of the head in front of the ear. The sublingual glands are under the tongue. The submandibular glands are under the mandible (lower jaw bone). Ducts from these glands bring saliva into the oral cavity.
Source: Pearson Education

Esophagus

The **esophagus** is a flexible, muscular tube that connects the pharynx to the stomach. It is lined with mucosa that produces mucus. With coordinated contractions of its wall—a process known as **peristalsis**—the esophagus moves food toward the stomach.

Stomach

The **stomach** (see Figure 3-4 ■) is a large, elongated sac in the upper abdominal cavity. It receives food from the esophagus. The stomach is divided into four regions: the **cardia**, **fundus**, **body**, and **pylorus**. The gastric mucosa is arranged in thick, deep folds, or **rugae**, that expand as the stomach fills with food. The stomach produces hydrochloric acid, pepsinogen, and gastrin to aid in the digestion of food. The mucosa produces mucus that protects the lining of the stomach from the hydrochloric acid.

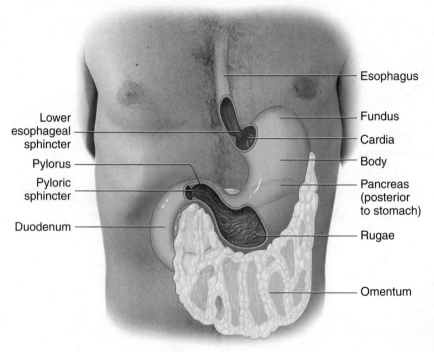

FIGURE 3-4 ■ Stomach.
The stomach has four regions. The cardia is a small area where the esophagus joins the stomach. The fundus is the rounded top of the stomach. The body is the large, curved part of the stomach. The pylorus is the narrowed canal at the end.
Source: Pearson Education

Two sphincters (muscular rings) keep food in the stomach. The **lower esophageal sphincter (LES)** is located at the distal end of the esophagus. The **pyloric sphincter** is located at the distal end of the stomach. **Chyme** is a semisolid mixture of partially digested food, saliva, digestive enzymes, and fluids in the stomach. An hour or so after eating, the pyloric sphincter opens and waves of peristalsis propel the chyme into the small intestine.

Small Intestine

The **small intestine** or **small bowel** is a long, hollow tube that receives chyme from the stomach. The small intestine produces three digestive enzymes: lactase, maltase, and sucrase. The small intestine consists of three parts: the duodenum, jejunum, and ileum (see Figure 3-5 ■). The **duodenum** is a 10-inch, C-shaped segment that begins at the stomach and ends at the jejunum. Digestive enzymes from the gallbladder and

---

Pronunciation/Word Parts

esophagus (eh-SAW-fah-gus)

esophageal (eh-saw-fah-JEE-al)
　esophag/o- *esophagus*
　-eal *pertaining to*

peristalsis (PAIR-ih-STAL-sis)
　peri- *around*
　stal/o- *contraction*
　-sis *condition; process*

gastric (GAS-trik)
　gastr/o- *stomach*
　-ic *pertaining to*
Gastric is the adjective form for *stomach*.

cardia (KAR-dee-ah)

fundus (FUN-dus)

pylorus (py-LOR-us)

pyloric (py-LOR-ik)
　pylor/o- *pylorus*
　-ic *pertaining to*

rugae (ROO-gee)
The singular form *ruga* is seldom used.

sphincter (SFINGK-ter)

chyme (KIME)

intestine (in-TES-tin)

intestinal (in-TES-tih-nal)
　intestin/o- *intestine*
　-al *pertaining to*
The combining form **enter/o-** also means *intestine*.

duodenum (DOO-oh-DEE-num)
(doo-AW-deh-num)

duodenal (DOO-oh-DEE-nal)
(doo-AW-deh-nal)
　duoden/o- *duodenum*
　-al *pertaining to*
Duodenum comes from a Latin word meaning *twelve*. Roman physicians studying the intestine noted that the duodenum was always 12 fingerbreadths (10 inches) in length.

pancreas flow through ducts into the duodenum. The **jejunum**, the second part of the small intestine, is an 8-foot segment that repeatedly twists and turns in the abdominal cavity. Digestion continues in the jejunum. Peristalsis slowly moves the chyme along for several hours until it reaches the ileum, the final part of the small intestine. The **ileum** is a 12-foot segment where absorption of nutrients is completed. The ileum contains **villi**, thousands of small, thin structures that project into the **lumen** (central, open area). The villi increase the amount of surface area to maximize the absorption of food nutrients and water through the intestinal wall and into the blood. The remaining undigested material (waste) and water move into the large intestine.

Pronunciation/Word Parts

jejunum (jeh-JOO-num)

jejunal (jeh-JOO-nal)
  jejun/o- *jejunum*
  -al *pertaining to*

ileum (IL-ee-um)

ileal (IL-ee-al)
  ile/o- *ileum*
  -al *pertaining to*

villi (VIL-eye)
The singular form *villus* is seldom used.

lumen (LOO-men)

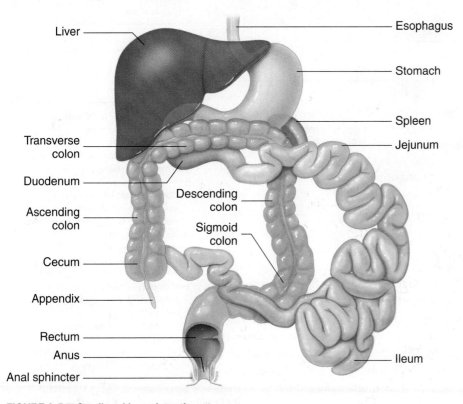

FIGURE 3-5 ■ Small and large intestines.
The small intestine consists of the duodenum, jejunum, and ileum. The large intestine consists of the cecum, colon, rectum, and anus. The colon can be divided into the ascending colon, transverse colon, descending colon, and sigmoid colon. The bends (flexures) in the colon are landmarks that are mentioned in x-ray reports. The bend near the liver is the hepatic flexure. The bend near the spleen is the splenic flexure.
Source: Pearson Education

cecum (SEE-kum)

cecal (SEE-kal)
  cec/o- *cecum*
  -al *pertaining to*

appendix (ah-PEN-diks)
  append/o- *appendix; small structure*
    hanging from a larger structure
  -ix *thing*

appendiceal (AP-en-DIH-see-al)
  appendic/o- *appendix*
  -eal *pertaining to*

haustra (HAW-strah)
The singular form *haustrum* is seldom used.

colon (KOH-lon)

colonic (koh-LAW-nik)
  colon/o- *colon*
  -ic *pertaining to*
The combining form **col/o-** also means *colon*.

Large Intestine

The **large intestine** or **large bowel** is a larger tube that receives undigested material and some water from the small intestine. The large intestine consists of the cecum, colon, rectum, and anus (see Figure 3-5). The **cecum** is a short sac. Hanging from its external wall is the **appendix**, a long, thin pouch that is closed at its distal end.

The walls of the large intestine contain **haustra** (puckered pouches) that can greatly expand as needed. Waves of peristalsis slowly move undigested wastes through the large intestine as water is absorbed through the intestinal wall and into the blood.

The **colon** is the longest part of the large intestine. It travels through all four quadrants of the abdomen as the **ascending colon, transverse colon, descending colon,** and

sigmoid colon (see Figure 3-5). As the ascending colon nears the liver, it bends at a right angle as the hepatic flexure. The transverse colon near the spleen bends at a right angle as the splenic flexure. The sigmoid colon bends toward the midline as an S-shaped curve that joins the rectum. The **rectum** is a short, straight segment that connects to the outside of the body. The **anus**, the external opening of the rectum, is located between the buttocks. The anal sphincter is a muscular ring whose opening and closing is under conscious, voluntary control.

DID YOU KNOW?

The appendix or vermiform appendix can be up to 8 inches in length. *Vermiform* is a Latin word meaning *wormlike*. The appendix plays no role in digestion.

CLINICAL CONNECTIONS

Immunology (Chapter 6). Some parts of the gastrointestinal system are also part of the body's immune response. Saliva contains antibodies that destroy microorganisms in the food we eat. Small areas on the walls of the intestines (Peyer's patches) as well as in the appendix contain lymphoid tissue and white blood cells that destroy microorganisms. However, large numbers of ingested microorganisms can still cause gastrointestinal illness.

Abdomen and Abdominopelvic Cavity

The anterior **abdominal wall** can be divided into four quadrants or nine regions (discussed in "The Body in Health and Disease," Chapter 2).

The **abdominopelvic cavity** contains the largest organs (viscera) of the gastrointestinal system. The **peritoneum** is a double-layer serous membrane. One layer lines the walls of the abdominopelvic cavity. The other layer surrounds each of the organs. The peritoneum secretes **peritoneal fluid**, a watery fluid that fills the spaces between the organs and allows them to slide past each other during the movements of digestion.

The peritoneum extends into the center of the abdominopelvic cavity as the **omentum** (see Figure 3-4). The omentum supports the stomach and hangs down as a broad, fatty apron to cover and protect the small intestine. The peritoneum also becomes the **mesentery**, a thick, fan-shaped sheet that supports the jejunum and ileum.

The blood supply to the stomach, small intestine, liver, gallbladder, and pancreas comes from the **celiac trunk** (a branch of the abdominal aorta, the largest artery in the body).

Accessory Organs of Digestion

The liver, gallbladder, and pancreas are accessory organs of digestion. They contribute to, but are not physically involved in, the process of digestion.

The **liver**, a large, dark red-brown organ, is located in the upper abdomen (see Figure 3-6 ■). Liver cells (**hepatocytes**) continuously produce **bile**, a yellow-green, bitter-tasting, thick fluid. Bile is a combination of bile acids, mucus, fluid, and two pigments: the yellow pigment **bilirubin** and the green pigment **biliverdin**. Bile produced by the liver flows through the common hepatic duct and into the common bile duct toward the duodenum. When that duct is full, bile then fills the cystic duct and gallbladder. All of the **bile ducts** collectively are known as the **biliary tree**.

Pronunciation/Word Parts

sigmoid (SIG-moyd)
Sigmoid is a combination of the *S*-shaped Greek letter *sigma* (Σ) and *-oid* (resembling). The combining form **sigmoid/o-** means *sigmoid colon*.

rectum (REK-tum)

rectal (REK-tal)
　rect/o- *rectum*
　-al *pertaining to*
The combining form **proct/o-** means *rectum and anus*.

anus (AA-nus)

anal (AA-nal)
　an/o- *anus*
　-al *pertaining to*

abdominal (ab-DAW-mih-nal)
　abdomin/o- *abdomen*
　-al *pertaining to*
The combining forms **celi/o-** and **lapar/o-** also mean *abdomen*.

abdominopelvic (ab-DAW-mih-noh-PEL-vik)
　abdomin/o- *abdomen*
　pelv/o- *hip bone; pelvis; renal pelvis*
　-ic *pertaining to*

peritoneum (PAIR-ih-toh-NEE-um)

peritoneal (PAIR-ih-toh-NEE-al)
　peritone/o- *peritoneum*
　-al *pertaining to*
The combining form **periton/o-** also means *peritoneum*.

omentum (oh-MEN-tum)

mesentery (MEZ-en-TAIR-ee)

mesenteric (MEZ-en-TAIR-ik)
　meso- *middle*
　enter/o- *intestine*
　-ic *pertaining to*
Delete the *o* in *meso-* before building the word.

celiac (SEE-lee-ak)
　celi/o- *abdomen*
　-ac *pertaining to*

liver (LIV-er)

hepatic (heh-PAT-ik)
　hepat/o- *liver*
　-ic *pertaining to*

hepatocyte (HEP-ah-toh-SITE)
　hepat/o- *liver*
　-cyte *cell*

bile (BILE)
The combining forms **bili/o-** and **chol/e-** mean *bile; gall*.

The **gallbladder** is a teardrop-shaped, dark green sac posterior to the liver (see Figure 3-6). It concentrates and stores bile. The presence of fatty chyme in the duodenum causes the gallbladder to contract, sending bile into the duodenum to digest fats.

The **pancreas** is a yellow gland shaped like an elongated triangle (see Figure 3-6). It is located posterior to the stomach. The presence of chyme in the duodenum causes the pancreas to secrete digestive enzymes (amylase, lipase, protein-digesting enzymes) through the pancreatic duct and into the duodenum. The pancreas also functions as an organ of the endocrine system (discussed in "Endocrinology," Chapter 14).

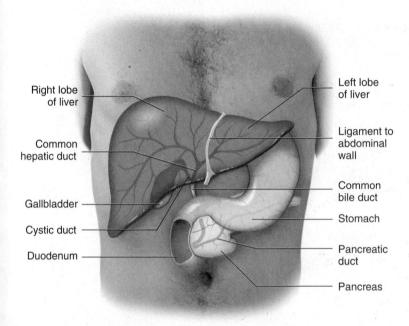

Right lobe of liver

Common hepatic duct

Gallbladder

Cystic duct

Duodenum

Left lobe of liver

Ligament to abdominal wall

Common bile duct

Stomach

Pancreatic duct

Pancreas

FIGURE 3-6 ■ Biliary tree.
Bile flows through hepatic ducts in the liver that merge to form the common hepatic duct. It joins the cystic duct from the gallbladder and becomes the common bile duct. Because of their branched appearance, these ducts are known as the *biliary tree*. The pancreatic duct joins the common bile duct just before it enters the duodenum.
Source: Pearson Education

Physiology of Digestion

The process of **digestion** begins in the oral cavity (see Figure 3-7 ■). There are two parts to digestion: mechanical and chemical.

Mechanical digestion involves mastication, deglutition, and peristalsis (mixing and moving food through the esophagus or moving chyme and undigested material through the stomach and intestines). Mechanical digestion also involves bile breaking apart fats in the duodenum. Fatty chyme stimulates the duodenum to secrete the hormone **cholecystokinin**, which stimulates the gallbladder to contract and release bile. Bile breaks apart fat during the process of **emulsification**.

Chemical digestion uses digestive **enzymes** and acid to break down foods. The enzyme amylase in saliva begins to break down carbohydrate foods in the mouth. The stomach secretes the following substances that continue the process of chemical digestion.

Pronunciation/Word Parts

bilirubin (BIL-ih-ROO-bin)
 bili/o- *bile; gall*
 rub/o- *red*
 -in *substance*
Rub/o- refers to red blood cells that break down and are used by the liver to make bilirubin.

biliverdin (BIL-ih-VER-din)
Verd/o- means *green*.

bile duct (BILE DUKT)
The combining form **cholangi/o-** means *bile duct* and **choledoch/o-** means *common bile duct*.

biliary (BIL-ee-AIR-ee)
 bili/o- *bile; gall*
 -ary *pertaining to*

gallbladder (GAWL-blad-er)
The combining form **cholecyst/o-** means *gallbladder*.

pancreas (PAN-kree-as)

pancreatic (PAN-kree-AT-ik)
 pancreat/o- *pancreas*
 -ic *pertaining to*

digestion (dy-JES-chun) (dih-JES-chun)
 digest/o- *break down food; digest*
 -ion *action; condition*

cholecystokinin (KOH-lee-SIS-toh-KY-nin)
 cholecyst/o- *gallbladder*
 kin/o- *movement*
 -in *substance*

emulsification (ee-MUL-sih-fih-KAY-shun)
 emulsific/o- *liquid with suspended particles*
 -ation *being; having; process*

enzyme (EN-zime)

- **Hydrochloric acid (HCl)**. This strong acid breaks down food fibers, converts pepsinogen to the digestive enzyme pepsin, and kills microorganisms in food.
- **Pepsinogen**. This inactive substance is converted by hydrochloric acid to **pepsin**, a digestive enzyme that breaks down protein foods into protein molecules.
- **Gastrin**. This hormone stimulates the release of more hydrochloric acid and pepsinogen.

Pronunciation/Word Parts

hydrochloric acid (HY-droh-KLOR-ik AS-id)
   hydr/o- *fluid; water*
   chlor/o- *chloride*
   -ic *pertaining to*

pepsinogen (pep-SIN-oh-jen)
   pepsin/o- *pepsin*
   -gen *that which produces*

pepsin (PEP-sin)
   peps/o- *digestion*
   -in *substance*

gastrin (GAS-trin)
   gastr/o- *stomach*
   -in *substance*

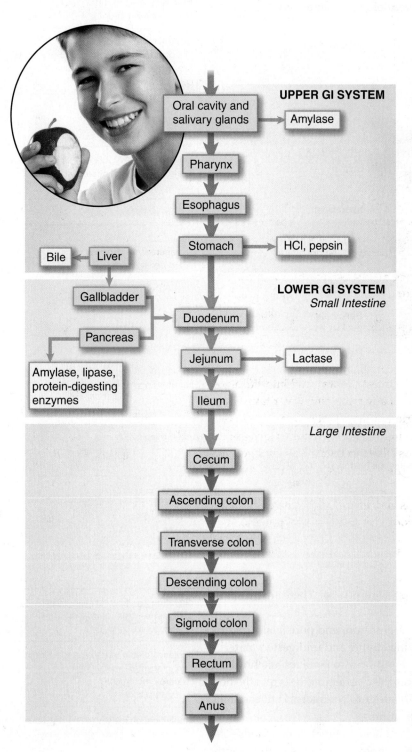

FIGURE 3-7 ■ Gastrointestinal system.
Everyone enjoys eating! The gastrointestinal system helps you taste and enjoy the food you eat and then uses mechanical and chemical digestion to break down that food into nutrients that nourish your body.
Source: Pearson Education; iPag/Fotolia

Chemical digestion continues in the small intestine as cholecystokinin from the duodenum stimulates the pancreas to secrete its digestive enzymes (amylase, lipase, protein-digesting enzymes) into the duodenum.

- **Amylase** from the pancreas continues the digestion of carbohydrates that was begun by amylase in the saliva. It breaks down carbohydrates and starches into sugars and food fibers.
- **Lipase** breaks down small fat globules into fatty acids.
- Protein-digesting enzymes break down protein molecules into peptide chains and then into amino acids.

The villi of the small intestine produce the digestive enzyme **lactase**. It breaks down the sugars in carbohydrates, starches, and milk to the simple sugar glucose, which is the only source of energy that body cells can use.

CLINICAL CONNECTIONS

Hematology (Chapter 6). The stomach plays an indirect role in the production of red blood cells. It secretes intrinsic factor that allows vitamin B_{12} (a building block of red blood cells) to be absorbed from the intestine into the blood. When the stomach does not produce enough intrinsic factor or when part of the stomach is removed (gastrectomy) because of a cancerous tumor, vitamin B_{12} is not absorbed; the red blood cells that are formed are very large, fragile, and die prematurely. This disease is known as *pernicious anemia*.

Dietetics. Individuals whose small intestine does not produce enough of the digestive enzyme lactase experience gas and bloating when they drink milk or eat dairy products. This is caused by undigested lactose (the sugar in milk).

Absorption of nutrients and water through the intestinal wall and into the blood takes place in the small intestine, while absorption of any remaining water takes place in the large intestine. Absorbed nutrients are carried in the blood of a large vein that goes to the liver. The liver plays an important role in regulating nutrients such as glucose and amino acids. Excess glucose in the blood is stored in the liver as glycogen and is released when the blood glucose level is low. The liver uses amino acids to build plasma proteins and clotting factors for the blood.

Elimination occurs when undigested materials and water are eliminated from the body in a solid waste form known as **feces** or **stool**. The process of elimination is a bowel movement or **defecation**.

A CLOSER LOOK

The large intestine is inhabited by millions of beneficial bacteria that produce vitamin K to supplement what is in the diet. These bacteria also change the yellow-green pigment in bile to the characteristic brown color of feces. Bacteria in the large intestine feed on undigested materials and produce intestinal gas or **flatus**.

Pronunciation/Word Parts

amylase (AM-ih-lays)
  amyl/o- *carbohydrate; starch*
  -ase *enzyme*

lipase (LIH-pays)
  lip/o- *fat; lipid*
  -ase *enzyme*

lactase (LAK-tays)
  lact/o- *milk*
  -ase *enzyme*

absorption (ab-SORP-shun)
  absorpt/o- *absorb; take in*
  -ion *action; condition*

elimination (ee-LIM-ih-NAY-shun)
The combining form **chez/o-** means *pass feces.*

feces (FEE-seez)

fecal (FEE-kal)
  fec/o- *feces; stool*
  -al *pertaining to*
The combining form **fec/a-** also means *feces; stool.*

stool (STOOL)

defecation (DEF-eh-KAY-shun)
  de- *reversal of; without*
  fec/o- *feces; stool*
  -ation *being; having; process*

flatus (FLAY-tus)

Vocabulary Review

Anatomy and Physiology

Word or Phrase	Description	Combining Forms
alimentary canal	Alternate name for the gastrointestinal system	**aliment/o-** *food; nourishment*
digestive system	Alternate name for the gastrointestinal system. It is also known as the **digestive tract**.	**digest/o-** *break down food; digest*
gastrointestinal system	Body system that includes the salivary glands, oral cavity (teeth, gums, palate, and tongue), pharynx, esophagus, stomach, small and large intestines, rectum, anus, and the accesssory organs of the liver, gallbladder, and pancreas. Its function is to digest food, absorb nutrients into the blood, and remove undigested material from the body. It is also known as the **gastrointestinal tract**, digestive system or tract, and **alimentary canal**.	**gastr/o-** *stomach* **intestin/o-** *intestine*

Oral Cavity and Pharynx

Word or Phrase	Description	Combining Forms
deglutition	Process of swallowing	**degluti/o-** *swallowing*
gustatory cortex	Area of the brain that receives and interprets tastes from the tongue	**gustat/o-** *sense of taste*
mastication	Process of chewing. This is part of the process of mechanical digestion.	**mastic/o-** *chewing*
mucosa	Mucous membrane that lines the gastrointestinal system and produces thin mucus	
oral cavity	Mouth. Hollow area that contains the hard palate, soft palate, uvula, tongue, gums, and teeth	**or/o-** *mouth* **stomat/o-** *mouth*
palate	The hard bone and posterior soft tissues that form the roof of the mouth	
pharynx	Throat. The passageway for both food and air	**pharyng/o-** *pharynx; throat*
salivary glands	Three pairs of glands (**parotid**, **sublingual**, and **submandibular**) that secrete saliva into the mouth. Saliva is a watery substance that contains the digestive enzyme amylase.	**saliv/o-** *saliva* **sial/o-** *saliva; salivary gland* **ot/o-** *ear* **mandibul/o-** *lower jaw; mandible* **lingu/o-** *tongue*
tongue	Large muscle that fills the oral cavity and assists with eating and talking. It contains receptors for the sense of taste.	**lingu/o-** *tongue* **gloss/o-** *tongue*
uvula	Fleshy hanging part of the soft palate. During swallowing, it initiates the gag reflex to prevent food from entering the pharynx before the epiglottis has sealed the opening to the larynx (voice box).	

Esophagus and Stomach

Word or Phrase	Description	Combining Forms
cardia	First part of the stomach just after the esophagus	
chyme	Semisolid mixture of partially digested food, saliva, digestive enzymes, and fluids in the stomach and small intestine	
esophagus	Flexible, muscular tube that moves food from the pharynx to the stomach	**esophag/o-** *esophagus*
fundus	Rounded, top part of the stomach	
lower esophageal sphincter (LES)	Muscular ring at the distal end of the esophagus. It keeps food in the stomach from going back into the esophagus.	**esophag/o-** *esophagus*

Word or Phrase	Description	Combining Forms
peristalsis	Coordinated contractions of smooth muscle that propel food, chyme, or wastes and water through the gastrointestinal tract	**stal/o-** *contraction*
pyloric sphincter	Muscular ring that closes to keep chyme in the stomach or opens to let chyme go into the duodenum	**pylor/o-** *pylorus*
pylorus	Narrowed, last part of the stomach just before it joins the duodenum. It contains the pyloric sphincter.	**pylor/o-** *pylorus*
rugae	Deep folds in the gastric mucosa that expand to accommodate food	
stomach	Organ of digestion between the esophagus and the small intestine. Areas of the stomach: cardia, fundus, body, and pylorus. The stomach secretes hydrochloric acid, pepsinogen, gastrin (to digest food) and intrinsic factor (to aid in the absorption of vitamin B$_{12}$).	**gastr/o-** *stomach*

Small and Large Intestines		
anus	External opening of the rectum. The anal sphincter is under voluntary control.	**an/o-** *anus*
appendix	Long, thin pouch on the exterior wall of the cecum. It does not play a role in digestion. It contains lymphatic tissue and is active in the body's immune response.	**appendic/o-** *appendix* **append/o-** *appendix; small structure hanging from a larger structure*
cecum	Short sac that is the first part of the large intestine. The appendix is attached to the cecum's external wall.	**cec/o-** *cecum*
colon	Longest part of the large intestine. It consists of the **ascending colon**, **transverse colon**, **descending colon**, and S-shaped **sigmoid colon**.	**col/o-** *colon* **colon/o-** *colon* **sigmoid/o-** *sigmoid colon*
duodenum	First part of the small intestine. It secretes the hormone cholecystokinin. Digestion takes place there, as well as some absorption of nutrients and water.	**duoden/o-** *duodenum*
haustra	Pouches in the wall of the large intestine that expand to accommodate the bulk of undigested materials	
ileum	Third part of the small intestine. It connects to the cecum of the large intestine. Some digestion takes place there. There is absorption of nutrients and water through the wall of the ileum into the blood.	**ile/o-** *ileum*
jejunum	Second part of the small intestine. Digestion takes place there, as well as some absorption of nutrients and water through the intestinal wall into the blood.	**jejun/o-** *jejunum*
large intestine	Organ of absorption between the small intestine and the anus. The large intestine includes the cecum, colon, rectum, and anus. It is also known as the **large bowel**.	**intestin/o-** *intestine*
lumen	Central, open area inside a tubular structure such as the esophagus, small intestine, and large intestine	
rectum	Short, straight segment that is the last part of the large intestine. It follows the sigmoid colon and connects to the outside of the body.	**rect/o-** *rectum* **proct/o-** *rectum and anus*

Word or Phrase	Description	Combining Forms
small intestine	Organ of digestion and absorption between the stomach and the large intestine. The duodenum, jejunum, and ileum are the three parts of the small intestine. It is also known as the **small bowel**.	**intestin/o-** *intestine* **enter/o-** *intestine*
villi	Microscopic projections of the mucosa in the small intestine. They produce the digestive enzyme lactase that breaks down sugar in carbohydrates, starches, and milk. The large combined surface area of the villi maximizes absorption of nutrients into the blood.	

Abdomen, Liver, Gallbladder, and Pancreas

Word or Phrase	Description	Combining Forms
abdominopelvic cavity	Continuous cavity within the **abdomen** and pelvis that contains the largest organs (viscera) of the gastrointestinal system	**abdomin/o-** *abdomen* **celi/o-** *abdomen* **lapar/o-** *abdomen* **pelv/o-** *hip bone; pelvis; renal pelvis*
bile	Bitter-tasting, thick fluid produced by the liver and stored in the gallbladder. It is released into the duodenum to digest fatty foods. It contains the yellow pigment **bilirubin** and the green pigment **biliverdin**.	**bili/o-** *bile; gall* **chol/e-** *bile; gall* **rub/o-** *red* **verd/o-** *green*
bile ducts	Bile produced by the liver flows through the hepatic ducts to the common hepatic duct. Then it goes into the common bile duct to the duodenum. When that duct is full, bile goes into the cystic duct and gallbladder. All of these ducts form the **biliary tree**, a branching structure.	**bili/o-** *bile; gall* **cholangi/o-** *bile duct* **choledoch/o-** *common bile duct*
celiac trunk	Part of the abdominal aorta where arteries branch off to take blood to the stomach, small intestine, liver, gallbladder, and pancreas	**celi/o-** *abdomen*
gallbladder	Teardrop-shaped, dark green sac posterior to the liver that stores and concentrates bile. Fatty chyme in the duodenum causes it to contract and release bile into the duodenum.	**cholecyst/o-** *gallbladder*
liver	Large, dark red-brown organ in the abdominal cavity. It contains **hepatocytes** that produce bile.	**hepat/o-** *liver*
mesentery	Thick, fan-shaped sheet of peritoneum that supports the jejunum and ileum	**enter/o-** *intestine*
omentum	Broad, fatty apron of peritoneum. It supports the stomach and protects the small intestine.	
pancreas	Yellow, elongated, triangular organ located posterior to the stomach. It secretes amylase, lipase, and protein-digesting enzymes into the duodenum.	**pancreat/o-** *pancreas*
peritoneum	Double-layer serous membrane that lines the abdominopelvic cavity and surrounds each gastrointestinal organ. It secretes peritoneal fluid to fill the spaces between the organs.	**peritone/o-** *peritoneum* **periton/o-** *peritoneum*

Digestion

Word or Phrase	Description	Combining Forms
absorption	Process by which digested nutrients move through villi of the small intestine and into the blood	**absorpt/o-** *absorb; take in*
amylase	Digestive enzyme in saliva that begins the digestion of carbohydrates in the mouth. It is also secreted by the pancreas to finish the digestion of carbohydrates in the small intestine.	**amyl/o-** *carbohydrate; starch*

Diseases

Eating		
Word or Phrase	**Description**	**Pronunciation/Word Parts**
anorexia	Decreased appetite because of disease or the gastrointestinal side effects of a drug. The patient is said to be **anorexic**. Treatment: Correct the underlying cause.	**anorexia** (AN-oh-REK-see-ah) **an-** *not; without* **orex/o-** *appetite* **-ia** *condition; state; thing* **anorexic** (AN-oh-REK-SIK)
	CLINICAL CONNECTIONS **Psychiatry (Chapter 17).** Anorexia nervosa is a psychiatric disorder in which patients have an obsessive desire to be thin. They decrease their food intake to the point of starvation, not because they have no appetite, but because they see themselves as being fat.	
dysphagia	Difficult or painful eating or swallowing. A stroke can make it difficult to coordinate the muscles for eating and swallowing. An oral infection, poorly fitted dentures, or radiation therapy to the mouth for cancer can cause painful eating. Treatment: Soft foods and thickened liquids. Antibiotic drug for a bacterial infection.	**dysphagia** (dis-FAY-jee-ah) **dys-** *abnormal; difficult; painful* **phag/o-** *eating; swallowing* **-ia** *condition; state; thing*
polyphagia	Excessive overeating due to an overactive thyroid gland, diabetes mellitus, or a psychiatric illness. Treatment: Correct the underlying cause.	**polyphagia** (PAW-lee-FAY-jee-ah) **poly-** *many; much* **phag/o-** *eating; swallowing* **-ia** *condition; state; thing*

Mouth and Lips		
cheilitis	Inflammation and cracking of the lips and corners of the mouth due to infection, allergies, or a nutritional deficiency. Treatment: Correct the underlying cause.	**cheilitis** (ky-LY-tis) **cheil/o-** *lip* **-itis** *infection of; inflammation of*
sialolithiasis	A stone (**sialolith**) that forms in the salivary gland and becomes lodged in the duct, blocking the flow of saliva. The salivary gland, mouth, and face become swollen. When the salivary gland contracts, the duct spasms, causing pain. Treatment: Surgical removal of the stone.	**sialolithiasis** (sy-AL-oh-lith-EYE-ah-sls) **sial/o-** *saliva; salivary gland* **lith/o-** *stone* **-iasis** *process; state* **sialolith** (sy-AL-oh-lith) **sial/o-** *saliva; salivary gland* **-lith** *stone*

Word or Phrase	Description	Pronunciation/Word Parts
stomatitis	Inflammation of the oral mucosa. Stomatitis can be caused by poorly fitted dentures or infection. **Aphthous stomatitis** consists of recurring outbreaks of small, painful ulcers (canker sores) on the lips or oral mucosa. Its cause is unknown. **Glossitis** is an inflammation that involves only the tongue (see Figure 3-8 ■). Treatment: Correct the underlying cause. 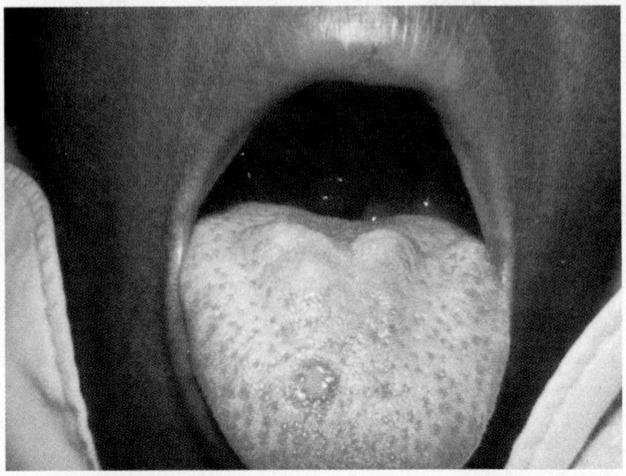	**stomatitis** (STOH-mah-TY-tis) **stomat/o-** *mouth* **-itis** *infection of; inflammation of* **aphthous** (AF-thus) **aphth/o-** *ulcer* **-ous** *pertaining to* **glossitis** (glaw-SY-tis) **gloss/o-** *tongue* **-itis** *infection of; inflammation of*

FIGURE 3-8 ■ Glossitis.
This inflammation of the tongue was caused by a viral infection. Other causes of glossitis include bacterial infection, food allergy, abrasive or spicy foods, or a vitamin B deficiency.
Source: Centers for Disease Control and Prevention (CDC)

Esophagus and Stomach

Word or Phrase	Description	Pronunciation/Word Parts
dyspepsia	**Indigestion** with mild, temporary epigastric pain, sometimes with gas or nausea. It can be caused by excess stomach acid or reflux of stomach acid into the esophagus, overeating, spicy foods, or stress. Treatment: Antacid drug. Avoid things that cause it.	**dyspepsia** (dis-PEP-see-ah) **dys-** *abnormal; difficult; painful* **peps/o-** *digestion* **-ia** *condition; state; thing*
esophageal varices	Swollen, protruding veins in the mucosa of the lower esophagus or stomach (see Figure 3-9 ■). When liver disease causes blood to back up in the large vein from the intestines to the liver, the blood is forced to take an alternate route through the gastroesophageal veins, but eventually these veins become engorged. Esophageal and gastric varices are easily irritated by passing food. They can hemorrhage suddenly, causing death. Treatment: Correct the underlying liver disease. Surgery: A drug is injected into the varix to harden it and block the blood flow.	**varix** (VAIR-iks) **varices** (VAIR-ih-seez) *Varix* is a Latin singular noun. Form the plural by changing *-ix* to *-ices*.

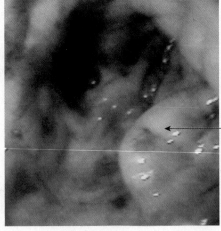

FIGURE 3-9 ■ Esophageal varix.
A varix is a dilated, swollen vein in the mucosa. This esophageal varix was seen through an endoscope passed through the mouth and into the esophagus. There are dark areas of old blood from previous bleeding.
Source: David M Martin/Science source

Word or Phrase	Description	Pronunciation/Word Parts
gastritis	Acute or chronic inflammation of the stomach due to spicy foods, excess acid production, or a bacterial infection. Treatment: Antacid drug, antibiotic drug for a bacterial infection.	**gastritis** (gas-TRY-tis) **gastr/o-** *stomach* **-itis** *infection of; inflammation of*
gastroenteritis	Acute inflammation or infection of the stomach and intestines due to a virus (flu) or bacterium (contaminated food). There is abdominal pain, nausea, vomiting, and diarrhea. Treatment: Antiemetic drug (to prevent vomiting), antidiarrheal drug, antibiotic drug for an infection.	**gastroenteritis** (GAS-troh-EN-ter-EYE-tis) **gastr/o-** *stomach* **enter/o-** *intestine* **-itis** *infection of; inflammation of*
gastroesophageal reflux disease (GERD)	Chronic inflammation and irritation due to **reflux** of stomach acid back into the esophagus because the lower esophageal sphincter does not close tightly. There is a sore throat, belching, and **esophagitis** with chronic inflammation. This can lead to esophageal ulcers or cancer of the esophagus. Treatment: Eat small, frequent meals, not large meals. Elevate the head of the bed while sleeping. Avoid alcohol and foods that stimulate acid secretion. Treatment: Antacid drug to neutralize acid, drug that decreases the production of acid. Surgery to repair the sphincter.	**gastroesophageal** (GAS-troh-eh-SAW-fah-JEE-al) **gastr/o-** *stomach* **esophag/o-** *esophagus* **-eal** *pertaining to* **reflux** (REE-fluks) **esophagitis** (eh-SAW-fah-JY-tis) **esophag/o-** *esophagus* **-itis** *infection of; inflammation of*
heartburn	Temporary inflammation of the esophagus due to reflux of stomach acid. It is also known as **pyrosis**. Treatment: Antacid drug.	**pyrosis** (py-ROH-sis) **pyr/o-** *burning; fire* **-osis** *condition; process*
hematemesis	Vomiting (emesis) of blood because of bleeding in the stomach or esophagus. This can be due to an esophageal or gastric ulcer or esophageal varices. Coffee-grounds emesis contains old, dark blood that has been partially digested by the stomach. Treatment: Correct the underlying cause.	**hematemesis** (HEE-mah-TEM-eh-sis) **hemat/o-** *blood* **eme/o-** *vomiting* **-sis** *condition; process* **Emet/o-** *also means vomiting.*
nausea and vomiting (N&V)	Nausea is an unpleasant, queasy feeling in the stomach that precedes the urge to vomit. The patient is said to be *nauseated*. It is caused by inflammation or infection of the stomach or by motion sickness. Vomiting or **emesis** is the expelling of food from the stomach through the mouth. It is triggered when impulses from the stomach or inner ear stimulate the vomiting center in the brain. Vomit or **vomitus** is the expelled food or chyme. Projectile vomiting is vomitus expelled with force and projected a distance from the patient. Retching (dry heaves) is continual vomiting when there is no longer anything in the stomach. **Regurgitation** is the reflux of small amounts of food and acid back into the mouth, but without vomiting. Treatment: Antiemetic drug. Treat the cause of inflammation or infection.	**nausea** (NAW-see-ah) (NAW-zha) **emesis** (EM-eh-sis) **vomitus** (VAW-mih-tus) **regurgitation** (ree-GER-jih-TAY-shun) **regurgitat/o-** *backward flow* **-ion** *action; condition*

CLINICAL CONNECTIONS

Obstetrics (Chapter 13). Morning sickness is the vomiting normally associated with early pregnancy. **Hyperemesis gravidarum** is excessive vomiting during the first months of pregnancy. These conditions are thought to be due to changes in hormone levels.

hyperemesis (HY-per-EM-eh-sis)

gravidarum (GRAV-ih-DAIR-um) *Gravidarum* means *of pregnancy*.

Word or Phrase	Description	Pronunciation/Word Parts

peptic ulcer disease (PUD)	Chronic irritation, burning pain, and erosion of the mucosa to form an ulcer (see Figure 3-10 ■). An esophageal ulcer, a gastric ulcer in the stomach, and a duodenal ulcer are all peptic ulcers. Gastric ulcers are most commonly caused by the bacterium *Helicobacter pylori*, which has been linked to cancer of the stomach. Ulcers can also be caused by excessive hydrochloric acid, stress, and drugs (such as aspirin) that irritate the mucosa. Treatment: Antibiotic drug to treat *H. pylori* infection. Drug to decrease acid production. Antacid drug. Avoid spicy foods, smoking, alcohol, caffeine, and aspirin-containing drugs.
	
	FIGURE 3-10 ■ Gastric ulcer.
	This gastric mucosa is raw and irritated with a large central ulcer crater. The bright red blood indicates a recent episode of bleeding from the ulcer.
	Source: David M. Martin, M.D./Science Source
		peptic (PEP-tik)
		  pept/o- *digestion*
		  -ic *pertaining to*
		
		ulcer (UL-ser)

stomach cancer	**Cancerous** tumor of the stomach that begins in glands in the gastric mucosa. It is categorized as an **adenocarcinoma**. It is caused by chronic irritation from a *Helicobacter pylori* infection. Treatment: Surgery to remove the cancer and part of the stomach (gastrectomy).	**cancer** (KAN-ser)
		cancerous (KAN-ser-us)
		  cancer/o- *cancer*
		  -ous *pertaining to*
		
		adenocarcinoma
		(AD-eh-noh-KAR-sih-NOH-mah)
		  aden/o- *gland*
		  carcin/o- *cancer*
		  -oma *mass; tumor*

Duodenum, Jejunum, Ileum

Word or Phrase	Description	Pronunciation/Word Parts

ileus	Abnormal absence of peristalsis in the small and large intestines. Obstipation, a tumor, adhesions, or a hernia can cause a mechanical obstruction. A severe infection in the intestine or abdominopelvic cavity, trauma, shock, or drugs can stop peristalsis and cause a paralytic ileus. **Postoperative ileus** occurs after the intestines are manipulated during abdominal surgery and peristalsis is slow to return. Treatment: Intravenous fluids for temporary nutritional support. Surgery (bowel resection and anastomosis) may be needed.	**ileus** (IL-ee-us)
		
		postoperative
		(post-AW-per-ah-TIV)
		  post- *after; behind*
		  operat/o- *perform a procedure; surgery*
		  -ive *pertaining to*

Word or Phrase	Description	Pronunciation/Word Parts
intussusception	Telescoping of one segment of intestine inside the lumen of the next segment (see Figure 3-11a ■). There is vomiting and abdominal pain. The cause is unknown. Treatment: Surgery (bowel resection and anastomosis).	**intussusception** (IN-tuh-suh-SEP-shun) **intussuscept/o-** *receive within* **-ion** *action; condition*

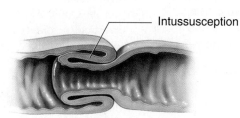
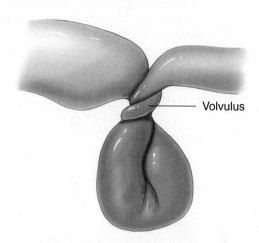

Intussusception

Volvulus

FIGURE 3-11 ■ Intussusception and volvulus of the intestine.
(a) In an intussusception, the intestine folds back on itself in the same way that one part of a telescope slides into the other. (b) In a volvulus, the intestine becomes twisted. Both of these conditions stop peristalsis and blood flow and can lead to tissue death.
Source: Pearson Education

Word or Phrase	Description	Pronunciation/Word Parts
volvulus	Twisting or rotating of the intestine around itself because of a structural abnormality of the mesentery (see Figure 3-11b). There is vomiting and abdominal pain. It is also known as **malrotation** of the intestines. It is caused by poor support of the intestine by the mesentery or by adhesions in the abdominal cavity. Treatment: Surgery (bowel resection and anastomosis).	**volvulus** (VAWL-vyoo-lus) **malrotation** (MAL-roh-TAY-shun) **mal-** *bad; inadequate* **rotat/o-** *rotate* **-ion** *action; condition*

	Cecum and Colon	
appendicitis	Inflammation and infection of the appendix. Undigested material becomes trapped in the lumen of the appendix. There is steadily increasing abdominal pain that finally localizes to the right lower quadrant. If the physician presses on that area and then quickly removes the hand and releases the pressure, the patient complains of severe rebound pain. An inflamed appendix can rupture (burst), spilling infection into the abdominopelvic cavity and causing peritonitis. Treatment: Surgery to remove the appendix (appendectomy).	**appendicitis** (ah-PEN-dih-SY-tis) **appendic/o-** *appendix* **-itis** *infection of; inflammation of*
colic	Common disorder in babies. There is crampy abdominal pain soon after eating. It can be caused by overfeeding, feeding too quickly, inadequate burping, or a food allergy to milk. Treatment: Correct the underlying cause.	**colic** (KAW-lik) **col/o-** *colon* **-ic** *pertaining to*
colon cancer	Cancerous tumor of the colon. It occurs when colonic polyps or ulcerative colitis become cancerous. It is also linked to a high-fat diet. There can be blood in the feces. It is also known as **colorectal adenocarcinoma**. Treatment: Preventive surgery to remove polyps before they become cancerous. Surgery to remove the cancer and the affected intestine (bowel resection) and reroute the colon to a new opening in the abdominal wall (colostomy).	**colorectal** (KOH-loh-REK-tal) **col/o-** *colon* **rect/o-** *rectum* **-al** *pertaining to* **adenocarcinoma** (AD-eh-noh-KAR-sih-NOH-mah) **aden/o-** *gland* **carcin/o-** *cancer* **-oma** *mass; tumor*

Word or Phrase	Description	Pronunciation/Word Parts

diverticulum	Weakness in the wall of the colon where the mucosa forms a pouch or tube. Diverticula can be caused by eating a low-fiber diet that forms small, compact feces. Then, increased intra-abdominal pressure and straining to pass those feces eventually creates diverticula. **Diverticulosis** or diverticular disease is the condition of multiple diverticula (see Figure 3-12 ■). If feces become trapped inside a diverticulum, this causes inflammation, infection, abdominal pain, and fever, a condition known as **diverticulitis** (see Figure 3-13 ■). Prevention: High-fiber diet. Treatment: Antibiotic drug to treat diverticulitis. Surgery (bowel resection and anastomosis) to remove the affected segment of intestine.	**diverticulum** (DY-ver-TIH-kyoo-lum)
		
		diverticula (DY-ver-TIH-kyoo-lah) *Diverticulum* is a Latin singular noun. Form the plural by changing *-um* to *-a*.
		
		diverticulosis (DY-ver-TIH-kyoo-LOH-sis)
		  diverticul/o- *diverticulum*
		  -osis *condition; process*
		
		diverticulitis (DY-ver-TIH-kyoo-LY-tis)
		  diverticul/o- *diverticulum*
		  -itis *infection of; inflammation of*

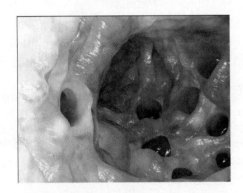

FIGURE 3-12 ■ Diverticula.
These openings in the wall of the colon lead to diverticular sacs where feces can become trapped.
Source: Juan Gärtner/123RF; Gastrolab, Photo Researchers, Inc. / Science Source

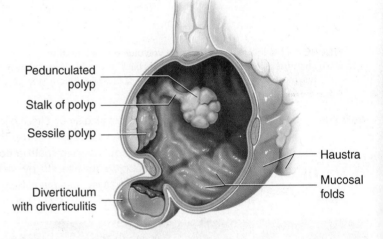

Pedunculated polyp
Stalk of polyp
Sessile polyp
Diverticulum with diverticulitis
Haustra
Mucosal folds

FIGURE 3-13 ■ Diverticulitis and polyposis.
This diverticulum has become infected from trapped feces. These polyps are irritated by the passage of feces and can become cancerous.
Source: Pearson Education

CLINICAL CONNECTIONS

Dietetics. Diverticular disease was unknown until the early 1900s, when refined flour began to replace whole wheat flour. Diverticular disease is common in countries where people eat a low-fiber diet, but is uncommon in third-world countries where there is a high-fiber diet. Fiber creates bulk and holds water to keep the feces soft.

Word or Phrase	Description	Pronunciation/Word Parts

dysentery	Bacterial infection caused by an unusual strain of *E. coli*, a common bacterium normally found in the large intestine. There is watery diarrhea mixed with blood and mucus. Treatment: Antibiotic drug.	**dysentery** (DIS-en-TAIR-ee)
		  dys- *abnormal; difficult; painful*
		  -entery *condition of the intestine*
		The ending *-entery* contains the combining form *enter/o-* and the one-letter suffix *-y*.

Word or Phrase	Description	Pronunciation/Word Parts
gluten sensitivity enteropathy	An autoimmune disorder and toxic reaction to the gluten found in certain grains (wheat, barley, rye, oats). The small intestine is damaged by the inflammatory response. It is also known as **celiac disease**. Treatment: Avoid eating foods and food products that contain gluten.	**gluten** (GLOO-ten) **enteropathy** (EN-ter-AW-pah-thee) **enter/o-** *intestine* **-pathy** *disease* **celiac** (SEE-lee-ak) **celi/o-** *abdomen* **-ac** *pertaining to*
inflammatory bowel disease (IBD)	Chronic inflammation of various parts of the small and large intestines. There is diarrhea, bloody feces, abdominal cramps, and fever. The cause is not known. There are two types of inflammatory bowel disease: (1) **Crohn's disease** (or **regional enteritis**) affects the ileum and colon (see Figure 3-14 ■). There are areas of normal mucosa ("skip areas") and then inflammation. There are ulcers and thickening of the intestinal wall that can cause a partial obstruction in the intestine. (2) **Ulcerative colitis** affects the colon and rectum and causes inflammation and ulcers. Treatment: Corticosteroid drug to decrease inflammation. Surgery (bowel resection) to remove the affected area and reroute the intestine to a new opening in the abdominal wall (ileostomy, colostomy).	**Crohn** (KROHN) **enteritis** (EN-ter-EYE-tis) **enter/o-** *intestine* **-itis** *infection of; inflammation of* **ulcerative** (UL-ser-ah-TIV) **ulcerat/o-** *ulcer* **-ive** *pertaining to* **colitis** (koh-LY-tis) **col/o-** *colon* **-itis** *infection of; inflammation of*

NORMAL ILEUM   **CROHN'S DISEASE**

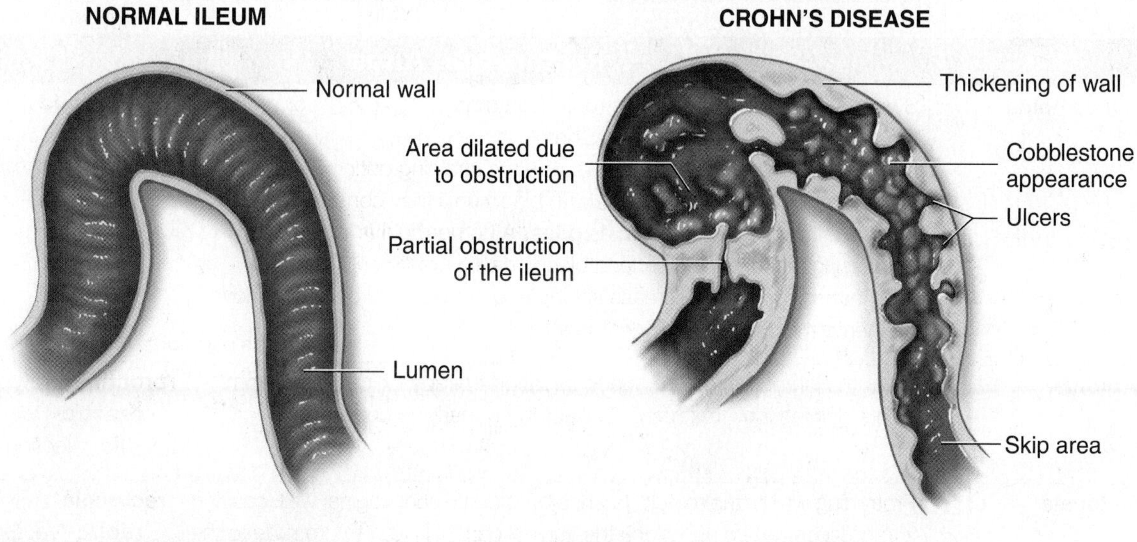

FIGURE 3-14 ■ Crohn's disease.
(a) This segment of normal intestine shows an open lumen throughout and an intestinal wall without thickening or ulcers.
(b) Crohn's disease shows thickening of the intestinal wall and ulcers. There is also a partial obstruction.

Source: Pearson Education

irritable bowel syndrome (IBS)	Disorder of the function of the colon, although the mucosa of the colon never shows any visible signs of inflammation. There is cramping, abdominal pain, bloating, diarrhea alternating with constipation, and excessive mucus. The cause is not known but may be related to lactose intolerance and emotional stress. It is also known as **spastic colon** or **mucous colitis**. Treatment: Antidiarrheal, antispasmodic, and antianxiety drugs. High-fiber diet and laxative drugs to prevent constipation.	**spastic** (SPAS-tik) **spast/o-** *spasm* **-ic** *pertaining to* **colitis** (koh-LY-tis) **col/o-** *colon* **-itis** *infection of; inflammation of*

Word or Phrase	Description	Pronunciation/Word Parts
polyp	Small, fleshy, benign or precancerous growth in the mucosa of the colon. A **pedunculated polyp** has a thin stalk that supports an irregular, ball-shaped top (see Figure 3-13). A **sessile polyp** is a mound with a broad base (see Figures 3-13 and 3-15 ■). **Benign familial polyposis** is an inherited condition in which family members have multiple colon polyps. Although polyps are benign, they can become cancerous. Treatment: Surgery to remove the polyps (polypectomy).	**polyp** (PAW-lip) **pedunculated** (peh-DUNG-kyoo-LAY-ted) **sessile** (SES-il) **benign** (bee-NINE) **polyposis** (PAW-lih-POH-sis) **polyp/o-** *polyp* **-osis** *condition; process*

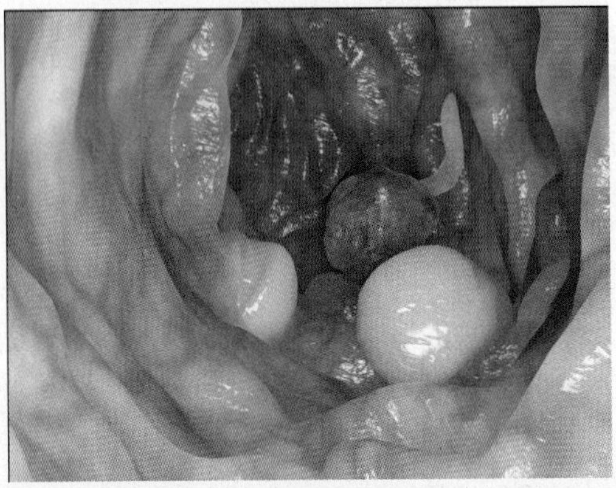

FIGURE 3-15 ■ Colonic polyps.
This patient has multiple sessile polyps protruding through the mucosal folds in the wall of the colon.
Source: Juan Gärtner/123 RF

Rectum and Anus

Word or Phrase	Description	Pronunciation/Word Parts
hemorrhoids	Swollen, protruding veins in the rectum (internal hemorrhoids) or on the skin around the anus (external hemorrhoids). They are caused by increased intra-abdominal pressure from straining during a bowel movement. This dilates the veins with blood until they constantly protrude. They are also known as **piles**. A hemorrhoid is irritated by passing feces, and its surface bleeds easily. Treatment: Topical corticosteroid drug to decrease itching and irritation. Surgery to remove the hemorrhoids (hemorrhoidectomy).	**hemorrhoid** (HEM-oh-royd) **hemorrh/o-** *flowing of blood* **-oid** *resembling*
proctitis	Inflammation of the rectum due to radiation therapy for cancer or from ulcers or infection. Treatment: Correct the underlying cause.	**proctitis** (prawk-TY-tis) **proct/o-** *rectum and anus* **-itis** *infection of; inflammation of*
rectocele	Protruding wall of the rectum pushes on the adjacent vaginal wall, causing it to collapse inward and block the vaginal canal or even to protrude to the outside of the body. Treatment: Surgery to repair the defect.	**rectocele** (REK-toh-seel) **rect/o-** *rectum* **-cele** *hernia*

Defecation and Feces

Word or Phrase	Description	Pronunciation/Word Parts
constipation	Failure to have regular, soft bowel movements. This can be due to decreased peristalsis, lack of dietary fiber, inadequate water intake, lack of exercise, or the side effect of a drug. The patient is said to be *constipated*. **Obstipation** is severe, unrelieved constipation that can lead to a mechanical obstruction of the bowel. The patient is said to be *obstipated*. A **fecalith** is hardened feces that becomes a stone-like mass. This can form in the appendix or in a diverticulum. It can be seen on an abdominal x-ray. Treatment: Laxative drug, a high-fiber diet, increased water intake, enemas.	**constipation** (CON-stih-PAY-shun) **constip/o-** *compacted feces* **-ation** *being; having; process* **obstipation** (AWB-stih-PAY-shun) **obstip/o-** *severe constipation* **-ation** *being; having; process* **fecalith** (FEE-kah-lith) **fec/a-** *feces; stool* **-lith** *stone*

Word or Phrase	Description	Pronunciation/Word Parts
diarrhea	Abnormally frequent, loose, and sometimes watery feces. It is caused by an infection (bacteria, viruses), irritable bowel syndrome, ulcerative colitis, lactose intolerance, or the side effect of a drug. There is increased peristalsis, and the feces move through the large intestine before the water can be absorbed. Treatment: Antidiarrheal drug, lactase enzyme supplement. Antibiotic drug to treat bacterial infections.	**diarrhea** (DY-ah-REE-ah) **dia-** *complete; completely through* **-rrhea** *discharge; flow* The ending *-rrhea* contains the combining form *rrhe/o-* and the one-letter suffix *-a*.
flatulence	Presence of excessive amounts of flatus (gas) in the stomach or intestines. It can be caused by milk (lactose intolerance), indigestion, or incomplete digestion of carbohydrates such as beans. Treatment: Lactase enzyme supplement, antigas drug.	**flatulence** (FLAT-yoo-lens) **flatul/o-** *flatus; gas* **-ence** *state*
hematochezia	Blood in the feces. The source of bleeding can be an ulcer, cancer, Crohn's disease, polyp, diverticulum, or hemorrhoid. Bright red blood indicates active bleeding in the lower gastrointestinal system. **Melena** is a dark, tar-like feces that contains digested blood from bleeding in the esophagus or stomach. Treatment: Correct the underlying cause of bleeding.	**hematochezia** (hee-MAH-toh-KEE-zha) **hemat/o-** *blood* **chez/o-** *pass feces* **-ia** *condition; state; thing* **melena** (meh-LEE-nah) **Melan/o-** *means black.*
incontinence	Inability to voluntarily control bowel movements. A patient with paralysis of the lower extremities lacks sensation and motor control of the external anal sphincter and is incontinent. Patients with dementia are unaware of a bowel movement. Treatment: None.	**incontinence** (in-CON-tih-nens) **in-** *in; not; within* **contin/o-** *hold together* **-ence** *state* Select the correct prefix meaning to get the definition of *incontinence*: *state (of) not hold(ing) together (feces).*
steatorrhea	Greasy, frothy, foul-smelling feces that contain undigested fats. There is not enough of the enzyme lipase because of pancreatic disease, cancer, or cystic fibrosis. Treatment: Correct the underlying cause.	**steatorrhea** (stee-AT-oh-REE-ah) **steat/o-** *fat* **-rrhea** *discharge; flow*

ACROSS THE LIFE SPAN

Pediatrics. Feces forms in the intestine while the fetus is in the uterus. Swallowed amniotic fluid and sloughed-off fetal skin cells mix with mucus and bile to form **meconium**, a thick, sticky, green-to-black stool that is passed after birth. In the newborn nursery, the nurse checks to see that the anus and rectum are **patent** (open). Occasionally, a newborn will have an **imperforate anus**. This is a congenital (present at birth) abnormality in which there is no anal opening. Treatment: Immediate surgery to open the anus and connect the rectum to the outside of the body.

Geriatrics. Constipation is a common complaint in older adults. A diet of refined foods with low fiber, lack of water intake, and inactivity contribute to the formation of small, hard feces. Narcotic drugs used to treat chronic, severe pain can cause constipation, and that can develop into a bowel obstruction in older adults. Some older patients are incontinent of feces (unable to voluntarily control their bowel movements). This can be due to a decrease in the size of the rectum because of a rectocele, impairment of anal sphincter function because of nerve damage, or mental impairment and dementia in which the patient is unaware that a bowel movement is occurring.

meconium (meh-KOH-nee-um)

patent (PAY-tent)

imperforate anus (im-PER-for-ate)
im- *not*
perfor/o- *opening*
-ate *composed of; pertaining to*

Abdominal Wall and Abdominal Cavity

Word or Phrase	Description	Pronunciation/Word Parts
adhesions	Fibrous bands that form after surgery in the abdominal cavity. They bind the intestines to each other or to other organs. They can bind so tightly that peristalsis and intestinal function are affected. Treatment: Surgery to cut the fibrous adhesions (lysis of adhesions).	**adhesion** (ad-HEE-zhun) **adhes/o-** *stick to* **-ion** *action; condition*
hernia	Weakness in the muscle of the diaphragm or the abdominal wall. The intestine bulges through that defect. There is swelling and pain. There is an inherited tendency to hernias, but hernias can also be caused by pregnancy, obesity, or heavy lifting. Treatment: Surgery to correct the hernia (herniorrhaphy). 1. Hernias are named according to how easily the intestine can move back into its normal position. A **sliding or reducible hernia** moves back and forth between the hernia sac and the abdominopelvic cavity (see Figure 3-16a ■). In an **incarcerated (irreducible) hernia**, the intestine swells within the hernia sac and becomes trapped. The intestine can no longer be pushed back into the abdomen. A **strangulated hernia** is an incarcerated hernia whose blood supply has been cut off (see Figure 3-16b). This leads to tissue death (necrosis). 2. Hernias are named according to their location. With a **hiatal hernia**, the stomach bulges up into the opening where the esophagus comes through the diaphragm. A **ventral hernia** occurs anywhere on the anterior abdominal wall (except at the umbilicus). An **umbilical hernia** is at the umbilicus (navel). An **omphalocele** is an umbilical hernia that is present at birth and is only covered with peritoneum, without any fat or abdominal skin (see Figure 3-16c). An **inguinal hernia** is in the groin. In a male patient with an inguinal hernia, the intestine can slide through the inguinal canal and into the scrotum. An **incisional hernia** is along the suture line of a prior abdominal surgical incision.	**hernia** (HER-nee-ah) **incarcerated** (in-KAR-ser-ᴀᴀ-ted) **incarcer/o-** *imprison* **-ated** *composed of; pertaining to a condition* **hiatal** (hy-ᴀᴀ-tal) **hiat/o-** *gap; opening* **-al** *pertaining to* **ventral** (VEN-tral) **ventr/o-** *abdomen; front* **-al** *pertaining to* **umbilical** (um-BIL-ih-kal) **umbilic/o-** *navel; umbilicus* **-al** *pertaining to* **omphalocele** (OM-fal-oh-ꜱᴇᴇʟ) **omphal/o-** *navel; umbilicus* **-cele** *hernia* **inguinal** (ING-gwih-nal) **inguin/o-** *groin* **-al** *pertaining to* **incisional** (in-SIH-zhun-al) **incis/o-** *cut into* **-ion** *action; condition* **-al** *pertaining to*

SLIDING HERNIA
Loop of intestine in
hernia sac

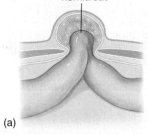

(a)

STRANGULATED HERNIA
Entrapped
loop of intestine

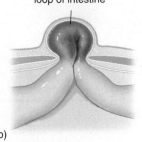

(b)

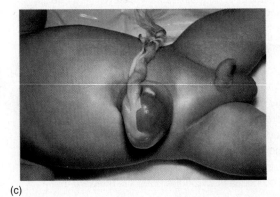

(c)

FIGURE 3-16 ■ Hernia.
(a) In a sliding hernia, the intestine moves in and out of the hernia sac. (b) In a strangulated hernia, the intestine is trapped in the hernia sac and its tissues begin to die. (c) This baby was born with an omphalocele, a hernia at the umbilicus. The hernia sac is only a layer of peritoneum with the intestine inside. This baby will have immediate surgery to correct the omphalocele and repair the abdominal wall defect.
Source: Pearson Education; Biophoto Associates / Science Source

Word or Phrase	Description	Pronunciation/Word Parts
peritonitis	Inflammation and infection of the peritoneum (see Figure 3-17 ■). It occurs when an ulcer, diverticulum, or cancerous tumor breaks through the wall of the stomach or intestines or when an inflamed appendix ruptures. Drainage and bacteria spill into the abdominopelvic cavity. Treatment: Surgery (exploratory laparotomy) to clean out the abdominal cavity. Correct the underlying cause. Antibiotic drug for bacterial infection. **FIGURE 3-17 ■ Peritonitis.** This patient developed peritonitis when a duodendal ulcer perforated the intestinal wall and spilled green bile and chyme into the abdominal cavity. The areas of white are large numbers of white blood cells (pus) that are fighting this infection. *Source*: Chanawit/Fotolia	**peritonitis** (PAIR-ih-toh-NY-tis) **periton/o-** *peritoneum* **-itis** *infection of; inflammation of*

Liver

Word or Phrase	Description	Pronunciation/Word Parts
ascites	Accumulation of **ascitic** fluid in the abdominopelvic cavity. Liver disease and congestive heart failure cause a backup of blood. This increases the blood pressure in the veins of the abdomen. This pressure pushes fluid out of the blood into the abdominopelvic cavity and grossly distends the abdomen. Treatment: Removal of ascitic fluid from the abdomen using a needle (abdominocentesis). Correct the underlying cause. Surgery: Permanent drainage of excess fluid via an implanted tube (shunt).	**ascites** (ah-SY-teez) **ascitic** (ah-SIT-ik) **ascit/o-** *ascites* **-ic** *pertaining to*

WORD ALERT

Sound-Alike Words

acidic   (adjective)   Pertaining to an acid, having a low pH
Example: Hydrochloric acid creates an acidic (low pH) environment in the stomach.

ascitic   (adjective)   Pertaining to ascites
Example: Ascitic fluid accumulates in the abdominopelvic cavity and causes the abdominal wall to bulge outward.

Word or Phrase	Description	Pronunciation/Word Parts
cirrhosis	Chronic, progressive inflammation and finally irreversible degeneration of the liver, with nodules and scarring (see Figure 3-18 ■). The cirrhotic liver is enlarged, and its function is severely impaired. There is nausea and vomiting, weakness, and jaundice. Cirrhosis is caused by alcoholism, viral hepatitis, or chronic obstruction of the bile ducts. Severe cirrhosis can progress to liver failure. Treatment: Correct the underlying cause. 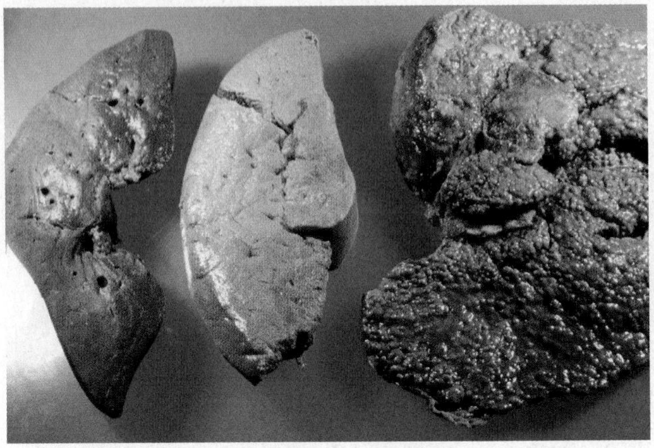 FIGURE 3-18 ■ **Fatty liver disease and cirrhosis of the liver.** The liver on the left is normal. The liver in the center shows fatty liver disease, which is common in alcoholics because the sugar in alcohol is converted to triglycerides (fats) and stored in the liver. Diabetes mellitus and lipid (fat) disorders also cause this yellow, fatty appearance. The liver on the right shows cirrhosis. It is deformed with nodules and scar tissue that affect liver function. *Source*: Arthur Glauberman / Science Source	**cirrhosis** (sih-ROH-sis) **cirrh/o-** *yellow* **-osis** *condition; process*
hepatitis	Inflammation and infection of the liver from the hepatitis virus. There is weakness, anorexia, nausea, fever, dark urine, and jaundice. It is also known as **viral hepatitis**. *(continued)*	**hepatitis** (HEP-ah-TY-tis) **hepat/o-** *liver* **-itis** *infection of; inflammation of* **viral** (VY-ral) **vir/o-** *virus* **-al** *pertaining to*

Word or Phrase	Description	Pronunciation/Word Parts

A CLOSER LOOK

Hepatitis is the most common chronic liver disease. There are five types of hepatitis.

- **Hepatitis A** is an acute but short-lived infection and most persons recover completely. There is no chronic form. It is caused by exposure to water or food that is contaminated with feces from a person who is infected with the hepatitis A virus (HAV). It is also known as **infectious hepatitis**. Treatment: Vaccination to prevent hepatitis A.
- **Hepatitis B** is an acute infection, but many persons recover completely. When it is chronic, there may be no symptoms for 20 years. During that time, however, the infected person is a carrier and can infect others. Hepatitis B is caused by exposure to the blood of a person who is already infected with the hepatitis B virus (HBV) (see Figure 3-19 ■). It is also spread during sexual activity by contact with saliva and vaginal secretions. An infected mother can pass hepatitis B to her fetus before birth or when breastfeeding. It is also known as **serum hepatitis**. Treatment: Vaccination. Healthcare workers are vaccinated because of their constant exposure to blood and body fluids.
- **Hepatitis C** begins as an acute infection that continues as a chronic infection. It is caused by exposure to contaminated needles or to the blood of a person who is already infected with the hepatitis C virus (HCV). Hepatitis C is not readily transmitted by sexual activity or from a mother to her fetus. Chronic hepatitis C is the main cause of chronic liver disease, cirrhosis, and liver cancer. Treatment: Antiviral drugs.
- **Hepatitis D** is a secondary infection caused by a mutated (changed) hepatitis virus. It only develops in patients who already have hepatitis B. It is also known as **delta hepatitis**.
- **Hepatitis E** is similar to hepatitis A, but rarely occurs in the United States.

infectious (in-FEK-shus)
  infect/o- *disease within*
  -ious *pertaining to*

serum (SEER-um)
Serum is the fluid portion of the blood (without the cells and clotting factors).

delta (DEL-tah)
The Greek word *delta* means *change*.

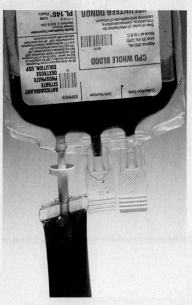

FIGURE 3-19 ■ Blood transfusion.
Receiving infected blood during a blood transfusion, coming in contact with blood-contaminated instruments, or the sharing of needles by drug addicts can result in hepatitis B or hepatitis C.
Source: Getty Photo Disc

| hepatomegaly | Enlargement of the liver due to cirrhosis, hepatitis, or cancer (see Figures 3-18 and 3-21). The enlarged liver can be felt on palpation of the abdomen. The degree of enlargement is measured as the number of fingerbreadths from the edge of the right rib cage to the inferior edge of the liver. **Hepatosplenomegaly** is enlargement of both the liver and the spleen. Treatment: Correct the underlying cause. | **hepatomegaly** (HEP-ah-toh-MEG-ah-lee) **hepat/o-** *liver* **-megaly** *enlargement*

 hepatosplenomegaly (HEP-ah-toh-SPLEN-oh-MEG-ah-lee) **hepat/o-** *liver* **splen/o-** *spleen* **-megaly** *enlargement* |

Word or Phrase	Description	Pronunciation/Word Parts
jaundice	Yellowish discoloration of the skin and whites of the eyes (the sclerae) (see Figure 3-20 ■). There is an increased level of unconjugated bilirubin in the blood. This bilirubin enters the tissues, giving them a yellow color. The patient is said to be *jaundiced*. If a patient does not have jaundice, he/she is **nonicteric**. Jaundice occurs: 1. If the liver is too diseased to conjugate bilirubin. 2. If the liver is too immature to conjugate bilirubin. This occurs in premature newborns. 3. If there is too much unconjugated bilirubin in the blood because of the destruction of large numbers of red blood cells. 4. If a gallstone is obstructing the flow of bile in the bile ducts (**obstructive jaundice**). Treatment: Correct the underlying cause.	**jaundice** (JAWN-dis) 　**jaund/o-** *yellow* 　**-ice** *quality; state* **nonicteric** (NAWN-ik-TAIR-ik) 　**non-** *not* 　**icter/o-** *jaundice* 　**-ic** *pertaining to* **obstructive** (awb-STRUK-tiv) 　**obstruct/o-** *blocked by a barrier* 　**-ive** *pertaining to*

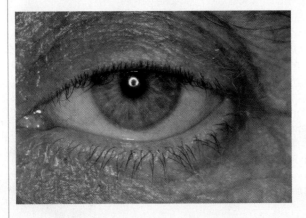

FIGURE 3-20 ■ Jaundice.
Jaundice can be seen as a yellow discoloration of the whites of the eyes (sclerae). The skin is also yellow, but skin pigmentation masks this to some extent.
Source: Dr. M.A. Ansary / Science Source

A CLOSER LOOK

Unconjugated (unjoined) bilirubin is produced when old red blood cells are broken down by the spleen and released into the blood. The liver joins this bilirubin to another substance to make conjugated (joined) bilirubin, which is used to make bile. When the liver is damaged, the amount of unconjugated bilirubin in the blood increases. When gallstones obstruct the flow of bile, conjugated bilirubin leaves the bile and moves into the blood.

Word or Phrase	Description	Pronunciation/Word Parts
liver cancer	Cancerous tumor of the liver (see Figure 3-21 ■). This is usually a secondary cancer that began in another place and spread (metastasized) to the liver. It is also known as a **hepatoma** or **hepatocellular carcinoma**. Treatment: Surgery to remove the tumor; chemotherapy drugs.	**hepatoma** (HEP-ah-TOH-mah) 　**hepat/o-** *liver* 　**-oma** *mass; tumor* **hepatocellular** (HEP-ah-toh-SEL-yoo-lar) 　**hepat/o-** *liver* 　**cellul/o-** *cell* 　**-ar** *pertaining to* **carcinoma** (KAR-sih-NOH-mah) 　**carcin/o-** *cancer* 　**-oma** *mass; tumor*

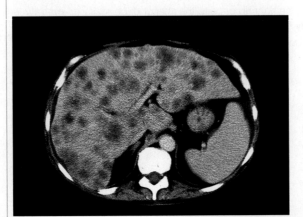

FIGURE 3-21 ■ Liver cancer.
This colored computerized tomography (CT scan) of the abdomen shows an enlarged (tan) liver, nearly filling the abdominal cavity, with many red-brown areas of cancer. A CT scan is read as if you were standing at the patient's feet, looking up, so the white area in the center bottom of the scan is the vertebra of the spine.
Source: Simon Fraser / Freeman Hospital, Newcastle upon Tyne / Science Source

Gallbladder and Bile Ducts

Word or Phrase	Description	Pronunciation/Word Parts
cholangitis	Acute or chronic inflammation of the bile ducts because of cirrhosis or gallstones. Treatment: Correct the underlying cause.	**cholangitis** (KOH-lan-JY-tis) **cholangi/o-** *bile duct* **-itis** *infection of; inflammation of* *Note*: The duplicated letter "i" is deleted when the word is formed.
cholecystitis	Acute or chronic inflammation of the gallbladder. Acute cholecystitis occurs when a gallstone blocks the cystic duct of the gallbladder. When the gallbladder contracts, the duct spasms, causing severe pain (**biliary colic**). Chronic cholecystitis occurs when a gallstone partially blocks the cystic duct, causing backup of bile and thickening of the gallbladder wall. Treatment: Avoid fatty foods that cause the gallbladder to contract. Drug to dissolve the gallstone. Surgery to remove the gallbladder (cholecystectomy).	**cholecystitis** (KOH-lee-sis-TY-tis) **cholecyst/o-** *gallbladder* **-itis** *infection of; inflammation of*
cholelithiasis	One or more gallstones in the gallbladder (see Figure 3-22 ■). When the bile is too concentrated, it forms a thick sediment (sludge) that gradually becomes small gallstones (gravel) and then larger gallstones. Cholelithiasis causes mild symptoms or can cause severe biliary colic when the gallbladder contracts or when a gallstone becomes lodged in a bile duct. **Choledocholithiasis** is a gallstone that is stuck in the common bile duct (see Figure 3-23 ■). Treatment: Avoid fatty foods that cause the gallbladder to contract. Drug to dissolve the gallstone. Surgery to remove the gallbladder (cholecystectomy) or to remove a gallstone from the common bile duct (choledocholithotomy).	**cholelithiasis** (KOH-lee-lith-EYE-ah-sis) **chol/e-** *bile; gall* **lith/o-** *stone* **-iasis** *process; state* **choledocholithiasis** (koh-LED-oh-KOH-lith-EYE-ah-sis) **choledoch/o-** *common bile duct* **lith/o-** *stone* **-iasis** *process; state*

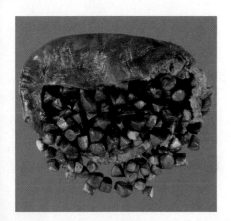

FIGURE 3-22 ■ Cholelithiasis.
This patient's gallbladder was removed during surgery. When it was opened by the pathologist, it contained numerous small and large gallstones.
Source: Encyclopedia/Corbis

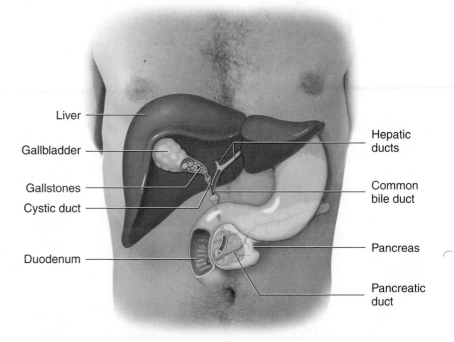

Liver
Gallbladder
Gallstones
Cystic duct
Duodenum
Hepatic ducts
Common bile duct
Pancreas
Pancreatic duct

FIGURE 3-23 ■ Gallstones in the biliary and pancreatic ducts.
A gallstone in the cystic duct causes bile to back up into the gallbladder. A gallstone in the upper common bile duct causes bile to back up into the gallbladder and liver. A gallstone in the lower common bile duct keeps pancreatic digestive enzymes from entering the duodenum.
Source: Pearson Education

Pancreas		
Word or Phrase	**Description**	**Pronunciation/Word Parts**
pancreatic cancer	Cancerous tumor (**adenocarcinoma**) of the pancreas. Most patients are in the advanced stage when they are diagnosed and so survival is usually less than one year. Treatment: Chemotherapy drugs; surgery to remove the tumor.	**adenocarcinoma** (AD-eh-noh-KAR-sih-NOH-mah) **aden/o-** *gland* **carcin/o-** *cancer* **-oma** *mass; tumor*
pancreatitis	Inflammation or infection of the pancreas. There is abdominal pain, nausea, and vomiting. Inflammation occurs when a gallstone blocks the lower common bile duct and the connecting pancreatic duct and pancreatic enzymes back up into the pancreas. Inflammation of the pancreas can also be due to chronic alcoholism. Infection in the pancreas is caused by bacteria or viruses. Treatment: Stop drinking alcohol. Antibiotic drug to treat a bacterial infection. Surgery to remove the gallstone (choledocholithotomy).	**pancreatitis** (PAN-kree-ah-TY-tis) **pancreat/o-** *pancreas* **-itis** *infection of; inflammation of*

Laboratory and Diagnostic Procedures

Blood Tests		
Word or Phrase	**Description**	**Pronunciation/Word Parts**
albumin	Test for albumin, the major protein molecule in the blood. Because albumin is produced by the liver, liver disease results in a low albumin level. The albumin level is also low in patients with malnutrition from poor protein intake.	**albumin** (al-BYOO-min)
alkaline phosphatase (ALP)	Test for the enzyme alkaline phosphatase that is found in both liver cells and bone cells. An elevated blood level is due to liver disease or bone disease.	**alkaline phosphatase** (AL-kah-lin FAWS-fah-tays)
ALT and AST	Test for the enzymes alanine transaminase (ALT) and aspartate transaminase (AST), which are mainly found in the liver. Elevated blood levels occur when damaged liver cells release these enzymes. Also known as *alanine transaminase* and *aspartate transaminase*. Formerly known as **SGPT** and **SGOT**.	
bilirubin	Test for unconjugated, conjugated, and total bilirubin levels. These levels are abnormal when there is liver disease or gallstones. Conjugated bilirubin is also known as **direct bilirubin** because it reacts directly with the reagent used to perform the lab test. Unconjugated bilirubin or **indirect bilirubin** only reacts when another substance is added to the reagent.	**bilirubin** (BIL-ih-ROO-bin)
GGT, GGTP	Test for the enzyme gamma-glutamyl transpeptidase, which is mainly found in the liver. An elevated blood level occurs when damaged liver cells release this enzyme into the blood.	
liver function tests (LFTs)	Panel of individual blood tests performed at the same time to give a comprehensive picture of liver function. It includes albumin, bilirubin, ALT, AST, and GGT, as well as prothrombin time (to evaluate blood clotting factors produced by the liver).	
Gastric and Feces Specimen Tests		
CLO test	Rapid screening test to detect the presence of the bacterium *Helicobacter pylori*. A biopsy of the patient's gastric mucosa is placed in urea. If *H. pylori* bacteria are present, they metabolize the urea to ammonia, and ammonia changes the color of the test pad.	**CLO** (KLOH) *CLO* stands for *Campylobacter-like organism* (because *H. pylori* used to be categorized with the genus Campylobacter).
culture and sensitivity (C&S)	Test that uses a culture to determine which bacterium is causing an intestinal infection and a sensitivity test to determine which antibiotic drugs it is sensitive to (see Figure 4-18). The patient's feces are swabbed onto a culture dish that contains a nutrient medium for growing bacteria. After the bacterium grows, it can be identified by the appearance of the colonies. Then disks of different antibiotic drugs are placed in the culture dish. If the bacteria are resistant to that antibiotic drug, there will only be a small zone of inhibition (no growth) around it. If the bacteria are sensitive to that antibiotic drug, there will be a medium or large zone of inhibition around that disk.	**sensitivity** (SEN-sih-TIV-ih-tee) **sensitiv/o-** *affected by; sensitive to* **-ity** *condition; state*

Word or Phrase	Description	Pronunciation/Word Parts
fecal occult blood test	Test for occult (hidden) blood in the feces. The feces are mixed with the chemical reagent guaiac. This is also known as a **stool guaiac test**. If blood is present, the guaiac will turn a blue color (guaiac-positive). Hemoccult and Coloscreen cards can be purchased by consumers for home testing. The results of these tests are heme positive or heme negative because they detect the heme molecule of hemoglobin from the blood.	**occult** (oh-KULT) **guaiac** (GWY-ak)
gastric analysis	Test to determine the amount of hydrochloric acid in the stomach. A nasogastric (NG) tube is inserted, and gastric fluid is collected. Then a drug is given to stimulate acid production, and another sample is collected.	
ova and parasites (O&P)	Test to determine if there is a parasitic infection in the gastrointestinal tract. Ova are the eggs of parasitic worms. They can be seen in the feces or by examining a sample under a microscope.	**ova** (OH-vah) *Ovum* is a Latin singular noun. Form the plural by changing *-um* to *-a*. **parasite** (PAIR-ah-site)

Radiologic Procedures		
barium enema (BE)	Procedure that uses liquid contrast medium (barium) inserted into the rectum and colon (see Figure 3-24 ■). Barium outlines and coats the intestinal walls, and an x-ray is then taken. This test is used to identify polyps, diverticula, ulcerative colitis, and colon cancer.	**barium** (BAIR-ee-um) **enema** (EN-eh-mah)

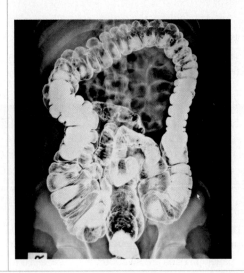

FIGURE 3-24 ■ Barium enema.
Barium contrast medium inserted through the rectum fills the sigmoid colon, descending colon, transverse colon, ascending colon, and cecum on this x-ray.
Source: Prakaymas Vitchitchalao/123 RF

Word or Phrase	Description	Pronunciation/Word Parts

cholangiography	Procedure that uses a contrast dye to outline the bile ducts. Then an x-ray is taken to show gallstones in the gallbladder and bile ducts or thickening of the gallbladder wall. The x-ray image is a **cholangiogram**.
	
	For an **intravenous cholangiography (IVC)**, the contrast dye is injected intravenously, travels through the blood to the liver, and is excreted with bile into the gallbladder.
	
	For a **percutaneous transhepatic cholangiography (PTC)**, a needle is passed through the abdominal wall, and the contrast dye is injected into the liver.
	
	For an **endoscopic retrograde cholangiopancreatography (ERCP)**, an endoscope is used and the contrast dye is injected by a catheter to visualize the common bile duct and pancreatic duct (see Figure 3-25 ■). *Retrograde* means the dye is injected in the opposite direction of the flow of bile. 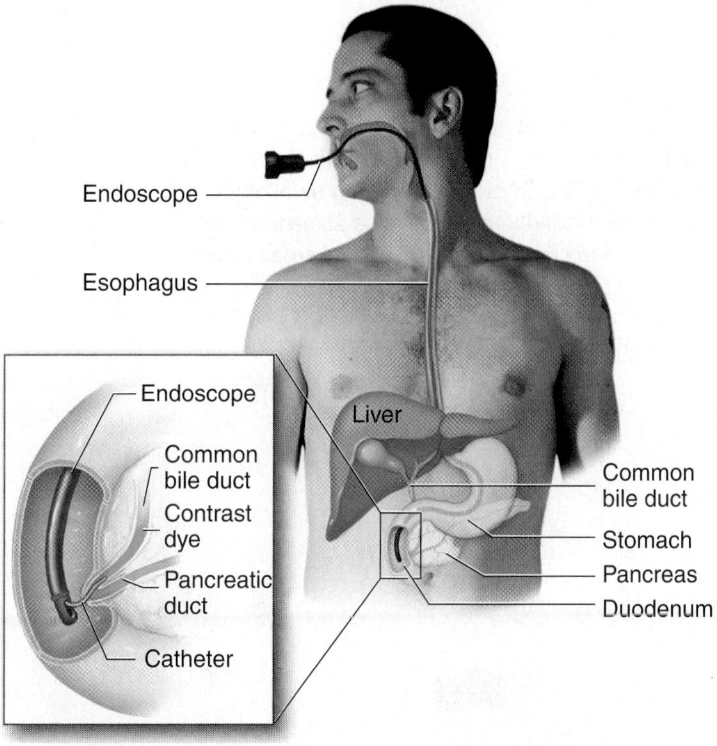
		cholangiography
		(koh-LAN-jee-AW-grah-fee)
		  cholangi/o- *bile duct*
		  -graphy *process of recording*
		
		cholangiogram
		(koh-LAN-jee-oh-GRAM)
		  cholangi/o- *bile duct*
		  -gram *picture; record*
		
		intravenous (IN-trah-VEE-nus)
		  intra- *within*
		  ven/o- *vein*
		  -ous *pertaining to*
		
		percutaneous
		(PER-kyoo-TAY-nee-us)
		  per- *through; throughout*
		  cutane/o- *skin*
		  -ous *pertaining to*
		
		transhepatic (TRANS-heh-PAT-ik)
		  trans- *across; through*
		  hepat/o- *liver*
		  -ic *pertaining to*
		
		endoscopic (EN-doh-SKAW-pik)
		  endo- *innermost; within*
		  scop/o- *examine with an instrument*
		  -ic *pertaining to*
		
		retrograde (REH-troh-grayd)
		  retro- *backward; behind*
		  -grade *pertaining to going*
		
		cholangiopancreatography
		(koh-LAN-jee-oh-PAN-kree-ah-TAW-grah-fee)
		  cholangi/o- *bile duct*
		  pancreat/o- *pancreas*
		  -graphy *process of recording*

Endoscope

Esophagus

Endoscope

Common bile duct

Contrast dye

Pancreatic duct

Catheter

Liver

Common bile duct

Stomach

Pancreas

Duodenum

FIGURE 3-25 ■ Endoscopic retrograde cholangiopancreatography.
In this procedure, an endoscope is passed through the mouth and into the duodenum. Then a catheter is passed through the endoscope, and contrast dye is injected to visualize the common bile duct and pancreatic duct.
Source: Pearson Education

Word or Phrase	Description	Pronunciation/Word Parts

computerized axial tomography (CAT, CT scan)	Procedure that uses x-rays to create images of abdominal organs and structures in many thin, successive "slices"	**tomography** (toh-MAW-grah-fee)
		  tom/o- *cut; layer; slice*
		  -graphy *process of recording*

flat plate of the abdomen	Procedure that uses an x-ray without contrast dye. The patient lies flat, in the supine position, on the x-ray table for this procedure.	

Word or Phrase	Description	Pronunciation/Word Parts

gallbladder ultrasound	Procedure that uses ultra high-frequency sound waves (not x-rays) to create images of the gallbladder. It is used to identify gallstones and thickening of the gallbladder wall. The image is a **gallbladder sonogram**.	**ultrasound** (UL-trah-sound)
		
		sonogram (SAW-noh-gram)
		  son/o- *sound*
		  -gram *picture; record*

magnetic resonance imaging (MRI)	Procedure that uses a strong magnetic field to align protons in the atoms of the patient's body. The protons emit signals to form very detailed images of abdominal organs and structures as thin, successive "slices."	**magnetic** (mag-NET-ik)
		  magnet/o- *magnet*
		  -ic *pertaining to*

oral cholecysto-graphy (OCG)	Procedure that uses tablets of iodinated contrast dye taken orally. The tablets dissolve in the small intestine. The contrast dye is absorbed into the blood, travels to the liver, and is excreted with bile into the gallbladder. An x-ray is taken to identify stones in the gallbladder and biliary ducts or thickening of the gallbladder wall. The x-ray image is an **oral cholecystogram**.	**cholecystography** (KOH-lee-sis-TAW-grah-fee)
		  cholecyst/o- *gallbladder*
		  -graphy *process of recording*
		
		cholecystogram (KOH-lee-SIS-toh-gram)
		  cholecyst/o- *gallbladder*
		  -gram *picture; record*

upper gastro-intestinal series (UGI)	Procedure that uses a liquid contrast medium (barium) that is swallowed (a barium meal). Barium coats and outlines the walls of the esophagus, stomach, and duodenum. It is also known as a **barium swallow**. Fluoroscopy (a continuously moving x-ray image on a screen) is used to follow the barium through the small intestine. This is a **small bowel follow-through**. Individual x-rays are taken at specific times throughout the procedure (see Figure 19-4). This test identifies ulcers, tumors, or obstruction in the esophagus, stomach, and small intestine.	

Medical and Surgical Procedures

Medical Procedures

Word or Phrase	Description	Pronunciation/Word Parts
insertion of nasogastric (NG) tube	Procedure to insert a long, flexible **nasogastric tube** through the nose into the stomach. It is used to drain secretions from the stomach, take a sample of gastric acid, or give feedings or drugs to the patient on a temporary basis (see Figure 3-26 ■).	**nasogastric** (NAY-zoh-GAS-trik) **nas/o-** *nose* **gastr/o-** *stomach* **-ic** *pertaining to*

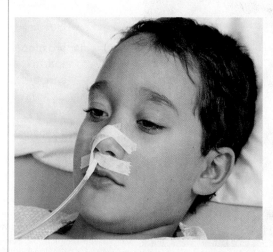

> **DID YOU KNOW?**
> The first nasogastric tube, developed in the late 1700s, was constructed from eel skin. It was used for several weeks to feed a patient who could not eat.

FIGURE 3-26 ■ Nasogastric tube.
This patient has a nasogastric (NG) tube. It was inserted into the nose and, as he swallowed, it was advanced through the esophagus and into the stomach and then taped to the skin to hold it in position. Only liquid feedings or liquid drugs can be given through an NG tube.
Source: Pearson Education

Surgical Procedures

Word or Phrase	Description	Pronunciation/Word Parts
abdominocentesis	Procedure to remove fluid from the abdomen using a needle and a vacuum container. It is done to relieve abdominal pressure from fluid produced by ascites. It is also done to see if there are cancer cells in the peritoneal fluid or to see if there is blood in the peritoneal fluid after abdominal trauma.	**abdominocentesis** (ab-DAW-mih-NOH-sen-TEE-sis) **abdomin/o-** *abdomen* **-centesis** *procedure to puncture*
appendectomy	Procedure to remove the appendix because of appendicitis	**appendectomy** (AP-en-DEK-toh-mee) **append/o-** *appendix; small structure hanging from a larger structure* **-ectomy** *surgical removal*
biopsy	Procedure to remove a small piece of tissue from an ulcer, polyp, mass, or tumor. It is examined under a microscope to look for abnormal or cancerous cells.	**biopsy** (BY-awp-see) **bi/o-** *life; living organism; living tissue* **-opsy** *process of viewing*
bowel resection and anastomosis	Procedure to remove a section of diseased intestine and rejoin the intestine. An end-to-end anastomosis joins the two cut ends of the intestine together. An end-to-side anastomosis joins one end to the side of another part of the intestine.	**resection** (ree-SEK-shun) **resect/o-** *cut out; remove* **-ion** *action; condition* **anastomosis** (ah-NAS-toh-MOH-sis) **anastom/o-** *create an opening between two structures* **-osis** *condition; process*

Word or Phrase	Description	Pronunciation/Word Parts
cholecystectomy	Procedure to remove the gallbladder. This is done as a minimally invasive **laparoscopic cholecystectomy** that uses a **laparoscope** (see Figure 3-27 ■).	**cholecystectomy** (KOH-lee-sis-TEK-toh-mee) **cholecyst/o-** *gallbladder* **-ectomy** *surgical removal* **laparoscopic** (LAP-ar-oh-SKAW-pik) **lapar/o-** *abdomen* **scop/o-** *examine with an instrument* **-ic** *pertaining to* **laparoscope** (LAP-ar-oh-SKOHP) **lapar/o-** *abdomen* **-scope** *instrument used to examine*

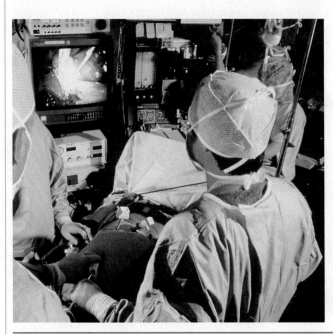

FIGURE 3-27 ■ Laparoscopic cholecystectomy.
Carbon dioxide gas is used to inflate the abdominal cavity and separate the organs. A laparoscope is inserted through one of several small incisions; it is used to visualize the gallbladder (on the computer screen), while other instruments grasp and remove the gallbladder.
Source: Geoff Tompkinson / Science Source

DID YOU KNOW?

At one time, a cholecystectomy to remove the gallbladder required a 5- to 7-inch abdominal incision, followed by a painful 6-week recovery. The first minimally invasive surgical procedure was performed in 1989 to remove a gallbladder. Minimally invasive surgery is done with laparoscopic instruments inserted through tiny incisions at various places on the abdominal wall.

Word or Phrase	Description	Pronunciation/Word Parts
choledocholitho-tomy	Procedure to make an incision in the common bile duct to remove a gallstone	**choledocholithotomy** (koh-LED-oh-KOH-lith-AW-toh-mee) **choledoch/o-** *common bile duct* **lith/o-** *stone* **-tomy** *process of cutting; process of making an incision*

TECHNOLOGY IN MEDICINE

Robots were first used to perform surgery in 1987 during a laparoscopic cholecystectomy. Now robots are used routinely for many different types of surgery, including prostatectomy and open heart surgery. The surgeon sits at a console in the surgical suite, sees a 3-D image of the operative site, and manipulates the robotic arms, which are computer activated or sometimes even voice activated.

Word or Phrase	Description	Pronunciation/Word Parts
colostomy	Procedure to remove the diseased part of the colon and create a new opening in the abdominal wall where feces can leave the body (see Figure 3-28 ■). The colon is brought out through the abdominal wall. The edges of the colon are rolled to make a mouth-like opening (**stoma**) and sutured to the abdominal wall. The patient wears a plastic disposable pouch that adheres to the abdominal wall to collect feces. If part of the ileum and colon are removed and a stoma created, the procedure is known as an **ileostomy**.	**colostomy** (koh-LAW-stoh-mee) **col/o-** *colon* **-stomy** *surgically created opening* **stoma** (STOH-mah) **ileostomy** (IL-ee-AW-stoh-mee) **ile/o-** *ileum* **-stomy** *surgically created opening*

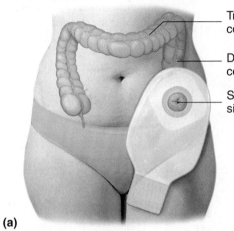

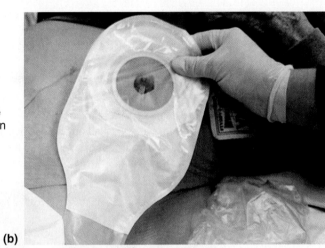

Transverse colon

Descending colon

Stoma of the sigmoid colon

(a)   (b)

FIGURE 3-28 ■ Colostomy and stoma.
(a) A colostomy is done in the transverse, descending, or sigmoid colon. The red mucosa of the colon is rolled back on itself to create a stoma, which is sutured to the abdominal wall. (b) The patient wears a plastic disposable bag that adheres to the skin and collects feces.
Source: Pearson Education

WORD ALERT

Sound-Alike Words

stoma	(noun) A surgically created opening like a mouth *Example: The colostomy patient wears a disposable pouch around the stoma on his abdominal wall.*
stomatitis	(noun) Inflammation of the oral mucosa of the mouth *Example: The patient was losing weight because of a painful stomatitis that prevented him from chewing his food.*

| endoscopy | Procedure that uses an **endoscope** (a flexible, fiberoptic scope with a magnifying lens and a light source) to internally examine the gastrointestinal tract. An endoscopic procedure can be coupled with another procedure such as a biopsy or removal of a polyp. | **endoscopy** (en-DAW-skoh-pee)
endo- *innermost; within*
-scopy *process of using an instrument to examine*

endoscope (EN-doh-skohp)
endo- *innermost; within*
-scope *instrument used to examine* |

Word or Phrase	Description	Pronunciation/Word Parts

A CLOSER LOOK

These procedures use an endoscope inserted through the nose or mouth.

- **esophagoscopy**:   visualization and examination of the esophagus
- **gastroscopy**:   visualization and examination of the stomach (after the endoscope first passes through the esophagus)
- **esophagogastroduodenoscopy (EGD)**:   visualization and examination of the esophagus first, followed by the stomach, and then the duodenum

The ileum, cecum, and ascending colon cannot be visualized with endoscopy. Instead, the patient swallows a capsule that contains a small camera. It uses wireless technology to transmit pictures until it is excreted from the body.

These procedures use an endoscope inserted through the rectum.

- **sigmoidoscopy**:   visualization and examination of the rectum and sigmoid colon using a sigmoidoscope
- **colonoscopy**:   visualization and examination of the entire colon after the **colonoscope** is passed through the rectum (see Figure 3-29 ■)

esophagoscopy
(eh-SAW-fah-GAW-skoh-pee)
  esophag/o- *esophagus*
  -scopy *process of using an instrument to examine*

gastroscopy (gas-TRAW-skoh-pee)
  gastr/o- *stomach*
  -scopy *process of using an instrument to examine*

esophagogastroduodenoscopy
(eh-SAW-fah-goh-GAS-troh-DOO-oh-den-AW-skoh-pee)
  esophag/o- *esophagus*
  gastr/o- *stomach*
  duoden/o- *duodenum*
  -scopy *process of using an instrument to examine*

sigmoidoscopy
(SIG-moyd-AW-skoh-pee)
  sigmoid/o- *sigmoid colon*
  -scopy *process of using an instrument to examine*

colonoscopy
(KOH-lon-AW-skoh-pee)
  colon/o- *colon*
  -scopy *process of using an instrument to examine*

colonoscope
(koh-LAW-noh-skohp)

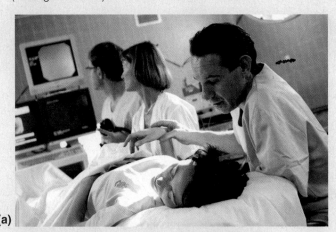

(a)

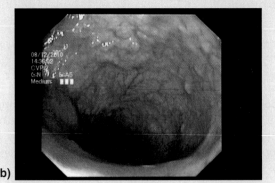

(b)

FIGURE 3-29 ■ Colonoscopy.
(a) A colonoscope with a camera is passed through the anus to examine the rectum and colon. (b) The images are transmitted to a computer screen for viewing and are also recorded for the patient's medical record.
Source: BURGER/PHANIE/phanie/Phanie Sarl/Corbis; R Diger Rebmann/123 RF

| **exploratory laparotomy** | Procedure that uses a long abdominal incision to open the abdominopelvic cavity widely so that it can be explored | **laparotomy** (LAP-ar-AW-toh-mee)
  lapar/o- *abdomen*
  -tomy *process of cutting; process of making an incision* |

Word or Phrase	Description	Pronunciation/Word Parts
gastrectomy	Procedure to remove all or part of the stomach because of a cancerous or benign tumor	**gastrectomy** (gas-TREK-toh-mee) **gastr/o-** *stomach* **-ectomy** *surgical removal*
gastroplasty	Procedure to treat severe obesity. Staples are used to make a small stomach pouch. A gastroplasty can be combined with a gastric bypass in which the stapled stomach pouch is anastomosed (connected) to the cut end of the jejunum. This bypasses the duodenum, where most fats are absorbed. It is also known as **gastric stapling** or **gastric bypass**.	**gastroplasty** (GAS-troh-PLAS-tee) **gastr/o-** *stomach* **-plasty** *process of reshaping by surgery*
gastrostomy	Procedure to create a temporary or permanent opening from the abdominal wall into the stomach to insert a gastrostomy feeding tube. This is done for patients who have had an NG tube for some time but still cannot eat on their own. For a **percutaneous endoscopic gastrostomy (PEG)**, a permanent PEG feeding tube is inserted through the abdominal wall. Then, under visual guidance from an endoscope that was previously passed through the mouth, the PEG tube is positioned in the stomach (see Figure 3-30 ■).	**gastrostomy** (gas-TRAW-stoh-mee) **gastr/o-** *stomach* **-stomy** *surgically created opening* **percutaneous** (PER-kyoo-TAY-nee-us) **per-** *through; throughout* **cutane/o-** *skin* **-ous** *pertaining to* **endoscopic** (EN-doh-SKAW-pik) **endo-** *innermost; within* **scop/o-** *examine with an instrument* **-ic** *pertaining to*

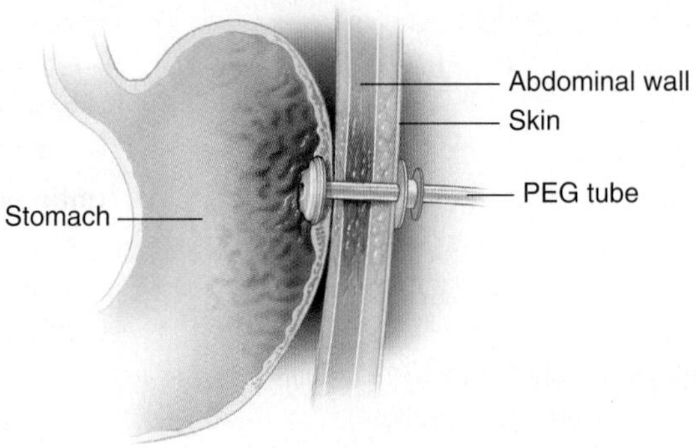

Abdominal wall
Skin
PEG tube
Stomach

FIGURE 3-30 ■ PEG tube.
This type of permanent feeding tube is inserted during a percutaneous endoscopic gastrostomy.
Source: Pearson Education

Word or Phrase	Description	Pronunciation/Word Parts
hemorrhoid-ectomy	Procedure to remove hemorrhoids from the rectum or around the anus	**hemorrhoidectomy** (HEM-oh-royd-EK-toh-mee) **hemorrhoid/o-** *hemorrhoid* **-ectomy** *surgical removal*
herniorrhaphy	Procedure that uses sutures to close a defect in the muscle wall where there is a hernia	**herniorrhaphy** (HER-nee-OR-ah-fee) **herni/o-** *hernia* **-rrhaphy** *procedure of suturing*
jejunostomy	Procedure to create a temporary or permanent opening from the abdominal wall into the jejunum to insert a jejunostomy feeding tube. For a **percutaneous endoscopic jejunostomy (PEJ)**, a PEJ tube is inserted through the abdominal wall. Then, under visual guidance from an endoscope that was previously passed through the mouth, the PEJ tube is positioned in the jejunum.	**jejunostomy** (JEH-joo-NAW-stoh-mee) **jejun/o-** *jejunum* **-stomy** *surgically created opening*
liver transplantation	Procedure to remove a severely damaged liver from a patient with end-stage liver disease and insert a new liver from a donor. The patient (the recipient) is matched by blood type and tissue type to the donor. Liver transplant patients must take immunosuppressant drugs for the rest of their lives to keep their bodies from rejecting the foreign tissue that is their new liver.	**transplantation** (TRANS-plan-TAY-shun) **transplant/o-** *move something across and put in another place* **-ation** *being; having; process*
polypectomy	Procedure to remove one or more polyps from the colon using forceps or a snare positioned around the thin stalk of a pedunculated polyp.	**polypectomy** (PAW-lih-PEK-toh-mee) **polyp/o-** *polyp* **-ectomy** *surgical removal*

Drugs

These drug categories and drugs are used to treat gastrointestinal diseases. The most common generic and trade name drugs in each category are listed.

Category	Indication	Examples	Pronunciation/Word Parts
antacid drugs	Treat heartburn by neutralizing acid in the stomach	Maalox, Mylanta, Tums	**antacid** (ant-AS-id) *Antacid* is a combination of *anti-* (against) and the word *acid*. The *i* in *anti-* is deleted.
antibiotic drugs	Treat gastrointestinal infections caused by bacteria. Helidac is a combination drug only used to treat an infection from *Helicobacter pylori*. Antibiotic drugs are not effective against viral gastrointestinal infections.	ciprofloxacin (Cipro), Helidac (bismuth, metronidazole, tetracycline), levofloxacin (Levaquin)	**antibiotic** (AN-tee-by-AW-tik) (AN-tih-by-AW-tik) **anti-** *against* **bi/o-** *life; living organism; living tissue* **-tic** *pertaining to*
antidiarrheal drugs	Treat diarrhea. They slow peristalsis and this increases water absorption from the feces.	loperamide (Imodium), Lomotil (atropine, diphenoxylate)	**antidiarrheal** (AN-tee-DY-ah-REE-al) **anti-** *against* **dia-** *complete; completely through* **rrhe/o-** *discharge; flow* **-al** *pertaining to*
antiemetic drugs	Treat nausea and vomiting and motion sickness	dimenhydrinate (Dramamine), meclizine (Antivert)	**antiemetic** (AN-tee-eh-MET-ik) **anti-** *against* **emet/o-** *vomiting* **-ic** *pertaining to*
drugs for gallstones	Dissolve gallstones (instead of surgical removal)	chenodiol (Chenodal), ursodiol (Actigall)	
H₂ blocker drugs	Treat gastroesophageal reflux disease (GERD) and peptic ulcers by blocking H₂ (histamine 2) receptors in the stomach that trigger the release of hydrochloric acid	cimetidine (Tagamet), famotidine (Pepcid), xranitidine (Zantac)	
laxative drugs	Treat constipation by softening the stool, adding dietary fiber, or directly stimulating the intestinal mucosa	docusate (Colace, Dulcolax, Surfak), lubiprostone (Amitiza), psyllium (Fiberall, Metamucil)	**laxative** (LAK-sah-tiv)
proton pump inhibitor drugs	Treat gastroesophageal reflux disease (GERD) and peptic ulcers by blocking the final step in the production of hydrochloric acid	esomeprazole (Nexium), omeprazole (Prilosec)	

DID YOU KNOW?

A **suppository** is a bullet-shaped capsule that contains a drug. It is inserted into the rectum, where it melts and releases the drug.

suppository (soo-PAW-zih-TOR-ee) **supposit/o-** *placed beneath* **-ory** *having the function of*

Abbreviations

ABD, abd	abdomen	**IBS**	irritable bowel syndrome
AC, a.c.	before meals (Latin, *ante cibum*)	**IVC**	intravenous cholangiogram; intravenous cholangiography
ALP	alkaline phosphatase	**LES**	lower esophageal sphincter
ALT	alanine aminotransferase; alanine transaminase	**LFTs**	liver function tests
AST	aspartate aminotransferase; aspartate transaminase	**LLQ**	left lower quadrant (of the abdomen)
		LUQ	left upper quadrant (of the abdomen)
BE	barium enema	**MRI**	magnetic resonance imaging
BM	bowel movement	**N&V**	nausea and vomiting
BRBPR	bright red blood per rectum	**NG**	nasogastric
BS	bowel sounds	**NPO, n.p.o.**	nothing by mouth (Latin, *nil per os*)
C&S	culture and sensitivity	**O&P**	ova and parasites
CAT	computerized axial tomography	**OCG**	oral cholecystogram; oral cholecystography
CBD	common bile duct	**PC, p.c.**	after meals (Latin, *post cibum*)
CLO	*Campylobacter*-like organism	**PEG**	percutaneous endoscopic gastrostomy
CT	computerized tomography	**PEJ**	percutaneous endoscopic jejunostomy
EGD	esophagogastroduodenoscopy	**PO, p.o.**	by mouth (Latin, *per os*)
ERCP	endoscopic retrograde cholangiopancreatography	**PTC**	percutaneous transhepatic cholangiography
		PUD	peptic ulcer disease
GERD	gastroesophageal reflux disease	**RLQ**	right lower quadrant (of the abdomen)
GGPT, GGT	gamma-glutamyl transpeptidase	**RUQ**	right upper quadrant (of the abdomen)
GI	gastrointestinal	**SGOT**	serum glutamic-oxaloacetic transaminase (older name for AST)
HAV	hepatitis A virus		
HBV	hepatitis B virus	**SGPT**	serum glutamic-pyruvic transaminase (older name for ALT)
HCl	hydrochloric acid		
HCV	hepatitis C virus	**UGI**	upper gastrointestinal (series)
IBD	inflammatory bowel disease		

WORD ALERT

Abbreviations

Abbreviations are commonly used in all types of medical documents; however, they can mean different things to different people and their meanings can be misinterpreted. Always verify the meaning of an abbreviation.

BS means *bowel sounds,* but it also means *breath sounds.*

PUD means *peptic ulcer disease,* but, when handwritten, the *U* can look like a *V*; *PVD* means *peripheral vascular disease.*

IT'S GREEK TO ME!

Did you notice that some words have two different combining forms? Combining forms from both Greek and Latin remain a part of medical language today.

Word	Greek	Latin	Medical Word Examples
abdomen	celi/o-	abdomin/o-	celiac trunk, celiac disease, abdominal
	lapar/o-	ventr/o-	laparoscopy, laparotomy, ventral
break down food; digest		digest/o-	digestive
digestion	peps/o-, pept/o-		pepsin, peptic
fat	steat/o-	lip/o-	steatorrhea, lipase
intestine	enter/o-	intestin/o-	enteropathy, gastroenteritis, intestinal, gastrointestinal
mouth	stomat/o-	or/o-	stomatitis, oral
navel; umbilicus	omphal/o-	umbilic/o-	omphalocele, umbilical
rectum	proct/o-	rect/o-	proctitis, rectal
saliva	sial/o-	saliv/o-	sialolith, salivary
tongue	gloss/o-	lingu/o-	glossitis, sublingual
yellow	icter/o-	jaund/o-	nonicteric, jaundice

CAREER FOCUS

Meet Patricia, a medical assistant

"The best part of my job as a medical assistant is dealing with the patients. I love coming to work and doing it every day. It's just very fulfilling to me. I love helping people. I love talking to them. I love learning about their families, and that's what you find in this kind of practice. This is a huge clinic. It has internal medicine, pediatrics, OB/GYN, and plastic surgery. We have a specialty department with ears, nose, and throat doctors. We have optometry; we have physical therapy. I work with patients. I bring them in, I weigh them, take their blood pressure, find out what their problem is, write down their problem, and go to the physician and tell why the patient is here. I definitely think medical assistants are the first line of defense for the doctor. I bring everything to the doctor. We work as a team. We have a great rapport together and with our patients."

Medical assistants are allied health professionals who perform and document a variety of clinical and laboratory procedures and assist the physician during medical procedures in the office or clinic.

    Gastroenterologists are physicians who practice in the medical specialty of gastroenterology. They diagnose and treat patients with diseases of the gastrointestinal system. Physicians can take additional training and become board certified in the subspecialty of pediatric gastroenterology. Cancerous tumors of the gastrointestinal system are treated medically by an **oncologist** or surgically by a general **surgeon**.

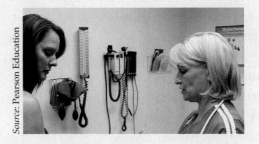

Source: Pearson Education

gastroenterologist
(GAS-troh-EN-ter-AW-loh-jist)
   gastr/o- *stomach*
   enter/o- *intestine*
   log/o- *study of; word*
   -ist *person who specializes in*

oncologist (ong-KAW-loh-jist)
   onc/o- *mass; tumor*
   log/o- *study of; word*
   -ist *person who specializes in*

surgeon (SER-jun)
   surg/o- *operative procedure*
   -eon *person who performs*

To see Patricia's complete video profile, log into MyMedicalTerminologyLab and navigate to the Multimedia Library for Chapter 3. Check the Video box, and then click the Career Focus - Medical Assistant link.

MyMedicalTerminologyLab™

3.8 Resear [] CF [] al Words

ON THE J [] NGE EXERCISE

On the job [] counter new medical words. Practice your medical language skills by researching the medical words in bold and writing [] tions on the lines.

OFFICE CHART NOTE

This is a 68-year-old white female with episodic abdominal pain, some head-aches, heartburn symptoms, **aerophagia** and **eructation**, obstipation, and **tenesmus**. The patient presented with a 3-day history of **singultus**, unrelieved by any medications. Her physical examination revealed **borborygmus** and a slightly tender abdomen, but no evidence of rebound.

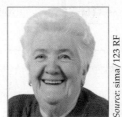

Source: sima / 123 RF

---

1. aerophagia _____

2. eructation _____

3. tenesmus _____

4. singultus _____

5. borborygmus _____

SOUND-ALIKE WORDS

Compare and contrast the medical meanings of sound-alike gastroenterology words.

1. *celiac trunk* and *celiac disease*

2. *acidic* and *ascitic*

3. *stoma* and *stomatitis*

3.9 Analyze Medical Reports

ELECTRONIC PATIENT RECORD #1

This report is an Office Visit SOAP Note. Read the note and answer the questions.

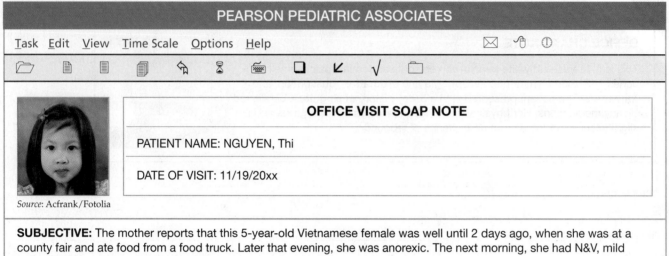

PEARSON PEDIATRIC ASSOCIATES

Task   Edit   View   Time Scale   Options   Help

OFFICE VISIT SOAP NOTE

PATIENT NAME: NGUYEN, Thi

DATE OF VISIT: 11/19/20xx

Source: Acfrank/Fotolia

SUBJECTIVE: The mother reports that this 5-year-old Vietnamese female was well until 2 days ago, when she was at a county fair and ate food from a food truck. Later that evening, she was anorexic. The next morning, she had N&V, mild dyspepsia, and then later diarrhea.

OBJECTIVE: Temperature 101, heart rate 160, respiratory rate 38, blood pressure 115/80. The child is flushed and sweaty and appears lethargic and slightly dehydrated. She complains of abdominal pain.

ASSESSMENT: Gastroenteritis.

PLAN: Increased fluid intake. Tylenol for fever. Call the office if not improved in 24 hours.

1. Divide these words into their word parts. Give the meanings of the word parts.

   anorexic   **dyspepsia**   **gastroenteritis**

2. What is the meaning of the abbreviation *N&V*?

3. What is the probable cause of the patient's gastroenteritis?

4. Research the meaning of these words.

   lethargic   **dehydrated**

ELECTRONIC PATIENT RECORD #2

This contains two related reports: an Admission History and Physical Examination and a Pathology Report. Read both reports and answer the questions.

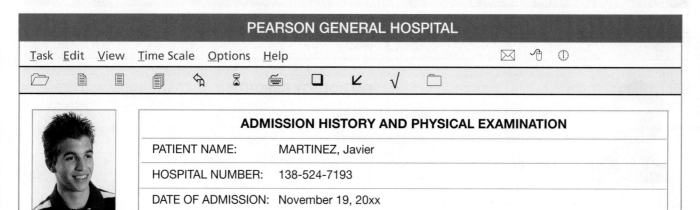

PEARSON GENERAL HOSPITAL

Task   Edit   View   Time Scale   Options   Help

ADMISSION HISTORY AND PHYSICAL EXAMINATION

PATIENT NAME:	MARTINEZ, Javier
HOSPITAL NUMBER:	138-524-7193
DATE OF ADMISSION:	November 19, 20xx

Source: yelo34/123 RF

HISTORY OF PRESENT ILLNESS
This is a 20-year-old Hispanic male who experienced severe abdominal pain beginning on the morning of admission. He was awakened at 6:00 A.M. by sharp pains in the stomach. Drinking a glass of milk, which usually helps this type of pain, was not effective. He also took his customary antacid, but with no relief. He went to college and ate lunch there and then developed nausea and vomiting. An hour later, he developed watery diarrhea with approximately 3–4 bowel movements over the next few hours. He denies any history of ulcerative colitis or Crohn's disease. By this evening, his pain was so severe that he came to the emergency room to be seen.

PHYSICAL EXAMINATION
Temperature 100.2, pulse 84, respiratory rate 30, blood pressure 132/88. He is alert and oriented, lying uncomfortably in bed. Abdominal examination: Abdomen is soft. There is rebound tenderness in the RLQ.

LABORATORY DATA
Labs drawn in the emergency room showed an elevated white blood cell count of 14.6. Bilirubin and amylase were within normal limits. Urinalysis was unremarkable.

IMPRESSION
Acute appendicitis. Possible peritonitis.

DISCUSSION
A detailed discussion was carried out with the patient and his parents. The dangers of waiting and observing his condition were discussed as well as the indications, possible risks, complications, and alternatives to an appendectomy. They agree with the plan to perform an appendectomy, and the patient will be taken to the operating room shortly.

James R. Rodgers, M.D.

James R. Rodgers, M.D.

JRR/bjg
D: 11/19/xx
T: 11/19/xx

ELECTRONIC PATIENT RECORD #3

PEARSON GENERAL HOSPITAL

Task   Edit   View   Time Scale   Options   Help   ✉ ↰ ①

🗁 📄 📃 📑 ↰ ⧗ ⌨ ☐ ↙ √ 🗀

PATHOLOGY REPORT

PATIENT NAME:	MARTINEZ, Javier
HOSPITAL NUMBER:	138-524-7193
DATE OF REPORT:	November 19, 20xx

Source: yelo34/123 RF

SPECIMEN
Appendix

GROSS EXAMINATION
The specimen identified as "appendix" is an inflamed, vermiform appendix with an attached piece of the mesoappendix. The appendix measures 6.5 cm in length and up to 1.3 cm in diameter. There is a yellow-gray exudate noted inside with marked hemorrhage of the mucosa. There is no evidence of tumor or fecalith.

PATHOLOGICAL DIAGNOSIS
Acute appendicitis.

Leona T. Parkins, M.D.

Leona T. Parkins, M.D.

LTP:rrg
D: 11/19/xx
T: 11/19/xx

1. The patient had sharp pains in his stomach. If you wanted to use the adjective form of *stomach*, you would say, "He had sharp _____ pains."

2. Divide *appendicitis* into its two word parts and give the meaning of each word part.

Word Part	**Meaning**
_____	_____
_____	_____

3. Divide *fecalith* into its two word parts and give the meaning of each word part.

Word Part	**Meaning**
_____	_____
_____	_____

4. What does the abbreviation *RLQ* mean? _____

5. What is the abbreviation for *nausea and vomiting*? _____

6. What is the name of the category of drug that neutralizes acid in the stomach?

   _____

7. What is another medical name for *vomiting*?

   _____

8. Ulcerative colitis and Crohn's disease both affect which part of the gastrointestinal system?

   _____

9. What does *vermiform* mean?

   _____

10. What is the medical word that means *surgical removal of the appendix*?

    _____

11. According to the pathology report on the specimen removed during surgery, what was the patient's diagnosis?

    _____

12. The patient has taken milk and an antacid in the past for his stomach pains. This suggests he has a previous history of what disease condition? Circle the correct answer.

    pyrosis   **colon cancer**   **hemorrhoids**

13. Acute symptoms of nausea and vomiting with diarrhea might lead you to think that the patient has what disease? Circle the correct answer.

    jaundice   **hematochezia**   **gastroenteritis**

14. An elevated white blood cell count is associated with an infection. Where was the site of this patient's infection?

    _____

15. The danger in waiting and observing the patient's condition was that he could develop a ruptured appendix that would lead to what condition? Circle the correct answer.

    peritonitis   **gastritis**   **cholecystitis**

16. The patient had a finding of "rebound tenderness" on the physical examination. Describe what a physician would do to check for rebound tenderness.

    _____

17. The patient's bilirubin was within normal limits. This tells you that he is not having any problems with which of these organs?

    stomach   **liver**   **pancreas**

18. The patient's amylase was within normal limits. This tells you that he is not having any problems with which of these organs?

    pancreas   **colon**   **esophagus**

19. What is peritonitis?

20. Describe why it might be present in a patient with acute appendicitis?

MyMedicalTerminologyLab™

MyMedicalTerminologyLab is a premium online homework management system that includes a host of features to help you study. Registered users will find:

- A multitude of quizzes and activities built within the MyLab platform

- Powerful tools that track and analyze your results—allowing you to create a personalized learning experience

- Videos and audio pronunciations to help enrich your progress

- Streaming lesson presentations (Guided Lectures) and self-paced learning modules

- A space where you and your instructor can check your progress and manage your assignments

Chapter 4
Pulmonology

Respiratory System

Pulmonology (PUL-moh-NAW-loh-jee) is the medical specialty that studies the anatomy and physiology of the respiratory system and uses laboratory and diagnostic procedures, medical and surgical procedures, and drugs to treat respiratory diseases.

 ## Learning Outcomes

After you study this chapter, you should be able to

4.1 Identify structures of the respiratory system.

4.2 Describe the process of respiration.

4.3 Describe common respiratory diseases, laboratory and diagnostic procedures, medical and surgical procedures, and drugs.

4.4 Form the plural and adjective forms of nouns related to pulmonology.

4.5 Give the meanings of word parts and abbreviations related to pulmonology.

4.6 Divide pulmonology words and build pulmonology words.

4.7 Spell and pronounce pulmonology words.

4.8 Research sound-alike and other pulmonology words.

4.9 Analyze the medical content and meaning of pulmonology reports.

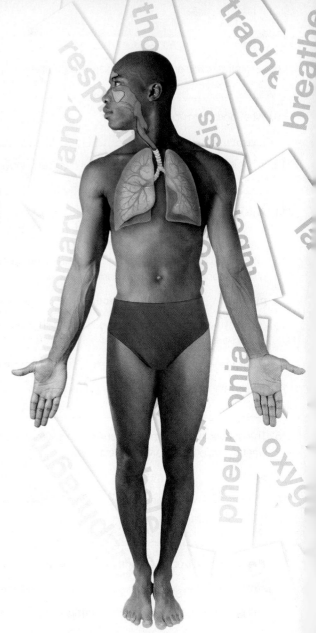

FIGURE 4-1 ■ Respiratory system.
The respiratory system consists of two main organs—the lungs–
and related structures connected to the lungs. These form a pathway through which air flows into and out of the body.

Source: Pearson Education

Medical Language Key

To unlock the definition of a medical word, break it into word parts. Give the meaning of each word part. Put the meanings of the word parts in order, beginning with the meaning of the suffix, then the prefix (if present), then the combining form(s).

	Word Part	Word Part Meaning
Suffix	**-logy**	*study of*
Combining Form	**pulmon/o-**	*lung*

Pulmonology: ▶ *Study of (the) lungs (and related structures).*

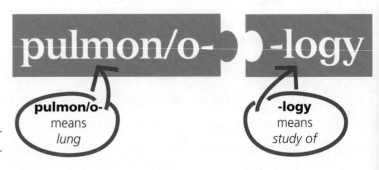

pulmon/o- means *lung*

-logy means *study of*

Anatomy and Physiology

Pronunciation/Word Parts

The **respiratory system** consists of the right and left lungs and the air passageways that connect the lungs to the outside of the body (see Figure 4-1 ■). The upper respiratory system in the head and neck includes the nose, nasal cavity, and pharynx (throat). The upper respiratory system shares these structures with the ears, nose, and throat system (discussed in "Otolaryngology," Chapter 16). The lower respiratory system includes the larynx (voice box) and trachea (windpipe) in the neck and the bronchi, bronchioles, and alveoli in the lungs. The lungs fill much of the thoracic cavity. The purpose of the respiratory system is to bring oxygen into the body and expel the waste product carbon dioxide.

respiratory (RES-pih-rah-TOR-ee)
(reh-SPY-rah-TOR-ee)
  re- again and again; backward; unable to
  spir/o- breathe; coil
  -atory pertaining to
Select the correct prefix meaning to get the definition of *respiratory*: pertaining to again and again (to) breathe.

WORD ALERT

The respiratory system is also known as the **respiratory tract**. A tract is a pathway. The adjective **cardiopulmonary** reflects the connection between the heart and the respiratory system. Without the heart, oxygen brought into the lungs would never reach the rest of the body, and carbon dioxide produced by the cells in the body would never reach the lungs to be exhaled.

cardiopulmonary
(KAR-dee-oh-PUL-moh-NAIR-ee)
  cardi/o- heart
  pulmon/o- lung
  -ary pertaining to

Anatomy of the Respiratory System

Nose and Nasal Cavity

The nose contains the **nasal cavity**, which is divided in the center by the **nasal septum**, a wall of cartilage and bone. On each side of the cavity are three long, bony projections: the superior, middle, and inferior **turbinates** or **nasal conchae** (see Figure 4-2 ■). These jut into the nasal cavity and slow down inhaled air. The nasal cavity is lined with **mucosa**, a **mucous membrane** that warms and humidifies the air and produces **mucus**. Mucus and hairs in the nose trap inhaled particles of dust, pollen, smoke, and bacteria and keep them from entering the lungs. The sinuses in the bones around the nose and elsewhere in the skull are discussed in "Otolaryngology," Chapter 16.

nasal (NAY-zal)
  nas/o- nose
  -al pertaining to
Nasal is the adjective for *nose*.

---

septum (SEP-tum)

---

septal (SEP-tal)
  sept/o- dividing wall; septum
  -al pertaining to

---

turbinate (TER-bih-nayt)
  turbin/o- scroll-like structure; turbinate
  -ate composed of; pertaining to

---

concha (CON-kah)

---

conchae (CON-kee)
Form the plural by changing *-a* to *-ae*.

---

mucosa (myoo-KOH-sah)

---

mucosal (myoo-KOH-sal)
  mucos/o- mucous membrane
  -al pertaining to

---

mucous (MYOO-kus)
  muc/o- mucus
  -ous pertaining to

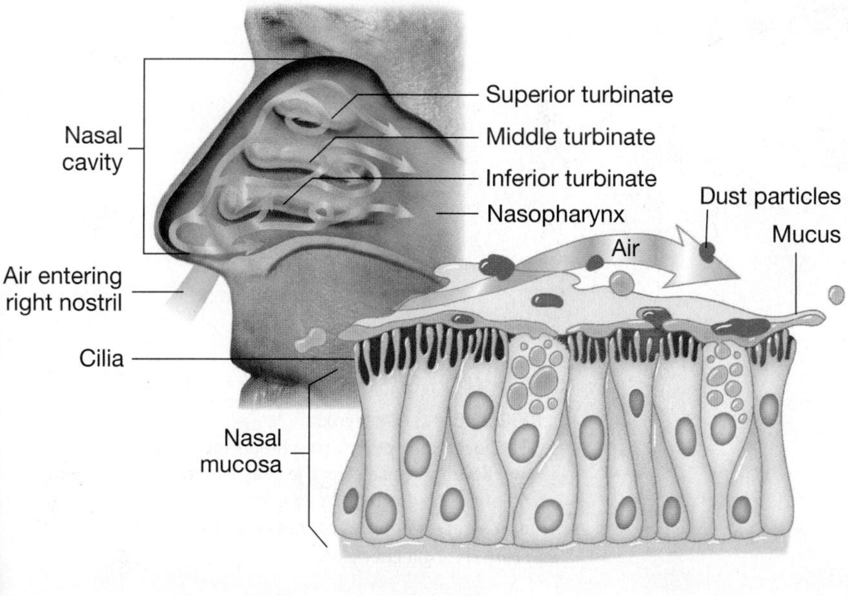

FIGURE 4-2 ■ Nasal cavity.
Air entering the nasal cavity swirls around the turbinates, allowing the mucosa to warm and moisten it before it goes to the lungs. This helps the body maintain its core temperature and keeps the tissues of the lungs from becoming dehydrated. The mucosa also produces mucus to trap inhaled particles and bacteria before they enter the lungs.
Source: Pearson Education

Pharynx

Posteriorly, the nasal cavity merges with the throat or **pharynx** (see Figure 4-3 ■). The **nasopharynx** is the area of the throat that is posterior to the nasal cavity, the **oropharynx** is the area of the throat that is posterior to the oral cavity, and the **laryngopharynx** is posterior to the larynx. The mucous membranes of the pharynx also warm and moisten inhaled air and trap particles. The pharynx is a common passageway for both air and food.

Larynx

At its inferior end, the pharynx divides into two parts: the larynx that leads to the trachea and the esophagus that leads to the stomach (see Figure 4-3). The **larynx**, or voice box, remains open during respiration and speech, allowing air to pass in and out through the vocal cords. During swallowing, muscles in the neck pull the larynx upward against the **epiglottis**, a lid-like structure, and that seals off the opening so that swallowed food goes into the esophagus, not into the trachea.

Trachea

Below the vocal cords, the larynx merges into the trachea. The **trachea** or windpipe is about 1 inch in diameter and 4 inches in length. It is a vertical passageway for inhaled and exhaled air (see Figure 4-4 ■). C-shaped rings of cartilage provide support to the trachea. On the posterior surface where there is no cartilage, the trachea is flexible and can flatten to make room when a large amount of swallowed food passes through the esophagus.

Pronunciation/Word Parts

pharynx (FAIR-ingks)

pharyngeal (fah-RIN-jee-al)
  pharyng/o- *pharynx; throat*
  -eal *pertaining to*

nasopharynx (NAY-soh-FAIR-ingks)
  nas/o- *nose*
  -pharynx *pharynx; throat*

oropharynx (OR-oh-FAIR-ingks)
  or/o- *mouth*
  -pharynx *pharynx; throat*

laryngopharynx (lah-RING-goh-FAIR-ingks)
  laryng/o- *larynx; voice box*
  -pharynx *pharynx; throat*

larynx (LAIR-ingks)

laryngeal (lah-RIN-jee-al)
  laryng/o- *larynx; voice box*
  -eal *pertaining to*

epiglottis (EP-ih-GLAW-tis)

epiglottic (EP-ih-GLAW-tik)
  epi- *above; upon*
  glott/o- *glottis of the larynx*
  -ic *pertaining to*

trachea (TRAY-kee-ah)

tracheal (TRAY-kee-al)
  trache/o- *trachea; windpipe*
  -al *pertaining to*

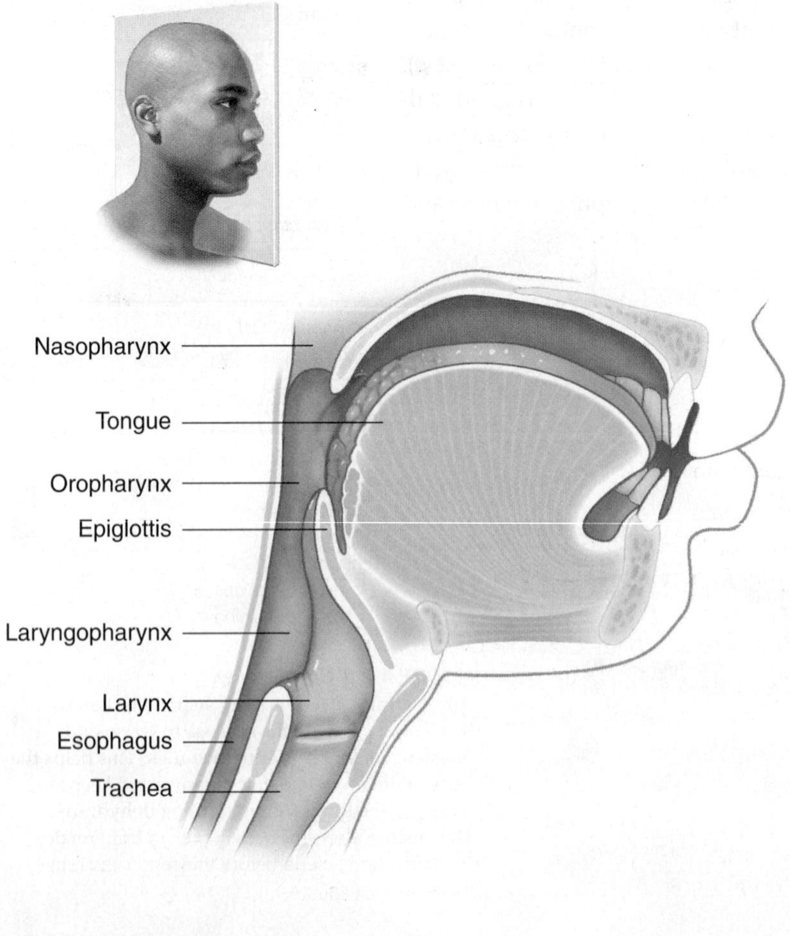

Nasopharynx

Tongue

Oropharynx

Epiglottis

Laryngopharynx

Larynx

Esophagus

Trachea

FIGURE 4-3 ■ Larynx.
The larynx is open during breathing but during swallowing muscles in the neck pull the larynx up to meet the epiglottis. The epiglottis covers the larynx so that swallowed food cannot enter the lungs.
Source: Pearson Education

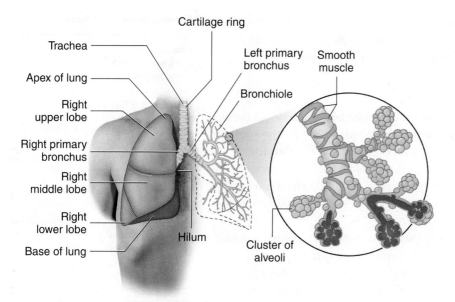

FIGURE 4-4 ■ Trachea, lung, bronchi, bronchioles, and alveoli.
The larger right lung has three lobes. The trachea divides into the right and left primary bronchi. A bronchus enters the lung at the hilum and then divides into bronchioles. Alveoli are clusters of microscopic air sacs at the end of each bronchiole where oxygen and carbon dioxide are exchanged.
Source: Pearson Education

Bronchi

The inferior end of the trachea splits to become the right and left primary **bronchi** (see Figure 4-4). The primary bronchi contain cartilage rings for support. Each primary bronchus enters a lung and branches into smaller **bronchioles**. The smallest bronchioles (with a diameter of 1 mm or less) have walls of smooth muscle, but no cartilage. The **lumen** is the central opening in the trachea, bronchi, and bronchioles through which air passes. **Bronchopulmonary** refers to the bronchi and the lungs.

The trachea, bronchi, and bronchioles look like the trunk and branches of an upside-down tree and are called the **bronchial tree**. The bronchial tree is lined with **cilia**, small hairs that flow in coordinated waves to move mucus and foreign particles toward the throat where they are expelled by coughing or are swallowed.

> **DID YOU KNOW?**
> Smoking immobilizes and eventually destroys the cilia. Without cilia, smoke particles easily enter the lung and are deposited there permanently. The normally pink lung tissue becomes gray in color with speckles of black.

Lungs

The **lungs** are spongy, air-filled structures. Each lung contains **lobes**, large divisions whose dividing lines are visible on the outer surface of the lung (see Figure 4-4). The right lung, which is larger, has three lobes: the right upper lobe (RUL), the right middle lobe (RML), and the right lower lobe (RLL). The left lung has two lobes: the left upper lobe (LUL) and the left lower lobe (LLL). The rounded top of each lung is the **apex**. The base of each lung lies along the diaphragm (see Figure 4-4). A bronchus enters the lung at the **hilum** (an indentation on the medial surface of the lung). The pulmonary arteries and pulmonary veins for each of the lobes also enter and exit there.

Inside the lung, the bronchus branches into bronchioles, which branch into alveoli. An **alveolus** is a hollow sphere of cells that expands and contracts with each breath (see Figure 4-4). Oxygen and carbon dioxide are exchanged between the alveolus and a nearby small blood vessel (capillary). The alveolus secretes **surfactant**, a protein–fat

Pronunciation/Word Parts

bronchus (BRONG-kus)

bronchi (BRONG-ki)
Form the plural by changing -*us* to -*i*.

bronchial (BRONG-kee-al)
   bronchi/o- *bronchus*
   -**al** *pertaining to*
The combining form **bronch/o-** also means *bronchus*.

bronchiole (BRONG-kee-ohl)
   bronchi/o- *bronchus*
   -**ole** *small thing*

bronchiolar (BRONG-kee-OH-lar)
   bronchiol/o- *bronchiole*
   -**ar** *pertaining to*

lumen (LOO-men)

bronchopulmonary
(BRONG-koh-PUL-moh-NAIR-ee)
   bronch/o- *bronchus*
   pulmon/o- *lung*
   -**ary** *pertaining to*

cilia (SIL-ee-ah)
Cilium is a Latin singular noun. Form the plural by changing -*um* to -*a*. The singular form *cilium* is seldom used.

pulmonary (PUL-moh-NAIR-ee)
   pulmon/o- *lung*
   -**ary** *pertaining to*
Pulmonary is the adjective for *lung*. The combining forms **pneum/o-** and **pneumon/o-** mean *air; lung*.

lobe (LOHB)

apex (AA-peks)

apices (AA-pih-seez)
Apex is a Latin singular noun. Form the plural by changing -*ex* to -*ices*.

hilum (HY-lum)

hila (HY-lah)
Hilum is a Latin singular noun. Form the plural by changing -*um* to -*a*.

compound that reduces surface tension and keeps the walls of the alveolus from collapsing with each exhalation. Collectively, the alveoli are the pulmonary **parenchyma**, the functional part of the lung, as opposed to the connective tissue framework.

Thoracic Cavity

The **thorax** is a bony cage that consists of the sternum (breast bone) anteriorly, the ribs laterally, and bones of the spine posteriorly. The thorax surrounds and protects the **thoracic cavity**. The lungs take up most of the space on either side of the thoracic cavity. Between the lungs lies the **mediastinum**, an irregularly shaped area that contains the trachea (and the heart and esophagus). The **diaphragm**, a sheet of skeletal muscle, lies along the inferior border of the thoracic cavity (see Figure 4-5 ■). The diaphragm is active during breathing.

Each lung is located within a **pleural cavity** that is surrounded by **pleura**, a double-layered serous membrane (see Figure 4-5). The **visceral pleura** is the layer next to the lung's surface, while the **parietal pleura** is the layer next to the wall of the thoracic cavity. The pleura secretes pleural fluid into the **pleural space**, the narrow space between its two layers. **Pleural fluid** is a slippery, watery fluid that allows the two layers to slide smoothly past each other as the lungs expand and contract during respiration.

Physiology of Respiration

Respiration consists of breathing in and breathing out. Breathing in is **inhalation** or **inspiration**. Breathing out is **exhalation** or **expiration**.

Breathing is normally an involuntary process that occurs without any conscious effort. **Respiratory control centers** in the brain regulate the depth and rate of respiration. Receptors in large arteries in the chest and neck send these centers information about the blood level of oxygen, and receptors in the brain send information about the blood level of carbon dioxide. Based on this information, the **respiratory control centers** control the rate of respiration by sending nerve impulses to the **phrenic nerve**,

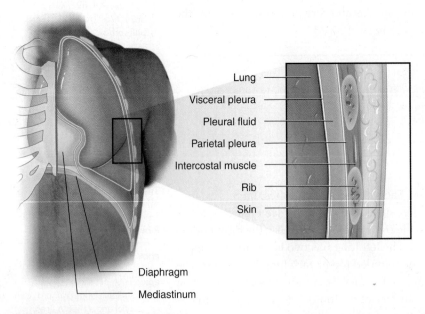

Lung
Visceral pleura
Pleural fluid
Parietal pleura
Intercostal muscle
Rib
Skin

Diaphragm
Mediastinum

FIGURE 4-5 ■ Diaphragm and pleura.
The diaphragm is the inferior border of the thoracic cavity. The pleura folds back on itself to make two layers. The visceral pleura covers the surface of the lungs. The parietal pleura lines the thoracic cavity. The pleural space between the two layers is filled with pleural fluid.
Source: Pearson Education

Pronunciation/Word Parts

hilar (HY-lar)
  hil/o- *indentation*
  -ar *pertaining to*

alveolus (al-VEE-oh-lus)

alveoli (al-VEE-oh-lie)
Alveolus is a Latin singular noun.
Form the plural by changing *-us* to *-i*.

alveolar (al-VEE-oh-lar)
  alveol/o- *air sac*
  -ar *pertaining to*

surfactant (ser-FAK-tant)
Surfactant is a combination of the words
surface and *active* plus the suffix *-ant*
(pertaining to).

parenchyma (pah-RENG-kih-mah)

thorax (THOR-aks)

thoracic (thor-AS-ik)
  thorac/o- *chest; thorax*
  -ic *pertaining to*
The combining forms **pector/o-** and
steth/o- mean *chest*.

mediastinum (MEE-dee-ah-STY-num)

diaphragm (DY-ah-fram)

diaphragmatic (DY-ah-frag-MAT-ik)
  diaphragmat/o- *diaphragm*
  -ic *pertaining to*

pleural (PLOOR-al)
  pleur/o- *lung membrane*
  -al *pertaining to*

pleura (PLOOR-ah)

visceral (VIS-eh-ral)
  viscer/o- *large internal organs*
  -al *pertaining to*

parietal (pah-RY-eh-tal)
  pariet/o- *wall of a cavity*
  -al *pertaining to*

respiration (RES-pih-RAY-shun)
  re- *again and again; backward; unable to*
  spir/o- *breathe; coil*
  -ation *being; having; process*
The combining form **pne/o-** means *breathing*.

inhalation (IN-hah-LAY-shun)
  in- *in; not; within*
  hal/o- *breathe*
  -ation *being; having; process*

inspiration (IN-spih-RAY-shun)
  in- *in; not; within*
  spir/o- *breathe; coil*
  -ation *being; having; process*

causing the diaphragm to contract. You can voluntarily control your respirations (when you hold your breath), but eventually involuntary control takes over, forcing you to breathe.

During inhalation, the diaphragm contracts and moves downward and the **intercostal muscles** between the ribs contract to pull the ribs up and out. This enlarges the thoracic cavity and creates negative internal pressure that causes air to flow into the lungs. During exhalation, the diaphragm and intercostal muscles relax, the thoracic cavity returns to its previous size, and air flows slowly out of the nose. A different set of intercostal muscles contracts to pull the ribs down and in to expel air during forceful exhalation (see Figure 4-6 ■). Having a normal depth and rate of respiration is known as **eupnea**.

Respiration involves five separate processes:

1. **Ventilation.** Movement of air in and out of the lungs.
2. **External respiration.** Movement of **oxygen** from inhaled air into the alveoli and then into the blood and the movement of **carbon dioxide** from the blood into the alveoli and then into exhaled air (see Figure 4-7 ■). External respiration is the exchange of these gases in the alveolus.
3. **Gas transport.** Transport of oxygen and carbon dioxide in the blood. Oxygen molecules in the blood bind with the hemoglobin in red blood cells to form the compound **oxyhemoglobin**. **Oxygenated** blood travels from the lungs to the heart, where it is pumped throughout the body to reach every cell. Carbon dioxide also binds with hemoglobin in the red blood cells and travels from body cells back to the lungs.
4. **Internal respiration.** Movement of oxygen from the blood into the cells and movement of carbon dioxide from the cells into the blood. Internal respiration is the exchange of these gases at the cellular level.
5. **Cellular respiration.** Oxygen is used by the cell to produce energy in the process of **metabolism**. Carbon dioxide is a gaseous waste product of cellular metabolism.

The respiratory system is solely responsible for process #1. The respiratory system and cardiovascular system share responsibility for process #2. The rest of the processes are done by the cardiovascular system and/or the individual cell.

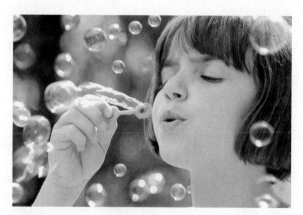

FIGURE 4-6 ■ Forceful exhalation.
When you want to forcefully exhale air, your brain tells one set of intercostal muscles between the ribs as well as the abdominal muscles to contract. This quickly decreases the size of the thoracic cavity and expels a large volume of air in just a few seconds—perfect for blowing bubbles, blowing up a balloon, or whistling.
Source: Gemphotography/Fotolia

Pronunciation/Word Parts

exhalation (EKS-hah-LAY-shun)
  ex- *away from; out*
  hal/o- *breathe*
  -ation *being; having; process*

expiration (EKS-pih-RAY-shun)
  ex- *away from; out*
  spir/o- *breathe; coil*
  -ation *being; having; process*
Delete the *s* from *spir/o-*; the prefix *ex-* already has an *s* sound.

phrenic (FREN-ik)
  phren/o- *diaphragm; mind*
  -ic *pertaining to*

intercostal (IN-ter-KAW-stal)
  inter- *between*
  cost/o- *rib*
  -al *pertaining to*

eupnea (YOOP-nee-ah)
  eu- *good; normal*
  -pnea *breathing*
The ending *-pnea* contains the combining form *pne/o-* and the one-letter suffix *-a*.

ventilation (VEN-tih-LAY-shun)
  ventil/o- *movement of air*
  -ation *being; having; process*

oxygen (AWK-seh-jen)
The combining forms **ox/i-, ox/o-,** and **ox/y-** mean *oxygen.*

carbon dioxide (KAR-bun dy-AWK-side)
The combining form **capn/o-** means *carbon dioxide.*

oxyhemoglobin
(AWK-see-HEE-moh-GLOH-bin)
  ox/y- *oxygen; quick*
  hem/o- *blood*
  glob/o- *comprehensive; shaped like a globe*
  -in *substance*

oxygenated (AWK-seh-jen-AA-ted)
  ox/y- *oxygen; quick*
  gen/o- *arising from; produced by*
  -ated *composed of; pertaining to a condition*

cellular (SEL-yoo-lar)
  cellul/o- *cell*
  -ar *pertaining to*

metabolism (meh-TAB-oh-lizm)
  metabol/o- *change; transformation*
  -ism *disease from a specific cause; process*

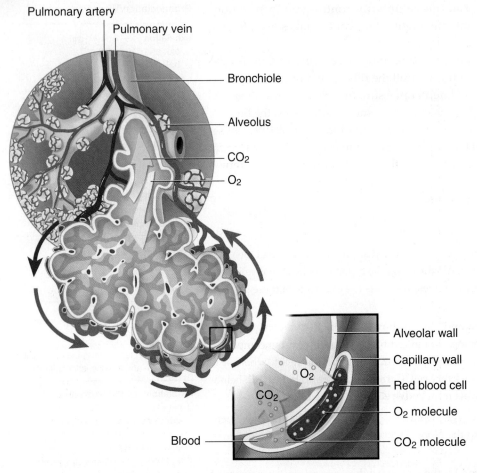

Pulmonary artery
Pulmonary vein
Bronchiole
Alveolus
CO₂
O₂
Alveolar wall
Capillary wall
Red blood cell
O₂ molecule
Blood
CO₂ molecule

FIGURE 4-7 ■ Gas exchange.
Oxygen moves from the alveolus into the blood, binds to hemoglobin in a red blood cell, and is carried to the cells of the body. Carbon dioxide comes from each cell as a waste product of metabolism. It dissolves in the blood or binds to hemoglobin and is carried to the lungs where it is exhaled.
Source: Pearson Education

WORD ALERT
Sound-Alike Words

breath   (noun)   the air that flows in and out of the lungs
(BRETH)   *Example: The breath of a diabetic patient can have a fruity odor to it.*

breathe   (verb)   the action of inhaling and exhaling
(BREETH)   *Example: If you ask an asthmatic patient to breathe deeply, you might hear a wheezing sound.*

mucosa   (noun)   a Latin word that means *mucous membrane*
(myoo-KOH-sah)   *Example: If a patient needs more oxygen, the oral mucosa might have a bluish color to it.*

mucous   (adjective)   pertaining to a membrane (the mucosa) that secretes mucus
(MYOO-kus)   *Example: Allergies make the mucous membranes of the nose swollen and inflamed.*

mucus   (noun)   a secretion from a mucous membrane
(MYOO-kus)   *Example: A chronic smoker coughs often and produces a significant amount of mucus.*

ACROSS THE LIFE SPAN

Pediatrics. In the uterus, the fetus does not breathe, and its lungs are collapsed. It receives oxygen from the mother's lungs via the placenta and umbilical cord. The lungs of the fetus do not function until the very first breath after birth. At that time, they must expand fully and stay expanded (which is helped by the presence of surfactant).

The normal respiratory rate for a newborn infant is 30–60 breaths per minute. The normal respiratory rate for an adult is 12–20 breaths per minute. One inhalation and one exhalation are counted as one respiration.

Geriatrics. As a person ages, some alveoli deteriorate. Because the body does not repair or replace alveoli, the total number of alveoli in the lungs continues to decline with age, and the remaining alveoli are less elastic. The thorax becomes stiff and less able to expand on inhalation. In addition, a lifetime of exposure to air pollution, chemical fumes, and smoke causes damage to the lungs. All of these changes decrease the pulmonary function in older adults.

Vocabulary Review

Anatomy and Physiology		
Word or Phrase	**Description**	**Combining Forms**
cardiopulmonary	Pertaining to the heart and lungs	*cardi/o-* heart *pulmon/o-* lung
respiratory system	Body system that brings oxygen into the body and expels carbon dioxide. The upper respiratory system includes the nose, nasal cavity, and pharynx (throat). The lower respiratory system includes the larynx (voice box) and trachea (windpipe) in the neck and the bronchi, bronchioles, and alveoli in the lungs. It is also known as the **respiratory tract**.	*spir/o-* breathe; coil

Upper Respiratory System		
mucosa	**Mucous membrane** that lines the entire respiratory system. It warms and humidifies incoming air. It produces **mucus** to trap foreign particles and bacteria.	*mucos/o-* mucous membrane *muc/o-* mucus
nasal cavity	Hollow area inside the nose	*nas/o-* nose
pharynx	The throat. A shared passageway for both air and food. The **nasopharynx** is posterior to the nasal cavity, the **oropharynx** is posterior to the oral cavity, and the **laryngopharynx** is posterior to the larynx.	*pharyng/o-* pharynx; throat *nas/o-* nose *or/o-* mouth *laryng/o-* larynx; voice box
septum	Center wall of cartilage and bone that divides the nasal cavity into right and left sides	*sept/o-* dividing wall; septum
turbinates	Three long, bony projections (superior, middle, and inferior) on either side of the nasal cavity. They break up and slow down inhaled air. They are also known as the **nasal conchae**.	*turbin/o-* scroll-like structure; turbinate

Lower Respiratory System		
alveolus	Hollow sphere of cells in the lungs where oxygen and carbon dioxide are exchanged	*alveol/o-* air sac
apex	Rounded top of each lung	
bronchiole	Small tubular air passageway that branches off from a bronchus and then branches into several alveoli. Its wall contains smooth muscle.	*bronchiol/o-* bronchiole
bronchus	Tubular air passageway supported by cartilage rings. It forms an inverted Y below the trachea. Each primary bronchus enters a lung and branches into bronchioles. The **bronchial tree** includes the trachea, bronchi, and bronchioles. **Bronchopulmonary** refers to the bronchi and the lungs.	*bronchi/o-* bronchus *bronch/o-* bronchus *pulmon/o-* lung
cilia	Small hairs that flow in waves to move mucus and foreign particles away from the lungs and toward the throat where they can be expelled	
epiglottis	Lidlike structure that seals off the opening to the larynx, so that swallowed food goes into the esophagus, not into the trachea	*glott/o-* glottis of the larynx

Word or Phrase	Description	Combining Forms
hilum	Indentation on the medial side of each lung where the bronchus, pulmonary arteries, and pulmonary veins enter and exit the lung.	**hil/o-** *indentation*
larynx	Structure that contains the vocal cords and is a passageway for inhaled and exhaled air. It is also known as the **voice box**.	**laryng/o-** *larynx; voice box*
lobe	Large division of a lung, whose dividing line is visible on the outer surface	
lumen	Central opening through which air flows inside the trachea, a bronchus, or a bronchiole	
lung	Organ of respiration that contains alveoli	**pneum/o-** *air; lung* **pneumon/o-** *air; lung* **pulmon/o-** *lung*
parenchyma	Functional part of the lung (i.e., the alveoli) as opposed to the connective tissue framework	
surfactant	Protein–fat compound that reduces surface tension and keeps the walls of the alveolus from collapsing with each exhalation	
trachea	Vertical tube with C-shaped rings of cartilage in it. It is an air passageway between the larynx and the bronchi. It is also known as the **windpipe**.	**trache/o-** *trachea; windpipe*
	**Thoracic Cavity**	
diaphragm	Sheet of skeletal muscle along the inferior border of the thoracic cavity. It divides the thoracic cavity from the abdominal cavity. It is active in breathing.	**diaphragmat/o-** *diaphragm*
intercostal muscles	Two sets of muscles between the ribs that contract to pull the ribs up and out during inhalation or down and in during forceful exhalation	**cost/o-** *rib*
mediastinum	Irregularly shaped area within the thoracic cavity. It contains the trachea (and the heart and esophagus).	
phrenic nerve	Nerve that, when stimulated by the respiratory control centers, causes the diaphragm to contract and move downward to expand the thoracic cavity during inspiration	**phren/o-** *diaphragm; mind*
pleura	Double-layered serous membrane. The **visceral pleura** is next to the lung's surface. The **parietal pleura** is next to the wall of the thoracic cavity. The pleura secretes **pleural fluid** into the **pleural space** (the space between the two layers of pleura).	**pleur/o-** *lung membrane* **viscer/o-** *large internal organs* **pariet/o-** *wall of a cavity*
pleural cavity	Area surrounded by pleura. Each pleural cavity contains a lung.	**pleur/o-** *lung membrane*
thoracic cavity	Hollow space within the bony thorax that contains the lungs and structures in the mediastinum	**thorac/o-** *chest; thorax*
thorax	Bony cage made of the sternum, ribs, and bones of the spine that surrounds and protects the lungs and other organs in the thoracic cavity	**thorac/o-** *chest; thorax* **pector/o-** *chest* **steth/o-** *chest*

Respiration

Word or Phrase	Description	Combining Forms
carbon dioxide	Exhaled gas that is a waste product of cellular metabolism. It is carried in the blood and by the hemoglobin in red blood cells.	**capn/o-** *carbon dioxide*
eupnea	Normal depth and rate of respiration	**pne/o-** *breathing*
exhalation	Breathing out. It is also known as **expiration**.	**hal/o-** *breathe* **spir/o-** *breathe; coil*
inhalation	Breathing in. It is also known as **inspiration**.	**hal/o-** *breathe* **spir/o-** *breathe; coil*
metabolism	Process of using oxygen to produce energy for cells. Metabolism produces carbon dioxide and other waste products.	**metabol/o-** *change; transformation*
oxygen	Inhaled gas that is used by each cell to produce energy in the process of metabolism. Oxygen is carried in the blood and by the hemoglobin in red blood cells. Blood that contains oxygen is **oxygenated**.	**ox/y-** *oxygen; quick* **ox/i-** *oxygen* **ox/o-** *oxygen* **gen/o-** *arising from; produced by*
oxyhemoglobin	Compound formed when oxygen combines with the hemoglobin in red blood cells	**ox/y-** *oxygen; quick* **hem/o-** *blood* **glob/o-** *comprehensive; shaped like a globe*
respiration	Consists of five processes: **ventilation** (movement of air in and out of the lungs), **external respiration** (exchange of oxygen and carbon dioxide between the alveoli and the blood), **gas transport** through the blood, **internal respiration** (exchange of oxygen and carbon dioxide between the blood and the cells), and **cellular respiration** (use of oxygen to produce energy in the cell and the production of carbon dioxide as a waste product of metabolism).	**spir/o-** *breathe; coil* **ventil/o-** *movement of air* **cellul/o-** *cell*
respiratory control centers	Centers in the brain that control the rate of respiration	**spir/o-** *breathe; coil*

Labeling Exercise

Match each anatomy word or phrase to its structure and write it in the numbered box. Be sure to check your spelling. Use the Answer Key at the end of the book to check your answers.

apex of lung	cluster of alveoli	lower lobe of lung	rib
bronchioles	diaphragm	nasal cavity	sternum
bronchus	larynx	pharynx	trachea

6.

7.

1.

8.

2.

9.

3.

10.

4.

11.

5.

12.

Source: Pearson Education

bronchiole	capillary wall	carbon dioxide	cluster of alveoli	oxygen	red blood cell

1.

2.

3.

4.

5.

6.

Source: Pearson Education

Give Word Part Meanings

Use the Answer Key at the end of the book to check your answers.

Combining Forms Exercise

Next to each combining form, write its meaning. The first one has been done for you.

Combining Form	Meaning	Combining Form	Meaning
1. **alveol/o-**	air sac	22. ox/i-	
2. bronchi/o-		23. ox/o-	
3. bronchiol/o-		24. ox/y-	
4. bronch/o-		25. pariet/o-	
5. capn/o-		26. pector/o-	
6. cardi/o-		27. pharyng/o-	
7. cellul/o-		28. phren/o-	
8. cost/o-		29. pleur/o-	
9. diaphragmat/o-		30. pne/o-	
10. gen/o-		31. pneum/o-	
11. glob/o-		32. pneumon/o-	
12. glott/o-		33. pulmon/o-	
13. hal/o-		34. sept/o-	
14. hem/o-		35. spir/o-	
15. hil/o-		36. steth/o-	
16. laryng/o-		37. thorac/o-	
17. metabol/o-		38. trache/o-	
18. muc/o-		39. turbin/o-	
19. mucos/o-		40. ventil/o-	
20. nas/o-		41. viscer/o-	
21. or/o-			

Build Medical Words

Combining Form and Suffix Exercise

Read the definition of the medical word. Look at the combining form that is given. Select the correct suffix from the Suffix List and write it on the blank line. Then build the medical word and write it on the line. (Remember: You may need to remove the combining vowel. Always remove the hyphens and slash.) Be sure to check your spelling. The first one has been done for you.

SUFFIX LIST

-al (pertaining to)	-ation (being; having; process)	-ism (disease from a specific cause; process)
-ar (pertaining to)	-eal (pertaining to)	-logy (study of)
-ary (pertaining to)	-ic (pertaining to)	-ole (small thing)

Definition of the Medical Word	Combining Form	Suffix	Build the Medical Word
1. Pertaining to (the) alveolus	alveol/o-)(-ar		alveolar

(You think *pertaining to* (-ar) + *alveolus* (alveol/o-). You change the order of the word parts to put the suffix last. You write *alveolar*.)

Definition of the Medical Word	Combining Form	Suffix	Build the Medical Word
2. Pertaining to (the) nose	nas/o-	_____	_____
3. Pertaining to (the) trachea	trache/o-	_____	_____
4. Pertaining to (the) lungs	pulmon/o-	_____	_____
5. Pertaining to (the nerve for the) diaphragm	phren/o-	_____	_____
6. Small thing (that comes from a) bronchus	bronchi/o-	_____	_____
7. Pertaining to (the) chest	thorac/o-	_____	_____
8. Study of (the) lung (and related structures)	pulmon/o-	_____	_____
9. Process (of) movement of air	ventil/o-	_____	_____
10. Process (of) change or transformation (that happens within a cell)	metabol/o-	_____	_____
11. Pertaining to (the) bronchus	bronchi/o-	_____	_____
12. Pertaining to (the) bronchiole	bronchiol/o-	_____	_____
13. Pertaining to (the) larynx	laryng/o-	_____	_____
14. Pertaining to (the) mucosa	mucos/o-	_____	_____
15. Pertaining to (the) diaphragm	diaphragmat/o-	_____	_____
16. Pertaining to (the) pharynx	pharyng/o-	_____	_____

Prefix Exercise

Read the definition of the medical word. Look at the medical word or partial word that is given (it already contains a combining form and suffix). Select the correct prefix from the Prefix List and write it on the blank line. Then build the medical word and write it on the line. Be sure to check your spelling. The first one has been done for you.

PREFIX LIST

epi- (above; upon)	in- (in; not; within)	re- (again and again; backward; unable to)
ex- (away from; out)	inter- (between)	

Definition of the Medical Word	Prefix	Word or Partial Word	Build the Medical Word
1. Process (to) in breathe	in-	spiration	inspiration
2. Pertaining to between (the) ribs	_____	costal	_____
3. Process (of) again and again breathe	_____	spiration	_____
4. Pertaining to above (the) glottis	_____	glottic	_____
5. Process (to) out breathe	_____	halation	_____
6. Having the function of again and again breathe	_____	spiratory	_____

Multiple Combining Forms and Suffix Exercise

Read the definition of the medical word. Select the correct suffix and combining forms. Then build the medical word and write it on the line. Be sure to check your spelling. The first one has been done for you.

SUFFIX LIST

-ary (pertaining to)
-ated (composed of; pertaining to a condition)
-in (substance)

COMBINING FORM LIST

bronch/o- (bronchus)
cardi/o- (heart)
gen/o- (arising from; produced by)
glob/o- (comprehensive; shaped like a globe)
hem/o- (blood)
ox/y- (oxygen; quick)
pulmon/o- (lung)

Definition of the Medical Word	Combining Form	Combining Form	Suffix	Build the Medical Word
1. Pertaining to (the) heart (and) lungs	cardi/o-	pulmon/o-	-ary	cardiopulmonary

(You think pertaining to (-ary) + heart (cardi/o-) + lungs (pulmon/o-). You change the order of the word parts to put the suffix last. You write cardiopulmonary.)

2. Pertaining to a condition (in which there is) oxygen arising from (the blood)	_____	_____	_____	_____
3. Pertaining to (the) bronchi (and) lungs	_____	_____	_____	_____
4. Substance (that carries oxygen in the) blood (and is) shaped like a globe	_____	_____	_____	_____

Diseases

Note: Most diseases of the nose, larynx, and pharynx are discussed in "Otolaryngology," Chapter 16.

Nose and Pharynx		
Word or Phrase	**Description**	**Pronunciation/Word Parts**

upper respiratory infection (URI)	Bacterial or viral infection of the nose and/or throat. It is also known as the **common cold** or a **head cold** (see Figure 4-8 ■). Treatment: Antibiotic drug for a bacterial infection.	**infection** (in-FEK-shun)
		  infect/o- *disease within*
		  -ion *action; condition*

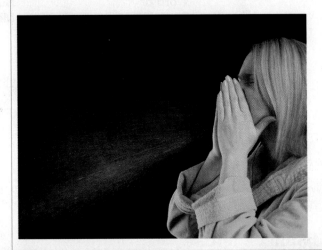

FIGURE 4-8 ■ Upper respiratory infection.
The common cold is an upper respiratory infection caused by a bacterium or virus. It spreads easily to others on unwashed hands or by droplets of mucus and saliva that are expelled into the air during sneezing and coughing.
Source: Rioblanco/123 RF

Trachea, Bronchi, and Bronchioles		

asthma	Hyperreactivity of the bronchi and bronchioles with **bronchospasm** (contraction of the smooth muscle). Inflammation and swelling severely narrow the lumens. Attacks are triggered by exposure to allergens, dust, mold, smoke, inhaled chemicals, exercise, cold air, or emotional stress. It is also known as **reactive airway disease**. There is severe shortness of breath, mucus production, coughing, audible wheezing, and difficulty exhaling. Patients with asthma are said to be **asthmatic**. **Status asthmaticus** is a prolonged, extremely severe, life-threatening asthma attack. Treatment: Avoid things that trigger asthma attacks. Corticosteroid drug, bronchodilator drug, and leukotriene receptor blocker drug to prevent attacks. Inhaled bronchodilator drug during attacks. Oxygen and epinephrine (Adrenalin) for severe attacks.	**asthma** (AZ-mah)
		
		bronchospasm (BRONG-koh-spazm)
		  bronch/o- *bronchus*
		  -spasm *sudden, involuntary muscle contraction*
		
		asthmatic (az-MAT-ik)
		  asthm/o- *asthma*
		  -atic *pertaining to*
		
		status asthmaticus (STAT-us az-MAT-ih-kus)

CLINICAL CONNECTIONS
Public Health. Asthma is prevalent in poor inner-city children. Researchers found that exposure to cockroaches appears to be a strong asthma trigger. Extermination of live cockroaches does not eliminate the problem because cockroach droppings and carcasses remain behind the walls of apartment buildings.

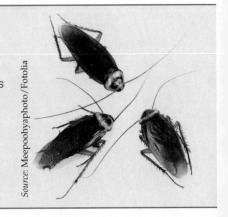

Source: Meepoohyaphoto/Fotolia

Word or Phrase	Description	Pronunciation/Word Parts
bronchitis	Acute or chronic inflammation or infection of the bronchi. Acute bronchitis with infection is due to bacteria or viruses. There is coughing, mucus production (**sputum**), wheezing, and a fever. Chronic bronchitis is due to pollution or smoking, and this causes a constant cough, mucus production, and wheezing. Chronic bronchitis is part of chronic obstructive pulmonary disease (COPD). Treatment: Bronchodilator drug, corticosteroid drug for inflammation. Antibiotic drug for a bacterial infection.	**bronchitis** (brong-KY-tis) **bronch/o-** *bronchus* **-itis** *infection of; inflammation of* **sputum** (SPYOO-tum)

DID YOU KNOW?

Pack-years are a standardized way to express as a single number the amount and duration of cigarette smoking. Pack-years equal the number of packs smoked per day multiplied by the number of years of smoking.

Word or Phrase	Description	Pronunciation/Word Parts
bronchiectasis	Chronic, permanent enlargement and loss of elasticity of the bronchioles. Chronic inflammation destroys the smooth muscle and allows secretions to accumulate. There is a large amount of mucus with coughing. It is often seen in patients with cystic fibrosis. Treatment: Bronchodilator drug. Oxygen therapy. Postural drainage and percussion.	**bronchiectasis** (BRONG-kee-EK-tah-sis) **bronchi/o-** *bronchus* **-ectasis** *condition of dilation*

Lungs

Word or Phrase	Description	Pronunciation/Word Parts
abnormal breath sounds	Normal inspiration sounds like a soft wind rushing through a tunnel. Abnormal breath sounds include a pleural friction rub, rales, rhonchi, stridor, or wheezes, as described below. Treatment: Correct the underlying cause.	

A CLOSER LOOK

Pleural friction rub: Creaking, grating, or rubbing sound when the two layers of inflamed pleura rub against each other during inspiration.

Rales: Irregular crackling or bubbling sounds during inspiration. Wet rales are caused by fluid or infection in the alveoli. Dry rales are caused by chronic irritation or fibrosis.

rales (RAWLZ)

Rhonchi: Humming, whistling, or snoring sounds during inspiration or expiration. They are caused by swelling, mucus, or a foreign body that partially obstructs the bronchi.

rhonchi (RONG-ki)

Stridor: High-pitched, harsh, crowing sound due to edema or obstruction in the trachea or larynx.

stridor (STRY-dor)

Wheezes: High-pitched whistling or squeaking sounds during inspiration or expiration. They are caused by extreme narrowing of the lumen due to bronchospasm from asthma.

wheezes (WHEE-zes)

Word or Phrase	Description	Pronunciation/Word Parts
adult respiratory distress syndrome (ARDS)	A severe infection, extensive burns, or injury to the lungs (aspiration of vomit or inhalation of chemical fumes) damages the alveoli (see Figure 4-9 ■). The alveoli are edematous (filled with fluid) and do not make surfactant; they collapse with each breath. Treatment: Oxygen therapy. Use of a respirator. Surfactant drug through an endotracheal tube. Correct the underlying cause.	

Poor blood flow

Air flow

Capillary

Fluid in alveoli

Edema of alveolar wall

Poor oxygenation of blood

Blood and fluid leak from capillary wall

Blood clot

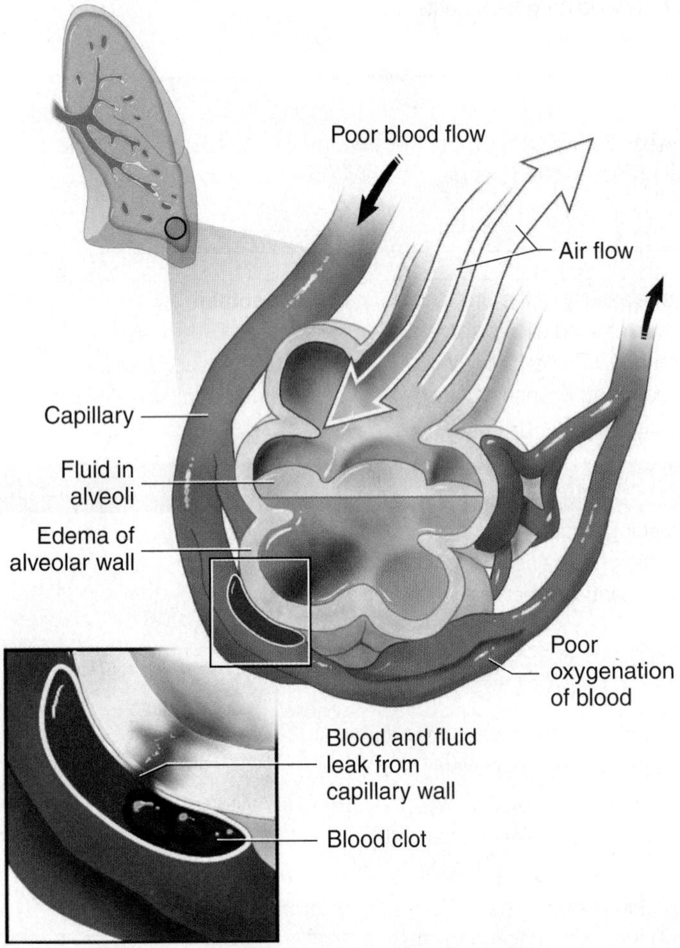

FIGURE 4-9 ■ Adult respiratory distress syndrome.
The alveolus is edematous and filled with fluid. There is poor blood flow in the capillary around the alveolus with some blood clots. The capillary walls leak fluid and blood into the alveolus. Capillary blood coming back to the heart (and going to the rest of the body) does not contain enough oxygen.
Source: Pearson Education

A CLOSER LOOK

Infant **respiratory distress syndrome (RDS)** develops in premature infants who produce too little surfactant because their lungs are not fully mature. There is nasal flaring (the nostrils flare with each breath to draw in more air), grunting (the larynx closes against the epiglottis to maintain pressure in the lungs and keep the alveoli from collapsing), and retractions. Sternal **retractions** bend the flexible breast bone inward. Intercostal retractions pull in the soft tissue and muscles between the ribs. It is also known as **hyaline membrane disease (HMD)**.

retraction (re-TRAK-shun)
  re- *again and again; backward; unable to*
  tract/o- *pulling*
  -ion *action; condition*
Select the correct prefix meaning to get the definition of *retraction*: *action (of) backward pulling (of the sternum).*

---

atelectasis	Incomplete expansion or collapse of part or all of a lung due to mucus, tumor, trauma, or a foreign body that blocks the bronchus. The lung is said to be **atelectatic**. It is also known as **collapsed lung**. This can develop postoperatively in patients who have shallow breathing and no cough reflex. It appears on a chest x-ray as a hazy, white patch. Treatment: Correct the underlying cause. Insert a chest tube to reinflate the lung.	**atelectasis** (AT-eh-LEK-tah-sis) **atel/o-** *incomplete* **-ectasis** *condition of dilation* **atelectatic** (AT-eh-lek-TAT-ik)

Word or Phrase	Description	Pronunciation/Word Parts
chronic obstructive pulmonary disease (COPD)	Combination of chronic bronchitis and **emphysema**. It is caused by chronic exposure to pollution or smoking. In emphysema, the alveoli become hyperinflated and often rupture, creating large air pockets in the lungs. Air can be inhaled but not exhaled. There is severe coughing, shortness of breath (dyspnea), sputum production, fatigue, and sometimes cyanosis. The chronic overexpansion of the lungs deforms the thorax (barrel chest). Treatment: Bronchodilator drug, corticosteroid drug. Oxygen therapy.	**chronic** (KRAW-nik) **chron/o-** *time* **-ic** *pertaining to* **obstructive** (awb-STRUK-tiv) **obstruct/o-** *blocked by a barrier* **-ive** *pertaining to* **emphysema** (EM-fih-SEE-mah) **em-** *in* **phys/o-** *distend; grow; inflate* **-ema** *condition* Add words to make a complete definition of *emphysema*: *condition (in the lungs of being) distended and inflated*.

DID YOU KNOW?

In healthy persons, an increased level of carbon dioxide stimulates breathing. Patients with COPD have a constantly increased level of carbon dioxide, so they depend on a decreased level of oxygen (hypoxic drive) to stimulate them to take a breath. Oxygen therapy for COPD patients must be carefully controlled so that it does not take away the hypoxic drive.

Word or Phrase	Description	Pronunciation/Word Parts
cystic fibrosis (CF)	Hereditary, eventually fatal disease caused by a recessive gene. Cystic fibrosis affects all the exocrine cells (those that secrete mucus, digestive enzymes, or sweat), but the respiratory system is particularly affected. Mucus is abnormally viscous (thick), and it blocks the alveoli, causing dyspnea. Constant coughing causes bronchiectasis. There are frequent bacterial infections in the lungs. The chronic lack of oxygen causes cyanosis and clubbing, a deformity of the fingertips (see Figure 4-10 ■). Mucus blocks pancreatic ducts and the secretion of pancreatic enzymes, and so fat is not digested properly. The patient has diarrhea and is undernourished. The pancreas develops cysts that become fibrous, hence the name *cystic fibrosis*. The sweat glands are overactive; the patient perspires excessively, losing large amounts of sodium. A sweat test shows increased amounts of sodium and chloride in the sweat. Treatment: Daily postural drainage (to let gravity help to drain the thick mucus) and chest percussion therapy (see Figure 4-11 ■) to remove mucus. Bronchodilator drug, corticosteroid drug, digestive enzymes, and a high-salt diet.	**cystic** (SIS-tik) **cyst/o-** *bladder; fluid-filled sac; semisolid cyst* **-ic** *pertaining to* Select the correct combining form meaning to get the definition of *cystic* (in *cystic fibrosis*): *pertaining to semisolid cysts (which are in the pancreas, not the lungs)*. **fibrosis** (fy-BROH-sis) **fibr/o-** *fiber* **-osis** *condition; process*

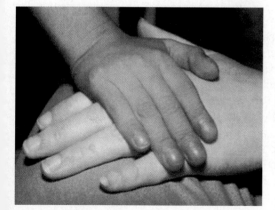

FIGURE 4-10 ■ Cystic fibrosis.
The hand of a child with cystic fibrosis compared to a normal adult hand (beneath). Cyanosis of the skin and clubbing of the fingertips are common in cystic fibrosis. A low level of oxygen causes blood in the arteries to be bluish rather than bright red, and the skin color is cyanotic. The chronic lack of oxygen causes the fingertips and fingernails to grow abnormally.
Source: Pearson Education/PH College

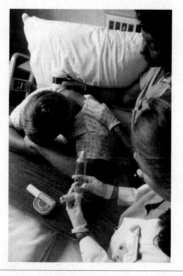

FIGURE 4-11 ■ Chest percussion therapy.
This young man with cystic fibrosis has been hospitalized. The respiratory therapist is using a vibrating device on his back to shake loose the thick mucus in his lungs so that he can cough it up. The nurse is preparing a drug for the patient to inhale.
Source: Will & Deni Mcintyre/Science Source/Getty Images

Word or Phrase	Description	Pronunciation/Word Parts
empyema	Localized collection of **purulent** material (pus) in the thoracic cavity from an infection in the lungs. It is also known as **pyothorax**. Treatment: Antibiotic drug. Surgery to drain the pus.	**empyema** (EM-py-EE-mah) **em-** *in* **py/o-** *pus* **-ema** *condition* Add words to make a complete definition of *empyema*: *condition in (the lungs of) pus.* **purulent** (PYOOR-yoo-lent) **purul/o-** *pus* **-ent** *pertaining to* **pyothorax** (PY-oh-THOR-aks) **py/o-** *pus* **-thorax** *chest; thorax*

WORD ALERT

Sound-Alike Words

emphysema   (noun)   Chronic, irreversibly damaged alveoli that are enlarged and trap air in the lungs.

Example: Emphysema caused this patient to have a barrel chest.

empyema   (noun)   Localized collection of pus in the thoracic cavity.

Example: She will be started immediately on intravenous antibiotic drugs for her empyema.

Word or Phrase	Description	Pronunciation/Word Parts
influenza	Acute viral infection of the upper and lower respiratory system. There is fever, severe muscle aches, and a cough. It is also known as *the flu*. It occurs most often in the fall and winter months. Influenza plus a secondary bacterial infection can cause pneumonia and death in older adults. Prevention: An annual flu vaccination. Treatment: Rest, analgesic drug, and fluids. Antibiotic drug for a secondary bacterial infection.	**influenza** (IN-floo-EN-zah)

CLINICAL CONNECTIONS

Pharmacology. There have been influenza epidemics in the past that killed thousands of people. Today, the most deadly strain of influenza is swine flu (H1N1 strain). (*Note*: For a discussion of flu shots, see the Clinical Connections feature box in the Drug Categories section.) The use of aspirin to relieve the symptoms of the flu can cause **Reye's syndrome**. The reason for this is not known. There is a very high level of ammonia in the blood and brain, with vomiting, seizures, and liver failure; it is sometimes fatal. Prevention: Use of acetaminophen (Tylenol) instead of aspirin to treat the symptoms of any viral infection.

Reye (RYE)

syndrome (SIN-drohm)
syn- *together*
-drome *a running*
The ending *-drome* contains the combining form *drom/o-* and the one-letter suffix *-e.*

Word or Phrase	Description	Pronunciation/Word Parts
legionnaires' disease	Severe, sometimes fatal, bacterial infection. There are flu-like symptoms, body aches, and fever, followed by severe pneumonia with liver and kidney degeneration. Treatment: Antibiotic drug that is effective against this bacterium.	**legionnaire** (LEE-jen-AIR)

DID YOU KNOW?

Legionnaires' disease was first identified in 1976 when many people at an American Legion convention in Philadelphia became sick. Physicians and epidemiologists from the Centers for Disease Control and Prevention (CDC) were called in to investigate this unknown disease. It was caused by an air conditioning system contaminated by a bacterium that is attracted to the lungs. The bacterium was named ***Legionella pneumophilia*** because of the American Legion, Philadelphia, and the bacterium's attraction to the lungs.

Legionella (LEE-jeh-NEL-ah)

pneumophilia (NOO-moh-FIL-ee-ah)
　pneum/o- *air; lung*
　phil/o- *attraction to; fondness for*
　-ia *condition; state; thing*

Word or Phrase	Description	Pronunciation/Word Parts
lung cancer	**Cancerous** tumor of the lungs that is more common in smokers (see Figure 4-12 ■) than nonsmokers. Lung cancer destroys normal tissue as it spreads (see Figure 4-13 ■). The different types of lung cancer are named for the characteristics of the original **malignant** cell or tissue: squamous cell **carcinoma**, **adenocarcinoma**, large cell carcinoma, small cell carcinoma, and oat cell carcinoma. Treatment: Surgery to remove a lobe of the lung (lobectomy) or the entire lung (pneumonectomy); chemotherapy drug or radiation therapy.	**cancer** (KAN-ser) **cancerous** (KAN-ser-us) 　**cancer/o-** *cancer* 　**-ous** *pertaining to* **malignant** (mah-LIG-nant) 　**malign/o-** *cancer; intentionally causing harm* 　**-ant** *pertaining to* **carcinoma** (KAR-sih-NOH-mah) 　**carcin/o-** *cancer* 　**-oma** *mass; tumor* **adenocarcinoma** (AD-eh-noh-KAR-sih-NOH-mah) 　**aden/o-** *gland* 　**carcin/o-** *cancer* 　**-oma** *mass; tumor*

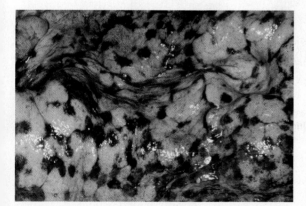

FIGURE 4-12 ■ Tar deposits in the lung.
This section of lung tissue shows hundreds of large and small deposits of black tar from years of smoking. Cigarette tar also contains carcinogens that can cause cancer.
Source: Spl/Science Source

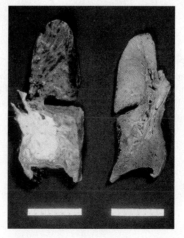

FIGURE 4-13 ■ Lung cancer.
These are two autopsy specimens of lungs. The normal lung on the right has some small darkened areas due to air pollution or smoking. The lung on the left shows a large, white cancerous tumor that has nearly destroyed the base of the lung, as well as darkened areas throughout due to heavy smoking.
Source: St Bartholomew's Hospital/Science Source

Word or Phrase	Description	Pronunciation/Word Parts
occupational lung diseases	Constant exposure to inhaled particles causes pulmonary fibrosis, and the alveoli lose their elasticity. **Anthracosis** (coal miner's lung or black lung disease) is caused by coal dust. **Asbestosis** is caused by asbestos fibers. **Pneumoconiosis** is a general word for any occupational lung disease caused by chronically inhaling some type of dust or particle. Treatment: Wear a filtering mask to prevent inhalation. Bronchodilator drug, corticosteroid drug.	**anthracosis** (AN-thrah-KOH-sis) anthrac/o- *coal* -osis *condition; process* Add words to make a complete definition of *anthracosis*: condition *(of the lungs from inhaling) coal (dust).*
	CLINICAL CONNECTIONS **Public Health.** Sick building syndrome consists of symptoms such as headache; eye, nose, or throat irritation; cough; dizziness; difficulty concentrating; and fatigue. These are not related to any specific illness, and the symptoms subside or disappear shortly after a person leaves that building. Sick building syndrome is caused by inadequate ventilation coupled with indoor pollutants released by carpeting, adhesives, paint that contains volatile organic compounds (VOCs), copy machines, cleaning agents, etc.	**asbestosis** (AS-bes-TOH-sis) asbest/o- *asbestos* -osis *condition; process* **pneumoconiosis** (NOO-moh-KOH-nee-OH-sis) pneum/o- *air; lung* coni/o- *dust* -osis *condition; process*
pneumonia	Infection of some or all of the lobes of the lungs (see Figure 4-14 ■). Fluid, microorganisms, and white blood cells fill the alveoli and air passages. There is difficulty breathing, with coughing and mucus production. Inflammation of the pleura causes pain on inspiration. Pneumonia is named according to its cause or its location in the lungs. Treatment: Antibiotic drug for bacterial pneumonia. Oxygen therapy and mechanical ventilation, if needed.	**pneumonia** (noo-MOHN-yah) pneumon/o- *air; lung* -ia *condition; state; thing*

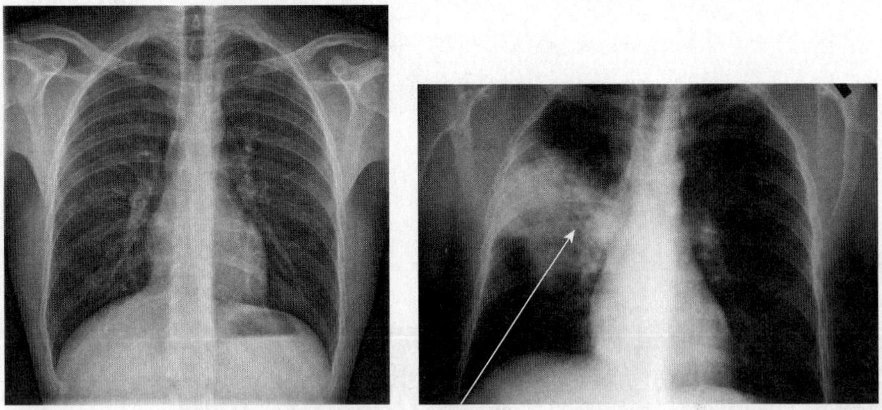

FIGURE 4-14 ■ Pneumonia.
(a) Compare the normal chest x-ray on the left with the chest x-ray on the right (b) that shows a dense gray-white area of pneumonia in the right upper and right middle lobes. Remember, when you look at the x-ray, the patient's right lung corresponds to your left side.
Source: Rvvelde/Fotolia; Joloei/Shutterstock

Word or Phrase	Description	Pronunciation/Word Parts
aspiration pneumonia	Caused by foreign matter (chemicals, vomit, etc.) that is inhaled into the lungs	**aspiration** (AS-pih-RAY-shun) aspir/o- *breathe in; suck in* -ation *being; having; process*

Word or Phrase	Description	Pronunciation/Word Parts
bacterial pneumonia	Caused by bacteria	**bacterial** (bak-TEER-ee-al) **bacteri/o-** *bacterium* **-al** *pertaining to*
broncho- pneumonia	Affects the bronchi, bronchioles, and alveoli in the lung	**bronchopneumonia** (BRONG-koh-noo-MOHN-yah) **bronch/o-** *bronchus* **pneumon/o-** *air; lung* **-ia** *condition; state; thing*
double pneumonia	Involves both lungs	
lobar pneumonia	Affects part or all of just one lobe of the lung. **Panlobar** pneumonia affects all of the lobes of one lung.	**lobar** (LOH-bar) **lob/o-** *lobe of an organ* **-ar** *pertaining to* **panlobar** (pan-LOH-bar) **pan-** *all* **lob/o-** *lobe of an organ* **-ar** *pertaining to*
pneumococcal pneumonia	Acute pneumonia caused by the bacterium *Streptococcus pneumoniae*. Prevention: Pneumococcal vaccination of at-risk patients (infants, older adults).	**pneumococcal** (NOO-moh-KAW-kal) **pneum/o-** *air; lung* **cocc/o-** *spherical bacterium* **-al** *pertaining to*
***Pneumocystis jiroveci* pneumonia**	Severe pneumonia caused by the fungus *Pneumocystis jiroveci*. Most people are infected with this microorganism in childhood. It causes a mild lung infection, and then lies dormant in small cysts. In patients with AIDS, it emerges from the cysts and causes disease. It is known as an **opportunistic infection** because it waits for an opportunity to cause disease in a person whose immune system is weakened. Treatment: Antifungal and antiprotozoal drugs.	***Pneumocystis jiroveci*** (NOO-moh-SIS-tis YEE-roh-VET-zee) **opportunistic** (AW-por-too-NIS-tik) **opportun/o-** *taking advantage of an opportunity; well timed* **-ist** *person who specializes in; thing that specializes in* **-ic** *pertaining to*
viral pneumonia	Caused by a virus	**viral** (VY-ral) **vir/o-** *virus* **-al** *pertaining to*
walking pneumonia	Mild form of pneumonia caused by the bacterium *Mycoplasma pneumoniae*. The patient does not feel well but can continue daily activities.	
pulmonary edema	Fluid (edema) collects in the alveoli. This is a result of backup of blood in the pulmonary circulation because of failure of the left side of the heart to adequately pump blood. There is dyspnea and orthopnea. Treatment: Correct the underlying heart failure. Oxygen therapy.	**edema** (eh-DEE-mah)

Word or Phrase	Description	Pronunciation/Word Parts
pulmonary embolism	Blockage of a pulmonary artery or one of its branches by an **embolus** (see Figure 4-15 ■). A patient on prolonged bedrest or one with an injury to the leg can develop a blood clot in the leg (deep vein thrombosis), or a fractured bone can release a fat globule. The embolus (blood clot or fat globule) travels in the circulatory system to a pulmonary artery where it is trapped and blocks the blood flow. There is decreased oxygenation of the blood and dyspnea. A large pulmonary embolus can be fatal. Treatment: Oxygen therapy, thrombolytic drug (to dissolve a blood clot), and anticoagulant drug (to prevent more blood clots from forming).	**embolism** (EM-boh-lizm) **embol/o-** *embolus; occluding plug* **-ism** *disease from a specific cause; process* **embolus** (EM-boh-lus)

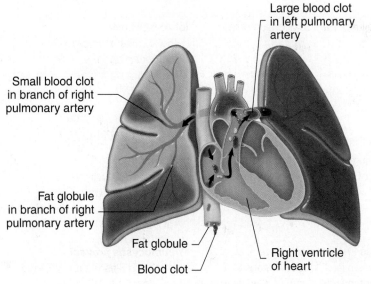

Large blood clot in left pulmonary artery

Small blood clot in branch of right pulmonary artery

Fat globule in branch of right pulmonary artery

Fat globule

Blood clot

Right ventricle of heart

FIGURE 4-15 ■ Pulmonary embolus.
An embolus (blood clot or fat globule) originates from veins anywhere in the body and travels to the heart. It easily goes through the large right ventricle of the heart, but becomes trapped when it leaves the heart and goes into the smaller branches of the pulmonary arteries. It blocks the flow of blood to the lung. The blood never reaches the alveoli to pick up oxygen. This lowers the overall oxygen content of the blood in the body. The alveoli collapse in that area of the lung.
Source: Pearson Education

Word or Phrase	Description	Pronunciation/Word Parts
severe acute respiratory syndrome (SARS)	Acute viral respiratory illness that can be fatal. There is fever, dyspnea, and cough, together with a history of travel in an airplane or close contact with another SARS patient. Chest x-ray shows pneumonia or adult respiratory distress syndrome. Treatment: Oxygen therapy and ventilator support. Antibiotic drugs are not effective against a viral illness.	
tuberculosis (TB)	Lung infection caused by the bacterium *Mycobacterium tuberculosis* and spread by airborne droplets and coughing. If the patient's immune system is strong, the bacteria remain dormant and cause no symptoms. If not, the bacteria multiply, producing **tubercles** (soft nodules of necrosis) in the lungs. There is fever, cough, weight loss, night sweats, and hemoptysis (coughing up blood). When this bacterium is stained in the laboratory, it holds an acid stain, and so it is known as an **acid-fast bacillus (AFB)**. Treatment: The waxy, external coating around this bacterium makes it resistant to regular antibiotic drugs. Several antitubercular drugs are used in combination for 9 months to treat tuberculosis.	**tuberculosis** (too-BER-kyoo-LOH-sis) **tubercul/o-** *nodule; tuberculosis* **-osis** *condition; process* **tubercle** (TOO-ber-kl) **tuber/o-** *nodule* **-cle** *small thing*

Pleura and Thorax

Word or Phrase	Description	Pronunciation/Word Parts
hemothorax	Presence of blood in the thoracic cavity, usually from trauma. Treatment: Thoracentesis or insertion of a chest tube to remove blood and fluid.	**hemothorax** (HEE-moh-THOR-aks) **hem/o-** *blood* **-thorax** *chest; thorax*

Word or Phrase	Description	Pronunciation/Word Parts
pleural effusion	Accumulation of fluid in the pleural space (between the two layers of pleura) due to inflammation or infection of the pleura and lungs. Treatment: Antibiotic drug for infection. Thoracentesis to remove the fluid.	**effusion** (ee-FYOO-zhun) **effus/o-** *pouring out* **-ion** *action; condition*
pleurisy	Inflammation or infection of the pleura due to pneumonia, trauma, or tumor. It is also known as **pleuritis**. The inflamed layers of pleura rub against each other, causing pain on inspiration. The rubbing sound heard through the stethoscope is a pleural friction rub. A patient with pleurisy is said to be pleuritic. Treatment: Correct the underlying cause.	**pleurisy** (PLOOR-ih-see) **pleur/o-** *lung membrane* **-isy** *condition of infection; condition of inflammation* **pleuritis** (ploor-EYE-tis) **pleur/o-** *lung membrane* **-itis** *infection of; inflammation of*
pneumothorax	Large volume of air in the pleural space. This increasingly separates the two layers of the pleura and compresses or collapses the lung. This is caused by a penetrating injury, or a spontaneous pneumothorax can occur when alveoli rupture from lung disease. *Note*: Air within the lung is normal; air within the pleural space is not. Treatment: Thoracentesis or insertion of a chest tube to remove the air.	**pneumothorax** (NOO-moh-THOR-aks) **pneum/o-** *air; lung* **-thorax** *chest; thorax*
	**Respiration**	
apnea	Brief or prolonged absence of spontaneous respirations due to respiratory failure or respiratory arrest. In premature infants, the immature central nervous system fails to maintain a consistent respiratory rate, and there are long pauses between periods of regular breathing. Middle-aged, obese patients who snore excessively have **obstructive sleep apnea**. They stop breathing as many as 30 times an hour during the night because of obstruction of the airway (by the soft palate or obesity of the neck), and then take a gasping breath that often awakens them. This causes sleep deprivation, fatigue, and difficulty concentrating during the day. Patients having an episode of apnea are said to be **apneic**. Treatment: Home apnea monitors for infants. Sleep apnea study to determine the cause in adults. A continuous positive airway pressure (CPAP) apparatus on the nose to give positive pressure to keep the airway open.	**apnea** (AP-nee-ah) **a-** *away from; without* **-pnea** *breathing* The ending *-pnea* contains the combining form *pne/o-* and the one-letter suffix *-a*. **apneic** (AP-nee-ik) **a-** *away from; without* **pne/o-** *breathing* **-ic** *pertaining to* **obstructive** (awb-STRUK-tiv) **obstruct/o-** *blocked by a barrier* **-ive** *pertaining to*
bradypnea	Abnormally slow rate of breathing (less than 10 breaths per minute in adults). This can be caused by a chemical imbalance in the blood or by brain damage that affects the respiratory control centers of the brain. Treatment: Correct the underlying cause.	**bradypnea** (BRAD-ip-NEE-ah) **brady-** *slow* **-pnea** *breathing*
cough	Protective mechanism to forcefully expel accidentally inhaled food, irritating particles (smoke, dust), or internally produced mucus. A cough may be nonproductive or productive of sputum. **Expectoration** is coughing up sputum from the lungs. **Hemoptysis** is coughing up blood-tinged sputum. Treatment: Expectorant drug for a productive cough, antitussive drug for a nonproductive cough. Correct the underlying cause.	**expectoration** (eks-PEK-toh-RAY-shun) **ex-** *away from; out* **pector/o-** *chest* **-ation** *being; having; process* Add words to make a complete definition of *expectoration*: *process (of expelling sputum) out (of the) chest*. **hemoptysis** (hee-MAWP-tih-sis) **hem/o-** *blood* **-ptysis** *condition of coughing up*

Word or Phrase	Description	Pronunciation/Word Parts
dyspnea	Difficult, labored, or painful respirations due to lung disease. It is also known as **shortness of breath (SOB)**. **Dyspnea on exertion (DOE)** occurs after brief activity in patients with severe chronic obstructive pulmonary disease (COPD). **Paroxysmal nocturnal dyspnea (PND)** is shortness of breath that occurs at night (nocturnal) because fluid builds up in the lungs while the patient is lying down. Patients are said to be **dyspneic**. Treatment: Sleeping propped up on pillows or in a chair. Oxygen therapy. Correct the underlying cause.	**dyspnea** (DISP-nee-ah) **dys-** *abnormal; difficult; painful* **-pnea** *breathing* **dyspneic** (DISP-nee-ik) **dys-** *abnormal; difficult; painful* **pne/o-** *breathing* **-ic** *pertaining to* **paroxysmal** (PAIR-awk-SIZ-mal) **paroxysm/o-** *sudden, sharp attack* **-al** *pertaining to*
orthopnea	The need to be propped in an upright or semi-upright position in order to breathe and sleep comfortably. Dyspnea and congestion occur if the patient lies down. The patient is said to be *orthopneic*. The severity of the orthopnea is expressed as the number of pillows that are needed (e.g., two-pillow orthopnea). Treatment: Oxygen therapy. Correct the underlying cause.	**orthopnea** (or-THAWP-nee-ah) **orth/o-** *straight* **-pnea** *breathing* Add words to make a complete definition of *orthopnea*: *breathing (that is only comfortable in a) straight (up position).*
tachypnea	Abnormally rapid rate of breathing (greater than 20 breaths per minute in adults) that is caused by lung disease. The patient is said to be **tachypneic**. Treatment: Oxygen therapy. Correct the underlying cause.	**tachypnea** (TAK-ip-NEE-ah) **tachy-** *fast* **-pnea** *breathing* **tachypneic** (TAK-ip-NEE-ik) **tachy-** *fast* **pne/o-** *breathing* **-ic** *pertaining to*

Oxygen and Carbon Dioxide Levels

Word or Phrase	Description	Pronunciation/Word Parts
anoxia	Complete lack (or a severely decreased level) of oxygen in the arterial blood and body tissues. It is caused by a lack of oxygen in the inhaled air or by an obstruction that prevents oxygen from reaching the lungs. The patient is said to be **anoxic**. Treatment: Oxygen therapy. Correct the underlying cause.	**anoxia** (an-AWK-see-ah) **an-** *not; without* **ox/o-** *oxygen* **-ia** *condition; state; thing* **anoxic** (an-AWK-sik)
asphyxia	The decrease in heart rate and blueness of the skin that occur because of an abnormally high level of carbon dioxide and an abnormally low level of oxygen. Asphyxia occurs if a person chokes, drowns, or suffocates. Treatment: Cardiopulmonary resuscitation.	**asphyxia** (as-FIK-see-ah)

CLINICAL CONNECTIONS

Obstetrics. Birth **asphyxia** occurs when the fetus in the uterus does not get enough oxygen through the umbilical cord and placenta before or during birth. This can be caused by premature separation of the placenta from the uterine wall, an umbilical cord that is wrapped tightly around the neck, or an umbilical cord that is compressed by the weight of the fetus during delivery.

Sudden infant death syndrome (SIDS) is an acute event in which an apparently healthy infant under 1 year of age suddenly dies. This was previously known as *crib death*. The cause is unknown; it may be due to respiratory arrest from vomiting and aspirating stomach contents, from asphyxiation from soft bedding blocking the nose, from sleep apnea, or from an imbalance of neurotransmitters in the brain. Parents are cautioned to position babies on their backs (or their sides) to sleep. The national campaign for this parental information was first known as "Back to Sleep."

Word or Phrase	Description	Pronunciation/Word Parts
cyanosis	Bluish-gray discoloration of the skin because of a very low level of oxygen and a very high level of carbon dioxide in the blood and tissues. It can be seen around the mouth (**circumoral cyanosis**) or in the nailbeds (see Figure 4-10). The patient is said to be **cyanotic**. Treatment: Oxygen therapy. Correct the underlying cause.	**cyanosis** (SY-ah-NOH-sis) **cyan/o-** *blue* **-osis** *condition; process* **cyanotic** (SY-ah-NAW-tik) **cyan/o-** *blue* **-tic** *pertaining to* **circumoral** (SIR-kum-OR-al) **circum-** *around* **or/o-** *mouth* **-al** *pertaining to*

CLINICAL CONNECTIONS

Forensic Science. When a person drowns or suffocates, there is a high level of carbon dioxide (CO_2) in the blood, and the skin shows cyanosis. However, when a person dies in a fire or from inhaling the fumes from car exhaust or a faulty space heater, there is a high level of carbon monoxide (CO) in the blood. Carbon monoxide binds to the same site on the hemoglobin molecule as oxygen does, and the hemoglobin is unable to carry any oxygen. Carbon monoxide poisoning causes a characteristic cherry red skin color.

Public Health. One new car in 1960 generated as much air pollution as 20 new cars today. According to the Foundation for Clean Air Progress, air pollution in the United States has decreased dramatically since 1970. The Air Quality Index is a numeral scale that rates the quality of the air daily. An AQI of 0–50 is good, over 100 is unhealthy for sensitive people, and over 300 is hazardous for everyone. Many states ban smoking in public places such as restaurants and bars because even secondhand smoke is a carcinogen, according to the Environmental Protection Agency. In children, exposure to it is linked to asthma, respiratory infections, and middle ear infections.

Word or Phrase	Description	Pronunciation/Word Parts
hypercapnia	Very high level of carbon dioxide (CO_2) in the arterial blood. Treatment: Oxygen therapy. Correct the underlying cause.	**hypercapnia** (HY-per-KAP-nee-ah) **hyper-** *above; more than normal* **capn/o-** *carbon dioxide* **-ia** *condition; state; thing*
hypoxemia	Very low level of oxygen in the arterial blood. **Hypoxia** is a very low level of oxygen in the cells. The patient is said to be **hypoxic**. Treatment: Oxygen therapy. Correct the underlying cause.	**hypoxemia** (HY-pawk-SEE-mee-ah) **hypo-** *below; deficient* **ox/o-** *oxygen* **-emia** *condition of the blood; substance in the blood* **hypoxia** (hy-PAWK-see-ah) **hypo-** *below; deficient* **ox/o-** *oxygen* **-ia** *condition; state; thing* **hypoxic** (hy-PAWK-sik)

Laboratory and Diagnostic Procedures

Word or Phrase	Description	Pronunciation/Word Parts
arterial blood gases (ABG)	Blood test to measure the partial pressure (P) of the gases oxygen (PO_2) and carbon dioxide (PCO_2) in a sample of arterial blood. The pH (how acidic or alkaline the blood is) is also measured. The higher the level of carbon dioxide, the more acidic the blood and the lower the pH.	**arterial** (ar-TEER-ee-al) **arteri/o-** *artery* **-al** *pertaining to*
carboxyhemo-globin	Blood test to measure the level of carbon monoxide in the blood of patients exposed to fires, smoke, or fumes in a closed, unventilated space. Carbon monoxide is carried by hemoglobin as carboxyhemoglobin. A blood level above 50% is fatal.	**carboxyhemoglobin** (kar-BAWK-see-HEE-moh-GLOH-bin) **carbox/y-** *carbon monoxide* **hem/o-** *blood* **glob/o-** *comprehensive; shaped like a globe* **-in** *substance*
oximetry	Procedure in which an **oximeter**, a small, noninvasive clip device, is placed on the patient's index finger or earlobe to measure the degree of oxygen saturation of the blood (see Figure 4-16 ■). It emits light waves that penetrate the skin and are absorbed or reflected by saturated hemoglobin (that is bound to oxygen) versus unsaturated hemoglobin. The oximeter calculates and displays a number for the oxygen saturation of the blood. It does not measure the CO_2 level. Some oximeters also measure the pulse rate; they are known as pulse oximeters.	**oximetry** (awk-SIM-eh-tree) **ox/i-** *oxygen* **-metry** *process of measuring* **oximeter** (awk-SIM-eh-ter) **ox/i-** *oxygen* **-meter** *instrument used to measure*

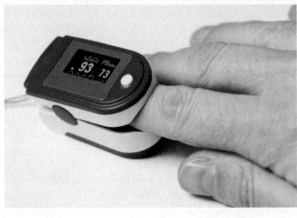

FIGURE 4-16 ■ Pulse oximeter.
This device is used in ambulances and in hospitals (at the patient's bedside) to provide a quick and accurate readout of the percentage of the patient's hemoglobin that is saturated with oxygen (%SO$_2$), 93%, and the pulse rate (PR), 73. Here, both of this patient's readings are within normal limits.
Source: Juanrvelasco/Fotolia

Word or Phrase	Description	Pronunciation/Word Parts
pulmonary function test (PFT)	Procedure to measure the capacity of the lungs and the volume of air during inhalation and exhalation (see Figure 4-17 ■). The FVC (forced vital capacity) measures the amount of air that can be forcefully exhaled from the lungs after inhaling fully. The FEV_1 (forced expiratory volume in 1 second) measures the volume of air that can be forcefully exhaled during the first second of measuring the FVC. **Spirometry** measures the FEV_1 and FVC and produces a tracing on a graph.	**spirometry** (spih-RAW-meh-tree) **spir/o-** *breathe; coil* **-metry** *process of measuring*

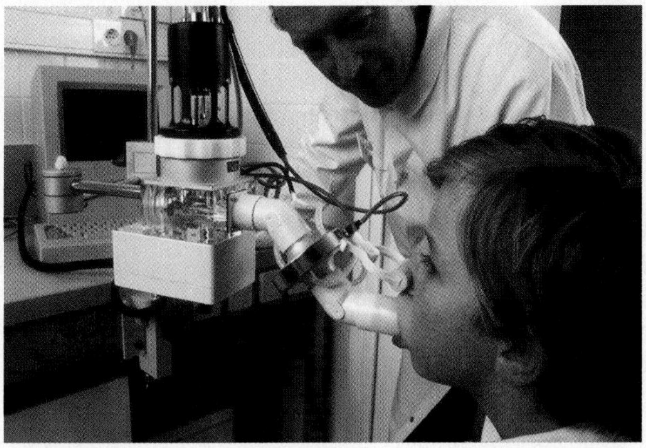

FIGURE 4-17 ■ Pulmonary function test.
This child who has asthma is having a pulmonary function test. The blue clip on his nose ensures that air only flows in and out of his mouth so that the volume of air in his lungs can be accurately measured.
Source: Edwige/BSIP/AGE Fotostock

Word or Phrase	Description	Pronunciation/Word Parts
sleep study	Procedure to determine if a patient has sleep apnea and what is causing it. Sensors record the patient's brain waves, eye movements, heart rate, breathing rate, blood pressure, movements of the extremities, and the oxygen level in the blood. This is also called **polysomnography**.	**polysomnography** (PAW-lee-sawm-NAW-grah-fee) **poly-** *many; much* **somn/o-** *sleep* **-graphy** *process of recording*
sputum culture and sensitivity (C&S)	Test to identify which bacterium is causing a pulmonary infection and to determine its sensitivity to various antibiotic drugs (see Figure 4-18 ■).	**sensitivity** (SEN-sih-TIV-ih-tee) **sensitiv/o-** *affected by; sensitive to* **-ity** *condition; state*

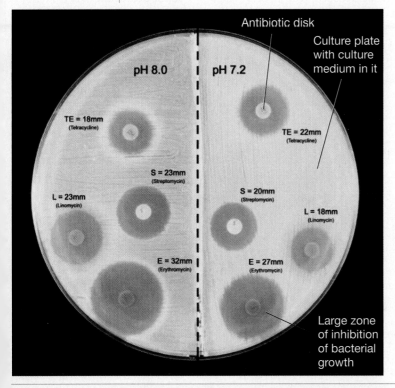

FIGURE 4-18 ■ Culture and sensitivity.
Disks containing various antibiotic drugs are placed on a culture plate. The plate contains a growth medium that has been swabbed with a specimen from the patient (sputum, wound fluid, etc.). If the bacteria in the specimen are resistant to that antibiotic drug, there will only be a small zone of inhibition (clear ring of no growth) around that disk. If the bacteria are sensitive to that antibiotic drug, there will be a medium or large clear zone of inhibition around that disk, and the physician may prescribe that drug to treat the patient's infection.
Source: Center for Disease Control (CDC)

Word or Phrase	Description	Pronunciation/Word Parts
tuberculosis tests	Test to determine if a patient has been exposed to tuberculosis. The **tine test** is a screening test that uses a four-pronged device (similar to the tines on a fork) to puncture the skin and introduce PPD (purified protein derivative), part of the bacterium *Mycobacterium tuberculosis*. The **Mantoux test** uses an intradermal injection of PPD. A raised skin reaction after 48 to 72 hours indicates a prior exposure to tuberculosis with antibodies to the tuberculosis bacterium. A positive Mantoux test is followed up with a chest x-ray to confirm whether or not the patient has active tuberculosis. A sputum specimen is smeared on a glass slide, stained, and examined under the microscope to look for acid-fast bacilli of *Mycobacterium tuberculosis*. Results of the smear can take 3 months and often miss a case of tuberculosis. The Xpert sputum test (the "while-you-wait" test) uses DNA technology, takes 100 minutes, is more accurate, and can detect TB that is already resistant to drugs.	**Mantoux** (man-TOO)

Radiology and Nuclear Medicine Procedure

Word or Phrase	Description	Pronunciation/Word Parts
chest radiography	Radiologic procedure that uses x-rays to create an image of the lungs. It is also known as a **chest x-ray (CXR)**. In an AP (anteroposterior) chest x-ray, the x-rays enter the patient's body through the anterior chest and then enter the x-ray plate. In a PA (posteroanterior) chest x-ray, the x-rays enter through the patient's back (see Figure 2-5). In a lateral chest x-ray, the x-rays enter through the patient's side. PA and lateral chest x-rays are often done during the same examination.	**radiography** (RAY-dee-AW-grah-fee) **radi/o-** *forearm bone; radiation; x-rays* **-graphy** *process of recording*
computerized axial tomography (CT), magnetic resonance imaging (MRI)	Radiologic procedures that scan a narrow slice of tissue and create an image. This process is known as **tomography**. A computer then assembles all of the "slices" into a three-dimensional image. A CT scan (which uses x-rays) and an MRI scan (which uses a magnetic field) are better at showing soft tissue structures than is radiography.	**tomography** (toh-MAW-grah-fee) **tom/o-** *cut; layer; slice* **-graphy** *process of recording*
lung scan	Nuclear medicine procedure that uses inhaled radioactive gas to show air flow (ventilation) in the lungs. Areas of decreased uptake ("cold spots") indicate pneumonia, atelectasis, or pleural effusion. A radioactive solution is given intravenously for the perfusion part of the scan. Areas of decreased uptake indicate poor blood flow to that part of the lung (and possible pulmonary embolus). It is also known as a **ventilation-perfusion (V/Q) scan**. The Q stands for *quotient*.	**ventilation** (VEN-tih-LAY-shun) **ventil/o-** *movement of air* **-ation** *being; having; process* **perfusion** (per-FYOO-zhun) **per-** *through; throughout* **fus/o-** *pouring* **-ion** *action; condition*

Medical and Surgical Procedures

Medical Procedures		
Word or Phrase	**Description**	**Pronunciation/Word Parts**
auscultation and percussion	Procedure that uses a **stethoscope** to listen to breath sounds (see Figures 2-20 and 4-21). Percussion uses the finger of one hand to tap over the finger of the other hand that is spread across the patient's back over a lobe of the lung (see Figure 2-21). After a few taps, the hand is moved over another lobe. The sound tells the physician if the lung is clear or if there is fluid or a tumor present.	**auscultation** (AWS-kul-TAY-shun)　**auscult/o-** *listening*　**-ation** *being; having; process*　　**percussion** (per-KUH-shun)　**percuss/o-** *tapping*　**-ion** *action; condition*　　**stethoscope** (STETH-oh-skohp)　**steth/o-** *chest*　**-scope** *instrument used to examine*
cardiopulmonary resuscitation (CPR)	Procedure to ventilate the lungs and circulate the blood if the patient has stopped breathing and the heart has stopped beating. In the past, mouth-to-mouth resuscitation involved forcing air into the patient's lungs; chest compressions pumped blood through the heart. In 2010, the American Heart Association changed its CPR guidelines to require only chest compressions because there is already enough oxygen in the blood and so just circulating the blood is all that is needed.	**cardiopulmonary** (KAR-dee-oh-PUL-moh-NAIR-ee)　**cardi/o-** *heart*　**pulmon/o-** *lung*　**-ary** *pertaining to*　　**resuscitation** (ree-SUS-ih-TAY-shun)　**resuscit/o-** *raise up again; revive*　**-ation** *being; having; process*

CLINICAL CONNECTIONS

Public Health. Many persons with chronic respiratory and other health problems wear a Medic Alert Foundation's emblem bracelet or necklace. The back of the emblem describes their disease or condition so that this information is available in an emergency even if they are unconscious.

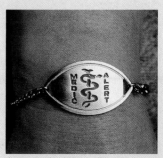

Source: Michael Heron Pearson Education/PH College

Word or Phrase	Description	Pronunciation/Word Parts
endotracheal intubation	Procedure in which an endotracheal tube (ETT) is inserted. A lighted **laryngoscope** helps visualize the vocal cords. The tube goes through the oral cavity and pharynx, between the vocal cords of the larynx, and into the trachea. This establishes an airway for a patient who is not breathing or needs a ventilator (see Figure 4-19 ■). This procedure is performed by paramedics in an ambulance, by physicians in the emergency department, or by anesthesiologists in the operating room prior to surgical procedures. Alternatively, a **nasotracheal tube** can be inserted through the nasopharynx to reach the trachea.	**endotracheal** (EN-doh-TRAY-kee-al) **endo-** *innermost; within* **trache/o-** *trachea; windpipe* **-al** *pertaining to* **intubation** (IN-too-BAY-shun) **in-** *in; not; within* **tub/o-** *tube* **-ation** *being; having; process* **laryngoscope** (lah-RING-goh-skohp) **laryng/o-** *larynx; voice box* **-scope** *instrument used to examine* **nasotracheal** (NAY-soh-TRAY-kee-al) **nas/o-** *nose* **trache/o-** *trachea; windpipe* **-al** *pertaining to*

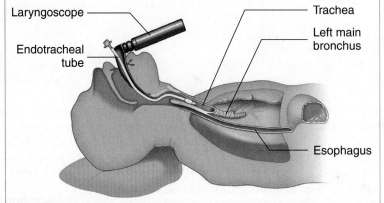

FIGURE 4-19 ■ Endotracheal intubation.
A laryngoscope is used to visualize the vocal cords prior to insertion of an endotracheal tube. The endotracheal tube is positioned in the trachea, just above the bronchi. A small balloon at the tip of the tube is inflated to hold the tube in place, and the external part of the tube is taped to the patient's cheek.
Source: Pearson Education

CLINICAL CONNECTIONS

Heimlich maneuver. Procedure to assist a choking victim with an airway obstruction. The rescuer stands behind the victim and places a fist on the victim's abdominal wall just below the diaphragm and, with both hands, gives a sudden push inward and upward. This generates an exhaled burst of air that pushes the obstruction into the mouth where it can be expelled.

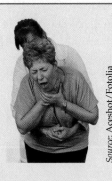

Source: Aceshot/Fotolia

Heimlich (HYM-lik)

Word or Phrase	Description	Pronunciation/Word Parts
incentive spirometry	Medical device to encourage patients to breathe deeply to prevent atelectasis. A **spirometer** is a portable plastic device with a mouthpiece. It contains balls that move, a visible incentive to the patient to inhale forcefully.	**spirometry** (spih-RAW-meh-tree) **spir/o-** *breathe; coil* **-metry** *process of measuring* **spirometer** (spih-RAW-meh-ter) **spir/o-** *breathe; coil* **-meter** *instrument used to measure*

Word or Phrase	Description	Pronunciation/Word Parts
oxygen therapy	Procedure to provide additional oxygen to patients with pulmonary disease. Room air is 21% oxygen. A patient can need amounts of oxygen ranging from 22% to 100%. Oxygen is delivered to the patient via a **nasal cannula** (see Figure 4-20 ■) or a face mask. An infant can receive oxygen through a rigid plastic hood placed over the head or in an oxygen tent. Oxygen is drying, and so patients who need a high flow of oxygen or prolonged oxygen therapy receive humidified oxygen (bubbled through water). A patient who requires respiratory assistance as well as oxygen is placed on a **ventilator (respirator)**, a mechanical device that breathes for the patient or assists with some breaths. Ventilators can provide up to 100% oxygen, as well as pressure to keep the alveoli from collapsing. An **Ambu bag** is a hand-held device that is used to manually breathe for the patient on a temporary basis. It is attached to a face mask or to an endotracheal tube and is squeezed to force air into the lungs (see Figure 4-21 ■). The patient is said to be being "bagged."	**cannula** (KAN-yoo-lah) **ventilator** (VEN-tih-LAY-tor) **ventil/o-** *movement of air* **-ator** *person who does; person who produces; thing that does; thing that produces* **respirator** (RES-pih-RAY-tor) **re-** *again and again; backward; unable to* **spir/o-** *breathe; coil* **-ator** *person who does; person who produces; thing that does; thing that produces* **Ambu** (AM-boo)

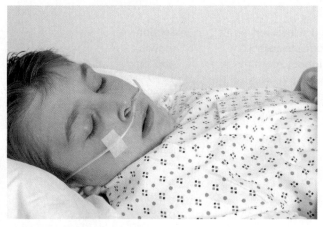

FIGURE 4-20 ■ Nasal cannula.
This patient is receiving oxygen therapy through a nasal cannula, a plastic tube with two short, flexible prongs that rest just inside the nostrils. A nasal cannula can provide an oxygen concentration up to 45%.
Source: Leah-Anne Thompson/Shutterstock

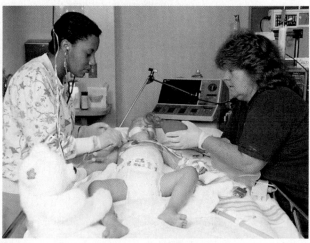

FIGURE 4-21 ■ Endotracheal tube and Ambu bag.
This infant in the pediatric intensive care unit has an endotracheal tube to assist with breathing. The nurse on the left is using a stethoscope to auscultate the breath sounds in the infant's right lung. The other nurse is squeezing a blue Ambu bag to breathe for the infant until the endotracheal tube is reconnected to the ventilator. The left chest is bandaged where a chest tube was inserted, and the yellow drainage tube for the chest tube is at the bottom right. The infant's pink skin color shows that the level of oxygen in the blood is adequate because of treatment with the ventilator and oxygen.
Source: Pearson Education/PH College

vital signs	Procedure during a physical examination in which the temperature, pulse, respirations (TPR), and blood pressure (BP) are measured. The respirations are measured for 1 minute by counting each rise and fall of the chest as one breath. An assessment of pain is often done as well, as the fifth vital sign.	

Surgical Procedures

Word or Phrase	Description	Pronunciation/Word Parts
bronchoscopy	Procedure that uses a lighted **bronchoscope** inserted through the mouth and larynx to examine the trachea and bronchi. Attachments on the bronchoscope can remove foreign bodies, suction thick mucus, or perform a biopsy.	**bronchoscopy** (brong-KAW-skoh-pee) **bronch/o-** *bronchus* **-scopy** *process of using an instrument to examine* **bronchoscope** (BRONG-koh-skohp) **bronch/o-** *bronchus* **-scope** *instrument used to examine*
chest tube insertion	Procedure that inserts a plastic tube between the ribs and into the thoracic cavity to remove accumulated air, fluid, pus, or blood due to trauma or infection. The tube is connected to a container (to measure the drainage) and to a suction device. A chest tube is used to treat pneumothorax, pyothorax, or hemothorax.	
lung resection	Procedure to remove part or all of a lung. A wedge resection removes a small wedge-shaped piece of lung tissue. A segmental resection removes a large piece or a segment of a lobe. A **lobectomy** removes an entire lobe (see Figure 4-22 ■). A **pneumonectomy** removes an entire lung. A lung resection is done as a biopsy procedure or to treat severe emphysema or lung cancer.	**resection** (ree-SEK-shun) **resect/o-** *cut out; remove* **-ion** *action; condition* **lobectomy** (loh-BEK-toh-mee) **lob/o-** *lobe of an organ* **-ectomy** *surgical removal* **pneumonectomy** (NOO-moh-NEK-toh-mee) **pneumon/o-** *air; lung* **-ectomy** *surgical removal*

LOBECTOMY

PREOPERATIVE

Emphysematous right upper lobe — Trachea

Right middle lobe

Right lower lobe

Surgical stapler

SURGERY

Lobe resected

POSTOPERATIVE

Bronchus stapled closed

Remaining lung tissue able to expand

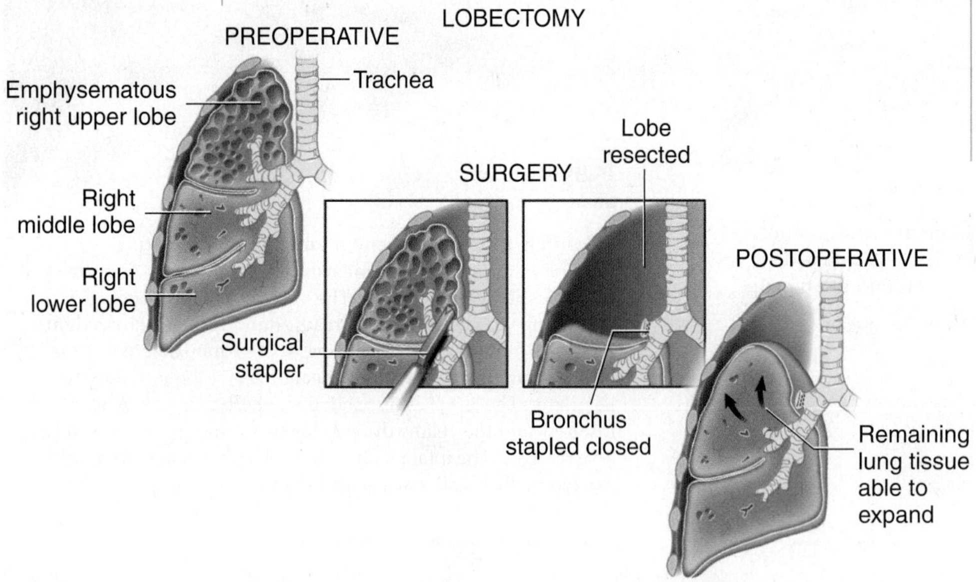

FIGURE 4-22 ■ Lobectomy.
A surgical stapler is used to staple and seal spongy lung tissue and the bronchus. Then the emphysematous right upper lobe is removed (resected). The remaining lung tissue has more room to normally expand with each breath.
Source: Pearson Education

Word or Phrase	Description	Pronunciation/Word Parts
thoracentesis	Procedure that uses a needle and a vacuum container to remove pleural fluid from the pleural space. It is used to treat a pleural effusion or obtain fluid for the diagnosis of lung cancer. It is also known as a **thoracocentesis**.	**thoracentesis** (THOR-ah-sen-TEE-sis) **thorac/o-** *chest; thorax* **-centesis** *procedure to puncture* *Note*: The duplicated "c" is deleted.
thoracotomy	Incision into the thoracic cavity. This is the first step of a surgical procedure involving the thoracic cavity and lungs.	**thoracotomy** (THOR-ah-KAW-toh-mee) **thorac/o-** *chest; thorax* **-tomy** *process of cutting; process of making an incision*

Word or Phrase	Description	Pronunciation/Word Parts
tracheostomy	Procedure that begins with an incision into the trachea (**tracheotomy**) to create an opening. A tracheostomy tube is then inserted to keep the opening from closing (see Figure 4-23 ■). A tracheostomy provides temporary or permanent access to the lungs in patients who need respiratory support, usually with a ventilator. The patient is said to have a "trach." 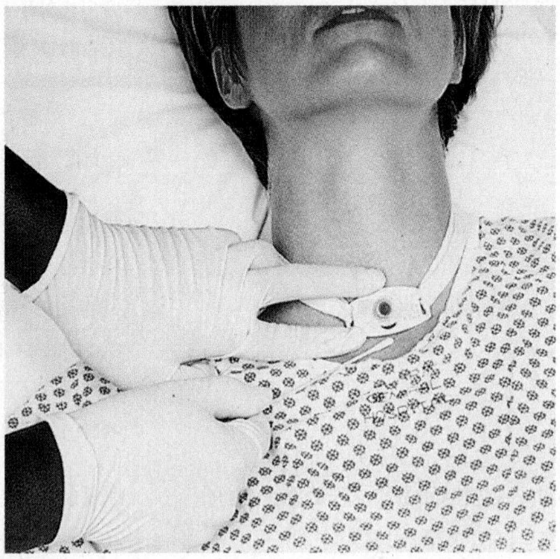	**tracheostomy** (TRAY-kee-AW-stoh-mee) **trache/o-** *trachea; windpipe* **-stomy** *surgically created opening* **tracheotomy** (TRAY-kee-AW-toh-mee) **trache/o-** *trachea; windpipe* **-tomy** *process of cutting; process of making an incision*

FIGURE 4-23 ■
Tracheostomy.
This patient has a permanent tracheostomy. The tracheostomy tube has a wide flange around it with slots where cotton tape can be inserted and tied around the patient's neck to secure the tube in the trachea. The nurse is cleansing the area to remove mucus.
Source: Jenny Thompson Pearson Education/PH College

Drugs

These drug categories and drugs are used to treat respiratory diseases. The most common generic and trade name drugs in each category are listed.

Category	Indication	Examples	Pronunciation/Word Parts
antibiotic drugs	Treat respiratory infections caused by bacteria. Antibiotic drugs are not effective against viral respiratory infections.	ampicillin (Principen), amoxicillin (Amoxil), ciprofloxacin (Cipro), ceftriaxone (Rocephin)	**antibiotic** (AN-tee-by-AW-tik) (AN-tih-by-AW-tik) **anti-** *against* **bi/o-** *life; living organism; living tissue* **-tic** *pertaining to*
antitubercular drugs	Treat tuberculosis. Several of these drugs must be used together in combination to be effective.	isoniazid (INH), ethambutol (Myambutol), rifampin (Rifadin)	**antitubercular** (AN-tee-too-BER-kyoo-lar) **anti-** *against* **tubercul/o-** *nodule; tuberculosis* **-ar** *pertaining to*
antitussive drugs	Suppress the cough center in the brain. They are used to treat chronic bronchitis and nonproductive coughs. Some of these contain a narcotic drug.	dextromethorphan (Robitussin), hydrocodone (Hycodan)	**antitussive** (AN-tee-TUS-iv) **anti-** *against* **tuss/o-** *cough* **-ive** *pertaining to*
antiviral drugs	Prevent and treat influenza virus infection in at-risk patients with asthma or lung disease.	oseltamivir (Tamiflu)	**antiviral** (AN-tee-VY-ral) **anti-** *against* **vir/o-** *virus* **-al** *pertaining to*
bronchodilator drugs	Dilate constricted airways by relaxing the smooth muscles that surround the bronchioles. They are used to treat asthma, COPD, emphysema, and cystic fibrosis. They are given orally or inhaled through a metered-dose inhaler (MDI) (see Figure 4-24 ■). When a bronchodilator drug is given through an inhaler to treat the symptoms of an acute asthma attack, it is known as a *rescue inhaler*.	albuterol (Proventil), salmeterol (Serevent), theophylline (Elixophyllin), tiotropium (Spiriva)	**bronchodilator** (BRONG-koh-DY-lay-tor) **bronch/o-** *bronchus* **dilat/o-** *dilate; widen* **-or** *person who does; person who produces; thing that does; thing that produces*

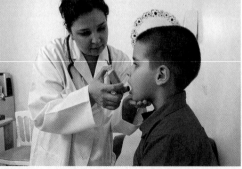

FIGURE 4-24 ■ Metered-dose inhaler.
A metered-dose inhaler (MDI) automatically delivers a premeasured dose of a bronchodilator drug or corticosteroid drug into the lungs as the patient inhales through the mouth. The dose is prescribed as the number of metered sprays or puffs. This healthcare professional is using a metered-dose inhaler device to administer a bronchodilator drug to this pediatric patient who has asthma symptoms.
Source: Levent Konuk/Shutterstock

Category	Indication	Examples	Pronunciation/Word Parts
corticosteroid drugs	Block the immune system from causing inflammation in the lung. They are used to treat asthma and COPD. They are given by a metered-dose inhaler, orally, or intravenously.	fluticasone (Flovent), mometasone (Asmanex), prednisolone (Orapred)	**corticosteroid** (KOR-tih-koh-STAIR-oyd) **cortic/o-** *cortex; outer region* **-steroid** *steroid* Corticosteroids are hormones secreted by the cortex (outer region) of the adrenal glands; they have a powerful, anti-inflammatory effect. Corticosteroid drugs have this same effect.
expectorant drugs	Reduce the thickness of sputum so that it can be coughed up. They are used to treat productive coughs.	guaifenesin (Mucinex)	**expectorant** (eks-PEK-toh-rant) **ex-** *away from; out* **pector/o-** *chest* **-ant** *pertaining to*
leukotriene receptor blocker drugs	Block leukotriene, which causes inflammation and edema. They are used to treat asthma.	montelukast (Singulair)	**leukotriene** (LOO-koh-TRY-een)
mast cell stabilizer drugs	Stabilize mast cells and prevent them from releasing histamine that causes bronchospasm during an allergic reaction. They are used to treat asthma.	cromolyn (Intal)	
stop smoking drugs	Bind to nicotine receptors and prevent them from being activated by nicotine from smoking (see Figure 4-25 ■).	nicotine (NicoDerm CQ) varenicline (Chanitx)	

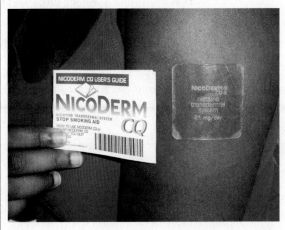

FIGURE 4-25 ■ Stop smoking drug.
This over-the-counter drug comes as a skin patch. It supplies nicotine in a gradually decreasing dose until the patient no longer needs nicotine and can stop smoking.
Source: Susan Turley

CLINICAL CONNECTIONS

Public Health. Flu shots are given to prevent influenza. Each February, the Centers for Disease Control and Prevention (CDC) selects those strains of influenza that are most prevalent in Asia and other parts of the world to include in the flu vaccine that will be offered in the United States the following fall before the start of flu season. Flu viruses mutate constantly, and so the influenza vaccine must be reformulated every year. Persons who get flu shots can still get the flu from other strains of influenza not included in the flu vaccine. The concern about a possible widespread epidemic and deaths from swine flu (H1N1 strain) has resulted in a massive public vaccination program to prevent infection from this specific strain of virus.

Abbreviations

A&P	auscultation and percussion		**MDI**	metered-dose inhaler
ABG	arterial blood gases		**MRI**	magnetic resonance imaging
AFB	acid-fast bacillus		**O_2**	oxygen
AP	anteroposterior		**PA**	posteroanterior
ARDS	acute respiratory distress syndrome; adult respiratory distress syndrome		**PCO_2, pCO_2**	partial pressure of carbon dioxide
BS	breath sounds		**PFT**	pulmonary function test
C&S	culture and sensitivity		**PND**	paroxysmal nocturnal dyspnea
CF	cystic fibrosis		**PO_2, pO_2**	partial pressure of oxygen
CO	carbon monoxide		**PPD**	packs per day (of cigarettes);
CO_2	carbon dioxide			purified protein derivative (TB test)
COPD	chronic obstructive pulmonary disease		**RA**	room air (no supplemental oxygen)
CPAP	continuous positive airway pressure (pronounced "SEE-pap")		**RDS**	respiratory distress syndrome
			RLL	right lower lobe (of the lung)
CPR	cardiopulmonary resuscitation		**RML**	right middle lobe (of the lung)
CT	computerized tomography		**RRT**	registered respiratory therapist
CXR	chest x-ray		**RUL**	right upper lobe (of the lung)
DOE	dyspnea on exertion		**SARS**	severe acute respiratory syndrome
ETT	endotracheal tube		**SIDS**	sudden infant death syndrome
FEV_1	forced expiratory volume (in one second)		**SOB****	shortness of breath
FiO_2	fraction (percentage) of inhaled oxygen		**TB**	tuberculosis
			TPR	temperature, pulse, and respiration
FVC	forced vital capacity		**URI**	upper respiratory infection
HMD	hyaline membrane disease		**V/Q**	ventilation-perfusion (scan)
LLL	left lower lobe (of the lung)			
LUL	left upper lobe (of the lung)			

**This abbreviation is still in use, but many hospitals have removed it from their official list of abbreviations because it also has an undesirable meaning that is unrelated to the respiratory system.

WORD ALERT

Abbreviations

Abbreviations are commonly used in all types of medical documents; however, they can mean different things to different people and their meanings can be misinterpreted. Always verify the meaning of an abbreviation.

A&P means *auscultation and percussion*, but it also means *anatomy and physiology*.

BS means *breath sounds*, but it also means *bowel sounds*.

C&S means *culture and sensitivity*, but it can be confused with the sound-alike abbreviation *CNS* (central nervous system).

PND means *paroxysmal nocturnal dyspnea*, but it also means *postnasal drip*.

RA means *room air*, but it also means *rheumatoid arthritis* or *right atrium*.

Word Part	Meaning	Word Part	Meaning
7. -atory	_____	33. -meter	_____
8. auscult/o-	_____	34. -metry	_____
9. brady-	_____	35. obstruct/o-	_____
10. carbox/y-	_____	36. -ole	_____
11. carcin/o-	_____	37. -osis	_____
12. circum-	_____	38. pan-	_____
13. cocc/o-	_____	39. percuss/o-	_____
14. coni/o-	_____	40. -pharynx	_____
15. cyan/o-	_____	41. -pnea	_____
16. dilat/o-	_____	42. -ptysis	_____
17. dys-	_____	43. purul/o-	_____
18. -eal	_____	44. py/o-	_____
19. -ectasis	_____	45. resect/o-	_____
20. -ectomy	_____	46. resuscit/o-	_____
21. -ema	_____	47. -scope	_____
22. embol/o-	_____	48. -scopy	_____
23. -gram	_____	49. -spasm	_____
24. -graphy	_____	50. -stomy	_____
25. hyper-	_____	51. tachy-	_____
26. hypo-	_____	52. therap/o-	_____
27. -ia	_____	53. -thorax	_____
28. -ion	_____	54. -tomy	_____
29. -ism	_____	55. tubercul/o-	_____
30. -isy	_____	56. tuber/o-	_____
31. -itis	_____	57. tuss/o-	_____
32. log/o-	_____		

RELATED COMBINING FORMS EXERCISE

Write the combining forms on the line. (Hint: See the It's Greek to Me feature box.)

1. Two combining forms that mean *breathe* _____

2. Three combining forms that mean *chest* _____

3. Three combining forms that mean *lung* _____

4.5B Define Abbreviations

MATCHING EXERCISE

Match each abbreviation to its description.

1. SOB	_____	Inhaler device used to give a bronchodilator drug
2. FVC	_____	Forced vital capacity
3. PFT	_____	Disease that includes chronic bronchitis and emphysema
4. TB	_____	Resuscitation
5. COPD	_____	Means the same as *dyspnea*
6. CXR	_____	Tuberculosis
7. MDI	_____	Radiology test of the chest
8. CPR	_____	Includes FVC and FEV_1

4.6A Divide Medical Words

DIVIDING WORDS EXERCISE

Separate these words into their component parts (prefix, combining form, suffix). Note: Some words do not contain all three word parts. The first one has been done for you.

Medical Word	Prefix	Combining Form	Suffix	Medical Word	Prefix	Combining Form	Suffix
1. inhalation	in-	hal/o-	-ation	13. auscultation			
2. pharyngeal				14. antitussive			
3. respiratory				15. thoracotomy			
4. hemoptysis				16. empyema			
5. circumoral				17. pneumonia			
6. bronchiectasis				18. bronchitis			
7. panlobar				19. expectorant			
8. pneumothorax				20. oximeter			
9. intercostal				21. cyanotic			
10. bronchiole				22. anoxia			
11. epiglottic				23. apneic			
12. pleurisy				24. therapist			

4.6B Build Medical Words

COMBINING FORM AND SUFFIX EXERCISE

Read the definition of the medical word. Select the correct suffix from the Suffix List. Select the correct combining form from the Combining Form List. Build the medical word and write it on the line. Be sure to check your spelling. The first one has been done for you.

SUFFIX LIST	COMBINING FORM LIST
-atic (pertaining to)	anthrac/o- (coal)
-ation (being; having; process)	asthm/o- (asthma)
-ator (person who does; person who produces; thing that does; thing that produces)	auscult/o- (listening)
-centesis (procedure to puncture)	bronchi/o- (bronchus)
-ectasis (condition of dilation)	bronch/o- (bronchus)
-ectomy (surgical removal)	cyan/o- (blue)
-ia (condition; state; thing)	hem/o- (blood)
-ist (person who specializes in)	laryng/o- (larynx; voice box)
-isy (condition of infection; condition of inflammation)	lob/o- (lobe of an organ)
-itis (infection of; inflammation of)	orth/o- (straight)
-meter (instrument used to measure)	ox/i- (oxygen)
-metry (process of measuring)	pleur/o- (lung membrane)
-osis (condition; process)	pneum/o- (air; lung)
-pnea (breathing)	pneumon/o- (air; lung)
-ptysis (condition of coughing up)	py/o- (pus)
-scope (instrument used to examine)	resuscit/o- (raise up again; revive)
-scopy (process of using an instrument to examine)	spir/o- (breathe; coil)
-spasm (sudden, involuntary muscle contraction)	steth/o- (chest)
-stomy (surgically created opening)	therap/o- (treatment)
-thorax (chest; thorax)	thorac/o- (chest; thorax)
-tomy (process of cutting; process of making an incision)	trache/o- (trachea; windpipe)
	ventil/o- (movement of air)

Definition of the Medical Word

Build the Medical Word

1. Pertaining to asthma — *asthmatic*
2. Infection of (or) inflammation of (the) bronchus
3. Thorax (that contains) pus
4. Process (of) listening (to the lung sounds)
5. Condition (of the skin being) blue
6. Surgically created opening (into the) trachea
7. Condition of coughing up blood
8. Surgical removal (of a) lung
9. Instrument used to examine (listen to the) chest
10. Sudden, involuntary muscle contraction (around the) bronchus
11. Condition of dilation (of the) bronchus
12. Instrument used to measure (the) oxygen (content of the blood)
13. Thing that produces movement of air
14. Instrument used to examine (the) larynx
15. Condition of infection (of the) pleura
16. Condition (of infection in the) lung
17. Condition (of having) coal (dust in the lungs)
18. Process of making an incision (into the) thorax
19. Process of using an instrument to examine (the) bronchus
20. Surgical removal (of a) lobe (of the lung)
21. Person who specializes in treatment
22. (Condition of the) thorax (having) air (in it)
23. Thorax (that contains) blood
24. Instrument used to measure (the volume that the patient) breathes
25. Process (to) revive or raise up again (a patient)
26. Process of measuring oxygen (in the blood)
27. Procedure to puncture (the) thorax (with a needle)
28. Breathing (in a) straight (up position)

PREFIX EXERCISE

Read the definition of the medical word. Look at the medical word or partial word that is given (it already contains a combining form and suffix). Select the correct prefix from the Prefix List and write it on the blank line. Then build the medical word and write it on the line. Be sure to check your spelling. The first one has been done for you.

PREFIX LIST			
an- (not; without)	em- (in)	hyper- (above; more than normal)	pan- (all)
anti- (against)	endo- (innermost; within)	in- (in; not; within)	tachy- (fast)
dys- (abnormal; difficult; painful)	ex- (away from; out)		

Definition of the Medical Word	Prefix	Word or Partial Word	Build the Medical Word
1. Process (of) within (the trachea putting a) tube	in-	tubation	intubation
2. Pertaining to difficult breathing		pneic	
3. Pertaining to all lobes (of the lung)		lobar	
4. Condition (of) more than normal carbon dioxide		capnia	

Definition of the Medical Word	Prefix	Word or Partial Word	Build the Medical Word
5. Pertaining to (a drug that is) against cough(ing)	_____	tussive	_____
6. Pertaining to fast breathing	_____	pneic	_____
7. Condition (of being) without oxygen	_____	oxia	_____
8. Condition in (the lung of) pus	_____	pyema	_____
9. Pertaining to within (the) trachea	_____	tracheal	_____
10. Pertaining to (a drug that takes sputum) out (of the) chest	_____	pectorant	_____

MULTIPLE COMBINING FORMS AND SUFFIX EXERCISE

Read the definition of the medical word. Select the correct suffix and combining forms. Then build the medical word and write it on the line. Be sure to check your spelling. The first one has been done for you.

SUFFIX LIST	COMBINING FORM LIST	
-al (pertaining to)	aden/o- (gland)	glob/o- (comprehensive; shaped like a globe)
-ia (condition; state; thing)	bronch/o- (bronchus)	hem/o- (blood)
-ic (pertaining to)	carbox/y- (carbon monoxide)	log/o- (study of; word)
-in (substance)	carcin/o- (cancer)	pneum/o- (air; lung)
-ist (person who specializes in)	cardi/o- (heart)	pneumon/o- (air; lung)
-oma (mass; tumor)	cocc/o- (spherical bacterium)	pulmon/o- (lung)
-or (person who does; person who produces; thing that does; thing that produces)	dilat/o- (dilate; widen)	thorac/o- (chest; thorax)

Definition of the Medical Word / Build the Medical Word

1. Pertaining to (the) heart (and) thorax — *cardiothoracic*
2. Tumor (of a) gland (that is a) cancer — _____
3. Thing (a drug) that produces (an effect to make the) bronchus widen — _____
4. Condition (of inflammation or infection of the) bronchi (and) lung — _____
5. Pertaining to (an infection in the) lung (that is caused by a) spherical bacterium — _____
6. Substance (that carries) carbon monoxide (in the) blood (and is) shaped like a globe — _____
7. Person who specializes in (the) lung (and the) study of (it) — _____

4.7A Spell Medical Words

HEARING MEDICAL WORDS EXERCISE

You hear someone speaking the medical words given below. Read each pronunciation and then write the medical word it represents. Be sure to check your spelling. The first one has been done for you.

1. an-AWK-see-ah — *anoxia*
2. az-MAT-ik — _____
3. AWS-kul-TAY-shun — _____
4. brong-KAW-skoh-pee — _____
5. EM-fih-SEE-mah — _____

6. hee-MAWP-tih-sis — _____
7. lah-RIN-jee-al — _____
8. loh-BEK-toh-mee — _____
9. NOO-moh-THOR-aks — _____
10. TRAY-kee-AW-stoh-mee — _____

ENGLISH AND MEDICAL WORD EQUIVALENTS EXERCISE

For each English word, write its equivalent medical word. Be sure to check your spelling. The first one has been done for you.

English Word	Medical Word	English Word	Medical Word
1. throat	pharynx	6. flu	
2. black lung disease		7. shortness of breath	
3. chest		8. common cold	
4. collapsed lung		9. voice box	
5. crib death		10. windpipe	

4.7B Pronounce Medical Words

PRONUNCIATION EXERCISE

Read the medical word and the syllables in its pronunciation. Circle the primary (main) accented syllable. The first one has been done for you.

1. bronchitis (brong-ky-tis)
2. bronchopulmonary (brong-koh-pul-moh-nair-ee)
3. cyanosis (sy-ah-noh-sis)
4. pneumonia (noo-mohn-yah)
5. respiration (res-pih-ray-shun)
6. thoracic (thor-as-ik)
7. tracheal (tray-kee-al)
8. tracheostomy (tray-kee-aw-stoh-mee)

4.8 Research Medical Words

ON THE JOB CHALLENGE EXERCISE

On the job, you will encounter new medical words. Practice your medical language skills by researching the phrases **cystic fibrosis** and **respiratory distress syndrome**. Did you find the complete definition under the first, second, or third word of the phrase? Which way of word searching is more effective? Write a word searching rule to help you remember how to look up these phrases.

1. cystic fibrosis

    Complete definition is under: **cystic**   **fibrosis**   (Circle one)

2. respiratory distress syndrome

    Complete definition is under: **respiratory**   **distress**   **syndrome**   (Circle one)

3. Wordsearching rule: _____

SOUND-ALIKE WORDS

Compare and contrast the medical meanings of these sound-alike pulmonology words.

1. *mucosa* and *mucous* and *mucus*
2. *larynx* and *pharnyx*
3. *emphysema* and *empyema*

4.9 Analyze Medical Reports

ELECTRONIC PATIENT RECORD #1

This is an office visit in the format of a SOAP note. Read the note and answer the questions.

PEARSON PRIMARY CARE ASSOCIATES

Task   Edit   View   Time Scale   Options   Help

OFFICE VISIT SOAP NOTE

PATIENT NAME: GUPTA, Priya

DATE OF VISIT: 11/19/xx

Source: sjenner 13/123 RF

SUBJECTIVE: This 45-year-old Indian American female has been followed in our office for reactive airway disease. She comes in today with shortness of breath and audible wheezing. This morning it was cold outside; she was in the city and was around someone who was smoking. She did not have her rescue inhaler with her.

OBJECTIVE: Temperature 98.2, heart rate 100, respiratory rate 30, blood pressure 130/80. Oximeter shows a %SO_2 of 85%. She appears anxious. Auscultation is positive for wheezing.

ASSESSMENT: Asthma attack.

PLAN: A bronchodilator drug was administered via a MDI and the symptoms subsided.

---

1. What is the other medical name for *reactive airway disease*?

2. Why is it important to note the temperature, location, and what others were doing in the location where the patient was this morning?

3. What instrument is needed to do auscultation?

4. Which result in the Objective section tells you that the patient was tachypneic?

5. Divide these words into their word parts and give the meaning of each word part.

   a. oximeter

   Word Part   **Meaning**

   _____   _____

   _____   _____

   b. auscultation

   Word Part   **Meaning**

   _____   _____

   _____   _____

6. What is a rescue inhaler and what is it used for?

7. What does the abbreviation *MDI* stand for?

ELECTRONIC PATIENT RECORD #2

This is a hospital Admission and Physical Examination report. Read the report and answer the questions.

PEARSON GENERAL HOSPITAL

Task   Edit   View   Time Scale   Options   Help

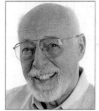

ADMISSION HISTORY AND PHYSICAL EXAMINATION

PATIENT NAME:	OTT, George
HOSPITAL NUMBER:	208-333-7943
DATE OF ADMISSION:	November 19, 20xx

Source: Lisa F. Young/Shutterstock

HISTORY OF PRESENT ILLNESS
This 65-year-old Caucasian male was evaluated by me in the emergency department on the above date, complaining of progressive shortness of breath, coughing, fever, and fatigue.

PAST HISTORY
The patient was a coal miner for 25 years before he retired on disability with black lung disease at age 55. He currently smokes 2 packs of cigarettes per day and has done so for the past 22 years. Surgical history of an appendectomy in the remote past. Chest x-ray done recently showed a suspicious lesion in the LLL; a bronchoscopy was performed and a biopsy was done, but the biopsy results were negative for malignancy.

PHYSICAL EXAMINATION
VITAL SIGNS: Pulse 110, respiratory rate 42 per minute, temperature 100.6, blood pressure 156/96.
GENERAL: The patient appears older than his stated age and quite tired at this time.
HEENT: Negative, except for slight cyanosis of the lips. The neck is supple and free of any masses.
CHEST: There is an increased anteroposterior diameter to the chest. There are no intercostal retractions during inspiration. There are diffuse expiratory wheezes, but no rales or rhonchi.
HEART: Normal heart sounds without murmur, gallop, or rub.
ABDOMEN: Soft and nontender.
EXTREMITIES: Normal with full range of motion noted. There was no clubbing of the fingers noted.

LABORATORY DATA
Complete blood count showed an elevated white blood cell count of 17,600 with 80 segs, 4 bands, and 2 lymphs. Oximeter showed 70% saturation. Sputum was sent for C&S. Chest x-ray: Patchy infiltrates from the apex to the midlung on the right with some consolidative changes involving the entire right lower lobe. There is no pleural fluid noted. There is a density seen in the left lower lobe posterolaterally, which extends to the pleural surface. It is most probably focal scarring or atelectasis from old inflammation.

IMPRESSION
1. Right-sided pneumonia.
2. Chronic obstructive pulmonary disease, secondary to anthracosis and smoking.

Linda C. Warren, M.D.

Linda C. Warren, M.D.

LCW: lcc
D: 11/19/xx
T: 11/19/xx

1. This patient has dyspnea. What phrase in the History of Present Illness says the same thing? _____ What is the medical abbreviation for this phrase? _____

2. If you wanted to use the adjective form of *dyspnea*, you would say, "The patient is _____."

3. Divide *bronchoscopy* into its two word parts and give the meaning of each word part.

   Word Part   **Meaning**

   _____   _____

   _____   _____

4. Divide *cyanosis* into its two word parts and give the meaning of each word part.

   Word Part   **Meaning**

   _____   _____

   _____   _____

5. What do these abbreviations stand for?

   a. C&S _____

   b. COPD _____

   c. LLL _____

6. What is the medical word for *black lung disease*?

   _____

7. What respiratory surgery did the patient have in the past?

   _____

8. What other surgery has the patient had in the past?

   _____

9. Circle all of the abnormalities that were seen on the patient's CXR.

   intercostal muscles   **consolidative changes**   **density in LLL**   **patchy infiltrates**

   atelectasis   **cyanosis**   **oximeter**   **pleural fluid**

10. Of the four medical complaints the patient had when he came to the emergency department, which one was directly related to an infection?

    _____

11. What is the descriptive name that laypersons give for the medical condition of increased anteroposterior diameter of the chest that is seen in patients with chronic obstructive pulmonary disease?

    _____

12. What method of examination would the physician use to hear the patient's expiratory wheezes? (Circle one)

    auscultation   **percussion**   **postural drainage**   **oximeter**

13. The patient has an elevated white blood cell count of 17,600, which indicates an infection. This is due to which of the two diagnoses listed in the Impression section?

    _____

14. Calculate the number of pack-years for this patient's history of smoking.

    _____

MyMedicalTerminologyLab™

MyMedicalTerminologyLab is a premium online homework management system that includes a host of features to help you study. Registered users will find:

- A multitude of quizzes and activities built within the MyLab platform

- Powerful tools that track and analyze your results—allowing you to create a personalized learning experience

- Videos and audio pronunciations to help enrich your progress

- Streaming lesson presentations (Guided Lectures) and self-paced learning modules

- A space where you and your instructor can check your progress and manage your assignments

Chapter 5
Cardiology

Cardiovascular System

Cardiology (KAR-dee-AW-loh-jee) is the medical specialty that studies the anatomy and physiology of the cardiovascular system and uses laboratory and diagnostic procedures, medical and surgical procedures, and drugs to treat cardiovascular diseases.

 ## Learning Outcomes

After you study this chapter, you should be able to

5.1 Identify structures of the cardiovascular system.

5.2 Describe the processes of circulation and a heartbeat.

5.3 Describe common cardiovascular diseases, laboratory and diagnostic procedures, medical and surgical procedures, and drugs.

5.4 Form the plural and adjective forms of nouns related to cardiology.

5.5 Give the meanings of word parts and abbreviations related to cardiology.

5.6 Divide cardiology words and build cardiology words.

5.7 Spell and pronounce cardiology words.

5.8 Research sound-alike and other cardiology words.

5.9 Analyze the medical content and meaning of cardiology reports.

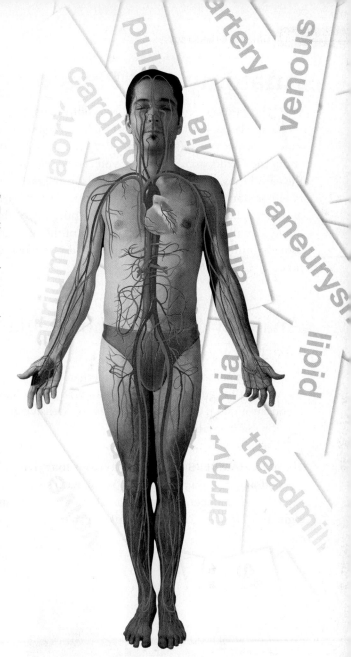

FIGURE 5-1 ■ Cardiovascular system.
The cardiovascular system consists of the heart and blood vessels connected in a continuous, circular pathway that carries blood to and from all parts of the body.
Source: Pearson Education

Medical Language Key

To unlock the definition of a medical word, break it into word parts. Give the meaning of each word part. Put the meanings of the word parts in order, beginning with the meaning of the suffix, then the prefix (if present), then the combining form(s).

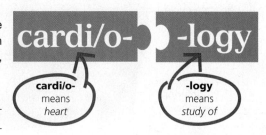

	Word Part	Word Part Meaning
Suffix	**-logy**	*study of*
Combining Form	**cardi/o-**	*heart*

Cardiology ▶ *Study of (the) heart (and related structures).*

Anatomy and Physiology

The **cardiovascular system** is a continuous, circular body system that includes the heart and the **vascular** structures (blood vessels such as arteries, capillaries, and veins) (see Figure 5-1 ■). It is also known as the **circulatory system**. To study the cardiovascular system, you can begin with the heart or you can begin with the capillaries, the tiniest blood vessels in the farthest parts of the body. Beginning at either starting point, you can go through every part of the cardiovascular system and arrive back where you began. The purpose of the cardiovascular system is to move (circulate) the blood to every part of the body as it transports oxygen, carbon dioxide, nutrients, and wastes. The blood is discussed in "Hematology and Immunology," Chapter 6.

Anatomy of the Cardiovascular System

Heart

The **heart** is perhaps the best-known organ in the body and certainly one of the most important. It is a muscular organ that contracts at least once every second to pump blood throughout the body. It also has an extensive electrical system that initiates and coordinates its contractions.

HEART CHAMBERS   The heart contains four chambers, two on the top and two on the bottom (see Figures 5-2 ■ and 5-3 ■). Each small upper chamber is an **atrium**. Each large lower chamber is a **ventricle**. The **septum**, a central wall, divides the heart into right and left sides. The inferior tip of the heart is the **apex**.

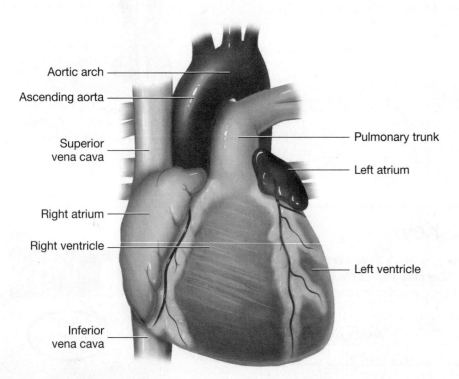

Aortic arch
Ascending aorta
Superior vena cava
Right atrium
Right ventricle
Inferior vena cava
Pulmonary trunk
Left atrium
Left ventricle

FIGURE 5-2 ■ Surface of the heart.
The boundaries of the internal chambers of the heart can be seen on the surface of the heart as elevated mounds and grooves that are filled with fat, blood vessels, and nerves.
Source: Pearson Education

Pronunciation/Word Parts

cardiovascular (KAR-dee-oh-VAS-kyoo-lar)
  cardi/o- *heart*
  vascul/o- *blood vessel*
  -ar *pertaining to*

vascular (VAS-kyoo-lar)
  vascul/o- *blood vessel*
  -ar *pertaining to*
The combining form **angi/o-** means *blood vessel; lymphatic vessel*. The combining form **vas/o-** means *blood vessel; vas deferens*.

circulatory (SIR-kyoo-lah-TOR-ee)
  circulat/o- *movement in a circular route*
  -ory *having the function of*

cardiac (KAR-dee-ak)
  cardi/o- *heart*
  -ac *pertaining to*
Cardiac is the adjective for *heart*. The Latin word *cor*, which means *heart*, is used in medical reports. The combining form **card/i-** also means *heart*.

atrium (AA-tree-um)

atria (AA-tree-ah)
Atrium is a Latin singular noun. Form the plural by changing *-um* to *-a*.

atrial (AA-tree-al)
  atri/o- *atrium; chamber that is open at the top*
  -al *pertaining to*

ventricle (VEN-trih-kl)

ventricular (ven-TRIH-kyoo-lar)
  ventricul/o- *chamber that is filled; ventricle*
  -ar *pertaining to*

septum (SEP-tum)

septal (SEP-tal)
  sept/o- *dividing wall; septum*
  -al *pertaining to*

apex (AA-peks)

apical (AP-ih-kal)
  apic/o- *apex; tip*
  -al *pertaining to*

WORD ALERT

Sound-Alike Words

The prefix *inter-* means *between*. The prefix *intra-* means *within*.

interventricular   (adjective) Pertaining to *between* the two ventricles
                        *Example: The interventricular septum is the dividing wall between the
                        right and left ventricles.*

intraventricular   (adjective) Pertaining to *within* the ventricle
                        *Example: Intraventricular blood is found within the right and left
                        ventricles.*

HEART VALVES   Four **valves** control the flow of blood through the heart. They are the tricuspid valve, pulmonary valve, mitral valve, and aortic valve (see Figure 5-3).

The **tricuspid valve** is between the right atrium and right ventricle. It has three triangular cusps (leaflets). As the right atrium contracts, the tricuspid valve opens to allow blood to flow into the right ventricle. Then it closes to prevent blood from flowing back into the right atrium.

The **pulmonary valve** is between the right ventricle and the pulmonary trunk. As the right ventricle contracts, the pulmonary valve opens to allow blood to flow into the pulmonary trunk and pulmonary arteries. Then it closes to prevent blood from flowing back into the right ventricle.

The **mitral valve** is between the left atrium and left ventricle. It has two cusps and is also known as the **bicuspid valve**. As the left atrium contracts, the mitral valve opens to allow blood to flow into the left ventricle. Then it closes to prevent blood from flowing back into the left atrium.

The **aortic valve** is between the left ventricle and the aorta (see Figure 5-4 ■). As the left ventricle contracts, the aortic valve opens to allow blood to flow into the aorta. Then it closes to prevent blood from flowing back into the left ventricle.

valve (VALV)

valvular (VAL-vyoo-lar)
  valvul/o- *valve*
  -ar *pertaining to*
The combining form **valv/o-** also means *valve*.

tricuspid (try-KUS-pid)
  tri- *three*
  cusp/o- *point; projection*
  -id *origin; resembling; source*

pulmonary (PUL-moh-NAIR-ee)
  pulmon/o- *lung*
  -ary *pertaining to*

mitral (MY-tral)
  mitr/o- *structure like a tall hat with two
    points*
  -al *pertaining to*

bicuspid (by-KUS-pid)
  bi- *two*
  cusp/o- *point; projection*
  -id *origin; resembling; source*

aortic (aa-OR-tik)
  aort/o- *aorta*
  -ic *pertaining to*

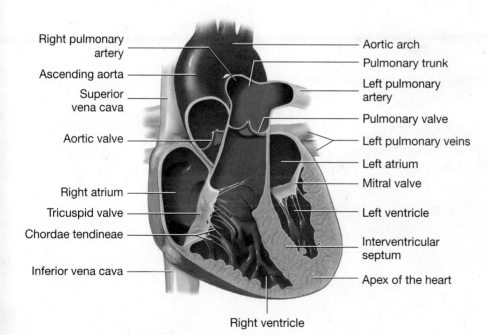

Right pulmonary artery
Ascending aorta
Superior vena cava
Aortic valve
Right atrium
Tricuspid valve
Chordae tendineae
Inferior vena cava

Aortic arch
Pulmonary trunk
Left pulmonary artery
Pulmonary valve
Left pulmonary veins
Left atrium
Mitral valve
Left ventricle
Interventricular septum
Apex of the heart

Right ventricle

FIGURE 5-3 ■ Chambers and valves of the heart.
The heart has four chambers: right atrium, right ventricle, left atrium, and left ventricle. The heart has four valves: tricuspid valve, pulmonary valve, mitral valve, and aortic valve.
Source: Pearson Education

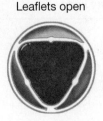

Leaflets open

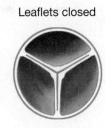

Leaflets closed

FIGURE 5-4 ■ Aortic valve.
With the three valve leaflets open, blood flows freely through the valve. When the valve leaflets close, their edges seal tightly against one another, preventing the backflow of blood.
Source: Pearson Education

Pronunciation/Word Parts

The tricuspid and mitral valves have **chordae tendineae**, rope-like strands attached to their valve leaflets (see Figure 5-3). The other end of the chordae tendineae is anchored to small muscles on the wall of the ventricles. When the ventricles contract, these small muscles also contract and pull on the chordae tendineae. This stabilizes the valve leaflets and keeps them firmly sealed together to keep blood from flowing back into the atria, even during the strong force of a ventricular contraction.

chordae tendineae
(KOR-dee TEN-dih-nee-ee)

The sounds of the valves closing are commonly known as "lubb-dupp" (a phonetic approximation of the actual sounds). The "lubb" is made as the tricuspid and mitral valves close. This first heart sound is abbreviated as S_1. The "dupp" is made as the pulmonary and aortic valves close. This second heart sound is abbreviated as S_2.

HEART MUSCLE   The **myocardium** is the muscular layer of the heart (see Figure 5-5 ■ and Table 5-1 ■). The myocardium is composed of cardiac muscle. Its muscle fibers (muscle cells) respond to electrical impulses generated by a node within the right atrium. This process is discussed in a later section.

myocardium (MY-oh-KAR-dee-um)
   my/o- *muscle*
   cardi/o- *heart*
   -um *period of time; structure*

myocardial (MY-oh-KAR-dee-al)
   my/o- *muscle*
   cardi/o- *heart*
   -al *pertaining to*

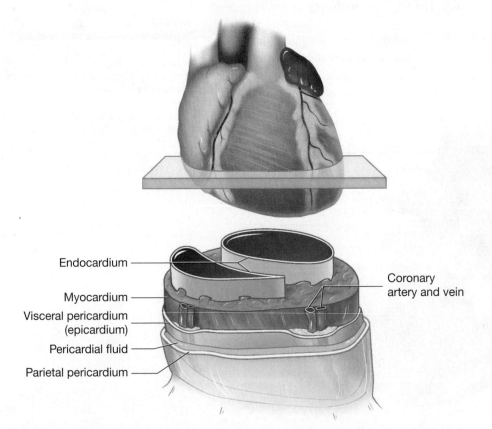

Endocardium

Myocardium

Visceral pericardium (epicardium)

Pericardial fluid

Parietal pericardium

Coronary artery and vein

FIGURE 5-5 ■ Layers and membranes of the heart.
The endocardium lines the four chambers and valves inside the heart. The myocardium is the muscular layer of the heart. The pericardium is the membrane around the pericardial sac that contains pericardial fluid.
Source: Pearson Education

Table 5–1 Layers and Membranes of the Heart

endocardium	Innermost layer that lines the atria, ventricles, and heart valves. (*Note*: This layer also extends into the blood vessels where it is known as the *endothelium* or *intima*.)
myocardium	Muscular layer of the heart
pericardium	Outermost layer. This membrane surrounds the heart as the **pericardial sac** and secretes pericardial fluid. The pericardial sac is U-shaped, and the heart is within the U. The part of the membrane that is next to the surface of the heart is the **visceral pericardium** or **epicardium** because it is upon the heart. The part that is the outer wall of the pericardial sac is the **parietal pericardium**. **Pericardial fluid** is a slippery, watery fluid that allows the two membranes to slide past each other as the heart contracts and relaxes.

The myocardium contracts in a coordinated way to pump blood. First the myocardium around the two atria contracts, forcing blood into the two ventricles. Then the myocardium around the two ventricles contracts. The blood in the right ventricle goes into the pulmonary trunk and the pulmonary arteries (that go to the lungs). The blood in the left ventricle goes into the aorta (that goes to the entire body). The myocardium is thickest on the left side of the heart because it is the left ventricle that must work the hardest to pump blood to the entire body.

Thoracic Cavity and Mediastinum

The **thoracic cavity** contains the lungs and the **mediastinum**, an irregularly shaped central area between the lungs (see Figure 5-6 ■). The mediastinum contains the heart and parts of the **great vessels** (aorta, superior vena cava, inferior vena cava, pulmonary arteries and veins), as well as the thymus, trachea, and the esophagus. The word **cardiothoracic** reflects the close relationship between the heart and the thoracic cavity.

Pronunciation/Word Parts

endocardium (EN-doh-KAR-dee-um)
  endo- *innermost; within*
  cardi/o- *heart*
  -um *period of time; structure*

pericardium (PAIR-ih-KAR-dee-um)
  peri- *around*
  cardi/o- *heart*
  -um *period of time; structure*

pericardial (PAIR-ih-KAR-dee-al)
  peri- *around*
  cardi/o- *heart*
  -al *pertaining to*

visceral (VIS-er-al)
  viscer/o- *large internal organs*
  -al *pertaining to*

epicardium (EP-ih-KAR-dee-um)
  epi- *above; upon*
  cardi/o- *heart*
  -um *period of time; structure*

parietal (pah-RY-eh-tal)
  pariet/o- *wall of a cavity*
  -al *pertaining to*

thoracic (thor-AS-ik)
  thorac/o- *chest; thorax*
  -ic *pertaining to*

mediastinum (MEE-dee-ah-STY-num)

mediastinal (MEE-dee-ah-STY-nal)
  mediastin/o- *mediastinum*
  -al *pertaining to*

cardiothoracic (KAR-dee-OH-thor-AS-ik)
  cardi/o- *heart*
  thorac/o- *chest; thorax*
  -ic *pertaining to*

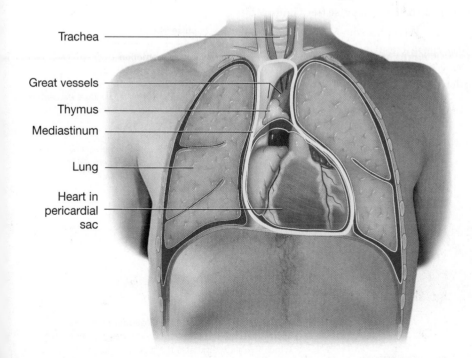

Trachea
Great vessels
Thymus
Mediastinum
Lung
Heart in pericardial sac

FIGURE 5-6 ■ Mediastinum.
The mediastinum holds the heart and pericardial sac, parts of the great vessels, as well as the thymus, trachea, and esophagus in place within the thoracic cavity.
Source: Pearson Education

Blood Vessels

The blood vessels are vascular channels through which blood circulates in the body. **Vasculature** refers to the blood vessels associated with a particular organ. Blood vessels have a central opening or **lumen** through which the blood flows. Blood vessels are lined with **endothelium**, a smooth inner lining that promotes the flow of blood. This layer is also known as the **intima**.

There are three kinds of blood vessels: arteries, capillaries, and veins. Each performs a different function in the circulatory system.

ARTERIES **Arteries** are large blood vessels that branch into smaller **arterioles**. All arteries share some important characteristics and functions.

1. All arteries carry blood away from the heart to the body or to the lungs.

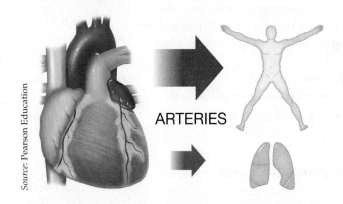

2. Most arteries carry bright red blood that has a high level of oxygen. The pulmonary arteries from the heart to the lungs carry dark red-purple blood that has a low level of oxygen.

3. Most arteries lie deep beneath the skin. A few, however, lie near the surface. Their walls bulge each time the heart contracts, and this can be felt as a **pulse** (see Figure 5-27).

4. All arteries have smooth muscle in their walls. When the smooth muscle contracts, the lumen of the artery decreases in size (**vasoconstriction**), and the pressure of the blood in the artery increases (see Figure 5-7 ■). When the smooth muscle relaxes, the lumen of the artery increases in size (**vasodilation**), and the pressure of the blood in the artery decreases.

Pronunciation/Word Parts

vasculature (VAS-kyoo-lah-CHUR)
  vascul/o- *blood vessel*
  -ature *system composed of*

lumen (LOO-men)

endothelium (EN-doh-THEE-lee-um)
  endo- *innermost; within*
  theli/o- *cellular layer*
  -um *period of time; structure*

intima (IN-tih-mah)

artery (AR-ter-ee)

arterial (ar-TEER-ee-al)
  arteri/o- *artery*
  -al *pertaining to*
The combining form **arter/o-** also means *artery*.

arteriole (ar-TEER-ee-ohl)
  arteri/o- *artery*
  -ole *small thing*

arteriolar (ar-TEER-ee-OH-lar)
  arteriol/o- *arteriole*
  -ar *pertaining to*

pulse (PULS)

vasoconstriction
(VAY-soh-con-STRIK-shun)
  vas/o- *blood vessel; vas deferens*
  constrict/o- *drawn together; narrowed*
  -ion *action; condition*

vasodilation (VAY-soh-dy-LAY-shun)
  vas/o- *blood vessel; vas deferens*
  dilat/o- *dilate; widen*
  -ion *action; condition*

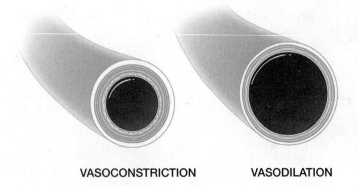

FIGURE 5-7 ■ Vasoconstriction and vasodilation.
Vasoconstriction and vasodilation of the arteries are important ways in which the body regulates the blood pressure.
Source: Pearson Education

CAPILLARIES   Capillaries are the smallest blood vessels in the body. The lumen of a capillary is so small that blood cells must pass through in single file. A network of capillaries connects the arterioles and venules. An arteriole branches into a network of capillaries that reaches each cell in the body and then the capillaries merge into a venule.

VEINS   Small veins, known as **venules**, combine to form a large **vein**. All veins share some important characteristics and functions.

1. All veins carry blood from the body and lungs to the heart.

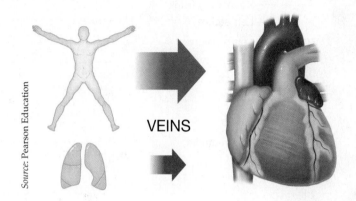

VEINS

Source: Pearson Education

2. Most veins carry dark red-purple blood that has a low level of oxygen. The pulmonary veins from the lungs to the heart carry bright red blood that has just picked up oxygen in the lungs.
3. The largest veins have valves that keep the blood flowing in one direction—back toward the heart (see Figure 5-8 ▇).
4. Many veins are near the surface of the body and can be seen just under the skin as bluish, sometimes bulging lines.

Pronunciation/Word Parts

capillary (KAP-ih-LAIR-ee)
   capill/o- *capillary; hair-like structure*
   -ary *pertaining to*

venule (VEN-yool)
   ven/o- *vein*
   -ule *small thing*

vein (VAYN)

venous (VEE-nus)
   ven/o- *vein*
   -ous *pertaining to*
The combining form **phleb/o-** also means *vein*.

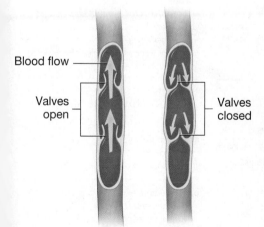

Blood flow

Valves open

Valves closed

FIGURE 5-8 ▇ Valves in a vein.
The heart pumps blood through the arteries, but not through the veins. As the large muscles in an arm or leg contract, they compress the vein and this moves blood through the vein. Valves in the vein then close to prevent gravity from pulling the blood back to its original location.
Source: Pearson Education

Blood Vessel Names and Locations

The names of many arteries and veins come from the names of nearby anatomical structures, such as bones or muscles. Capillaries are not named.

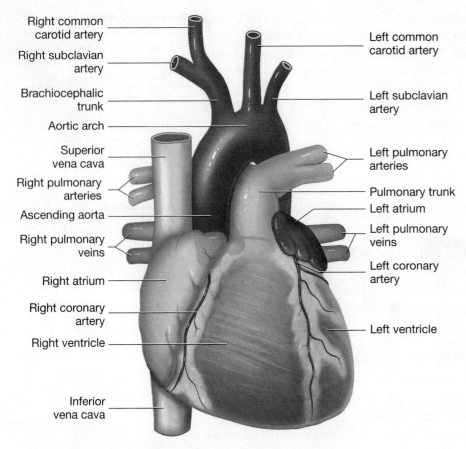

Right common carotid artery

Right subclavian artery

Brachiocephalic trunk

Aortic arch

Superior vena cava

Right pulmonary arteries

Ascending aorta

Right pulmonary veins

Right atrium

Right coronary artery

Right ventricle

Inferior vena cava

Left common carotid artery

Left subclavian artery

Left pulmonary arteries

Pulmonary trunk

Left atrium

Left pulmonary veins

Left coronary artery

Left ventricle

FIGURE 5-9 ■ **Arteries and veins around the heart.**
The aorta is the largest artery in the body. The coronary arteries to the heart are the first to receive oxygenated blood directly from the aorta. The aortic arch contains the first three major branches of arteries. The superior vena cava and inferior vena cava are the largest veins in the body.
Source: Pearson Education

ASCENDING AORTA AND ARTERIAL BRANCHES   The **aorta** is the largest artery in the body (see Figures 5-9 ■ and 5-10 ■). It receives oxygenated blood from the left ventricle of the heart. The **ascending aorta** travels from the heart in a superior direction. The **coronary arteries** to the myocardium are the first arteries to branch off from the ascending aorta.

aorta (aa-OR-tah)

coronary (KOR-oh-NAIR-ee)
   coron/o- *structure that encircles like a crown*
   -ary *pertaining to*

> **DID YOU KNOW?**
> Even though the chambers of the heart are filled with blood, the myocardium cannot use this blood. It must get its oxygen from blood that flows through the coronary arteries. Before oxygenated blood goes to any other part of the body, it goes through the coronary arteries to the myocardium. This is because of the primary role that the heart muscle plays in maintaining life.

aortic (aa-OR-tik)
   aort/o- *aorta*
   -ic *pertaining to*

carotid (kah-RAW-tid)
   carot/o- *sleep; stupor*
   -id *origin; resembling; source*

   The ascending aorta then becomes the **aortic arch**, an inverted, U-shaped segment. Three major arteries branch off from the aortic arch (see Figure 5-9): the brachiocephalic trunk (that branches into the right common carotid artery and right subclavian artery), the left common carotid artery, and the left subclavian artery. The **carotid arteries** bring oxygenated blood to the neck, face, head, and brain (see Figure 5-10). The **subclavian arteries** bring oxygenated blood to the shoulders. Each subclavian artery goes underneath the clavicle (collar bone) and then continues as the **axillary artery** (in the area of

subclavian (sub-KLAY-vee-an)
   sub- *below; underneath*
   clav/o- *clavicle; collar bone*
   -ian *pertaining to*

axillary (AK-zih-LAIR-ee)
   axill/o- *armpit*
   -ary *pertaining to*

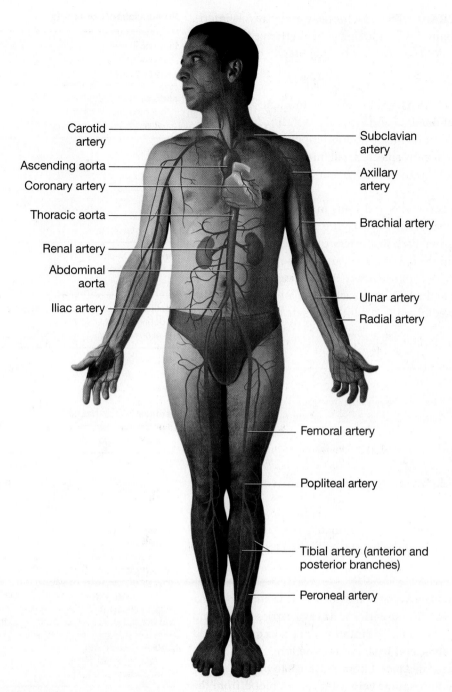

FIGURE 5-10 ■ Arteries in the body.
Arteries branch off from the aorta and carry oxygenated blood to the head, arms, chest, abdomen, pelvis, and legs.
Source: Pearson Education

the armpit). The axillary artery divides into the **brachial artery**, which brings oxygenated blood to the upper arm, and then into the **radial artery**, which bring oxygenated blood to the thumb side of the lower arm, and the **ulnar artery**, which brings oxygenated blood to the little finger side.

DID YOU KNOW?

The brachial artery takes its name from the biceps brachii muscle of the upper arm. The radial and ulnar arteries take their names from the radius (the bone on the thumb side of the lower arm) and the ulna (the bone on the little finger side of the lower arm).

brachial (BRAY-kee-al)
  brachi/o- *arm*
  -al *pertaining to*

radial (RAY-dee-al)
  radi/o- *forearm bone; radiation; x-rays*
  -al *pertaining to*
Select the correct combining form meaning to get the definition of *radial*: *pertaining to the forearm bone.*

ulnar (UL-nar)
  uln/o- *forearm bone; ulna*
  -ar *pertaining to*

THORACIC AORTA AND ARTERIAL BRANCHES   The **thoracic aorta** travels inferiorly through the thoracic cavity (see Figure 5-10). It branches into arteries that bring oxygenated blood to the esophagus, muscles between the ribs, diaphragm, upper spinal cord, and back.

ABDOMINAL AORTA AND ARTERIAL BRANCHES   As the thoracic aorta goes through the diaphragm, it becomes the **abdominal aorta** (see Figure 5-10). The abdominal aorta brings oxygenated blood to organs in the abdominopelvic cavity. These include the stomach, liver, gallbladder, pancreas, spleen, small intestine, large intestine, adrenal glands, kidneys (the **renal arteries**), ovaries (in a woman), testes (in a man), and the lower spinal cord.

In the pelvic cavity, the abdominal aorta ends and splits in two (a bifurcation) to form the inverted Y of the right and left iliac arteries (see Figure 5-10). The **iliac arteries** bring oxygenated blood to the hip and groin. Each iliac artery continues as the **femoral artery**, which brings oxygenated blood to the upper leg. Near the knee joint, the femoral artery becomes the **popliteal artery**. The popliteal artery then divides into the **tibial artery**, which brings oxygenated blood to the front and back of the lower leg, and the **peroneal artery**, which brings oxygenated blood to the little toe side of the lower leg along the fibula bone.

DID YOU KNOW?

The femoral artery takes its name from the femur (the bone in the upper leg). The popliteal artery takes its name from the popliteus, a small muscle at the back of the knee. The tibial artery takes its name from the tibia (the main bone in the lower leg). The peroneal artery goes along the fibula (the smaller bone in the lower leg). *Peroneal* is the adjective for *fibula*.

PULMONARY ARTERIES   The **pulmonary arteries** originate from the pulmonary trunk, which comes from the right ventricle of the heart (see Figure 5-9). They carry deoxygenated blood to the lungs.

VENAE CAVAE AND VEINS   The two major veins of the body are the superior vena cava and inferior vena cava (see Figure 5-9). The **superior vena cava** carries blood from the head, neck, arms, and chest to the right atrium. The **inferior vena cava** carries blood from the rest of the body (abdomen, pelvis, and legs, but not the lungs) to the right atrium. The **pulmonary veins** carry oxygenated blood from the lungs to the left atrium of the heart. Other major veins include the **jugular vein** (that carries blood from the head to the superior vena cava), the **portal vein** (that carries blood from the intestines to the liver), and the **saphenous vein** and **femoral vein** (that carry blood from the leg to the groin).

DID YOU KNOW?

The jugular vein takes its name from a Latin word that means *neck*. The portal vein takes its name from the porta hepatis, the Latin phrase for the portal or site where the vein enters the liver. (*Hepatis* is a Latin word meaning *of the liver*.) The saphenous vein takes its name from a Latin word that means *clearly visible*, as this vein often can be seen through the skin of the posterior lower leg.

Pronunciation/Word Parts

thoracic (thor-AS-ik)
 thorac/o- *chest; thorax*
 -ic *pertaining to*

abdominal (ab-DAW-mih-nal)
 abdomin/o- *abdomen*
 -al *pertaining to*

renal (REE-nal)
 ren/o- *kidney*
 -al *pertaining to*

iliac (IL-ee-ak)
 ili/o- *hip bone; ilium*
 -ac *pertaining to*

femoral (FEM-oh-ral)
 femor/o- *femur; thigh bone*
 -al *pertaining to*

popliteal (pop-LIT-ee-al) (POP-lih-TEE-al)
 poplite/o- *back of the knee*
 -al *pertaining to*

tibial (TIB-ee-al)
 tibi/o- *shin bone; tibia*
 -al *pertaining to*

peroneal (PAIR-oh-NEE-al)
 perone/o- *fibula; lower leg bone*
 -al *pertaining to*

pulmonary (PUL-moh-NAIR-ee)
 pulmon/o- *lung*
 -ary *pertaining to*

vena cava (VEE-nah KAY-vah)
 Vena is a Latin singular noun. Form the plural by changing -*a* to -*ae*. Example: The superior and inferior venae cavae.

jugular (JUG-yoo-lar)
 jugul/o- *jugular; throat*
 -ar *pertaining to*

portal (POR-tal)
 port/o- *point of entry*
 -al *pertaining to*

saphenous (sah-FEE-nus)
 saphen/o- *clearly visible*
 -ous *pertaining to*

Circulation

Circulation of the blood occurs through two different pathways (see Figure 5-11 ■): the systemic circulation and the pulmonary circulation.

1. **Systemic circulation.** Arteries, arterioles, capillaries, venules, and veins everywhere in the body, except in the lungs.

2. **Pulmonary circulation**. Arteries, arterioles, capillaries, venules, and veins going to, within, and coming from the lungs. The word **cardiopulmonary** reflects the close connection between the heart and the lungs.

Now let's trace the route that blood takes as it travels through the systemic and pulmonary circulations to complete one trip through the whole body.

Pronunciation/Word Parts

circulation (SIR-kyoo-LAY-shun)
  circulat/o- *movement in a circular route*
  -ion *action; condition*

systemic (sis-TEM-ik)
  system/o- *body as a whole*
  -ic *pertaining to*

cardiopulmonary
(KAR-dee-oh-PUL-moh-NAIR-ee)
  cardi/o- *heart*
  pulmon/o- *lung*
  -ary *pertaining to*

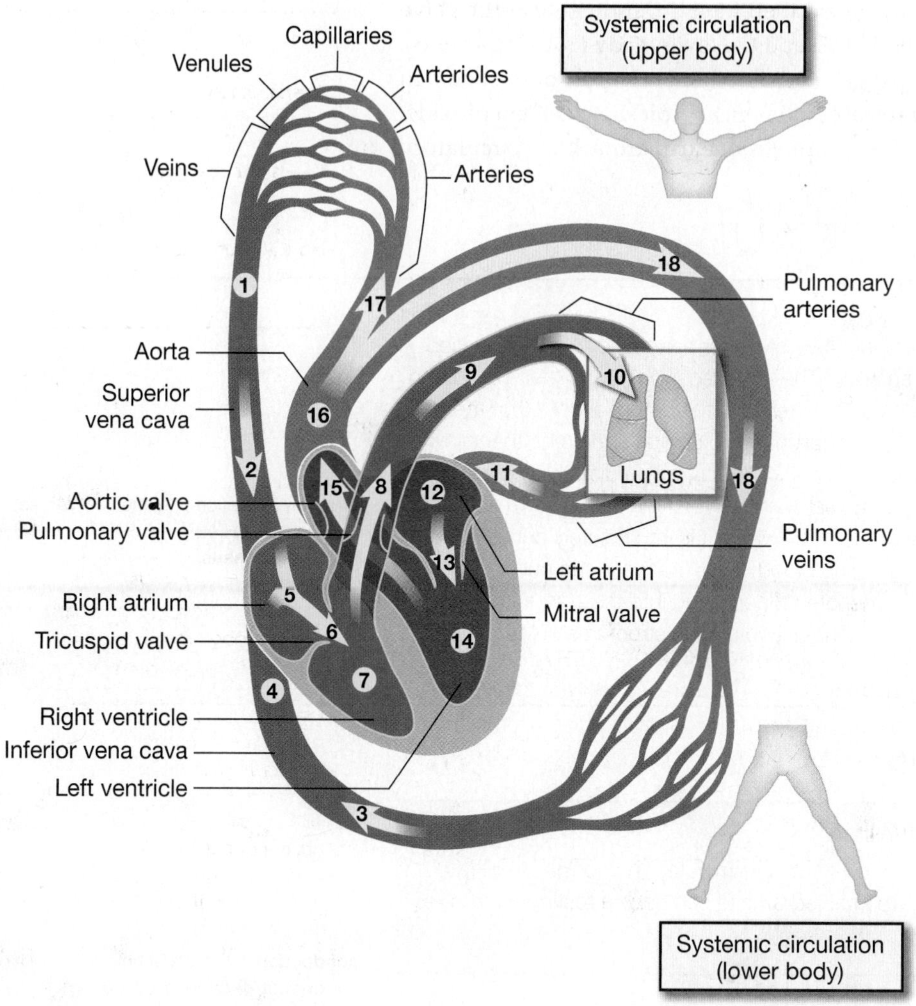

FIGURE 5-11 ■ Circulation of the blood.

Blood low in oxygen in veins from the upper body (1) and the lower body (3) comes into the heart via the superior vena cava (2) and the inferior vena cava (4). Each time the heart contracts, it pumps blood from the right atrium (5), through the tricuspid valve (6), into the right ventricle (7), then through the pulmonary valve (8), pulmonary trunk (9) and the pulmonary arteries (10) to the lungs. At the same time, the heart receives oxygenated blood from the lungs via the pulmonary veins (11). This blood comes into the left atrium (12), goes through the mitral valve (13) and into the left ventricle (14) and then goes through the aortic valve (15), into the aorta (16) to the upper body (17) and to the lower body (18).

Source: Pearson Education

Pronunciation/Word Parts

SYSTEMIC CIRCULATION THROUGH THE VEINS   Blood coming from the cells is dark red-purple in color because it has a low level of oxygen. Blood coming from cells in the upper body (1) travels through capillaries, venules, and veins to the superior vena cava (2). Blood coming from cells in the lower body (3) travels through capillaries, venules, and veins to the inferior vena cava (4). Then this blood travels through the right atrium (5), tricuspid valve (6), and right ventricle (7).

PULMONARY CIRCULATION   At this point, the blood enters the pulmonary circulation. The blood travels through the pulmonary valve (8), pulmonary trunk (9), and pulmonary arteries (10) and arterioles to the capillaries in the lungs. In a capillary beside an alveolus, the blood releases carbon dioxide, picks up oxygen, and becomes bright red in color. The blood then travels through the pulmonary veins (11) to the left atrium (12) of the heart.

SYSTEMIC CIRCULATION THROUGH THE ARTERIES   At this point, the blood is back in the systemic circulation. From the left atrium (12), the blood travels through the mitral valve (13) and left ventricle (14). The blood then travels through the aortic valve (15) and into the aorta (16) to the upper body (17) and the lower body (18). The arteries, arterioles, and capillaries distribute this oxygenated blood to every part of the body. In a capillary beside a body cell, the blood releases oxygen, and picks up carbon dioxide, and becomes dark red-purple in color. This completes one trip around the circulatory system.

CLINICAL CONNECTIONS

Neonatology. The fetal heart begins to beat just 4 weeks after conception. The circulation of blood in a fetus is different from that of an adult. The fetus receives oxygenated blood and nutrients from the mother through the placenta, via arteries in the umbilical cord that merge with the inferior vena cava of the fetus. The fetal heart has two unique structures that allow this oxygenated blood to bypass the (not-yet functioning) lungs and go directly to the body. The **foramen ovale**, a small, oval opening in the septum between the atria, allows some of the oxygenated blood to enter the left side of the heart where it is immediately pumped out to the body. The **ductus arteriosus**, a connecting blood vessel between the pulmonary trunk and the aorta, allows the rest of the oxygenated blood to go into the right ventricle and pulmonary trunk but then diverts it to the aorta. These two unique structures in the fetal heart close automatically within 24 hours after birth.

foramen ovale (foh-RAY-men oh-VAL-ee)

ductus arteriosus (DUK-tus ar-TEER-ee-OH-sus)

DID YOU KNOW?

The normal heart rate for a newborn is 110–150 beats per minute. The normal heart rate for an adult is 70–80 beats per minute. A well-trained athlete can have a resting heart rate lower than 60 beats per minute.

conduction (con-DUK-shun)
  conduct/o- *carrying; conveying*
  -ion *action; condition*

sinoatrial (SY-noh-AA-tree-al)
  sin/o- *channel; hollow cavity*
  atri/o- *atrium; chamber that is open at the top*
  -al *pertaining to*

node (NOHD)

Physiology of a Heartbeat

The heart contracts and relaxes in a regular rhythm that is coordinated by the **conduction system** of the heart (see Figure 5-12 ■). The **sinoatrial node (SA node)** (in the wall of the right atrium), is the pacemaker of the heart. It initiates the electrical impulse that begins each heartbeat. This impulse causes both atria to contract simultaneously.

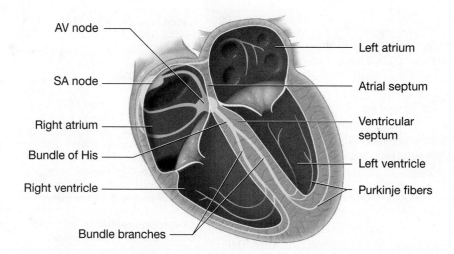

FIGURE 5-12 ■ Conduction system of the heart.
The SA node (pacemaker) initiates an electrical impulse that travels through the AV node, the bundle of His, the right and left bundle branches, and then to the Purkinje fibers, causing the atria and then the ventricles to contract.
Source: Pearson Education

The electrical impulse then travels through the **atrioventricular node (AV node)** (in the right atrium near the septum), through the **bundle of His**, and into the right and left **bundle branches** that end in a network of nerves (the **Purkinje fibers**). Then both ventricles contract simultaneously. A contraction is known as **systole**, and the resting period between contractions is known as **diastole**.

Pronunciation/Word Parts

atrioventricular
(AA-tree-OH-ven-TRIH-kyoo-lar)
  atri/o- atrium; chamber that is open at the top
  ventricul/o- chamber that is filled; ventricle
  -ar pertaining to

bundle of His (HISS)

Purkinje (per-KIN-jee)

systole (SIS-toh-lee)

systolic (sis-TAW-lik)
  systol/o- contracting
  -ic pertaining to

diastole (dy-AS-toh-lee)

diastolic (DY-ah-STAW-lik)
  diastol/o- dilating
  -ic pertaining to

epinephrine (EH-pih-NEF-rin)

CLINICAL CONNECTIONS

Neurology. The heart rate is controlled by the SA node, as well as by the parasympathetic and sympathetic divisions of the nervous system. The SA node continually generates an impulse of 80–100 beats each minute, but this is faster than the body needs. So the parasympathetic division (through the vagal nerve) releases the neurotransmitter acetylcholine; this slows the heart to its normal resting heart rate of 70–80 beats each minute. The sympathetic division (through spinal cord nerves) releases the neurotransmitter norepinephrine to increase the heart rate. So, fine adjustments in the heart rate are possible from moment to moment. When the heart needs to beat much faster during exercise (see Figure 5-13 ■) or to escape danger (the "fight-or-flight" response), the sympathetic division stimulates the adrenal gland to secrete the hormone **epinephrine**. It travels through the blood to the heart, overrides the normal sinus rhythm, and causes the heart to beat much faster.

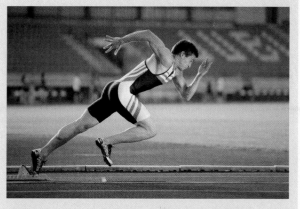

FIGURE 5-13 ■ Exercise increases the heart rate.
During exercise, epinephrine secreted by the adrenal glands increases the heart rate, constricts the arteries to increase the blood pressure, and dilates the bronchi to increase the flow of air into the lungs.
Source: Peter Bernick/Shutterstock

When the SA node controls the heart beat, the heart is in **normal sinus rhythm (NSR)**. Besides the SA node, several other areas in the atria and ventricles can produce electrical impulses on their own. These impulses are usually too weak to override the SA node. However, if the SA node fails to produce impulses, if the SA node impulses are blocked, or if these other areas become hyperexcited (from excessive amounts of caffeine or smoking), then these **ectopic** sites can take over and produce an abnormal heart rhythm.

sinus (SIGH-nus)
The SA node is in a sinus (a recessed area or channel) in the right atrium.

ectopic (ek-TAW-pik)
  ectop/o- outside
  -ic pertaining to

A CLOSER LOOK

Electrical Activity of the Heart. On a molecular level, an elegant and intricate system allows the heart to contract tirelessly, approximately 100,000 times each day. An electrical impulse from the SA node changes the permeability of a myocardial cell. Sodium ions (Na^+) outside the cell move through the cell membrane, followed by calcium ions (Ca^{++}). This gives the inside of the cell a positive electrical charge, which triggers the release of calcium ions stored inside the cell. This process is known as **depolarization** because it reverses the normal, slightly negative electrical state of the cell. The calcium ions cause the myocardial cell to contract. As one cell depolarizes and contracts, it triggers the next myocardial cell to do the same.

A contraction ends when potassium ions (K^+) move out of the cell, while tiny molecular pumps move sodium ions and some calcium ions out of the cell and move the rest of the calcium ions back into storage within the cell. This process is known as **repolarization**. This restores the normal, slightly negative electrical state of a resting myocardial cell. The myocardial cell is now ready for another impulse from the SA node.

A myocardial cell cannot respond to another electrical impulse from the SA node until the full cycle of depolarization and repolarization is complete. This very short period of unresponsiveness is known as the **refractory period**.

Pronunciation/Word Parts

depolarization (dee-POH-lar-ih-ZAY-shun)
  de- *reversal of; without*
  polar/o- *negative state; positive state*
  -ization *process of creating; process of inserting; process of making*

repolarization (ree-POH-lar-ih-ZAY-shun)
  re- *again and again; backward; unable to*
  polar/o- *negative state; positive state*
  -ization *process of creating; process of inserting; process of making*

refractory (ree-FRAK-tor-ee)
  re- *again and again; backward; unable to*
  fract/o- *bend; break up*
  -ory *having the function of*
Select the correct prefix meaning to get the definition of *refractory*: having the function of (being) unable to break up.

WORD ALERT

cardia   (noun)   Small region of the stomach where the esophagus enters
  Example: *The cardia is the first part of the stomach to receive food from the esophagus.*

cardiac   (adjective)   Pertaining to the heart
  Example: *During a cardiac arrest, the heart stops beating.*

cardiac valve   (noun)   Structure between two chambers of the heart (or between a heart chamber and a blood vessel). It opens and closes to regulate the flow of blood.

  Example: *A stethoscope allows you to hear the sound that a cardiac valve makes as it opens and closes.*

Vocabulary Review

Anatomy and Physiology		
Word or Phrase	**Description**	**Combining Forms**
cardiopulmonary	Pertaining to the heart and lungs	**cardi/o-** *heart* **pulmon/o-** *lung*
cardiothoracic	Pertaining to the heart and thoracic cavity	**cardi/o-** *heart* **thorac/o-** *chest; thorax*
cardiovascular system	Body system that includes the heart and the blood vessels (vascular structures)	**cardi/o-** *heart* **vascul/o-** *blood vessel*
circulatory system	Continuous, circular pathway that the blood takes as it moves through the body. **Circulation** is the process of moving the blood through the system. The circulatory system consists of the systemic circulation and the pulmonary circulation.	**circulat/o-** *movement in a circular route*
mediastinum	Irregularly shaped, central area in the **thoracic cavity** that lies between the lungs. It contains the heart, parts of the great vessels, as well as the thymus, trachea, and esophagus.	**mediastin/o-** *mediastinum* **thorac/o-** *chest; thorax*
pulmonary circulation	The arteries, arterioles, capillaries, venules, and veins going to, within, and coming from the lungs	**pulmon/o-** *lung*
systemic circulation	The arteries, arterioles, capillaries, venules, and veins everywhere in the body, except in the lungs	**system/o-** *body as a whole*

Heart		
aortic valve	Heart valve between the left ventricle and the aorta	**aort/o-** *aorta* **valvul/o-** *valve*
atrium	Each of the two upper chambers of the heart	**atri/o-** *atrium; chamber that is open at the top*
chordae tendineae	Rope-like strands that support the tricuspid and mitral valve leaflets and keep them tightly closed when the ventricles are contracting	
ductus arteriosus	Temporary blood vessel in the fetal heart that connects the pulmonary trunk to the aorta. It closes within 24 hours after birth.	
endocardium	Innermost layer that lines the atria, ventricles, and valves of the heart	**cardi/o-** *heart*
foramen ovale	Temporary, oval-shaped opening in the interatrial septum of the fetal heart. It closes within 24 hours after birth.	
heart	Organ that pumps blood throughout the body. It contains four chambers, the **septum** (a center wall), and four valves. The lower tip of the heart is the **apex**. The adjective for *heart* is *cardiac*.	**cardi/o-** *heart* **card/i-** *heart* **sept/o-** *dividing wall; septum* **apic/o-** *apex; tip*
mitral valve	Heart valve between the left atrium and the left ventricle. It is also known as the **bicuspid valve**. It has two (*bi-*) **leaflets** or **cusps**.	**mitr/o-** *structure like a tall hat with two points* **valvul/o-** *valve* **cusp/o-** *point; projection*
myocardium	Muscular layer of the heart	**my/o-** *muscle* **cardi/o-** *heart*

Word or Phrase	Description	Combining Forms
pericardium	Membrane that surrounds the heart as the **pericardial sac** and is filled with **pericardial fluid**. The part of the membrane next to the surface of the heart is the **visceral pericardium** or **epicardium**. The part in the outer wall of the pericardial sac is the **parietal pericardium**.	**cardi/o-** heart **viscer/o-** large internal organs **pariet/o-** wall of a cavity
pulmonary valve	Heart valve between the right ventricle and the pulmonary trunk	**pulmon/o-** lung **valvul/o-** valve
tricuspid valve	Heart valve between the right atrium and right ventricle. It has three (*tri-*) **leaflets** or **cusps**.	**cusp/o-** point; projection **valvul/o-** valve
valve	Structure that opens and closes to control the flow of blood. Heart valves include the tricuspid valve, pulmonary valve, mitral valve, and aortic valve. There are also valves in some of the large veins to prevent backflow of blood.	**valvul/o-** valve **valv/o-** valve
ventricle	Each of the two large, lower chambers of the heart	**ventricul/o-** chamber that is filled; ventricle
Blood Vessels		
aorta	Largest artery. It receives oxygenated blood from the left ventricle. It includes the **ascending aorta**, the **aortic arch**, the **thoracic aorta**, and the **abdominal aorta**.	**aort/o-** aorta **thorac/o-** chest; thorax **abdomin/o-** abdomen
arteriole	Smallest branch of an artery	**arteriol/o-** arteriole
artery	Blood vessel that carries oxygenated blood away from the heart to the body. This bright red blood has a high level of oxygen. (The pulmonary arteries carry blood from the heart to the lungs. They carry dark red-purple blood with a low level of oxygen.)	**arteri/o-** artery **arter/o-** artery
axillary artery	Artery that carries oxygenated blood to the axilla (armpit) area	**axill/o-** armpit
blood vessels	Large and small channels through which the blood circulates throughout the body. These include arteries, arterioles, capillaries, venules, and veins that are also known as **vascular structures**. The **lumen** is the central opening inside a blood vessel through which the blood flows.	**angi/o-** blood vessel; lymphatic vessel **vascul/o-** blood vessel **vas/o-** blood vessel; vas deferens
brachial artery	Artery that carries oxygenated blood to the upper arm	**brachi/o-** arm
capillary	Smallest blood vessel in the body. A capillary network connects the arterioles to the venules. The exchange of oxygen and carbon dioxide takes place in the capillaries.	**capill/o-** capillary; hair-like structure
carotid artery	Artery that carries oxygenated blood to the neck, face, head, and brain. If these arteries are compressed, the lack of blood to the brain will cause a person to become unconscious.	**carot/o-** sleep; stupor
coronary artery	Artery that carries oxygenated blood to the myocardium (heart muscle)	**coron/o-** structure that encircles like a crown
endothelium	Smooth layer that lines the inner wall of a blood vessel. It is also known as the **intima**.	**theli/o-** cellular layer
femoral artery	Artery that carries oxygenated blood to the upper leg	**femor/o-** femur; thigh bone
great vessels	Collective phrase for the aorta (the largest artery), the superior and inferior venae cavae (the largest veins), and the pulmonary trunk, pulmonary arteries, and pulmonary veins	

Word or Phrase	Description	Combining Forms
iliac artery	Artery that carries oxygenated blood to the hip and groin area	**ili/o-** *hip bone; ilium*
jugular vein	Vein that carries blood from the head to the superior vena cava	**jugul/o-** *jugular; throat*
peroneal artery	Artery that carries oxygenated blood to the little toe side of the lower leg (along the fibula bone)	**perone/o-** *fibula; lower leg bone*
popliteal artery	Artery that carries oxygenated blood to the back of the knee and then branches into the tibial and peroneal arteries	**poplite/o-** *back of the knee*
portal vein	Vein that carries blood from the intestines to the liver	**port/o-** *point of entry*
pulmonary artery	Artery that carries blood away from the heart to the lungs. The pulmonary artery is the only artery that carries blood that has a low level of oxygen.	**pulmon/o-** *lung*
pulmonary vein	Vein that carries oxygenated blood from the lungs to the heart. The pulmonary vein is the only vein that carries blood that has a high level of oxygen.	**pulmon/o-** *lung*
pulse	The bulging of the wall of an artery located near the surface as blood is pumped by the heart	
radial artery	Artery that carries oxygenated blood to the thumb side of the lower arm (along the radius bone)	**radi/o-** *forearm bone; radiation; x-rays*
renal artery	Artery that carries oxygenated blood to the kidney	**ren/o-** *kidney*
saphenous vein	Vein that carries blood from the leg to the groin	**saphen/o-** *clearly visible*
subclavian artery	Artery that carries oxygenated blood to the shoulder. It goes underneath *(sub-)* the clavicle (collar bone).	**clav/o-** *clavicle; collar bone*
tibial artery	Artery that carries oxygenated blood to the front and back of the lower leg	**tibi/o-** *shin bone; tibia*
ulnar artery	Artery that carries oxygenated blood to the little finger side of the lower arm (along the ulna bone)	**uln/o-** *forearm bone; ulna*
vasculature	Blood vessels associated with a particular organ	**vascul/o-** *blood vessel*
vasoconstriction	Constriction of smooth muscle in the wall of a blood vessel that causes the lumen to decrease in size	**vas/o-** *blood vessel; vas deferens* **constrict/o-** *drawn together; narrowed*
vasodilation	Relaxation of smooth muscle in the wall of a blood vessel that causes the lumen to increase in size	**vas/o-** *blood vessel; vas deferens* **dilat/o-** *dilate; widen*
vein	Blood vessel that carries blood from the body back to the heart. This blood has a low level of oxygen and a high level of carbon dioxide and waste products of cellular metabolism from the cells. The exception is the pulmonary veins that carry blood that has a high level of oxygen from the lungs back to the heart.	**ven/o-** *vein* **phleb/o-** *vein*
venae cavae	The two major veins. The **superior vena cava** carries blood from the head, neck, arms, and chest back to the right atrium of the heart. The **inferior vena cava** carries blood from the abdomen, pelvis, and legs back to the right atrium.	
venule	Smallest branch of a vein	**ven/o-** *vein*

Conduction System		
Word or Phrase	**Description**	**Combining Forms**
atrioventricular (AV) node	Small area of tissue between the right atrium near the septum. The AV node is part of the conduction system of the heart and receives electrical impulses from the SA node.	**atri/o-** *atrium; chamber that is open at the top* **ventricul/o-** *chamber that is filled; ventricle*
bundle branches	Part of the conduction system of the heart after the bundle of His. At the apex of the heart, the branches split into the right bundle branch to the right ventricle and the left bundle branch to the left ventricle. Then, each divides into the **Purkinje fibers** that spread across the ventricles.	
bundle of His	Part of the conduction system of the heart after the AV node. It splits into the right and left bundle branches.	
conduction system	System that carries the electrical impulse that makes the heart beat. It consists of the SA node, AV node, bundle of His, bundle branches, and Purkinje fibers.	**conduct/o-** *carrying; conveying*
depolarization	To begin a contraction of the heart, an impulse from the SA node changes the permeability of the myocardial cell membrane. Positive sodium ions, then positive calcium ions, outside the cell move through the cell membrane, and more calcium ions stored in the cell are released. This reverses the normally negative state in a resting myocardial cell and causes a contraction.	**polar/o-** *negative state; positive state*
diastole	Resting period between contractions	**diastol/o-** *dilating*
ectopic site	Area within the heart that can produce an electrical impulse but is not part of the conduction system. It sometimes overrides the impulse of the SA node and produces an abnormal heart rhythm.	**ectop/o-** *outside*
refractory period	Short period of time when the myocardium is unresponsive to electrical impulses	**fract/o-** *bend; break up*
repolarization	To end a contraction of the heart, positive potassium ions diffuse out of the cell, while molecular pumps move positive sodium and some calcium ions out of the cell and move the rest of the calcium ions into storage within the cell. This restores the slightly negative state of a resting myocardial cell.	**polar/o-** *negative state; positive state*
sinoatrial node	Pacemaker of the heart. Small area of tissue in the posterior wall of the right atrium. The SA node originates the electrical impulse for the entire conduction system of the heart.	**sin/o-** *channel; hollow cavity* **atri/o-** *atrium; chamber that is open at the top*
systole	Contraction of the atria or the ventricles	**systol/o-** *contracting*

Give Word Part Meanings

Use the Answer Key at the end of the book to check your answers.

Combining Forms Exercise

Next to each combining form, write its meaning. The first one has been done for you.

Combining Form	Meaning	Combining Form	Meaning
1. axill/o-	armpit	29. mitr/o-	
2. abdomin/o-		30. my/o-	
3. angi/o-		31. pariet/o-	
4. aort/o-		32. perone/o-	
5. apic/o-		33. phleb/o-	
6. arteri/o-		34. polar/o-	
7. arteriol/o-		35. poplite/o-	
8. arter/o-		36. port/o-	
9. atri/o-		37. pulmon/o-	
10. brachi/o-		38. radi/o-	
11. capill/o-		39. ren/o-	
12. card/i-		40. saphen/o-	
13. cardi/o-		41. sept/o-	
14. carot/o-		42. sin/o-	
15. circulat/o-		43. system/o-	
16. clav/o-		44. systol/o-	
17. conduct/o-		45. theli/o-	
18. constrict/o-		46. thorac/o-	
19. coron/o-		47. tibi/o-	
20. cusp/o-		48. uln/o-	
21. diastol/o-		49. valv/o-	
22. dilat/o-		50. valvul/o-	
23. ectop/o-		51. vascul/o-	
24. femor/o-		52. vas/o-	
25. fract/o-		53. ven/o-	
26. ili/o-		54. ventricul/o-	
27. jugul/o-		55. viscer/o-	
28. mediastin/o-			

Build Medical Words

Combining Form and Suffix Exercise

Read the definition of the medical word. Look at the combining form that is given. Select the correct suffix from the Suffix List and write it on the blank line. Then build the medical word and write it on the line. (Remember: You may need to remove the combining vowel. Always remove the hyphens and slash.) Be sure to check your spelling. The first one has been done for you.

SUFFIX LIST

-ac (pertaining to)	-ary (pertaining to)	-ion (action; condition)	-ous (pertaining to)
-al (pertaining to)	-ature (system composed of)	-ole (small thing)	-ule (small thing)
-ar (pertaining to)	-ic (pertaining to)	-ory (having the function of)	

	Definition of the Medical Word	Combining Form	Suffix	Build the Medical Word
1.	Pertaining to (the) chest	thorac/o-	-ic	thoracic

(You think *pertaining to* (-ic) + *chest* (thorac/o-). You change the order of the word parts to put the suffix last. You write *thoracic*.)

2.	Pertaining to (an) artery	arteri/o-	_____	_____
3.	Pertaining to (a) valve	valvul/o-	_____	_____
4.	Action (of) movement in a circular route	circulat/o-	_____	_____
5.	Pertaining to (the) heart	cardi/o-	_____	_____
6.	Pertaining to (a) hair-like structure (blood vessel)	capill/o-	_____	_____
7.	Pertaining to (a) vein	ven/o-	_____	_____
8.	Pertaining to (the) body as a whole	system/o-	_____	_____
9.	Pertaining to (the) atrium	atri/o-	_____	_____
10.	Pertaining to (the) arm	brachi/o-	_____	_____
11.	Small thing (that is an) artery	arteri/o-	_____	_____
12.	Pertaining to (a vein that is) clearly visible	saphen/o-	_____	_____
13.	Pertaining to (the) aorta	aort/o-	_____	_____
14.	System composed of blood vessel(s)	vascul/o-	_____	_____
15.	Pertaining to contracting	systol/o-	_____	_____
16.	Having the function of movement in a circular route	circulat/o-	_____	_____
17.	Pertaining to (the) ventricle	ventricul/o-	_____	_____
18.	Small thing (that is a) vein	ven/o-	_____	_____

Multiple Combining Forms and Suffix Exercise

Read the definition of the medical word. Look at the correct suffix that is given. Select the two correct combining forms from the Combining Form List. Then build the medical word and write it on the line. Be sure to check your spelling. The first one has been done for you.

COMBINING FORM LIST

atri/o- (atrium; chamber that is open at the top)	dilat/o- (dilate; widen)	vascul/o- (blood vessel)
	my/o- (muscle)	vas/o- (blood vessel; vas deferens)
cardi/o- (heart)	pulmon/o- (lung)	ventricul/o- (chamber that is filled;
constrict/o- (drawn together; narrowed)	sin/o- (channel; hollow cavity)	ventricle)

Definition of the Medical Word	Combining Form	Combining Form	Suffix	Build the Medical Word
1. Condition (of) blood vessel(s being) dilated	vas/o-	dilat/o-	-ion	vasodilation
(You think *condition* (-ion) + *blood vessel* (vas/o-) + *dilated* (dilat/o-). You change the order of the word parts to put the suffix last. You write *vasodilation*.)				
2. Pertaining to (the) heart (and) lungs	_____	_____	-ary	_____
3. Pertaining to (the) heart (and) blood vessel(s)	_____	_____	-ar	_____
4. Pertaining to (the) SA (node)	_____	_____	-al	_____
5. Condition (of) blood vessel(s being) narrowed	_____	_____	-ion	_____
6. Pertaining to (the) muscle (of the) heart	_____	_____	-al	_____
7. Pertaining to (the) atrium (and) ventricle	_____	_____	-ar	_____

Diseases

Myocardium		
Word or Phrase	**Description**	**Pronunciation/Word Parts**
acute coronary syndrome	Syndrome that includes acute **ischemia** of the myocardium (because of a blood clot or atherosclerosis blocking blood flow through a coronary artery) and unstable angina pectoris. Treatment: Nitroglycerin drug, thrombolytic drug, oxygen therapy.	**ischemia** (is-KEE-mee-ah) **isch/o-** *block; keep back* **-emia** *condition of the blood; substance in the blood*
angina pectoris	Mild-to-severe chest pain caused by ischemia of the myocardium. Atherosclerosis blocks the flow of oxygenated blood through the coronary arteries to the myocardium. **Anginal** pain is a crushing, squeezing, heaviness, or pressure-like sensation in the chest, with pain extending up into the jaw, teeth, neck, or down the left arm, often with extreme sweating (diaphoresis) and a sense of doom. Angina pectoris can occur during exercise, stress, after a heavy meal, or while resting. It is a warning sign of an impending myocardial infarction. Treatment: Nitroglycerin drug, oxygen therapy.	**angina** (AN-jih-nah) (an-JY-nah) **pectoris** (PEK-toh-ris) The combining form **pector/o-** means *chest*. **anginal** (AN-jih-nal) (an-JY-nal) **angin/o-** *angina* **-al** *pertaining to*

> **DID YOU KNOW?**
>
> For many years, newspaper and magazine articles described the classic symptoms of angina pectoris in order to raise public awareness and encourage those with angina to promptly seek medical help. Now it is known that those symptoms occur in men, but women most often experience angina as indigestion, nausea, anxiety, extreme fatigue, or trouble sleeping.

cardiomegaly	Enlargement of the heart, usually due to congestive heart failure. Treatment: Correct the underlying cause.	**cardiomegaly** (KAR-dee-oh-MEG-ah-lee) **cardi/o-** *heart* **-megaly** *enlargement*
cardiomyopathy	Any disease condition of the heart muscle that includes heart enlargement and heart failure. In **dilated cardiomyopathy**, the left ventricle is dilated and the myocardium is so stretched that it can no longer contract to pump blood. **Idiopathic cardiomyopathy** has an unknown cause. Treatment: Correct the underlying cause, if known.	**cardiomyopathy** (KAR-dee-OH-my-AW-pah-thee) **cardi/o-** *heart* **my/o-** *muscle* **-pathy** *disease* **idiopathic** (ID-ee-oh-PATH-ik) **idi/o-** *individual; unknown* **path/o-** *disease* **-ic** *pertaining to*

Word or Phrase	Description	Pronunciation/Word Parts
congestive heart failure (CHF)	Inability of the heart to pump sufficient amounts of blood. It is caused by coronary artery disease or hypertension. During early CHF, the myocardium undergoes **hypertrophy** (enlargement). This temporarily improves blood flow, and the patient is in **compensated** heart failure. In the later stages of CHF, the heart can no longer enlarge. Instead, the myocardium becomes flabby and loses its ability to contract, and the patient is in **decompensated** heart failure. Either side or both sides of the heart may fail. In right-sided congestive heart failure, the right ventricle is unable to adequately pump blood. Blood backs up in the superior vena cava, causing **jugular venous distention** (dilated jugular veins in the neck). Blood also backs up in the inferior vena cava, causing hepatomegaly (enlargement of the liver) and **peripheral edema** in the legs, ankles, and feet (see Figure 5-14 ■). Lung disease and increased pressure in the lungs cause the right ventricle to become enlarged; this condition is **cor pulmonale**. In left-sided congestive heart failure, the left ventricle is unable to adequately pump blood. The blood backs up into the lungs, causing pulmonary congestion and edema that can be seen on a chest x-ray. There is also shortness of breath, cough, and an inability to sleep while lying flat. Treatment: Diuretic drug, digitalis drug, and antihypertensive drug. Severe left-sided heart failure is life-threatening; it may require surgery for a heart transplant or a left ventricular assist device (LVAD). 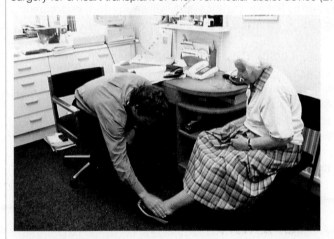 **FIGURE 5-14 ■ Peripheral edema.** This patient is complaining of ankle swelling. The physician knows that fluid-filled soft tissues in the feet and lower legs can be a sign of right-sided congestive heart failure. He will also examine the neck veins to look for jugular venous distention, another sign of right-sided congestive heart failure. He will use a stethoscope to listen to the lungs to detect pulmonary edema, a sign of left-sided heart failure. *Source*: Antonia Reeve/Science Source	**congestive** (con-JES-tiv) 　**congest/o-** *accumulation of fluid* 　**-ive** *pertaining to* **hypertrophy** (hy-PER-troh-fee) 　**hyper-** *above; more than normal* 　**-trophy** *process of development* The ending *-trophy* contains the combining form **troph/o-** and the one-letter suffix *-y*. **compensated** (KAWM-pen-SAY-ted) 　**compens/o-** *compensate; counterbalance* 　**-ated** *composed of; pertaining to a condition* **decompensated** (dee-KAWM-pen-SAY-ted) 　**de-** *reversal of; without* 　**compens/o-** *compensate; counterbalance* 　**-ated** *composed of; pertaining to a condition* **peripheral** (peh-RIF-eh-ral) 　**peripher/o-** *outer aspects* 　**-al** *pertaining to* **edema** (eh-DEE-mah) **cor pulmonale** (KOR PUL-moh-NAL-ee) *Cor* is the Latin word for *heart*.
myocardial infarction (MI)	Death of myocardial cells due to severe ischemia. The flow of oxygenated blood in a coronary artery is blocked by a blood clot or atherosclerosis. The patient may experience severe angina pectoris, may have mild symptoms similar to indigestion, or may have no symptoms at all (a silent MI). The infarcted area of myocardium has dead tissue or **necrosis**. If the area of necrosis is small, it will eventually be replaced by scar tissue. If the area is large, the heart muscle may be unable to contract and the patient will die. Also known as a **heart attack**. Treatment: Baby aspirin taken to prevent an MI or at the first sign of an MI. Thrombolytic drug to dissolve a clot during an MI.	**myocardial** (MY-oh-KAR-dee-al) 　**my/o-** *muscle* 　**cardi/o-** *heart* 　**-al** *pertaining to* **infarction** (in-FARK-shun) 　**infarct/o-** *small area of dead tissue* 　**-ion** *action; condition* **necrosis** (neh-KROH-sis) 　**necr/o-** *dead body; dead cells; dead tissue* 　**-osis** *condition; process*

Heart Valves and Layers of the Heart

Word or Phrase	Description	Pronunciation/Word Parts
endocarditis	Inflammation and bacterial infection of the endocardium lining a heart valve. This occurs in patients who have a structural defect of the valve. Bacteria from an infection elsewhere in the body travel through the blood, are trapped by the structural defect, and cause infection. Acute endocarditis causes a high fever and shock, while **subacute bacterial endocarditis (SBE)** causes fever, fatigue, and aching muscles. Treatment: Antibiotic drug.	**endocarditis** (EN-doh-kar-DY-tis) **endo-** *innermost; within* **card/i-** *heart* **-itis** *infection of; inflammation of* The combining vowel *i* of *card/i-* is deleted before it is joined to the suffix *-itis*. **subacute** (SUB-ah-KYOOT)
mitral valve prolapse (MVP)	Structural abnormality in which the leaflets of the mitral valve do not close tightly. This can be a congenital condition or can occur if the valve is damaged by infection. There is **regurgitation** as blood flows back into the left atrium with each contraction. A slight prolapse is a common condition and does not require treatment. Treatment: Valvoplasty, mitral valve ring implant, or valve replacement surgery.	**prolapse** (PROH-laps) **regurgitation** (ree-GER-jih-TAY-shun) **regurgitat/o-** *backward flow* **-ion** *action; condition*

CLINICAL CONNECTIONS

Neonatology. Congenital abnormalities can occur in the fetal heart as it develops:

1. **Coarctation of the aorta.** The aorta is abnormally narrow.
2. **Atrial septal defect (ASD).** There is a permanent hole in the interatrial septum.
3. **Ventricular septal defect (VSD).** There is a permanent hole in the interventricular septum.
4. **Tetralogy of Fallot.** There are four defects: a ventricular septal defect, narrowing of the pulmonary trunk, hypertrophy of the right ventricle, and abnormal position of the aorta.
5. **Transposition of the great vessels.** The aorta incorrectly comes from the right ventricle, and the pulmonary trunk incorrectly comes from the left ventricle.

coarctation (KOH-ark-TAY-shun)
coarct/o- *pressed together*
-ation *being; having; process*

tetralogy (teh-TRAL-oh-jee)
tetr/a- *four*
-logy *study of*

Fallot (fah-LOH)

The following abnormalities occur at the time of birth during the change from fetal circulation to normal newborn circulation:

1. **Patent ductus arteriosus (PDA).** The ductus arteriosus fails to close.
2. **Patent foramen ovale.** The foramen ovale fails to close.

patent (PAY-tent)
pat/o- *open*
-ent *pertaining to*

Word or Phrase	Description	Pronunciation/Word Parts
murmur	Abnormal heart sound created by turbulence as blood leaks through a defective heart valve. Murmurs are described according to their volume (soft or loud), their sound, and when they occur. Functional murmurs are mild murmurs that are not associated with disease and are not clinically significant. Treatment: Surgery to correct a severely defective heart valve (valvuloplasty).	**murmur** (MER-mer)

DID YOU KNOW?

Heart murmurs can sound like the call of a sea gull, blowing wind, the clatter of machinery, high-pitched musical notes, or like churning, humming, or clicking.

Word or Phrase	Description	Pronunciation/Word Parts

pericarditis	Inflammation or infection of the pericardial sac with an excessive accumulation of pericardial fluid. When the fluid compresses the heart and prevents it from beating, this is **cardiac tamponade**. Treatment: Antibiotic drug. Surgery to remove the fluid (pericardiocentesis).	**pericarditis** (PAIR-ee-kar-DY-tis)
		  peri- *around*
		  card/i- *heart*
		  -itis *infection of; inflammation of*
		
		tamponade (tam-poh-NAYD)
		  tampon/o- *stop up*
		  -ade *action; process*

rheumatic heart disease	Autoimmune response to a noncardiac streptococcal infection, such as strep throat. Rheumatic heart disease occurs most often in children and is known as rheumatic fever. The body makes antibodies to fight the bacteria, but the antibodies attack connective tissue in the body, particularly in the joints and/or the heart. The joints become swollen with fluid and inflamed. The mitral and aortic valves of the heart become inflamed and damaged. **Vegetations** (irregular collections of platelets, fibrin, and bacteria) form on the valves (see Figure 5-15 ■). The valves become scarred and narrowed, a condition known as **stenosis**. Treatment: Antibiotic drug to treat the initial infection. After rheumatic heart disease has occurred, a prophylactic (preventive) antibiotic drug is given prior to any dental or surgical procedure that might release bacteria that could further damage the valves. Valve replacement surgery.	**rheumatic** (roo-MAT-ik)
		  rheumat/o- *watery discharge*
		  -ic *pertaining to*
		
		vegetation (VEJ-eh-TAY-shun)
		  vegetat/o- *growth*
		  -ion *action; condition*
		
		stenosis (steh-NOH-sis)
		  sten/o- *constriction; narrowness*
		  -osis *condition; process*

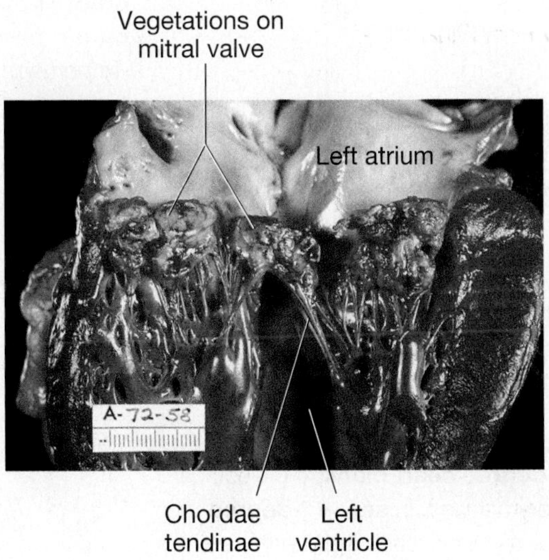

FIGURE 5-15 ■ Vegetation on the mitral valve.
There are irregular, yellow vegetations growing on the otherwise smooth surface of the mitral valve. The multiple rope-like strands below are the normal chordae tendineae that stabilize the valve leaflets.
Source: Science Source/Getty Images

Conduction System

Word or Phrase	Description	Pronunciation/Word Parts
arrhythmia	Any type of irregularity in the rate or rhythm of the heart. It is also known as **dysrhythmia**. Arrhythmias include bradycardia, fibrillation, flutter, heart block, premature contraction, sick sinus syndrome, and tachycardia. Electrocardiography is performed to diagnose the type of arrhythmia (see Figure 5-16 ■). Treatment: Antiarrhythmic drug, cardioversion, or implanting a pacemaker in the chest, depending on the type of arrhythmia. Bradycardia Normal sinus rhythm Ventricular tachycardia Ventricular fibrillation Asystole **FIGURE 5-16 ■ Arrhythmias on an ECG tracing.** (a) Bradycardia with a heart rate of 60 beats per minute. (b) A normal heart rate at 80 beats per minute. (c) Ventricular tachycardia at 150 beats per minute. (d) Ventricular fibrillation. (e) Asystole is not an arrhythmia because there is no heartbeat. *Source*: Pearson Education	**arrhythmia** (aa-RITH-mee-ah) **a-** *away from; without* **rrhythm/o-** *rhythm* **-ia** *condition; state; thing* **dysrhythmia** (dis-RITH-mee-ah) **dys-** *abnormal; difficult; painful* **rhythm/o-** *rhythm* **-ia** *condition; state; thing* Select the correct prefix meaning to get the definition of *dysrhythmia*: *condition of an abnormal rhythm*. Note that *arrhythmia* is spelled with two r's, and *dysrhythmia* is spelled with one r.
bradycardia	Arrhythmia in which the heart beats too slowly (see Figure 5-16). A patient with bradycardia is **bradycardic**. Treatment: Intravenous atropine (drug). Surgery to insert a pacemaker.	**bradycardia** (BRAD-ee-KAR-dee-ah) **brady-** *slow* **card/i-** *heart* **-ia** *condition; state; thing* **bradycardic** (BRAD-ee-KAR-dik) **brady-** *slow* **card/i-** *heart* **-ic** *pertaining to*
fibrillation	Arrhythmia in which there is a very fast, uncoordinated quivering of the myocardium (see Figure 5-16). It can affect the atria or ventricles. Ventricular fibrillation ("V fib"), a life-threatening emergency in which the heart is unable to pump blood, can progress to cardiac arrest. Treatment: Defibrillation.	**fibrillation** (FIB-rih-LAY-shun) **fibrill/o-** *muscle fiber; nerve fiber* **-ation** *being; having; process*
flutter	Arrhythmia in which there is a very fast but regular rhythm (250 beats per minute) of the atria or ventricles. The chambers of the heart do not have time to completely fill with blood before the next contraction. Flutter can progress to fibrillation. Treatment: Antiarrhythmic drug; cardioversion.	
heart block	Arrhythmia in which electrical impulses cannot travel normally from the SA node to the Purkinje fibers. In **first-degree heart block**, the electrical impulses reach the ventricles but are very delayed. In **second-degree heart block**, only some of the electrical impulses reach the ventricles. In **third-degree heart block** (complete heart block), no electrical impulses reach the ventricles. In **right or left bundle branch block**, the electrical impulses are unable to travel down the right or left bundle of His. Treatment: Antiarrhythmic drug. Surgery to insert a pacemaker.	

Word or Phrase	Description	Pronunciation/Word Parts
arrhythmia (continued) **premature contraction**	Arrhythmia in which there are one or more extra contractions in between systole and diastole. This is also known as an **extrasystole**. There are two types of premature contractions: **premature atrial contractions (PACs)** and **premature ventricular contractions (PVCs)**. A repeating pattern of one premature contraction followed by one normal contraction is **bigeminy**. A repeating pattern of one premature contraction followed by two normal contractions is **trigeminy**. Two premature contractions occurring together is a **couplet**. Treatment: Antiarrhythmic drug. Surgery to insert a pacemaker.	**contraction** (con-TRAK-shun) **contract/o-** *pull together* **-ion** *action; condition* **extrasystole** (EKS-trah-SIS-toh-lee) **extra-** *outside* **-systole** *contraction* The ending *-systole* contains the combining form **systol/o-** and the one-letter suffix *-e*. **bigeminy** (by-JEM-ih-nee) The prefix **bi-** means *two*. **trigeminy** (try-JEM-ih-nee) The prefix **tri-** means *three*.
sick sinus syndrome	Arrhythmia in which bradycardia alternates with tachycardia. It occurs when the sinoatrial node and an ectopic site elsewhere in the myocardium take turns being the heart's pacemaker. Treatment: Antiarrhythmic drug. Surgery to insert a pacemaker.	
tachycardia	Arrhythmia in which there is a fast but regular rhythm (up to 200 beats/minute) (see Figure 5-16). A patient with tachycardia is **tachycardic**. **Sinus tachycardia** occurs because of an abnormality in the sinoatrial (SA) node. Atrial tachycardia occurs when an ectopic site somewhere in the atrium produces an electrical impulse that overrides the SA node rhythm. **Supraventricular tachycardia** occurs when an ectopic site above (superior to) the ventricles produces an electrical impulse. **Paroxysmal tachycardia** is an episode of tachycardia that occurs suddenly and then goes away without treatment. Treatment: Antiarrhythmic drug. Cardioversion. Surgery to insert a pacemaker.	**tachycardia** (TAK-ih-KAR-dee-ah) **tachy-** *fast* **card/i-** *heart* **-ia** *condition; state; thing* **tachycardic** (TAK-ih-KAR-dik) **tachy-** *fast* **card/i-** *heart* **-ic** *pertaining to* **supraventricular** (SOO-prah-ven-TRIH-kyoo-lar) **supra-** *above* **ventricul/o-** *chamber that is filled; ventricle* **-ar** *pertaining to* **paroxysmal** (PAIR-awk-SIZ-mal)
asystole	Complete absence of a heartbeat (see Figure 5-16). This is also known as **cardiac arrest**. Treatment: Cardiopulmonary resuscitation (CPR).	**asystole** (aa-SIS-toh-lee) **a-** *away from; without* **-systole** *contraction*
palpitation	An uncomfortable sensation felt in the chest during a premature contraction of the heart. It is often described as a "thump." Treatment: None, unless it becomes an arrhythmia.	**palpitation** (PAL-pih-TAY-shun) **palpit/o-** *throb* **-ation** *being; having; process*

WORD ALERT

Sound-Alike Words

palpation   (noun)   A process of touching and feeling.

Example: *Palpation allowed the physician to identify a tumor in the abdomen.*

palpitation   (noun)   Being or having (the heart) throb

Example: *Her occasional palpitations concerned the patient until the physician reassured her.*

Blood Vessels

Word or Phrase	Description	Pronunciation/Word Parts

aneurysm	Area of dilation and weakness in the wall of an artery (see Figure 5-17 ■). This can be congenital or where arteriosclerosis has damaged the artery. With each heartbeat, the weakened artery wall balloons outward. An aneurysm can rupture without warning. A **dissecting aneurysm** is one that enlarges by tunneling between the layers of the artery wall. Treatment: Placement of a metal clip on the neck (narrowest part) of a small **aneurysmal** dilation to occlude the blood flow. Surgical removal of a large aneurysm and replacement with a synthetic tubular graft.	**aneurysm** (AN-yoor-izm)
		
		dissecting (dy-SEK-ting)
		   dissect/o- *cut apart*
		   -ing *doing*
		
		aneurysmal (AN-yoor-IZ-mal)
		   aneurysm/o- *aneurysm; dilation*
		   -al *pertaining to*

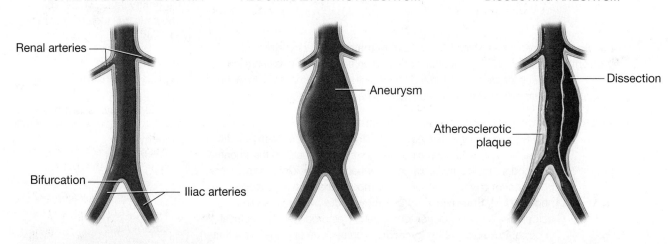

NORMAL ABDOMINAL AORTA   ABDOMINAL AORTIC ANEURYSM   DISSECTING ANEURYSM

Renal arteries

Bifurcation

Iliac arteries

Aneurysm

Dissection

Atherosclerotic plaque

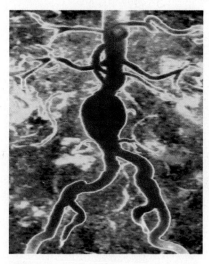

FIGURE 5-17 ■ Aneurysm.

(a) A normal abdominal aorta, a large abdominal aortic aneurysm, and a dissecting aneurysm that has tunneled between and separated the atherosclerotic plaque from the artery wall. (b) This x-ray image is an arteriogram. Contrast dye shows a large dissecting abdominal aortic aneurysm above the bifurcation where the right and left iliac arteries begin in the pelvic area.

Source: Pearson Education; Zephyr/Science Photo Library/Getty Images

Word or Phrase	Description	Pronunciation/Word Parts

arteriosclerosis	Progressive degenerative changes that produce a narrowed, hardened artery. The process begins with a small tear in the endothelium caused by chronic hypertension. Then low-density lipoproteins (LDLs) in the blood deposit cholesterol and form an **atheroma** or **atheromatous plaque** inside the artery (see Figure 5-18 ■). Collagen fibers form underneath the plaque, so that the artery wall becomes hard and nonelastic. An artery with arteriosclerosis is said to be **arteriosclerotic.** This is also known as **arteriosclerotic cardiovascular disease (ASCVD).**
	
	Fatty plaque deposits enlarge more rapidly in patients who eat high-fat diets, have diabetes mellitus, or have a genetic predisposition (family history). As plaque grows on an artery wall, it makes the lumen narrower and narrower (see Figure 5-19 ■). This condition is **atherosclerosis.** Pieces of atheromatous plaque easily break off, travel through the blood, and block other arteries. The rough edges of the plaque can trap red blood cells and form a blood clot.
	
	Severe atherosclerosis completely blocks the artery (see Figure 5-19). In the carotid arteries to the brain, this can cause a stroke. In the coronary arteries to the heart muscle, this can cause angina pectoris and a myocardial infarction. In the renal arteries to the kidney, this can cause kidney failure. Treatment: Lipid-lowering drug. Surgery: Angioplasty or stent to press down the plaque or endarterectomy to remove the plaque.
		arteriosclerosis
		(ar-TEER-ee-OH-skleh-ROH-sis)
		    arteri/o- *artery*
		    scler/o- *hard; sclera of the eye*
		    -osis *condition; process*
		
		atheroma (ATH-eh-ROH-mah)
		    ather/o- *soft, fatty substance*
		    -oma *mass; tumor*
		
		atheromatous
		(ATH-eh-ROH-mah-tus)
		    atheromat/o- *fatty deposit; fatty mass*
		    -ous *pertaining to*
		
		plaque (PLAK)
		
		arteriosclerotic
		(ar-TEER-ee-OH-skleh-RAW-tik)
		    arteri/o- *artery*
		    scler/o- *hard; sclera of the eye*
		    -tic *pertaining to*
		
		atherosclerosis
		(ATH-eh-ROH-skleh-ROH-sis)
		    ather/o- *soft, fatty substance*
		    scler/o- *hard; sclera of the eye*
		    -osis *condition; process*

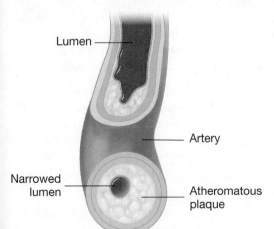

FIGURE 5-18 ■ Mild, moderate, and severe atheromatous plaque.
These segments of aorta show varying degrees of plaque formation. The dark openings are where arteries branch off from the aorta, bringing oxygenated blood to the body. In the middle specimen, moderate plaque narrows these artery openings. In the specimen on the right, severe plaque formation occludes these openings and decreases blood flow through the aorta itself.
Source: Biophoto Associates/Science Source/Getty Images

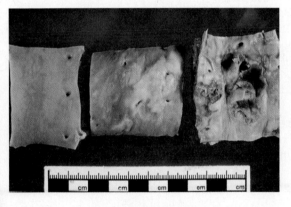

Lumen

Artery

Narrowed lumen

Atheromatous plaque

FIGURE 5-19 ■ Severe atherosclerotic plaque in an artery.
The lumen of the artery is so narrow that little blood can flow through it.
Source: Pearson Education

Word or Phrase	Description	Pronunciation/Word Parts
arteriosclerosis (*continued*)	**CLINICAL CONNECTIONS** **Dietetics.** The body produces its own supply of cholesterol to make bile, neurotransmitters, and male and female sexual hormones. The diet contains additional cholesterol in foods from animal sources. An excessive amount of animal fat in the diet increases the cholesterol level in the blood. An excessive amount of sugar in the diet is converted by the body to triglycerides, and this causes an increased triglyceride level in the blood and increased storage as adipose tissue (fat). Lipoproteins are carrier molecules produced in the liver. They transport lipids (fats such as cholesterol and triglycerides) in the blood. There are three types of lipoproteins. High-density lipoprotein (HDL) carries cholesterol to the liver where it is excreted in the bile. HDL is known by laypersons as "good cholesterol," and an increased level of HDL is beneficial. Low-density lipoprotein (LDL) carries cholesterol but deposits it on the walls of the arteries, and so it is known as "bad cholesterol." Very low-density lipoprotein (VLDL) carries triglycerides and deposits them on the walls of the arteries.	
bruit	A harsh, rushing sound made by blood passing through an artery narrowed and roughened by atherosclerosis. The bruit can be heard when a stethoscope is placed over the artery. Treatment: Correct the underlying cause.	**bruit** (BROO-ee)
coronary artery disease (CAD)	Arteriosclerosis of the coronary arteries. They are filled with atheromatous plaque, and their narrowed lumens cannot carry enough oxygenated blood to the myocardium. This results in angina pectoris. Severe atherosclerosis (or a blood clot that forms on an atherosclerotic plaque) can completely block the lumen of a coronary artery. This causes a myocardial infarction. Treatment: Lipid-lowering drug. Surgery: Percutaneous transluminal coronary angioplasty (PTCA) or coronary artery bypass grafting (CABG). **CLINICAL CONNECTIONS** **Public Health.** There are many factors that contribute to the development of coronary artery disease. These are known as **cardiac risk factors.** They include demographic factors (heredity, gender, age), medical factors (hypertension, hypercholesterolemia, diabetes mellitus, obesity), and lifestyle factors (smoking, lack of exercise, poor diet, stress, alcoholism).	
hyperlipidemia	Elevated levels of lipids (fats) in the blood. Lipids include cholesterol and triglycerides. **Hypercholesterolemia** is an elevated level of cholesterol in the blood. **Hypertriglyceridemia** is an elevated level of triglycerides in the blood. Normal levels are below 200 mg/dL for cholesterol and below 150 mg/dL for triglycerides. Treatment: Lipid-lowering drug.	**hyperlipidemia** (HY-per-LIP-ih-DEE-mee-ah) **hyper-** *above; more than normal* **lipid/o-** *fat; lipid* **-emia** *condition of the blood; substance in the blood* **hypercholesterolemia** (HY-per-koh-LES-ter-awl-EE-mee-ah) **hyper-** *above; more than normal* **cholesterol/o-** *cholesterol* **-emia** *condition of the blood; substance in the blood* **hypertriglyceridemia** (HY-per-try-GLIS-eh-ry-DEE-mee-ah) **hyper-** *above; more than normal* **triglycerid/o-** *triglyceride* **-emia** *condition of the blood; substance in the blood*

Word or Phrase	Description	Pronunciation/Word Parts
hypertension (HTN)	Elevated blood pressure. A normal blood pressure reading in an adult is less than 120/80 mm Hg. Readings between 120/80 mm Hg and 140/90 mm Hg are categorized as **prehypertension**. Blood pressures above 140/90 mm Hg are categorized as hypertension, and the patient is said to be **hypertensive**. Several blood pressure readings, not just one, are needed to make a diagnosis. Essential hypertension, the most common type of hypertension, is one in which the exact cause is not known. Secondary hypertension has a known cause, such as kidney disease. Treatment: Lifestyle changes (decreased salt intake, increased exercise, weight loss) followed by an antihypertensive drug.	**hypertension** (HY-per-TEN-shun) **hyper-** *above; more than normal* **tens/o-** *pressure; tension* **-ion** *action; condition* **prehypertension** (pree-HY-per-TEN-shun) **pre-** *before; in front of* **hyper-** *above; more than normal* **tens/o-** *pressure; tension* **-ion** *action; condition* **hypertensive** (HY-per-TEN-siv) **hyper-** *above; more than normal* **tens/o-** *pressure; tension* **-ive** *pertaining to*

DID YOU KNOW?

Some people have increased blood pressure readings just because they are nervous about being in a doctor's office. This is known as *white-coat hypertension*. This is not a true hypertension because as soon as they leave the doctor's office, their blood pressure returns to normal.

Word or Phrase	Description	Pronunciation/Word Parts
hypotension	Blood pressure lower than 90/60 mm Hg, usually because of a loss of blood volume. A patient with hypotension is **hypotensive**. Orthostatic **hypotension** is the sudden, temporary, but self-correcting decrease in systolic blood pressure that occurs when the patient changes from a lying to a standing position and experiences lightheadedness. Treatment: Change positions slowly to avoid dizziness.	**hypotension** (HY-poh-TEN-shun) **hypo-** *below; deficient* **tens/o-** *pressure; tension* **-ion** *action; condition* **hypotensive** (HY-poh-TEN-siv) **hypo-** *below; deficient* **tens/o-** *pressure; tension* **-ive** *pertaining to* **orthostatic** (OR-thoh-STAT-ik) **orth/o-** *straight* **stat/o-** *standing still; staying in one place* **-ic** *pertaining to*
peripheral artery disease (PAD)	Atherosclerosis of the arteries in the legs. Blood flow (**perfusion**) to the extremities is poor, and there is ischemia of the tissues. While walking, the patient experiences pain in the calf (intermittent **claudication**). In severe PAD, the feet and toes remain cool and cyanotic and may become **necrotic** as the tissues die. Treatment: Lipid-lowering drug. Surgery: Angioplasty and stent in the iliac or femoral artery. Possible amputation of the foot.	**peripheral** (peh-RIF-eh-ral) **peripher/o-** *outer aspects* **-al** *pertaining to* **perfusion** (per-FYOO-zhun) **per-** *through; throughout* **fus/o-** *pouring* **-ion** *action; condition* **claudication** (KLAW-dih-KAY-shun) **claudicat/o-** *limping pain* **-ion** *action; condition* **necrotic** (neh-KRAW-tik) **necr/o-** *dead body; dead cells; dead tissue* **-tic** *pertaining to*
peripheral vascular disease (PVD)	Any disease of the arteries of the extremities. It includes peripheral artery disease as well as Raynaud's disease. Treatment: See *peripheral artery disease* and *Raynaud's disease*.	**peripheral** (peh-RIF-eh-ral) **peripher/o-** *outer aspects* **-al** *pertaining to*

Word or Phrase	Description	Pronunciation/Word Parts
phlebitis	Inflammation of a vein, usually accompanied by infection. The area around the vein is painful, and the skin overlying the vein may show a red streak. A severe inflammation can partially occlude the vein and slow the flow of blood. **Thrombophlebitis** is phlebitis with the formation of a thrombus (blood clot). Treatment: Analgesic drug for pain, anti-inflammatory drug for inflammation. Antibiotic drug. Thrombolytic drug to dissolve a blood clot.	**phlebitis** (fleh-BY-tis) **phleb/o-** *vein* **-itis** *infection of; inflammation of* **thrombophlebitis** (THRAWM-boh-fleh-BY-tis) **thromb/o-** *blood clot* **phleb/o-** *vein* **-itis** *infection of; inflammation of*
Raynaud's disease	Sudden, severe vasoconstriction and spasm of the arterioles in the fingers and toes, often triggered by cold or emotional upset. They become white or cyanotic and numb for minutes or hours until the attack passes. This can lead to necrosis. Treatment: Vasodilator drug.	**Raynaud** (ray-NO)
varicose veins	Damaged or incompetent valves in a vein that allow blood to flow backward and collect in the preceding section of vein. The vein becomes distended with blood, twisting and bulging under the surface of the skin (see Figure 5-20 ■). There is pain and aching; the legs feel heavy and leaden. Varicose veins can be caused by phlebitis, injury, long periods of sitting with the legs crossed, or occupations that require constant standing. Also, during pregnancy, pressure from the enlarging uterus restricts the flow of blood in the lower extremities and can cause varicose veins. There is a family tendency to develop varicose veins. Treatment: Injecting a sclerosing solution or foam to harden and occlude the vein (sclerotherapy). Laser or radiowaves to destroy the vein. These procedures redirect the blood into deeper veins.	**varicose** (VAIR-ih-kohs) **varic/o-** *varicose vein; varix* **-ose** *full of*

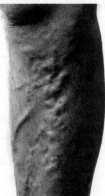

FIGURE 5-20 ■ **Severe varicose veins in the leg.**
Superficial, protruding varicose veins are unsightly and easily injured. Patients often have varicose veins treated for an improved cosmetic appearance, but this also helps decrease the chance of injury and thrombophlebitis.
Source: Audie/Shutterstock

CLINICAL CONNECTIONS
Gastroenterology (Chapter 3). Varicose veins of the esophagus and stomach are known as esophageal and gastric *varices*. Varicose veins of the rectum are known as *hemorrhoids*.

Laboratory and Diagnostic Procedures

Blood Tests		
Word or Phrase	**Description**	**Pronunciation/Word Parts**
cardiac enzymes	Test to measure the levels of enzymes that are released into the blood when myocardial cells die during a myocardial infarction. (These enzymes are not released during angina pectoris.) The higher the levels, the more severe the myocardial infarction and the larger the area of infarct. **Creatine kinase (CK)** is found in all muscle cells, but a specific form of it (CK-MB) is only found in myocardial cells. The CK-MB level begins to rise 2–6 hours after a myocardial infarction. It is also known as **creatine phosphokinase (CPK)**. **Lactate dehydrogenase (LDH)** is found in many different cells, including the heart. The LDH level begins to rise 12 hours after a myocardial infarction. An elevated LDH can support the CK-MB results but cannot be the only basis for a diagnosis of myocardial infarction. Cardiac enzymes are measured every few hours for several days. This test is done in conjunction with troponin.	**enzyme** (EN-zime) The suffix **-ase** means *enzyme*. **creatine kinase** (KREE-ah-teen KY-nays) **creatine phosphokinase** (KREE-ah-teen FAWS-foh-KY-nays) **lactate dehydrogenase** (LAK-tayt dee-HY-droh-JEH-nays)
C-reactive protein (CRP)	Test to measure the level of inflammation in the body. Inflammation from sites other than the cardiovascular system (such as inflammation of the gums or from a chronic urinary tract infection) can produce inflammation of the walls of the blood vessels. This can lead to blood clot formation and a myocardial infarction. The high-sensitivity CRP test can detect a lower blood level of CRP and is used to predict a healthy person's risk of developing cardiovascular disease.	
homocysteine	Test included as part of a cardiac risk assessment. This amino acid damages the blood vessel walls. An elevated level increases the patient's risk of arteriosclerosis and a blood clot that can cause a heart attack or stroke.	**homocysteine** (HOH-moh-SIS-teen)
lipid profile	Test that provides a comprehensive picture of the blood levels of cholesterol and triglycerides and their **lipoprotein** carriers (HDL, LDL, VLDL).	**lipid** (LIP-id) **lip/o-** *fat; lipid* **-id** *origin; resembling; source* **lipoprotein** (LIH-poh-PROH-teen)
troponin	Test to measure the level of two proteins that are released into the blood when myocardial cells die. Troponin I and troponin T are only found in the myocardium. The troponin levels begin to rise 4–6 hours after a myocardial infarction. More importantly, they remain elevated for up to 10 days, so they can be used to diagnose a myocardial infarction many days after it occurred. Troponin levels are done in conjunction with cardiac enzyme levels.	**troponin** (troh-POH-nin)
Diagnostic Procedures		
cardiac catheterization	Procedure performed to study the anatomy and pressures in the heart. During a right heart catheterization, a catheter is inserted into the femoral or brachial vein and threaded to the right atrium. The catheter is used to record right heart pressures. Then a radiopaque contrast dye is injected through the catheter to outline the chambers of the heart to diagnose congenital heart defects. During a left heart catheterization, a catheter is inserted into the femoral or brachial artery and threaded to the left atrium. Then radiopaque contrast dye is injected to outline the coronary arteries and show narrowed or blocked areas. If blockage of a coronary artery is present, an angioplasty can be performed at that time. This procedure is also referred to as a *cardiac cath*.	**catheterization** (KATH-eh-TER-ih-ZAY-shun) **catheter/o-** *catheter* **-ization** *process of creating; process of inserting; process of making*

Word or Phrase	Description	Pronunciation/Word Parts
cardiac exercise stress test	Procedure performed to evaluate the heart's response to exercise in patients with chest pain, palpitations, or arrhythmias (see Figure 5-21 ■). The patient walks on a motorized treadmill (**treadmill exercise stress test**) or rides a stationary bicycle while an ECG is performed. The speed of the treadmill and the steepness of its incline (or the resistance of the bicycle) are gradually increased while the patient's heart rate, blood pressure, and ECG are monitored. The procedure is stopped if the patient complains of angina, palpitations, shortness of breath, or tiredness, or if the ECG pattern becomes abnormal. The patient's resting heart rate and maximum heart rate are compared to standards for other people of the same age and sex. Any abnormality in the ECG pattern is analyzed.	

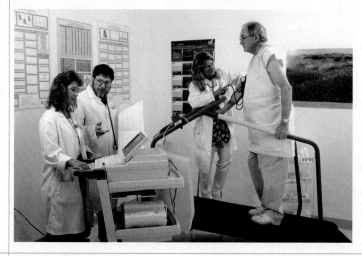

FIGURE 5-21 ■ Treadmill exercise stress test.
This patient is exercising on a treadmill. Electrode patches on his chest pick up the electrical impulses of the heart. The cardiologist watches the computer screen for any arrhythmias. The nurse periodically checks the patient's blood pressure.
Source: Brownie Harris/Flirt/Corbis

Word or Phrase	Description	Pronunciation/Word Parts
electrocardiography (ECG, EKG)	Procedure that records the electrical activity of the heart (see Figure 5-22 ■). Electrodes (metal pieces in adhesive patches) are placed on the limbs (both arms and one leg) to send the electrical impulses of the heart to the ECG machine. These are the three limb leads (leads I–III). Electrodes placed on the chest are known as the precordial leads (V_1–V_6). A 12-lead ECG records the electrical activity between different combinations of electrodes to give an electrical picture of the heart from 12 different angles. Samples of each of these 12 tracings are printed out and mounted on a backing for an **electrocardiogram**. A longer sample of just a single lead tracing (usually lead II) is known as a *rhythm strip*.	**electrocardiography** (ee-LEK-troh-KAR-dee-AW-grah-fee) **electr/o-** *electricity* **cardi/o-** *heart* **-graphy** *process of recording* **electrocardiogram** (ee-LEK-troh-KAR-dee-oh-GRAM) **electr/o-** *electricity* **cardi/o-** *heart* **-gram** *picture; record*

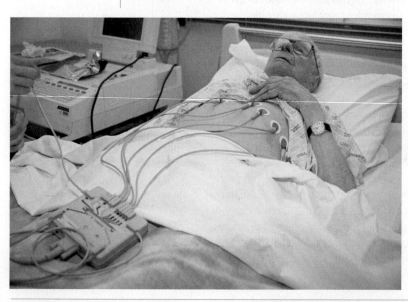

FIGURE 5-22 ■ Electrocardiography.
This portable ECG machine has been brought to the patient's bedside. Electrode patches attached to wire leads pick up the electrical impulses of the heart. Interpretation of an ECG includes the heart rate and rhythm and identifying abnormalities in the shape of the electrical pattern.
Source: Antonia Reeve/Science Source

Word or Phrase	Description	Pronunciation/Word Parts
electrocardiography (ECG, EKG) (*continued*)		

A CLOSER LOOK

ECG Interpretation. The electrical image generated by the contraction and relaxation of the heart has a characteristic pattern of waves and a spike (see Figure 5-23 ■). The P wave corresponds to depolarization of the SA node and contractions of both atria. The QRS complex corresponds to depolarization of the septum and contractions of both ventricles. The T wave corresponds to repolarization of the ventricles. (*Note*: The wave that corresponds to repolarization of the atria is hidden by the QRS complex.)

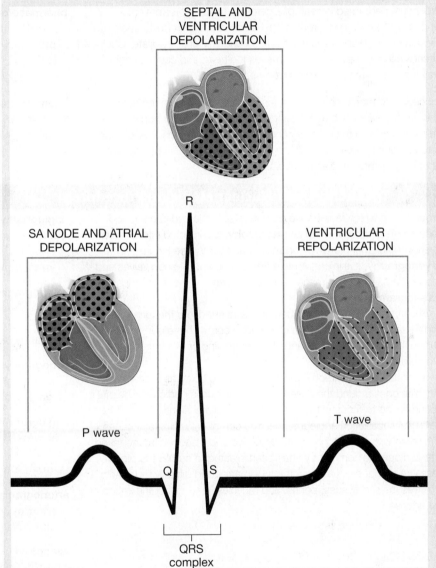

SEPTAL AND VENTRICULAR DEPOLARIZATION

SA NODE AND ATRIAL DEPOLARIZATION

VENTRICULAR REPOLARIZATION

R

Q   S

P wave

T wave

QRS complex

FIGURE 5-23 ■ ECG tracing. On an ECG, a normal tracing shows a P wave, QRS complex, and T wave that correspond to depolarization (large dots) and repolarization (small dots) changes going on in the heart. These are so named to create a simple and universal reference. *Source*: Pearson Education

DID YOU KNOW?

The *K* in the abbreviation *EKG* comes from the Greek word *kardia* (heart).

| **electrophysiologic study (EPS)** | Procedure to map the heart's conduction system in a patient with an arrhythmia. While an ECG is performed, catheters are inserted into the femoral vein and subclavian vein. X-rays are used to guide the catheters to the heart. The catheters send out electrical impulses to stimulate the heart and try to cause an arrhythmia to pinpoint the ectopic site where the arrhythmia is coming from. | **electrophysiologic** (ee-LEK-troh-FIZ-ee-oh-LAW-jik) **electr/o-** *electricity* **physi/o-** *physical function* **log/o-** *study of; word* **-ic** *pertaining to* |

Word or Phrase	Description	Pronunciation/Word Parts
Holter monitor	Procedure during which the patient's heart rate and rhythm are continuously monitored as an outpatient for 24 hours. The patient wears electrodes attached to a small portable ECG monitor (carried in a vest or placed in a pocket). The patient also keeps a diary of activities, meals, and symptoms. A Holter monitor procedure is used to document infrequently occurring arrhythmias and to link them to activities or symptoms such as chest pain.	**Holter** (HOL-ter)
pharmacologic stress test	Procedure performed instead of a cardiac stress test for patients who cannot exercise vigorously. The vasodilator drug dipyridamole (Persantine) is given to cause normal coronary arteries to dilate. Occluded arteries cannot dilate, and this stresses the heart and causes angina in a way that is similar to an exercise stress test.	**pharmacologic** (FAR-mah-koh-LAW-jik) **pharmac/o-** *drug; medicine* **log/o-** *study of; word* **-ic** *pertaining to*
telemetry	Procedure to monitor a patient's heart rate and rhythm in the hospital. The patient wears electrodes connected to a device that continuously transmits an ECG tracing to a central monitoring station in the coronary care unit or intensive care unit. A nurse at the station constantly watches all of the patients' cardiac monitors.	**telemetry** (teh-LEM-eh-tree) **tele/o-** *distance* **-metry** *process of measuring*

Radiology and Nuclear Medicine Procedures

angiography	Procedure in which radiopaque contrast dye is injected into a blood vessel to fill and outline it. In **arteriography**, it is injected into an artery to show blockage, narrowed areas, or aneurysms (see Figure 5-17). In **venography**, it is injected into a vein to show weakened valves and dilated walls. The x-ray image is an **angiogram** or, more specifically, an **arteriogram** or **venogram**. In coronary angiography, a catheter is inserted into the femoral artery and threaded to the aorta. The radiopaque contrast dye is injected to outline the coronary arteries and show narrowing or blockage. The x-ray is a coronary angiogram. In rotational angiography, multiple x-rays are taken as the x-ray machine goes around the patient. This technique is particularly helpful in documenting tortuous blood vessels in three dimensions. Digital subtraction angiography (DSA) combines two x-ray images, one taken without radiopaque contrast dye and a second image taken after radiopaque contrast dye has been injected to outline the blood vessel. A computer compares the two images and digitally "subtracts" or removes the soft tissues, bones, and muscles, leaving just the image of the arteries.	**angiography** (AN-jee-AW-grah-fee) **angi/o-** *blood vessel; lymphatic vessel* **-graphy** *process of recording* **arteriography** (ar-TEER-ee-AW-grah-fee) **arteri/o-** *artery* **-graphy** *process of recording* **venography** (vee-NAW-grah-fee) **ven/o-** *vein* **-graphy** *process of recording* **angiogram** (AN-jee-oh-GRAM) **angi/o-** *blood vessel; lymphatic vessel* **-gram** *picture; record* **arteriogram** (ar-TEER-ee-oh-GRAM) **arteri/o-** *artery* **-gram** *picture; record* **venogram** (VEE-noh-gram) **ven/o-** *vein* **-gram** *picture; record*

Word or Phrase	Description	Pronunciation/Word Parts

echocardiography	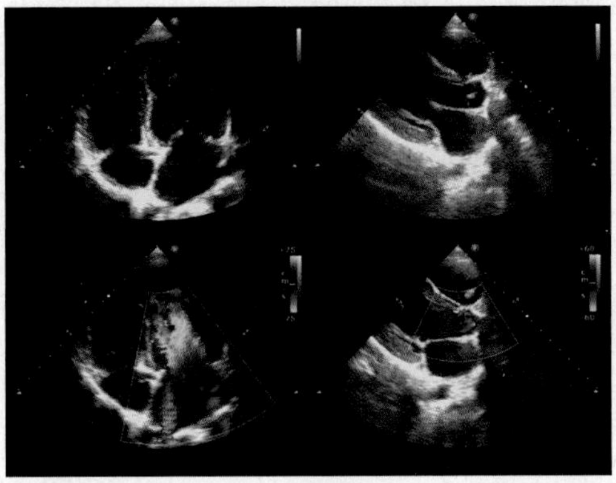 Procedure that uses a transducer to produce ultra high-frequency sound waves (ultrasound) that are bounced off the heart to create an image. **Two-dimensional echocardiography** (2-D echo) creates a real-time picture of the heart and its chambers and valves as it contracts and relaxes. The image is an **echocardiogram** (see Figure 5-24 ■)	**echocardiography**
		(EK-oh-KAR-dee-AW-grah-fee)
		  ech/o- *echo of a sound wave*
		  cardi/o- *heart*
		  -graphy *process of recording*
		
		echocardiogram
		(EK-oh-KAR-dee-oh-GRAM)
		  ech/o- *echo of a sound wave*
		  cardi/o- *heart*
		  -gram *picture; record*

FIGURE 5-24 ■ Echocardiogram.
These images were taken while a two-dimensional echocardiography produced real-time, moving images of the heart on the display screen. Echocardiography uses sound waves to create images.
Source: Kalewa/Shutterstock

Transesophageal echocardiography (TEE) may be ordered when a standard echocardiogram has a poor-quality image. For a TEE, the patient swallows an endoscopic tube that contains a tiny, sound-emitting transducer. This is positioned in the esophagus directly behind, and closer to, the heart.

Doppler ultrasonography images the flow of blood in an artery or vein (see Figure 5-25 ■). The two-dimensional ultrasound image shows blockages or clots in the blood vessel. Doppler technology shows how fast blood is traveling in that artery or vein. Doppler technology is also used in automatic blood pressure machines, in hand-held devices that give the heart rate if placed on the skin over an artery, and in fetal monitors that, when placed on the mother's abdomen, give the heart rate of the fetus. **Color flow duplex ultrasonography** combines the ultrasound image with a color-coded Doppler image. Variations in blood flow and turbulence are shown, with faster flow in red and slower flow In blue. Color flow duplex ultrasonography is the "gold standard" for evaluating tortuous varicose veins.

transesophageal
(TRANS-eh-SAW-fah-JEE-al)
  trans- *across; through*
  esophag/o- *esophagus*
  -eal *pertaining to*

Doppler (DAW-pler)

ultrasonography
(UL-trah-soh-NAW-grah-fee)
  ultra- *beyond; higher*
  son/o- *sound*
  -graphy *process of recording*

duplex (DOO-pleks)

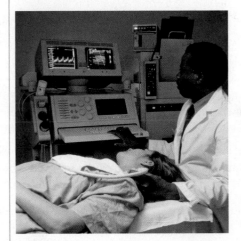

FIGURE 5-25 ■ Doppler ultrasonography.
This radiologic technologist has positioned an ultrasound transducer over the left carotid artery in the patient's neck. He moves the transducer to obtain the clearest image on the computer screen and then records this permanent image for the electronic patient record.
Source: Ouellette Theroux/Publiphoto/ Science Source

Word or Phrase	Description	Pronunciation/Word Parts
multiple-gated acquisition (MUGA) scan	Nuclear medicine procedure that uses the radioactive tracer technetium-99m. First, pyrophosphate is injected intravenously to allow red blood cells to bind with technetium-99m. Then technetium-99m is injected. A gamma camera records gamma rays emitted by the technetium-99m bound to red blood cells. The camera is coordinated (gated) with the patient's ECG so that images of the heart chambers (with blood—and red blood cells—in them) are taken at various times. A MUGA scan also calculates the ejection fraction (how much blood the ventricle can eject with one contraction). The ejection fraction is the most accurate indicator of overall heart function. This procedure is also known as a **radionuclide ventriculography (RNV)** or **gated blood pool scan**.	**radionuclide** (RAY-dee-oh-NOO-klide) **radi/o-** *forearm bone; radiation; x-rays* **nucle/o-** *nucleus of an atom; nucleus of a cell* **-ide** *chemically modified structure* **ventriculography** (ven-TRIH-kyoo-LAW-grah-fee) **ventricul/o-** *chamber that is filled; ventricle* **-graphy** *process of recording*
myocardial perfusion scan	Nuclear medicine procedure that combines a cardiac exercise stress test with intravenous injections of a radioactive tracer. The radioactive tracer collects in those parts of the myocardium that have the best perfusion (blood flow). A gamma camera records gamma rays emitted by the radioactive tracer and creates a two-dimensional image of the heart. Areas of decreased uptake ("cold spots") indicate poor perfusion from a blocked coronary artery. The artery must be about 70% blocked before any abnormality is evident on the image. Areas of no uptake indicate dead tissue from a previous myocardial infarction. Technetium-99m is joined to a synthetic molecule (sestamibi). The combination of technetium-99m with sestamibi is the drug Cardiolite, so this test is also known as a **Cardiolite stress test**. In a **thallium stress test**, thallium-201 is the radioactive tracer, or thallium-201 and technetium-99m can be used. Myocardial perfusion PET scans are used to image the metabolism of the heart.	**perfusion** (per-FYOO-zhun) **per-** *through; throughout* **fus/o-** *pouring* **-ion** *action; condition* **Cardiolite** (KAR-dee-oh-LITE) **thallium** (THAL-ee-um)
single-photon emission computed tomography (SPECT) scan	Procedure that is a variation of a myocardial perfusion scan or a MUGA scan. Instead of being stationary above the patient's chest, the gamma camera is moved in a circle around the patient. The computer creates many individual images or "slices" (tomography) and compiles them into a three-dimensional image of the heart.	**photon** (FOH-tawn) A photon is another name for a gamma ray. **tomography** (toh-MAW-grah-fee) **tom/o-** *cut; layer; slice* **-graphy** *process of recording*

Medical and Surgical Procedures

Medical Procedures		
Word or Phrase	**Description**	**Pronunciation/Word Parts**
auscultation	Procedure that uses a **stethoscope** to listen to the heart sounds. The stethoscope is placed at the **point of maximum impulse (PMI)**, which is at the apex of the heart. Auscultation can determine the heart rate and detect arrhythmias and murmurs.	**auscultation** (AWS-kul-TAY-shun) **auscult/o-** *listening* **-ation** *being; having; process* **stethoscope** (STETH-oh-skohp) **steth/o-** *chest* **-scope** *instrument used to examine*

Word or Phrase	Description	Pronunciation/Word Parts
cardiopulmonary resuscitation (CPR)	Procedure to circulate the blood and ventilate the lungs after a patient has stopped breathing and the heart has stopped. This procedure was already described in Chapter 4 Pulmonology.	**cardiopulmonary** (KAR-dee-oh-PUL-moh-NAIR-ee) **cardi/o-** *heart* **pulmon/o-** *lung* **-ary** *pertaining to*
cardioversion	Procedure to treat an arrhythmia (atrial flutter, atrial fibrillation, or ventricular tachycardia) that cannot be controlled with antiarrhythmic drugs. Two large, hand-held paddles are placed on either side of the patient's chest. The machine generates an electrical shock coordinated with the QRS complex of the patient's heart to restore the heart to a normal rhythm. For a patient with ventricular fibrillation, the same machine is used (it is now called a **defibrillator**) to give a much stronger electrical shock (see Figure 5-26 ■). An automatic implantable cardioverter/defibrillator (AICD) is a small device that is implanted in a patient who is at high risk for developing a serious arrhythmia. The AICD is implanted under the skin of the chest. It has leads (wires) that go to the heart, sense its rhythm, and deliver an electrical shock, if needed. An automatic external defibrillator (AED) is a portable computerized device kept on emergency response vehicles and in public places such as airports. It analyzes the patient's heart rhythm and delivers an electrical shock to stimulate the heart in cardiac arrest. An AED is designed to be used by nonmedical persons.	**cardioversion** (KAR-dee-oh-VER-zhun) **cardi/o-** *heart* **vers/o-** *travel; turn* **-ion** *action; condition* **defibrillator** (dee-FIB-rih-LAY-tor) **de-** *reversal of; without* **fibrill/o-** *muscle fiber; nerve fiber* **-ator** *person who does; person who produces; thing that does; thing that produces*

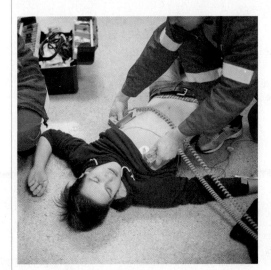

FIGURE 5-26 ■ Defibrillation.
This emergency medical technician has applied defibrillator paddles to the patient's chest to convert a life-threatening ventricular fibrillation. The defibrillator unit and an emergency drug box are on the ground next to the patient.
Source: Mika/Comet/Corbis

Word or Phrase	Description	Pronunciation/Word Parts
sclerotherapy	Procedure in which a sclerosing drug (liquid or foam) is injected into a varicose vein. The drug causes irritation and inflammation that later becomes fibrosis that occludes the vein. The blood flow is redirected to another, deeper vein, and the varicose vein is no longer distended.	**sclerotherapy** (SKLAIR-oh-THAIR-ah-pee) **scler/o-** *hard; sclera of the eye* **-therapy** *treatment* Add words to make a complete definition of *sclerotherapy*: *treatment (to make a vein) hard(en)*.

Word or Phrase	Description	Pronunciation/Word Parts
vital signs	Procedure during a physical examination to measure the temperature, heart rate (pulse), and respirations (TPR) as well as the blood pressure (BP). Sometimes an evaluation of pain is included and it is known as the fourth vital sign. 　　The heart rate is measured by counting the pulse. The pulse can be felt in several different parts of the body (see Figure 5-27 ■). Pulse points include the carotid pulse in the neck, apical pulse on the anterior chest, axillary pulse in the armpit, brachial pulse at the inner elbow, radial pulse at the wrist, femoral pulse in the inguinal area (groin), popliteal pulse at the back of the knee, posterior tibial pulse at the back of the lower leg, and the dorsalis pedis pulse on the dorsum of the foot. The **radial pulse** in the wrist is the most commonly used site. In an emergency, the **carotid pulse** is used (see Figure 5-28 ■) because, if the patient is in shock, there is less blood flowing to the extremities. The **apical pulse** (at the apex of the heart) can be heard with a stethoscope and is also used to evaluate the heart rhythm and heart sounds. The presence of peripheral vascular disease can be determined by comparing the strength of the pulse in the right leg to the same pulse on the left.	

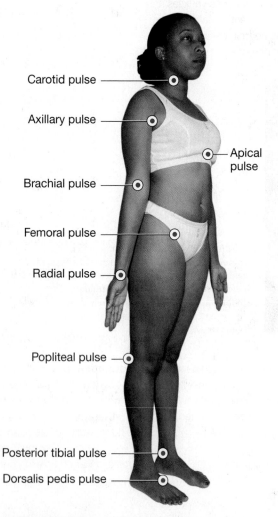

Carotid pulse

Axillary pulse

Apical pulse

Brachial pulse

Femoral pulse

Radial pulse

Popliteal pulse

Posterior tibial pulse

Dorsalis pedis pulse

FIGURE 5-27 ■ Pulse points.
A pulse point is where the pulse of an artery can be felt on the surface of the body. Pulse points are used to determine the heart rate and the amount of flow through the artery.
Source: Pearson Education

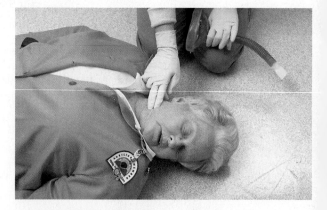

FIGURE 5-28 ■ Carotid pulse.
The pulse of the carotid artery can be felt easily in the neck. This emergency medical technician is using this site to quickly assess a patient's heart rate.
Source: Pearson Education

Word or Phrase	Description	Pronunciation/Word Parts

vital signs
 (*continued*)
	The blood pressure is measured with a **sphygmomanometer** and a stethoscope. The sphygmomanometer consists of a thin, inflatable cuff that wraps around the arm (or leg), a hand bulb that is pumped to increase the pressure in the cuff, a regulating valve that is opened to slowly release pressure from the cuff, and a calibrated gauge to read the pressure (see Figure 5-29 ■). The stethoscope is placed at the inner elbow over the brachial pulse. As pressure increases in the cuff, it cuts off the flow of blood. The cuff pressure is decreased. When the cuff pressure is lower than the pressure in the artery, the blood spurts through and creates the first sound. This is the **systolic pressure**, the top number in a blood pressure reading, which represents the force of the contraction of the ventricles. When the cuff pressure reaches the resting pressure in the artery, this is the **diastolic pressure**. A blood pressure measurement is recorded as two numbers: the systolic pressure over the diastolic pressure. Blood pressure is measured in millimeters of mercury (example: 120/80 mm Hg). Blood pressure cuffs come in several different sizes to accommodate very thin to very large arms. There are even blood pressure cuffs for newborn and premature infants. The correct size blood pressure cuff must be used or the blood pressure reading will be either too high or too low.	**sphygmomanometer**
		 (SFIG-moh-mah-NAW-meh-ter)
		   sphygm/o- *pulse*
		   man/o- *frenzy; thin*
		   -meter *instrument used to measure*
		 Add words to make a complete definition of *sphygmomanometer*: *instrument used to measure (the pressure of the) pulse (by using a) thin (inflatable cuff).*
		
		 systolic (sis-TAW-lik)
		   systol/o- *contracting*
		   -ic *pertaining to*
		
		 diastolic (DY-ah-STAW-lik)
		   diastol/o- *dilating*
		   -ic *pertaining to*

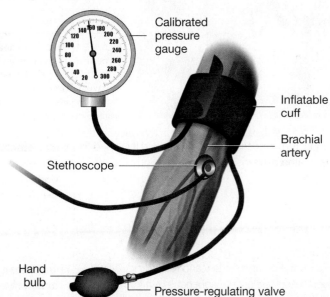

Calibrated pressure gauge

Inflatable cuff

Brachial artery

Stethoscope

Hand bulb

Pressure-regulating valve

FIGURE 5-29 ■ Measuring the blood pressure.
A sphygmomanometer and a stethoscope are used to measure the blood pressure. This is most commonly done at the brachial artery.

Source: Pearson Education

	Surgical Procedures	

aneurysmectomy	Procedure to remove an aneurysm and repair the defect in the artery wall. If an aneurysm involves a large segment of artery, a flexible, tubular synthetic graft is used to replace the segment.	**aneurysmectomy**
		 (AN-yoor-iz-MEK-toh-mee)
		   aneurysm/o- *aneurysm; dilation*
		   -ectomy *surgical removal*

Word or Phrase	Description	Pronunciation/Word Parts
cardiopulmonary bypass	Procedure used during open heart surgery (see Figure 5-30 ■) in which the patient's blood is rerouted through a cannula in the femoral vein to a heart-lung machine. There, the blood is oxygenated, carbon dioxide and waste products are removed, and the blood is pumped back into the patient's body through a cannula in the femoral artery. Cardiopulmonary bypass takes over the functions of the heart and lungs during the surgery.	**cardiopulmonary** (KAR-dee-oh-PUL-moh-NAIR-ee) **cardi/o-** *heart* **pulmon/o-** *lung* **-ary** *pertaining to*

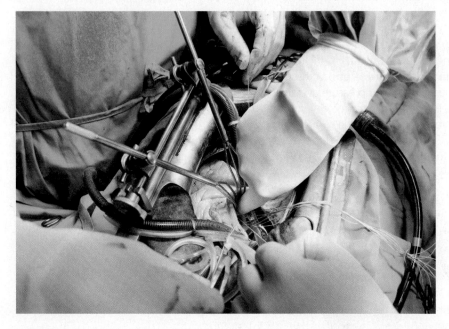

FIGURE 5-30 ■ Open heart surgery.
To perform open heart surgery, the sternum is cut in half lengthwise. Metal retractors are used to pull the two halves apart to create an operative field that allows access to the heart.
Source: pirke/Fotolia LLC

Word or Phrase	Description	Pronunciation/Word Parts
carotid endarterectomy	Procedure to remove plaque from an occluded carotid artery. It is used to treat carotid stenosis due to atherosclerosis.	**endarterectomy** (END-ar-ter-EK-toh-mee) **endo-** *innermost; within* **arter/o-** *artery* **-ectomy** *surgical removal* The *o* in *endo-* is deleted when the word parts are combined.
coronary artery bypass graft (CABG)	Procedure to bypass an occluded coronary artery and restore blood flow to the myocardium. A blood vessel (either the saphenous vein from the leg or the internal mammary artery from the chest) is used as the bypass graft. If the saphenous vein is used, it must be placed in a reversed position so that its valves will not obstruct the flow of blood. The suturing of one blood vessel to another is an **anastomosis**. Oxygenated blood flows through the graft, around the blockage in the coronary artery, and back into the coronary artery. The abbreviation CABG is pronounced "cabbage."	**anastomosis** (ah-NAS-toh-MOH-sis) **anastom/o-** *create an opening between two structures* **-osis** *condition; process*
heart transplantation	Procedure to remove a severely damaged heart from a patient with end-stage heart failure and insert a new heart from a **donor** (a person who has recently died). The patient is matched by blood type and tissue type to the donor. Heart transplant patients must take immunosuppressant drugs for the rest of their lives to keep their bodies from rejecting the foreign tissue of their new heart. Some patients receive an artificial heart made of plastic, metal, and other synthetic materials.　　While awaiting a donor heart, the patient may have a left ventricular assist device (LVAD) temporarily implanted. This battery- or pneumatic-powered pump is placed in the abdomen and connected by tubes to the left ventricle and the aorta. In some patients, it becomes a permanent solution.	**transplantation** (TRANS-plan-TAY-shun) **transplant/o-** *move something across and put in another place* **-ation** *being; having; process* **donor** (DOH-nor)

Word or Phrase	Description	Pronunciation/Word Parts
pacemaker insertion	Procedure in which an automated device is implanted to control the heart rate and rhythm in a patient with an arrhythmia (see Figure 5-31 ■). A pacemaker uses a wire positioned on the heart to coordinate the heartbeat with an electrical impulse.	

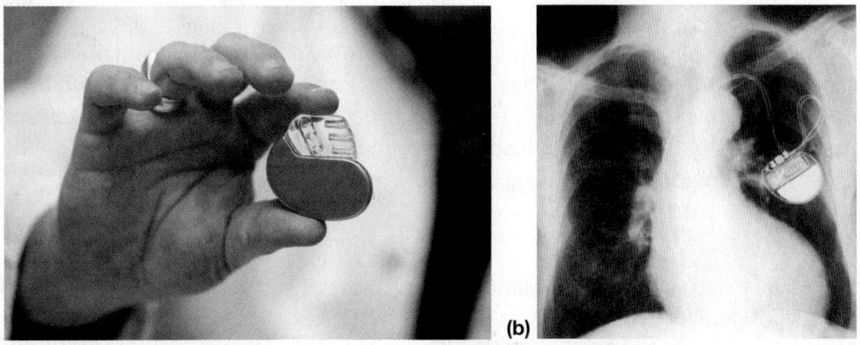

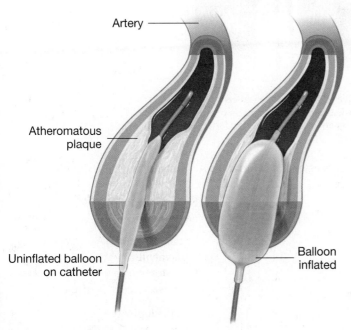

FIGURE 5-31 ■ Pacemaker.
(a) This pacemaker (programmable pulse generator) is placed under the skin of the anterior chest. (b) This chest x-ray shows the position of an implanted pacemaker and the pacemaker wires on the heart.
Source: Picsfive/Shutterstock; Dario Sabljak/Shutterstock

Word or Phrase	Description	Pronunciation/Word Parts
percutaneous transluminal coronary angioplasty (PTCA)	Procedure to reconstruct a coronary artery that is narrowed because of atherosclerosis. A catheter is inserted into the femoral artery and threaded to the site of the stenosis. Also known as **percutaneous coronary intervention (PCI)**. During a **balloon angioplasty**, a balloon within the catheter is inflated. It compresses the atheromatous plaque and widens the lumen of the artery. Then the balloon is deflated and the catheter is removed (see Figure 5-32 ■). Alternatively, an intravascular stainless steel mesh **stent** (unexpanded) can be inserted on the catheter (see Figure 5-33 ■). The stent is expanded, the catheter is removed, and the expanded stent remains in the artery.	**percutaneous** (PER-kyoo-TAY-nee-us) **per-** *through; throughout* **cutane/o-** *skin* **-ous** *pertaining to* **transluminal** (trans-LOO-mih-nal) **trans-** *across; through* **lumin/o-** *lumen; opening* **-al** *pertaining to* **angioplasty** (AN-jee-oh-PLAS-tee) **angi/o-** *blood vessel; lymphatic vessel* **-plasty** *process of reshaping by surgery*

Artery

Atheromatous plaque

Uninflated balloon on catheter

Balloon inflated

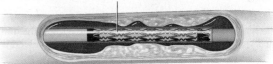
Unexpanded stent on catheter

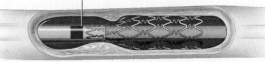
Sheath removed from stent

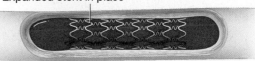
Expanded stent in place

FIGURE 5-32 ■ Balloon angioplasty.
The inflated balloon compresses atheromatous plaque in the artery to open the lumen and increase the blood flow. Then the balloon is deflated and the catheter is withdrawn.
Source: Pearson Education

FIGURE 5-33 ■ Stent.
A stent is expanded inside the artery to compress the atheromatous plaque and increase the blood flow. The stent is left in place as the catheter is withdrawn. It provides continuing support to keep the lumen of the artery open over time.
Source: Pearson Education

Word or Phrase	Description	Pronunciation/Word Parts
pericardiocentesis	Procedure that uses a needle to puncture the pericardium and withdraw inflammatory fluid accumulated in the pericardial sac. It is used to treat pericarditis and cardiac tamponade.	**pericardiocentesis** (PAIR-ih-KAR-dee-OH-sen-TEE-sis) **peri-** *around* **cardi/o-** *heart* **-centesis** *procedure to puncture*
radiofrequency ablation (RFA)	Procedure to destroy ectopic areas in the heart that are emitting electrical impulses and producing arrhythmias. A catheter is inserted into the heart. Radiofrequency electrical current is used to produce enough heat to kill the cells causing the arrhythmia. **Radiofrequency catheter occlusion** uses heat to collapse and seal large varicose veins.	**ablation** (ah-BLAY-shun) **ablat/o-** *destroy; take away* **-ion** *action; condition* **occlusion** (oh-KLOO-zhun) **occlus/o-** *close against* **-ion** *action; condition*
valve replacement	Procedure to replace a severely damaged or prolapsed heart valve with an artificial valve, or **prosthesis** (see Figure 5-34 ■). There are several types of **prosthetic** heart valves that can be used. If the replacement heart valve comes from an animal, it is known as a **xenograft**.	**prosthesis** (praws-THEE-sis) **prosthetic** (praws-THET-ik) **prosthet/o-** *artificial part* **-ic** *pertaining to* **xenograft** (ZEN-oh-graft) **xen/o-** *foreign* **-graft** *tissue for implant; tissue for transplant*

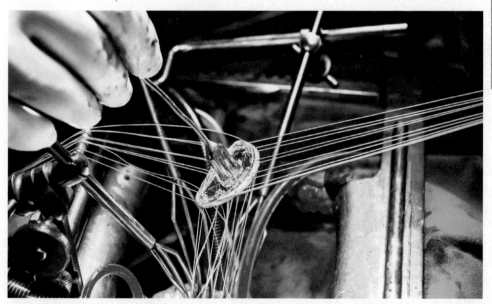

FIGURE 5-34 ■ Surgery for mitral valve regurgitation.
A white artificial ring is implanted in the heart to encircle the mitral valve and pull the two leaflets together. Many sutures are used to attach the ring so that blood will not leak around the edges. In other cases, the entire valve is replaced.

Source: Pirke/Fotolia

Word or Phrase	Description	Pronunciation/Word Parts
valvoplasty	Procedure to reconstruct a heart valve to correct stenosis or prolapse. A **valvulotome** is used to cut the valve. This procedure is also known as a **valvuloplasty**.	**valvoplasty** (VAL-voh-PLAS-tee) **valv/o-** *valve* **-plasty** *process of reshaping by surgery* **valvulotome** (VAL-vyoo-loh-TOHM) **valvul/o-** *valve* **-tome** *area with distinct edges; instrument used to cut* **valvuloplasty** (VAL-vyoo-loh-PLAS-tee) **valvul/o-** *valve* **-plasty** *process of reshaping by surgery*

Drugs

These drug categories and drugs are used to treat cardiovascular diseases. The most common generic and trade name drugs in each category are listed.

Category	Indication	Examples	Pronunciation/Word Parts
ACE (angiotensin-converting enzyme) inhibitor drugs	Treat congestive heart failure and hypertension. ACE inhibitor drugs produce vasodilation and decrease the blood pressure by blocking an enzyme that converts angiotensin I to angiotensin II (a vasoconstrictor).	captopril (Capoten), lisinopril (Prinivil, Zestril), trandolapril (Mavik)	**angiotensin** (AN-jee-oh-TEN-sin) **angi/o-** *blood vessel; lymphatic vessel* **tens/o-** *pressure; tension* **-in** *substance*
antiarrhythmic drugs	Treat arrhythmias	Intravenous atropine for heart block, intravenous lidocaine (Xylocaine) for ventricular fibrillation. Some beta-blocker drugs and calcium channel blocker drugs are used to treat ventricular tachycardia.	**antiarrhythmic** (AN-tee-aa-RITH-mik) **anti-** *against* **a-** *away from; without* **rrhythm/o-** *rhythm* **-ic** *pertaining to*
anticoagulant drugs	Prevent a blood clot from forming in patients with arteriosclerosis, atrial fibrillation, previous myocardial infarction, or an artificial heart valve	heparin, warfarin (Coumadin), clopidogrel (Plavix)	**anticoagulant** (AN-tee-koh-AG-yoo-lant) (AN-tih-koh-AG-yoo-lant) **anti-** *against* **coagul/o-** *clotting* **-ant** *pertaining to*
antihypertensive drugs	Treat hypertension	See *ACE inhibitor drugs, beta-blocker drugs, calcium channel blocker drugs,* and *diuretic drugs.*	**antihypertensive** (AN-tee-HY-per-TEN-siv) **anti-** *against* **hyper-** *above; more than normal* **tens/o-** *pressure; tension* **-ive** *pertaining to*
aspirin	Prevents heart attacks. Prevents blood clots from forming by keeping platelets from sticking together.	aspirin (81 mg)	
beta-blocker drugs	Treat angina pectoris and hypertension. Beta-blocker drugs decrease the heart rate and dilate the arteries by blocking beta receptors.	atenolol (Tenormin), nadolol (Corgard), propranolol (Inderal), metoprolol (Lopressor)	
calcium channel blocker drugs	Treat angina pectoris and hypertension. These drugs block the movement of calcium ions into myocardial cells and smooth muscle cells of the artery walls, causing the heart rate and blood pressure to decrease.	amlodipine (Norvasc), diltiazem (Cardizem), nifedipine (Adalat, Procardia), verapamil (Calan)	

Category	Indication	Examples	Pronunciation/Word Parts
digitalis drugs	Treat congestive heart failure. Digitalis drugs decrease the heart rate and strengthen the heart's contractions (see Figure 5-35 ■).	digoxin (Lanoxin)	**digitalis** (DIJ-ih-TAL-is)

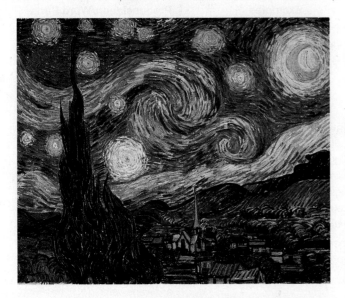

FIGURE 5-35 ■ The Starry Night.
Vincent van Gogh's "The Starry Night" (1889) is believed by some physicians to show evidence of digitalis toxicity in the way the Dutch painter depicted yellow-green halos around the stars. Van Gogh (1853–1890) suffered from mania and epilepsy and may have been given digitalis for lack of a more specific drug therapy. Digitalis can easily reach a toxic level in the blood. Symptoms of toxicity include nausea and vomiting, decreased heart rate, and sometimes visual halos. Van Gogh may simply have painted what he actually saw because of digitalis toxicity.

SOURCE: Vincent van Gogh (1853–1890), "The Starry Night." 1889. Oil on canvas, 29 × 36 1/4" (73.7 × 92.1 cm). Acquired through the Lillie P. Bliss Bequest. (472.1941). The Museum of Modern Art, New York, NY, U.S.A./Digital Image © The Museum of Modern Art/Licensed by SCALA/Art Resource, NY.

DID YOU KNOW?

Digitalis drugs come from *Digitalis* (foxglove plant). Its flowers were thought to resemble fingerlike projections or digits.

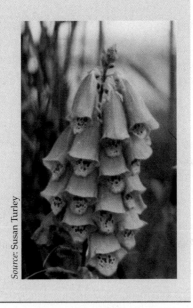

Source: Susan Turley

Category	Indication	Examples	Pronunciation/Word Parts
diuretic drugs	Block sodium from being absorbed from the tubule (of the nephron of the kidney) back into the blood. As the sodium is excreted in the urine, it brings water and potassium with it because of osmotic pressure. This process is known as *diuresis*. This decreases the volume of blood and is used to treat hypertension and congestive heart failure. Laypersons call these drugs "water pills."	furosemide (Lasix), hydrochlorothiazide (HCTZ)	**diuretic** (DY-yoor-EH-tik) **dia-** *complete; completely through* **ur/o-** *urinary system; urine* **-etic** *pertaining to* The *a* in *dia-* is dropped when the word is formed.

Category	Indication	Examples	Pronunciation/Word Parts
drugs for cardiac arrest	Treat a nonbeating heart (asystole) by stimulating it to contract	intracardiac epinephrine (Adrenalin)	
drugs for hyperlipidemia	Treat hypercholesterolemia. They are often referred to as "statin drugs" because of the common ending of the generic drug names.	atorvastatin (Lipitor), lovastatin (Mevacor), rosuvastatin (Crestor), simvastatin (Zocor)	
nitrate drugs	Treat angina pectoris. Nitrate drugs dilate the veins (to decrease the amount of work that the heart must do) and dilate the arteries (to decrease the blood pressure)	isosorbide (Isordil), nitroglycerin (Nitro-Dur)	**nitrate** (NY-trayt)

DID YOU KNOW?

In the mid-1890s, physicians observed that the pain of angina pectoris seemed to be relieved in patients who worked in dynamite and gunpowder factories where nitroglycerin was an ingredient. This led to the practice of prescribing nitroglycerin for angina pectoris.

Category	Indication	Examples	Pronunciation/Word Parts
thrombolytic drugs	Treat a blood clot that is blocking blood flow through an artery. Thrombolytic drugs lyse (break apart) a clot.	alteplase (Activase)	**thrombolytic** (THRAWM-boh-LIT-ik) **thromb/o-** *blood clot* **lyt/o-** *break down; destroy* **-ic** *pertaining to*

Abbreviations

AAA	abdominal aortic aneurysm		**LVH**	left ventricular hypertrophy
ACE	angiotensin-converting enzyme		**MI**	myocardial infarction
ACS	acute coronary syndrome		**mm Hg**	millimeters of mercury
AED	automatic external defibrillator		**MR**	mitral regurgitation
AI	aortic insufficiency; apical impulse		**MUGA**	multiple-gated acquisition (scan) (pronounced "MUG-ah")
AICD	automatic implantable cardiac defibrillator; automatic implantable cardioverter-defibrillator		**MVP**	mitral valve prolapse
			NSR	normal sinus rhythm
			P	pulse (rate)
AMI	acute myocardial infarction		**PAC**	premature atrial contraction
AS	aortic stenosis		**PAD**	peripheral artery disease
ASCVD	arteriosclerotic cardiovascular disease		**PCI**	percutaneous coronary intervention
ASD	atrial septal defect		**PDA**	patent ductus arteriosus
ASHD	arteriosclerotic heart disease		**PMI**	point of maximum impulse
AV	atrioventricular		**PTCA**	percutaneous transluminal coronary angioplasty
BP	blood pressure			
BPM, bpm	beats per minute		**PVC**	premature ventricular contraction
CABG	coronary artery bypass graft (pronounced "cabbage")		**PVD**	peripheral vascular disease
			RA	right atrium
CAD	coronary artery disease		**RBBB**	right bundle branch block
CCU	coronary care unit		**RFA**	radiofrequency ablation
CHF	congestive heart failure		**RNV**	radionuclide ventriculography
CK-MB	creatine kinase-MB (band)		**RV**	right ventricle
CPK-MB	creatine phosphokinase-MB (band)		S_1	first heart sound
CPR	cardiopulmonary resuscitation		S_2	second heart sound
CRP	C-reactive protein		S_3	third heart sound
CV	cardiovascular		S_4	fourth heart sound
DSA	digital subtraction angiography		**SA**	sinoatrial
ECG	electrocardiogram; electrocardiography		**SBE**	subacute bacterial endocarditis
EKG	electrocardiogram; electrocardiography		**SPECT**	single-photon emission computerized tomography
HDL	high-density lipoprotein			
HTN	hypertension		**SVT**	supraventricular tachycardia
JVD	jugular venous distention		**TEE**	transesophageal echocardiogram; transesophageal echocardiography
LA	left atrium			
LBBB	left bundle branch block		**TPR**	temperature, pulse, and respiration
LDH	lactic dehydrogenase		**V fib**	ventricular fibrillation (short form)
LDL	low-density lipoprotein		**VLDL**	very low-density lipoprotein
LV	left ventricle		**VSD**	ventricular septal defect
LVAD	left ventricular assist device		**V tach**	ventricular tachycardia (short form)

Word Part	Meaning	Word Part	Meaning
83. ili/o-		129. poplite/o-	
84. -in		130. port/o-	
85. infarct/o-		131. pre-	
86. -ion		132. prosthet/o-	
87. isch/o-		133. pulmon/o-	
88. -ist		134. radi/o-	
89. -itis		135. re-	
90. -ive		136. regurgitat/o-	
91. -ization		137. ren/o-	
92. jugul/o-		138. rheumat/o-	
93. lipid/o-		139. rrhythm/o-	
94. lip/o-		140. saphen/o-	
95. log/o-		141. scler/o-	
96. -logy		142. -scope	
97. lumin/o-		143. sept/o-	
98. lyt/o-		144. sin/o-	
99. man/o-		145. son/o-	
100. mediastin/o-		146. sphygm/o-	
101. -megaly		147. sten/o-	
102. -meter		148. sub-	
103. -metry		149. supra-	
104. mitr/o-		150. system/o-	
105. my/o-		151. -systole	
106. necr/o-		152. systol/o-	
107. occlus/o-		153. tachy-	
108. -ole		154. tampon/o-	
109. -oma		155. techn/o-	
110. -ory		156. tele/o-	
111. -ose		157. tens/o-	
112. -osis		158. tetr/a-	
113. -ous		159. theli/o-	
114. palpit/o-		160. -therapy	
115. pariet/o-		161. thorac/o-	
116. path/o-		162. thromb/o-	
117. -pathy		163. tibi/o-	
118. pat/o-		164. -tic	
119. pector/o-		165. -tome	
120. per-		166. tom/o-	
121. peri-		167. trans-	
122. peripher/o-		168. transplant/o-	
123. perone/o-		169. tri-	
124. pharmac/o-		170. triglycerid/o-	
125. phleb/o-		171. -trophy	
126. physi/o-		172. -ule	
127. -plasty		173. uln/o-	
128. polar/o-		174. ultra-	

Word Part	Meaning	Word Part	Meaning
175. -um	_____	182. vegetat/o-	_____
176. ur/o-	_____	183. ven/o-	_____
177. valv/o-	_____	184. ventricul/o-	_____
178. valvul/o-	_____	185. vers/o-	_____
179. varic/o-	_____	186. viscer/o-	_____
180. vas/o-	_____	187. xen/o-	_____
181. vascul/o-	_____		

RELATED COMBINING FORMS EXERCISE

Write the combining forms on the line provided. (Hint: See the It's Greek to Me feature box.)

1. Three combining forms that mean *blood vessel*. _____

2. Two combining forms that mean *heart*. _____

3. Two combining forms that mean *vein*. _____

5.5B Define Abbreviations

MATCHING EXERCISE

Match each abbreviation to its description.

1. LVAD	_____	"Good cholesterol," a high-density lipoprotein
2. AAA	_____	High blood pressure
3. SBE	_____	Bacterial infection inside the heart
4. CRP	_____	Type of aneurysm
5. mm Hg	_____	Test to detect inflammation in the heart
6. HTN	_____	Hole in the septum between the ventricles
7. TPR	_____	Vital signs
8. TEE	_____	Measurement of blood pressure
9. VSD	_____	Heart test that goes into the esophagus
10. DL	_____	May be used instead of heart transplantation

5.6A Divide Medical Words

DIVIDING WORDS EXERCISE

Separate these words into their component parts (prefix, combining form, suffix). Note: Some words do not contain all three word parts. The first one has been done for you.

Medical Word	Prefix	Combining Form	Suffix	Medical Word	Prefix	Combining Form	Suffix
1. circulation	_____	circulat/o-	-ion	6. bradycardia	_____	_____	_____
2. depolarization	_____	_____	_____	7. aneurysmal	_____	_____	_____
3. ischemia	_____	_____	_____	8. hyperlipidemia	_____	_____	_____
4. endocarditis	_____	_____	_____	9. angioplasty	_____	_____	_____
5. arrhythmia	_____	_____	_____	10. transluminal	_____	_____	_____

5.6B Build Medical Words

COMBINING FORM AND SUFFIX EXERCISE

Read the definition of the medical word. Select the correct suffix from the Suffix List. Select the correct combining form from the Combining Form List. Build the medical word and write it on the line. Be sure to check your spelling. The first one has been done for you.

SUFFIX LIST	COMBINING FORM LIST
-ation (being; having; process)	aneurysm/o- (aneurysm; dilation)
-ectomy (surgical removal)	angi/o- (blood vessel; lymphatic vessel)
-ent (pertaining to)	arteri/o- (artery)
-gram (picture; record)	ather/o- (soft, fatty substance)
-graphy (process of recording)	auscult/o- (listening)
-ion (action; condition)	cardi/o- (heart)
-itis (infection of; inflammation of)	claudicat/o- (limping pain)
-megaly (enlargement)	fibrill/o- (muscle fiber; nerve fiber)
-metry (process of measuring)	infarct/o- (small area of dead tissue)
-oma (mass; tumor)	necr/o- (dead body; dead cells; dead tissue)
-osis (condition; process)	palpit/o- (throb)
-plasty (process of reshaping by surgery)	pat/o- (open)
-scope (instrument used to examine)	phleb/o- (vein)
-therapy (treatment)	scler/o- (hard; sclera of the eye)
-tic (pertaining to)	sten/o- (constriction; narrowness)
-tome (area with distinct edges; instrument used to cut)	steth/o- (chest)
	tele/o- (distance)
	valvul/o- (valve)

Definition of the Medical Word

Build the Medical Word

1. Pertaining to dead cells (or) dead tissue — *necrotic*

2. Enlargement (of the) heart

3. Mass (composed of a) soft, fatty substance

4. Having limping pain (in the calf of the leg)

5. Surgical removal (of an) aneurysm

6. Condition (of) constriction or narrowness (of a blood vessel)

7. Condition (of having a) small area of dead tissue (in the heart)

8. Process of reshaping by surgery (of a) blood vessel

9. Process (of) listening (to the heart)

10. Treatment (that makes a varicose vein) hard

11. Process of measuring (the heart rate and rhythm from a) distance

12. Inflammation of (or) infection of (a) vein

13. Pertaining to (a blood vessel being) open

14. Having (a very fast, uncoordinated twitching of the) muscle fibers (of the heart)

15. Process of recording (the image of a) blood vessel

16. Instrument used to cut (a heart) valve

17. Having (the heart) throb (or "thump")

18. Picture or record (of an) artery

19. Process of reshaping by surgery (of a) valve

20. Instrument used to examine (and listen to the) chest (and heart)

PREFIX EXERCISE

Read the definition of the medical word. Look at the medical word or partial word that is given (it already contains a combining form and a suffix). Select the correct prefix from the Prefix List and write it on the blank line. Then build the medical word and write it on the line. Be sure to check your spelling. The first one has been done for you.

PREFIX LIST

a- (away from; without)	hyper- (above; more than normal)	tachy- (fast)
brady- (slow)	hypo- (below; deficient)	trans- (across; through)
de- (reversal of; without)	peri- (around)	
endo- (innermost; within)	supra- (above)	

Definition of the Medical Word	Prefix	Word or Partial Word	Build the Medical Word
1. Substance in the blood (of a) more than normal (level of) cholesterol	hyper-	cholesterolemia	hypercholesterolemia
2. Pertaining to (a) fast heart (rate)	_____	cardic	_____
3. Condition (of) more than normal pressure (of the blood)	_____	tension	_____
4. Pertaining to a condition (of) reversal of (a) compensated (heart)	_____	compensated	_____
5. Procedure to puncture (the membrane that is) around (the) heart	_____	cardiocentesis	_____
6. Pertaining to through (the) lumen (of a blood vessel)	_____	luminal	_____
7. Condition (of a) slow heart (rate)	_____	cardia	_____
8. Substance in the blood (of a) more than normal (level of) fat	_____	lipidemia	_____
9. Pertaining to (an area) above (the) ventricle	_____	ventricular	_____
10. Condition (of the heart being) without rhythm	_____	rrhythmia	_____
11. Inflammation of (the membrane that is) around (the) heart	_____	carditis	_____
12. Surgical removal (of plaque from) within (an) artery	_____	arterectomy	_____
13. Pertaining to below (normal blood) pressure	_____	tensive	_____
14. Inflammation of (or) infection of (the) innermost (lining of the) heart	_____	carditis	_____

MULTIPLE COMBINING FORMS AND SUFFIX EXERCISE

Read the definition of the medical word. Select the correct suffix and combining forms. Then build the medical word and write it on the line. Be sure to check your spelling. The first one has been done for you.

SUFFIX LIST

COMBINING FORM LIST

SUFFIX LIST	COMBINING FORM LIST	
-al (pertaining to)	arteri/o- (artery)	my/o- (muscle)
-graphy (process of recording)	ather/o- (soft, fatty substance)	path/o- (disease)
-ic (pertaining to)	cardi/o- (heart)	phleb/o- (vein)
-ion (action; condition)	ech/o- (echo of a sound wave)	scler/o- (hard; sclera of the eye)
-itis (infection of; inflammation of)	electr/o- (electricity)	sphygm/o- (pulse)
-meter (instrument used to measure)	idi/o- (individual; unknown)	thromb/o- (blood clot)
-osis (condition; process)	lyt/o- (break down; destroy)	vers/o- (travel; turn)
-pathy (disease)	man/o- (frenzy; thin)	

Definition of the Medical Word

Build the Medical Word

1. Condition (of the) artery (with) hard(ness)

arteriosclerosis

2. Pertaining to (the) muscle (of the) heart

_____

3. Process of recording (the) echo of a sound wave (from the) heart

_____

4. Pertaining to (a drug that takes a) blood clot (and) breaks down and destroys (it)

_____

5. Condition (of a) soft, fatty substance (as well as) hard(ness in an artery)

_____

Definition of the Medical Word

6. Process of recording (the) electrical (impulses of the) heart

7. Inflammation of (or) infection of (a) blood clot (in a) vein

8. Disease (of the) heart muscle

9. Instrument used to measure (the) pulse (of the blood pressure using a) thin (cuff)

10. Pertaining to (an) unknown (cause of a) disease

11. Action (done to the) heart (to) turn (it away from an arrhythmia)

Build the Medical Word

_____

_____

_____

_____

_____

_____

5.7A Spell Medical Words

PROOFREADING AND SPELLING EXERCISE

Read the following paragraph. Identify each misspelled medical word and write the correct spelling of it on the line provided.

The nurse used a sphigmomanometer to take the patient's blood pressure. He had hypertension in the past. He had a caroted endarterectomy because of an atherometous plaque in his artery. He has also had an arhythmia in the past with ventricular takycardia. He just developed congestive heart failure and takes a dijitalis drug for that. We are considering this patient for an angoplasty in the future to keep him from having a myocardal infarcktion. His cardiomegalee is becoming more severe.

1. _____   6. _____

2. _____   7. _____

3. _____   8. _____

4. _____   9. _____

5. _____   10. _____

YOU WRITE THE MEDICAL REPORT

You are a healthcare professional interviewing a patient. Listen to the patient's statements and then enter them in the patient's medical record using medical words and phrases. Be sure to check your spelling. The first one has been done for you.

1. The patient says, "Last night, I had severe pain in my chest that was like a crushing sensation and bad sweating and I felt like something really bad was happening."

   You write: Last night, the patient experienced severe _angina_ _pectoris_ with the pain feeling like a crushing sensation. He also had _diaphoresis_ and a sense of doom.

2. The patient says, "Last year, I went to the emergency room and my heart rate was about 200. They brought this machine in and it had two paddles and they gave me a shock and then my heart rhythm was normal. Today, I could feel my heart do some "thumps" and then be okay. But the last time this happened, they did hook me up to those electrodes and took a tracing of my heart."

   You write: The patient states that last year she went to the emergency room with ventricular _____ with a rate of about 200. They did a _____, and her heart rhythm returned to normal. The patient says she felt some _____ today, and so we will have an _____ done in the office today.

3. The patient says, "I know I have a history of my arteries being hard and clogged with fatty stuff, but now I have this new problem and I get on-and-off pain in the calf of my leg when I try to walk very far. My podiatrist said my one toe does not get enough blood to it and the tissue might die."

   You write: The patient has a history of _____, but now she has a new problem of experiencing _____ when she tries to walk very far. Her podiatrist noted a lack of perfusion to one toe and feels it might become _____.

4. The nurse's note in the patient's medical record shows that the patient's blood pressure today is 130/88. Previous office visits have shown similar BP results. The patient says, "I am trying to stay on my low-salt diet."

   You write: Based on serial blood pressure measurements today and over the past 3 months, the patient's blood pressure remains in the range of 130/88, and she now has a diagnosis of _____. She has been on a low-salt diet, and we will now add the _____ drug furosemide for treatment to lower her blood pressure.

HEARING MEDICAL WORDS EXERCISE

You hear someone speaking the medical words given below. Read each pronunciation and then write the medical word it represents. Be sure to check your spelling. The first one has been done for you.

1. KAR-dee-ac   cardiac _____
2. AN-yoor-izm   _____
3. KAR-DEE-oh-THOR-AS-IK   _____
4. MY-oh-KAR-dee-um   _____
5. KOR-oh-NAIR-ee AR-ter-ee   _____
6. VAY-soh-con-STRIK-shun   _____

7. KAR-dee-oh-MEG-ah-lee   _____
8. aa-RITH-mee-ah   _____
9. ATH-eh-ROH-skleh-ROH-sis   _____
10. EK-oh-KAR-dee-oh-GRAM   _____
11. AN-jee-oh-PLAS-tee   _____
12. SFIG-moh-mah-NAW-meh-ter   _____

5.7B Pronounce Medical Words

PRONUNCIATION EXERCISE

Read the medical word and the syllables in its pronunciation. Circle the primary (main) accented syllable. The first one has been done for you.

1. cardiac (kar-dee-ac)
2. coronary (kor-oh-nair-ee)
3. vasodilation (vay-soh-dy-lay-shun)
4. cardiopulmonary (kar-dee-oh-pul-moh-nair-ee)
5. pericarditis (pair-ee-kar-dy-tis)
6. myocardial infarction (my-oh-kar-dee-al in-fark-shun)
7. fibrillation (fib-rih-lay-shun)
8. atherosclerosis (ath-eh-roh-skleh-roh-sis)
9. auscultation (aws-kul-tay-shun)
10. angioplasty (an-jee-oh-plas-tee)

5.8 Research Medical Words

SOUND-ALIKE WORDS

Compare and contrast the meanings of these sound-alike cardiology words.

1. *cardiac* and *cardia* (Chapter 3)
2. *stress test* and *nonstress test* (Chapter 13)
3. *palpation* (Chapter 2) and *palpitation*

5.9 Analyze Medical Reports

ELECTRONIC PATIENT RECORD #1

This is a hospital Admission History and Physical Examination report. Read the report and answer the questions.

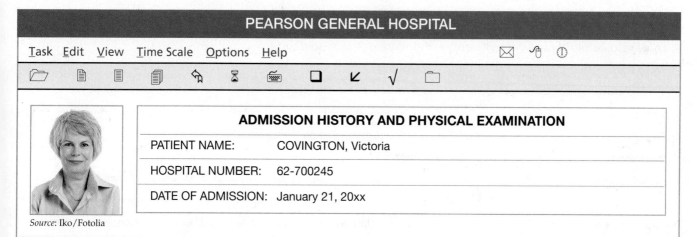

PEARSON GENERAL HOSPITAL

Task   Edit   View   Time Scale   Options   Help

ADMISSION HISTORY AND PHYSICAL EXAMINATION

PATIENT NAME:	COVINGTON, Victoria
HOSPITAL NUMBER:	62-700245
DATE OF ADMISSION:	January 21, 20xx

Source: Iko/Fotolia

HISTORY OF PRESENT ILLNESS

The patient is a 66-year-old white female who was transferred from home via ambulance to this emergency department. Apparently, the patient had just finished eating breakfast when her family noticed that she was standing in the middle of the hallway with her walker and seemed dazed. She was assisted to her bed, but rest did not improve her mental status. The family stated that she continued to be confused, incoherent, and unable to answer simple questions. At that point, the family called 911.

PAST MEDICAL HISTORY

The past medical history was obtained from the patient's daughter-in-law. The patient has a history of CHF, which has been slowly worsening over about the past 8 years. She also has a history of hypertension. The patient has been diagnosed with type 2 diabetes mellitus. The daughter-in-law remembers that the patient's last fasting blood sugar in the doctor's office last month was over 250. She is usually noncompliant with her diet, eating foods that are high in fat and calories. The patient does not take a pill or insulin for her diabetes. In the past week, the patient has had no appetite, has eaten little, but reportedly gained 2 pounds anyway. The daughter-in-law does not know the names of all of the patient's medications, except for Lasix. The patient smokes 1 pack of cigarettes per day and has done so for the past 40+ years. The patient has no known allergies.

PHYSICAL EXAMINATION

The patient is an obese female, lying in bed. She is stuporous, opening her eyes to commands but she is unable to answer questions. Heart: Regular rate and rhythm. The neck veins are slightly distended. The breath sounds reveal congestion in both lungs bilaterally. The abdomen is soft with hypoactive bowel sounds. Physical examination of the lower extremities shows severe edema in both feet and legs.

COURSE IN THE EMERGENCY DEPARTMENT

The patient was placed on a cardiac monitor and given a stat dose of intravenous Lasix. Labs were sent for CBC with WBC differential, electrolytes, CK-MB, troponin, and glucose. An arterial blood gas was drawn. Portable chest x-ray in the emergency department showed cardiomegaly with LVH. There was significant pulmonary congestion. While awaiting the results of the blood chemistries, the patient suddenly went into cardiac arrest. CPR was initiated. She responded to aggressive drug intervention, and we were able to establish a normal sinus rhythm. The patient was then transferred to the intensive care unit in critical condition, intubated, and on a ventilator.

Alfred P. Molina, M.D.

Alfred P. Molina, M.D.

APM:mtt
D: 01/21/xx
T: 01/21/xx

1. What is the medical abbreviation for hypertension? _____

2. The patient has hypertension. If you wanted to use the adjective form of *hypertension*, you would say, "The patient is
_____."

3. What do these abbreviations stand for?

   a. CHF _____

   b. CK-MB _____

   c. CPR _____

   d. LVH _____

4. Divide *vascular* into its two word parts and give the meaning of each word part.

   Word Part   **Meaning**

   _____   _____

   _____   _____

5. Divide *cardiomegaly* into its two word parts and give the meaning of each word part.

   Word Part   **Meaning**

   _____   _____

   _____   _____

6. These medical words were not covered in this chapter, but you need to know their meanings in order to understand this medical
report. Research these words and write their definitions.

   Word   **Meaning**

   bilaterally   _____

   incoherent   _____

   stuporous   _____

7. What is the normal range of the heart rate in beats per minute for an adult?

   _____

8. Besides hypertension, what other two diagnoses did the patient have before this hospitalization?

   a. _____

   b. _____

9. Resuscitation was used to treat what condition? (Circle one)

   cardiomegaly   **hypertension**   **cardiac arrest**   **diabetes mellitus**

10. Circle the two lab tests that were done to check to see if the patient had had a myocardial infarction.

    troponin   **portable chest x-ray**   **blood glucose**   **CK-MB**   **intubation**

11. The patient had a cardiac arrest. What is the medical word for having no heartbeat?

    _____

12. The severe edema in the patient's lower extremities reflected backup of blood due to failure of which side of the heart?

    _____

13. The pulmonary congestion seen on the chest x-ray reflected failure of which side of the heart?

    _____

14. Lasix is a diuretic drug that removes fluid from the body by excreting it in the urine. For which of the patient's medical conditions
was this drug prescribed? (Circle one)

    congestive heart failure   **lack of appetite**   **obesity**   **confusion**

15. If the patient ate little food in the past week, why did she gain 2 pounds?

    _____

ELECTRONIC PATIENT RECORD #2

This is an Office Visit SOAP Note. Read the note and answer the questions.

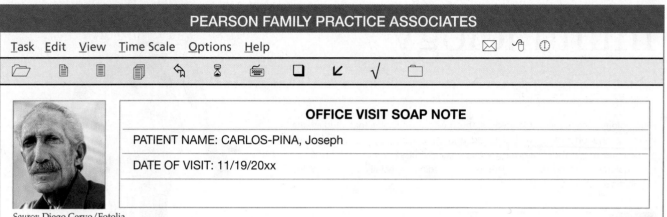

PEARSON FAMILY PRACTICE ASSOCIATES

Task   Edit   View   Time Scale   Options   Help

OFFICE VISIT SOAP NOTE

PATIENT NAME: CARLOS-PINA, Joseph

DATE OF VISIT: 11/19/20xx

Source: Diego Cervo/Fotolia

SUBJECTIVE: The patient is a 85-year-old Hispanic male who drove himself to our office and is complaining of chest discomfort since last evening. He lives alone and is a widower. He has a past history of an episode of asystole and 6 years ago was resuscitated by the paramedics doing CPR.

OBJECTIVE: Temperature 98.8 F, respiratory rate 30, blood pressure 150/100. The heart rate is irregular with runs of atrial fibrillation. The patient is alert and oriented, but in some distress.

ASSESSMENT: Atrial fibrillation and hypertension.

PLAN: An ambulance was called, and the patient was sent to the Emergency Department. His family was notified and will join him there.

1. What is the medical description of atrial fibrillation?
2. Which vital sign reading led to a diagnosis of hypertension?
3. What is the medical description of asystole and how is it treated medically?
4. What does the abbreviation *CPR* mean?

Chapter 6
Hematology and Immunology

Blood and Lymphatic System

Hematology (HEE-mah-TAW-loh-jee) is the medical specialty that studies the anatomy and physiology of the blood and uses laboratory and diagnostic procedures, medical and surgical procedures, and drugs to treat blood diseases. Immunology (IH-myoo-NAW-loh-jee) is the medical specialty related to the lymphatic system and the immune response.

Learning Outcomes

After you study this chapter, you should be able to

6.1 Identify structures of the blood and lymphatic system.

6.2 Describe the processes of blood clotting and the immune response.

6.3 Describe common blood, lymphatic system, and immune response diseases, laboratory and diagnostic procedures, medical and surgical procedures, and drugs.

6.4 Form the plural and adjective forms of nouns related to hematology and immunology.

6.5 Give the meanings of word parts and abbreviations related to hematology and immunology.

6.6 Divide hematology and immunology words and build hematology and immunology words.

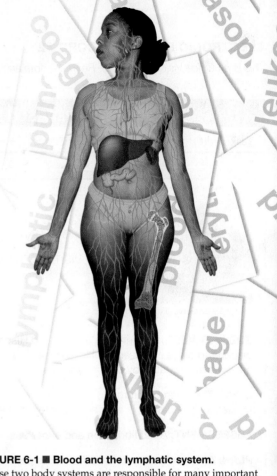

FIGURE 6-1 ■ Blood and the lymphatic system.
These two body systems are responsible for many important body functions: producing blood cells, clotting the blood, and coordinating the body's immune response.
Source: Pearson Education

6.7 Spell and pronounce hematology and immunology words.

6.8 Research sound-alike and other hematology and immunology words.

6.9 Analyze the medical content and meaning of hematology and immunology reports.

Medical Language Key

To unlock the definition of a medical word, break it into word parts. Give the meaning of each word part. Put the meanings of the word parts in order, beginning with the meaning of the suffix, then the prefix (if present), then the combining form(s).

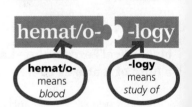

hemat/o- means *blood*

-logy means *study of*

	Word Part	Word Part Meaning
Suffix	**-logy**	*study of*
Combining Form	**hemat/o-**	*blood*

Hematology: ▶ *Study of (the) blood.*

	Word Part	Word Part Meaning
Suffix	**-logy**	*study of*
Combining Form	**immun/o-**	*immune response*

Immunology: ▶ *Study of (the) immune response.*

Anatomy and Physiology

Blood is categorized as connective tissue because its formed elements (blood cells and blood cell fragments) are produced by the bone marrow of the skeletal system (see Figure 6-1 ■). Blood contains blood cells and blood cell fragments, water, and other substances (proteins, clotting factors, etc.). Blood travels in the blood vessels of the cardiovascular system (discussed in "Cardiology," Chapter 5). The purpose of the blood is to transport oxygen, carbon dioxide, nutrients, and the waste products of metabolism. The blood can stop its own flow at the site of an injury. Some blood cells also function as part of the immune response of the lymphatic system.

The lymphatic system (see Figure 6-1) consists of the lymphatic vessels, lymph nodes, lymph fluid, lymphoid tissues, and lymphoid organs. The lymphatic system forms a pathway throughout the body that is separate from that of the cardiovascular system; however, some cells in the blood function as part of the immune response of the lymphatic system. The purpose of the lymphatic system is to defend the body against microorganisms, foreign particles, and cancerous cells by means of the immune response.

Anatomy of the Blood

Plasma

Plasma is a clear, straw-colored liquid that makes up 55% of the blood (see Figure 6-2 ■). The formed elements of the blood (erythrocytes, leukocytes, thrombocytes) are suspended in the plasma. The plasma contains nutrients from digested foods: amino acids, cholesterol, triglycerides, electrolytes, glucose, minerals, and vitamins. Also in the plasma are substances produced by the liver or glands: albumin, conjugated bilirubin, unconjugated bilirubin, hormones, complement proteins, and clotting factors. Finally, the plasma contains creatinine and urea, the waste products of cellular metabolism. Plasma is about 90% water, but this percentage can change if there is a decreased intake of water or an increased loss of water (from diarrhea, increased urination, excessive sweating, etc.).

plasma (PLAZ-mah)
The combining form **plasm/o-** means *plasma*.

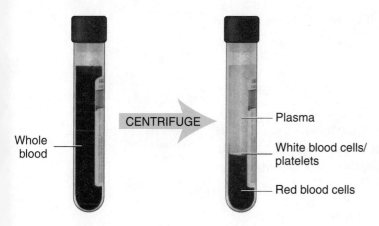

Whole blood — CENTRIFUGE → Plasma

White blood cells/platelets

Red blood cells

FIGURE 6-2 ■ Plasma.
Blood is composed of plasma and formed elements (red blood cells, white blood cells, platelets). When a specimen of whole blood is placed in a centrifuge and spun quickly, the heavier parts (the formed elements) settle to the bottom, and the clear, straw-colored plasma remains on the top.
Source: Pearson Education

A CLOSER LOOK

Plasma proteins, the most abundant of which is **albumin**, are molecules that are too large to pass through the wall of a blood vessel. They stay in the plasma and exert an osmotic pressure that keeps water in the blood from moving out into the surrounding tissues.

albumin (al-BYOO-min)

WORD ALERT
Sound-Alike Words

albumen	(noun)	the white of an egg
		Example: Albumen in egg whites is a good source of dietary protein.
albumin	(noun)	protein molecule in the blood
		Example: Albumin is an important protein in the plasma.

Electrolytes are elements that carry a positive or negative electrical charge. Electrolytes in the plasma include sodium (Na^+), potassium (K^+), calcium (Ca^{++}), chloride (Cl^-), and bicarbonate (HCO_3^-). Sodium plays an important role in maintaining the volume and pressure of the blood. Sodium, potassium, and calcium are important in the contraction of the heart and skeletal muscles. Calcium is also important during blood clotting and in the formation of bone. Bicarbonate acts as a buffer to maintain the normal pH (acidity versus alkalinity) of the blood.

Pronunciation/Word Parts

electrolyte (ee-LEK-troh-lite)
  electr/o- *electricity*
  -lyte *dissolved substance*

DID YOU KNOW?

Blood tastes salty because the electrolytes sodium and chloride in the plasma are the same ingredients that make up table salt.

Hematopoiesis

Hematopoiesis is the process by which all of the formed elements in the blood are produced. Hematopoiesis occurs in the red marrow of long bones or flat bones (such as the sternum, ribs, hip bones, bones of the spinal column, and bones of the legs). Every type of blood cell (erythrocyte, leukocyte) and blood cell fragment (thrombocyte) begins in the bone marrow as a very immature cell known as a **stem cell** (see Figure 6-3 ■).

hematopoiesis (HEE-mah-TOH-poy-EE-sis)
  hemat/o- *blood*
  -poiesis *process of formation*

Erythrocytes

Erythrocytes are the most numerous of the formed elements suspended in the plasma. An **erythrocyte** or **red blood cell (RBC)** is a round, somewhat flattened, red disk. Its depressed center (where the cell is not as thick) is paler in color (see Figure 6-4 ■). Erythrocytes are unique because, unlike other body cells, they have no cell nucleus when they are mature.

erythrocyte (eh-RITH-roh-site)
  erythr/o- *red*
  -cyte *cell*

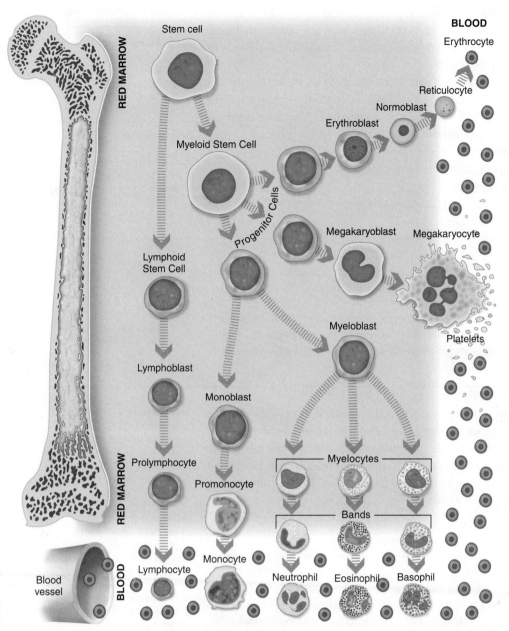

BLOOD

Stem cell

Erythrocyte

RED MARROW

Reticulocyte

Normoblast

Myeloid Stem Cell

Erythroblast

Progenitor Cells

Megakaryoblast

Megakaryocyte

Lymphoid Stem Cell

Platelets

Lymphoblast

Myeloblast

Monoblast

Myelocytes

Prolymphocyte

Bands

Promonocyte

RED MARROW

Blood vessel

BLOOD

Lymphocyte

Monocyte

Neutrophil

Eosinophil

Basophil

FIGURE 6-3 ■ **Hematopoiesis.**
All of the formed elements of the blood begin in the red bone marrow as stem cells that progress to mature cells.

Source: Pearson Education

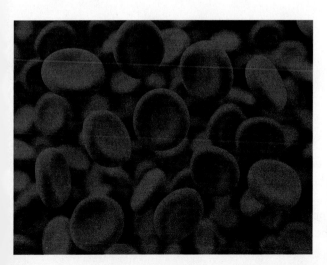

FIGURE 6-4 ■ **Erythrocytes.**
Notice the characteristic red color of erythrocytes (red blood cells) and their unique "donut" shape. Each erythrocyte has a depressed center and no cell nucleus. Because there is no nucleus, an erythrocyte deteriorates and dies after 120 days.

Source: Mihalis A/Fotolia

Erythrocytes contain **hemoglobin**, a red, iron-containing molecule. It is this molecule that binds to and carries oxygen from the lungs to every cell in the body. Hemoglobin bound to oxygen is known as **oxyhemoglobin**. Hemoglobin also binds to and carries carbon dioxide from the cells back to the lungs.

Erythrocytes develop in the red marrow from stem cells that become **erythroblasts** and then **normoblasts**. They are released into the blood in a slightly immature form known as **reticulocytes**. Within a day, the reticulocyte becomes a mature erythrocyte, which has no nucleus. The body produces several million erythrocytes every second. Any time the body experiences a significant blood loss, the kidneys secrete **erythropoietin**, a hormone that dramatically increases the speed at which erythrocytes are produced and become mature.

Pronunciation/Word Parts

hemoglobin (HEE-moh-GLOH-bin)
(HEE-moh-GLOH-bin)
hem/o- *blood*
glob/o- *comprehensive; shaped like a globe*
-in *substance*

oxyhemoglobin
(AWK-see-HEE-moh-GLOH-bin)
ox/y- *oxygen; quick*
hem/o- *blood*
glob/o- *comprehensive; shaped like a globe*
-in *substance*

CLINICAL CONNECTIONS

Forensic Science. When a person drowns or suffocates, there is a high level of carbon dioxide (CO_2) in the blood. This causes the skin to have a deep bluish-purple color known as *cyanosis*. However, when a person dies in a fire or from inhaling the fumes from car exhaust or a faulty space heater, there is a high level of carbon monoxide (CO) in the blood. Unlike oxygen and carbon dioxide, **carbon monoxide** binds so tightly and irreversibly that the hemoglobin is unable to carry any other molecule. Carbon monoxide poisoning causes a characteristic cherry red skin color.

carbon monoxide
(KAR-bon mawn-AWK-side)
Mon/o- is a combining form meaning *one; single.*

Because an erythrocyte does not have a nucleus, it is unable to divide or repair itself. It lasts 120 days and then begins to deteriorate. The spleen removes old erythrocytes from the blood, breaking down their hemoglobin into heme and globin molecules. Iron is stripped from the heme molecule and stored in the liver and spleen; it is released to build more erythrocytes if the diet does not contain enough iron. The rest of the heme molecule becomes bilirubin. The globin molecule is broken down into amino acids that are used by the body to build cells.

erythroblast (eh-RITH-roh-blast)
erythr/o- *red*
-blast *immature cell*

normoblast (NOR-moh-blast)
norm/o- *normal; usual*
-blast *immature cell*

reticulocyte (reh-TIH-kyoo-loh-SITE)
reticul/o- *small network*
-cyte *cell*
A reticulocyte has a network of ribosomes in its cytoplasm.

erythropoietin (eh-RITH-roh-POY-eh-tin)
erythr/o- *red*
-poietin *substance that forms*
Add words to make a correct definition of *erythropoietin: substance that forms red (blood cells).*

CLINICAL CONNECTIONS

Gastroenterology (Chapter 3). Bilirubin is used by the liver to make bile. Bilirubin is a yellow pigment that gives bile its characteristic yellow-green appearance. The combining form *rub/o-* (red) indicates that bilirubin comes from the breakdown of red blood cells, not that it is red in color. Bilirubin also plays an important role as an antioxidant, protecting body cells from damage by free radicals.

DID YOU KNOW?

Erythrocytes and leukocytes are also known as red corpuscles and white corpuscles. *Corpuscle* is a Latin word meaning *a little body*.

Leukocytes

Leukocytes or **white blood cells (WBCs)** include five types of cells, each of which plays a unique role in the body's immune response. Leukocytes include neutrophils, eosinophils, basophils, lymphocytes, and monocytes (see Table 6-1 ■).

You can identify each type of leukocyte by the presence or absence of granules in its cytoplasm and by the shape of its nucleus. These differences can be seen when leukocytes are stained and examined under a microscope.

leukocyte (LOO-koh-site)
leuk/o- *white*
-cyte *cell*

Table 6-1 Leukocyte Types and Characteristics

Leukocyte	Category		Cytoplasm	Nucleus	Function
neutrophil segmented neutrophil, segmenter, seg, polymorphonuclear leukocyte (PMN), poly	granulocyte	*Source:* Pearson Education	many large, pale granules that do not stain either red or blue	three or more lobes	engulf and destroy bacteria
eosinophil eo	granulocyte	*Source:* Pearson Education	many large granules that stain bright pink to red	two lobes	release chemicals to destroy foreign cells (pollen, animal dander, dust, etc.) and kill parasites
basophil baso	granulocyte	*Source:* Pearson Education	many large granules that stain dark blue to purple	more than one lobe	release histamine at the site of tissue injury; release heparin to limit the size of a forming blood clot
lymphocyte lymph	agranulocyte	*Source:* Pearson Education	few or no granules	one that is round	produce antibodies (immunoglobulins); produce toxic granules to destroy cells infected with a virus
monocyte mono	agranulocyte	*Source:* Pearson Education	few or no granules	one that is kidney bean–shaped	engulf and destroy microorganisms, cancerous cells, dead leukocytes, and cellular debris

Any leukocyte with many large granules in its cytoplasm is categorized as a granulocyte. **Granulocytes** include neutrophils, eosinophils, and basophils. Any leukocyte with few or no granules in its cytoplasm is categorized as an agranulocyte. **Agranulocytes** include lymphocytes and monocytes.

GRANULOCYTES

1. **Neutrophils** are the most common leukocyte. They make up 54–62% of the leukocytes in the blood. A neutrophil has many large, pale-colored granules in its cytoplasm, and its nucleus has many segments or lobes (see Figure 6-5 ■ and Table 6-1). A neutrophil

Pronunciation/Word Parts

granulocyte (GRAN-yoo-loh-SITE)
  granul/o- *granule*
  -cyte *cell*

agranulocyte (aa-GRAN-yoo-loh-SITE)
  a- *away from; without*
  granul/o- *granule*
  -cyte *cell*

neutrophil (NOO-troh-fil)
  neutr/o- *not taking part*
  -phil *attraction to; fondness for*

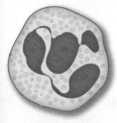

FIGURE 6-5 ■ **Neutrophil.**
A neutrophil has many large, pale granules in its cytoplasm. These granules are "neutral" in that they do not stain well with either a red, acidic dye (eosin) or with a blue, alkaline dye (hematoxylin). Neutrophils get their name from their neutral reaction to these dyes.
Source: Pearson Education

is also known as a *segmented neutrophil, segmenter, seg,* **polymorphonuclear leukocyte (PMN)**, or *poly*.

Neutrophils develop in the red marrow from **stem cells** that become **myeloblasts**, then **myelocytes**, and then **bands** (see Figure 6-3). A band is an immature neutrophil that has a nucleus shaped like a curved band. Bands are also known as **stabs** (the German word for *band*). There are always a few bands present in the blood, but, during a severe bacterial infection, the number of bands rises as the need for more neutrophils increases.

Neutrophils are blood cells, but they are also part of the immune response of the lymphatic system because they are **phagocytes** that engulf and destroy bacteria. This process is known as **phagocytosis**. Neutrophils only live a few days or even just a few hours if they are actively destroying bacteria. One neutrophil can destroy about 10 bacteria before it dies.

2. **Eosinophils** make up just 1–3% of the leukocytes in the blood. An eosinophil has many large, red-pink granules in its cytoplasm, and its nucleus has two lobes (see Figure 6-6 ■ and Table 6-1). Eosinophils are also known as *eos*.

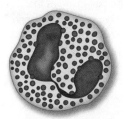

FIGURE 6-6 ■ Eosinophil.
An eosinophil has many large granules in its cytoplasm. These granules stain bright pink to red with a red, acidic dye (eosin). Eosinophils get their name from their reaction to this dye.
Source: Pearson Education

Eosinophils develop in the red marrow from stem cells (see Figure 6-3). Eosinophils are blood cells, but they are also part of the immune response of the lymphatic system because they release chemicals to destroy foreign cells (pollen, animal dander, dust, etc.) and kill parasites.

3. **Basophils** are the least common leukocyte. They make up just 0.5–1% of the leukocytes in the blood. A basophil has many large, purple granules in its cytoplasm, and its nucleus has more than one lobe (see Figure 6-7 ■ and Table 6-1). Basophils are also known as *basos*.

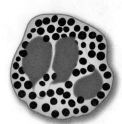

FIGURE 6-7 ■ Basophil.
A basophil has many large granules in its cytoplasm. These granules stain dark blue to purple with a blue, alkaline dye (hematoxylin). (Something that is alkaline is known as a base, which is the opposite of an acid.) Basophils get their name from their reaction to this dye, which is a base.
Source: Pearson Education

Basophils develop in the red marrow from stem cells (see Figure 6-3). Basophils are blood cells, but they are also part of the immune response of the lymphatic system because they go to the site of tissue injury and release histamine. Histamine dilates blood vessels and increases inflammation. Basophils are also part of the blood clotting process because they release heparin (an anticoagulant) that limits the size of a blood clot at the site of tissue injury.

AGRANULOCYTES

1. **Lymphocytes** make up 25–33% of the leukocytes in the blood. Lymphocytes are the smallest leukocytes. A lymphocyte has just a thin ring of cytoplasm that contains few or no granules, and its nucleus is round and nearly fills the cell (see Figure 6-8 ■ and Table 6-1).

Pronunciation/Word Parts

polymorphonuclear
(PAW-lee-MOR-foh-NOO-klee-ar)
  poly- *many; much*
  morph/o- *shape*
  nucle/o- *nucleus of an atom; nucleus of a cell*
  -ar *pertaining to*

myeloblast (MY-eh-loh-BLAST)
  myel/o- *bone marrow; myelin; spinal cord*
  -blast *immature cell*

myelocyte (MY-eh-loh-SITE)
  myel/o- *bone marrow; myelin; spinal cord*
  -cyte *cell*

phagocyte (FAG-oh-site)
  phag/o- *eating; swallowing*
  -cyte *cell*

phagocytosis (FAG-oh-sy-TOH-sis)
  phag/o- *eating; swallowing*
  cyt/o- *cell*
  -osis *condition; process*

eosinophil (EE-oh-SIN-oh-fil)
  eosin/o- *eosin; red acidic dye*
  -phil *attraction to; fondness for*

basophil (BAY-soh-fil)
  bas/o- *alkaline; base of a structure*
  -phil *attraction to; fondness for*

lymphocyte (LIM-foh-site)
  lymph/o- *lymph; lymphatic system*
  -cyte *cell*

FIGURE 6-8 ■ Lymphocyte.
A lymphocyte has few or no granules, little cytoplasm, and a round nucleus.
Source: Pearson Education

Some lymphocytes live for just a few days, while others live for many years. Lymphocytes are also known as *lymphs*.

Lymphocytes develop in the red marrow from stem cells that become **lymphoblasts** (see Figure 6-3). Lymphoblasts that mature in the red marrow of the bones become B lymphocytes (B cells) (*B* for *bone*) or NK (natural killer) cells. Other lymphoblasts migrate to the thymus and become T lymphocytes (T cells) (*T* for *thymus*). Lymphocytes are blood cells, but they are also part of the immune response of the lymphatic system. B lymphocytes produce antibodies (immunoglobulins). The different types of T lymphocytes and their functions are discussed in the section on the immune response.

2. **Monocytes** make up 3–7% of the leukocytes in the blood. They are the largest leukocytes. A monocyte has a large amount of cytoplasm that contains few or no granules, and its nucleus is large and kidney bean–shaped (see Figure 6-9 ■ and Table 6-1). Monocytes are also known as *monos*.

Monocytes develop in the red marrow from stem cells that become **monoblasts** and then mature monocytes (see Figure 6-3). Monocytes are blood cells, but they are also part of the immune response of the lymphatic system because they are phagocytes that engulf and destroy microorganisms, cancerous cells, dead leukocytes, and cellular debris. Monocytes in the lymph nodes, intestine, liver, pancreas, thymus, spleen, bone, and skin are known as **macrophages**.

lymphoblast (LIM-foh-blast)
　lymph/o- *lymph; lymphatic system*
　-blast *immature cell*

monocyte (MAW-noh-site)
　mon/o- *one; single*
　-cyte *cell*
Add words to make a complete definition of *monocyte*: *cell (that has) one (lobe in its nucleus)*.

monoblast (MAW-noh-blast)
　mon/o- *one; single*
　-blast *immature cell*

macrophage (MAK-roh-fayj)
　macr/o- *large*
　-phage *thing that eats; thing that swallows*

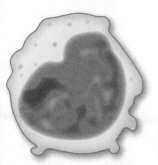

FIGURE 6-9 ■ Monocyte.
A monocyte has few or no granules, a large amount of cytoplasm, and a large, kidney bean–shaped nucleus.
Source: Pearson Education

DID YOU KNOW?

Of the 5–6 quarts of blood in the body, leukocytes make up 1½ fluid ounce and thrombocytes make up only 1 teaspoonful.

Thrombocytes

A **thrombocyte** or **platelet** is different from other blood cells because it is only a cell fragment. Thrombocytes are active in the blood clotting process. Within seconds of an injury, they form clumps to decrease the loss of blood. Thrombocytes also contain some clotting factors that begin the formation of a blood clot.

An individual thrombocyte begins in the red marrow as a stem cell that becomes a **megakaryoblast** (see Figure 6-3). Then it matures into a **megakaryocyte**, a very large cell with a great deal of cytoplasm. The cytoplasm of the megakaryocyte breaks away at the edges to form cell fragments (thrombocytes) that are released into the blood. When all of the cytoplasm has broken off, the nucleus of the megakaryocyte is recycled to build other cells.

thrombocyte (THRAWM-boh-site)
　thromb/o- *blood clot*
　-cyte *cell*

platelet (PLAYT-let)

megakaryoblast
(MEG-ah-KAIR-ee-oh-BLAST)
　mega- *large*
　kary/o- *nucleus of a cell*
　-blast *immature cell*

megakaryocyte (MEG-ah-KAIR-ee-oh-SITE)
　mega- *large*
　kary/o- *nucleus of a cell*
　-cyte *cell*

Blood Type

Erythrocytes contain inherited genetic material that determines a person's blood type. The most important blood types are the ABO and Rh blood groups, although there are 22 other minor blood groups. Each blood group is named for its **antigen** (protein molecule on the cell membrane of the erythrocyte).

The **ABO blood group** contains A, B, AB, and O antigens (see Table 6-2 ■). A person with type A blood has A antigens on their erythrocytes and so forth. A person with type O blood has neither A nor B antigens on their erythrocytes. In addition, each person's plasma contains antibodies against blood types other than its own.

The **Rh blood group** has 47 different antigens. As a group, they are known as the **Rh factor**. When these antigens are present on a person's erythrocytes, the blood type is Rh positive. When these antigens are not present, the blood type is Rh negative.

The ABO and the Rh blood groups are always considered together. For example, type A blood is either A positive (Rh positive) or A negative (Rh negative).

Pronunciation/Word Parts

antigen (AN-tih-jen)
 anti- *against*
 -gen *that which produces*
Antigen is a combination of part of the word *antibody* and the suffix *-gen* (that which produces).

Table 6-2 ABO Blood Group

Blood Type	Antigen on the Erythrocyte	Antibodies in Plasma
A	A antigen	anti-B antibodies
B	B antigen	anti-A antibodies
AB	A and B antigens	none
O	none	anti-A and anti-B antibodies

Type O negative blood is known as the *universal donor* because it can be given to patients with any other blood type without causing a transfusion reaction. Blood is collected and stored in units (see Figure 6-10 ■).

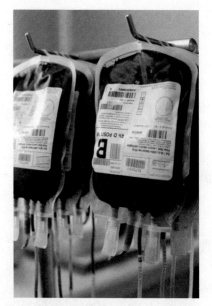

FIGURE 6-10 ■ Unit of blood.
This donated unit of blood is blood type B positive. A donated unit of blood contains 500 cc. This is nearly the same as 1 pint. That is why people talk of donating "a pint" of blood. There are approximately 10–12 pints of blood in the body. A unit of blood is hung upside down when it is given to the patient through an intravenous line.
Source: Scott Camazine/Science Source; Li Wa/Shutterstock

Physiology of Blood Clotting

When the body is injured, the injured blood vessel constricts to decrease the loss of blood. Thrombocytes stick to the damaged blood vessel wall and form clumps that slow the flow of blood. This process is known as platelet **aggregation**. The platelets also release several clotting factors. Damage to the blood vessel also activates **clotting factors** in the plasma. The clotting factors make strands of **fibrin** that trap erythrocytes and form a **thrombus** or blood clot (see Figure 6-11 ■). This process is known as **coagulation**, and the cessation of bleeding is known as **hemostasis**. The final size of a blood clot is limited by the action of heparin, a natural anticoagulant released from basophils.

aggregation (AG-reh-GAY-shun)
  aggreg/o- *crowding together*
  -ation *being; having; process*

fibrin (FY-brin)
  fibr/o- *fiber*
  -in *substance*

thrombus (THRAWM-bus)

thrombi (THRAWM-by)
Thrombus is a Latin singular noun. Form the plural by changing *-us* to *-i*.

coagulation (koh-AG-yoo-LAY-shun)
  coagul/o- *clotting*
  -ation *being; having; process*

hemostasis (HEE-moh-STAY-sis)
  hem/o- *blood*
  -stasis *standing still; staying in one place*

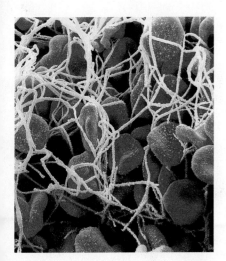

FIGURE 6-11 ■ Blood clot.
These strands of fibrin trap many erythrocytes to form a blood clot or thrombus.
Source: Susumu Nishinaga/Science Source

All of the clotting factors must be present and be at normal levels for the blood to clot. There are 12 clotting factors (see Table 6-3 ■), numbered as Roman numerals I through XIII (there is no factor VI). Although the clotting factors are listed in numeral order, they are not activated in this order.

When clotting factors in the plasma are activated to form a blood clot, the fluid portion of plasma that remains is known as **serum**.

serum (SEER-um)

Table 6-3 Blood Clotting Factors

Factor Number and Name	Source	Pronunciation/Word Parts
I **fibrinogen**	liver	**fibrinogen** (fy-BRIN-oh-jen) **fibrin/o-** *fibrin* **-gen** *that which produces*
II **prothrombin**	liver	**prothrombin** (proh-THRAWM-bin) **pro-** *before* **thromb/o-** *blood clot* **-in** *substance* Prothrombin is the clotting factor that is activated just before the thrombus is formed.
III tissue factor (**thromboplastin**)	injured tissue	**thromboplastin** (THRAWM-boh-PLAS-tin) **thromb/o-** *blood clot* **plast/o-** *formation; growth* **-in** *substance*
IV calcium	platelets	
V prothrombin accelerator	liver	
VII prothrombin conversion accelerator	liver	
VIII antihemophilic factor	platelets	
IX plasma thromboplastin factor	liver	
X Stuart-Prower factor	liver	
XI plasma thromboplastin antecedent	liver	
XII Hageman factor	liver	
XIII fibrin-stabilizing factor	liver and platelets	

Anatomy of the Lymphatic System

Lymphatic Vessels, Lymph, and Lymph Nodes

Lymphatic vessels are similar in structure to blood vessels, but with several important differences. Lymphatic vessels have a beginning point (as tiny lymphatic capillaries in the tissues) and an end point at lymphatic ducts that empty into large veins in the neck. Tissue fluid enters a lymphatic capillary and becomes **lymph** (lymphatic fluid) that then flows through the lymphatic system. Lymphatic capillaries have large openings in their walls that allow microorganisms and cancerous cells to enter. Lymphatic capillaries become larger lymphatic vessels that bring lymph to the lymph nodes. Like large veins in the cardiovascular system, large lymphatic vessels have valves that keep the lymph flowing in one direction.

Lymph nodes are encapsulated pieces of lymphoid tissue that are round, oval, or bean shaped. They range in size from the head of a pin to 1 inch. The lymph node filters the lymph, and then macrophages in the lymph node destroy any microorganisms or cancerous cells that are present.

Lymph nodes are grouped together in chains in areas where there is a high risk of invasion by microorganisms or cancerous cells (see Figure 6-12 ■).

Pronunciation/Word Parts

lymphatic (lim-FAT-ik)
 lymph/o- *lymph; lymphatic system*
 -atic *pertaining to*

lymph (LIMF)

node (NOHD)
 Lymph gland is an alternate phrase for *lymph node*, although lymph nodes are not really glands. The combining form *aden/o-* means *gland*.

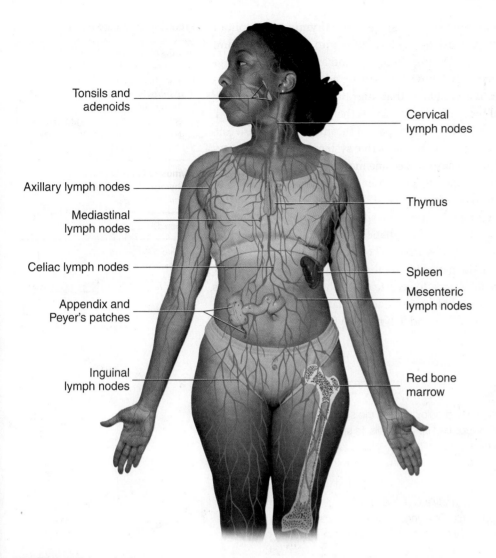

Tonsils and adenoids

Cervical lymph nodes

Axillary lymph nodes

Mediastinal lymph nodes

Thymus

Celiac lymph nodes

Spleen

Mesenteric lymph nodes

Appendix and Peyer's patches

Inguinal lymph nodes

Red bone marrow

FIGURE 6-12 ■ Lymphatic system.
The lymphatic system consists of lymphatic vessels, lymph nodes, lymph fluid, lymphoid tissues (tonsils and adenoids in the throat, and Peyer's patches and appendix in the intestines), and lymphoid organs (thymus and spleen). Blood cells produced by the red bone marrow are part of the immune response of the lymphatic system.
Source: Pearson Education

WORD ALERT		
Sound-Alike Words		
lymph	(noun)	Fluid that flows through lymphatic vessels and lymph nodes
lymphs	(noun)	Another name for lymphocytes

Lymphoid Tissues and Lymphoid Organs

Lymphoid tissues and lymphoid organs contain lymphocytes and macrophages that are active in the immune response. **Lymphoid tissues** include the tonsils and adenoids in the posterior oral cavity (discussed in "Otolaryngology," Chapter 16) and Peyer's patches and the appendix in the intestines (discussed in "Gastroenterology," Chapter 3) (see Figure 6-12).

lymphoid (LIM-foyd)
lymph/o- *lymph; lymphatic system*
-oid *resembling*

Lymphoid organs include the thymus and the spleen. The **thymus**, a lymphoid organ with a pink color and a grainy consistency, is located within the mediastinum, posterior to the sternum (see Figure 6-12). During childhood and adolescence, the thymus gland is large because it is very active; however, during adulthood, it becomes much smaller. The thymus receives lymphoblasts that migrate from the red marrow and helps them mature into several types of T lymphocytes (helper T cells, memory T cells, cytotoxic T cells, and suppressor T cells) that are part of the immune response (the T stands for *thymus*). The thymus is also part of the endocrine system because it secretes hormones (**thymosins**) that cause lymphoblasts to become mature T lymphocytes.

The **spleen**, a rounded lymphoid organ, is located in the left upper quadrant of the abdomen, posterior to the stomach (see Figure 6-12). The spleen is surrounded by a firm splenic capsule, but has a soft, pulpy interior. The spleen functions as part of the blood and as part of the immune response of the lymphatic system. The spleen removes and recycles old erythrocytes, as previously described. The spleen also acts as a storage area for whole blood. During times of danger or injury, the sympathetic division of the nervous system stimulates the adrenal glands to secrete epinephrine, and this causes the spleen to contract and release its stored blood into the circulatory system. The lymphoid tissue in the spleen contains mature B and T lymphocytes that are part of the immune response.

Pronunciation/Word Parts

thymus (THY-mus)

thymic (THY-mik)
  thym/o- *rage; thymus*
  -ic *pertaining to*
Select the correct combining form meaning to get the definition of *thymic*: *pertaining to the thymus.*

thymosins (thy-MOH-sins)
  thym/o- *rage; thymus*
  -sin *substance*

spleen (SPLEEN)

splenic (SPLEH-nik)
  splen/o- *spleen*
  -ic *pertaining to*

CLINICAL CONNECTIONS

Sports Medicine. Because of its location and pulpy center, the spleen can rupture from sports trauma (or car accidents). A ruptured spleen spills its stored blood into the abdominal cavity. This can cause shock and death unless surgery is done to stop the bleeding, remove the blood from the abdominal cavity, and remove the damaged spleen (splenectomy).

Dermatology (Chapter 7). The skin is the body's first line of defense. Intact skin acts as a protective barrier that stops microorganisms. Openings in the skin (the nose, ears, mouth, urethra, rectum, vagina) are high-risk areas where microorganisms can enter the body, and so lymph nodes are concentrated in these areas.

Physiology of the Immune Response

The **immune response** involves a coordinated effort between the blood and the lymphatic system to identify and destroy microorganisms or foreign cells that invade the body and cancerous cells that are produced within the body.

The immune response begins with the detection of an invading microorganism. Microorganisms (bacteria, viruses, protozoa, fungi, yeasts, etc.) that cause disease are known as **pathogens**. Once a pathogen or a cancer cell is detected in the blood or lymphatic system, the body attacks it in several different ways.

immune (ih-MYOON)

pathogen (PATH-oh-jen)
  path/o- *disease*
  -gen *that which produces*

1. **Neutrophils.** Neutrophils engulf and destroy bacteria that have been coated with antibodies.

2. **Eosinophils.** Eosinophils release chemicals that destroy foreign cells (pollen, animal dander, dust, etc.) and kill parasites.

3. **Basophils.** Basophils release histamine at the site of tissue injury. **Histamine** dilates blood vessels and increases blood flow, which causes redness and also brings more leukocytes to the area. Histamine also changes the permeability of the blood vessel walls, allowing large protein molecules and water to leak out into the tissues; this causes edema (swelling). Redness and edema are both signs of inflammation or infection associated with the presence of microorganisms.

histamine (HIS-tah-meen)

4. **Lymphocytes**

   a. **NK (natural killer) cells** recognize a cancer cell or a cell infected with a virus and release chemicals to destroy it. NK cells can recognize these cells even before they are coated with antibodies.

   b. **B cells** are inactive until a monocyte presents them with fragments from an eaten pathogen. Then the B cell changes into a plasma cell and produces antibodies that coat that pathogen. B cells also activate helper T cells.

   c. **T cells** (lymphocytes that matured in the thymus) have four different subsets:

   - **Cytotoxic T cells** produce toxic granules to kill cells infected with a virus.

   - **Helper T cells** produce interleukin and stimulate the production of cytotoxic T cells. Helper T cells (known as **CD4 cells** because of a protein marker on their cell membranes) also produce memory T cells.

   - **Memory T cells** are created when a helper T cell is exposed to a virus. Memory T cells are inactive until the next time that virus enters the body. Then they remember the virus and become cytotoxic T cells.

   - **Suppressor T cells** limit the extent and duration of the immune response by inhibiting B cells and cytotoxic T cells. Suppressor T cells are known as **CD8 cells** because of a protein marker on their cell membranes.

5. **Monocytes.** Monocytes have several jobs. They engulf and destroy pathogens that have been coated with antibodies. They eat dead leukocytes and cellular debris. They take fragments of the pathogens they have eaten and present them to B cell and T cell lymphocytes. Monocytes also produce interferon, interleukin, and tumor necrosis factor.

   a. **Interferon** is produced by monocytes that have engulfed a virus. Interferon stimulates other cells to produce an antiviral substance that prevents a virus from entering them and reproducing itself. This keeps viral infections from spreading through the body. Interferon also stimulates NK (natural killer) cells to attack cells already infected with viruses.

   b. **Interleukin** stimulates B cell and T cell lymphocytes and NK cells. It also produces the fever associated with inflammation and infection. An increased body temperature stimulates leukocyte activity. Interleukin is also produced by helper T cell lymphocytes.

   c. **Tumor necrosis factor (TNF)** destroys **endotoxins** produced by certain bacteria. It also destroys cancer cells.

6. **Antibodies.** Antibodies coat the outside of a bacterium or a virus (or a cancer cell or a cell infected with a virus that has not been destroyed by NK cells) and mark it to be destroyed. The antibody coating attracts phagocytes (neutrophils, monocytes) to come and engulf the bacterium, virus, cancer cell, or infected cell and destroy it. Antibodies are also known as **immunoglobulins**.

7. **Complement proteins.** Complement is a group of nine proteins (C1–C9) that activate each other. When antibodies coat a bacterium, virus, cancer cell, or infected cell, complement proteins attach to the antibodies to "complement" their effect and drill holes in the bacterium or virus.

Pronunciation/Word Parts

cytotoxic (SY-toh-TAWK-sik)
   cyt/o- *cell*
   tox/o- *poison*
   -ic *pertaining to*

suppressor (soo-PRES-or)
   suppress/o- *press down*
   -or *person who does; person who produces; thing that does; thing that produces*

interferon (IN-ter-FEER-on)

interleukin (IN-ter-LOO-kin)
   inter- *between*
   leuk/o- *white*
   -in *substance*

endotoxin (EN-doh-TAWK-sin)
   endo- *innermost; within*
   tox/o- *poison*
   -in *substance*

antibody (AN-tih-BAW-dee)
The prefix *anti-* means *against*.

immunoglobulin
(IH-myoo-noh-GLAW-byoo-lin)
   immun/o- *immune response*
   globul/o- *shaped like a globe*
   -in *substance*

complement (COM-pleh-ment)

WORD ALERT
Sound-Alike Words

globin   (noun)   Breakdown product of hemoglobin
             Example: The spleen breaks down old erythrocytes into heme and globin molecules.

globulin   (noun)   Protein molecule in an immunoglobulin
             Example: Globulin is used by a plasma cell to build antibodies.

A CLOSER LOOK

There are five classes of **antibodies** or **immunoglobulins**: immunoglobulin A (IgA), immunoglobulin D (IgD), immunoglobulin E (IgE), immunoglobulin G (IgG), and immunoglobulin M (IgM).

Class	Description
IgA	IgA is in body secretions (tears; saliva; mucus in the nose, lungs, and intestines) and on the surface of the skin. IgA is in colostrum, the first milk produced by the mother; this maternal IgA provides **passive immunity** to the breastfeeding baby for all of the diseases that the mother has had, until 18 months of age when the infant begins to make its own antibodies.
IgD	IgD is on the surface of a B cell lymphocyte and activates it to become a plasma cell.
IgE	IgE is on the surface of a basophil and causes it to release heparin and histamine during inflammatory and allergic reactions.
IgG	IgG is the most abundant of all the immunoglobulins. It provides **active immunity,** the body's response and defense against pathogens it has seen before. IgG is also the smallest immunoglobulin. It can pass from the mother's blood through the placenta, where it provides passive immunity to the fetus.
IgM	IgM is the largest immunoglobulin. It is produced the first time the body encounters a pathogen. IgM also is the immunoglobulin that reacts to incompatible blood types during a blood transfusion reaction.

immunity (ih-MYOO-nih-tee)
immun/o- *immune response*
-ity *condition; state*

ACROSS THE LIFE SPAN

Pediatrics. Childhood immunizations against measles, mumps, rubella, polio, diphtheria, pertussis, and tetanus use a vaccine made of dead or weakened pathogens or inactivated endotoxins. The vaccination causes B lymphocytes to become plasma cells and produce antibodies, and this gives active immunity without exposure to the actual disease.
The meningococcal meningitis vaccine is recommended for college students living in dormitories.

Adult immunizations include annual vaccinations for influenza (the flu) and periodic boosters for tetanus.

Geriatrics. The influenza (the flu) and pneumococcal pneumonia vaccinations are recommended for older adults.

Vocabulary Review

Blood		
Word or Phrase	**Description**	**Combining Forms**
ABO blood group	Category that includes blood types A, B, AB, and O. Blood types are inherited. Each blood type has its own **antigens** on the erythrocytes and antibodies in the plasma against other blood types.	
agranulocyte	Category of leukocytes with few or no granules in the cytoplasm. It includes lymphocytes and monocytes.	granul/o- *granule*
albumin	Most abundant plasma protein. Plasma proteins contribute to the osmotic pressure of the blood.	
band	Immature neutrophil in the blood. It has a nucleus shaped like a curved band. It is also known as a **stab**.	
basophil	Type of leukocyte. It is categorized as a granulocyte because it has many large granules in its cytoplasm, and they stain dark blue to purple with basic dye. Basophils release histamine and heparin at the site of tissue injury. Basophils are also known as *basos*.	bas/o- *alkaline; base of a structure, basic*
blood	Type of connective tissue that contains formed elements (blood cells and blood cell fragments), water, proteins, and clotting factors. The blood transports oxygen, carbon dioxide, nutrients, and waste products of metabolism.	hem/o- *blood* hemat/o- *blood*
electrolytes	Molecules that carry a positive or negative electrical charge: sodium (Na^+), potassium (K^+), calcium (Ca^{++}), chloride (Cl^-), and bicarbonate (HCO_3^-). They are in the plasma.	electr/o- *electricity*
eosinophil	Type of leukocyte. It is categorized as a granulocyte because it has many large granules in its cytoplasm, and they stain bright pink to red with eosin dye. The nucleus has two lobes. Eosinophils release chemicals to destroy foreign cells (pollen, animal dander, dust, etc.) and kill parasites. Eosinophils are also known as *eos*.	eosin/o- *eosin; red, acidic dye*
erythrocyte	A mature red blood cell. An **erythroblast** is a very immature form that comes from a stem cell in the red marrow. It matures into a **normoblast**, which becomes a **reticulocyte**, a nearly mature erythrocyte that is released into the blood. An erythrocyte has no nucleus. Erythrocytes contain hemoglobin.	erythr/o- *red* norm/o- *normal; usual* reticul/o- *small network*
erythropoietin	Hormone secreted by the kidneys to increase the speed at which erythrocytes are produced and become mature	erythr/o- *red*
granulocyte	Category of leukocytes with many large granules in the cytoplasm. It includes neutrophils, eosinophils, and basophils.	granul/o- *granule*
hematopoiesis	Process by which all of the formed elements in the blood are produced in the red marrow	hemat/o- *blood*
hemoglobin	Red, iron-containing molecule in an erythrocyte that contains a heme molecule and globin chains. The heme molecule contains iron that gives erythrocytes their red color. **Oxyhemoglobin** is a compound of hemoglobin that carries oxygen from the lungs to the cells and carries carbon dioxide from the cells to the lungs.	hem/o- *blood* glob/o- *comprehensive; shaped like a globe* ox/y- *oxygen; quick*

Word or Phrase	Description	Combining Forms
leukocyte	A white blood cell. There are five different types of mature leukocytes: neutrophils, eosinophils, basophils, lymphocytes, and monocytes.	leuk/o- *white*
lymphocyte	Second most abundant leukocyte, but the smallest in size. It is categorized as an agranulocyte as there are few or no granules in its cytoplasm. The cytoplasm is only a thin ring next to the round nucleus. A **lymphoblast** is an immature form that develops from a stem cell in the red marrow. Lymphocytes in the red marrow become NK cells or become B lymphocytes that produce antibodies. Lymphocytes in the thymus become T lymphocytes that produce toxic granules to destroy cells infected with a virus. Lymphocytes are also known as *lymphs*.	lymph/o- *lymph; lymphatic system*
monocyte	The largest leukocyte. It is categorized as an agranulocyte as there are few or no granules in its cytoplasm. The nucleus is shaped like a kidney bean. A **monoblast** is an immature form that comes from a stem cell in the red marrow. Monocytes are phagocytes that engulf and destroy microorganisms, cancerous cells, dead leukocytes, and cellular debris. They also produce interferon, interleukin, and tumor necrosis factor. Monocytes are also known as *monos*. In the tissues, they are known as **macrophages**.	mon/o- *one; single* macr/o- *large*
myelocyte	Immature cell that comes from a **myeloblast** in the red marrow and develops into either a neutrophil, eosinophil, or basophil	myel/o- *bone marrow; myelin; spinal cord*
neutrophil	Most numerous type of leukocyte. It is categorized as a granulocyte because it has many large, pale granules in its cytoplasm, and they do not easily stain red or blue, but remain neutral in color. The nucleus has several segmented lobes. Neutrophils are phagocytes that engulf and destroy bacteria. Neutrophils are also known as *segmented neutrophils, segmenters, segs,* **polymorphonuclear leukocytes**, *polys,* or *PMNs*.	neutr/o- *not taking part* morph/o- *shape* nucle/o- *nucleus of an atom; nucleus of a cell*
plasma	Clear, straw-colored liquid portion of the blood that carries formed elements (blood cells and blood cell fragments) and contains nutrients from digested foods (amino acids, cholesterol, triglycerides, electrolytes, glucose, minerals, and vitamins)—as well as substances provided by the liver or glands (albumin, bilirubin, hormones, complement proteins, clotting factors), and waste products of cellular metabolism (creatinine and urea) produced by the body.	plasm/o- *plasma*
Rh blood group	Category of blood type. When the Rh factor is present, the blood is Rh positive. Without the Rh factor, the blood is Rh negative.	
stem cell	Extremely immature cell in the red marrow that is the precursor to all types of blood cells	
thrombocyte	A **platelet**. A **megakaryoblast** is a very immature form that develops from a stem cell in the red marrow. A **megakaryocyte** is a very large, mature cell with a large amount of cytoplasm that breaks away in individual pieces as thrombocytes. A thrombocyte is a cell fragment that does not have a nucleus. Thrombocytes are active in the blood clotting process.	thromb/o- *blood clot* kary/o- *nucleus of a cell*

Blood Clotting

Word or Phrase	Description	Combining Forms
aggregation	Process of thrombocytes (platelets) sticking to a damaged blood vessel wall and forming clumps	**aggreg/o-** *crowding together*
clotting factors	A series of 12 substances that are released either from platelets or injured tissue or are produced by the liver. They activate each other in a series of steps that form fibrin strands that trap erythrocytes and form a blood clot.	
coagulation	Formation of a blood clot by platelets, erythrocytes, and clotting factors	**coagul/o-** *clotting*
fibrin	Strands formed by the activation of clotting factors. Fibrin traps erythrocytes to form a blood clot.	**fibr/o-** *fiber*
fibrinogen	Blood clotting factor I	**fibrin/o-** *fibrin*
hemostasis	The cessation of bleeding	**hem/o-** *blood*
prothrombin	Blood clotting factor II. It is activated just before the thrombus (blood clot) is formed.	**thromb/o-** *blood clot*
serum	Fluid portion of the plasma that remains after the clotting factors are activated to form a blood clot	
thromboplastin	Blood clotting factor III. It is also known as *tissue factor* because it is released when tissue is injured.	**thromb/o-** *blood clot* **plast/o-** *formation; growth*
thrombus	A blood clot	**thromb/o-** *blood clot*

Lymphatic System and Immune Response

active immunity	The body's continuing immune response and defense against pathogens it has seen before. It is provided by immunoglobulin G. For the fetus, IgG passes from the mother's blood through the placenta to provide active immunity.	**immun/o-** *immune response*
antibody	Produced by a B cell when it becomes a plasma cell. It is also known as an *immunoglobulin*.	
antigen	Protein marker on the cell membrane of an erythrocyte that indicates the blood type. Also, a protein marker on the cell wall of a pathogen or on a cancerous cell that allows the immune system to recognize it as foreign.	
B cell	Type of lymphocyte that matures in the red marrow of the bone. B cells are activated when a monocyte presents them with fragments from an eaten pathogen. Then the B cells become **plasma cells** that make antibodies. B cells also activate helper T cells.	
complement proteins	Group of nine proteins in the plasma (C1–C9). When antibodies coat a bacterium, virus, cancer cell, or infected cell, complement proteins kill it by drilling holes in it.	
endotoxin	Toxic substance produced by some bacteria. It acts as a poison in the body, causing chills, fever, and shock. Endotoxins are destroyed by tumor necrosis factor.	**tox/o-** *poison*

Word or Phrase	Description	Combining Forms
histamine	Released by basophils. It dilates blood vessels and increases blood flow to damaged tissue, which produces redness. It also allows protein molecules and water to leak out of blood vessels into the tissue, which produces edema (swelling).	
IgA	Immunoglobulin A. Antibody present in body secretions (tears, saliva, mucus, and breast milk) and on the surface of the skin. It gives passive immunity to a breastfeeding infant.	
IgD	Immunoglobulin D. Antibody present on the surface of B cells. It activates the B cell to become a plasma cell.	
IgE	Immunoglobulin E. Antibody present on the surface of basophils. It causes them to release histamine and heparin during allergic and inflammatory reactions.	
IgG	Immunoglobulin G. Antibody that provides active immunity. It is the smallest of all the immunoglobulins, but also the most abundant. During pregnancy, it crosses the placenta and provides passive immunity to the fetus.	
IgM	Immunoglobulin M. Antibody that is produced by plasma cells during the initial exposure to a pathogen. IgM also reacts to incompatible blood types during a blood transfusion. It is the largest of the immunoglobulins.	
immune response	Coordinated effort between the blood and lymphatic system to identify and destroy invading microorganisms or foreign particles, or cancerous cells produced within the body	immun/o- *immune response*
immunoglobulins	**Antibodies**. There are five classes of immunoglobulins: IgA, IgD, IgE, IgG, and IgM.	immun/o- *immune response* globul/o- *shaped like a globe*
interferon	Substance produced by monocytes that have engulfed a virus. It stimulates other cells to produce an antiviral substance that prevents the virus from entering them to reproduce itself.	
interleukin	Substance produced by monocytes that stimulates B cell and T cell lymphocytes and NK cells. It also produces fever.	leuk/o- *white*
lymph	Fluid that flows through the lymphatic system	
lymph nodes	Small, encapsulated pieces of lymphoid tissue. They are grouped together in chains in areas where there is a high rate of invasion by microorganisms or cancer cells. Macrophages in the lymph nodes destroy pathogens and cancerous cells in the lymph fluid. They are also known as **lymph glands**.	aden/o- *gland*
lymphatic system	Body system that includes a network of lymphatic vessels, lymph fluid, lymph nodes, the **lymphoid organs** (thymus, spleen), and **lymphoid tissues** (tonsils and adenoids, appendix, and Peyer's patches).	lymph/o- *lymph; lymphatic system*
lymphatic vessels	Vessels that begin as capillaries, carry lymph, continue through lymph nodes, and end at ducts that empty into large veins in the neck.	lymph/o- *lymph; lymphatic system*
macrophage	A large monocyte in the lymph nodes, intestine, liver, pancreas, thymus, spleen, bone, and skin	macr/o- *large* phag/o- *eating; swallowing*
natural killer (NK) cell	Type of lymphocyte that matures in the red marrow and, without the help of antibodies or complement proteins, recognizes and destroys cancer cells or cells infected with a virus	

Word or Phrase	Description	Combining Forms
passive immunity	Immune response and defense against pathogens that is conveyed by the mother's antibodies via colostrum to the breastfeeding baby. These maternal antibodies provide protection from all the diseases the mother has had.	**immun/o-** *immune response*
pathogen	Microorganism that causes a disease. Pathogens include bacteria, viruses, and protozoa, as well as plant cells such as fungi or yeast.	**path/o-** *disease*
phagocyte	Type of leukocyte that engulfs microorganisms, foreign cells, cancerous cells, and cellular debris and destroys them with digestive enzymes. Phagocytes include neutrophils and monocytes. **Phagocytosis** is the process by which a phagocyte engulfs and destroys a pathogen.	**phag/o-** *eating; swallowing* **cyt/o-** *cell*
spleen	Lymphoid organ located in the left upper quadrant of the abdomen, posterior to the stomach. The spleen removes old erythrocytes, breaking their hemoglobin into heme and globin chains. It also acts as a storage area for whole blood. Its lymphoid tissue contains B cell and T cell lymphocytes.	**splen/o-** *spleen*
T cell	Type of lymphocyte that matures in the thymus. There are four subsets of T cells: helper T cells (CD4 cells), memory T cells, **cytotoxic** T cells, and **suppressor** T cells (CD8 cells).	**cyt/o-** *cell* **tox/o-** *poison* **suppress/o-** *press down*
thymus	Lymphoid organ in the mediastinum. As an endocrine gland, it secretes thymosins, which are hormones that cause lymphoblasts in the thymus to mature into T cell lymphocytes.	**thym/o-** *rage; thymus*
tumor necrosis factor (TNF)	Substance that destroys endotoxins produced by certain bacteria. It also destroys cancerous cells.	

Labeling Exercise

Match each anatomy word or phrase to its structure and write it in the numbered box. Be sure to check your spelling. Use the Answer Key at the end of the book to check your answers.

basophil	eosinophil	lymphocyte	monocyte	neutrophil

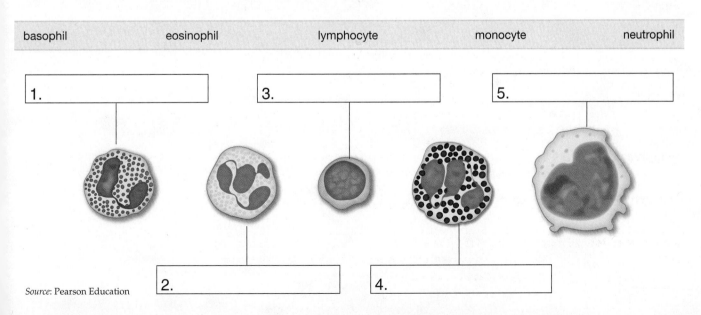

1.   3.   5.

2.   4.

Source: Pearson Education

appendix and Peyer's patches
axillary lymph nodes
celiac lymph nodes

cervical lymph nodes
inguinal lymph nodes
mesenteric lymph nodes

mediastinal lymph nodes
red bone marrow
spleen

thymus
tonsils and adenoids

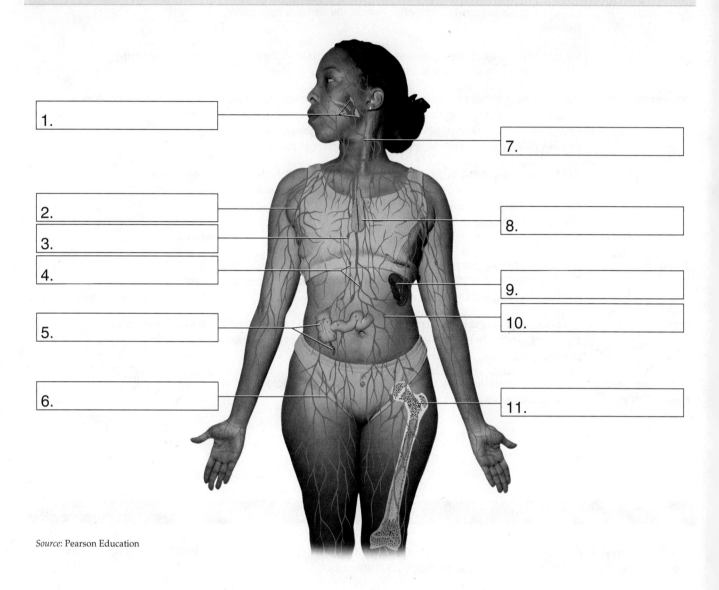

1.

2.

3.

4.

5.

6.

7.

8.

9.

10.

11.

Source: Pearson Education

Give Word Part Meanings

Use the Answer Key at the end of the book to check your answers.

Combining Forms Exercise

Next to each combining form, write its meaning. The first one has been done for you.

Combining Form	Meaning		Combining Form	Meaning
1. **aggreg/o-**	*crowding together*	20.	macr/o-	
2. aden/o-		21.	mon/o-	
3. bas/o-		22.	morph/o-	
4. coagul/o-		23.	myel/o-	
5. cyt/o-		24.	neutr/o-	
6. electr/o-		25.	norm/o-	
7. eosin/o-		26.	nucle/o-	
8. erythr/o-		27.	ox/y-	
9. fibrin/o-		28.	path/o-	
10. fibr/o-		29.	phag/o-	
11. glob/o-		30.	plasm/o-	
12. globul/o-		31.	plast/o-	
13. granul/o-		32.	reticul/o-	
14. hemat/o-		33.	splen/o-	
15. hem/o-		34.	suppress/o-	
16. immun/o-		35.	thromb/o-	
17. kary/o-		36.	thym/o-	
18. leuk/o-		37.	tox/o-	
19. lymph/o-				

Build Medical Words

Combining Form and Suffix Exercise

Read the definition of the medical word. Look at the combining form that is given. Select the correct suffix from the Suffix List and write it on the blank line. Then build the medical word and write it on the line. (Remember: You may need to remove the combining vowel. Always remove the hyphens and slash.) Be sure to check your spelling. The first one has been done for you.

SUFFIX LIST

-atic (pertaining to)	-ic (pertaining to)	-phage (thing that eats)
-ation (being; having; process)	-ity (condition; state)	-phil (attraction to; fondness for)
-blast (immature cell)	-logy (study of)	-poiesis (process of formation)
-cyte (cell)	-lyte (dissolved substance)	-poietin (substance that forms)
-gen (that which produces)	-oid (resembling)	

	Definition of the Medical Word	Combining Form	Suffix	Build the Medical Word
		hemat/o-	-poiesis	
1.	Process of formation (of) blood			hematopoiesis
	(You think *process of formation* (-poiesis) + *blood* (hemat/o-). You change the order of the word parts to put the suffix last. You write *hematopoiesis*.)			
2.	Cell (in the blood that is) white	leuk/o-	_____	_____
3.	Process (of blood) clotting	coagul/o-	_____	_____
4.	Pertaining to (the) spleen	splen/o-	_____	_____
5.	Cell (that is) eating	phag/o-	_____	_____
6.	Resembling (the) lymph or lymphatic system	lymph/o-	_____	_____
7.	Study of (the) blood	hemat/o-	_____	_____
8.	Substance that forms red (blood cells)	erythr/o-	_____	_____
9.	(Cell with an) attraction to eosin (a red, acidic dye)	eosin/o-	_____	_____
10.	That which produces disease	path/o-	_____	_____
11.	Cell (that helps to form a) blood clot	thromb/o-	_____	_____
12.	Immature cell (in the) bone marrow	myel/o-	_____	_____
13.	Dissolved substance (that conducts) electricity	electr/o-	_____	_____
14.	State (of readiness of the) immune response	immun/o-	_____	_____
15.	Process (of platelets) crowding together (and forming a clump)	aggreg/o-	_____	_____
16.	Pertaining to (the) lymph (system)	lymph/o-	_____	_____
17.	Cell (that has) granules (in its cytoplasm)	granul/o-	_____	_____
18.	Cell (in the blood that is) red	erythr/o-	_____	_____
19.	(Cell with an) attraction to alkaline (dye)	bas/o-	_____	_____
20.	Thing (cell) that eats (other cells and is) large	macr/o-	_____	_____

Prefix Exercise

Read the definition of the medical word. Look at the medical word or partial word that is given (it already contains a combining form and a suffix). Select the correct prefix from the Prefix List and write it on the blank line. Then build the medical word and write it on the line. Be sure to check your spelling. The first one has been done for you.

PREFIX LIST				
a- (away from; without)	endo- (innermost; within)	mega- (large)	poly- (many; much)	pro-(before)

Definition of the Medical Word	Prefix	Word or Partial Word	Build the Medical Word
1. Substance within (some bacteria that is) poison (to body cells)	**endo-**	**toxin**	*endotoxin*
2. Cell without granules (in its cytoplasm)	_____	granulocyte	_____
3. Pertaining to (a) many-shaped nucleus	_____	morphonuclear	_____
4. Substance (that comes) before (a) blood clot	_____	thrombin	_____
5. Cell (that has a) large (amount of cytoplasm around the) nucleus of the cell	_____	karyocyte	_____

Multiple Combining Forms and Suffix Exercise

Read the definition of the medical word. Select the correct suffix and combining forms. Then build the medical word and write it on the line. Be sure to check your spelling. The first one has been done for you.

SUFFIX LIST	COMBINING FORM LIST	
-cyte (cell)	cyt/o- (cell)	phag/o- (eating; swallowing)
-ic (pertaining to)	globul/o- (shaped like a globe)	plast/o- (formation; growth)
-in (substance)	immun/o- (immune response)	thromb/o- (blood clot)
-osis (condition; process)	kary/o- (nucleus of a cell)	tox/o- (poison)

Definition of the Medical Word	Combining Form	Combining Form	Suffix	Build the Medical Word
1. Pertaining to (a) cell (that is) poison (to pathogens)	**cyt/o-**	**tox/o-**	**-ic**	*cytotoxic*
(You think *pertaining to* (-ic) + *cell* (cyt/o-) + *poison* (tox/o-). You change the order of the word parts to put the suffix last. You write *cytotoxic*.)				
2. Substance (needed for) blood clot formation and growth	_____	_____	_____	_____
3. Substance (that is part of the) immune response (and is) shaped like a globe	_____	_____	_____	_____
4. Process (of) eating (done by a certain type of) cell	_____	_____	_____	_____

Diseases

Blood		
Word or Phrase	**Description**	**Pronunciation/Word Parts**
blood dyscrasia	Any disease involving blood cells. Treatment: Correct the underlying cause.	**dyscrasia** (dis-KRAY-zha) **dys-** *abnormal; difficult; painful* **-crasia** *condition of a mixing*
hemorrhage	Loss of a large amount of blood, externally or internally. Injury to an artery causes a forceful spurting of a large amount of bright red blood. Treatment: Tourniquet, pressure, or suturing to stop the bleeding.	**hemorrhage** (HEM-oh-rij) **hem/o-** *blood* **-rrhage** *excessive discharge; excessive flow*
pancytopenia	Decreased numbers of all types of blood cells due to failure of the bone marrow to produce stem cells. Treatment: Correct the underlying cause.	**pancytopenia** (PAN-sy-toh-PEE-nee-ah) **pan-** *all* **cyt/o-** *cell* **-penia** *condition of deficiency*
septicemia	Severe bacterial infection of the tissues that spreads to the blood and then the entire body. Both the bacteria and their endotoxins cause severe systemic symptoms. It is also known as **sepsis** or **blood poisoning**. Treatment: Antibiotic drug.	**septicemia** (SEP-tih-SEE-mee-ah) **septic/o-** *infection* **-emia** *condition of the blood; substance in the blood*
Erythrocytes		
abnormal red blood cell morphology	Category that includes any type of abnormality in the size, shape, or color of erythrocytes, such as anisocytosis, poikilocytosis, microcytic cells, or hypochromic cells. Treatment: Correct the underlying cause.	**morphology** (mor-FAW-loh-jee) **morph/o-** *shape* **-logy** *study of*
anemia	Decrease in the number of erythrocytes due to: 1. Insufficient amounts of amino acids, folic acid, iron, vitamin B_6, or vitamin B_{12} in the diet. 2. Disease, cancer, radiation therapy, or chemotherapy drugs that have damaged or destroyed the red marrow. 3. Hemolysis or increased cell fragility. 4. Hemorrhage, excessive menstruation, or chronic blood loss. Anemias can be categorized by the cause of the anemia or by the size, shape, or color of their erythrocytes. A patient with anemia is said to be **anemic**. Treatment: Correct the underlying cause.	**anemia** (ah-NEE-mee-ah) **an-** *not; without* **-emia** *condition of the blood; substance in the blood* Add words to make a complete definition of *anemia*: *condition of the blood (of) not (enough red blood cells).* **anemic** (ah-NEE-mik) **an-** *not; without* **-emic** *pertaining to a condition of the blood; pertaining to a substance in the blood*
aplastic anemia	Anemia caused by failure of the bone marrow to produce erythrocytes because it has been damaged by disease, cancer, radiation therapy, or chemotherapy drugs. The number of erythrocytes is decreased, but each erythrocyte is normocytic (normal in size) and normochromic (normal in color). Treatment: Blood transfusion, erythropoietin drug to stimulate erythrocyte production, or bone marrow transplantation.	**aplastic** (aa-PLAS-tik) **a-** *away from; without* **plast/o-** *formation; growth* **-ic** *pertaining to*

Word or Phrase	Description	Pronunciation/Word Parts
folic acid deficiency anemia	Anemia caused by a deficiency of folic acid in the diet. This anemia is seen in malnourished patients (older adults, those who are poor, people with alcoholism), those who have malabsorption diseases, and pregnant women. Each erythrocyte is abnormally large (**macrocytic**). Treatment: Balanced diet, folic acid supplements.	**macrocytic** (MAK-roh-SIT-ik) **macr/o-** *large* **cyt/o-** *cell* **-ic** *pertaining to*
iron deficiency anemia	Anemia caused by a deficiency of iron in the diet or increased loss of iron from menstruation, hemorrhage, or chronic blood loss. The patient has pale skin and mucous membranes because iron gives erythrocytes their color. Each erythrocyte is **microcytic** (small in size) and **hypochromic** (pale in color) (see Figure 6-13 ■). Compare to normal red blood cells (see Figure 6-4). Treatment: Infant formula with iron, dietary iron supplements, correction of blood loss. **FIGURE 6-13 ■ Microcytic, hypochromic erythrocytes.** Under a microscope, this blood smear shows small, pale erythrocytes that are characteristic of iron deficiency anemia. *Source*: Joaquin Carrillo Farga/Science Source	**microcytic** (MY-kroh-SIT-ik) **micr/o-** *one millionth; small* **cyt/o-** *cell* **-ic** *pertaining to* **hypochromic** (HY-poh-KROH-mik) **hypo-** *below; deficient* **chrom/o-** *color* **-ic** *pertaining to*
pernicious anemia	Anemia caused by a lack of vitamin B_{12} in the diet or a lack of intrinsic factor in the stomach. As a person ages, the stomach produces less hydrochloric acid and intrinsic factor; both of these must be present in order to absorb vitamin B_{12}. Untreated, this anemia can cause permanent damage to the nerves. Each erythrocyte is abnormally large and immature (megaloblast). Treatment: Intramuscular injection or nasal spray of vitamin B_{12} drug.	**pernicious** (per-NIH-shus)
sickle cell anemia	Anemia caused by an inherited genetic abnormality of an amino acid in hemoglobin. If one amino acid is abnormal, the patient has sickle cell trait and is a carrier for sickle cell disease, but does not have the disease. If two amino acids are abnormal, the patient has sickle cell disease. In patients with sickle cell disease, when there is a low level of oxygen in the blood, an erythrocyte distorts to become a crescent or sickle shape (see Figures 6-14 ■ and 6-15 ■). Treatment: Pain medication, avoidance of situations that lower the blood oxygen level. Hydroxyurea (a drug that stimulates the production of fetal hemoglobin and erythrocytes that do not sickle).	

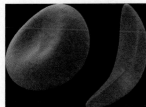

FIGURE 6-14 ■ Sickle cell.
The abnormal crescent shape and sharp edges of this sickled erythrocyte are very different from the smooth, rounded contour of a normal erythrocyte. Repeated sickling causes these fragile erythrocytes to have a shortened life span, resulting in anemia.
Source: Sebastian Kaulitzki/Fotolia

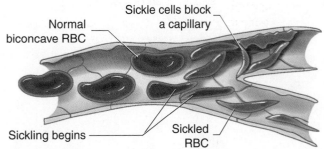

FIGURE 6-15 ■ Sickle cells in a capillary.
Sickle cells do not move easily through the capillaries. They become tangled and block the flow of blood. This causes severe pain and blood clots, particularly in the joints and abdomen.
Source: Pearson Education

Word or Phrase	Description	Pronunciation/Word Parts
anisocytosis	Erythrocytes that are unequal in size, either too large or too small. A **macrocyte** is an abnormally large erythrocyte (seen in folic acid anemia and pernicious anemia). A **microcyte** is an abnormally small erythrocyte (seen in iron deficiency anemia). Treatment for pernicious anemia or iron deficiency anemia.	**anisocytosis** (an-EYE-soh-sy-TOH-sis) anis/o- *unequal* cyt/o- *cell* -osis *condition; process* **macrocyte** (MAK-roh-site) macr/o- *large* -cyte *cell* **microcyte** (MY-kroh-site) micr/o- *one millionth; small* -cyte *cell*
poikilocytosis	Erythrocytes that have irregular shapes. A sickle cell is a crescent-shaped erythrocyte (seen in sickle cell anemia). Erythrocytes can also be in the shape of spheres (spherocytes), ovals, teardrops, or have spike-like projections on their surface. Treatment: None, as these are genetic defects.	**poikilocytosis** (POY-kih-LOH-sy-TOH-sis) poikil/o- *irregular* cyt/o- *cell* -osis *condition; process*
polycythemia vera	Increased number of erythrocytes due to uncontrolled production by the red marrow. The cause is unknown. The viscosity (thickness) of the blood increases and the blood volume is increased. There is dizziness, headache, fatigue, and splenomegaly. Patients are prone to develop blood clots and high blood pressure. Treatment: Periodic phlebotomy to remove blood to keep the blood volume and number of erythrocytes at a normal level.	**polycythemia vera** (PAW-lee-sy-THEE-mee-ah VAIR-ah) poly- *many; much* cyt/o- *cell* hem/o- *blood* -ia *condition; state; thing*
thalassemia	Inherited genetic abnormality that affects the globin chains in hemoglobin. The erythrocytes are small (microcytic), pale (hypochromic), and of variable size (anisocytosis). Target cells (erythrocytes with a central dark spot) are seen. There is anemia, weakness, and splenomegaly. Thalassemia major is the severe form of the disease; thalassemia minor produces fewer symptoms and signs. Treatment: Blood transfusions.	**thalassemia** (THAL-ah-SEE-mee-ah)
transfusion reaction	Reaction that occurs when a patient receives a transfusion with an incompatible blood type. Antibodies in the patient's serum attack antigens on the erythrocytes of the donor blood, causing **hemolysis** of the donor erythrocytes—a **hemolytic reaction**. Fever, chills, and hypotension occur almost immediately. The patient has flank pain because hemolyzed erythrocytes clog the filtering membrane of the kidneys and cause kidney failure. Transfusion reactions can be fatal. Treatment: Stop the transfusion immediately and treat the patient's symptoms and signs.	**transfusion** (trans-FYOO-shun) trans- *across; through* fus/o- *pouring* -ion *action; condition* **hemolysis** (hee-MAW-lih-sis) hem/o- *blood* -lysis *process to break down; process to destroy* **hemolytic** (HEE-moh-LIT-ik) hem/o- *blood* lyt/o- *break down; destroy* -ic *pertaining to*

Leukocytes

Word or Phrase	Description	Pronunciation/Word Parts
acquired immunodeficiency syndrome (AIDS)	Severe infection caused by the human immunodeficiency virus (HIV), a retrovirus. AIDS is a sexually transmitted disease (from sexual intercourse with an infected partner), but is also transmitted by shared needles (in drug abusers), accidental needlesticks or exposure to infected blood (in healthcare professionals), blood transfusions, and via the placenta to a fetus or via breast milk from an infected mother to a nursing baby. Initially, there is fever, night sweats, weight loss, enlarged lymph nodes, and diarrhea. A patient with antibodies against HIV is said to be *HIV positive.* HIV uses helper T cells (CD4 lymphocytes) to reproduce itself (see Figure 6-16 ▪). As large numbers of helper T cells are infected and destroyed, the action of suppressor T cells (CD8 lymphocytes) is unopposed. This suppresses the normal immune response and leaves the patient **immunocompromised** and defenseless against infection and cancer. Treatment: Antiretroviral drugs.	**immunodeficiency** (IH-myoo-NOH-deh-FIH-shun-see) **immun/o-** *immune response* **defici/o-** *inadequate; lacking* **-ency** *condition of being; condition of having* **immunocompromised** (IH-myoo-noh-KAWM-proh-myzd) **immun/o-** *immune response* **compromis/o-** *exposed to danger* **-ed** *pertaining to*

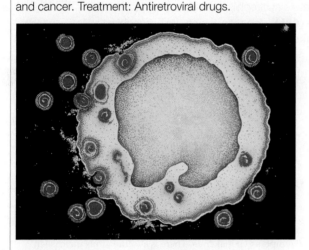

FIGURE 6-16 ▪ Human immunodeficiency virus.
This color-enhanced photograph taken with an electron microscope shows a helper T cell (CD4 lymphocyte) being invaded by many small human immunodeficiency viruses. Like all viruses, HIV cannot reproduce itself. It must enter a lymphocyte and use that cell's DNA to replicate itself. Then, the lymphocyte is destroyed as the new viruses are released.
Source: Chris Bjornberg/Science Source

A CLOSER LOOK

A diagnosis of AIDS is made when the CD4 cell count is below 200 (normal is 500–1,500 cells/mm^3) and there is an **opportunistic infection** such as *Pneumocystis jiroveci* pneumonia, oral or esophageal candidiasis (see Figure 16-16), cytomegalovirus retinitis, or unusual cancers such as Kaposi's sarcoma (see Figure 7-21). AIDS wasting syndrome is characterized by weight loss and loss of muscle mass and strength. There is no cure for AIDS. The universal symbol for AIDS is a red ribbon.

opportunistic (AW-por-too-NIS-tik)
opportun/o- *taking advantage of an opportunity; well timed*
-ist *person who specializes in; thing that specializes in*
-ic *pertaining to*

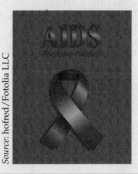

Source: hofred/Fotolia LLC

Word or Phrase	Description	Pronunciation/Word Parts

leukemia	**Cancer** of the leukocytes. Excessive numbers of leukocytes crowd out other cells in the bone marrow, causing anemia (from too few erythrocytes), easy bruising and hemorrhages (from too few thrombocytes), fever, and susceptibility to infection (from too few mature leukocytes). Leukemia is named according to the type of immature or mature leukocyte and whether the onset of symptoms is acute or chronic. Leukemia can be caused by exposure to radiation or toxic chemicals and drugs. Patients with chronic myelogenous leukemia have an abnormal chromosome known as the Philadelphia chromosome. Most cases of leukemia occur in persons over age 60. The most common leukemia in children is acute lymphocytic leukemia.
	
	acute myelogenous leukemia (AML)—too many immature myeloblasts and myelocytes
	chronic myelogenous leukemia (CML)—too many immature myeloblasts, myelocytes, but mature neutrophils, eosinophils, and basophils
	acute lymphocytic leukemia (ALL)—too many immature lymphoblasts
	chronic lymphocytic leukemia (CLL)—too many mature lymphocytes
	
	The diagnosis is made by examination of the blood (see Figure 6-17 ■) and by performing a bone marrow aspiration to look at blood cells in the bone marrow. Treatment: Chemotherapy drugs, radiation therapy, bone marrow transplantation or stem cell transplantation.
	
	FIGURE 6-17 ■ Acute lymphocytic leukemia.
	This blood smear was taken from a patient with acute lymphocytic leukemia. There is a tremendous increase in the number of immature lymphoblasts with some mature lymphocytes present in the blood. The pale cells in the background are erythrocytes.
	Source: Suthep Kukhunthod / 123 RF
		leukemia (loo-KEE-mee-ah)
		  leuk/o- *white*
		  -emia *condition of the blood; substance in the blood*
		Add words to make a complete definition of *leukemia*: *condition of the blood (with too many) white (blood cells)*.
		
		cancer (KAN-ser)
		
		myelogenous (MY-eh-LAW-jeh-nus)
		  myel/o- *bone marrow; myelin; spinal cord*
		  gen/o- *arising from; produced by*
		  -ous *pertaining to*
		
		lymphocytic (LIM-foh-SIT-ik)
		  lymph/o- *lymph; lymphatic system*
		  cyt/o- *cell*
		  -ic *pertaining to*

mononucleosis	Infectious disease caused by the Epstein-Barr virus (EBV). There is lymphadenopathy, fever, and fatigue. It is often called the "kissing disease" because it commonly affects young adults and is transmitted through contact with saliva that contains the virus. It is also known as *mono*. Treatment: Rest. (There is no antiviral drug that is effective against mononucleosis. Antibiotic drugs are not effective against viruses.)	**mononucleosis** (MAW-noh-NOO-klee-OH-sis)
		  mon/o- *one; single*
		  nucle/o- *nucleus of an atom; nucleus of a cell*
		  -osis *condition; process*
		Add words to make a complete definition of *mononucleosis*: *condition (of monocytes that have) one (unlobed) nucleus of a cell*.

multiple myeloma	Cancer of the B cells (lymphocytes) that normally become plasma cells and produce antibodies. There is weakness, anemia, and increased susceptibility to infections. Multiple tumors in the bone destroy the red marrow and cause pain, fractures, and **hypercalcemia** (as calcium is released from destroyed bone). Bence Jones protein, an immunoglobulin produced by the abnormal B cells, can be detected in the urine. Treatment: Radiation therapy and chemotherapy drugs.	**myeloma** (MY-eh-LOH-mah)
		  myel/o- *bone marrow; myelin; spinal cord*
		  -oma *mass; tumor*
		
		hypercalcemia (HY-per-kal-SEE-mee-ah)
		  hyper- *above; more than normal*
		  calc/o- *calcium*
		  -emia *condition of the blood; substance in the blood*

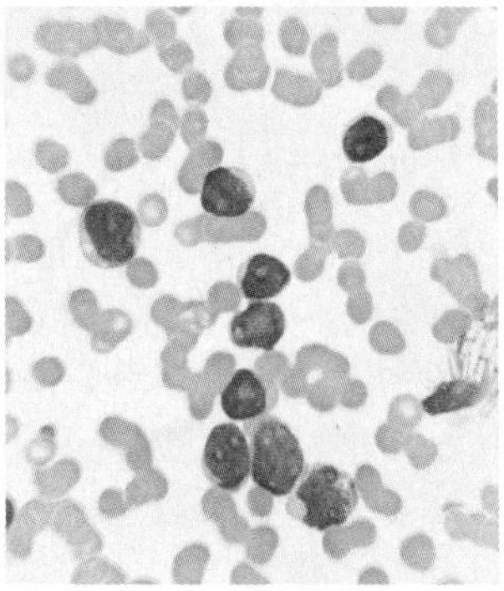

Thrombocytes and Blood Clotting

Word or Phrase	Description	Pronunciation/Word Parts
coagulopathy	Any disease that affects the ability of the blood to clot normally. Treatment: Correct the underlying cause.	**coagulopathy** (koh-AG-yoo-LAW-pah-thee) **coagul/o-** *clotting* -**pathy** *disease*
deep venous thrombosis (DVT)	A **thrombus** (blood clot) in one of the deep veins of the lower leg, often after surgery or in patients who are immobile or on bedrest. Lack of exercise causes the blood to pool in the veins (**venous stasis**) and form a blood clot (see Figure 6-18 ■). Sometimes a thrombus from a deep vein becomes an **embolus** that travels to the heart but then becomes trapped in a branch of the pulmonary artery to the lung. It blocks the blood flow, and the blood never reaches the lung to pick up oxygen. This condition is known as a pulmonary **embolism**. Treatment: Anticoagulant drug to prevent another thrombus from forming; thrombolytic drug to dissolve the embolus.	**thrombosis** (thrawm-BOH-sis) **thromb/o-** *blood clot* -**osis** *condition; process* **thrombus** (THRAWM-bus) **thrombi** (THRAWM-by) **stasis** (STAY-sis) **embolus** (EM-boh-lus) **embolism** (EM-boh-LIZ-em) **embol/o-** *embolus; occluding plug* -**ism** *disease from a specific cause; process*

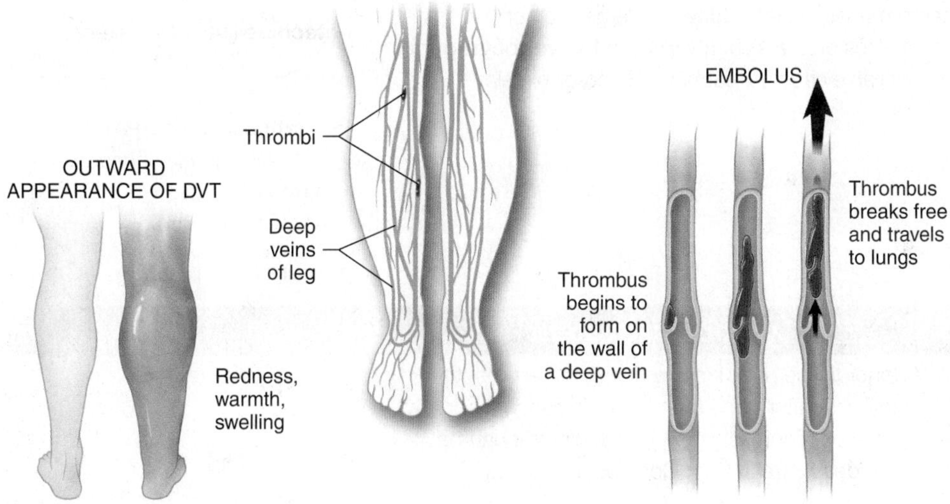

OUTWARD APPEARANCE OF DVT

Thrombi

Deep veins of leg

Redness, warmth, swelling

EMBOLUS

Thrombus begins to form on the wall of a deep vein

Thrombus breaks free and travels to lungs

FIGURE 6-18 ■ Deep venous thrombosis.
(a) When a blood clot (thrombus) forms in a deep vein, there is swelling as the blood flow is impaired, and redness and warmth as the tissues become inflamed. (b) A thrombus can become an embolus that travels to other parts of the body.
Source: Pearson Education

disseminated intravascular coagulation (DIC)	Severe disorder of clotting in which multiple small thrombi are formed throughout the body. These thrombi use up platelets and fibrinogen from the plasma to such an extent that there is spontaneous bleeding from the nose, mouth, IV sites, and incisions. DIC can be triggered by severe injuries, burns, cancer, or systemic infections. Treatment: Intravenous fibrinogen and platelets.	**disseminated** (dih-SEM-ih-NAY-ted) **dissemin/o-** *scattered throughout the body* -**ated** *composed of; pertaining to a condition* **intravascular** (IN-trah-VAS-kyoo-lar) **intra-** *within* **vascul/o-** *blood vessel* -**ar** *pertaining to* **coagulation** (koh-AG-yoo-LAY-shun) **coagul/o-** *clotting* -**ation** *being; having; process*

Word or Phrase	Description	Pronunciation/Word Parts
hemophilia	Inherited genetic abnormality that causes a lack or a deficiency of a specific clotting factor. The abnormal gene is carried by a female on the X chromosome, but she does not have the disease. If a male inherits the abnormal gene, it causes hemophilia. A patient who has hemophilia is a **hemophiliac**. Hemophilia A, the most common type, is due to a lack of clotting factor VIII. Hemophilia B is due to a lack of factor IX. Hemophilia C is due to a lack of factor XI. When injured, hemophiliac patients continue to bleed for long periods of time. Minor injuries produce large hematomas under the skin and bleeding inside body cavities, joints, and organs. Treatment: Intravenous administration of the specific clotting factor that is lacking.	**hemophilia** (HEE-moh-FIL-ee-ah) **hem/o-** *blood* **phil/o-** *attraction to; fondness for* **-ia** *condition; state; thing* Add words to make a complete definition of *hemophilia*: *condition (of the) blood (in which it has a) fondness for (not clotting).* **hemophiliac** (HEE-moh-FIL-ee-ak) **hem/o-** *blood* **phil/o-** *attraction to; fondness for* **-iac** *pertaining to*
thrombocytopenia	Deficiency in the number of thrombocytes due to exposure to radiation, chemicals, or drugs that damage stem cells in the red bone marrow. It also occurs when leukemia cells crowd out the stem cells in the red marrow that produce thrombocytes. Also, some patients have antibodies that destroy their own thrombocytes. Thrombocytopenia results in small, pinpoint hemorrhages or **petechiae** and larger hemorrhages or **ecchymoses** and bruises on the skin. **Idiopathic thrombocytopenia purpura** has no identifiable cause. Treatment: Blood or platelet transfusion.	**thrombocytopenia** (THRAWM-boh-SY-toh-PEE-nee-ah) **thromb/o-** *blood clot* **cyt/o-** *cell* **-penia** *condition of deficiency* **petechiae** (peh-TEE-kee-ee) **ecchymoses** (EK-ih-MOH-seez) **idiopathic** (ID-ee-oh-PATH-ik) **idi/o-** *individual; unknown* **path/o-** *disease* **-ic** *pertaining to* **purpura** (PER-peh-rah)

Lymphatic System

graft-versus-host disease (GVHD)	Immune reaction of donor tissue or a donor organ (graft) against the patient (host). This can occur after bone marrow transplantation or any type of organ transplantation. There is a rash and fever, or it can be severe enough to cause death. Treatment: Corticosteroid drug.	
lymphadenopathy	Enlarged lymph nodes. Lymph nodes in the neck, axillae, and groin can be felt easily if they are enlarged. A sore throat causes lymph nodes in the neck to enlarge (see Figure 6-19 ■). A severe infection or cancer will cause the lymph nodes in that area to become enlarged. Treatment: Correct the underlying cause.	**lymphadenopathy** (lim-FAD-eh-NAW-pah-thee) **lymph/o-** *lymph; lymphatic system* **aden/o-** *gland* **-pathy** *disease*

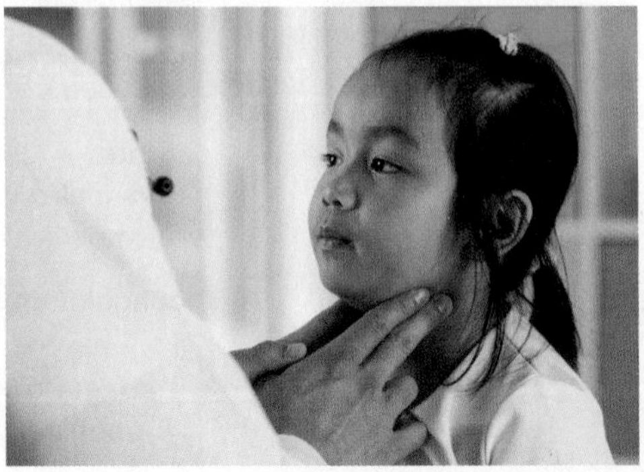

FIGURE 6-19 ■ Lymphadenopathy.
The pediatrician is palpating the cervical lymph nodes of this patient. Macrophages in the lymph nodes trap and destroy pathogens or cancerous cells from the nose, mouth, or throat, but large numbers of pathogens or cancerous cells can cause enlarged lymph nodes and a complaint of sore throat or difficulty swallowing.
Source: Photographee.eu/Fotolia

Word or Phrase	Description	Pronunciation/Word Parts
lymphedema	Generalized swelling of an arm or leg that occurs after surgery when a chain of lymph nodes has been removed. Tissue fluid in that area cannot drain into the lymphatic vessels at the normal rate, and this causes edema. Treatment: Elevation of the body part to promote drainage.	**lymphedema** (LIMF-eh-DEE-mah) **lymph/o-** *lymph; lymphatic system* **-edema** *swelling*
lymphoma	**Cancerous** tumor of lymphocytes in the lymph nodes or lymphoid tissue. A lymphoma that originates in a lymph node should not be confused with a metastasis to a lymph node from a primary site of cancer located elsewhere. Treatment: Radiation therapy, chemotherapy drugs.	**lymphoma** (lim-FOH-mah) **lymph/o-** *lymph; lymphatic system* **-oma** *mass; tumor* **cancerous** (KAN-ser-us) **cancer/o-** *cancer* **-ous** *pertaining to*
Hodgkin's lymphoma	Most common type of lymphoma. It occurs most often in young adults and is discovered on physical examination as a painless, enlarged cervical lymph node in the neck. There is fever, weakness, weight loss, and splenomegaly. A biopsy of the lymph node shows abnormal lymphocytes known as Reed-Sternberg cells. It is also known as **Hodgkin's disease**.	**Hodgkin** (HAWJ-kin)
non-Hodgkin's lymphoma	A group of more than 20 different types of lymphomas that occur in older adults and do not show Reed-Sternberg cells.	
splenomegaly	Enlargement of the spleen, as felt on palpation of the abdomen. It can be caused by mononucleosis, Hodgkin's disease, hemolytic anemia, polycythemia vera, or leukemia. Treatment: Correct the underlying cause.	**splenomegaly** (SPLEH-noh-MEG-ah-lee) **splen/o-** *spleen* **-megaly** *enlargement*
thymoma	Tumor of the thymus that is usually benign. It may cause a cough and chest pain. It is often seen in patients who already have an autoimmune disorder such as myasthenia gravis. Treatment: Thymectomy.	**thymoma** (thy-MOH-mah) **thym/o-** *rage; thymus* **-oma** *mass; tumor*

Autoimmune Disorders

Word or Phrase	Description	Pronunciation/Word Parts
autoimmune disorders	Disorders in which the body makes antibodies against its own tissues, causing pain and loss of function. The following autoimmune disorders are described in other chapters: **Autoimmune Disorder** — **Area Affected** diabetes mellitus, type 1 — pancreas gluten sensitivity enteropathy — intestines Graves' disease — thyroid gland Hashimoto's thyroiditis — thyroid gland inflammatory bowel disease — intestines multiple sclerosis — nerves myasthenia gravis — muscles psoriasis — skin rheumatoid arthritis — joints scleroderma — skin and blood vessels systemic lupus erythematosus — connective tissue, skin, kidneys, lungs	**autoimmune** (AW-toh-ih-MYOON) **aut/o-** *self* **-immune** *immune response*

Laboratory and Diagnostic Procedures

Blood Cell Tests		
Word or Phrase	**Description**	**Pronunciation/Word Parts**
blood type	Blood test to determine the blood type (A, B, AB, or O) and Rh factor (positive or negative) of the patient's blood. **Type and crossmatch** is done when a patient needs to receive a blood transfusion. The donor's blood type was determined when it was stored in the blood bank. The patient's (recipient's) blood type is determined. Then the patient's plasma is crossmatched by mixing it with the donor's red blood cells. If the donor's red blood cells clump together (**agglutination**), the blood types are not compatible.	**agglutination** (ah-GLOO-tih-NAY-shun) **agglutin/o-** *clumping; sticking* **-ation** *being; having; process*
complete blood count (CBC) with differential	Group of blood tests that are performed automatically by machine to determine the number, type, and characteristics of various cells in the blood (see Table 6-4 ▪). This is also known as a *CBC with diff*.	**differential** (DIF-er-EN-shal) **different/o-** *different; distinct* **-ial** *pertaining to*
	A CLOSER LOOK A severe bacterial infection will increase the number of bands in the differential count as the body tries to meet the increased demand for neutrophils by releasing immature bands from the red marrow. This is known as a **shift to the left**. It refers to a time when the differential count was done by hand with a column on the tally sheet for each type of leukocyte. While counting the leukocytes under the microscope, the laboratory technician put tally marks in the appropriate columns. The column to the far left was for bands. When there were more tally marks in that column than usual, the differential count was said to show a shift to the left.	
peripheral blood smear	Blood test done manually to examine the characteristics of erythrocytes and leukocytes under a microscope. A drop of blood is spread as a thin smear on a glass slide. Then hematoxylin and eosin dyes are used to stain the blood cells. A blood smear is used to investigate abnormal blood cells discovered on the automated CBC, or a blood smear can be ordered by the physician when there is reason to suspect blood cell abnormalities.	**peripheral** (peh-RIF-eh-ral) **peripher/o-** *outer aspects* **-al** *pertaining to* *Peripheral* refers to blood that is taken from an extremity (usually by venipuncture from a vein in the arm).

Table 6-4 Complete Blood Count (CBC) with Differential		
Test Name	**Description**	**Pronunciation/Word Parts**
erythrocytes (red blood cells, RBCs)	Number in millions per milliliter (mL) of blood	
hematocrit (HCT)	Percentage of RBCs in a blood sample	**hematocrit** (hee-MAT-oh-krit) **hemat/o-** *blood* **-crit** *separation of*
hemoglobin (Hgb)	Amount in grams per deciliter (g/dL) of blood	

red blood cell **indices**
  mean cell volume (MCV)
  mean cell hemoglobin (MCH)
  mean cell hemoglobin concentration (MCHC)
	
	Average volume of one RBC
	Average weight of hemoglobin in one RBC
	
	Average concentration of hemoglobin in one RBC
		indices (IN-dih-seez)
		Index is a Latin singular noun. Form the plural by changing *–ex* to *–ices*.
		
		mean (MEEN)
		Mean is an arithmetic word that means *the average*.

(continued)

Table 6-4   Complete Blood Count (CBC) with Differential *(continued)*

Test Name	Description	Pronunciation/Word Parts
leukocytes (white blood cells, WBCs)	Number in thousands per milliliter (k/mL) of blood	The *k* in *k/mL* stands for *kilo-*, a prefix meaning *one thousand*.

WBC differential
  neutrophils
  eosinophils
  basophils
  lymphocytes
  monocytes
	Percentage of each type of WBC per 100 WBCs	

thrombocytes (platelets)	Number in thousands per milliliter (k/mL) of blood	

Coagulation Tests

Word or Phrase	Description	Pronunciation/Word Parts
activated clotting time (ACT)	Blood test to monitor the effectiveness of the anticoagulant drug heparin when it is given in high doses. A prolonged (rather than normal) activated clotting time would be expected.	
partial thromboplastin time (PTT)	Blood test to monitor the effectiveness of the anticoagulant drug heparin when it is given in regular doses. A prolonged (rather than normal) PTT would be expected. An activated partial thromboplastin time (aPTT) test uses a chemical activator to get faster test results.	
prothrombin time (PT)	Blood test to evaluate the effectiveness of the anticoagulant drug Coumadin. A prolonged (rather than normal) PT would be expected. The **international normalized ratio (INR)** reports the PT value in a standardized way, regardless of which laboratory performed the test.	

Other Blood Tests

blood chemistries	Blood test used to determine the levels of various substances in the blood (see Figure 6-20 ■). These include electrolytes, albumin, total protein, ALT, AST, BUN, creatinine, bilirubin, glucose, LDH, total cholesterol, uric acid, and alkaline phosphatase. A Chem-20 includes 20 individual chemistry tests performed at the same time. This is also called a **metabolic panel**.	

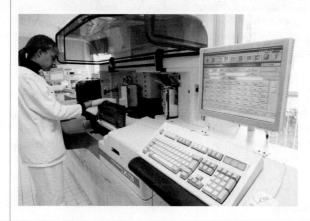

FIGURE 6-20 ■ Blood chemistry analyzer.
This clinical laboratory scientist is performing a blood chemistry analysis, the results of which are displayed on the computer screen. Multiple tests can be performed together automatically on this computerized equipment.
Source: BSIP/Science Source

Word or Phrase	Description	Pronunciation/Word Parts

ferritin	Blood test that indirectly measures the amount of iron (ferritin) stored in the body by measuring the small amount that is always present in the blood. **The total iron-binding capacity (TIBC)** measures the level of **transferrin**, a protein that carries iron in the blood. These tests are used to diagnose iron deficiency anemia.	**ferritin** (FAIR-ih-tin)
		  ferrit/o- *iron*
		  -in *substance*
		
		transferrin (trans-FAIR-in)
		  trans- *across; through*
		  ferr/o- *iron*
		  -in *substance*

human immunodeficiency virus (HIV) tests	Blood tests that detect infection with HIV. HIV tests are reported as either HIV negative or HIV positive.	
ELISA	First screening test done for HIV. It can be done on blood, urine, or saliva samples. The test uses two antibodies. The first binds to HIV, forming a complex; the second reacts to an enzyme in that complex. However, this test can also be positive if the patient has antibodies against lupus erythematosus, Lyme disease, or syphilis. *ELISA* stands for *enzyme-linked immunosorbent assay.* The test results are available in 1–2 weeks; however, the SUDS (Single-Use Diagnostic System) test, which uses ELISA methods, is a rapid HIV test that gives results in 10 minutes. OraSure is a quick screening test done in a doctor's office or clinic to detect antibodies to HIV in the saliva.	
Western blot	Used to confirm a positive ELISA and make a diagnosis of HIV infection. A positive ELISA and a positive Western blot together are 99.9% accurate in diagnosing HIV infection.	
viral RNA load test	Measures tiny amounts of RNA (from HIV) that are in the blood during the 6 weeks before antibodies against HIV can be detected. This test is also used to monitor the progression of the disease and the patient's response to antiretroviral drugs.	
p24 antigen test	Detects p24, a protein in HIV. The results are reported as a titer. This test is also used to screen donated units of blood for HIV.	
CD4 count	Measures the number of CD4 lymphocytes (helper T cells). It is used to monitor the progression of the disease and the patient's response to antiretroviral drugs. The CD4:CD8 ratio is also monitored.	
Serum Tests		

MonoSpot test	Rapid test that uses the patient's serum mixed with horse erythrocytes. If the patient has infectious mononucleosis, **heterophil antibodies** in the patient's serum cause the horse's erythrocytes to clump. It is also called the **heterophil antibody test**.	**heterophil** (HET-er-oh-FIL)
		  heter/o- *other*
		  -phil *attraction to; fondness for*

serum protein electrophoresis (SPEP)	Immunoglobulin electrophoresis test that determines the amount of each immunoglobulin (IgA, IgD, IgE, IgG, and IgM) in the blood. A sample of serum is placed in a gel with an electrical current. The immunoglobulins become charged and move toward the positive or negative electrode. Each immunoglobulin travels a different distance and direction through the gel, depending on its size and charge, and it appears as a spike in a different area on the graph paper. The size of the spike corresponds to how much immunoglobulin is present.	**electrophoresis**
		(ee-LEK-troh-foh-REE-sis)
		  electr/o- *electricity*
		  phor/o- *bear; carry; range*
		  -esis *condition; process*
		Add words to make a complete definition of *electrophoresis*: *process (of using) electricity (to) carry (immunoglobulins in a gel).*

Urine Tests

Word or Phrase	Description	Pronunciation/Word Parts
Bence Jones protein	Urine test, also known as **urine protein electrophoresis (UPEP)**, that is used to monitor the course of multiple myeloma. The cancerous plasma cells produce this abnormal immunoglobulin that can be detected in the urine.	
Schilling test	Urine test used to diagnose pernicious anemia. It measures the amount of radioactive vitamin B_{12} excreted in the urine. The patient swallows a capsule that contains intrinsic factor and vitamin B_{12} labeled with a radioactive tracer. The patient swallows a second capsule that contains vitamin B_{12} labeled with a different radioactive tracer but no intrinsic factor. If the patient has pernicious anemia, only the capsule that contained vitamin B_{12} and intrinsic factor will be absorbed into the blood and then excreted in the urine.	

Radiologic Procedures

Word or Phrase	Description	Pronunciation/Word Parts
lymphangiography	Radiologic procedure in which a radiopaque contrast dye is injected into a lymphatic vessel. X-rays are taken as the dye travels through the lymphatic vessels and lymph nodes. It shows enlarged lymph nodes, lymphomas, and areas of blocked lymphatic drainage. The x-ray image is a **lymphangiogram**.	**lymphangiography** (lim-FAN-jee-AW-grah-fee) **lymph/o-** *lymph; lymphatic system* **angi/o-** *blood vessel; lymphatic vessel* **-graphy** *process of recording* **lymphangiogram** (lim-FAN-jee-oh-GRAM) **lymph/o-** *lymph; lymphatic system* **angi/o-** *blood vessel; lymphatic vessel* **-gram** *picture; record*

Medical and Surgical Procedures

Medical Procedures

Word or Phrase	Description	Pronunciation/Word Parts
bone marrow aspiration	Procedure to remove red bone marrow from the posterior iliac crest of the hip bone. This is done to diagnose leukemia, lymphoma, and unusual types of anemia by examining the different stages of blood cell development (stem cell to mature cell). It is also done to harvest bone marrow from a healthy donor to give to a patient who needs a bone marrow transplantation.	**aspiration** (AS-pih-RAY-shun) **aspir/o-** *breathe in; suck in* **-ation** *being; having; process*
phlebotomy	Procedure for drawing a sample of venous blood into a vacuum tube. This is also known as **venipuncture**. The vacuum tubes have different-colored rubber stoppers that indicate which additive or anticoagulant is in the tube; this determines what blood test can be performed on the blood in that tube (see Figure 6-21 ■).	**phlebotomy** (fleh-BAW-toh-mee) **phleb/o-** *vein* **-tomy** *process of cutting;* *process of making an incision* **venipuncture** (VEE-nih-PUNK-chur) **ven/i-** *vein* **punct/o-** *hole; perforation* **-ure** *result of; system*

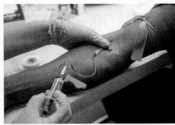

FIGURE 6-21 ■ Phlebotomy.
This patient is having blood drawn. The phlebotomist placed a tourniquet around the patient's upper arm to distend the veins in the lower arm. The patient's arm is supported to keep the elbow straight so that the needle goes into the lumen of the vein, not through it. A vacuum tube is placed into the plastic holder and the vacuum draws blood into the tube. The tubes of blood are sent to a laboratory for testing.
Source: Andrew Aitchison/In Pictures/Corbis News/Corbis

Word or Phrase	Description	Pronunciation/Word Parts
vaccination	Procedure that injects a vaccine into the body. The **vaccine** consists of killed or **attenuated** (weakened) bacterial or viral cells or cell fragments. The body produces antibodies and memory B lymphocytes specific to that pathogen. If the vaccinated patient encounters that pathogen again, the patient will have mild or no symptoms of the disease. Vaccinations are routinely used to provide active immunity to diseases that could be fatal or cause serious disability (polio, diphtheria, tetanus, etc.). Immunoglobulins (antibodies) against some diseases (rabies or tetanus) can be given to provide passive immunity if the person has just been exposed. Vaccination is also known as **immunization**.	**vaccination** (VAK-sih-NAY-shun) **vaccin/o-** *vaccine* **-ation** *being; having; process* **vaccine** (vak-SEEN) **attenuated** (ah-TEN-yoo-AA-ted) **attenu/o-** *weakened* **-ated** *composed of; pertaining to a condition* **immunization** (IH-myoo-nih-ZAY-shun) **immun/o-** *immune response* **-ization** *process of creating; process of inserting; process of making*

> **A CLOSER LOOK**
>
> The principles of vaccination were established in 1796 by Edward Jenner, an English physician. He noticed that milkmaids did not get the serious disease smallpox because they first contracted cowpox, a viral disease of cows. Jenner took fluid from the skin sores of a milkmaid with cowpox. He made cuts in the skin of a young boy and introduced the fluid, and the boy later developed cowpox. Later, Jenner gave the boy the smallpox virus, and the boy did not develop smallpox. This procedure was successful, but it horrified people. Cartoonists drew pictures of patients with cow parts coming out of their bodies. However, several years later, most doctors were using Jenner's technique to protect their patients from smallpox.

Blood Donation and Tranfusion Procedures

Word or Phrase	Description	Pronunciation/Word Parts
blood donation	Procedure in which a unit of whole blood is collected from a donor. The unit is tested and labeled as to blood type and stored in a refrigerated blood bank. A unit of whole blood can be given as a transfusion, or the unit can be divided into its component parts (erythrocytes, platelets, plasma), and just that part can be given as a transfusion to meet the needs of a specific patient.	**donation** (doh-NAY-shun) **donat/o-** *gift; giving* **-ion** *action; condition*

CLINICAL CONNECTIONS

Public Health. All donated blood must be tested for syphilis, hepatitis, and HIV. The Food and Drug Administration (FDA) is responsible for the safety of blood and blood products used in the United States. The FDA has banned people from donating blood if they lived in or visited Europe for a certain length of time because of the possibility of contamination with the microorganism that causes mad cow disease in cows and new variant Creutzfeldt-Jakob disease in humans, a fatal neurologic disease.

Word or Phrase	Description	Pronunciation/Word Parts
blood transfusion	Procedure in which whole blood, blood cells, or plasma is given by intravenous transfusion. Transfusions of whole blood provide a complete correction of blood loss. Packed red blood cells (PRBCs) are a concentrated preparation of RBCs in a small amount of plasma. Transfusion with PRBCs avoids fluid overload in patients with congestive heart failure or in premature infants. Platelets are given to patients with thrombocytopenia or leukemia and to cancer patients whose bone marrow is depressed after radiation therapy or chemotherapy drugs. Plasma is given to hemophiliac patients who need clotting factors.	**transfusion** (trans-FYOO-shun) **trans-** *across; through* **fus/o-** *pouring* **-ion** *action; condition*

A CLOSER LOOK

Patients scheduled to have certain types of surgery may be asked to donate a unit of their own blood in advance so they can receive it during surgery. This is known as an **autologous blood transfusion**. It is also called this when blood in the operative field is suctioned, collected, filtered, and returned to the patient during the surgery. At the conclusion of every surgery, the surgeon estimates the amount of blood loss and records this in the patient's operative report.

autologous (aw-TAW-loh-gus)
 aut/o- *self*
 log/o- *study of; word*
 -ous *pertaining to*

Word or Phrase	Description	Pronunciation/Word Parts
bone marrow transplantation (BMT)	Procedure used to treat patients with leukemia and lymphoma. Red marrow is harvested by aspirating it from the hip bone of a matched donor. The patient is treated with chemotherapy drugs or radiation to destroy all cancerous cells (this also destroys all the cells in the red marrow). The donor marrow is then filtered and given to the patient intravenously. The donated bone marrow cells travel through the blood to the bones where they implant. After 2–4 weeks, the patient's red marrow begins to produce normal blood cells.	**transplantation** (TRANS-plan-TAY-shun) **transplant/o-** *move something across and put in another place* **-ation** *being; having; process*

A CLOSER LOOK

Unlike blood transfusions where donor blood and patient blood are crossmatched for compatibility of the ABO and Rh blood groups, bone marrow donors and recipient patients are matched for a different set of proteins called human leukocyte-associated (HLA) antigens. In **autologous transplants**, patients provide their own bone marrow or stem cells (which are treated to destroy any cancerous cells). In **allogeneic transplants**, patients receive bone marrow or stem cells donated by another person.

allogeneic (AL-oh-jeh-NEE-ik)
  all/o- *other; strange*
  gene/o- *gene*
  -ic *pertaining to*
Add words to make a complete definition of *allogeneic*: *pertaining to (someone) other (than the patient and his or her) genes.*

Word or Phrase	Description	Pronunciation/Word Parts
plasmapheresis	Procedure in which plasma is separated from the blood cells. A donor gives a unit of blood, which is rapidly spun in a centrifuge. Centrifugal force pulls the blood cells to the bottom of the unit of blood. The plasma portion at the top is siphoned off. The blood cells are given back to the donor. Then the plasma is processed and pooled with plasma from other donors to make fresh frozen plasma, albumin, or clotting factors.	**plasmapheresis** (PLAZ-mah-feh-REE-sis) **plasm/o-** *plasma* **apher/o-** *withdrawal* **-esis** *condition; process*
stem cell transplantation	Procedure to treat leukemia and lymphoma. Stem cells from the patient or from a matched donor are collected. Matched stem cells from umbilical cord blood can also be used. The stem cells are given intravenously. They migrate to the red marrow and begin producing normal blood cells.	

TECHNOLOGY IN MEDICINE

Tissue Engineering. In 2001, the first embryonic stem cell (see Figure 6-22 ■) was made into a mature blood cell. This ignited a controversy over the use of human embryos in stem cell research. In 2009, the first human clinical trial of embryonic stem cell therapy was done on patients with recent spinal cord injuries. Then the technology was developed to use a patient's own stem cells. In 2010, a patient's stem cells were used to repair his damaged cornea. In 2012, a plastic framework and stem cells were used to create a new trachea for a cancer patient. In 2012, doctors injected stem cells to heal a severely damaged heart in a patient with congestive heart failure.

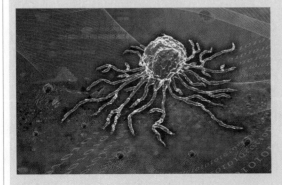

FIGURE 6-22 ■ Stem cell.
Source: Krishnacreations/Fotolia

Surgical Procedures

Word or Phrase	Description	Pronunciation/Word Parts
lymph node biopsy	Procedure that uses a fine needle to aspirate tissue from a lymph node. The lymph node may also be completely removed by doing an **excisional biopsy**. This is done to look for cancer cells.	**biopsy** (BY-awp-see) **bi/o-** *life; living organism; living tissue* **-opsy** *process of viewing* **excisional** (ek-SIH-zhun-al) **excis/o-** *cut out* **-ion** *action; condition* **-al** *pertaining to*
lymph node dissection	Procedure to remove several or all of the lymph nodes in a lymph node chain during extensive surgery for cancer.	**dissection** (dy-SEK-shun) **dissect/o-** *cut apart* **-ion** *action; condition*
splenectomy	Procedure to remove the spleen when it has ruptured due to trauma.	**splenectomy** (spleh-NEK-toh-mee) **splen/o-** *spleen* **-ectomy** *surgical removal*

WORD ALERT

Sound-Alike Words

spleen	*(noun)*	organ of the lymphatic system
splenectomy	*(noun)*	surgical removal of the spleen
splenic	*(adjective)*	pertaining to the spleen
splenomegaly	*(noun)*	enlargement of the spleen

Word or Phrase	Description	Pronunciation/Word Parts
thymectomy	Procedure to remove the thymus because of a benign or cancerous tumor or to treat myasthenia gravis.	**thymectomy** (thy-MEK-toh-mee) **thym/o-** *rage; thymus* **-ectomy** *surgical removal*

CLINICAL CONNECTIONS

Orthopedics (Muscular) (Chapter 9). A thymectomy is also performed in patients with the muscular disease myasthenia gravis. This disease causes severe muscle weakness as the body's antibodies destroy acetylcholine receptors on the muscles. In these patients, the thymus contains abnormal cells that may cause this autoimmune reaction. After a thymectomy, the number of antibodies against acetylcholine receptors decreases.

Drugs

These drug categories and drugs are used to treat blood and lymphatic diseases. The most common generic and trade name drugs in each category are listed.

Category	Indication	Examples	Pronunciation/Word Parts
anticoagulant drugs	Prevent blood clots from forming by inhibiting the clotting factors (heparin drug) or by inhibiting vitamin K that is needed to make the clotting factors (warfarin drug)	heparin (subcutaneous or intravenous), warfarin (Coumadin) (oral)	**anticoagulant** (AN-tee-koh-AG-yoo-lant) (AN-tih-koh-AG-yoo-lant) **anti-** *against* **coagul/o-** *clotting* **-ant** *pertaining to*
corticosteroid drugs	Anti-inflammatory drugs that suppress the immune response and decrease inflammation. Also given to organ transplant patients to prevent rejection of the donor organ.	methylprednisolone (Medrol), prednisone	**corticosteroid** (KOR-tih-koh-STAIR-oyd) **cortic/o-** *cortex; outer region* **-steroid** *steroid*
erythropoietin	Stimulates the red marrow to make erythrocytes	epoetin alfa (Epogen, procrit)	**erythropoietin** (eh-RITH-roh-POY-eh-tin) **erythr/o-** *red* **-poietin** *substance that forms*
immuno-suppressant drugs	Suppress the immune response. Prevent rejection of a transplanted organ.	cyclosporine (Sandimmune)	**immunosuppressant** (IH-myoo-NOH-soo-PRES-ant) **immun/o-** *immune response* **suppress/o-** *press down* **-ant** *pertaining to*
nucleoside reverse transcriptase inhibitor drugs	Antiretroviral drugs that inhibit reverse transcriptase, an enzyme that HIV needs to reproduce itself	lamivudine (Epivir), telbivudine (Tyzeka), zidovudine (Retrovir)	**nucleoside** (NOO-klee-oh-SIDE) **transcriptase** (trans-KRIP-tays)
platelet aggregation inhibitor drugs	Prevent platelets from aggregating (clumping together), the first step in forming a blood clot	aspirin, clopidogrel (Plavix), abciximab (ReoPro)	**inhibitor** (in-HIB-ih-tor) **inhibit/o-** *block; hold back* **-or** *person who does; person who produces; thing that does; thing that produces*
protease inhibitor drugs	Antiretroviral drugs that inhibit protease, an enzyme that HIV needs to reproduce itself	indinavir (Crixivan), nelfinavir (Viracept), ritonavir (Norvir)	**protease** (PROH-tee-ays) **prote/o-** *protein* **-ase** *enzyme*
thrombolytic enzyme drugs	Break fibrin strands to dissolve a blood clot that has already formed	urokinase (Abbokinase). The suffix *-ase* indicates that the drug is an enzyme.	**thrombolytic** (THRAWM-boh-LIT-ik) **thromb/o-** *blood clot* **lyt/o-** *break down; destroy* **-ic** *pertaining to*
tissue plasminogen activator (TPA) drugs	Activate plasminogen by converting it to an enzyme that breaks fibrin strands and dissolves a blood clot that has already formed	alteplase (Activase), reteplase (Retavase)	**plasminogen** (plaz-MIN-oh-jen)
vitamin B$_{12}$ drugs	Used to treat pernicious anemia. They are given by intramuscular injection or by nasal spray.	cyanocobalamin (Nascobal)	

A CLOSER LOOK

Some **antiretroviral** drugs used to treat HIV exert their action on reverse transcriptase. Reverse transcriptase in the virus tells the DNA in a human cell to make more viral RNA and more viruses. This is backward (*retro-*) from the normal process in which human DNA tells its own RNA what to produce.

antiretroviral (AN-tee-REH-troh-VY-ral)
(AN-tih-REH-troh-VY-ral)
　anti- *against*
　retro- *backward; behind*
　vir/o- *virus*
　-al *pertaining to*

Abbreviations

A	blood type A in the ABO blood group		**IgD**	immunoglobulin D
AB	blood type AB in the ABO blood group		**IgE**	immunoglobulin E
ACT	activated clotting time		**IgG**	immunoglobulin G
AIDS	acquired immunodeficiency syndrome		**IgM**	immunoglobulin M
ALL	acute lymphocytic leukemia		**INR**	international normalized ratio
AML	acute myelogenous leukemia		**lymphs**	lymphocytes (short form)
aPTT	activated partial thromboplastin time		**MCH**	mean cell hemoglobin
B	blood type B in the ABO blood group		**MCHC**	mean cell hemoglobin concentration
basos	basophils (short form)		**MCV**	mean cell volume
BMT	bone marrow transplantation		**mm3**	cubic millimeter
CBC	complete blood count		**mono**	mononucleosis (short form)
CD4	helper T cell		**monos**	monocytes (short form)
CD8	suppressor T cell		**O**	blood type O in the ABO blood group
CLL	chronic lymphocytic leukemia		**PMN**	polymorphonuclear (leukocyte)
CML	chronic myelogenous leukemia		**polys**	polymorphonuclear leukocytes (short form)
cmm	cubic millimeter		**PRBCs**	packed red blood cells
DIC	disseminated intravascular coagulation		**pro time**	prothrombin time (short form)
DVT	deep venous thrombosis		**PT**	prothrombin time
EBV	Epstein-Barr virus		**PTT**	partial thromboplastin time
ELISA	enzyme-linked immunosorbent assay		**RBC**	red blood cell
eos	eosinophils (short form)		**segs**	segmented neutrophils (short form)
GVHD	graft-versus-host disease		**SPEP**	serum protein electrophoresis (pronounced "S-pep")
H&H	hemoglobin and hematocrit			
HCT	hematocrit		**TIBC**	total iron-binding capacity
HGB, Hgb	hemoglobin		**TNF**	tumor necrosis factor
HIV	human immunodeficiency virus		**TPA**	tissue plasminogen activator (drug)
HLA	human leukocyte antigen		**UPEP**	urine protein electrophoresis (pronounced "U-pep")
IgA	immunoglobulin A		**WBC**	white blood cell

WORD ALERT

Abbreviations

Abbreviations are commonly used in all types of medical documents; however, they can mean different things to different people and their meanings can be misinterpreted. Always verify the meaning of an abbreviation.

Monos is a short form that means *monocytes,* but the short form *mono* means *mononucleosis.*

PT means *prothrombin time,* but it also means *physical therapist* or *physical therapy.*

IT'S GREEK TO ME!

Did you notice that some words have two different combining forms? Combining forms from both Greek and Latin remain a part of medical language today.

Word	Greek	Latin	Medical Word Examples
cell	cyt/o-	cellul/o-	pancytopenia, cellular
nucleus	kary/o-	nucle/o-	megakaryocyte, polymorphonuclear
red	erythr/o-	rub/o-	erythrocyte, bilirubin
vein	phleb/o-	ven/o-	phlebotomy, venous

CAREER FOCUS

Meet Adriana, a phlebotomist in a hospital

"A phlebotomist's job description is to draw blood, the collection of blood. On a daily basis, I draw blood from about 30 to 50 patients. Every time it's someone different, so every time it's a different challenge. That's why I love it."

Phlebotomists are allied health professionals who use venipuncture techniques to draw blood. They follow procedures for storing and transporting blood specimens for diagnostic testing in the laboratory.

Hematologists are physicians who practice in the medical specialty of hematology. They diagnose and treat patients with diseases of the blood. Malignancies of the blood and lymphatic system are treated medically by an oncologist or surgically by a general surgeon.

Immunologists are physicians or they are scientists who have a Ph.D. in cellular biology or pharmacology. They practice in the medical specialty of immunology. Clinical immunologists diagnose and treat patients who have autoimmune diseases, immunodeficiency diseases, cancer, or who are undergoing transplantation (organ, bone marrow, or stem cell).

Oncologists are physicians who treat patients with cancer of the blood or immune system.

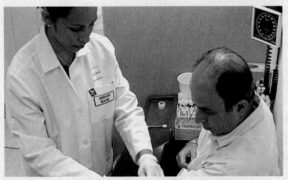

Source: Dan Frank for Pearson Education/PH College

phlebotomist (fleh-BAW-toh-mist)
  phleb/o- *vein*
  tom/o- *cut; layer; slice*
  -ist *person who specializes in; thing that specializes in*

hematologist (HEE-mah-TAW-loh-jist)
  hemat/o- *blood*
  log/o- *study of; word*
  -ist *person who specializes in; thing that specializes in*

immunologist (IH-myoo-NAW-loh-jist)
  immun/o- *immune response*
  log/o- *study of; word*
  -ist *person who specializes in; thing that specializes in*

MyMedicalTerminologyLab™   To see Adriana's complete video profile, log into MyMedicalTerminologyLab and navigate to the Multimedia Library for Chapter 6. Check the Video box, and then click the Career Focus - Phlebotomist] link.

6.6B Build Medical Words

COMBINING FORM AND SUFFIX EXERCISE

Read the definition of the medical word. Select the correct suffix from the Suffix List. Select the correct combining form from the Combining Form List. Build the medical word and write it on the line. Be sure to check your spelling. The first one has been done for you.

SUFFIX LIST	COMBINING FORM LIST
-ated (composed of; pertaining to a condition)	agglutin/o- (clumping; sticking)
-ation (being; having; process)	attenu/o- (weakened)
-cyte (cell)	aut/o- (self)
-ectomy (surgical removal)	coagul/o- (clotting)
-edema (swelling)	embol/o- (embolus; occluding plug)
-emia (condition of the blood)	lymph/o- (lymph; lymphatic system)
-immune (immune response)	micr/o- (one millionth; small)
-ism (disease from a specific cause; process)	morph/o- (shape)
-logy (study of)	myel/o- (bone marrow; myelin; spinal cord)
-megaly (enlargement)	phleb/o- (vein)
-oma (mass; tumor)	septic/o- (infection)
-osis (condition; process)	splen/o- (spleen)
-pathy (disease)	thromb/o- (blood clot)
-rrhage (excessive discharge; excessive flow)	thym/o- (rage; thymus)
-tomy (process of cutting; process of making an incision)	vaccin/o- (vaccine)

Definition of the Medical Word

Build the Medical Word

1. (Red blood) cell (that is abnormally) small — *microcyte*
2. Excessive flow (of) blood
3. Condition of the blood (of too many) white (blood cells)
4. Disease (of blood) clotting
5. Disease from a specific cause (of an) embolus (occluding plug)
6. Tumor (of a) lymph (node)
7. Condition of the blood (having) infection
8. Study of (the) shape (of red blood cells)
9. Condition (of having a) blood clot
10. Tumor (of the) bone marrow
11. Process of cutting (into a) vein (to draw blood)
12. Process (of giving a) vaccine
13. Surgical removal (of the) spleen
14. Swelling (because the) lymph (is not draining well)
15. Immune response (directed at one's own) self (and body)
16. Process (of platelets) clumping or sticking (together)
17. Enlargement (of the) spleen
18. Tumor (of the) thymus
19. Composed of weakened (bacteria in a vaccine)

PREFIX EXERCISE

Read the definition of the medical word. Look at the medical word or partial word that is given (it already contains a combining form and a suffix). Select the correct prefix from the Prefix List and write it on the blank line. Then build the medical word and write it on the line. Be sure to check your spelling. The first one has been done for you.

PREFIX LIST

a- (away from; without)	hyper- (above; more than normal)	intra- (within)	trans- (across; through)
anti- (against)	hypo- (below; deficient)	pan- (all)	

Definition of the Medical Word	Prefix	Word or Partial Word	Build the Medical Word
1. Pertaining to without formation or growth (of blood cells)	a-	plastic	aplastic
2. Pertaining to (red blood cells with) deficient color	_____	chromic	_____
3. Condition of deficiency (of) all (blood) cell(s)	_____	cytopenia	_____
4. Action (of) through (a vein) pouring (in a unit of blood)	_____	fusion	_____
5. Pertaining to (a drug that acts) against (blood) clotting	_____	coagulant	_____
6. Condition of the blood (of) more than normal calcium	_____	calcemia	_____
7. Pertaining to within (the) blood vessel	_____	vascular	_____

MULTIPLE COMBINING FORMS AND SUFFIX EXERCISE

Read the definition of the medical word. Select the correct suffix and combining forms. Then build the medical word and write it on the line. Be sure to check your spelling. The first one has been done for you.

SUFFIX LIST	COMBINING FORM LIST	
-ency (condition of being; condition of having)	aden/o- (gland)	lymph/o- (lymph; lymphatic system)
-esis (condition; process)	angi/o- (blood vessel; lymphatic vessel)	lyt/o- (break down; destroy)
-graphy (process of recording)	anis/o- (unequal)	mon/o- (one; single)
-ia (condition; state; thing)	cyt/o- (cell)	norm/o- (normal; usual)
-ic (pertaining to)	defici/o- (inadequate; lacking)	nucle/o- (nucleus of a cell)
-ist (person who specializes in)	electr/o- (electricity)	phil/o- (attraction to; fondness for)
-osis (condition; process)	hemat/o- (blood)	phor/o- (bear; carry; range)
-pathy (disease)	hem/o- (blood)	poikil/o- (irregular)
-penia (condition of deficiency)	immun/o- (immune response)	punct/o- (hole; perforation)
-ure (result of; system)	log/o- (study of; word)	thromb/o- (blood clot)
		ven/i- (vein)

Definition of the Medical Word

1. Condition (of) irregular (shapes of red blood) cell(s)
2. Condition (in which the) blood (has a) fondness for (bleeding)
3. Disease (of the lymph) gland
4. Condition (that affects monocytes that have) one (unlobed) nucleus
5. Pertaining to (a) normal (size of red blood) cell
6. Condition of deficiency (in the number of) blood clot (making) cell(s)
7. Condition of having (an) immune response (that is) inadequate or lacking
8. Process (that uses) electricity (to) carry (immunoglobulins in a gel)
9. Pertaining to (a drug that acts on a) blood clot (to) break down and destroy (it)

Build the Medical Word

poikilocytosis

_____

_____

_____

_____

_____

_____

_____

_____

Definition of the Medical Word

Build the Medical Word

10. Process of recording lymph (and a) lymphatic vessel (by using contrast dye)

_____

11. Condition (of) unequal (sizes of red blood) cell(s)

_____

12. System (for creating in a) vein (a) hole (to withdraw blood)

_____

13. Person who specializes in blood (and the) study of (it)

_____

6.7A Spell Medical Words

HEARING MEDICAL WORDS EXERCISE

You hear someone speaking the medical words given below. Read each pronunciation and then write the medical word it represents. Be sure to check your spelling. The first one has been done for you.

1. ah-NEE-mee-ah   anemia _____

2. AW-toh-ih-MYOON   _____

3. EM-boh-LIZ-em   _____

4. HEE-mah-TAW-loh-jist   _____

5. HEM-oh-rij   _____

6. IH-myoo-noh-GLAW-byoo-lin   _____

7. loo-KEE-mee-ah   _____

8. lim-FAN-jee-oh-GRAM   _____

9. MAW-noh-NOO-klee-OH-sis   _____

10. fleh-BAW-toh-mee   _____

6.7B Pronounce Medical Words

PRONUNCIATION EXERCISE

Read the medical word and the syllables in its pronunciation. Circle the primary (main) accented syllable. The first one has been done for you.

1. leukocyte (⟨loo⟩-koh-site)

2. erythrocyte (eh-rith-roh-site)

3. eosinophil (ee-oh-sin-oh-fil)

4. lymphatic (lim-fat-ik)

5. coagulation (koh-ag-yoo-lay-shun)

6. pathogen (path-oh-jen)

7. septicemia (sep-tih-see-mee-ah)

8. hemophilia (hee-moh-fil-ee-ah)

9. phlebotomy (fleh-baw-toh-mee)

10. splenectomy (spleh-nek-toh-mee)

6.8 Research Medical Words

SOUND-ALIKE WORDS

Compare and contrast the medical meanings of these sound-alike hematology and immunology words.

1. _albumen_ and _albumin_

2. _lymph_ and _lymphs_

3. _mono_ and _monos_

6.9 Analyze Medical Reports

ELECTRONIC PATIENT RECORD #1

This is a laboratory report. Read the report and answer the questions.

PEARSON OUTPATIENT LABORATORY REPORT

Task   Edit   View   Time Scale   Options   Help

ACCESSION NUMBER:	309-019	PATIENT NAME:	THOMAS, Irene
DATE DRAWN:	11/19/xx	PATIENT ID NUMBER:	365-14-3972
DATE RECEIVED:	11/19/xx	DATE OF BIRTH:	07/29/xx
TIME RECEIVED:	0900	SEX:	Female

Source: Jeffrey Banke/Fotolia

Test	Result	Normal Range	Technician
Complete Blood Count (CBC)			
RBC	4.7 m/mL	4.2–5.7 m/mL	JRT
Hemoglobin	14.7 g/dL	12.6–16.6 g/dL	JRT
Hematocrit	42.9%	38.0–50.0%	JRT
MCV	91.2 fL	80–100 fL	JRT
MCH	31.3 pg	28.0–33.0 pg	JRT
MCHC	34.3 g/dL	32–36 g/dL	JRT
WBC	7.7 k/mL	4.3–10.5 k/mL	JRT
Platelets	130 k/mL	150–450 k/mL	JRT

1. What is the name of the group of tests done on this patient? _____

2. What unit of measurement is used to report erythrocytes? _____

3. Write out this unit of measurement in words. _____

4. What individual test result was not within the normal range of values? _____

5. What does the *k* stand for in the unit of measurement k/mL? _____

ELECTRONIC PATIENT RECORD #2

Read this Emergency Department Report and answer the questions.

PEARSON GENERAL HOSPITAL

Task   Edit   View   Time Scale   Options   Help   ✉ ⌖ ◑

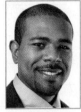

EMERGENCY DEPARTMENT REPORT	
PATIENT NAME:	JONES, Jerome
HOSPITAL NUMBER:	635-64-46223
DATE OF REPORT:	November 19, 20xx

Source: Konstantin Sutyagin/123 RF

HISTORY OF PRESENT ILLNESS
This 42-year-old black male presented to the emergency room today with complaints of dysphagia, extreme weakness, fevers, diarrhea, and weight loss.

PAST MEDICAL HISTORY
He has a prior history of intravenous heroin use for many years and was diagnosed with HIV about 6 years ago. At that time, he tested HIV positive, but was asymptomatic. His CD4 count then was 500. He was subsequently lost to follow-up until recently. In the last few months, his health has deteriorated rapidly, but he refused to seek medical attention. Last month, however, he was admitted to this hospital through the emergency department in respiratory distress with a CD4 count of 100 and was diagnosed with *Pneumocystis jiroveci* pneumonia and AIDS. He was given a 14-day course of intravenous pentamidine. He was discharged on a triple-drug regimen of Retrovir, Epivir, and Crixivan. He was also given a prescription for aerosolized pentamidine to prevent future episodes of this pneumonia. Today he states that he has been noncompliant with his drug therapy, stating that he does not take his AIDS drugs on a regular basis.

PHYSICAL EXAMINATION
General: Physical examination today showed a black male appearing much older than his stated age. Temperature 101.2, pulse 100, respirations 26, blood pressure 110/76. Height: 5 feet 11 inches. Weight: 128 pounds. HEENT exam: Normocephalic, atraumatic. Eyes: Sclerae and conjunctivae pale and nonicteric. Mouth: White plaque coating on the tongue and underneath is beefy red and bleeds slightly. Neck: The neck is supple. There is cervical lymphadenopathy.

HEART: Regular rate and rhythm.

CHEST: Clear.

ABDOMEN: Soft, nontender, with normal bowel sounds.

EXTREMITIES: Wasting of the extremities. Extreme weakness with muscle strength decreased on both sides. Deep tendon reflexes intact bilaterally. The skin shows no evidence of Kaposi's sarcoma.

DIAGNOSES
1. Oral candidiasis.
2. Wasting syndrome, secondary to acquired immunodeficiency syndrome (AIDS).
3. Acquired immunodeficiency syndrome (AIDS).
4. Past history of *Pneumocystis jiroveci* pneumonia.

PLAN
Bloodwork was sent for CBC and differential and CD4 total count. The patient was restarted on his antiretroviral three-drug regimen of Retrovir 300 mg b.i.d., Epivir 150 mg b.i.d., and Crixivan 800 mg every 8 hours. He was given nystatin oral suspension 5 cc q.i.d., swish and swallow, to treat his oral candidiasis. He will be started on Megace oral suspension, 20 mg/0.5 cc, to stimulate his appetite and help him gain weight.

Joseph K. McAdams, M.D.

Joseph K. McAdams, M.D.

JKM:ltt
D: 11/19/xx
T: 11/19/xx

1. Six years ago, the patient was "asymptomatic," which means that _____

   a. he did not have an HIV infection

   b. he did not have any symptoms of an HIV infection

   c. he was healthy

2. The patient has now and did have last month what two opportunistic infections?

   _____

3. What was the patient's CD4 count 6 years ago? _____

   What was the patient's CD4 count when he was diagnosed with AIDS? _____

   Which CD4 count is more desirable to have? _____

4. What three drugs (triple-drug regimen) were prescribed for the patient's AIDS?

   _____

5. What laboratory test was ordered to show the current number of helper T lymphocytes? _____

6. What does the physical examination show about the patient's lymph nodes in his neck? _____

7. What is the probable source of the patient's HIV infection? _____

8. Which of these symptoms would be related to the patient's oral candidiasis?

   a. extreme weakness

   b. fevers

   c. dysphagia

   d. diarrhea

9. When the patient was admitted to the hospital last month with *Pneumocystis jiroveci* pneumonia, why was his diagnosis changed from HIV positive to AIDS? _____

10. The patient is diagnosed with wasting syndrome due to AIDS. What three pieces of information support this diagnosis?

    a. Hint: Look for a phrase at the beginning of the History of Present Illness.

    _____

    b. Hint: Look for a measurement in the "General" section of the Physical Examination.

    _____

    c. Hint: Look for a phrase in the "Extremities" section of the Physical Examination.

    _____

MyMedicalTerminologyLab™

MyMedicalTerminologyLab is a premium online homework management system that includes a host of features to help you study. Registered users will find:

- A multitude of quizzes and activities built within the MyLab platform

- Powerful tools that track and analyze your results—allowing you to create a personalized learning experience

- Videos and audio pronunciations to help enrich your progress

- Streaming lesson presentations (Guided Lectures) and self-paced learning modules

- A space where you and your instructor can check your progress and manage your assignments

Chapter 7
Dermatology

Integumentary System

Dermatology (DER-mah-TAW-loh-jee) is the medical specialty that studies the anatomy and physiology of the integumentary system and uses laboratory and diagnostic procedures, medical and surgical procedures, and drugs to treat integumentary diseases.

Learning Outcomes

After you study this chapter, you should be able to

7.1 Identify structures of the integumentary system.

7.2 Describe the process of an allergic reaction.

7.3 Describe common integumentary diseases, laboratory and diagnostic procedures, medical and surgical procedures, and drugs.

7.4 Form the plural and adjective forms of nouns related to dermatology.

7.5 Give the meanings of word parts and abbreviations related to dermatology.

7.6 Divide dermatology words and build dermatology words.

7.7 Spell and pronounce dermatology words.

7.8 Research sound-alike and other dermatology words.

7.9 Analyze the medical content and meaning of a dermatology report.

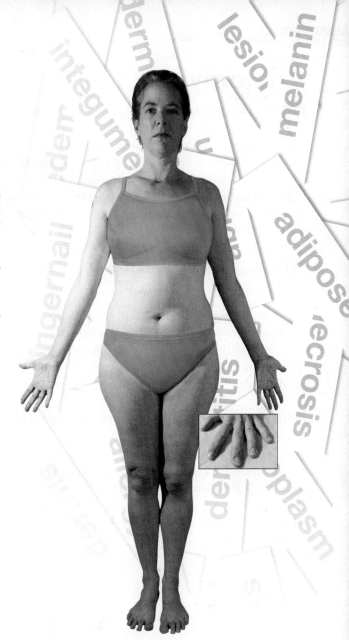

FIGURE 7-1 ■ Integumentary system.
The integumentary system covers the entire surface of the body and consists of the skin, hair, and nails. The skin is the largest organ in the body.
Source: Pearson Education

Medical Language Key

To unlock the definition of a medical word, break it into word parts. Give the meaning of each word part. Put the meanings of the word parts in order, beginning with the meaning of the suffix, then the prefix (if present), then the combining form(s).

	Word Part	Word Part Meaning
Suffix	**-logy**	*study of*
Combining Form	**dermat/o-**	*skin*

Dermatology: ▶ *Study of (the) skin (and related structures).*

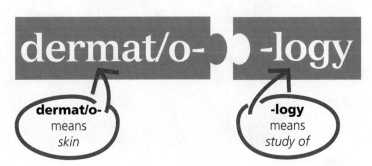

dermat/o- means skin

-logy means study of

Anatomy and Physiology

The **integumentary system** (see Figure 7-1 ■) is an extremely large, flat, flexible body system that covers the entire surface of the body. The integumentary system includes the skin (epidermis and dermis), sebaceous glands, sweat glands, hair, and nails. In addition, this chapter discusses the subcutaneous tissue, a layer of connective tissue that is beneath the skin. The purpose of the integumentary system is to protect the body; it is the body's first line of defense against invading microorganisms. The sense of touch is also part of the integumentary system.

Anatomy of the Integumentary System

Skin

The skin or **integument** consists of two different layers: the epidermis and the dermis. The epidermis is categorized as **epithelium** or **epithelial tissue**. The epithelium covers the external surface of the body, but also includes the mucous membranes that line the walls of internal cavities that connect to the outside of the body. The dermis is categorized as connective tissue.

EPIDERMIS   The **epidermis** is the thin, outermost layer of the skin (see Figure 7-2 ■). The most superficial part of the epidermis contains dead cells that have no nuclei and are filled with **keratin**, a hard, fibrous protein. These cells form a protective layer, but they are dead cells, and so they are constantly being shed or sloughed off. This process is known as **exfoliation**. In contrast, the deepest part or **basal layer** of the epidermis is composed of living cells that are constantly dividing and moving to the surface. The epidermis does not contain any blood vessels. It receives nutrients and oxygen from the blood vessels in the dermis.

Pronunciation/Word Parts

integumentary (in-TEH-gyoo-MEN-tair-ee)
  integument/o- *skin*
  -ary *pertaining to*

cutaneous (kyoo-TAY-nee-us)
  cutane/o- *skin*
  -ous *pertaining to*
Cutaneous is another adjective for *skin.*
The combining forms **cut/i-**, **derm/a-**,
dermat/o-, and **derm/o-** also mean *skin.*

integument (in-TEH-gyoo-ment)
  integu/o- *cover*
  -ment *action; state*

epithelium (EP-ih-THEE-lee-um)
  epi- *above; upon*
  theli/o- *cellular layer*
  -um *period of time; structure*

epithelial (EP-ih-THEE-lee-al)
  epi- *above; upon*
  theli/o- *cellular layer*
  -al *pertaining to*

epidermis (EP-ih-DER-mis)

epidermal (EP-ih-DER-mal)
  epi- *above; upon*
  derm/o- *skin*
  -al *pertaining to*

keratin (KAIR-ah-tin)
  kerat/o- *cornea of the eye; hard, fibrous
    protein*
  -in *substance*

exfoliation (eks-FOH-lee-AA-shun)
  ex- *away from; out*
  foli/o- *leaf*
  -ation *being; having; process*
Add words to make a complete definition
of *exfoliation*: *process (of skin cells moving)
away from (the body like a) leaf (falling off
a tree).*

basal (BAY-sal)
  bas/o- *alkaline; base of a structure*
  -al *pertaining to*

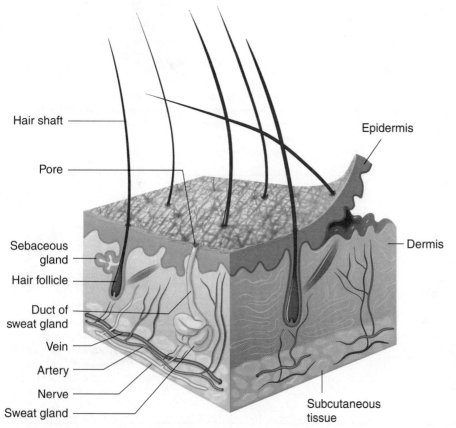

Hair shaft

Pore

Sebaceous gland

Hair follicle

Duct of sweat gland

Vein

Artery

Nerve

Sweat gland

Epidermis

Dermis

Subcutaneous tissue

FIGURE 7-2 ■ Epidermis and dermis.
The skin is composed of the epidermis and the dermis. The epidermis contains dead protective cells on its surface and living, actively dividing cells at its base. The dermis contains hair follicles, sebaceous glands, and sweat glands. The subcutaneous tissue, a type of connective tissue, lies beneath the dermis.
Source: Pearson Education

The epidermis also contains **melanocytes**, pigment cells that produce **melanin**, a dark brown or black pigment. Melanin in the epidermis absorbs ultraviolet light from the sun to protect the DNA in skin cells from undergoing genetic mutations.

DID YOU KNOW?

All races of people have the same number of melanocytes in the skin. Differences in skin color occur because of differing levels of melanin production. Dark-skinned people produce more melanin than fair-skinned people. Albinos have a normal number of melanocytes in their skin, but the cells do not produce any melanin. Exposure to the sun's ultraviolet rays increases the rate of melanin production in all people and causes a suntan. During prolonged sun exposure, the melanin is unable to absorb all of the ultraviolet light, and the result is a sunburn.

CLINICAL CONNECTIONS

Dietetics. The sun's ultraviolet rays convert cholesterol in the epidermis to a compound that is then made into vitamin D. The amount of vitamin D produced depends on the time of day and the season of the year. About 20–45 minutes of sunlight per week produces sufficient amounts of vitamin D. Vitamin D is stored in fat cells in the subcutaneous tissue. It helps the body absorb and use the calcium and phosphorus from foods. Vitamin D also protects the entire body against many types of cancer.

DERMIS The **dermis** is a thicker layer beneath the epidermis (see Figure 7-2). It is both firm and elastic because it contains **collagen** fibers (firm, white protein) and **elastin** fibers (elastic, yellow protein). The dermis contains arteries, veins, and nerves, as well as hair follicles, sebaceous glands, and sweat glands.

A **dermatome** is a specific area on the skin that sends sensory information through a nerve to the spinal cord (see Figure 7-3 ■).

Pronunciation/Word Parts

melanocyte (meh-LAN-oh-SITE) (MEL-ah-noh-SITE)
  melan/o- *black*
  -cyte *cell*
Add words to make a complete definition of *melanocyte*: cell (in the skin that produces a dark brown or) black (pigment).

melanin (MEL-ah-nin)
  melan/o- *black*
  -in *substance*

dermis (DER-mis)

dermal (DER-mal)
  derm/o- *skin*
  -al *pertaining to*

collagen (KAW-lah-jen)
  coll/a- *fibers that hold together*
  -gen *that which produces*

elastin (ee-LAS-tin)
  elast/o- *flexing; stretching*
  -in *substance*

dermatome (DER-mah-tohm)
  derm/a- *skin*
  -tome *area with distinct edges; instrument used to cut*

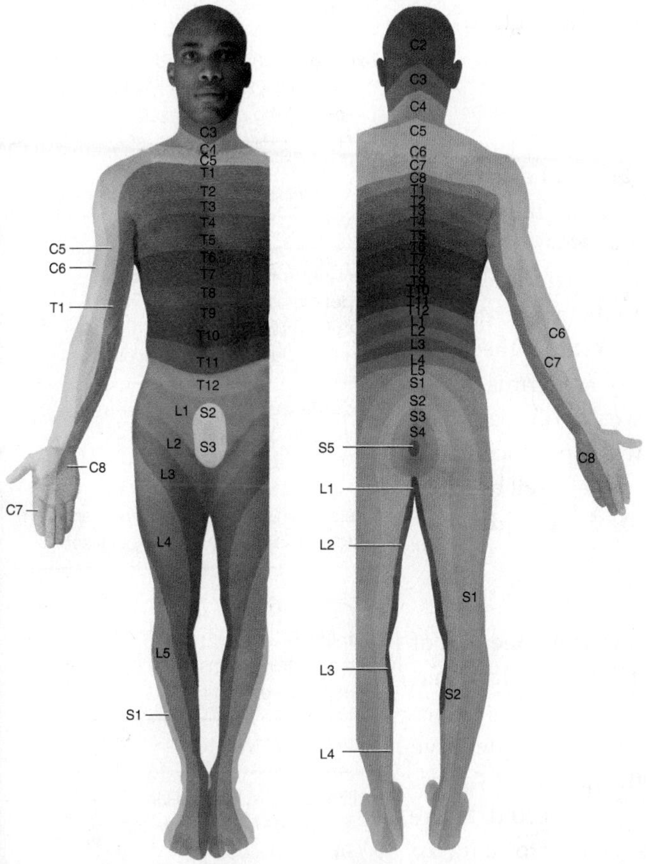

FIGURE 7-3 ■ **Dermatomes of the body.**
One of the functions of the skin is the sense of touch. A dermatome is a specific area of the skin that sends sensory information from the skin to a spinal nerve and the spinal cord. Each dermatome is named according to the level at which the spinal nerve enters the spinal cord. C stands for the spinal cord at the level of the neck (the combining form *cervic/o-* means *neck*). T stands for the spinal cord at the level of the thorax. L stands for the spinal cord at the level of the lumbar area (lower back). S stands for the spinal cord at the level of the sacrum (last bone in the spine). The skin of the face sends sensory information through the cranial nerves to the brain.
Source: Pearson Education

CLINICAL CONNECTIONS

Neurology. Nerves in the dermis are stimulated by light touch, pressure, vibration, pain, and temperature. When you touch something hot, the sensation is carried as sensory information by the nerve from the skin to the spinal cord. The spinal cord immediately sends a motor command to a muscle for you to move your hand away from the heat. This takes place without any conscious input from the brain. It is only after your hand has already moved that your brain finally receives that sensory information and thinks "That was hot!"

A CLOSER LOOK

The skin is the body's first line of defense against disease and injury. The dead cells of the outer epidermis present a dry and slightly acidic environment that discourages the growth of microorganisms. The constant shedding of epidermal cells prevents microorganisms from multiplying and invading the dermis. Sweat and sebum (oil) contain antibodies and enzymes that kill bacteria. **Normal skin flora** (bacteria that are able to thrive under these conditions) do not cause disease, and they inhibit the growth of disease-causing microorganisms by competing with them for space and nutrients.

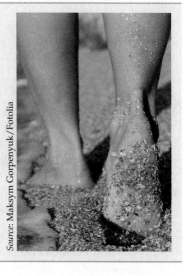

Source: Maksym Gorpenyuk/Fotolia

Sebaceous Glands

The **sebaceous glands** in the dermis are a type of **exocrine gland**. They secrete **sebum** through a duct that goes into a hair follicle (see Figure 7-2). Sebum consists of oil that coats and protects the hair shaft to keep it from becoming brittle. Sebaceous glands are also known as **oil glands**.

sebaceous (seh-BAY-shus)
  sebace/o- *oil; sebum*
  -ous *pertaining to*

exocrine (EKS-oh-krin) (EKS-oh-krine)
  ex/o- *away from; external; outward*
  -crine *thing that secretes*

sebum (SEE-bum)
The combining form **seb/o-** means *oil; sebum.*

Sweat Glands

The **sweat glands** in the dermis are also exocrine glands. The sweat gland duct opens onto the surface of the skin through a pore (see Figure 7-2). Sweat contains water, sodium, and small amounts of body wastes (ammonia, creatinine, urea). It is sodium that gives sweat its salty taste. Sweating helps to regulate the body temperature. When the body is hot, temperature receptors in the skin send impulses to the hypothalamus in the brain, which then signals the sweat glands to secrete sweat. Water in the sweat evaporates from the skin and cools the body. Also, blood vessels in the dermis dilate, and heat from the blood is radiated out from the body. Although sweat is odorless, bacteria on the surface of the skin digest sebum and sweat, and their waste products cause the odor associated with sweat. The process of sweating and the sweat itself are both known as **perspiration**. The sweat glands are also known as the **sudoriferous glands**.

perspiration (PER-spih-RAY-shun)
  per- *through; throughout*
  spir/o- *breathe; coil*
  -ation *being; having; process*

sudoriferous (soo-doh-RIF-er-us)
  sudor/i- *sweat*
  fer/o- *bear*
  -ous *pertaining to*
The combining forms **diaphor/o-** and **hidr/o-** also mean *sweating* or *sweat.*

Hair

Hair covers most of the body, although its consistency and color vary from one part of the body to another and from one person to the next. Additional facial, axillary, and pubic hairs appear during puberty.

Each hair forms in a hair **follicle** in the dermis (see Figure 7-2). Melanocytes give color to the hair. Hair cells are filled with keratin, which makes the hair shaft strong. Usually, the hair lies flat on the surface of the skin, but when the skin is cold, a tiny erector muscle at the base of the hair follicle contracts and causes the hair to stand up

hair (HAIR)
The combining forms **pil/o-** and **trich/o-** both mean *hair.*

follicle (FAW-lih-kl)

follicular (foh-LIH-kyoo-lar)
  follicul/o- *follicle; small sac*
  -ar *pertaining to*

(**piloerection**). The contracted muscle forms a goosebump. In furry animals, the erect hairs create an insulating layer and trap heat near the skin, but this effect is insignificant in humans.

> **DID YOU KNOW?**
> The scalp contains about 100,000 hairs. Dark hair contains melanin, but blond hair and red hair contain a variant of melanin that contains more sulfur, so the hair is more yellow or orange. As a person ages, melanocytes stop producing melanin, and the hair appears gray or white. Hair grows fastest during the daytime and during the summer.

Nails

The nails cover and protect the distal ends of the fingers and toes because these areas are easily traumatized. Each nail consists of several parts (see Figure 7-4 ■). The outer layer—the hard, opaque **nail plate**—is composed of dead cells that contain keratin. The nail plate rests on the **nail bed**, a layer of living tissue that contains nerves and blood vessels. Blood vessels in the nail bed give the nail plate its color—normally pink (but bluish-purple if the oxygen level in the blood is low). The nail bed is also known as the *quick*. The **cuticle** is an edge of dead cells, arising from the epidermis along the proximal end of the nail. The cuticle is adherent to the nail plate to prevent microorganisms from entering the nail root. The **lunula**, the whitish half-moon, is the visible, white part of the nail root. The **nail root**, which is located beneath the skin of the finger, produces keratin-containing cells that form the nail plate. These cells are white at first (in the lunula), but gradually become opaque as the nail plate grows. Trauma to or infection of the nail root causes a misshapen nail plate.

Subcutaneous Tissue

The **subcutaneous tissue** is a loose, connective tissue (see Figure 7-2). It is not considered to be part of the integumentary system, but because it is directly beneath the dermis of the skin, it is discussed here. It is composed of **adipose tissue** or fat that contains **lipocytes**. These cells store fat as an energy reserve. The amount of fat in adipose tissue usually far exceeds any energy needs the body might have! The subcutaneous tissue also provides a layer of insulation to conserve internal body heat. Depending on a

Pronunciation/Word Parts

piloerection (PY-loh-ee-REK-shun)
  pil/o- *hair*
  erect/o- *stand up*
  -ion *action; condition*

ungual (UNG-gwal)
  ungu/o- *fingernail; toenail*
  -al *pertaining to*
Ungual is the adjective form for *nail*.
The combining form **onych/o-** also means *fingernail; toenail*.

cuticle (KYOO-tih-kl)
  cut/i- *skin*
  -cle *small thing*

lunula (LOO-nyoo-lah)
  lun/o- *moon*
  -ula *small thing*

subcutaneous (SUB-kyoo-TAY-nee-us)
  sub- *below; underneath*
  cutane/o- *skin*
  -ous *pertaining to*

adipose (AD-ih-pohs)
  adip/o- *fat*
  -ose *full of*

lipocyte (LIP-oh-site)
  lip/o- *fat; lipid*
  -cyte *cell*

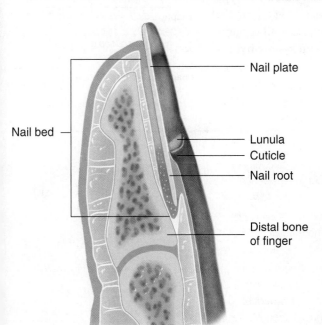

Nail plate

Nail bed

Lunula
Cuticle
Nail root

Distal bone of finger

FIGURE 7-4 ■ Nail.
The nail is composed of both living and dead cells. The nail root produces keratin-containing cells that form the lunula. As the nail plate grows, these cells die and harden to form a protective covering for the distal end of the finger.
Source: Pearson Education

person's metabolism, dietary intake of sugars and fats, and the amount of fat stored in the lipocytes, the subcutaneous tissue can be thin or as thick as several inches. The subcutaneous layer also acts as a cushion to protect the bones and internal organs.

CLINICAL CONNECTIONS

Forensic Science. Oil from the sebaceous glands leaves a fingerprint when a person touches something. Each person's fingerprints are a unique combination of whorls, loops, or arches that can be matched to fingerprints on file in a database. Cells from a hair follicle can be analyzed for DNA. Hair can be tested for evidence of toxins or poisons. White horizontal bands on the fingernails indicate arsenic poisoning. Criminal investigators know that, if a body was buried in moist dirt, adipose tissue decomposes and forms a characteristic waxy substance known as **adipocere** (grave wax).

adipocere (AD-ih-poh-SEER)
  adip/o- *fat*
  -cere *waxy substance*

Physiology of an Allergic Reaction

An **allergy** or **allergic reaction** is an individually unique **hypersensitivity** response to certain types of antigens known as *allergens*. **Allergens** include cells from plant and animal sources (foods, pollens, molds, animal dander), as well as dust, chemicals, and drugs. The basis of all allergic reactions is the release of **histamine** from basophils in the blood and from **mast cells** in the connective tissue. Allergic reactions anywhere in the body almost always involve the skin or mucous membranes.

A **local reaction** occurs when an allergen touches the skin or mucous membranes of a hypersensitive individual. Histamine released in that area causes inflammation and redness (erythema), swelling (edema), irritation, and itching (pruritus). Examples: Chemicals in deodorant applied to the skin or pollen in the air that touches the mucous membranes in the nose.

A **systemic reaction** occurs when allergens are inhaled by, ingested by, or injected into a hypersensitive person, causing symptoms in several body systems. Histamine constricts the bronchioles, dilates the blood vessels throughout the body, and causes hives on the skin. Examples: Inhaled pollens, molds, or dust trigger asthma attacks; ingested foods or drugs cause hives on the skin. **Anaphylaxis** is a severe systemic allergic reaction that can be life threatening. Symptoms include respiratory distress, hypotension, and shock. Examples: Eating peanuts, being stung by a bee, taking a drug that has caused a past allergic reaction, or being exposed to latex gloves are all common causes of anaphylaxis in hypersensitive individuals. This is also known as **anaphylactic shock.**

allergy (AL-er-jee)
  all/o- *other; strange*
  -ergy *activity; process of working*

allergic (ah-LER-jik)
  all/o- *other; strange*
  erg/o- *activity; work*
  -ic *pertaining to*

hypersensitivity (HY-per-SEN-sih-TIV-ih-tee)
  hyper- *above; more than normal*
  sensitiv/o- *affected by; sensitive to*
  -ity *condition; state*

allergen (AL-er-jen)
  all/o- *other; strange*
  erg/o- *activity; work*
  -gen *that which produces*
Note: The duplicated letter "g" is deleted before forming the word.

histamine (HIS-tah-meen)

local (LOH-kal)
  loc/o- *one place*
  -al *pertaining to*

systemic (sis-TEM-ik)
  system/o- *body as a whole*
  -ic *pertaining to*

anaphylaxis (AN-ah-fih-LAK-sis)
  ana- *apart; excessive*
  -phylaxis *condition of guarding; condition of protecting*

anaphylactic (AN-ah-fih-LAK-tik)
  ana- *apart; excessive*
  phylact/o- *guarding; protecting*
  -ic *pertaining to*

ACROSS THE LIFE SPAN

Pediatrics. The skin of an infant is smooth and very flexible. It has no wrinkles because of the large amount of elastin in the dermis and the thick layer of fat in the subcutaneous tissue. This fat layer conserves body heat and protects the internal organs as the infant learns to walk.

In persons who smoke, the nicotine in cigarettes decreases oxygen levels in the skin and destroys the collagen fibers. This causes deep wrinkles and gives a leathery quality to the skin, even in middle age.

Geriatrics. In older adults, the amount of elastin decreases, and the skin develops sags and wrinkles. The fat in the subcutaneous layer thins, the skin appears translucent, and arteries and veins—especially in the hands—become obvious. There is a simultaneous underproduction and overproduction of melanin that gives the skin a mottled, irregular appearance.

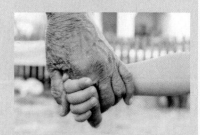

Source: Family Business/Fotolia LLC

Vocabulary Review

Anatomy and Physiology		
Word or Phrase	**Description**	**Combining Forms**
integumentary system	Body system that covers the entire surface of the body and consists of the skin, hair, and nails	**integument/o-** *skin*
subcutaneous tissue	Loose, connective tissue beneath the dermis. It is composed of **adipose tissue** that contains **lipocytes** that store fat. When a dead body is buried in moist dirt, adipose tissue becomes **adipocere**. The subcutaneous tissue is near to, but not part of, the integumentary system.	**cutane/o-** *skin* **adip/o-** *fat* **lip/o-** *fat; lipid*

Skin, Hair, and Nails		
collagen	Firm, white protein fibers throughout the dermis	**coll/a-** *fibers that hold together*
cutaneous	Pertaining to the skin	**cutane/o-** *skin*
cuticle	Edge of dead cells arising from the epidermis along the proximal end of the nail. It keeps microorganisms from entering the nail root.	**cut/i-** *skin*
dermatome	Area of the skin that sends sensory information through a nerve to the spinal cord	**derm/a-** *skin*
dermis	Layer of skin beneath the epidermis. It contains collagen and elastin fibers. It contains arteries, veins, nerves, hair follicles, sebaceous glands, and sweat glands.	**derm/o-** *skin*
elastin	Elastic, yellow protein fibers in the dermis	**elast/o-** *flexing; stretching*
epidermis	Thin, outermost layer of skin. The most superficial part of the epidermis consists of dead cells filled with keratin. The deepest part or **basal layer** contains constantly dividing cells and melanocytes.	**derm/o-** *skin* **bas/o-** *alkaline; base of a structure*
epithelium	Tissue category that includes the epidermis and all of its structures. It also includes the mucous membranes that line the walls of internal cavities that connect to the outside of the body. It is also known as **epithelial tissue**.	**theli/o-** *cellular layer*
exfoliation	Normal process of the constant shedding of dead cells from the most superficial part of the epidermis	**foli/o-** *leaf*
exocrine gland	Type of gland that secretes substances through a duct. Examples: Sebaceous (oil) glands and sudoriferous (sweat) glands in the dermis.	**ex/o-** *away from; external; outward*
follicle	Site where a hair is formed. Hair follicles are located in the dermis.	**follicul/o-** *follicle; small sac*
hair	Structure that grows as a shaft from a follicle in the dermis	**pil/o-** *hair* **trich/o-** *hair*
integument	The skin	**integu/o-** *cover*
keratin	Hard protein found in the cells of the outermost part of the epidermis and in the nails and hair	**kerat/o-** *cornea of the eye; hard, fibrous protein*
lipocyte	Cell in the subcutaneous tissue that stores fat	**lip/o-** *fat; lipid*
lunula	Whitish half-moon under the proximal portion of the nail plate. It is the visible white part of the nail root.	**lun/o-** *moon*

melanocyte	Pigment-containing cell in the epidermis that produces **melanin**, a dark brown or black pigment that gives color to the skin and hair	**melan/o-** *black*
nail bed	Layer of living tissue beneath the nail plate. It is also known as the *quick*.	
nail plate	Hard, opaque protective covering over the distal end of each finger and toe. It is composed of dead cells that contain keratin. It is also known as the *nail*.	**ungu/o-** *fingernail; toenail* **onych/o-** *fingernail; toenail*
nail root	Produces cells that form the lunula and nail plate	
perspiration	Process of sweating and the sweat itself. Sweat is secreted by sudoriferous glands. It contains sodium and body wastes. As its water content evaporates from the skin, it cools the body.	**spir/o-** *breathe; coil*
piloerection	Process in which an erector muscle contracts (to form a goosebump) and the body hair becomes erect when the skin is cold.	**pil/o-** *hair* **erect/o-** *stand up*
sebaceous gland	Exocrine gland in the dermis. It secretes **sebum** through a duct. The duct joins with a hair follicle, and sebum coats the hair shaft. It is also known as an **oil gland**.	**sebace/o-** *oil; sebum* **seb/o-** *oil; sebum*
skin	Tissue covering of the body that consists of two layers (epidermis and dermis). The skin is one part of the integumentary system.	**cutane/o-** *skin* **cut/i-** *skin* **derm/a-** *skin* **dermat/o-** *skin* **derm/o-** *skin* **integument/o-** *skin*
sudoriferous gland	Exocrine gland in the dermis. It secretes sweat through a duct that opens at a pore on the surface of the skin. It is also known as a **sweat gland**.	**sudor/i-** *sweat* **fer/o-** *bear* **hidr/o-** *sweat* **diaphor/o-** *sweating*

Allergic Reaction

allergen	Cells from plants or animals (foods, pollens, molds, animal dander), as well as dust, chemicals, and drugs that cause an allergic reaction in a hypersensitive person	**all/o-** *other; strange*
allergic reaction	Response to an allergen in a hypersensitive person. An allergic reaction is based on the release of **histamine**. It is also known as an **allergy**.	**all/o-** *other; strange* **erg/o-** *activity; work*
anaphylaxis	Severe systemic allergic reaction characterized by respiratory distress, hypotension, and shock. It is also known as **anaphylactic shock**.	**phylact/o-** *guarding; protecting*
basophils	Blood cells that release histamine during an allergic reaction	
hypersensitivity	Individually unique response to an allergen that provokes an allergic response in some people	**sensitiv/o-** *affected by; sensitive to*
local reaction	Allergic reaction that takes place in a hypersensitive person on an area of the skin or mucous membranes that was exposed to an allergen	**loc/o-** *one place*
mast cells	Cells in the connective tissue that release histamine during an allergic reaction	
systemic reaction	Allergic reaction that takes place throughout the body in a hypersensitive person after contact with an allergen that was ingested, inhaled, or injected	**system/o-** *body as a whole*

Build Medical Words

Combining Form and Suffix Exercise

Read the definition of the medical word. Look at the combining form that is given. Select the correct suffix from the Suffix List and write it on the blank line. Then build the medical word and write it on the line. (Remember: You may need to remove the combining vowel. Always remove the hyphens and slash.) Be sure to check your spelling. The first one has been done for you.

SUFFIX LIST

-al (pertaining to)	-in (substance)	-tome (area with distinct edges; instrument used to cut)
-ary (pertaining to)	-ment (action; state)	-ula (small thing)
-cyte (cell)	-ose (full of)	
-gen (that which produces)	-ous (pertaining to)	

Definition of the Medical Word	Combining Form	Suffix	Build the Medical Word
1. Substance (that does) flexing and stretching	elast/o-	-in	*elastin*

(You think *substance* (-in) + *flexing and stretching* (elast/o-). You change the order of the word parts to put the suffix last. You write *elastin*.)

Definition of the Medical Word	Combining Form	Suffix	Build the Medical Word
2. Pertaining to (the) nail	ungu/o-	_____	_____
3. Area with distinct edges (on the) skin	derm/a-	_____	_____
4. Substance (of) hard, fibrous protein	kerat/o-	_____	_____
5. That which produces fibers that hold together	coll/a-	_____	_____
6. Full of fat (tissue)	adip/o-	_____	_____
7. Cell (that makes dark brown and) black (pigment)	melan/o-	_____	_____
8. Pertaining to (the) skin	cutane/o-	_____	_____
9. Pertaining to oil and sebum	sebace/o-	_____	_____
10. Cell (that stores) fat	lip/o-	_____	_____
11. Pertaining to (the) skin	integument/o-	_____	_____
12. Small thing (shaped like a) moon	lun/o-	_____	_____
13. State (of something that acts to) cover	integu/o-	_____	_____

Prefix Exercise

Read the definition of the medical word. Look at the medical word or partial word that is given (it already contains a combining form and a suffix). Select the correct prefix from the Prefix List and write it on the blank line. Then build the medical word and write it on the line. Be sure to check your spelling. The first one has been done for you.

PREFIX LIST

epi- (above; upon)	ex- (away from; out)	per- (through; throughout)	sub- (below; underneath)

Definition of the Medical Word	Prefix	Word or Partial Word	Build the Medical Word
1. Process (of skin cells moving) away from (the body like a) leaf	ex-	foliation	*exfoliation*
2. Pertaining to above (the) dermis	_____	dermal	_____
3. Pertaining to underneath (the) skin	_____	cutaneous	_____
4. Process (of) through (the skin to) breathe	_____	spiration	_____

Diseases

	General	
Word or Phrase	**Description**	**Pronunciation/Word Parts**
dermatitis	Any condition caused by disease or injury that results in inflammation or infection of the skin. Treatment: Correct the underlying cause.	**dermatitis** (DER-mah-TY-tis) **dermat/o-** *skin* **-itis** *infection of; inflammation of*
edema	Excessive amounts of fluid move from the blood into the dermis or subcutaneous tissue and cause swelling (see Figure 7-5 ■). Localized areas of edema occur with inflammation, allergic reactions, and infections. Large areas of edema occur with cardiovascular or urinary system diseases. Treatment: Correct the underlying cause.	**edema** (eh-DEE-mah)

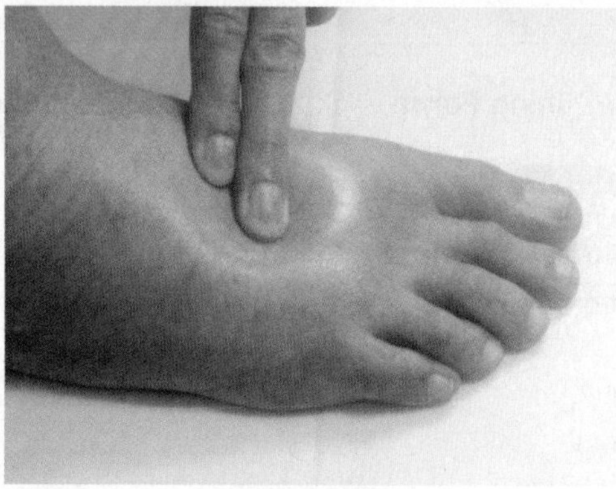

FIGURE 7-5 ■ Edema.
Fingertip pressure on an area of severe edema displaces the fluid and produces a deep indentation in the tissues. This is known as *pitting edema.*
Source: Pearson Education

hemorrhage	Trauma to the skin releases a small or large amount of blood. **Extravasation** is when the blood flows into the surrounding tissues. **Petechiae** are pinpoint hemorrhages in the skin from ruptured capillaries. A **contusion** is any size of hemorrhage under the skin that was caused by trauma. An **ecchymosis** is a hemorrhage under the skin that is 3 cm in diameter or larger. A contusion and an ecchymosis are both commonly known as a **bruise**. A **hematoma** is an elevated, localized collection of blood under the skin. Treatment: None.	**hemorrhage** (HEM-oh-rij) **hem/o-** *blood* **-rrhage** *excessive discharge; excessive flow*
		extravasation (eks-TRAV-ah-SAY-shun) **extra-** *outside* **vas/o-** *blood vessel; vas deferens* **-ation** *being; having; process*
		petechia (peh-TEE-kee-ah)
		petechiae (peh-TEE-kee-ee) *Petechia* is a Latin singular noun. Form the plural by changing *-a* to *-ae.*
		contusion (con-TOO-zhun) **contus/o-** *bruising* **-ion** *action; condition*
		ecchymosis (EK-ih-MOH-sis) **ecchym/o-** *blood in the tissue* **-osis** *condition; process*
		ecchymoses (EK-ih-MOH-seez) *Ecchymosis* is a Greek singular noun. Form the plural by changing *-is* to *-es.*
		ecchymotic (EK-ih-MAW-tik)
		hematoma (HEE-mah-TOH-mah) **hemat/o-** *blood* **-oma** *mass; tumor*

Word or Phrase	Description	Pronunciation/Word Parts

lesion	Any visible damage to or variation from normal of the skin, whether it is from disease or injury (see Figure 7-6 ■). Treatment: Correct the underlying cause.	**lesion** (LEE-zhun)
		
		cyst (SIST)
		
		fissure (FIH-shur)
		  fiss/o- *splitting*
		  -ure *result of; system*
		
		macule (MAK-yool)
		
		papule (PAP-yool)
		
		pustule (PUS-tyool)
		
		vesicle (VEH-sih-kl)
		  vesic/o- *bladder; fluid-filled sac*
		  -cle *small thing*
		
		vesicular (veh-SIH-kyoo-lar)
		  vesicul/o- *bladder; fluid-filled sac*
		  -ar *pertaining to*
		
		wheal (HWEEL)

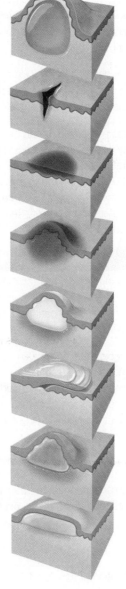

LESION	DESCRIPTION	COLOR	CONTENTS	EXAMPLE
Cyst	Elevated circular mound	Skin color or erythema	Semisolid or partly fluid filled	Acne sebaceous cyst
Fissure	Small, cracklike crevice	Erythema	None; some fluid exudate	Dry, chapped skin
Macule	Flat circle	Pigmented brown or black	None	Freckle, age spot
Papule	Elevated	Skin color or erythema	Solid	Acne pimple
Pustule	Elevated	White top	Pus	Acne whitehead
Scale	Flat to slightly elevated, thin flake	White	None	Dandruff, psoriasis
Vesicle	Elevated with pointed top	Erythema with a transparent top	Clear fluid	Herpes, chickenpox, shingles
Wheal	Elevated with broad, flat top	Erythema with a pale top	Clear fluid	Insect bites, urticaria

FIGURE 7-6 ■ Types of skin lesions.
Source: Pearson Education

Word or Phrase	Description	Pronunciation/Word Parts

neoplasm	Any **benign** or **malignant** new growth that occurs on or in the skin. Treatment: Excision of a benign neoplasm; excision and chemotherapy drugs or radiation therapy for a malignant neoplasm.	**neoplasm** (NEE-oh-plazm)
		  ne/o- *new*
		  -plasm *formed substance; growth*
		
		benign (bee-NINE)
		
		malignant (mah-LIG-nant)
		  malign/o- *cancer; intentionally causing harm*
		  -ant *pertaining to*

Word or Phrase	Description	Pronunciation/Word Parts

pruritus	Itching. Pruritus is associated with many skin diseases. It is also part of an allergic reaction because of the release of histamine. A patient with pruritus is said to be **pruritic**. Treatment: Topical or oral antihistamine drug or corticosteroid drug.	**pruritus** (proo-RY-tus)
		
		pruritic (proo-RIH-tik)
		  prurit/o- *itching*
		  -ic *pertaining to*

rash	Any type of skin lesion that is pink to red, flat or raised, pruritic or nonpruritic. Certain systemic diseases (chickenpox, measles) have characteristic rashes. Treatment: Topical or oral antihistamine drug or corticosteroid drug.	
wound	Any area of visible damage to the skin that is caused by physical means (such as rubbing, trauma, etc.). Treatment: Apply a protective covering and topical antibiotic drug to prevent infection.	

xeroderma	Excessive dryness of the skin. It can be caused by aging, cold weather with low humidity, vitamin A deficiency, or dehydration.
	The level of hydration can be assessed by testing the **skin turgor**. A fold of skin pinched between the thumb and fingertips should flatten out immediately when released. Dehydration causes the skin to remain elevated (tenting of the skin) or to flatten out very slowly. Treatment: Correct the underlying cause.
		xeroderma (ZEER-oh-DER-mah)
		  xer/o- *dry*
		  -derma *skin*
		
		turgor (TER-gor)

Changes in Skin Color		

albinism	A lack of pigment in the skin, hair, and iris of the eye. This is a genetic mutation in which there is a normal number of melanocytes, but they do not produce melanin. The patient is said to be an **albino**. Treatment: None.	**albinism** (AL-by-NIZ-em)
		  albin/o- *white*
		  -ism *disease from a specific cause; process*

cyanosis	Bluish-purple discoloration of the skin and nails due to a decreased level of oxygen in the blood (see Figure 4-10). It is caused by cardiac or respiratory disease. The patient is said to be **cyanotic**. In healthy persons, areas of skin exposed to the cold temporarily exhibit cyanosis. Treatment: Correct the underlying cause.	**cyanosis** (SY-ah-NOH-sis)
		  cyan/o- *blue*
		  -osis *condition; process*
		
		cyanotic (SY-ah-NAW-tik)
		  cyan/o- *blue*
		  -tic *pertaining to*

erythema	Reddish discoloration of the skin. It can be confined to one area of local inflammation or infection, or it can affect large areas of the skin surface, as in sunburn. The area is said to be **erythematous**. Treatment: Correct the underlying cause.	**erythema** (AIR-ih-THEE-mah)
		
		erythematous (AIR-ih-THEM-eh-tus)
		  erythemat/o- *redness*
		  -ous *pertaining to*

jaundice	Yellowish discoloration of the skin, mucous membranes, and whites of the eyes (see Figure 3-20). It is associated with liver disease. The liver cannot process bilirubin, and high levels of unconjugated bilirubin in the blood move into the tissues and color the skin yellow. It is also known as **icterus**. The patient is said to be *jaundiced* or **icteric**. A patient without jaundice is said to be *anicteric*. Treatment: Correct the underlying cause.	**jaundice** (JAWN-dis)
		
		icterus (IK-ter-us)
		
		icteric (ik-TAIR-ik)
		  icter/o- *jaundice*
		  -ic *pertaining to*

Word or Phrase	Description	Pronunciation/Word Parts
necrosis	Gray-to-black discoloration of the skin in areas where the tissue has died (see Figure 7-7 ■). **Necrotic** tissue can occur in a burn, decubitus ulcer, wound, or any tissue with a poor blood supply. Necrosis with subsequent bacterial invasion and decay is **gangrene**, and the area is said to be **gangrenous**. Treatment: Correct the underlying cause.	**necrosis** (neh-KROH-sis) **necr/o-** *dead body; dead cells; dead tissue* **-osis** *condition; process* **necrotic** (neh-KRAW-tik) **necr/o-** *dead body; dead cells; dead tissue* **-tic** *pertaining to* **gangrene** (GANG-green) **gangrenous** (GANG-greh-nus) **gangren/o-** *gangrene* **-ous** *pertaining to*

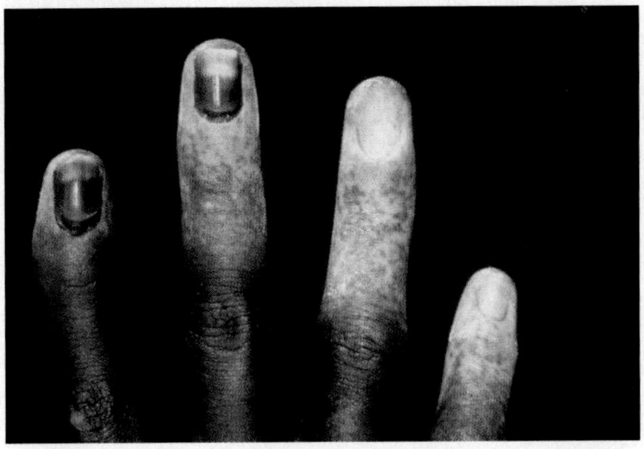

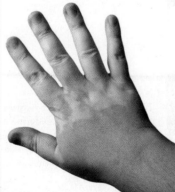

FIGURE 7-7 ■ Necrosis and pallor.
This patient's hand shows necrosis and pallor due to severe frostbite. The fingernails of the first two fingers show necrosis. Those fingertips may need to be amputated. The third and fourth fingers show pallor, indicating poor blood flow, which may eventually lead to tissue death and necrosis.
Source: Southern Illinois University/Science Source

Word or Phrase	Description	Pronunciation/Word Parts
pallor	Unnatural paleness due to a lack of blood supply to the tissue (see Figure 7-7). This is caused by blockage of an artery, hypotension, or severe exposure to the cold. Treatment: Correct the underlying cause.	**pallor** (PAL-or)
vitiligo	An autoimmune disorder in which the melanocytes are slowly destroyed in irregular and ever-enlarging areas. There are white patches of **depigmentation** interspersed with normal skin (see Figure 7-8 ■). Treatment: None.	**vitiligo** (VIT-ih-LY-goh) **depigmentation** (dee-PIG-men-TAY-shun) **de-** *reversal of; without* **pigment/o-** *pigment* **-ation** *being; having; process*

FIGURE 7-8 ■ Vitiligo.
This patient has areas of depigmentation on the hand due to vitiligo, a progressive autoimmune disorder.
Source: Axel Bueckert/Fotolia

CLINICAL CONNECTIONS

Obstetrics (Chapter 13). Melanocyte-stimulating hormone (from the anterior pituitary gland in the brain) can become overactive during pregnancy, causing dark, hyperpigmented areas on the face (**chloasma** or the mask of pregnancy) and/or a vertical dark line on the skin of the abdomen from the umbilicus downward (**linea nigra**).

Stretch marks (**striae**) in the skin of the abdomen and buttocks are the result of small tears in the dermis as the skin stretches to accommodate the pregnant uterus. These are irregular, reddened lines that later become lighter and shiny as they heal as scar tissue.

chloasma (kloh-AZ-mah)	
linea nigra (LIN-ee-ah NY-grah)	
striae (STRY-ee)	

Skin Injuries

Word or Phrase	Description	Pronunciation/Word Parts
abrasion	Sliding or scraping injury that mechanically removes the epidermis. It is also known as a **brush burn**. Treatment: Apply a protective covering.	**abrasion** (ah-BRAY-zhun) **abras/o-** *scrape off* **-ion** *action; condition*
blister	Repetitive rubbing injury that mechanically separates the epidermis from the dermis and releases tissue fluid. A blister is a fluid-filled sac with a thin, transparent covering of epidermis. Blisters often form on the heel from walking in poorly fitting shoes or on the hand from rubbing with constant use of a tool. Treatment: Apply a protective covering before the activity.	**blister** (BLIS-ter)
burns	Heat (fire, hot objects, steam, boiling water), electrical current (lightning, electrical outlets or cords), chemicals, and radiation or x-rays (sunshine or prescribed radiation therapy) can cause a burn to the epidermis or dermis. Treatment: Topical anti-infective drug to prevent infection. Second-degree burns over a large area and all third-degree burns require debridement and skin grafting.	
first-degree burn	This burn involves only the epidermis and causes erythema, pain, and swelling, but not blisters.	
second-degree burn	This burn involves the epidermis and the upper part of the dermis. It causes erythema, pain, and swelling. There are small blisters or larger **bullae** that form as the epidermis detaches from the dermis and the space between fills with tissue fluid (see Figure 7-9 ■). This is also known as a **partial-thickness burn**.	**bulla** (BUL-ah) **bullae** (BUL-ee) *Bulla* is a Latin singular noun. Form the plural by changing *-a* to *-ae*.

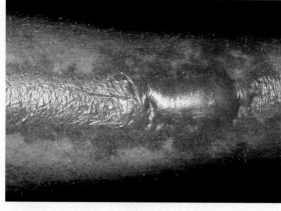

FIGURE 7-9 ■ Second-degree burn of the leg.
The burn caused the epidermis to separate from the dermis. Tissue fluid caused the epidermis to swell into a large, fluid-filled bulla.
Source: Dr. P. Marazzi/Science Source

Word or Phrase	Description	Pronunciation/Word Parts
third-degree burn	This burn involves the epidermis and entire dermis, and sometimes the subcutaneous tissue and muscle layer beneath may be involved. The area is black where the skin is charred. If nerves in the dermis are destroyed, there is local **anesthesia** (no sensation of pain). This is also known as a **full-thickness burn**. An **eschar** is a thick, crusty scar of necrotic tissue that forms on a third-degree burn. Eschar is removed because it traps fluid, delays healing, and can become infected. A fourth-degree burn affects muscles and bones.	**anesthesia** (AN-es-THEE-zha) **an-** *not; without* **esthes/o-** *feeling; sensation* **-ia** *condition; state; thing* **eschar** (ES-kar)
callus	Repetitive rubbing injury that causes the epidermis to gradually thicken into a wide, elevated pad. A **corn** is a callus with a hard central area with a pointed tip that causes pain and inflammation. Treatment: Removal.	**callus** (KAL-us)

Word or Phrase	Description	Pronunciation/Word Parts

cicatrix	Fibrous tissue composed of collagen that forms as an injury heals. It is also known as a **scar**. A **keloid** is a very firm, abnormally large scar that is bigger than the original injury. It is caused by an overproduction of collagen (see Figure 7-10 ■). Unlike a scar, a keloid does not fade or decrease in size over time. Treatment: Surgical removal of a keloid, although they often grow back.	**cicatrix** (SIK-ah-triks)
		
		keloid (KEE-loyd)
		  kel/o- *tumor*
		  -oid *resembling*

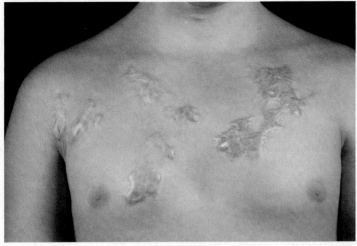

FIGURE 7-10 ■ Keloid.
A keloid is a scar that continues to grow until it is larger than the original injury. Depending on its location and size, a keloid can be cosmetically unacceptable.
Source: Biophoto Associates/Science Source/ Getty Images

Word or Phrase	Description	Pronunciation/Word Parts
decubitus ulcer	Constant pressure to a particular area of the skin restricts the blood flow to those tissues. The epidermis and then dermis break down and slough off, resulting in a shallow or deep ulcer (see Figure 7-11 ■). Decubitus ulcers most often occur at pressure points overlying bony prominences such as the hip or sacrum. They are also known as **pressure sores** or **bed sores**. Treatment: Frequent repositioning, increased protein intake to rebuild tissue, and debridement of any necrotic tissue to promote healing.	**decubitus** (dee-KYOO-bih-tus) **decubiti** (dee-KYOO-bih-tie) *Decubitus* is a Latin singular noun. Form the plural by changing -*us* to -*i*. **ulcer** (UL-ser)

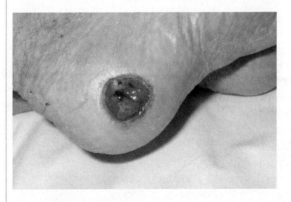

FIGURE 7-11 ■ Decubitus ulcer.
This decubitus ulcer was caused by prolonged pressure on the heel from lying on the back for long periods of time.
Source: Mediscan/Alamy

A CLOSER LOOK

Decreased fat in the subcutaneous tissue, poor nutrition, long-standing circulatory problems, and confinement to a bed or wheelchair predispose older patients to developing decubitus ulcers. Frequent repositioning of the patient and keeping the skin free of urine help prevent decubitus ulcers. The level of protein (albumin) in the blood indicates whether the patient is able to build healthy tissue and heal an existing decubitus ulcer. A low level of albumin is treated nutritionally by offering the patient high-protein snacks.

Word or Phrase	Description	Pronunciation/Word Parts

excoriation	Superficial injury with a sharp object such as a fingernail, animal claw, or thorn that creates a linear **scratch** in the skin. Treatment: Topical antibiotic drug to prevent infection.	**excoriation** (eks-KOR-ee-AA-shun)
		  excori/o- *take out skin*
		  -ation *being; having; process*

Word or Phrase	Description	Pronunciation/Word Parts

laceration	Deep, penetrating wound. It can have clean-cut or torn, ragged skin edges (see Figure 7-12 ■). Treatment: Layered closure with sutures.	**laceration** (LAS-er-AA-shun)
		  lacer/o- *tearing*
		  -ation *being; having; process*

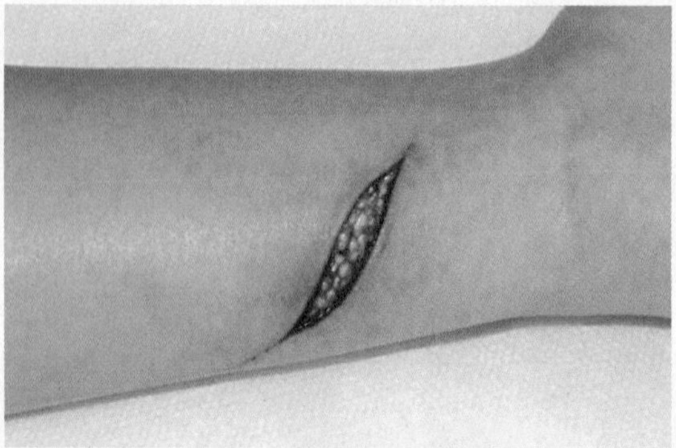

FIGURE 7-12 ■ Laceration.
This deep laceration of the forearm was caused by a piece of glass that penetrated through the epidermis and dermis to expose the adipose tissue in the subcutaneous layer.
Source: Susan Turley

Skin Infections

Word or Phrase	Description	Pronunciation/Word Parts
abscess	Localized, pus-containing pocket under the skin caused by a bacterial infection. The infection is usually caused by *Staphylococcus aureus*, a common bacterium on the skin. A **furuncle** is a localized, elevated abscess around a hair follicle and the skin is inflamed and painful. It is also known as a **boil**. A **carbuncle** is composed of large furuncles with connecting channels through the subcutaneous tissue or to the skin surface. Treatment: Incision and drainage, oral antibiotic drug.	**abscess** (AB-ses) **furuncle** (FYOOR-ung-kl) **carbuncle** (KAR-bung-kl)

cellulitis	Spreading inflammation and infection of the connective tissues of the skin and muscle. It develops from a superficial cut, scratch, insect bite, blister, or splinter that becomes infected. The infecting bacteria produce enzymes that allow the infection to spread between the tissue layers. There is erythema (often as a red streak), warmth, and pain. Treatment: Oral antibiotic drug.	**cellulitis** (SEL-yoo-LY-tis)
		  cellul/o- *cell*
		  -itis *infection of; inflammation of*

herpes	Skin infection caused by the herpes virus. There are clustered vesicles, erythema, edema, and pain. The vesicles rupture, releasing clear fluid that forms crusts. Treatment: Topical or oral antiviral drug. **Herpes simplex virus (HSV) type 1** occurs on the lips. These lesions tend to recur during illness and stress. They are also known as **cold sores** or **fever blisters**. **Herpes simplex virus (HSV) type 2** is a sexually transmitted disease that causes vesicles in the genital area. These lesions tend to recur during illness and stress. This is also known as **genital herpes**. **Herpes whitlow** is a herpes simplex infection at the base of the fingernail from contact with herpes simplex type 1 of the mouth or type 2 of the genitals. The virus enters through a small tear in the cuticle. **Herpes varicella-zoster** causes the skin rash of chickenpox during childhood. The virus then remains dormant in the nerve roots until it is activated in later life by illness or stress. Then it forms painful vesicles and crusts along a dermatome. This is also known as **shingles** (see Figure 7-13 ■).	**herpes** (HER-peez) **herpes simplex** (HER-peez SIM-pleks) **herpes whitlow** (HER-peez WHIT-loh) **herpes varicella-zoster** (HER-peez VAIR-ih-SEH-lah ZAW-ster) **shingles** (SHING-glz)

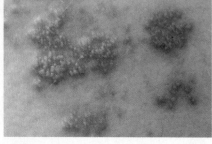

FIGURE 7-13 ■ Shingles.
The vesicles and crusts of shingles. The lesions occur along a dermatome (an area of skin associated with a nerve from the spinal cord).
Source: CLS Design/Shutterstock

Word or Phrase	Description	Pronunciation/Word Parts
tinea	Skin infection caused by a fungus that feeds on epidermal cells. It multiplies quickly in the warm, moist environment of body creases and areas enclosed by clothing or shoes. There is severe itching and burning with red, scaly lesions. Because some lesions are round, it was originally thought to be caused by a worm, and was (and still is) called **ringworm**. Tinea is named according to where it occurs on the body. **Tinea capitis** occurs on the scalp and causes hair loss. **Tinea corporis** occurs on the trunk and extremities (see Figure 7-14 ■). **Tinea cruris** occurs in the groin and genital areas and is known as **jock itch**. **Tinea pedis** occurs on the feet and is known as **athlete's foot**. Treatment: Topical antifungal drug.	**tinea** (TIN-ee-ah) **capitis** (KAP-ih-tis) **corporis** (KOR-por-is) **cruris** (KROOR-is) **pedis** (PEE-dis)

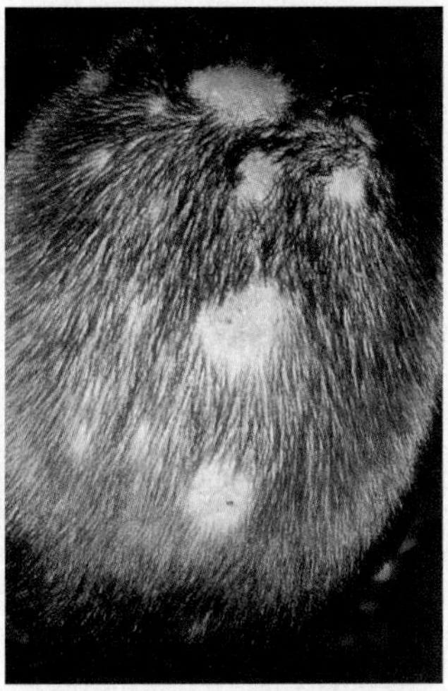

FIGURE 7-14 ■ Tinea capitis.
This fungal infection, known as *ringworm*, occurs on the scalp. The Latin word *corporis* means *of the head*. This infection causes itching and hair loss. Because the skin lesions are often round, it was originally thought to be caused by a worm, hence the name "ringworm."
Source: Centers for Disease Control and Prevention (CDC)

Word or Phrase	Description	Pronunciation/Word Parts
verruca	Irregular, rough skin lesion caused by the human papillomavirus. It is usually on the hand, fingers, or the sole of the foot (plantar wart). It is also known as a **wart**. Treatment: Topical keratolytic drug to break down the keratin in the wart. Cryosurgery or electrosurgery, if needed.	**verruca** (veh-ROO-kah) **verrucae** (veh-ROO-kee) *Verruca* is a Latin singular noun. Form the plural by changing -a to -ae.

Skin Infestations

Word or Phrase	Description	Pronunciation/Word Parts
pediculosis	Infestation of lice and their eggs (nits) in the scalp, hair, eyelashes, or genital hair. Lice are easily transmitted from one person to another by combs or hats. Treatment: Shampoo and skin lotion to kill lice.	**pediculosis** (peh-DIH-kyoo-LOH-sis) **pedicul/o-** *lice* **-osis** *condition; process*
scabies	Infestation of parasitic mites that tunnel under the skin and produce vesicles that are itchy. Treatment: Shampoo and skin lotion to kill mites.	**scabies** (SKAY-beez)

Allergic Skin Conditions

Word or Phrase	Description	Pronunciation/Word Parts
contact dermatitis	Local reaction to physical contact with a substance that is an allergen or an irritant. Examples: Chemicals (deodorant, soaps, detergents, makeup, urine), metals, synthetic products (latex gloves, Spandex bathing suit or girdle), plants (poison ivy), or animals (see Figure 7-15 ■). The skin becomes inflamed and irritated. Small vesicles may also appear. Treatment: Topical or oral antihistamine drug or corticosteroid drug.	**dermatitis** (DER-mah-TY-tis) **dermat/o-** *skin* **-itis** *infection of; inflammation of*

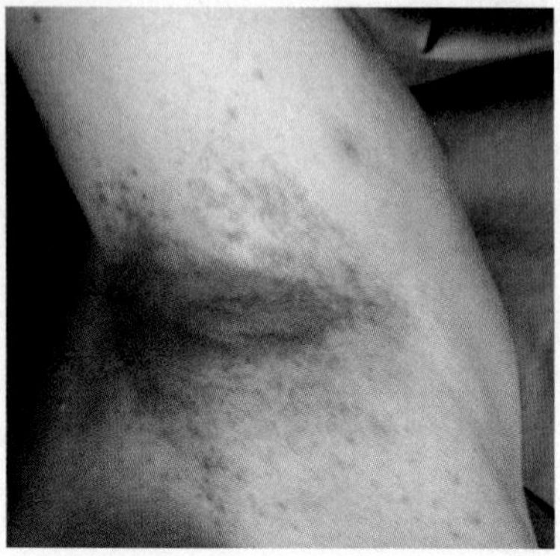

FIGURE 7-15 ■ Severe contact dermatitis.
This skin reaction was caused by the application of a new deodorant whose chemical ingredients caused irritation.
Source: Susan M. Turley

CLINICAL CONNECTIONS
Infection Control. According to the National Institute for Occupational Safety and Health, there has been an increase in the number of healthcare professionals who have allergic reactions to latex rubber gloves. This causes skin rashes, hives, itching, and asthma. Nonlatex gloves should be used instead to protect and to prevent the spread of infection.

Word or Phrase	Description	Pronunciation/Word Parts
urticaria	Condition of raised areas of redness and edema that appear suddenly and may also disappear rapidly. There is itching (pruritus), and scratching tends to cause the areas to enlarge. Urticaria is caused by an allergic reaction to food, plants, animals, insect bites, or drugs. It is also known as **hives**. Each individual area is known as a **wheal**. A large wheal is a **welt**. Treatment: Topical or oral antihistamine drug or corticosteroid drug.	**urticaria** (ER-tih-KAIR-ee-ah) **wheal** (HWEEL)

Benign Skin Markings and Neoplasms

Word or Phrase	Description	Pronunciation/Word Parts
actinic keratoses	Raised, irregular, rough areas of skin that are dry and feel like sandpaper. These develop in middle-aged persons in areas chronically exposed to the sun. They can become squamous cell carcinoma. They are also known as **solar keratoses**. Treatment: Avoid more sun exposure.	**actinic** (ak-TIN-ik) **actin/o-** *rays of the sun* **-ic** *pertaining to* **keratosis** (KAIR-ah-TOH-sis) **kerat/o-** *cornea of the eye; hard, fibrous protein* **-osis** *condition; process* **keratoses** (KAIR-ah-TOH-seez) **solar** (SOH-lar)
freckle	**Benign**, pigmented, flat macule that develops after sun exposure. Freckles contain groups of melanocytes. Freckles fade over time without continued sun exposure. Treatment: None.	**freckle** (FREH-kl) **benign** (bee-NINE)

Word or Phrase	Description	Pronunciation/Word Parts

hemangioma	Congenital growth composed of a mass of superficial, dilated blood vessels (see Figure 7-16 ◼). Treatment: Most hemangiomas disappear without treatment by age 3. 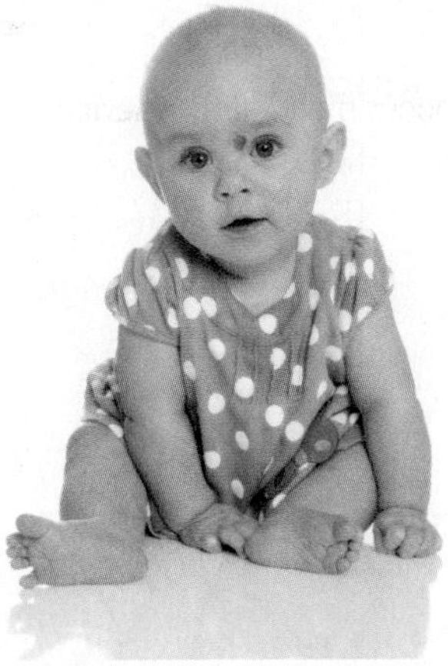
	
	FIGURE 7-16 ◼ Hemangioma. The bright red color of this skin lesion comes from the large number of dilated blood vessels.
	Source: Julie DeGuia/Shutterstock
		hemangioma
		(hee-MAN-jee-OH-mah)
		  hem/o- *blood*
		  angi/o- *blood vessel; lymphatic vessel*
		  -oma *mass; tumor*

lipoma	Benign growth of adipose tissue in the subcutaneous layer. It makes a soft, rounded, nontender fatty elevation in the skin. Treatment: Excision, if desired.	**lipoma** (ly-POH-mah)
		  lip/o- *fat; lipid*
		  -oma *mass; tumor*

nevus	Benign skin lesion that is present at birth and comes in a variety of colors and shapes. It is also known as a **mole** (see Figure 7-17 ◼). A port-wine stain is another type of nevus; it is slightly elevated, red to purple, and irregularly shaped. It can cover large areas of skin on the face and neck. Its shape and color resemble a puddle of spilled wine. It is also known as a **birthmark**. A **dysplastic nevus** has irregular edges and variations in color. It can develop into a malignant melanoma. Treatment: Excision of a mole if clothing irritates it; laser treatment to remove port-wine stains; observe a dysplastic nevus for change. 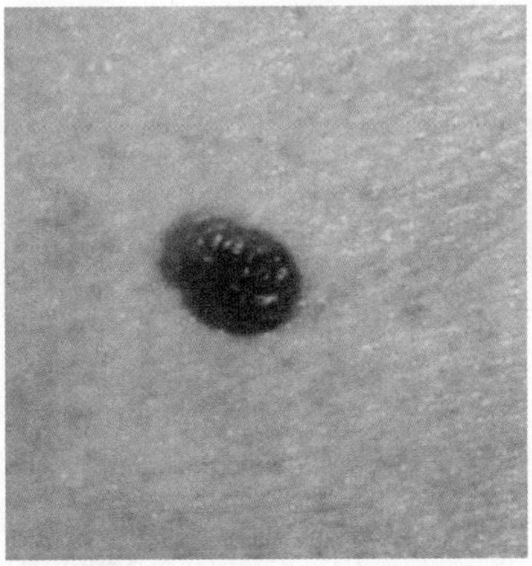
	
	FIGURE 7-17 ◼ Nevus. This mole is a pigmented nevus that is round and elevated. Other moles are flat, darker in color, and can contain a hair.
	Source: Susan M. Turley
		nevus (NEE-vus)
		nevi (NEE-vi)
		Nevus is a Latin singular noun. Form the plural by changing *-us* to *-i*.
		
		dysplastic (dis-PLAS-tik)
		  dys- *abnormal; difficult; painful*
		  plast/o- *formation; growth*
		  -ic *pertaining to*

papilloma	Small, soft, flesh-colored growth of epidermis and dermis that protrudes outwardly. It comes in a variety of shapes: irregular mounds, globes, flaps, or polyps with rounded tops on slender stalks. It occurs on the eyelid, neck, or trunk of the body. It is also known as a **skin tag**. Treatment: Removal by cryotherapy, electrocautery, or surgical excision, if desired.	**papilloma** (PAP-ih-LOH-mah)
		  papill/o- *elevated structure*
		  -oma *mass; tumor*

Word or Phrase	Description	Pronunciation/Word Parts
premalignant skin lesions	Abnormal skin lesions that are not yet cancerous. Over time and with continued exposure to sunlight or irritation, these lesions can become cancerous. Treatment: None; observe for changes.	**premalignant** (PREE-mah-LIG-nant) **pre-** *before; in front of* **malign/o-** *cancer; intentionally causing harm* **-ant** *pertaining to*
senile lentigo	Light-to-dark brown macules with irregular edges. They occur most often on the hands and face, areas that are chronically exposed to the sun (see Figure 7-18 ■). Treatment: None. 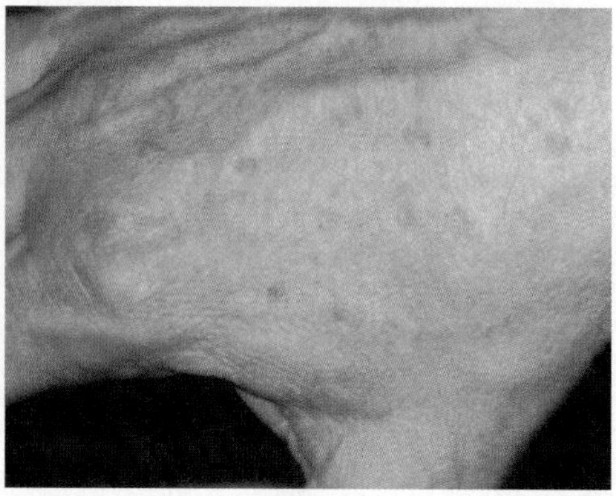 **FIGURE 7-18 ■ Senile lentigo.** *These light brown macules occur with age and are called* age spots *or* liver spots. *Source*: Anita Hylton/Pearson	**senile** (SEE-nile) **sen/o-** *old age* **-ile** *pertaining to* **lentigo** (len-TY-goh)
syndactyly	Congenital abnormality in which the skin and soft tissues are joined between the fingers or toes (see Figure 7-19 ■). In some cases the fingernails or toenails are also joined. **Polydactyly** is a congenital abnormality in which there are extra fingers or toes. Treatment: Surgical correction, if desired. 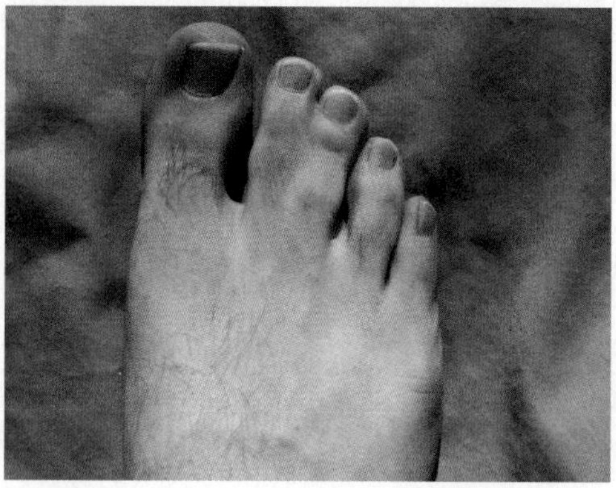 **FIGURE 7-19 ■ Syndactyly.** *The skin and soft tissues of the second and third toes are fused together in this patient with syndactyly.* *Source*: Susan M. Turley	**syndactyly** (sin-DAK-tih-lee) **syn-** *together* **-dactyly** *condition of fingers; condition of toes* The ending *-dactyly* contains the combining form *dactyl/o-* and the one-letter suffix *-y*. **polydactyly** (PAW-lee-DAK-tih-lee) **poly-** *many; much* **-dactyly** *condition of fingers; condition of toes*
xanthoma	Benign growth that is a yellow nodule or plaque on the hands, elbows, knees, or feet. It is seen in patients who have a high level of lipids in the blood or have diabetes mellitus. A xanthoma that occurs on the eyelid is known as a **xanthelasma**. Treatment: Excision, if desired.	**xanthoma** (zan-THOH-mah) **xanth/o-** *yellow* **-oma** *mass; tumor* **xanthelasma** (ZAN-thel-AZ-mah) **xanth/o-** *yellow* **-elasma** *plate-like structure*

Malignant Neoplasms of the Skin

Word or Phrase	Description	Pronunciation/Word Parts
cancer of the skin	A **cancerous** lesion or **malignancy** in areas of the skin that are chronically exposed to ultraviolet light radiation from the sun. Skin cancer is more common in older adults (because of a lifetime of sun exposure) and in fair-skinned persons (because there is less melanin to absorb radiation). Treatment: Moh's surgery to remove the cancer, chemotherapy drugs, photodynamic therapy.	**cancer** (KAN-ser) **cancerous** (KAN-ser-ous) **cancer/o-** *cancer* **-ous** *pertaining to* **malignancy** (mah-LIG-nan-see) **malign/o-** *cancer; intentionally causing harm* **-ancy** *state*
basal cell carcinoma	Skin cancer that begins in the basal layer of the epidermis. It is the most common type of skin cancer. It often appears as a raised, pearly bump. It is a slow-growing cancer that does not metastasize to other parts of the body.	**carcinoma** (KAR-sih-NOH-mah) **carcin/o-** *cancer* **-oma** *mass; tumor*

malignant melanoma	Skin cancer that begins in melanocytes in the epidermis (see Figure 7-20 ■). It grows quickly and metastasizes to other parts of the body. Malignant melanomas have these four characteristics:
	  A Asymmetry. One side of the lesion has a different shape than the other side.
	  B Border or edge is irregular or ragged.
	  C Color varies from black to brown (or to red) within the same lesion.
	  D Diameter is greater than 6 mm (1/4 inch).
		malignant (mah-LIG-nant)
		malign/o- *cancer; intentionally causing harm*
		-ant *pertaining to*
		
		melanoma (MEL-ah-NOH-mah)
		melan/o- *black*
		-oma *mass; tumor*
		Add words to make a complete definition of *melanoma*: *tumor (whose color is brown or) black.*

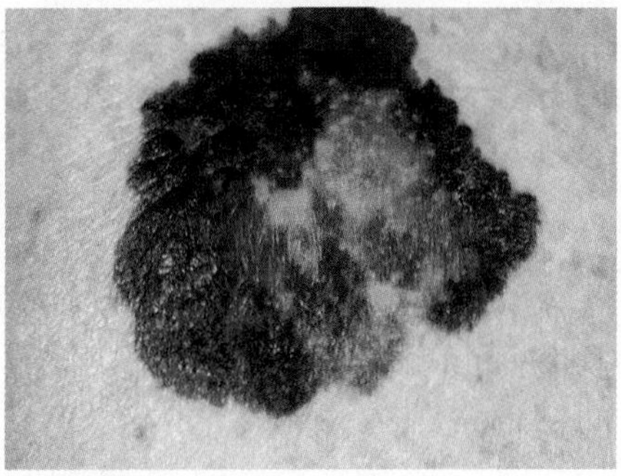

FIGURE 7-20 ■ Malignant melanoma.
This lesion reveals three of the four typical characteristics of a malignant melanoma: asymmetry, irregular edges, and varying shades of color. The fourth characteristic—an increase in size—would be noted over time.
Source: Centers for Disease Control Public Heath Image Library

CLINICAL CONNECTIONS
Public Health. Depletion of the earth's ozone layer has led to many cases of malignant melanoma. The use of sunscreen and avoiding prolonged sun exposure, particularly during midday, helps to decrease this risk. Self-examination of the skin should be done regularly. Irregular or changing skin lesions should be examined by a dermatologist.

Word or Phrase	Description	Pronunciation/Word Parts
squamous cell carcinoma	Skin cancer that begins in the flat squamous cells of the superficial layer of the epidermis. It often begins as an actinic keratosis. It most often appears as a red bump or an ulcer. It is the second most common type of skin cancer, but it grows slowly.	**squamous** (SKWAY-mus) **squam/o-** *scale-like cell* **-ous** *pertaining to*
Kaposi's sarcoma	Skin cancer that begins in connective tissue or lymph nodes. Tumors on the skin are elevated, irregular, and dark reddish-blue. This previously rare cancer is now commonly seen in AIDS patients because of their impaired immune response. The cancer involves the skin, mucous membranes, and internal organs. Treatment: Excision of single lesions, radiation therapy for multiple lesions.	**Kaposi** (kah-POH-see) **sarcoma** (sar-KOH-mah) **sarc/o-** *connective tissue* **-oma** *mass; tumor*

Autoimmune Disorders with Skin Symptoms

Word or Phrase	Description	Pronunciation/Word Parts
psoriasis	Autoimmune disorder that produces an excessive number of epidermal cells. The skin lesions are itchy, red, and covered with silvery scales and plaques. They usually occur on the scalp, elbows, hands, and knees (see Figure 7-21 ■). Illness and stress cause flare-ups, and psoriasis has a hereditary component. Treatment: Topical coal tar drug, vitamin A drug, vitamin D drug, and corticosteroid drug; light therapy with a psoralen drug and ultraviolet light A (PUVA) or ultraviolet light B (UVB). 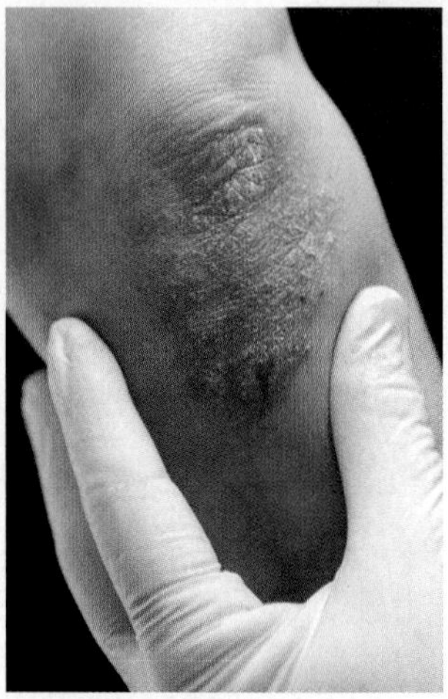 **FIGURE 7-21** ■ **Psoriasis.** Psoriasis produces characteristic elevated, erythematous lesions that are topped by silvery scales and plaques. The elbows and the knees are common sites of psoriasis. *Source*: Hriana/Fotolia	**psoriasis** (sor-EYE-ah-sis) **psor/o-** *itching* **-iasis** *process; state* **psoriatic** (SOR-ee-AT-ik) **psor/o-** *itching* **-iatic** *pertaining to a process; pertaining to a state*
scleroderma	Autoimmune disorder that causes the skin and internal organs to progressively harden due to deposits of collagen. Treatment: Oral corticosteroid drug.	**scleroderma** (SKLAIR-oh-DER-mah) **scler/o-** *hard; sclera of the eye* **-derma** *skin*
systemic lupus erythematosus (SLE)	Autoimmune disorder with deterioration of collagen in the skin and connective tissues. There is joint pain, sensitivity to sunlight, and fatigue. Often there is a characteristic butterfly-shaped, erythematous rash over the bridge of the nose that spreads out over the cheeks. Treatment: Oral corticosteroid drug.	**systemic** (sis-TEM-ik) **system/o-** *body as a whole* **-ic** *pertaining to* **lupus erythematosus** (LOO-pus AIR-eh-THEM-ah-TOH-sus)

Diseases of the Sebaceous Glands

Word or Phrase	Description	Pronunciation/Word Parts
acne vulgaris	During puberty, the sebaceous glands produce large amounts of sebum, particularly on the forehead, nose, chin, shoulders, and back. Excess sebum builds up around the hair shaft, hardens, and blocks the follicle. The blocked secretions elevate the skin and form a reddish papule. In other hair follicles, the oily sebum traps dirt and enlarges the pore. The sebum turns black as its oil is oxidized from exposure to the air. This forms a **comedo** or **blackhead**. As bacteria feed on the sebum, they release irritating substances that produce inflammation. The bacteria also produce infection, drawing white blood cells to the area and forming pustules or **whiteheads** (see Figure 7-22 ■ and Table 7-1 ■). In severe cystic acne, the papules enlarge to form deep, pus-filled cysts. Treatment: Topical cleansing drug, topical or oral antibiotic drug to kill skin bacteria; oral vitamin A–type drug for severe cystic acne.	**acne vulgaris** (AK-nee vul-GAIR-is) **comedo** (KOH-meh-doh) (koh-MEE-doh) **comedones** (KOH-meh-dohns)

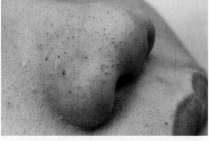

FIGURE 7-22 ■ Acne vulgaris.
This adolescent boy has acne vulgaris with small and large comedos on his nose and a pustule by the side of his nose. Increased secretions of the sebaceous glands during puberty trigger the onset of acne vulgaris.
Source: ThamKC/Fotolia

CLINICAL CONNECTIONS

Pharmacology. Severe cystic acne is frequently treated with the vitamin A–type drug isotretinoin. This drug has been linked to the unusual and severe adverse effects of fetal deformities in pregnant women and suicide, and this warning must be included on the drug's package and information sheet.

Word or Phrase	Description	Pronunciation/Word Parts

acne rosacea	Chronic skin condition of the face in middle-aged patients. The sebaceous glands secrete excessive amounts of sebum. There is blotchy erythema, dilated superficial blood vessels, and edema that is made worse by heat, cold, stress, emotions, certain foods, alcoholic beverages, and sunlight (see Figure 7-23 ■ and Table 7-1). Men can develop **rhinophyma**, an erythematous, irregular enlargement of the nose. Treatment: Topical antibacterial or antiprotozoal drug; laser surgery to destroy small, superficial blood vessels.	**acne rosacea**
		(AK-nee roh-ZAY-shee-ah)
		
		rhinophyma (RY-noh-FY-mah)
		  rhin/o- *nose*
		  -phyma *growth; tumor*

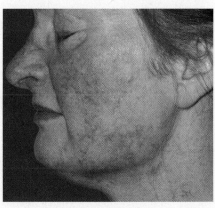

FIGURE 7-23 ■ Acne rosacea.
This patient's face shows the blotchy, rose-colored erythema and dilated superficial blood vessels of acne rosacea. Even the eyelids and neck are affected.
Source: Susan M. Turley

Table 7-1 Comparison of Acne Vulgaris and Acne Rosacea

	Site	Comedones	Pustules and Papules	Dilated Blood Vessels	Age
Acne vulgaris	face, shoulders, back	yes	yes	no	adolescence
Acne rosacea	face, neck	no	no	yes	middle age

Word or Phrase	Description	Pronunciation/Word Parts
seborrhea	Overproduction of sebum, particularly on the face and scalp, that occurs at a time other than puberty. In seborrheic dermatitis, oily areas are interspersed with patches of dry, scaly skin and dandruff. There can also be erythema and crusty, yellow exudates from leaking tissue fluids. In adults, seborrheic dermatitis often appears after illness or stress. It can be caused by allergies. It is called **cradle cap** in infants and **eczema** in children and adults. Treatment: Topical corticosteroid drug, medicated shampoo.	**seborrhea** (SEB-oh-REE-ah) **seb/o-** *oil; sebum* **-rrhea** *discharge; flow* **eczema** (EK-zeh-mah)

Diseases of the Sweat Glands

Word or Phrase	Description	Pronunciation/Word Parts
anhidrosis	Congenital absence of the sweat glands and inability to tolerate heat. Treatment: Avoid overheating.	**anhidrosis** (AN-hy-DROH-sis) **an-** *not; without* **hidr/o-** *sweat* **-osis** *condition; process*
diaphoresis	Profuse sweating. Although a high fever, emotional stress, strenuous exercise, or the hot flashes of menopause can cause profuse sweating, these are *not* referred to as diaphoresis. Diaphoresis is caused by an underlying condition such as myocardial infarction, hyperthyroidism, hypoglycemia, or withdrawal from narcotic drugs. The patient is said to be **diaphoretic**. Treatment: Correct the underlying cause.	**diaphoresis** (DY-ah-foh-REE-sis) **diaphor/o-** *sweating* **-esis** *condition; process* **diaphoretic** (DY-ah-foh-RET-ik) **diaphor/o-** *sweating* **-etic** *pertaining to*

Diseases of the Hair

Word or Phrase	Description	Pronunciation/Word Parts
alopecia	Acute or chronic loss of scalp hair. Acute alopecia can be caused by chemotherapy drugs that attack rapidly dividing cancer cells, but also affect rapidly dividing hair cells. Skin diseases of the scalp can also cause acute hair loss. Chronic hair loss usually begins in early middle age, although inherited tendencies can make it occur sooner. In men, a decreasing testosterone level and decreased blood flow to the scalp cause the hair follicles to shrink. The hair on the top of the scalp thins and disappears, leaving a fringe of hair at the back of the head. This is known as **male pattern baldness**. In women, menopause causes the level of estradiol from the ovaries to be lower than the male hormone androgen (produced by the adrenal cortex), and this hormonal change causes the hair to thin. Treatment: Topical drug to dilate the arteries in the scalp or oral drug to block the effect of DHT (substance that is increased in the balding scalp).	**alopecia** (AL-oh-PEE-sha) **alopec/o-** *bald* **-ia** *condition; state; thing*

Word or Phrase	Description	Pronunciation/Word Parts
folliculitis	Inflammation or infection of the hair follicle. It occurs after shaving, plucking, or removing hair with hot wax. Treatment: Topical corticosteroid or antibiotic drug.	**folliculitis** (foh-LIH-kyoo-LY-tis) **follicul/o-** *follicle; small sac* **-itis** *infection of; inflammation of*
hirsutism	The presence of excessive, dark hair on the forearms and over the upper lip of a woman. It is due to too much of the male hormone androgen caused by a tumor in the adrenal cortex. Treatment: Correct the underlying cause.	**hirsutism** (HER-soo-tizm) **hirsut/o-** *hairy* **-ism** *disease from a specific cause; process*
pilonidal sinus	An abnormal passageway (**fistula**) that begins as a large, abnormal hair follicle that contains a hair that is never shed. The follicle is visible as a pit or dimple on the skin in the sacral area of the back. Irritation causes the hair follicle to become infected, eventually creating a sinus into the subcutaneous tissue, with erythema, tenderness, and purulent discharge. Treatment: Incision and drainage of the sinus.	**pilonidal** (PY-loh-NY-dal) **pil/o-** *hair* **nid/o-** *focus; nest* **-al** *pertaining to* **sinus** (SY-nus) **fistula** (FIS-tyoo-lah)

DID YOU KNOW? Even the condition of split ends on hairs has a medical name: **schizotrichia**.		**schizotrichia** (SKIZ-oh-TRIH-kee-ah) **schiz/o-** *split* **trich/o-** *hair* **-ia** *condition; state; thing*

Diseases of the Nails

Word or Phrase	Description	Pronunciation/Word Parts
clubbing and cyanosis	Abnormal downward curved and bluish fingernails and stunted growth of the finger associated with a chronic lack of oxygen in patients with cystic fibrosis (see Figure 4-10). Treatment: Correct the underlying cause.	
onychomycosis	Fungal infection of the fingernails or toenails. It infects the nail root and deforms the nail as it grows (see Figure 7-24 ■). Treatment: Topical or oral antifungal drug; treatment with a laser.	**onychomycosis** (ON-ih-KOH-my-KOH-sis) **onych/o-** *fingernail; toenail* **myc/o-** *fungus* **-osis** *condition; process*

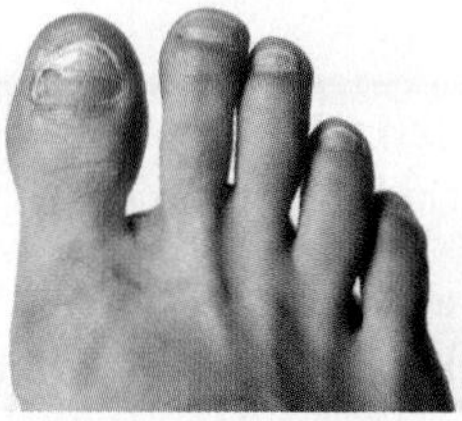

FIGURE 7-24 ■ Onychomycosis.
A fungal infection can involve one or all of the nails of the hands or feet. The nails become discolored, misshapen, thickened, and raised up from the nail bed.
Source: Melinda Nagy/Fotolia

Word or Phrase	Description	Pronunciation/Word Parts
paronychia	Bacterial infection of the skin next to the cuticle. It can be caused by an injury, nail biting, or a manicure that trims the cuticle. There is tenderness, erythema, and swelling, and sometimes an abscess with pus. Treatment: A topical or oral antibiotic drug.	**paronychia** (PAR-oh-NIH-kee-ah) **par-** *beside* **onych/o-** *fingernail; toenail* **-ia** *condition; state; thing*

Laboratory and Diagnostic Procedures

Word or Phrase	Description	Pronunciation/Word Parts
allergy skin testing	Test in which antigens (animal dander, foods, plants, pollen, etc.) in a liquid form are given by **intradermal** injections into the skin. If the patient is allergic to a particular antigen, a wheal will form at the site of that injection (see Figure 7-25 ■). Alternatively, the antigen is scratched into the skin, and the procedure is known as a **scratch test**.	**intradermal** (IN-trah-DER-mal) **intra-** *within* **derm/o-** *skin* **-al** *pertaining to*

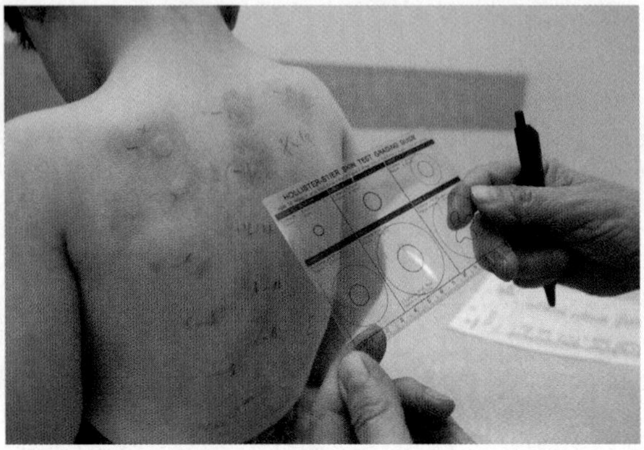

FIGURE 7-25 ■ Allergy skin testing.
This patient's back shows a number of wheals where the body's immune response was triggered by the injected antigens. The size of the wheal corresponds to the degree of allergy to that antigen. No wheal formation means that the patient is not allergic to that antigen.
Source: Joseph Songco / Alamy

Word or Phrase	Description	Pronunciation/Word Parts
culture and sensitivity (C&S)	Test in which a specimen of the **exudates** from an ulcer, wound, burn, or laceration or the pus from an infection is cultured in a Petri dish. The bacterium in it grows into colonies, is identified to make a diagnosis, and is tested to determine its sensitivity to specific antibiotic drugs.	**sensitivity** (SEN-sih-TIV-ih-tee) **sensitiv/o-** *affected by; sensitive to* **-ity** *condition; state* **exudate** (EKS-yoo-dayt) **exud/o-** *oozing fluid* **-ate** *composed of; pertaining to*
RAST	Blood test that measures the amount of IgE produced each time the blood is mixed with a specific allergen. It shows which of many allergens the patient is allergic to and how severe the allergy is. RAST stands for *radioallergosorbent test*. A newer, more sensitive test is the ImmunoCAP Specific IgE test.	
skin scraping	Test in which a skin scraping is done with the edge of a scalpel to obtain cellular material from a skin lesion. It is examined under a microscope to make a diagnosis of ringworm.	
Tzanck test	Test in which a skin scraping is done to obtain fluid from a vesicle. A smear of the fluid is placed on a slide, stained, and examined under a microscope. Herpes virus infections and shingles show characteristic giant cells with viruses in them.	**Tzanck** (TSANGK)
Wood's lamp or light	Test that uses ultraviolet light to highlight areas of skin abnormality. In a darkened room, ultraviolet light makes vitiligo appear bright white and tinea capitus (ringworm) appear blue-green because the fungus fluoresces (glows).	

Medical and Surgical Procedures

Medical Procedures		
Word or Phrase	**Description**	**Pronunciation/Word Parts**
Botox injections	Procedure in which the drug Botox is injected into the muscle to release deep wrinkle lines on the face (see Figure 7-26 ■). The drug keeps the muscle from contracting and wrinkling the skin. This treatment is only effective for several months.	**Botox** (BOH-tawks)
collagen injections	Procedure in which a liquid containing collagen is injected into wrinkles or acne scars. This plumps the skin and decreases the depth of the wrinkle or scar. The collagen is from cow or human sources.	
cryosurgery	Procedure in which liquid nitrogen is sprayed or painted onto a wart, mole, or other benign lesion, or onto a small malignant lesion. The liquid nitrogen freezes and destroys the lesion.	**cryosurgery** (KRY-oh-SER-jer-ee) **cry/o-** cold **surg/o-** operative procedure **-ery** process
curettage	Procedure that uses a **curet** to scrape off a superficial skin lesion. A curet is a metal instrument that ends in a small, circular or oval ring with a sharp edge. Curettage is often combined with electrodesiccation for complete removal of a lesion.	**curettage** (kyoor-eh-TAWZH) **curet** (kyoor-ET)
debridement	Procedure in which necrotic tissue is debrided (removed) from a burn, wound, or ulcer. This is done to prevent infection from developing, to assess the extent or depth of a wound, or to create a clean, raw surface that is ready to heal or receive a skin graft. Mechanical debridement consists of putting on a wet dressing, letting it dry, removing the dressing, and pulling off necrotic tissue with it. Topical enzyme drugs debride by chemically dissolving necrotic tissue. Surgical debridement is done under anesthesia using a scalpel, scissors, or curet.	**debridement** (deh-BREED-maw) *Note:* This pronunciation reflects the French origin of this word.

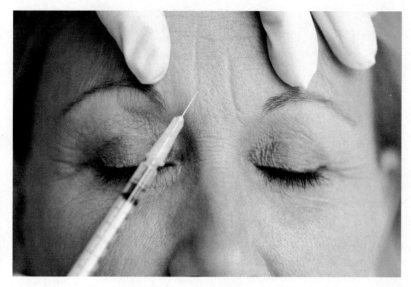

FIGURE 7-26 ■ Botox injection.
The drug Botox is actually a diluted neurotoxin from the bacterium *Clostridium botulinum* type A that causes food poisoning (botulism) and is present in canned goods with bulging ends.
Source: Alamy

Word or Phrase	Description	Pronunciation/Word Parts

electrosurgery	Procedure that involves the use of electrical current to remove a nevus, wart, skin tag, or small malignant lesion. The electrical current passes through an electrode and evaporates the intracellular contents of the lesion.
	
	In **fulguration**, the electrode is held away from the skin and transmits a spark to the skin surface. In **electrodesiccation**, the electrode is touched to or inserted into the skin or lesion. **Electrosection** uses a wire loop electrode to cut out the lesion.
		electrosurgery
		(ee-LEK-troh-SER-jer-ee)
		  electr/o- *electricity*
		  surg/o- *operative procedure*
		  -ery *process*
		
		fulguration (FUL-gyoor-AA-shun)
		  fulgur/o- *spark of electricity*
		  -ation *being; having; process*
		
		electrodesiccation
		(ee-LEK-troh-DES-ih-KAY-shun)
		  electr/o- *electricity*
		  desicc/o- *dry up*
		  -ation *being; having; process*
		
		electrosection
		(ee-LEK-troh-SEK-shun)
		  electr/o- *electricity*
		  sect/o- *cut*
		  -ion *action; condition*

incision and drainage (I&D)	Procedure to treat a cyst or abscess. A scalpel is used to make an incision, and the fluid or pus inside is expressed manually or allowed to drain out.	**incision** (in-SIH-zhun)
		  incis/o- *cut into*
		  -ion *action; condition*

laser surgery	Procedure that uses pulses of laser light to remove birthmarks, tattoos, enlarged superficial blood vessels (acne rosacea), or unwanted hair. A tunable laser has a specific wavelength of light that only reacts with certain colors (the dark red of a birthmark, the black pigment of a tattoo, etc.) to break up that color and the structure that contains it. Surrounding tissue of a different color is unharmed.	**laser** (LAY-zer) *Laser* is an acronym, a word made from the first letters of the phrase *l*ight *a*mplification by *s*timulated *e*mission of *r*adiation.
skin examination	Procedure to examine all of the patient's skin or just one skin lesion, rash, or tumor. The dermatologist uses a lens to magnify the area (see Figure 7-27 ■).	

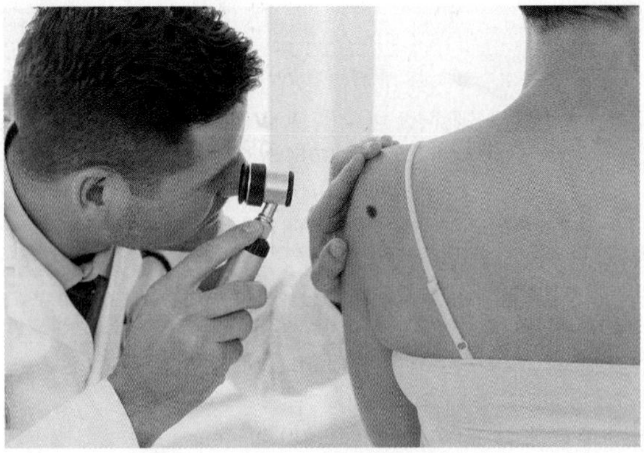

FIGURE 7-27 ■ **Skin examination.**
This dermatologist is using a magnifying lens to examine a lesion on this patient's skin. The area may need to be biopsied to obtain a diagnosis.
Source: Wavebreakmedia/Shutterstock

Word or Phrase	Description	Pronunciation/Word Parts
skin resurfacing	Procedure that removes superficial or deep acne scars, fine or deep wrinkles, or tattoos, or corrects large pores and skin tone irregularities to promote the regrowth of smooth skin	
chemical peel	Skin resurfacing that uses an acid liquid to remove the epidermis. The strongest chemical peels are done in surgery.	
dermabrasion	Skin resurfacing that uses a rapidly spinning wire brush or diamond surface to mechanically abrade (scrape away) the epidermis.	**dermabrasion** (DER-mah-BRAY-zhun) **derm/o-** *skin* **abras/o-** *scrape off* **-ion** *action; condition*
laser skin resurfacing	Skin resurfacing that uses a computer-controlled laser to vaporize the epidermis and some of the dermis. It is also known as a **laser peel**.	
microderm-abrasion	Skin resurfacing that uses aluminum oxide crystals to abrade and remove the epidermis	**microdermabrasion** (MY-kroh-DER-mah-BRAY-zhun) **micr/o-** *one millionth; small* **derm/o-** *skin* **abras/o-** *scrape off* **-ion** *action; condition*
suturing	Procedure that uses sutures to bring the edges of the skin together after a laceration or other injury or at the end of a surgical procedure (see Figure 7-28 ■)	

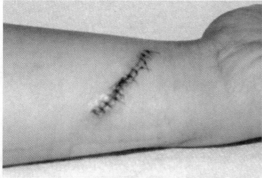

FIGURE 7-28 ■ Layered closure with sutures.
After an anesthetic drug was given to numb the area, this laceration in the forearm was sewn closed with two layers of sutures, the first in the deeper tissues and the second to close the skin edges. After a week, the skin sutures were removed. The deeper sutures, which were made of a material that was absorbed by the body, did not need to be removed.
Source: Susan M. Turley

Surgical Procedures

Word or Phrase	Description	Pronunciation/Word Parts
biopsy (Bx)	Procedure done in a dermatologist's office or the hospital to remove all or part of a skin lesion or tumor (see Figure 7-29 ■). The biopsy specimen is sent to the pathology department for examination under a microscope to obtain a diagnosis.	**biopsy** (BY-awp-see) **bi/o-** *life; living organism; living tissue* **-opsy** *process of viewing*
excisional biopsy	Procedure that uses a scalpel to remove an entire skin lesion or tumor	**excisional** (ek-SIH-zhun-al) **excis/o-** *cut out* **-ion** *action; condition* **-al** *pertaining to*
incisional biopsy	Procedure that uses a scalpel to make an incision to remove part of a skin lesion or tumor	**incisional** (in-SIH-zhun-al) **incis/o-** *cut into* **-ion** *action; condition* **-al** *pertaining to*

Word or Phrase	Description	Pronunciation/Word Parts
needle aspiration	Procedure that uses a needle to aspirate the fluid and cells from a cyst	**aspiration** (AS-pih-RAY-shun) **aspir/o-** *breathe in; suck in* **-ation** *being; having; process*
punch biopsy	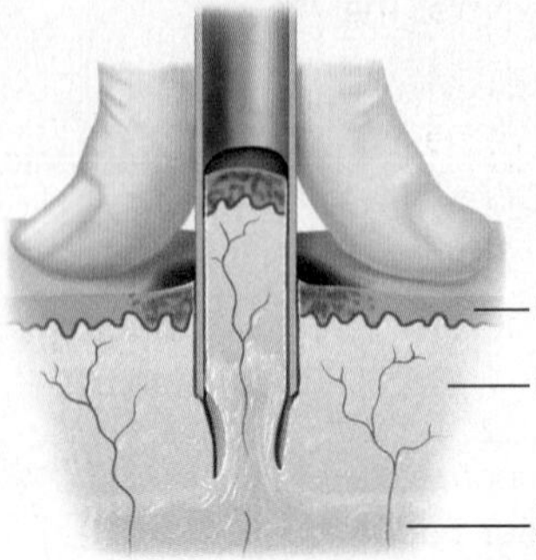 FIGURE 7-29 ■ **Punch biopsy.** A punch biopsy uses a circular metal cutter to remove a plug-shaped core that includes the epidermis, dermis, and subcutaneous tissue. *Source*: Pearson Education	
shave biopsy	Procedure that uses a scalpel or razor blade to shave off a superficial lesion in the epidermis or dermis	
dermatoplasty	Procedure of any type that requires plastic surgery to the skin, such as skin grafting, removal of a keloid, facelift, etc.	**dermatoplasty** (DER-mah-toh-PLAS-tee) **dermat/o-** *skin* **-plasty** *process of reshaping by surgery*
liposuction	Procedure to remove excessive adipose tissue deposits from the breasts, abdomen, hips, legs, or buttocks. A cannula inserted through a small incision is used to suction out the subcutaneous tissue (see Figure 7-30 ■). Ultrasonic-assisted liposuction uses ultrasonic waves to break up the fatty tissue before it is removed. This is also known as **suction-assisted lipectomy**. 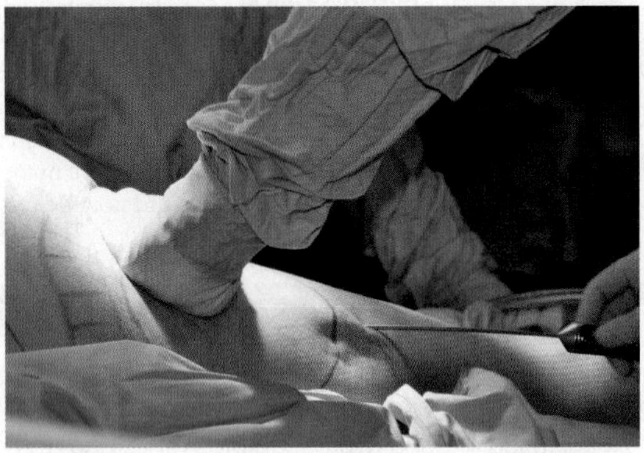 FIGURE 7-30 ■ **Liposuction.** This plastic surgeon is performing liposuction to remove fat from the thigh. Lines drawn on the skin show the areas of greatest fat deposit. Both legs will be done to achieve a symmetrical result. *Source*: Daleen Loest/Shutterstock	**liposuction** (LIP-oh-SUK-shun) **lip/o-** *fat; lipid* **suct/o-** *suck* **-ion** *action; condition* **lipectomy** (ly-PEK-toh-mee) **lip/o-** *fat; lipid* **-ectomy** *surgical removal*
Mohs' surgery	Procedure to remove skin cancer, particularly tumors with irregular shapes and depths. An operating microscope is used during the surgery to examine each layer of excised tissue. If the tissue shows cancerous cells, more tissue is removed until no trace of cancer remains.	**Mohs'** (MOHZ)
rhytidectomy	Procedure to remove wrinkles and tighten loose, aging skin on the face and neck. It is also known as a **facelift**. A **blepharoplasty**, the removal of fat and drooping skin from around the eyelids, is often done at the same time.	**rhytidectomy** (RIH-tih-DEK-toh-mee) **rhytid/o-** *wrinkle* **-ectomy** *surgical removal* **blepharoplasty** (BLEF-ah-roh-PLAS-tee) **blephar/o-** *eyelid* **-plasty** *process of reshaping by surgery*

Word or Phrase	Description	Pronunciation/Word Parts
skin grafting	Procedure that uses human, animal, or artificial skin to provide a temporary covering or a permanent layer of skin over a burn or wound. A **dermatome** is used to remove (harvest) a thin layer of skin to be used as a graft. A split-thickness skin graft contains the epidermis and part of the dermis. A full-thickness skin graft contains the epidermis and all of the dermis. Tiny holes can be cut in the skin graft to make a mesh that can stretch and cover a larger area. These holes allow draining tissue fluid to flow out and provide spaces into which the new skin can grow.	**dermatome** (DER-mah-tohm) **derm/a-** *skin* **-tome** *area with distinct edges; instrument used to cut*
allograft	Skin graft that is taken from a cadaver. It is frozen and stored in a skin bank until needed. This is a temporary skin graft to protect the skin and prevent infection and fluid loss.	**allograft** (AL-oh-graft) **all/o-** *other; strange* **-graft** *tissue for implant; tissue for transplant*
autograft	Skin graft that is taken from another part of the patient's own body. This is a permanent skin graft.	**autograft** (AW-toh-graft) **aut/o-** *self* **-graft** *tissue for implant; tissue for transplant*
synthetic skin graft	Skin graft that is made from collagen fibers arranged in a lattice pattern. The patient's body does not reject synthetic skin, and healing skin grows into it as the graft gradually disintegrates.	
xenograft	Skin graft of just the dermis that is taken from an animal (pig). This is a temporary skin graft to protect the skin and prevent infection and fluid loss.	**xenograft** (ZEN-oh-graft) **xen/o-** *foreign* **-graft** *tissue for implant; tissue for transplant*

WORD ALERT

HOMONYMS

dermatome   (noun)   a specific area of the skin that sends sensory information to the spinal cord

   Example: The patient had shingles on the chest and back along the T6 dermatome.

dermatome   (noun)   a surgical instrument used to make a shallow, continuous cut to form a skin graft

   Example: After the donor site was prepped and draped, a dermatome was used to obtain a split-thickness skin graft.

DID YOU KNOW?

The skin of frogs and lizards were used as skin grafts in the 1600s.

Drugs

These drug categories and drugs are used to treat integumentary diseases. The most common generic and trade name drugs in each category are listed.

Category	Indication	Examples	Pronunciation/Word Parts
anesthetic drugs	Provide temporary numbness of the skin to treat injuries and skin diseases or to remove skin lesions. They are applied topically or injected.	lidocaine (Lidoderm, Xylocaine)	**anesthetic** (AN-es-THEH-tik) **an-** *not; without* **esthet/o-** *feeling; sensation* **-ic** *pertaining to*
antibiotic drugs	Treat bacterial infections of the skin or acne vulgaris. They are applied topically or given orally.	bacitracin, neomycin, erythromycin (Emgel, Eryderm); oral tetracycline (Sumycin)	**antibiotic** (AN-tee-by-AW-tik) (AN-tih-by-AW-tik) **anti-** *against* **bi/o-** *life; living organism; living tissue* **-tic** *pertaining to*
antifungal drugs	Treat ringworm (tinea) when applied topically. Treat fungal infections of the nails when applied topically or given orally.	clotrimazole (Cruex, Desenex, Lotrimin AF), efinaconazole (Jublia), tavaborole (Kerydin), tolnaftate (Aftate, Tinactin); oral ketoconazole (Nizoral)	**antifungal** (AN-tee-FUN-gal) (AN-tih-FUN-gal) **anti-** *against* **fung/o-** *fungus* **-al** *pertaining to*
antipruritic drugs	Decrease itching. They are applied topically or given orally.	diphenhydramine (Benadryl); topical colloidal oatmeal (Aveeno)	**antipruritic** (AN-tee-proo-RIH-tik) (AN-tih-proo-RIH-tik) **anti-** *against* **prurit/o-** *itching* **-ic** *pertaining to*
antiviral drugs	Treat herpes simplex virus infections. They are applied topically or given orally.	docosanol (Abreva), acyclovir (Zovirax); oral famciclovir (Famvir)	**antiviral** (AN-tee-VY-ral) (AN-tih-VY-ral) **anti-** *against* **vir/o-** *virus* **-al** *pertaining to*
coal tar drugs	Treat psoriasis. They cause the epidermal cells to multiply more slowly and decrease itching. Coal tar is a by-product of the processing of bituminous coal. It contains more than 10,000 different chemicals. It is applied topically.	coal tar (Balnetar, Neutrogena T/Gel, Zetar)	
corticosteroid drugs	Treat skin inflammation from contact dermatitis, psoriasis, and eczema. They are applied topically or given orally.	fluocinonide (Lidex), hydrocortisone (Dermolate); oral prednisone	**corticosteroid** (KOR-tih-koh-STAIR-oyd) **cortic/o-** *cortex; outer region* **-steroid** *steroid*
drugs for alopecia	Applied topically to dilate the arteries in the scalp to increase blood flow and hair growth. Given orally to block the production of DHT.	topical minoxidil (Rogaine); oral finasteride (Propecia)	
drugs for infestations	Treat scabies (mites) and pediculosis (lice). Lotion and shampoo.	lindane, malathion (Ovide)	

Category	Indication	Examples	Pronunciation/Word Parts
photodynamic therapy (PDT)	Treats cancer of the skin with laser light and a photosensitizing drug.	porfimer (Photofrin)	**photodynamic** (FOH-toh-dy-NAM-ik) **phot/o-** *light* **dynam/o-** *movement; power* **-ic** *pertaining to*
psoralen drugs	Treat psoriasis. Psoralen sensitizes the skin to ultraviolet light therapy and it damages cellular DNA and decreases the rate of cell division. This combination is known as PUVA (psoralen drug and ultraviolet A light)	methoxsalen (Oxsoralen)	**psoralen** (SOR-ah-len)
vitamin A–type drugs	Treat acne vulgaris or severe cystic acne. They cause the epidermal cells to multiply rapidly to keep the pores from becoming clogged. Applied topically or given orally.	topical tretinoin (Retin-A); oral isotretinoin	

CLINICAL CONNECTIONS

Pharmacology. The administration of drugs often involves the skin. **Topical** drugs such as creams, lotions, and ointments are absorbed into the skin for a local drug effect. **Transdermal** drug patches release small amounts of a drug over time that are absorbed through the skin and exert a systemic effect. The **intradermal** route uses a needle inserted just beneath the epidermis. This is used for the Mantoux tuberculosis test and allergy testing. Other types are **hypodermic** injections because the needle goes below the dermis and into the subcutaneous tissue (see Figure 7-31 ■) or the muscle.

topical (TOP-ih-kal)
  topic/o- *specific area*
  -al *pertaining to*

transdermal (trans-DER-mal)
  trans- *across; through*
  derm/o- *skin*
  -al *pertaining to*

intradermal (IN-trah-DER-mal)
  intra- *within*
  derm/o- *skin*
  -al *pertaining to*

hypodermic (HY-poh-DER-mik)
  hypo- *below; deficient*
  derm/o- *skin*
  -ic *pertaining to*

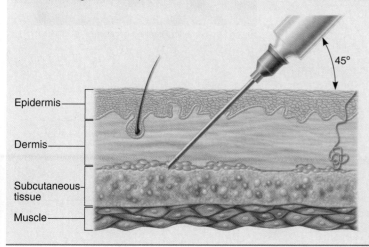

Epidermis
Dermis
Subcutaneous tissue
Muscle
45°

FIGURE 7-31 ■ Subcutaneous injection.
Source: Pearson Education

Abbreviations

BX, Bx	biopsy	**PUVA**	psoralen (drug and) ultraviolet A (light therapy)
C&S	culture and sensitivity	**SLE**	systemic lupus erythematosus
Ca	cancer (pronounced "c-a")	**SQ*■**	subcutaneous
Derm	dermatology (short form)	**subcu**	subcutaneous (short form)
HSV	herpes simplex virus	**subQ■**	subcutaneous (short form)
I&D	incision and drainage	**UVB**	ultraviolet light B
PDT	photodynamic therapy		

*According to The Joint Commission and ■ the Institute for Safe Medication Practices (ISMP), this abbreviation should not be used. Because it is still used by some healthcare professionals, it is included here.

IT'S GREEK TO ME!

Did you notice that some words have two different combining forms? Combining forms from both Greek and Latin remain a part of medical language today.

Word	Greek	Latin	Medical Word Examples
fat	lip/o-	adip/o-	lipocyte, adipose tissue, adipocere
hair or hairy	trich/o-	hirsut/o-, pil/o-	schizotrichia, hirsutism, pilonidal cyst, piloerection
itching	psor/o-	prurit/o-	psoriasis, pruritic
nail	onych/o-	ungu/o-	onychomycosis, ungual
skin	derm/a-, derm/o-	cutane/o-, cut/i-	dermatome, dermal, subcutaneous, cuticle
	dermat/o-	integument/o-	dermatologist, integumentary
sweating or sweat	diaphor/o-	hidr/o-, sudor/i-	diaphoresis, anhidrosis, sudoriferous gland

CAREER FOCUS

Meet Toral, a physician's assistant in a cosmetic surgeon's office

"Growing up, I always knew I would be in medicine. At first, I entertained the idea of becoming a nurse. Then I entertained the idea of becoming a physician. Being a physician's assistant allows me to see my own patients, treat and diagnose, write my own prescriptions, care for patients, and advise them. I also assist in laser procedures and all surgical procedures. Our everyday language is medical terminology—from talking to the physician, talking to your coworkers, to charting in the charts. With so many patients being Internet-savvy, they come in talking in medical terminology!"

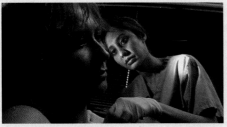

Source: Dan Frank for Pearson Education/PH College

Physician's assistants are physician extenders who are licensed to perform basic medical care while under the supervision of a physician. They perform physical examinations, prescribe drugs, and perform minor surgery. They can assist the physician during more extensive surgery. They work in physicians' offices, clinics, and hospitals.

Dermatologists are physicians who practice in the medical specialty of dermatology. They diagnose and treat patients with diseases of the skin. Physicians can take additional training and become board certified in the subspecialty of pediatric dermatology. Malignancies of the skin are treated medically by an oncologist or surgically by a dermatologist, a general surgeon, or a plastic surgeon.

Plastic surgeons are physicians who perform plastic and reconstructive surgery to reshape the body. They remove lesions and scars and perform liposuction and other procedures that reshape the skin and subcutaneous tissue.

dermatologist (DER-mah-TAW-loh-jist)
  dermat/o- *skin*
  log/o- *study of; word*
  -ist *person who specializes in; thing that specializes in*

plastic (PLAS-tik)
  plast/o- *formation; growth*
  -ic *pertaining to*

surgeon (SER-jun)
  surg/o- *operative procedure*
  -eon *person who performs*

MyMedicalTerminologyLab™ To see Toral's complete video profile, log into MyMedicalTerminologyLab and navigate to the Multimedia Library for Chapter 7. Check the Video box, and then click the Career Focus - Physician Assistant link.

Definition of the Medical Word   **Build the Medical Word**

6. Tumor (of the cell that produces) black (pigment) _____

7. Condition (of the skin being) blue _____

8. Infection of (or) inflammation of (the) skin _____

9. Pertaining to itching _____

10. Tumor (of) fat _____

11. Growth (that is) new _____

12. Pertaining to redness (of the skin) _____

13. Pertaining to dead cells or dead tissue _____

14. Condition (of having) lice _____

15. (Scar that becomes larger until it is) resembling (a) tumor _____

16. Condition (of) bruising _____

17. Composed of oozing fluid _____

18. Process (on the skin that uses a) spark of electricity _____

19. Process of (removing and) viewing living tissue
    (with a microscope) _____

20. Surgical removal (of) fat _____

21. Instrument used to cut (the) skin _____

22. Process of reshaping by surgery (the) eyelid(s) _____

23. Surgical removal (of) wrinkle(s) _____

24. Tissue for implant or transplant (that is taken from one's own) self _____

PREFIX EXERCISE

Read the definition of the medical word. Look at the medical word or partial word that is given (it already contains a combining form and a suffix). Select the correct prefix from the Prefix List and write it on the blank line. Then build the medical word and write it on the line. Be sure to check your spelling. The first one has been done for you.

PREFIX LIST		
an- (not; without)	de- (reversal of; without)	intra- (within)
anti- (against)	dys- (abnormal; difficult; painful)	pre- (before; in front of)

Definition of the Medical Word	Prefix	Word or Partial Word	Build the Medical Word
1. Pertaining to (a drug that is) against fungus	anti-	fungal	antifungal
2. Pertaining to (an) abnormal formation or growth	_____	plastic	_____
3. Condition (of being) without feeling or sensation	_____	esthesia	_____
4. Process (of having) reversal of pigment (in the skin)	_____	pigmentation	_____
5. Condition (of being) without sweat	_____	hidrosis	_____
6. Pertaining to within (the) skin	_____	dermal	_____
7. Pertaining to (being) before cancer	_____	malignant	_____
8. Pertaining to (a drug that is) against itching	_____	pruritic	_____

7.7A Spell Medical Words

ENGLISH AND MEDICAL WORD EQUIVALENTS EXERCISE

For each English word or phrase, write its equivalent medical word. Be sure to check your spelling. The first one has been done for you.

English Word	Medical Word	English Word	Medical Word
1. cradle cap	*eczema*	8. infestation with lice	
2. age spots or liver spots		9. infestation with mites	
3. baldness		10. port-wine stain	
4. bed sore		11. ringworm	
5. boil		12. skin tag	
6. brush burn		13. wart	
7. hives			

HEARING MEDICAL WORDS EXERCISE

You hear someone speaking the medical words given below. Read each pronunciation and then write the medical word it represents. Be sure to check your spelling. The first one has been done for you.

1. AK-nee vul-GAIR-is	*acne vulgaris*	6. deh-BREED-maw	
2. AN-ah-fih-LAK-sis		7. DER-mah-TAW-loh-jist	
3. BLEF-ah-roh-PLAS-tee		8. AIR-eh-THEM-ah-tus	
4. KRY-oh-SER-jer-ee		9. proo-RY-tus	
5. SY-ah-NOH-sis		10. sor-EYE-ah-sis	

7.7B Pronounce Medical Words

PRONUNCIATION EXERCISE

Read the medical word and the syllables in its pronunciation. Circle the primary (main) accented syllable. The first one has been done for you.

1. abrasion (ah-**bray**-zhun)
2. adipose (ad-ih-pohs)
3. alopecia (al-oh-pee-sha)
4. biopsy (by-awp-see)
5. cellulitis (sel-yoo-ly-tis)
6. hematoma (hee-mah-toh-mah)
7. liposuction (lip-oh-suk-shun)
8. neoplasm (nee-oh-plazm)
9. psoriasis (sor-eye-ah-sis)
10. subcutaneous (sub-kyoo-tay-nee-us)

7.8 Research Medical Words

ON THE JOB CHALLENGE EXERCISE

On the job, you will encounter new medical words. Practice your medical language skills by looking up the medical words in bold and writing their definitions on the lines.

OFFICE CHART NOTE

This 11-year-old young lady was brought in by her mother. The mother states that the patient continually bites her fingernails despite all attempts to discourage her. Her fingernails are always bitten to the quick, and the skin around them is frequently bloody. The patient states she is unable to stop. When the mother stepped out of the examining room, the patient became tearful as she related pressure at school and an impending divorce between her parents.

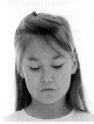
Source: Iko/Fotolia

On examination, the fingernails show evidence of chronic biting, right hand greater than left. The patient is right handed. Examination of the feet also shows evidence of nail biting. There is erythema and swelling of the tissue along the medial nail groove of her right great toe where the nail was bitten away and is growing back but is ingrown. The skin on the lower arms bilaterally shows aggressive scratching of small, isolated insect bites. The scalp shows some small, patchy areas where there is an absence of hair. The patient admits to some hair-pulling.

DIAGNOSES

1. Onychophagia.

2. Onychocryptosis.

3. Trichotillomania.

Plan: The medial side of the nail on the right great toe was trimmed with clippers. The patient's mother was given a prescription for a 7-day course of an antibiotic drug. The patient's mother was also given a referral for the patient to see a child psychologist for counseling.

---

1. onychophagia _____

2. onychocryptosis _____

3. trichotillomania _____

SOUND-ALIKE WORDS

Compare and contrast the medical meanings of these sound-alike dermatology words.

1. The two meanings of *dermatome*

2. *adipose tissue* and *adipocere*

3. *excoriation* and *exfoliation*

7.9 Analyze Medical Reports

ELECTRONIC PATIENT RECORD

This is an Office Visit Note. Read the note and answer the questions.

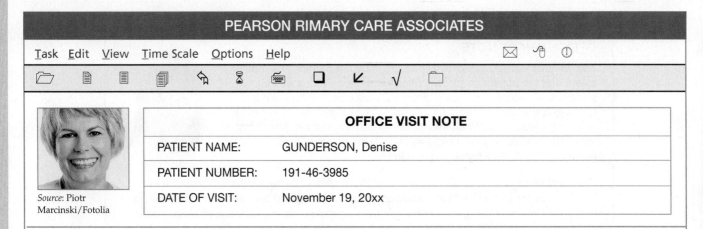

PEARSON RIMARY CARE ASSOCIATES

Task   Edit   View   Time Scale   Options   Help

OFFICE VISIT NOTE

PATIENT NAME:	GUNDERSON, Denise
PATIENT NUMBER:	191-46-3985
DATE OF VISIT:	November 19, 20xx

Source: Piotr Marcinski/Fotolia

HISTORY

The patient has been on the antibiotic drug Zithromax for a severe skin flare-up of erythema nodosum following an untreated strep throat. This caused swelling and edema in her right foot, but it then spread to her right leg, areas on her chest, left knee, and her left foot. These areas were extremely painful, erythematous, and her right knee developed a large, painful nodule under the skin. Her right foot was so painful and edematous that it was nearly impossible for her to walk. Then the dorsum of her right foot developed cellulitis, and she was placed on the antibiotic drug Zithromax. Today, she had just taken her last scheduled dose of Zithromax when she describes that she suddenly had a very itchy scalp. When she scratched her scalp, she could feel multiple raised areas. About 20 minutes later, there were about twice as many raised areas on her scalp, and now she could see wheals on her cheeks and on her chest. When the wheals on her face became large welts, she became concerned about not being able to breathe and took two antihistamine tablets (Benadryl). One hour later, she had to take two more Benadryl. After that, the welts and itching began to subside. Although she was feeling better, she decided to come to the office today to be examined.

PHYSICAL EXAMINATION

Integumentary system: There are a few small, scattered hives still visible on her trunk and arms. The welts on her scalp and face have completely disappeared. The cellulitis of her right foot has cleared up and the smaller nodules from the erythema nodosum have disappeared. The largest nodule over her right knee is slowly resolving.

ASSESSMENT

1. Severe urticaria, secondary to an allergic drug reaction to azithromycin (Zithromax).
2. Right foot cellulitis, resolved.
3. Resolving erythema nodosum following an untreated strep throat.

PLAN

A note has been made in the patient's medical record that she is allergic to Zithromax. The acute phase of this allergic reaction is past. The patient has been instructed to never take that antibiotic drug again. Follow-up as needed for her resolving erythema nodosum.

Bonnie R. Grant, M.D.

Bonnie R. Grant, M.D.

BRG: smt
D: 11/19/xx
T: 11/19/xx

1. Divide *cellulitis* into word parts and give the meaning of each word part.

   Word Part   **Meaning**

   cellul/o-   cell

   -itis   infection of, inflammation of

2. The patient has erythema on her legs. If you wanted to use the adjective form of *erythema*, you would say, "She has erythematous areas on her legs."

3. What is the medical word for *itching*? pruritis

4. Circle the word that means reddened: (**edematous,** **erythematous,** **flare-up**)

5. Which are larger—welts or wheals? welts

6. In the Physical Examination section of this chart note, which body system is examined? Integumentary

7. The patient's urticaria was due to a (**cellulitis,** **drug reaction,** **strep throat**).

8. What four symptoms of urticaria did this patient have?

   hives

   welts

   cellulitis

   erythema nodosum

9. What skin condition did the patient develop after having an untreated strep throat? erythema nodosum

---

MyMedicalTerminologyLab™

MyMedicalTerminologyLab is a premium online homework management system that includes a host of features to help you study. Registered users will find:

- A multitude of quizzes and activities built within the MyLab platform

- Powerful tools that track and analyze your results—allowing you to create a personalized learning experience

- Videos and audio pronunciations to help enrich your progress

- Streaming lesson presentations (Guided Lectures) and self-paced learning modules

- A space where you and your instructor can check your progress and manage your assignments

Chapter 8
Orthopedics

Skeletal System

Orthopedics (OR-thoh-PEE-diks) is the medical specialty that studies the anatomy and physiology of the skeletal and muscular systems and uses laboratory and diagnostic procedures, medical and surgical procedures, and drugs to treat skeletal and muscular diseases. In this chapter, you will study orthopedics from the perspective of the skeletal system. In Chapter 9, you will study the muscular system.

 ## Learning Outcomes

After you study this chapter, you should be able to

8.1 Identify structures of the skeletal system.

8.2 Describe the process of growth.

8.3 Describe common skeletal diseases, laboratory and diagnostic procedures, medical and surgical procedures, and drugs.

8.4 Form the plural and adjective forms of nouns related to orthopedics (skeletal).

8.5 Give the meanings of word parts and abbreviations related to orthopedics (skeletal).

8.6 Divide orthopedic (skeletal) words and build orthopedic (skeletal) words.

8.7 Spell and pronounce orthopedic (skeletal) words.

8.8 Research sound-alike and other orthopedic (skeletal) words.

8.9 Analyze the medical content and meaning of an orthopedic (skeletal) report.

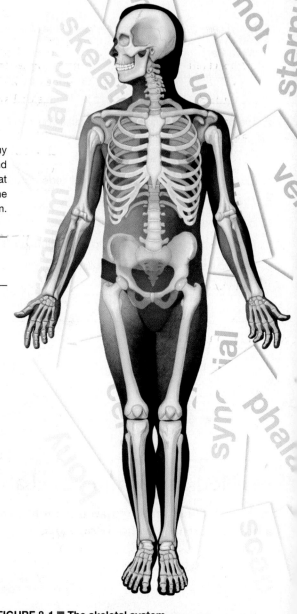

FIGURE 8-1 ■ The skeletal system.
The skeletal system is a widespread, connected system that consi of 206 bones and other structures. It stretches throughout the boc from the top of the head to the tips of the fingers and toes.
Source: Pearson Education

Medical Language Key

To unlock the definition of a medical word, break it into word parts. Give the meaning of each word part. Put the meanings of the word parts in order, beginning with the meaning of the suffix, then the prefix (if present), then the combining form(s).

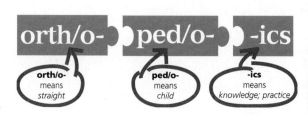

	Word Part	Word Part Meaning
Suffix	-ics	*knowledge; practice*
Combining Form	orth/o-	*straight*
Combining Form	ped/o-	*child*

Orthopedics: ▸ *Knowledge and practice (of producing) straight(ness of the bones and muscles in a) child (or adult).*

Anatomy and Physiology

The **skeletal system** is the **bony** framework on which the body is built. The **skeleton** is composed of 206 bones as well as cartilage and ligaments (see Figure 8-1 ■). The purpose of the skeletal system is to provide structural support for the body, work with the muscles to maintain body posture and produce movement, and protect the body's internal organs. The skeletal system is also known as the **skeletomuscular system** or **musculoskeletal system** because of the close working relationship between the bones and muscles.

Anatomy of the Skeletal System

Axial and Appendicular Skeleton

The skeleton can be divided into two areas: the axial skeleton and the appendicular skeleton. The **axial skeleton** forms the central bony structure of the body around which other parts move. It consists of the bones of the head, chest, and back. The **appendicular skeleton** consists of the bones of the shoulders, upper extremities, hips, and lower extremities.

Bones of the Head

The **skull** is the bony structure of the head. It includes both the cranium and facial bones.

CRANIUM The **cranium** is the domelike bone at the top of the head. Within the cranium is the **cranial cavity**, which contains the brain and other structures. There are eight bones in the cranium (see Figure 8-2 ■ and Figure 8-3 ■). A **suture** is the joint where two cranial bones meet. The **frontal bone** forms the forehead and top of the cranium and ends at the **coronal suture** (see Figure 8-14). The two **parietal bones** form the upper sides and posterior parts of the cranium. Between these bones is the sagittal suture, which runs from front to back. The **occipital bone** forms the posterior base of the cranium. It contains the **foramen magnum**, a large, round opening through which the spinal cord passes to join the brain. The two **temporal bones** form the lower sides of the cranium. Each temporal bone contains an opening for the external ear canal. The **mastoid process** is a projection from the temporal bone just behind the ear. The inferior temporal bone ends in the sharp **styloid process**, a point of attachment for ligaments to the hyoid bone in the anterior neck. The **sphenoid bone**, a large, irregularly shaped bone, forms part of the central base and sides of the cranium and the posterior walls of

Pronunciation/Word Parts

skeletal (SKEL-eh-tal)
　skelet/o- *skeleton*
　-al *pertaining to*

bony (BOH-nee)
Osseous and *osteal* are also adjectives for *bone*. The combining forms **osse/o-** and **oste/o-** mean *bone*.

skeleton (SKEL-eh-ton)

skeletomuscular
(SKEL-eh-toh-MUS-kyoo-lar)
　skelet/o- *skeleton*
　muscul/o- *muscle*
　-ar *pertaining to*

musculoskeletal
(MUS-kyoo-loh-SKEL-eh-tal)
　muscul/o- *muscle*
　skelet/o- *skeleton*
　-al *pertaining to*

axial (AK-see-al)
　axi/o- *axis*
　-al *pertaining to*

appendicular (AP-en-DIH-kyoo-lar)
　appendicul/o- *limb; small attached part*
　-ar *pertaining to*

skull (SKUHL)

cranium (KRAY-nee-um)

cranial (KRAY-nee-al)
　crani/o- *cranium; skull*
　-al *pertaining to*

suture (SOO-chur)

frontal (FRUN-tal)
　front/o- *front*
　-al *pertaining to*

parietal (pah-RY-eh-tal)
　pariet/o- *wall of a cavity*
　-al *pertaining to*

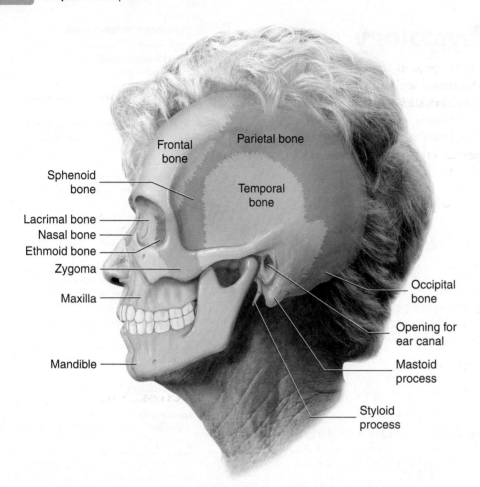

FIGURE 8-2 ■ Lateral view of the bones of the skull.
All of the cranial bones and most of the facial bones (except the vomer and palatine bones) can be seen in this lateral view.
Source: Pearson Education

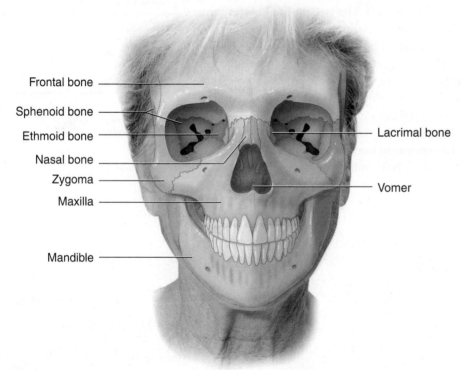

FIGURE 8-3 ■ Frontal view of the bones of the skull.
The facial bones connect to each other and to the bones of the cranium.
Source: Pearson Education

Pronunciation/Word Parts

occipital (awk-SIH-pih-tal)
  occipit/o- *back of the head; occiput*
  -al *pertaining to*

foramen magnum
(foh-RAY-min MAG-num)

temporal (TEM-poh-ral)
  tempor/o- *side of the head; temple*
  -al *pertaining to*

process (PRAW-ses)

styloid (STY-loyd)
  styl/o- *stake*
  -oid *resembling*

mastoid (MAS-toyd)
  mast/o- *breast; mastoid process*
  -oid *resembling*
This rounded, downward-pointing bone was thought to resemble a breast.

sphenoid (SFEE-noyd)
  sphen/o- *wedge shape*
  -oid *resembling*

the eye sockets. A bony cup in the sphenoid bone holds the pituitary gland (discussed in "Endocrinology," Chapter 14). The **ethmoid bone** forms the posterior nasal septum that divides the nasal cavity into right and left sides and forms the medial walls of the eye sockets. The frontal bone, sphenoid bones, and ethmoid bones all contain hollow sinuses (discussed in "Otolaryngology," Chapter 16).

FACIAL BONES   The facial bones support the nose, cheeks, and lips and protect the eyes and internal structures of the nose, mouth, and upper throat. There are 12 bones in the face (see Figures 8-2 and 8-3). The two **nasal bones** form the bridge of the nose and the roof of the nasal cavity. The **vomer** is a narrow wall of bone that forms the inferior part of the nasal septum and continues posteriorly to join the sphenoid bone. The two **lacrimal bones** are small, flat bones within the eye sockets, near the lacrimal (tear) glands. Each **zygoma** or **zygomatic bone** is a cheek bone that goes to the edge of the eye socket. The **maxilla** is the upper jaw bone. It contains the roots of the upper teeth and two hollow maxillary sinuses. The maxilla consists of two **maxillary bones** fused at the midline. The two **palatine bones** are small, flat bones that form the posterior hard palate. The **mandible** is the lower jaw bone. It is the only movable bone in the skull. The roots of the lower teeth are in the mandible. Each side of the mandible ends in two bony tips; one tip is under the zygoma, while the other tip forms a movable joint (the temporomandibular joint) with the temporal bone just in front of the ear.

CLINICAL CONNECTIONS

Neonatology. When a fetus is in the uterus, the bones of the cranium have large areas of fibrous connective tissue between them. These are **fontanels** (laypersons call these "soft spots") (see Figure 8-4 ■). Fontanels allow the cranial bones to move together as the head goes through the birth canal and move apart as the brain grows during childhood. The bony edges finally fuse together at a suture line, and the cranial bones become immobile in early adulthood.

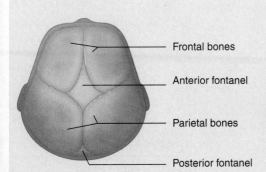

Frontal bones

Anterior fontanel

Parietal bones

Posterior fontanel

FIGURE 8-4 ■ Fontanel.
This fetal cranium shows a large open space (the anterior fontanel) between the two frontal bones and the two parietal bones. The translucent yellow membrane in the fontanel is fibrous connective tissue.
Source: Pearson Education

OTHER BONES OF THE HEAD   There are also three tiny bones in each middle ear: the malleus, incus, and stapes. Collectively, these are known as the **ossicles** or the ossicular chain because they are arranged in a row. They are active in the process of hearing (discussed in "Otolaryngology," Chapter 16).

The **hyoid bone** is a flat, U–shaped bone in the anterior neck. It does not connect directly to any other bones. It is attached by ligaments to the styloid process of each temporal bone.

Pronunciation/Word Parts

ethmoid (ETH-moyd)
   ethm/o- *sieve*
   -oid *resembling*
The ethmoid bone has many small, hollow spaces like a sieve.

nasal (NAY-zal)
   nas/o- *nose*
   -al *pertaining to*

vomer (VOH-mer)

lacrimal (LAK-rih-mal)
   lacrim/o- *tears*
   -al *pertaining to*

zygoma (zy-GOH-mah)

zygomatic (ZY-goh-MAT-ik)

maxilla (mak-SIL-ah)

maxillary (MAK-sih-LAIR-ee)
   maxill/o- *maxilla; upper jaw*
   -ary *pertaining to*

palatine (PAL-ah-tyne)
   palat/o- *palate*
   -ine *pertaining to; thing pertaining to*

mandible (MAN-dih-bl)

mandibular (man-DIH-byoo-lar)
   mandibul/o- *lower jaw; mandible*
   -ar *pertaining to*

fontanel (FAWN-tah-NEL)

ossicle (AW-sih-kl)

hyoid (HY-oyd)
   hy/o- *U-shaped structure*
   -oid *resembling*

Bones of the Chest

The chest contains the **thorax** or **rib cage** (see Figure 8-5 ■). Within the thorax is the **thoracic cavity**, which contains the heart, lungs, and other structures. The **sternum** or **breast bone** is in the center of the anterior thorax. It consists of the triangular-shaped **manubrium**, the body of the sternum, and the inferior tip or **xiphoid process**.

There are 12 pairs of **ribs**. Rib pairs 1–7 (true ribs) are attached to the vertebrae posteriorly and to the sternum anteriorly by **costal cartilage**. Cartilage is a smooth, firm, but flexible connective tissue. The **costochondral joint** is where the cartilage meets the rib. Rib pairs 8–10 (false ribs) are attached to the vertebrae posteriorly, but are only indirectly attached to the sternum by long lengths of costal cartilage. Rib pairs 11 and 12 (floating ribs) are attached to the vertebrae posteriorly but are not attached to the sternum.

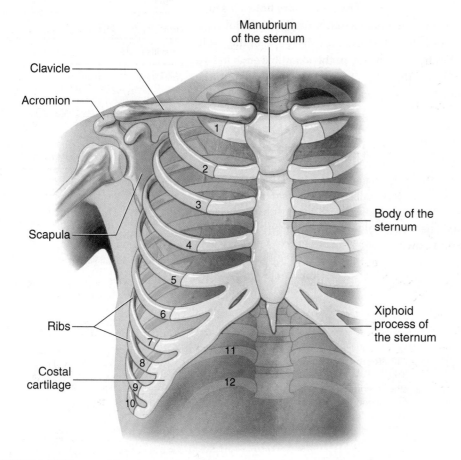

FIGURE 8-5 ■ Bones of the chest and shoulder.
The sternum and ribs form the thorax, a bony cage that protects the heart and lungs. The clavicle and scapula are part of the bones of each shoulder.
Source: Pearson Education

Bones of the Back

The **spine** or **backbone** is a vertical column of bones. It is also known as the **vertebral column** or **spinal column** (see Figure 8-6 ■). The vertebral column supports the weight of the head, neck, and trunk of the body and protects the spinal cord.

The vertebral column contains 24 individual vertebrae, plus the sacrum and coccyx. It is divided into five regions: the cervical vertebrae, the thoracic vertebrae, the lumbar vertebrae, the sacrum, and the coccyx. The **cervical vertebrae** (C1–C7) are in the neck.

Pronunciation/Word Parts

thorax (THOR-aks)

thoracic (thor-AS-ik)
  thorac/o- *chest; thorax*
  -ic *pertaining to*

sternum (STER-num)

sternal (STER-nal)
  stern/o- *breast bone; sternum*
  -al *pertaining to*

manubrium (mah-NOO-bree-um)

xiphoid (ZY-foyd)
  xiph/o- *sword*
  -oid *resembling*

costal (KAW-stal)
  cost/o- *rib*
  -al *pertaining to*
Costal is the adjective for *rib*.

cartilage (KAR-tih-lij)

cartilaginous (KAR-tih-LAJ-ih-nus)
  cartilagin/o- *cartilage*
  -ous *pertaining to*

costochondral (KAW-stoh-CON-dral)
  cost/o- *rib*
  chondr/o- *cartilage*
  -al *pertaining to*

spine (SPYN)

spinal (SPY-nal)
  spin/o- *backbone; spine*
  -al *pertaining to*

vertebral (VER-teh-bral)
  vertebr/o- *vertebra*
  -al *pertaining to*
The combining form **spondyl/o-** also means *vertebra*.

vertebra (VER-teh-brah)

vertebrae (VER-teh-bree)
Vertebra is a Latin singular noun. Form the plural by changing -a to -ae.

cervical (SER-vih-kal)
  cervic/o- *cervix; neck*
  -al *pertaining to*

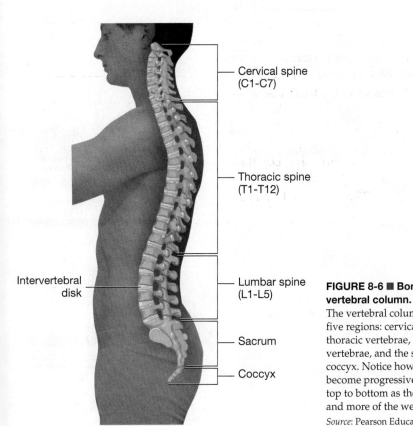

Cervical spine (C1-C7)

Thoracic spine (T1-T12)

Lumbar spine (L1-L5)

Intervertebral disk

Sacrum

Coccyx

FIGURE 8-6 ■ Bones of the vertebral column.
The vertebral column consists of five regions: cervical vertebrae, thoracic vertebrae, lumbar vertebrae, and the sacrum and coccyx. Notice how the vertebrae become progressively larger from top to bottom as they bear more and more of the weight of the body.
Source: Pearson Education

The first cervical vertebra (C1, the **atlas**) is directly below the occipital bone of the cranium. Its appearance is different from the other cervical vertebrae because it must form a joint that allows the head to move up and down. The second cervical vertebra (C2, the **axis**) fits into the atlas to form a joint that allows the head to move from side to side. The **thoracic vertebrae** (T1–T12) are in the chest. Each thoracic vertebra joins with one pair of the 12 pairs of ribs. The **lumbar vertebrae** (L1–L5) are in the lower back. The lumbar vertebrae are larger than the cervical or thoracic vertebrae because they bear the weight of the head, neck, and trunk of the body. The **sacrum** is a group of five fused vertebrae that are not individually numbered, except for the first sacral vertebra (S1). The sacrum joins with the hip bones in the posterior pelvis. The **coccyx** or **tail bone** is a group of several small, fused vertebrae that are not individually numbered.

DID YOU KNOW?
Atlas was the name given to the mythological Greek god who was forced to hold the world on his shoulders. A person's head was imagined as a round globe and therefore the first vertebra was named the *atlas*.

Many of the vertebrae share common features (see Figure 8-8 ■): a vertebral body (circular, flat area), a **spinous process** (a long, bony projection that juts out in the midline along a person's back), two **transverse processes** (bony projections to each side), and a vertebral **foramen** (the hole through which the spinal cord passes). Between most vertebrae are **intervertebral disks**. The outer wall of each disk is fibrocartilage, and the inside is filled with **nucleus pulposus**, a gelatinous substance. The disks act as cushions to absorb the impact during body movements.

atlas (AT-las)

axis (AK-sis)

thoracic (thor-AS-ik)
  thorac/o- *chest; thorax*
  -ic *pertaining to*

lumbar (LUM-bar)
  lumb/o- *area between the ribs and pelvis; lower back*
  -ar *pertaining to*

sacrum (SAY-krum)

sacral (SAY-kral)
  sacr/o- *sacrum*
  -al *pertaining to*

coccyx (KAWK-siks)

coccygeal (kawk-SIH-jee-al)
  coccyg/o- *coccyx; tail bone*
  -eal *pertaining to*

spinous (SPY-nus)
  spin/o- *backbone; spine*
  -ous *pertaining to*

process (PRAW-ses)

transverse (trans-VERS)
  trans- *across; through*
  -verse *travel; turn*
The ending *-verse* contains the combining form *vers/o-* and the one-letter suffix *-e*.

foramen (foh-RAY-min)

intervertebral (IN-ter-VER-teh-bral)
  inter- *between*
  vertebr/o- *vertebra*
  -al *pertaining to*

disk (DISK)

nucleus pulposus
(NOO-klee-us pul-POH-sis)
The nucleus is the central part of an intervertebral disk. *Pulposus* refers to the pulpy consistency of the contents.

DID YOU KNOW?

Andreas Vesalius (1514–1564) was born in Belgium and was educated in medical universities in France and Italy. At that time, medical textbooks contained almost no illustrations. He studied and illustrated a human skeleton by taking down a dead body after a public hanging and dissecting it. His masterpiece, *De Humani Corporis Fabrica (The Structure of the Human Body)*, was published in 1543. Its illustrations showed dissected bodies in natural poses with scenery in the background. These beautiful, highly detailed, anatomically correct, and occasionally whimsical illustrations educated many generations of physicians (see Figure 8-7 ■).

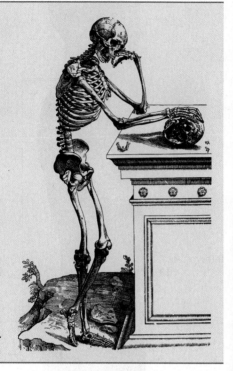

FIGURE 8-7 ■ The skeleton.
An anatomical illustration of the skeleton by Andreas Vesalius.
Source: Pearson Education

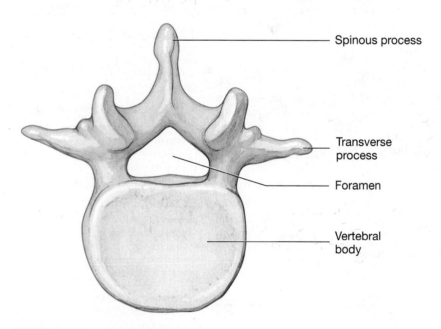

Spinous process

Transverse process

Foramen

Vertebral body

FIGURE 8-8 ■ Lumbar vertebra.
This vertebra shows the wide, flat surface that is characteristic of lumbar vertebrae. The lumbar vertebrae support the weight of the entire upper body.
Source: Andreas Vesalius

Bones of the Shoulders

The shoulder bones include a clavicle and a scapula on the right and left sides (see Figures 8-5 and 8-9 ■). The **clavicle** or **collar bone** is a thin, rod-like bone on each side of the anterior neck. It connects to the manubrium of the sternum and laterally to the scapula. The **scapula** or **shoulder blade** is a triangular-shaped bone on either side of the vertebral column in the upper back. It has a long, bony blade across its upper half that ends in a flat projection (the **acromion**) that connects to the clavicle. The **glenoid fossa**, a shallow depression, is where the head of the humerus (upper arm bone) joins the scapula to make the shoulder joint.

Pronunciation/Word Parts

clavicle (KLAV-ih-kl)

clavicular (klah-VIH-kyoo-lar)
  clavicul/o- *clavicle; collar bone*
  -ar *pertaining to*

scapula (SKAP-yoo-lah)

scapulae (SKAP-yoo-lee)
Scapula is a Latin singular noun. Form the plural by changing *-a* to *-ae*.

scapular (SKAP-yoo-lar)
  scapul/o- *scapula; shoulder blade*
  -ar *pertaining to*

acromion (ah-KROH-mee-on)

glenoid (GLEH-noyd)
  glen/o- *socket of a joint*
  -oid *resembling*

fossa (FAW-sah)

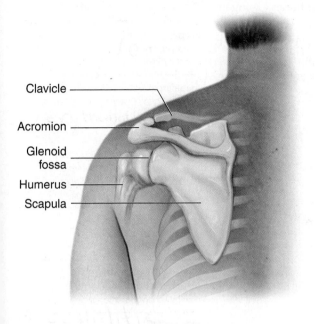

Clavicle

Acromion

Glenoid
fossa

Humerus

Scapula

FIGURE 8-9 ■ Bones of the shoulder.
This posterior view shows the scapula joining the humerous (upper arm bone) at the glenoid fossa. The acromion of the scapula is connected to the clavicle. The scapula itself is not connected to the ribs or vertebral column. This allows it to move freely in several directions as the shoulder moves.
Source: Pearson Education

Bones of the Upper Extremities

UPPER AND LOWER ARM   The upper extremity contains the upper arm and lower arm (forearm) (see Figure 8-10 ■). The **humerus** is the long bone in the upper arm. The head of the humerus fits into the glenoid fossa of the scapula to form the shoulder joint. At its distal end, the humerus joins with both the radius and the ulna to form the elbow joint.

DID YOU KNOW?

The "funny bone" is not a bone at all. The ulnar nerve travels across a rounded, bony projection (medial epicondyle) on the distal humerus. When you accidentally bump this area, you hit the ulnar nerve and send a shock wave (that is in no way "funny") through your entire upper extremity.

The **radius** is one of the two bones in the forearm. It lies on the thumb side of the forearm. At its distal end, it connects to the bones of the wrist. The **ulna** lies on the little finger side of the forearm. At its proximal end is the **olecranon**, a large, square projection that forms the point of the elbow. At its distal end, the ulna also connects to the bones of the wrist.

humerus (HYOO-mer-us)

humeri (HYOO-mer-eye)
Humerus is a Latin singular noun. Form the plural by changing *-us* to *-i.*

humeral (HYOO-mer-al)
  humer/o- *humerus; upper arm bone*
  -al *pertaining to*

radius (RAY-dee-us)

radii (RAY-dee-eye)
Radius is a Latin singular noun. Form the plural by changing *-us* to *-i.*

radial (RAY-dee-al)
  radi/o- *forearm bone; radiation; x-rays*
  -al *pertaining to*
Select the correct combining form meaning to get the definition of *radial: pertaining to the forearm bone (radius).*

ulna (UL-nah)

ulnae (UL-nee)
Ulna is a Latin singular noun. Form the plural by changing *-a* to *-ae.*

ulnar (UL-nar)
  uln/o- *forearm bone; ulna*
  -ar *pertaining to*

olecranon (oh-LEH-krah-non)

WORD ALERT
Sound-Alike Words

humerus	(noun)	bone of the upper arm
		Example: The patient sustained a fracture of the humerus.
humorous	(adjective)	descriptive English word meaning *funny*
		Example: It is not very humorous when you fracture a bone.
humeral	(adjective)	descriptive word for the bone of the upper arm
		Example: The x-ray showed a humeral fracture.
humoral	(adjective)	descriptive word for immunity to infection that comes from antibodies in the blood
		Example: Humoral immunity from infection occurs when B cell lymphocytes attack pathogens.

203
BONE
BANK

PLEASE,
NO MORE
HUMERUS
JOKES

WRIST, HAND, AND FINGERS   The wrist contains eight small **carpal bones** arranged in two rows (see Figure 8-10). One row connects to the radius and ulna. The other row connects to the bones of the hand. Each hand contains five **metacarpal bones**, one for each finger. Each finger contains three **phalangeal bones** or **phalanges** (except the thumb, which contains two), arranged end to end. The distal **phalanx** is the final bone at the very tip of each finger. The fingers are also known as **digits** or **rays**. The metacarpophalangeal (MCP) joint is between a metacarpal bone of the hand and a phalanx. The distal interphalangeal (DIP) joint is between the last two phalanges.

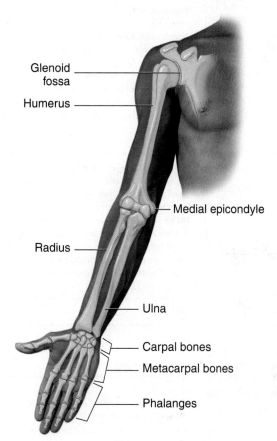

Glenoid fossa
Humerus
Medial epicondyle
Radius
Ulna
Carpal bones
Metacarpal bones
Phalanges

FIGURE 8-10 ■ Bones of the upper extremity.
The humerus of the upper arm joins with both the radius and the ulna, the bones of the forearm. The radius and ulna rotate around each other to allow the hand to turn palm up or palm down. The carpal bones in the wrist are connected to the metacarpal bones in the hand. Each finger contains three phalangeal bones; the thumb contains only two.
Source: Pearson Education

Bones of the Hips

The **pelvis** includes the hip bones as well as the sacrum and coccyx of the vertebral column. The hip bones include an ilium, ischium, and pubis on each side of the vertebral column (see Figure 8-11 ■). The **ilium**, the most superior of the hip bones, has a broad, flaring rim known as the **iliac crest**. Posteriorly, each ilium joins to the sacrum. The ilium contains the **acetabulum** (the cup-shaped, deep socket of the hip joint). The **ischium** is the most inferior of the hip bones. Each ischium is one of the "seat bones" that you sit on. The **pubis** or **pubic bone**, a small bridgelike bone, is the most anterior of the hip bones. Its two halves meet in the midline, where they form the **pubic symphysis**, a nearly immobile joint that has a cartilage pad between the bone ends. The pubis also forms the inferior part of the acetabulum.

Pronunciation/Word Parts

carpal (KAR-pal)
  carp/o- *wrist*
  -al *pertaining to*

metacarpal (MET-ah-KAR-pal)
  meta- *after; change; subsequent to; transition*
  carp/o- *wrist*
  -al *pertaining to*
Select the correct combining form meaning to get the definition of *metacarpal*: *pertaining to (bones that are) after or subsequent to (the) wrist.*

phalangeal (fah-LAN-jee-al)
  phalang/o- *digit; finger; toe*
  -eal *pertaining to*

phalanges (fah-LAN-jeez)
Phalanx is a Greek singular noun. Form the plural by changing *-x* to *-ges.*

phalanx (FAY-langks)
The combining form **dactyl/o-** also means *digit; finger; toe.*

digit (DIJ-it), **ray** (RAY)
Digits go from the hand like rays of the sun.

pelvis (PEL-vis)

pelvic (PEL-vik)
  pelv/o- *hip bone; pelvis; renal pelvis*
  -ic *pertaining to*

ilium (IL-ee-um)
Ilium is a Latin singular noun. There are two ilia, but the plural form is seldom used.

iliac (IL-ee-ak)
  ili/o- *hip bone; ilium*
  -ac *pertaining to*

acetabulum (AS-eh-TAB-yoo-lum)

acetabular (AS-eh-TAB-yoo-lar)
  acetabul/o- *hip socket*
  -ar *pertaining to*

ischium (IS-kee-um)
Ischium is a Latin singular noun. There are two ischia, but the plural form is seldom used.

ischial (IS-kee-al)
  ischi/o- *hip bone; ischium*
  -al *pertaining to*

pubis (PYOO-bis)

pubic (PYOO-bik)
  pub/o- *hip bone; pubis*
  -ic *pertaining to*

symphysis (SIM-fih-sis)
  sym- *together; with*
  -physis *state of growing*
The ending *-physis* contains the combining form *phys/o-* and the two-letter suffix *-is.*

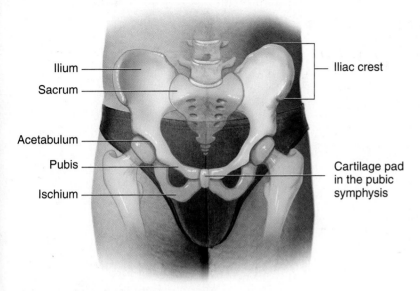

FIGURE 8-11 ■ Bones of the hip.
The ilium, ischium, and pubis on each side of the hip flow into each other without visible sutures or joints. However, the main part of each bone can be identified by its bony landmarks.
Source: Pearson Education

Labels: Ilium, Sacrum, Acetabulum, Pubis, Ischium, Iliac crest, Cartilage pad in the pubic symphysis

---

WORD ALERT
Sound-Alike Words

ilium	(noun)	the superior flaring part of the hip bone
		Example: During the car accident, she sustained a hip fracture that involved the ilium.
ileum	(noun)	the third part of the small intestine
		Example: Inflammation in the ileum can also extend to other parts of the small bowel.
ileus	(noun)	abnormal absence of contractions in the small intestine
		Example: A postoperative ileus can occur after extensive abdominal surgery.

Bones of the Lower Extremities

UPPER AND LOWER LEG   The lower extremity contains the upper leg (thigh) and the lower leg (see Figure 8-12 ■). The **femur** or **thigh bone** is the long, weight-bearing bone in the upper leg. The head of the femur fits into the acetabulum to form the hip joint.

The **tibia** or **shin bone** is the large bone on the medial (great toe) side of the lower leg. At its distal end, it has a bony prominence known as the **medial malleolus**. The **fibula** is the very thin bone on the lateral (little toe) side of the lower leg. Its proximal end connects to the tibia, not to the femur, and it is not a weight-bearing bone in the leg. Its distal end has a bony prominence known as the **lateral malleolus**. The malleoli are often mistakenly called the *ankle bones*. The **patella** or **kneecap** is a thick, round bone anterior to the knee joint. It is most prominent in thin people and when the knee is partially bent.

---

femur (FEE-mur)

femora (FEM-oh-rah)
Femur is a Latin singular noun. The plural form is *femora.*

femoral (FEM-oh-ral)
  femor/o- *femur; thigh bone*
  -al *pertaining to*

tibia (TIB-ee-ah)

tibiae (TIB-ee-ee)
Tibia is a Latin singular noun. Form the plural by changing -a to -ae.

tibial (TIB-ee-al)
  tibi/o- *shin bone; tibia*
  -al *pertaining to*

malleolus (mah-LEE-oh-lus)

malleoli (mah-LEE-oh-lie)
Malleolus is a Latin singular noun. Form the plural by changing -us to -i.

fibula (FIH-byoo-lah)

fibulae (FIH-byoo-lee)
Fibula is a Latin singular noun. Form the plural by changing -a to -ae.

fibular (FIH-byoo-lar)
  fibul/o- *fibula; lower leg bone*
  -ar *pertaining to*
The combining form **perone/o-** means *fibula; lower leg bone*, and *peroneal* is an adjective for *fibula.*

patella (pah-TEL-ah)

patellae (pah-TEL-ee)
Patella is a Latin singular noun. Form the plural by changing -a to -ae.

patellar (pah-TEL-ar)
  patell/o- *kneecap; patella*
  -ar *pertaining to*

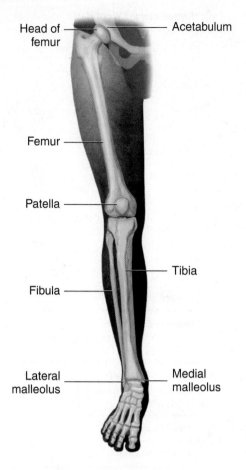

Head of femur

Acetabulum

Femur

Patella

Tibia

Fibula

Lateral malleolus

Medial malleolus

FIGURE 8-12 ■ Bones of the lower extremity.
The femur of the upper leg joins the tibia of the lower leg to support the weight of the body. The fibula, the smaller of the two bones in the lower leg, is on the little toe side. The patella is a small, round bone that protects the anterior knee joint.
Source: Pearson Education

ANKLE, FOOT, AND TOES Each ankle contains seven **tarsal bones** (see Figure 8-13 ■). The talus is the first tarsal bone, and the **calcaneus** or **heel bone** is the largest tarsal bone. The midfoot contains five **metatarsal bones**, one for each toe. The instep or arch of the foot contains both tarsal bones and metatarsal bones. Each toe or digit contains three phalangeal bones or phalanges (except the great toe, which contains two). The distal phalanx is at the very tip of the toe. The toes are also known as **digits** or **rays.** The great toe is known as the **hallux.**

tarsal (TAR-sal)
  tars/o- *ankle*
  -al *pertaining to*

calcaneus (kal-KAY-nee-us)

calcaneal (kal-KAY-nee-al)
  calcane/o- *calcaneus; heel bone*
  -al *pertaining to*

metatarsal (MET-ah-TAR-sal)

hallux (HAL-uks)

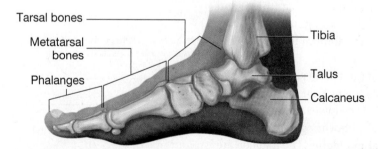

Tarsal bones

Metatarsal bones

Phalanges

Tibia

Talus

Calcaneus

FIGURE 8-13 ■ Bones of the ankle and foot.
The tarsal bones in the ankle are connected to the metatarsal bones in the midfoot. Each toe contains three phalangeal bones; the great toe or hallux contains only two. In all, each foot contains 26 bones and 150 ligaments.
Source: Pearson Education

Joints, Cartilage, and Ligaments

A **joint** or **articulation** is where two bones come together. There are three types of joints: suture, symphysis, and synovial.

1. A **suture joint** between two cranial bones is immovable and contains no cartilage (see Figure 8-14 ■).

2. A **symphysis joint**, such as the pubic symphysis or the joints between the vertebrae, is a slightly movable joint with a cartilage pad or disk between the bones (see Figures 8-6 and 8-11).

3. A **synovial joint** is a fully movable joint (see Figure 8-15 ■). There are two kinds of synovial joints: hinge joints (elbow and knee) that allow motion in two directions and ball-and-socket joints (shoulder and hip) that allow motion in many directions. A synovial joint joins two bones whose ends are covered with **articular cartilage**.

Pronunciation/Word Parts

joint (JOYNT)

articulation (ar-TIH-kyoo-LAY-shun)
  articul/o- *joint*
  -ation *being; having; process*
The combining form **arthr/o-** also means *joint.*

suture (SOO-chur)

symphysis (SIM-fih-sis)

synovial (sih-NOH-vee-al)
  synovi/o- *joint membrane; synovium*
  -al *pertaining to*
The combining form **synov/o-** also means *joint membrane; synovium*

articular (ar-TIH-kyoo-lar)
  articul/o- *joint*
  -ar *pertaining to*

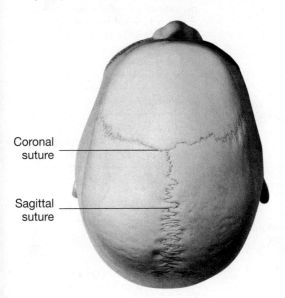

Coronal suture

Sagittal suture

FIGURE 8-14 ■ Suture joint.
In an adult, the coronal suture is an immoveable joint that joins the frontal and parietal bones. The parietal suture joins the two parietal bones on either side of the cranium. A suture is not a straight line, as the two bones grow together faster in some areas than in others.
Source: Susan Turley

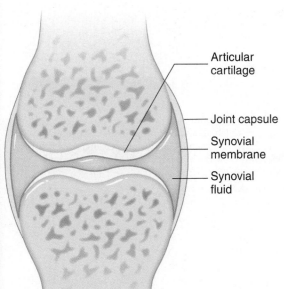

Articular cartilage

Joint capsule

Synovial membrane

Synovial fluid

FIGURE 8-15 ■ Synovial joint.
Unlike other types of joints, synovial joints are fully movable. They have a joint capsule and a synovial membrane that makes synovial fluid. Hinge joints (elbows and knees) allow motion in two directions. Ball-and-socket joints (shoulders and hips) allow motion in many directions.
Source: Pearson Education

Ligaments are strong fibrous bands of connective tissue that hold the two bones together in a synovial joint. The entire joint is encased in a **joint capsule** that has a fibrous outer layer and an inner membrane. This inner **synovial membrane** produces **synovial fluid**, a clear, thick fluid that lubricates the joint. A **meniscus** is a crescent-shaped cartilage pad found in some synovial joints, such as the knee.

The Structure of Bone

Bone or **osseous tissue** is a type of connective tissue. The surface of a bone is covered with **periosteum**, a thick, fibrous membrane (see Figure 8-16 ■). A long bone such as the humerus or femur has a straight shaft or **diaphysis** and two widened ends—the proximal **epiphysis** and the distal epiphysis. It is at the **epiphyseal plates** that bone growth takes place.

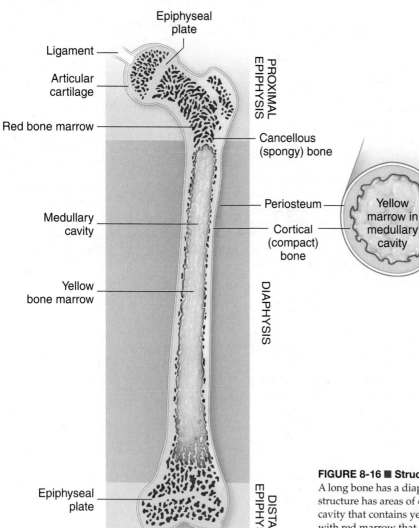

FIGURE 8-16 ■ Structure of a bone.
A long bone has a diaphysis (shaft) and epiphyses (ends). The internal structure has areas of dense cortical bone for weight bearing, a medullary cavity that contains yellow marrow, and bone ends of cancellous bone filled with red marrow that produces blood cells.
Source: Pearson Education

Pronunciation/Word Parts

ligament (LIG-ah-ment)

ligamentous (LIG-ah-MEN-tus)
  ligament/o- *ligament*
  -ous *pertaining to*

meniscus (meh-NIS-kus)

menisci (meh-NIS-ki)
Meniscus is a Latin singular noun. Form the plural by changing *-us* to *-i*.

osseous (AW-see-us)
  osse/o- *bone*
  -ous *pertaining to*

periosteum (PAIR-ee-AW-stee-um)

periosteal (PAIR-ee-AW-stee-al)
  peri- *around*
  oste/o- *bone*
  -al *pertaining to*

diaphysis (dy-AF-ih-sis)

diaphyses (dy-AF-ih-seez)
Diaphysis is a Greek singular noun. Form the plural by changing *-is* to *-es*.

diaphyseal (DY-ah-FIZ-ee-al)
  diaphys/o- *shaft of a bone*
  -eal *pertaining to*

epiphysis (eh-PIF-ih-sis)

epiphyses (eh-PIF-ih-seez)
Epiphysis is a Greek singular noun. Form the plural by changing *-is* to *-es*.

epiphyseal (EP-ih-FIZ-ee-al)
  epiphys/o- *enlarged area at the end of a long bone*
  -eal *pertaining to*

Along the diaphysis is a layer of dense compact **cortical bone** for weight bearing. Inside this is the **medullary cavity**, which is filled with yellow bone marrow that contains fatty tissue. In each epiphysis is **cancellous bone** or spongy bone. It is less dense than compact bone, and the spaces in it are filled with red bone marrow. There are small foramina (openings) in the bones where the blood vessels go through to the bone marrow.

Pronunciation/Word Parts

cortical (KOR-tih-kal)
    cortic/o- *cortex; outer region*
    -al *pertaining to*

medullary (MEH-dyoo-LAIR-ee)
    medull/o- *inner region; medulla*
    -ary *pertaining to*

cancellous (kan-SEL-us)
    cancell/o- *lattice structure*
    -ous *pertaining to*

CLINICAL CONNECTIONS

Hematology and Immunology (Chapter 6). Red bone marrow produces stem cells that eventually mature, become erythrocytes, leukocytes, etc., and enter the blood. Red bone marrow is found in the ends of the long bones and in the skull, clavicles, sternum, ribs, vertebrae, and hip bones.

Physiology of Bone Growth

Ossification is the gradual replacing of cartilage with bone that takes place during childhood and adolescence. In addition, new bone is formed along the epiphyseal growth plates at the ends of long bones as the body grows taller. Although mature bone is a hard substance, it is also a living tissue that undergoes change. About 10% of the entire skeleton is broken down and rebuilt each year. This process occurs in areas that are damaged or subjected to mechanical stress. **Osteoclasts** break down areas of old or damaged bone. **Osteoblasts** deposit new bone tissue in those areas. **Osteocytes** maintain and monitor the mineral content (calcium, phosphorus) of the bone. Almost all of the body's calcium is stored in the bones, but calcium is also needed to help the heart and skeletal muscles contract. Calcium comes from foods but is also released into the blood as osteoclasts break down old or damaged bone.

ossification (AW-sih-fih-KAY-shun)
    ossificat/o- *changing into bone*
    -ion *action; condition*

osteoclast (AW-stee-oh-KLAST)
    oste/o- *bone*
    -clast *cell that breaks down substances*

osteoblast (AW-stee-oh-BLAST)
    oste/o- *bone*
    -blast *immature cell*

osteocyte (AW-stee-oh-SITE)
    oste/o- *bone*
    -cyte *cell*

CLINICAL CONNECTIONS

Endocrinology (Chapter 14). The calcium level in the blood is constantly controlled and balanced by parathyroid hormone secreted by the parathyroid glands and calcitonin hormone secreted by the thyroid gland. Parathyroid hormone raises the calcium level by stimulating osteoclasts to break down bone. Calcitonin has the opposite effect. Estradiol and other hormones stimulate bone formation. Growth hormone from the pituitary gland influences the rate of bone growth.

Space Medicine. Astronauts who live in a weightless environment for prolonged periods of time lose bone mass. The lack of weight-bearing stress on the bones decreases new bone formation while the rate of bone breakdown remains the same. The astronauts have regular exercise programs that include resistance exercises that exert weight-bearing force on the bones.

ACROSS THE LIFE SPAN

Pediatrics. During birth, it is not unusual for the clavicle to break as the baby goes through the birth canal. This fracture does not need to be treated, as it heals by itself within a matter of days because of the high rate of bone growth. Babies are born without kneecaps! These bones develop between 2 and 6 years of age. From childhood through adolescence, new bone formation exceeds bone breakdown, as cartilage is continuously replaced by mature bone. The height and weight of a child are important indicators of health and are measured at regular intervals by the pediatrician and recorded on a standardized pediatric growth chart in the child's electronic health record (see Figure 8-17 ■).

During adolescence, the rate of bone growth accelerates (a "growth spurt") because of growth hormone secreted by the anterior pituitary gland.

During adulthood, the rate of new bone formation equals the rate of bone breakdown. In all stages of life, formation of new bone is dependent on having enough calcium and phosphorus in the diet.

Geriatrics. In older adults, the rate of bone breakdown is faster than new bone formation, and bones can become fragile and prone to fracture. Patients confined to bed who are unable to do any weight-bearing exercise to stimulate new bone formation have an increased rate of bone loss.

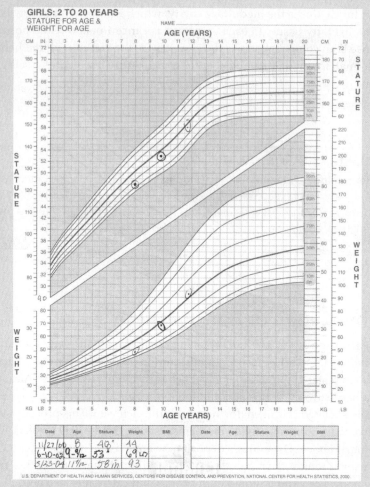

FIGURE 8-17 ■ Pediatric growth chart.
This chart tracks height and weight for girls ages 2–20 years and assigns percentiles. On the initial visit to her pediatrician, this 8-year-old child had a diagnosis of malnutrition and was in about the 15th percentile for both height (stature) and weight. After 3 years of good nutrition, her visit at age 11 years, 7 months, showed that she was in the 40th percentile for height and the 55th percentile for weight.

Source: Susan M. Turley

Vocabulary Review

Anatomy and Physiology		
Word or Phrase	**Description**	**Combining Forms**
appendicular skeleton	The bones of the shoulders, upper extremities, hips, and lower extremities	**appendicul/o-** *limb; small attached part*
axial skeleton	The bones of the head, chest, and back	**axi/o-** *axis*
bones	The framework on which the body is built. The 206 individual pieces of the skeleton. Bone is known as **osseous tissue**. *Bony* and *osteal* are also adjectives for *bone*.	**osse/o-** *bone* **oste/o-** *bone*
skeletal system	Body system that consists of all of the bones, cartilage, ligaments, and joints in the body	**skelet/o-** *skeleton*
skeletomuscular system	The combined systems of the bones and muscles. The bones provide structural support for the body, and the muscles produce movement. It is also known as the **musculoskeletal system**.	**skelet/o-** *skeleton* **muscul/o-** *muscle*
skeleton	Bony framework of the body that consists of all 206 bones, plus cartilage and ligaments	**skelet/o-** *skeleton*

Bones of the Head		
cranium	Domelike bone at the top of the head that contains the **cranial cavity** and the brain and other structures	**crani/o-** *cranium; skull*
ethmoid bone	Bone that forms the posterior nasal septum and the medial walls of the eye sockets. It contains many small, hollow spaces.	**ethm/o-** *sieve*
fontanel	"Soft spot" on a baby's head where the cranial sutures are still open and there is only fibrous connective tissue	
foramen	A hole in a bone. The **foramen magnum** is the largest. The spinal cord passes through it to join with the brain. There is a foramen in each vertebra where the spinal cord passes through. There are small foramina in the bones where blood vessels go through to the bone marrow.	
frontal bone	Bone that forms the forehead and top of the cranium and ends at the coronal suture. It contains the frontal sinuses.	**front/o-** *front*
hyoid bone	U-shaped bone in the anterior neck. It is attached by ligaments to the styloid process of the temporal bone.	**hy/o-** *U–shaped structure*
lacrimal bones	Facial bones within the eye socket. They are small, flat bones near the lacrimal glands, which produce tears.	**lacrim/o-** *tears*
mandible	Facial bone that is the lower jaw bone and contains the roots of the lower teeth. It is the only movable bone in the skull and forms a joint in front of the ear with the temporal bone (the temporomandibular joint).	**mandibul/o-** *lower jaw; mandible*
maxilla	Facial bone that is the immovable upper jaw bone. It contains the roots of the upper teeth and the maxillary sinuses. The maxilla consists of two fused **maxillary bones**.	**maxill/o-** *maxilla; upper jaw*

Word or Phrase	Description	Combining Forms
nasal bones	Facial bones that form the bridge of the nose and the roof of the nasal cavity	**nas/o-** *nose*
occipital bone	Bone that forms the posterior base of the cranium. It contains the large opening, the foramen magnum.	**occipit/o-** *back of the head; occiput*
ossicles	Three tiny bones in the middle ear that function in the process of hearing. They are also known as the *ossicular chain.*	
palatine bones	Facial bones that are small and flat and form the posterior hard palate	**palat/o-** *palate*
parietal bones	Bones that form the upper sides and posterior of the cranium. They join at the sagittal suture.	**pariet/o-** *wall of a cavity*
skull	Bony structure of the head that consists of the cranium and facial bones	
sphenoid bone	Large, irregular bone that forms the central base and sides of the cranium and the posterior walls of the eye sockets. It contains the sphenoid sinuses. A bony cup in the sphenoid bone holds the pituitary gland.	**sphen/o-** *wedge shape*
suture	Joint where one cranial bone meets another. A suture is an immovable joint that contains no cartilage. Examples: Coronal suture, sagittal suture	
temporal bones	Bones that form the lower sides of the cranium. They contain the openings for the external ear canals. Bony landmarks include the **mastoid process** behind the ear and the pointed **styloid process**, a point of attachment for ligaments to the hyoid bone.	**tempor/o-** *side of the head; temple* **mast/o-** *breast; mastoid process* **styl/o-** *stake*
vomer	Facial bone that forms the inferior part of the nasal septum and continues posteriorly to join the sphenoid bone	
zygoma	Facial bone that is a cheek bone and goes to the edge of the eye socket. Also known as the **zygomatic bone**.	

Bones of the Chest

costal cartilage	Firm, but flexible segments of connective tissue that join the ribs to the sternum. The area where the costal cartilage meets the rib is the **costochondral joint**.	**cost/o-** *rib* **chondr/o-** *cartilage* **cartilagin/o-** *cartilage*
ribs	Twelve pairs of bones that form the sides of the thorax. There are true ribs, false ribs, and floating ribs.	**cost/o-** *rib*
sternum	Vertical bone of the anterior thorax to which the clavicle and ribs are attached. It is also known as the **breast bone**. The **manubrium** is the triangular-shaped superior part of the sternum, while the **xiphoid process** is the inferior pointed tip.	**stern/o-** *breastbone; sternum* **xiph/o-** *sword*
thorax	Bony cage of the chest that contains the **thoracic cavity** with the heart, lungs, and other structures. It is also known as the **rib cage**.	**thorac/o-** *chest; thorax*

Bones of the Back

Word or Phrase	Description	Combining Forms
cervical vertebrae	Vertebrae C1–C7 of the vertebral column in the neck. C1 is the **atlas**; C2 is the **axis**.	**cervic/o-** *cervix; neck*
coccyx	Group of several small, fused vertebrae inferior to the sacrum. It is also known as the **tail bone**.	**coccyg/o-** *coccyx; tail bone*
intervertebral disk	Disk between two vertebrae. It consists of an outer wall of fibrocartilage and an inner gelatinous substance, the **nucleus pulposus**, that acts as a cushion.	**vertebr/o-** *vertebra*
lumbar vertebrae	Vertebrae L1–L5 of the verteral column in the lower back	**lumb/o-** *area between the ribs and pelvis; lower back*
sacrum	Group of five fused vertebrae inferior to the lumbar vertebrae. The first one is S1.	**sacr/o-** *sacrum*
spine	Bony column of vertebrae. It is also known as the **vertebral column**, **spinal column**, or **backbone**. It is divided into five regions: cervical vertebrae, thoracic vertebrae, lumbar vertebrae, sacrum, and coccyx. *Spine* also refers to a bony projection, such as the spinous process on a vertebra.	**spin/o-** *backbone; spine* **vertebr/o-** *vertebra*
thoracic vertebrae	Vertebrae T1–T12 of the vertebral column in the area of the chest. Each vertebra joins with one pair of ribs.	**thorac/o-** *chest; thorax*
vertebrae	Bony structure in the spine. Most vertebrae have a vertebral body (flat, circular area), **spinous process** (bony projection along the midback), two **transverse processes** (bony projections to the side), and a **foramen** (hole where the spinal cord passes through).	**vertebr/o-** *vertebra* **spondyl/o-** *vertebra* **spin/o-** *backbone; spine*

Bones of the Shoulders

clavicle	Rod-like bone on each side of the anterior neck. It joins with the manubrium of the sternum and the acromion of the scapula. It is also known as the **collar bone**.	**clavicul/o-** *clavicle; collar bone*
glenoid fossa	Shallow depression in the scapula where the head of the humerus joins the scapula to make the shoulder joint	**glen/o-** *socket of a joint*
scapula	Triangular-shaped bone on each side of the upper back. It is also known as the **shoulder blade**. It contains the **acromion**, a bony projection that connects to the clavicle.	**scapul/o-** *scapula; shoulder blade*

Bones of the Upper Extremities

carpal bones	The eight small bones of the wrist joint	**carp/o-** *wrist*
humerus	Long bone of the upper arm. The head of the humerus fits into the glenoid fossa of the scapula to make the shoulder joint.	**humer/o-** *humerus; upper arm bone*
metacarpal bones	The five bones of the hand, one corresponding to each finger. They connect the carpal bones to the phalanges.	**carp/o-** *wrist*
phalanx	One of the individual bones of a finger or toe. A finger or toe is a **digit** or a **ray**.	**phalang/o-** *digit; finger; toe* **dactyl/o-** *digit; finger; toe*

Word or Phrase	Description	Combining Forms
radius	Forearm bone located along the thumb side of the lower arm	**radi/o-** *forearm bone; radiation; x-rays*
ulna	Forearm bone located along the little finger side of the lower arm. The **olecranon** (point of the elbow) is a large, square, bony projection on the proximal ulna.	**uln/o-** *forearm bone; ulna*
Bones of the Hips		
acetabulum	Cup-shaped, deep socket of the hip joint. It is in the ilium and the pubic bone. It is where the head of the femur fits to make the hip joint.	**acetabul/o-** *hip socket*
ilium	Most superior hip bone. It has a broad, flaring **iliac crest**. Posteriorly, each ilium joins the sacrum. The ilium contains the acetabulum, the deep, cup-shaped socket of the hip joint.	**ili/o-** *hip bone; ilium*
ischium	Most inferior hip bone. Each ischium is one of the "seat bones."	**ischi/o-** *hip bone; ischium*
pelvis	The hip bones as well as the sacrum and coccyx of the vertebral column	**pelv/o-** *hip bone; pelvis; renal pelvis*
pubis	Small bridgelike bone that is the most anterior hip bone. The **pubic symphysis** is a nearly immobile joint between the two **pubic bones**.	**pub/o-** *hip bone; pubis*
Bones of the Lower Extremities		
calcaneus	Largest of the ankle bones. It is also known as the **heel bone**.	**calcane/o-** *calcaneus; heel bone*
femur	Long bone of the upper leg. It is also known as the **thigh bone**. The head of the femur fits into the acetabulum to make the hip joint.	**femor/o-** *femur; thigh bone*
fibula	Thin bone in the lower leg, located on the little toe side. The adjectives *fibular* and *peroneal* mean *fibula*.	**fibul/o-** *fibula; lower leg bone* **perone/o-** *fibula; lower leg bone*
hallux	The great toe	
malleolus	Bony projection of the distal tibia (**medial malleolus**) or the distal fibula (**lateral malleolus**). Often mistakenly called the *ankle bones*.	
metatarsal bones	The five bones of the midfoot, one corresponding to each toe. They connect the ankle bones to the phalanges.	**tars/o-** *ankle*
patella	Thick, round bone anterior to the knee joint. It is also known as the **kneecap**.	**patell/o-** *kneecap; patella*
phalanx	(See Bones of the Upper Extremities, page 379)	
tarsal bones	The seven bones in the ankle joint. The first is the tarsus; the largest is the calcaneus.	**tars/o-** *ankle*
tibia	Large, weight-bearing bone of the lower leg located on the great toe side. It is also known as the **shin bone**.	**tibi/o-** *shin bone; tibia*

Build Medical Words

Combining Form and Suffix Exercise

Read the definition of the medical word. Look at the combining form that is given. Select the correct suffix from the Suffix List and write it on the blank line. Then build the medical word and write it on the line. (Remember: You may need to remove the combining vowel. Always remove the hyphens and slash.) Be sure to check your spelling. The first one has been done for you.

SUFFIX LIST

-al (pertaining to)
-ar (pertaining to)
-ation (being; having; process)
-clast (cell that breaks down substances)

-cyte (cell)
-eal (pertaining to)
-ic (pertaining to)

-ion (action; condition)
-oid (resembling)
-ous (pertaining to)

Definition of the Medical Word	Combining Form	Suffix	Build the Medical Word
1. Pertaining to (the) cranium	**crani/o-** **-al**		*cranial*
(You think *pertaining to* (-al) + *cranium* (crani/o-). You change the order of the word parts to put the suffix last. You write *cranial*.)			
2. Pertaining to (the) thorax	thorac/o-	_____	_____
3. Pertaining to (the) rib	cost/o-	_____	_____
4. Pertaining to (the) mandible	mandibul/o-	_____	_____
5. Pertaining to (a) ligament	ligament/o-	_____	_____
6. Pertaining to (the) pelvis	pelv/o-	_____	_____
7. Pertaining to (a) finger or toe	phalang/o-	_____	_____
8. Pertaining to bone	osse/o-	_____	_____
9. Being or having (a) joint	articul/o-	_____	_____
10. Cell that breaks down substances (like) bone	oste/o-	_____	_____
11. Pertaining to (the) vertebra	vertebr/o-	_____	_____
12. Pertaining to (the) lower back	lumb/o-	_____	_____
13. Pertaining to (the) ulna	uln/o-	_____	_____
14. Pertaining to (the) fibula	fibul/o-	_____	_____
15. Action (of) changing into bone	ossificat/o-	_____	_____
16. (A bone) resembling (a) sieve	ethm/o-	_____	_____
17. Pertaining to (the) sternum	stern/o-	_____	_____
18. Pertaining to (the) neck	cervic/o-	_____	_____
19. Pertaining to (the) clavicle	clavicul/o-	_____	_____
20. Pertaining to (the) humerus	humer/o-	_____	_____
21. Pertaining to (the) pubis	pub/o-	_____	_____
22. Pertaining to (the) wrist	carp/o-	_____	_____
23. Pertaining to (the) kneecap	patell/o-	_____	_____
24. Cell (that maintains the mineral content of) bone	oste/o-	_____	_____

Diseases

Diseases of the Bones and Cartilage		
Word or Phrase	**Description**	**Pronunciation/Word Parts**
avascular necrosis	Death of cells in the epiphysis of a long bone, often the femur. This is caused by an injury, fracture, or dislocation that damages nearby blood vessels or by a blood clot that interrupts the blood supply to the bone. Treatment: Surgery to remove the dead bone, then a bone graft. For large areas of avascular necrosis, joint replacement surgery is done.	**avascular** (aa-VAS-kyoo-lar) a- *away from; without* vascul/o- *blood vessel* -ar *pertaining to* **necrosis** (neh-KROH-sis) necr/o- *dead body; dead cells; dead tissue* -osis *condition; process*
bone tumor	**Osteoma** is a benign tumor of the bone. **Osteosarcoma** is a cancerous bone tumor in which osteoblasts, the cells that form new bone, multiply uncontrollably. It is also known as **osteogenic sarcoma**. **Ewing's sarcoma** is a cancerous bone tumor that occurs mainly in young men. Treatment: Surgical removal of a benign tumor. Amputation of the limb followed by radiation therapy or chemotherapy drugs for a cancerous tumor.	**osteoma** (AW-stee-OH-mah) oste/o- *bone* -oma *mass; tumor* **osteosarcoma** (AW-stee-OH-sar-KOH-mah) oste/o- *bone* sarc/o- *connective tissue* -oma *mass; tumor* **osteogenic** (AW-stee-oh-JEN-ik) oste/o- *bone* gen/o- *arising from; produced by* -ic *pertaining to* **Ewing** (YOO-ing)
chondroma	Benign tumor of the cartilage. Treatment: Surgical removal, if large.	**chondroma** (con-DROH-mah) chondr/o- *cartilage* -oma *mass; tumor*
chondromalacia patellae	Abnormal softening of the patella because of thinning and uneven wear. The thigh muscle pulls the patella in a crooked path that wears away the underside of the bone. Treatment: Strengthening of the thigh muscle to correct the direction of its contraction.	**chondromalacia** (CON-droh-mah-LAY-sha) chondr/o- *cartilage* malac/o- *softening* -ia *condition; state; thing* **patellae** (pah-TEL-ee)

Word or Phrase	Description	Pronunciation/Word Parts

fracture	Broken bone due to an accident, injury, or disease process. Fractures are categorized according to how the bone breaks (see Figure 8-18 ■ and Table 8-1 ■). A fracture caused by force or torsion during an accident or sports activity is a **stress fracture**. A fracture caused by a disease process such as osteoporosis, bone cancer, or metastases to the bone is a **pathologic fracture**. Fractures that are allowed to heal without treatment often show malunion or **malalignment** of the fracture fragments. Treatment: Closed reduction and manipulation to align the fracture pieces, application of a cast. Surgery: Open reduction and internal fixation using wires, pins, screws, or plates.
	
	FIGURE 8-18 ■ **Bone fracture.** This x-ray shows two views of an oblique, displaced fracture of the radius and ulna in the forearm.
	Source: Oceandigital/Fotolia
		fracture (FRAK-chur)
		  fract/o- *bend; break up*
		  -ure *result of; system*
		
		pathologic (PATH-oh-LAW-jik)
		  path/o- *disease*
		  log/o- *study of; word*
		  -ic *pertaining to*
		
		malalignment (MAL-ah-LINE-ment)
		  mal- *bad; inadequate*
		  align/o- *arranged in a straight line*
		  -ment *action; state*

Table 8-1 Fracture Names and Descriptions

Fracture Name	Description	Illustration	Pronunciation/Word Parts
closed fracture	Broken bone does not break through the overlying skin		
open fracture	Broken bone breaks through the overlying skin. It is also known as a **compound fracture**.		
nondisplaced fracture	Broken bone remains in its normal anatomical alignment	 Nondisplaced fracture Displaced fracture	**nondisplaced** (non-dis-PLAYSD) The prefix *non-* means *not.* The prefix *dis-* means *away from.*

(continued)

Table 8-1 Fracture Names and Descriptions *(continued)*

Fracture Name	Description	Illustration	Pronunciation/Word Parts
displaced fracture	Broken bone is pulled out of its normal anatomical alignment		**displaced** (dis-PLAYSD)
Colles' fracture	Distal radius is broken by falling onto an outstretched hand	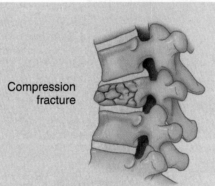 Colles' fracture	**Colles' fracture** (KOH-leez)
comminuted fracture	Bone is crushed into several small pieces	Comminuted fracture	**comminuted** (COM-ih-NYOO-ted) **comminut/o-** *break into small pieces* **-ed** *pertaining to*
compression fracture	Vertebrae are compressed together when a person falls onto the buttocks or when a vertebra collapses in on itself because of disease	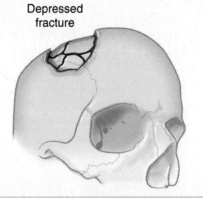 Compression fracture	**compression** (com-PREH-shun) **compress/o-** *press together* **-ion** *action; condition*
depressed fracture	Cranium is fractured inward toward the brain	Depressed fracture	**depressed** (dee-PRESD) **depress/o-** *press down* **-ed** *pertaining to*
greenstick fracture	Bone is broken on only one side. This occurs in children because part of the bone is still flexible cartilage.	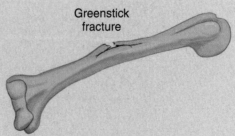 Greenstick fracture	

Fracture Name	Description	Illustration	Pronunciation/Word Parts
hairline fracture	Very thin fracture line with the bone pieces still together. It is difficult to detect except on an x-ray.	Hairline fracture	
oblique fracture	Bone is broken on an oblique angle (see Figure 8-18)	Oblique fracture	**oblique** (oh-BLEEK)
spiral fracture	Bone is broken in a spiral because of a twisting force	Spiral fracture	**spiral** (SPY-ral) **spir/o-** *breathe; coil* **-al** *pertaining to*
transverse fracture	Bone is broken in a transverse plane perpendicular to its long axis	Transverse fracture	**transverse** (trans-VERS) **trans-** *across; through* **-verse** *travel; turn* The ending *-verse* contains the combining form *vers/o-* and the one-letter suffix *–e*.

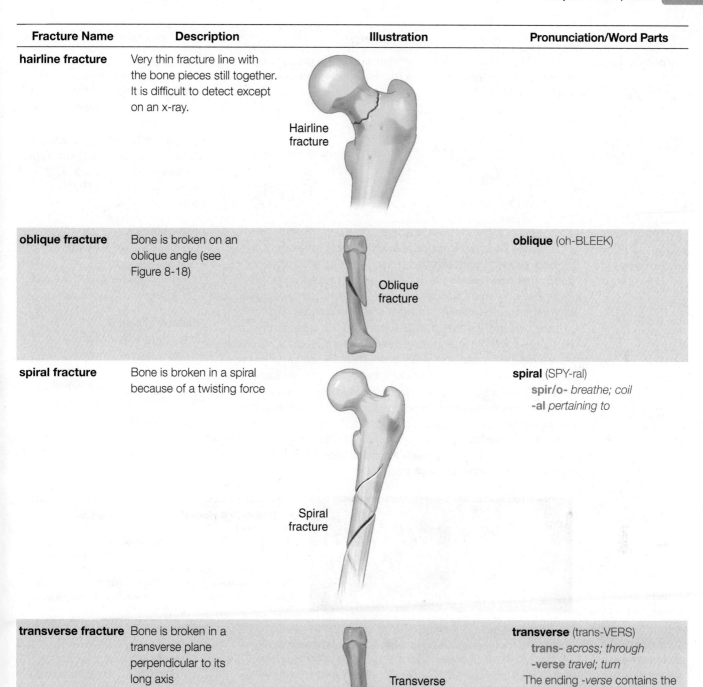

Word or Phrase	Description	Pronunciation/Word Parts
osteomalacia	Abnormal softening of the bones due to a deficiency of vitamin D in the diet or inadequate exposure to the sun whose rays make vitamin D in the skin. In children, this causes rickets with bone pain and fractures. Treatment: Vitamin D supplement, sun exposure.	**osteomalacia** (AW-stee-OH-mah-LAY-sha) **oste/o-** *bone* **malac/o-** *softening* **-ia** *condition; state; thing*

Word or Phrase	Description	Pronunciation/Word Parts
osteomyelitis	Infection in the bone and the bone marrow. Bacteria enter the bone following an open fracture, crush injury, or surgical procedure. Treatment: Antibiotic drug.	**osteomyelitis** (AW-stee-oh-MY-eh-LY-tis) **oste/o-** *bone* **myel/o-** *bone marrow; myelin; spinal cord* **-itis** *infection of; inflammation of* Select the correct combining form meaning to get the definition of *osteomyelitis*: *infection of the bone and bone marrow.*
osteoporosis	Abnormal thinning of the bone structure. When bone breakdown exceeds new bone formation, calcium and phosphorus are lost, and the bone becomes osteoporotic (porous) with many small areas of **demineralization** (see Figure 8-19 ■). This can cause a compression fracture as a vertebra collapses in on itself. The vertebral column decreases in height, the patient becomes shorter, and there is an abnormal curvature of the upper back and shoulders (dowager's hump). Osteoporosis can also cause a spontaneous fracture (pathologic fracture) of the hip or femur. Sometimes it is unclear whether an older patient fell and fractured the bone or whether the osteoporotic bone itself spontaneously fractured and caused the patient to fall. Osteoporosis occurs in postmenopausal women and older men. Estradiol in women stimulates bone formation, and loss of estradiol at menopause leads to osteoporosis. A lack of dietary calcium and a lack of exercise contribute to the process. Treatment: Bone density test for diagnosis; drug to decrease the rate of bone resorption or drug to activate estradiol receptors, and calcium supplement.	**osteoporosis** (AW-stee-OH-poh-ROH-sis) **oste/o-** *bone* **por/o-** *pores; small openings* **-osis** *condition; process* **demineralization** (dee-MIN-er-AL-ih-ZAY-shun) **de-** *reversal of; without* **mineral/o-** *electrolyte; mineral* **-ization** *process of creating; process of inserting; process of making*

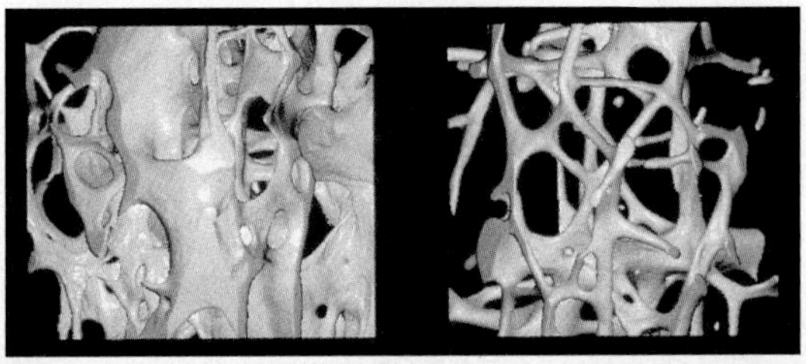

FIGURE 8-19 ■ Normal bone versus bone with osteoporosis.
Viewed under a microscope, the bone on the left shows normal mineralization and density. The bone on the right shows demineralization, large holes, and loss of density from osteoporosis. This bone is extremely prone to fracture.
Source: European Synchrotron Radiation Facility/Creatis/Science Source

Diseases of the Vertebrae

Word or Phrase	Description	Pronunciation/Word Parts
ankylosing spondylitis	Chronic inflammation of the vertebrae that leads to fibrosis, fusion, and restriction of movement of the spine. Treatment: Nonsteroidal anti-inflammatory drug.	**ankylosing** (ANG-kih-LOH-sing) **ankyl/o-** *fused together; stiff* **-osing** *condition of making* **spondylitis** (SPAWN-dih-LY-tis) **spondyl/o-** *vertebra* **-itis** *infection of; inflammation of*
kyphosis	Abnormal, excessive, posterior curvature of the thoracic spine. It is also known as **humpback** or **hunchback**. The back is said to have a **kyphotic** curvature. **Kyphoscoliosis** is a complex curvature with components of both kyphosis and scoliosis. Treatment: Back brace or surgery to fuse and straighten a severely curved spine.	**kyphosis** (ky-FOH-sis) **kyph/o-** *bent; humpbacked* **-osis** *condition; process* **kyphotic** (ky-FAW-tik) **kyph/o-** *bent; humpbacked* **-tic** *pertaining to* **kyphoscoliosis** (KY-foh-SKOH-lee-OH-sis) **kyph/o-** *bent; humpbacked* **scoli/o-** *crooked; curved* **-osis** *condition; process*

Word or Phrase	Description	Pronunciation/Word Parts

lordosis	Abnormal, excessive, anterior curvature of the lumbar spine. It is also known as **swayback**. The back is said to have a **lordotic** curvature. Treatment: Back brace or surgery to fuse and straighten a severely curved spine.	**lordosis** (lor-DOH-sis)
		  lord/o- *swayback*
		  -osis *condition; process*
		
		lordotic (lor-DAW-tik)
		  lord/o- *swayback*
		  -tic *pertaining to*

scoliosis	Abnormal, excessive, C-shaped or S-shaped lateral curvature of the spine (see Figure 8-20 ■). The back is said to have a **scoliotic** curvature. A **dextroscoliosis** curves to the patient's right, while a **levoscoliosis** curves to the patient's left. Scoliosis can be congenital but most often the cause is unknown. It develops during childhood and may continue to progress during adolescence. It impairs movement, posture, and breathing. An x-ray shows the degree of curvature. Treatment: Back brace or surgery to fuse and straighten a severely curved spine.	**scoliosis** (SKOH-lee-OH-sis)
		  scoli/o- *crooked; curved*
		  -osis *condition; process*
		
		scoliotic (SKOH-lee-AW-tik)
		  scoli/o- *crooked; curved*
		  -tic *pertaining to*
		
		dextroscoliosis
		(DEKS-troh-SKOH-lee-OH-sis)
		  dextr/o- *right; sugar*
		  scoli/o- *crooked; curved*
		  -osis *condition; process*
		
		levoscoliosis
		(LEE-voh-SKOH-lee-OH-sis)
		  lev/o- *left*
		  scoli/o- *crooked; curved*
		  -osis *condition; process*

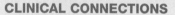

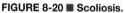

FIGURE 8-20 ■ Scoliosis.
A patient with moderate scoliosis of the spine shows the characteristic tilt of the shoulders and hips, uneven scapulae, and a difference in arm lengths.
Source: Sciepro/Science Photo Library/Corbis

CLINICAL CONNECTIONS
Public Health. Scoliosis screening is routinely done by a school nurse for all elementary school children (see Figure 8-21 ■). The child's back is observed while standing and then while bending over. Some cases of scoliosis become more apparent with bending over as one side of the back becomes noticeably higher and one scapula sticks out.

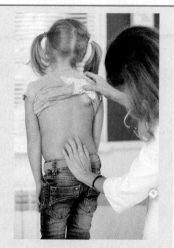

FIGURE 8-21 ■ School examination.
This school nurse is evaluating this elementary school child for signs of scoliosis.
Source: Dmytro Panchenko/Fotolia

Word or Phrase	Description	Pronunciation/Word Parts

spondylolisthesis	Degenerative condition of the spine in which one vertebra moves anteriorly and slips out of proper alignment due to degeneration of the intervertebral disk. It can also occur because of a sports injury or a compression fracture of the vertebra from osteoporosis. Treatment: Back brace or surgery to relieve a pinched spinal nerve. Analgesic drug, nonsteroidal anti-inflammatory drug. Intra-articular injection of a corticosteroid drug.	**spondylolisthesis**
		(SPAWN-dih-LOH-lis-THEE-sis)
		  spondyl/o- *vertebra*
		  olisthe/o- *slipping*
		  -esis *condition; process*

Diseases of the Joints and Ligaments

arthralgia	Pain in the joint from injury, inflammation, or infection from various causes. Treatment: Correct the underlying cause.	**arthralgia** (ar-THRAL-jah)
		  arthr/o- *joint*
		  alg/o- *pain*
		  -ia *condition; state; thing*

arthropathy	Disease of a joint from any cause. Treatment: Correct the underlying cause.	**arthropathy** (ar-THRAW-pah-thee)
		  arthr/o- *joint*
		  -pathy *disease*

dislocation	Displacement of the end of a bone from its normal position within a joint. This is usually caused by injury or trauma. **Congenital dislocation of the hip (CDH)** is present at birth because the acetabulum is poorly formed or the ligaments are loose. Treatment: Manipulate and return the bone to its normal position. Congenital dislocation of the hip is treated with a splint or with surgery to correct the shape of the acetabulum or looseness of the ligaments.	**dislocation** (DIS-loh-KAY-shun)
		  dis- *away from*
		  locat/o- *place*
		  -ion *action; condition*
		
		congenital (con-JEN-ih-tal)
		  congenit/o- *present at birth*
		  -al *pertaining to*

gout	Metabolic disorder that occurs most often in men. There is a high level of uric acid in the blood. An acute attack causes sudden, severe pain after uric acid moves from the blood into the soft tissues and forms crystals known as **tophi**. Historically, patients with gout have been pictured with throbbing big toes, although tophi can form in any joint in the feet or hands. Tophi in the joints causes **gouty arthritis**. Treatment: Avoid foods that increase the uric acid level. Drug to decrease the uric acid level.	**gout** (GOWT)
		
		tophus (TOH-fus)
		
		tophi (TOH-fi)
		Tophus is a Latin singular noun. Form the plural by changing *-us* to *-i*.
		
		gouty (GOW-tee)
		
		arthritis (ar-THRY-tis)
		  arthr/o- *joint*
		  -itis *infection of; inflammation of*

hemarthrosis	Blood in the joint cavity from blunt trauma or a penetrating wound. It also occurs spontaneously in hemophiliac patients. Treatment: Temporary immobilization of the joint, aspiration of blood from the joint cavity, corticosteroid drug. Surgery: Arthroscopy.	**hemarthrosis**
		(HEE-mar-THROH-sis)
		  hem/o- *blood*
		  arthr/o- *joint*
		  -osis *condition; process*

Lyme disease	Arthritis caused by a bacterium in the bite of an infected deer tick. There is an erythematous rash that expands outward from the bite for several weeks (bull's-eye rash) but is not itchy; there is joint pain, fever, chills, and fatigue. If untreated, Lyme disease can cause severe fatigue and affect the nervous system (numbness, severe headache) and the heart. Treatment: Antibiotic drug.	**Lyme** (LIME)

osteoarthritis	Chronic inflammatory disease of the joints, particularly the large weight-bearing joints (knees, hips) and joints that move repeatedly (shoulders, neck, hands). Osteoarthritis (OA) usually begins in middle age, but can develop sooner in a joint that has been overused or injured. There is joint pain and stiffness. There is inflammation from constant wear and tear, and this is worsened if the patient is overweight. The normally smooth cartilage becomes roughened and then wears away in spots (see Figure 8-22 ■). The bone ends rub against each other, causing additional inflammation and **crepitus**, a grinding sound. New bone sometimes forms abnormally as an **osteophyte**, a sharp bone spur that causes pain. Osteoarthritis is also known as **degenerative joint disease (DJD)**. Treatment: Analgesic drug, nonsteroidal anti-inflammatory drug. Intra-articular injection of a corticosteroid drug. Surgery for a joint replacement.	**osteoarthritis**
		(AW-stee-OH-ar-THRY-tis)
		  oste/o- *bone*
		  arthr/o- *joint*
		  -itis *infection of; inflammation of*
		
		crepitus (KREP-ih-tus)
		
		osteophyte (AW-stee-oh-FITE)
		  oste/o- *bone*
		  -phyte *growth*
		
		degenerative (dee-JEN-er-ah-TIV)
		  de- *reversal of; without*
		  gener/o- *creation; production*
		  -ative *pertaining to*

Word or Phrase	Description	Pronunciation/Word Parts

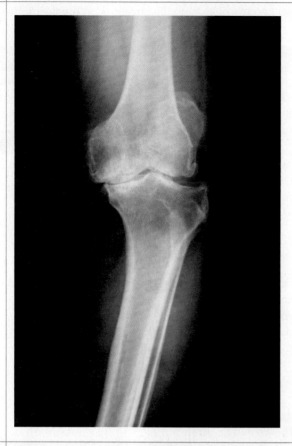

FIGURE 8-22 ■ Osteoarthritis.
This patient's knee shows loss of the articular cartilage and narrowing of the joint space between the bone ends on one side more than the other. This narrowing is characteristic of degenerative joint disease.
Source: Puwadol Jaturawutthichai/123RF

rheumatoid arthritis	Acute and chronic inflammatory disease of connective tissue, particularly of the joints. RA is an autoimmune disorder in which the patient's own antibodies attack cartilage and connective tissue. Patients are usually young to middle-aged females. There is redness and swelling of the joints, most often of the hands and feet. The joint cartilage is slowly destroyed by inflammation. The symptoms flare and subside over time, and there is progressive deformity of the joints (see Figure 8-23 ■). Treatment: Corticosteroid drug. Surgery: Joint replacement surgery.	**rheumatoid** (ROO-mah-toyd)
		  rheumat/o- *watery discharge*
		  -oid *resembling*
		
		arthritis (ar-THRY-tis)
		  arthr/o- *joint*
		  -itis *infection of; inflammation of*

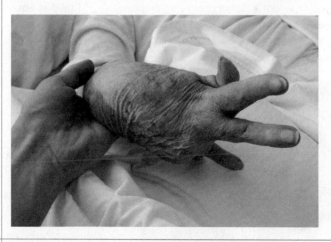

FIGURE 8-23 ■ Rheumatoid arthritis.
This patient has severe joint deformities of the hand that are characteristic of rheumatoid arthritis.
Source: Gines Romero/Shutterstock

sprain	Overstretching or tearing of a ligament around a joint. Treatment: Rest or surgery to repair the ligament.	**sprain** (SPRAYN)

Word or Phrase	Description	Pronunciation/Word Parts
torn meniscus	Tear of the cartilage pad of the knee because of an injury. Treatment: Arthroscopy and repair.	**meniscus** (meh-NIS-kus)

Diseases of the Bony Thorax

pectus excavatum	Congenital deformity of the bony thorax in which the sternum, particularly the xiphoid process, is bent inward, creating a hollow depression in the anterior chest. Treatment: Surgical correction, if severe.	**pectus excavatum** (PEK-tus EKS-kah-VAH-tum)

Diseases of the Bones of the Legs and Feet

genu valgum	Congenital deformity in which the knees are rotated toward the midline and are abnormally close together and the lower legs are bent laterally. This is also known as **knock-knee**. Treatment: Surgical correction, if severe.	**genu valgum** (JEE-noo VAL-gum)
genu varum	Congenital deformity in which the knees are rotated laterally away from each other and the lower legs are bent toward the midline. This is also known as **bowleg**. Treatment: Surgical correction, if severe.	**genu varum** (JEE-noo VAR-um)
hallux valgus	Deformity in which the great toe is angled laterally toward the other toes (see Figure 8-24 ■). Often a **bunion** develops at the base of the great toe with swelling and inflammation. This is a common deformity in women who wear pointy-toed shoes. Treatment: Wear wide-toed shoes; bunionectomy.	**hallux valgus** (HAL-uks VAL-gus) **bunion** (BUN-yun)

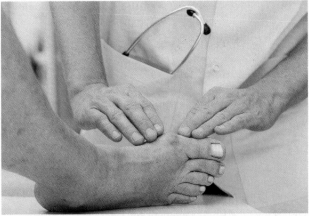

FIGURE 8-24 ■ Hallux valgus and bunion.
This patient's great toe is angled away from the midline, and there is a reddened, enlarged, and painful bunion on the medial side of the foot.
Source: Photographee.eu/Fotolia

talipes equinovarus	Congenital deformity in which the foot is pulled downward and toward the midline. This is also known as **clubfoot**. One or both feet can be affected (see Figure 8-25 ■). Treatment: Casts applied to progressively straighten the foot. Surgical correction, if severe.	**talipes equinovarus** (TAY-lih-peez ee-KWY-noh-VAR-us)

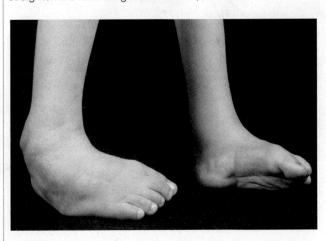

FIGURE 8-25 ■ Bilateral clubfeet.
This child was born with bilateral clubfeet. Although all newborns' feet are rotated medially due to the confining environment of the uterus, their feet can easily be moved into an anatomically correct position. In this child, the position of the feet cannot be corrected and remains this way throughout childhood and adulthood.
Source: Biophoto Associates/Science Source/Getty Images

Laboratory and Diagnostic Procedures

Laboratory Tests		
Word or Phrase	**Description**	**Pronunciation/Word Parts**
rheumatoid factor (RF)	Blood test that is usually positive in patients with rheumatoid arthritis. Anti-CCP blood test measures the level of antibodies and is always increased in patients with rheumatoid arthritis.	
uric acid	Blood test that has an elevated level in patients with gout and gouty arthritis	**uric acid** (YOOR-ik AS-id)

Radiology and Nuclear Medicine Procedures		

arthrography	Procedure that uses a radiopaque contrast dye that is injected into a joint. It coats and outlines the bone ends and joint capsule. An x-ray, CT scan, or MRI scan is done. MRI arthrography uses a strong magnetic field to align protons in the atoms of the patient's body. The protons emit signals to form a series of thin, successive images or "slices" of the joint. An MRI can be done with or without contrast dye. The x-ray, CT, or MRI image is an **arthrogram**.	**arthrography** (ar-THRAW-grah-fee)
		   arthr/o- *joint*
		   -graphy *process of recording*
		
		arthrogram (AR-throh-gram)
		   arthr/o- *joint*
		   -gram *picture; record*

bone density tests	Procedure that measures the bone mineral density (BMD) to determine if demineralization from osteoporosis has occurred (see Figure 8-26 ■). The heel or wrist bone can be tested, but the hip and spine bones give a more accurate result. This is also known as **bone densitometry**. There are two types of bone density tests: **DEXA (or DXA) scan** and **quantitative computerized tomography (QCT)**. A DEXA scan (dual-energy x-ray absorptiometry) uses two (dual) x-ray beams with different energy levels to create a two-dimensional image. This scan can detect as little as a 1% loss of bone. Quantitative computerized tomography uses an x-ray beam and a CT scan to create a three-dimensional image. QCT is able to measure the density of both cancellous and cortical bone. Cancellous bone is the first to be affected by osteoporosis and the first to respond to therapy.	**densitometry** (DEN-sih-TAW-meh-tree)
		   densit/o- *density*
		   -metry *process of measuring*
		
		DEXA scan (DEK-sah)
		DEXA stands for dual-energy x-ray absorptiometry.
		
		tomography (toh-MAW-grah-fee)
		   tom/o- *cut; layer; slice*
		   -graphy *process of recording*

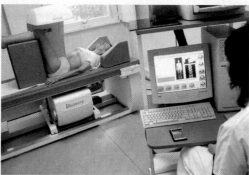

FIGURE 8-26 ■ Bone density test.
This patient is having a bone mineral density test performed, and the technician is viewing the results on the computer screen.
Source: Véronique Burger/Science Source

DID YOU KNOW?

A standard x-ray is not used to measure bone density because patients must lose at least 30% of their bone mass before the loss can be detected on an x-ray image. Both older men and postmenopausal women lose bone mass. After menopause, a woman can lose 1–2 percent of her bone mass each year.

Word or Phrase	Description	Pronunciation/Word Parts
bone scintigraphy	Nuclear medicine procedure in which a phosphate compound is tagged with the radioactive tracer technetium-99m. This is injected intravenously and is taken up into the bone. A gamma scintillation camera detects gamma rays from the radioactive tracer. Areas of increased uptake ("hot spots") indicate arthritis, fracture, osteomyelitis, cancerous tumors of the bone, or areas of bony metastasis. The nuclear medicine image is a **scintigram**.	**scintigraphy** (sin-TIH-grah-fee) **scint/i-** *point of light* **-graphy** *process of recording* **scintigram** (SIN-tih-gram) **scint/i-** *point of light* **-gram** *picture; record*
x-ray	Procedure that uses x-rays to diagnose bony abnormalities in any part of the body. X-rays are the primary means for diagnosing fractures, dislocations, and bone tumors.	**x-ray** (EKS-ray)

Medical and Surgical Procedures

Medical Procedures

cast	Procedure in which a cast of plaster or fiberglass is applied around a fractured bone and adjacent areas to immobilize the fracture in a fixed position to facilitate healing (see Figures 8-27 ■ and 8-28 ■). For fractures of the leg, the physician may order the patient to be nonweight bearing (putting no weight on the affected leg), toe touch (partial weight bearing), or full weight bearing (with a walking cast). Patients with leg casts are instructed in the use of crutches.	**cast** (KAST)

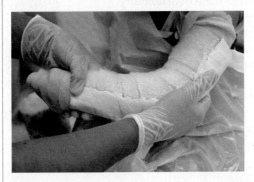

FIGURE 8-27 ■ Application of a cast.
This patient sustained several fractures during a dirt-bike accident. His fractured wrist (Colles' fracture) and fractured radius were immobilized in a long-arm cast to above the elbow.
Source: ChameleonsEye/Shutterstock

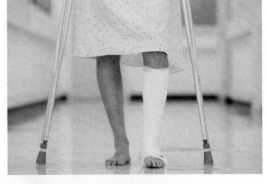

FIGURE 8-28 ■ Cast and crutches.
When one or both of the bones of the lower leg are fractured, the patient is taught how to use crutches to walk and how to care for the cast. After the fracture is healed and the cast is removed, he may need to have physical therapy to regain range of motion.
Source: ERproductions Ltd/Blend Images/Corbis

closed reduction	Procedure in which manual manipulation of a displaced fracture is performed so that the bone ends go back into normal alignment without the need for surgery. Then a cast is applied.	**reduction** (ree-DUK-shun) **reduct/o-** *bring back; decrease* **-ion** *action; condition*
extracorporeal shock wave therapy (ESWT)	Procedure in which sound waves produced outside the body (extracorporeal) are used to break up bone spurs and treat other minor but painful problems of the foot	**extracorporeal** (EKS-trah-kor-POR-ee-al) **extra-** *outside* **corpor/o-** *body* **-eal** *pertaining to*

Word or Phrase	Description	Pronunciation/Word Parts

goniometry	Procedure in which a **goniometer** is used to measure the angle of a joint and its range of motion (ROM) (see Figure 8-29 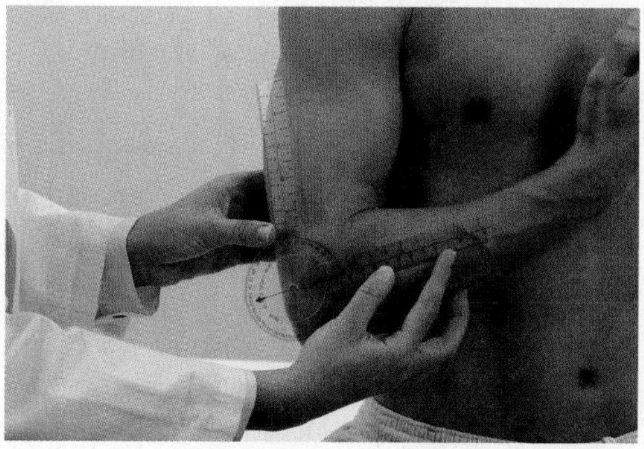 ■)
	
	FIGURE 8-29 ■ Goniometer.
	The two arms of the goniometer are positioned to correspond to body parts on either side of the joint. A scale on the goniometer measures (in degrees) how much motion of the joint is possible.
	Source: Patrick Watson for Pearson Education/PH College
		goniometry (GOH-nee-AW-meh-tree)
		  goni/o- *angle*
		  -metry *process of measuring*
		
		goniometer (GOH-nee-AW-meh-ter)
		  goni/o- *angle*
		  -meter *instrument used to measure*

orthosis	Orthopedic device such as a brace, splint, or collar that is used to immobilize a body part and keep it straight or correct an orthopedic problem. It is often custom-made to fit the patient.	**orthosis** (or-THOH-sis)
		  orth/o- *straight*
		  -osis *condition; process*

physical therapy	Procedure that uses exercises to improve a patient's range of motion, joint mobility, strength, and balance. Active exercises are done by the patient. Passive exercises are done by the therapist who moves the patient's body.	**physical** (FIZ-ih-kal)
		  physic/o- *body*
		  -al *pertaining to*
		
		therapy (THAIR-ah-pee)
		The combining form **therap/o-** means *treatment*.

prosthesis	Orthopedic device such as an artificial leg for a patient who has had amputation of a limb (see Figure 8-30 ■). It is known as a **prosthetic device**. An implanted artificial joint is also a prosthetic device. 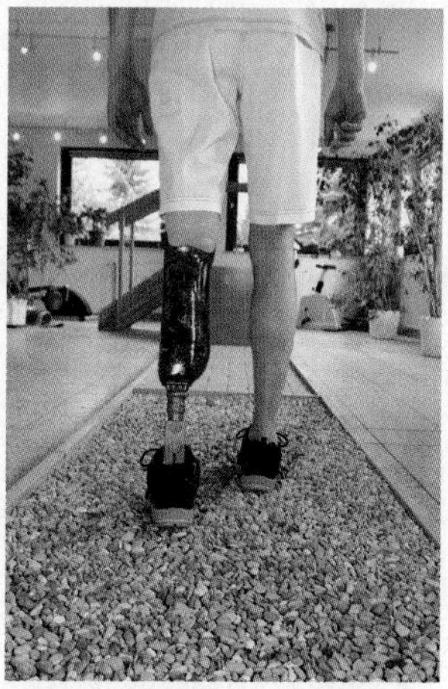
	
	FIGURE 8-30 ■ Leg prosthesis.
	Each prosthesis is custom-built for the patient, using computer-aided design. It is built according to the patient's height and weight (to match the other leg) and according to where the leg was amputated. This young man is learning to walk with his prosthetic leg on the uneven surface of a gravel path in a rehab center.
	Source: Belushi/Shutterstock
		prosthesis (praws-THEE-sis)
		
		prosthetic (praws-THET-ik)
		  prosthet/o- *artificial part*
		  -ic *pertaining to*

traction	Procedure that uses a weight to pull the bone ends of a fracture into correct alignment. Skin traction uses elastic wraps, straps, halters, or skin adhesives connected to a pulley and a weight. Skeletal traction uses pins, wires, or tongs inserted into the bone during surgery. Halo traction uses pins inserted into the cranium and attached to a circular metal frame that forms a halo around the patient's head (see Figure 10-32). Bars connect the halo to a rigid vest that immobilizes the chest and back while exerting upward traction on the head to straighten a fracture of the spine.	**traction** (TRAK-shun)
		  tract/o- *pulling*
		  -ion *action; condition*

Surgical Procedures

Word or Phrase	Description	Pronunciation/Word Parts
amputation	Procedure to remove all or part of an extremity because of trauma, cardiovascular disease, or diabetes mellitus. A below-the-knee amputation (BKA) is at the level of the tibia and fibula. An above-the-knee amputation (AKA) is at the level of the femur. A muscle flap is wrapped over the end of the amputated limb to provide a cushion and bulk so the patient can be fitted with an artificial limb (prosthesis). A patient who has had an amputation is an **amputee**.	**amputation** (AM-pyoo-TAY-shun) **amputat/o-** *cut off* **-ion** *action; condition* _____ **amputee** (AM-pyoo-tee) **amput/o-** *cut off* **-ee** *person who is the object of an action; person who receives; thing that is the object of an action; thing that receives*
arthrocentesis	Procedure to remove an accumulation of fluid from an injured joint by using a needle inserted into the joint space. It is also done to inject a drug to control inflammation and pain.	**arthrocentesis** (AR-throh-sen-TEE-sis) **arthr/o-** *joint* **-centesis** *procedure to puncture*
arthrodesis	Procedure to fuse the bones in a degenerated, unstable joint	**arthrodesis** (AR-throh-DEE-sis) **arthr/o-** *joint* **-desis** *procedure to fuse together*
arthroscopy	Procedure that uses an **arthroscope** inserted into the joint to visualize structures inside the joint (see Figure 8-31 ■). Other instruments can be inserted through the arthroscope to scrape or cut damaged cartilage or smooth sharp bone edges.	**arthroscopy** (ar-THRAW-skoh-pee) **arthr/o-** *joint* **-scopy** *process of using an instrument to examine* _____ **arthroscope** (AR-throh-skohp) **arthr/o-** *joint* **-scope** *instrument used to examine* _____ **arthroscopic** (AR-throh-SKAW-pik) **arthr/o-** *joint* **scop/o-** *examine with an instrument* **-ic** *pertaining to*

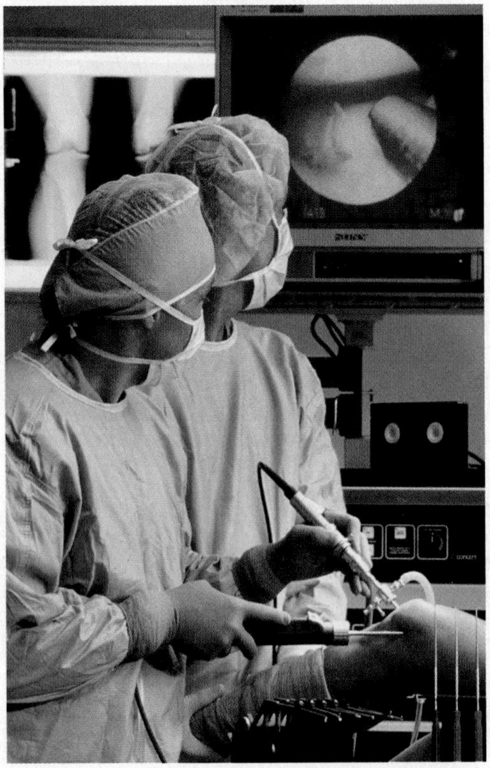

FIGURE 8-31 ■ Arthroscopic surgery.
The arthroscope was inserted into the knee joint through a surgically created portal (opening in the skin). Other portals were used to insert other instruments. A fiberoptic light and magnifying lens on the arthroscope allow the surgeon to see inside the joint, and the image is also displayed on a computer screen in the operating room.
Source: Ted Horowitz/Flirt/Corbis

Word or Phrase	Description	Pronunciation/Word Parts
bone graft	Procedure that uses whole bone or bone chips to repair fractures with extensive bone loss or defects due to bone cancer. Bone taken from the patient's own body is an **autograft**. Frozen or freeze-dried bone taken from a cadaver is an **allograft**.	**graft** (GRAFT) **autograft** (AW-toh-graft) aut/o- *self* -graft *tissue for implant; tissue for transplant* **allograft** (AL-oh-graft) all/o- *other; strange* -graft *tissue for implant; tissue for transplant*
bunionectomy	Procedure to remove the prominent part of the metatarsal bone that is causing a bunion in patients with hallux valgus.	**bunionectomy** (BUN-yun-EK-toh-mee) bunion/o- *bunion* -ectomy *surgical removal*
cartilage transplantation	Procedure that replaces damaged cartilage as an alternative to a total knee replacement. It is used to treat middle-aged adults (as opposed to older adults) with degenerative joint disease of the knee who have an active lifestyle.	**transplantation** (TRANS-plan-TAY-shun) transplant/o- *move something across and put in another place* -ation *being; having; process*

> **DID YOU KNOW?**
> Active people walk 1–3 million steps each year! The average person walks 4 miles each day.

Word or Phrase	Description	Pronunciation/Word Parts
external fixation	Procedure used to treat a complicated fracture. An external fixator orthopedic device has metal pins that are inserted into the bone on either side of the fracture and connected to a metal frame. This immobilizes the fracture. A similar device is used to perform a **leg lengthening** to treat a congenitally short leg. It has screws that are turned daily, pulling the cut ends of bone apart so new bone grows in the gap and lengthens the leg.	**external** (eks-TER-nal) extern/o- *outside* -al *pertaining to* **fixation** (fik-SAY-shun) fixat/o- *make stable; make still* -ion *action; condition*
joint replacement surgery	Procedure to replace a joint that has been destroyed by disease or osteoarthritis. A metal or plastic joint prosthesis is inserted (see Figure 8-32 ■). This surgery is done on the hips as a **total hip replacement (THR)**, or on the knees, shoulders, or even on the small joints of the fingers. For a total hip replacement, the head of the femur is sawn off. The stem (long metal projection) of the prosthesis is hammered into the cut end of the femur. The head (ball) of the prosthesis is matched to the size of the patient's acetabulum. The cup of the prosthesis is used to replace the acetabulum, and the ball is inserted into the cup. This is also known as an **arthroplasty**.	**arthroplasty** (AR-throh-PLAS-tee) arthr/o- *joint* -plasty *process of reshaping by surgery*

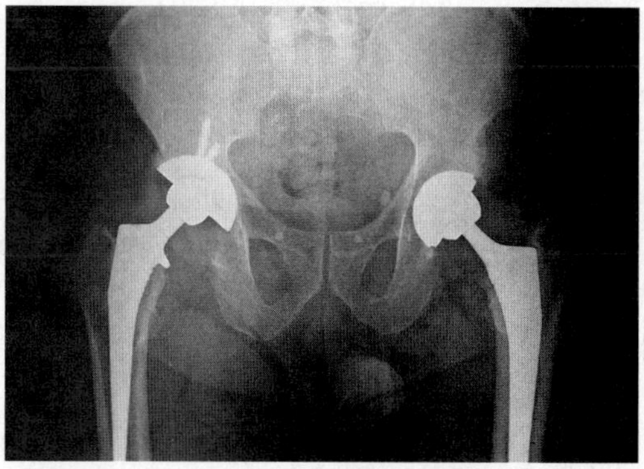

FIGURE 8-32 ■ Hip prostheses.
This patient has had two total hip replacement surgeries and received a different style of hip prosthesis each time. The metal components of a prosthesis stand out clearly on an x-ray.
Source: Nicolas Larento/Fotolia

Word or Phrase	Description	Pronunciation/Word Parts
open reduction and internal fixation (ORIF)	Procedure to treat a complicated fracture. An incision is made to open the skin and visualize the fracture, the fracture is reduced (realigned), and an internal fixation procedure is done using screws, nails, or plates to hold the fracture fragments in correct anatomical alignment (see Figure 8-33 ■).	**reduction** (ree-DUK-shun) **reduct/o-** *bring back; decrease* **-ion** *action; condition*

DID YOU KNOW?

Orthopedic surgery is not unlike carpentry, but instead of wood, it works on bone. Surgical orthopedic instruments include hammers, nails, screws, metal plates, chisels, mallets, gouges, and saws. An **osteotome** is used to cut bone. A **rongeur** is a forceps that is used to remove small bone fragments.

osteotome (AW-stee-oh-TOHM)
  oste/o- *bone*
  -tome *area with distinct edges; instrument used to cut*

rongeur (rawn-ZHER)

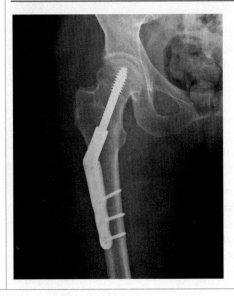

FIGURE 8-33 ■ Orthopedic plate and screws.
This fracture of the tibia was surgically repaired with an open reduction and internal fixation using a metal plate and multiple screws to stabilize the bone fragments. The plate and a larger screw extend up into the head of the femur.
Source: Nicolas Larento/Fotolia

Drugs

These drug categories and drugs are used to treat skeletal diseases. The most common generic and trade name drugs in each category are listed.

Category	Indication	Examples	Pronunciation/Word Parts
analgesic drugs	Over-the-counter drugs aspirin and acetaminophen decrease mild-to-moderate inflammation and pain. They are used to treat minor injuries and osteoarthritis. Prescription narcotic drugs are used to treat severe pain.	aspirin (Bayer, Ecotrin), acetaminophen (Tylenol); prescription narcotic drugs: meperidine (Demerol), oxycodone (OxyContin), morphine sulfate (MS Contin)	**analgesic** (AN-al-JEE-zik) **an-** *not; without* **alges/o-** *sensation of pain* **-ic** *pertaining to*
bone resorption inhibitor drugs	Inhibit osteoclasts from breaking down bone. They are used to prevent and treat osteoporosis.	alendronate (Fosamax), ibandronate (Boniva), zoledronic acid (Reclast, Zometa)	**resorption** (ree-SORP-shun) **re-** *again and again; backward; unable to* **sorb/o-** *suck up* **-tion** *being; having; process* The "b" in *sorb/o-* (absorb) is changed to a "p".

Category	Indication	Examples	Pronunciation/Word Parts
corticosteroid drugs	Decrease severe inflammation. They are given orally to treat osteoarthritis and rheumatoid arthritis. Some are given by **intra-articular** injection into the joint.	dexamethasone, hydrocortisone (Cortef, Solu-Cortef), prednisone; intra-articular injection: betamethasone (Celestone), methylprednisolone (Depo-Medrol), triamcinolone (Aristospan, Kenalog) *Note*: This is often referred to as a "cortisone shot," even though it is not the drug cortisone (which is only available as a tablet).	**corticosteroid** (KOR-tih-koh-STAIR-oyd) **cortic/o-** *cortex; outer region* **-steroid** *steroid* **intra-articular** (IN-trah-ar-TIH-kyoo-lar) **intra-** *within* **articul/o-** *joint* **-ar** *pertaining to*
gold compound drugs	Inhibit the immune response that attacks the joints and connective tissue in patients with rheumatoid arthritis. These drugs actually contain gold.	auranofin (Ridaura)	
nonsteroidal anti-inflammatory drugs (NSAIDs)	Decrease mild-to-moderate inflammation and pain. They are used to treat osteoarthritis and orthopedic injuries. Celebrex is a COX-2 inhibitor drug, a type of NSAID that blocks the COX-2 enzyme that produces prostaglandins that cause pain.	celecoxib (Celebrex), diclofenac (Cataflam, Voltaren), ibuprofen (Advil, Motrin), naproxen (Aleve, Naprosyn)	**nonsteroidal** (NON-stair-OYD-al) **non-** *not* **steroid/o-** *steroid* **-al** *pertaining to* **anti-inflammatory** (AN-tee-in-FLAM-ah-TOR-ee) **anti-** *against* **inflammat/o-** *redness and warmth* **-ory** *having the function of*

Abbreviations

AKA	above-the-knee amputation
anti-CCP	anti-cyclic citrullinated peptide
AP	anteroposterior
BKA	below-the-knee amputation
BMD	bone mineral density
C1–C7	cervical vertebrae
Ca, Ca++	calcium
CDH	congenital dislocation of the hip
DEXA, DXA	dual-energy x-ray absorptiometry
DIP	distal interphalangeal (joint)
DJD	degenerative joint disease
ESWT	extracorporeal shock wave therapy
FX, Fx	fracture
L1–L5	lumbar vertebrae
LLE	left lower extremity
LUE	left upper extremity
MCP	metacarpophalangeal (joint)

NSAID	nonsteroidal anti-inflammatory drug
OA	osteoarthritis
ORIF	open reduction and internal fixation
ortho	orthopedics (short form)
P	phosphorus
PIP	proximal interphalangeal (joint)
PT	physical therapist; physical therapy
QCT	quantitative computerized tomography
RA	rheumatoid arthritis
RF	rheumatoid factor
RLE	right lower extremity
ROM	range of motion
RUE	right upper extremity
S1	first sacral vertebra
T1–T12	thoracic vertebrae
THR	total hip replacement
tib-fib	tibia-fibula (short form)

WORD ALERT
Abbreviations

Abbreviations are commonly used in all types of medical documents; however, they can mean different things to different people and their meanings can be misinterpreted. Always verify the meaning of an abbreviation.

AKA means *above-the-knee amputation,* but it also means the English phrase *also known as.*
Ca means *calcium,* but it also means *cancer.*
OA means *osteoarthritis,* but it also means *Overeaters Anonymous.*
PT means *physical therapist* and *physical therapy,* but it also means *prothrombin time.*
RA means *rheumatoid arthritis,* but it also means *right atrium* (of the heart) or *room air.*
ROM means *range of motion,* but it also means *rupture of membranes* (before the birth of a baby).

IT'S GREEK TO ME!

Did you notice that some words have two different combining forms? Combining forms from both Greek and Latin remain a part of medical language today.

Word	Greek	Latin	Medical Word Examples
bone	oste/o-	osse/o-	osteoarthritis, osseous
cartilage	chondr/o-	cartilagin/o-	costochondral, cartilaginous
fibula	perone/o-	fibul/o-	peroneal, fibular
joint	arthr/o-	articul/o-	arthroscopy, articulation
vertebra	spondyl/o-	vertebr/o-	spondylolisthesis, vertebral

Definition of the Medical Word

1. Disease (of a) joint
2. Tumor (of the) cartilage
3. Condition (of) humpback
4. Inflammation of (a) joint
5. Pertaining to (a condition that is) present at birth
6. Process of measuring (the) density (of bone)
7. Tumor (of the) bone
8. Pertaining to (an) artificial part (arm or leg)
9. Instrument used to measure (the) angle (of a joint)
10. Surgical removal (of a) bunion
11. Procedure to fuse together (a) joint
12. Instrument used to examine (a) joint
13. Person who is the object of an action (that is to) cut off (a body part)
14. Pertaining to break into small pieces
15. Condition (of) swayback

Build the Medical Word

arthropathy

PREFIX EXERCISE

Read the definition of the medical word. Look at the medical word or partial word that is given (it already contains a combining form and suffix). Select the correct prefix from the Prefix List and write it on the blank line. Then build the medical word and write it on the line. Be sure to check your spelling. The first one has been done for you.

PREFIX LIST

a- (away from; without)
an- (not; without)

de- (reversal of; without)
dis- (away from)

intra- (within)
mal- (bad; inadequate)

Definition of the Medical Word	Prefix	Word or Partial Word	Build the Medical Word
1. Pertaining to without blood vessels (and blood to a bone)	a-	vascular	avascular
2. Process (of making the bone to be) without minerals		mineralization	
3. Pertaining to within (the) joint		articular	
4. Action (of moving a bone) away from (its normal) place		location	
5. State (of a bone being in a) bad arrangement in a straight line		alignment	
6. Pertaining to (the) reversal of (the) production (of bone)		generative	
7. Pertaining to (a drug that makes you be) without (the) sensation of pain		algesic	

MULTIPLE COMBINING FORMS AND SUFFIX EXERCISE

Read the definition of the medical word. Select the correct suffix and combining forms. Then build the medical word and write it on the line. Be sure to check your spelling. The first one has been done for you.

SUFFIX LIST

-ia (condition; state; thing)
-ics (knowledge; practice)
-itis (infection of; inflammation of)
-oma (mass; tumor)
-osis (condition; process)

alg/o- (pain)
arthr/o- (joint)
chondr/o- (cartilage)
dextr/o- (right)
hem/o- (blood)
lev/o- (left)
malac/o- (softening)
myel/o- (bone marrow; myelin; spinal cord)

COMBINING FORM LIST

orth/o- (straight)
oste/o- (bone)
ped/o- (child)
por/o- (pores; small openings)
sarc/o- (connective tissue)
scoli/o- (crooked; curved)

Definition of the Medical Word

1. Condition (of a) left-(turning) curved (spine)
2. Condition (of) cartilage softening
3. Condition (of) bone (having) small openings
4. Knowledge and practice (of producing) straight(ness of the bones and muscles in a) child (or adult)
5. Condition (of) blood (in the) joint
6. Condition of right-(turning) curved (spine)
7. Condition (of) joint pain
8. Infection of (the) bone and bone marrow
9. Tumor (of the) bone (and) connective tissue

Build the Medical Word

levoscoliosis

_____

_____

_____

_____

_____

_____

_____

_____

8.7A Spell Medical Words

ENGLISH AND MEDICAL WORD EQUIVALENTS EXERCISE

For each English word, write its equivalent medical word. Be sure to check your spelling. The first one has been done for you.

English Word	Medical Word	English Word	Medical Word
1. top of the skull	*cranium*	12. thigh bone	
2. cheek bone		13. kneecap	
3. soft spot		14. shin bone	
4. upper jaw		15. heel bone	
5. lower jaw		16. hunchback	
6. shoulder blade		17. swayback	
7. breast bone		18. bowleg	
8. collar bone		19. knock-knee	
9. point of the elbow		20. clubfoot	
10. finger or toe		21. bone spur	
11. tail bone		22. great toe/big toe	

HEARING MEDICAL WORDS EXERCISE

You hear someone speaking the medical words given below. Read each pronunciation and then write the medical word it represents. Be sure to check your spelling. The first one has been done for you.

1. ar-THRY-tis — *arthritis*
2. ar-THRAW-grah-fee — _____
3. con-DROH-mah — _____
4. COM-ih-NYOO-ted FRAK-chur — _____
5. DEKS-troh-SKOH-lee-OH-sis — _____
6. MUS-kyoo-loh-SKEL-eh-tal — _____
7. OR-thoh-PEE-dist — _____
8. AW-stee-OH-poh-ROH-sis — _____
9. FAY-langks — _____
10. praws-THEE-sis — _____

8.7B Pronounce Medical Words

PRONUNCIATION EXERCISE

Read the medical word and the syllables in its pronunciation. Circle the primary (main) accented syllable. The first one has been done for you.

1. amputation (am-pyoo-⟨tay⟩-shun)
2. arthralgia (ar-thral-jah)
3. arthroscopy (ar-thraw-skoh-pee)
4. cartilaginous (kar-tih-laj-ih-nus)
5. hemarthrosis (hee-mar-throh-sis)
6. humeral (hyoo-mer-al)
7. kyphosis (ky-foh-sis)
8. mandibular (man-dih-byoo-lar)
9. metacarpal (met-ah-kar-pal)
10. osteoarthritis (aw-stee-oh-ar-thry-tis)

8.8 Research Medical Words

TEST YOURSELF

Three of these words are related in some way to each other. Define each word. Then circle the word that is not related.

1. osteoblast _____
2. osteoclast _____
3. osteocyte _____
4. osteophyte _____
5. Three of these words are related in some way to the others. Which word is not related? _____

SOUND-ALIKE WORDS

Compare and contrast the medical meanings of these sound-alike orthopedic (skeletal) words.

1. *ileum* (Chapter 3) and *ilium*
2. *malleolus* and *malleus* (Chapter 16)
3. *humerus* and *humorous*
4. *perineal* (Chapter 13) and *peroneal*

ON THE JOB CHALLENGE EXERCISE

On the job, you will often have to talk with patients and explain medical words to them. Research the meanings of these sound-alike phrases.

1. closed fracture _____
2. closed reduction of a fracture _____
3. open fracture _____
4. open reduction and internal fixation of a fracture _____

8.9 Analyze Medical Reports

ELECTRONIC PATIENT RECORD

This is an Office Visit Note. Read the note and answer the questions.

PEARSON PRIMARY CARE ASSOCIATES

Task   Edit   View   Time Scale   Options   Help

OFFICE VISIT NOTE

PATIENT NAME:	LOWE, James
PATIENT NUMBER:	63-1004
DATE OF VISIT:	November 19, xx

Source: Elena Elissiva/123 RF

HISTORY

This is a 20-year-old male who has been having problems with intermittent low back pain for several years now. He leads an active lifestyle and his job requires him to do a lot of lifting and walking. The pain is getting worse, and he would like to get some definitive treatment at this time. He has been told in the past by a physician that his pelvis is tilted up on the left. However, he does not believe this was ever diagnosed as a leg-length discrepancy. He denies any radiation of the pain to his buttocks or legs, and he says he has not noticed any tingling in his lower extremities.

PHYSICAL EXAMINATION

Left leg: The leg length from the iliac crest to the medial malleolus is 106 cm. Right leg: The leg length from the iliac crest to the medial malleolus is 103 cm. Examination of his back reveals diffuse tenderness over the spinous processes in the lumbar region. I also noticed a dextroscoliosis in the lower thoracic region, which seemed to be significant. Neurologically, the patient had normal reflexes and normal strength in the lower extremities.

ASSESSMENT

Chronic back pain due to a significant leg-length discrepancy. He also has a dextroscoliosis, although the exact number of degrees of curvature was not measured.

PLAN

1. Refer to an orthopedist for a definitive diagnosis and measurement of the scoliosis.

2. Prescription for Motrin 600 mg tablet, 1 tablet, 3 times a day.

Samantha P. Campbell, M.D.

Samantha P. Campbell, M.D.

SPC: lcc
D: 11/19/xx
T: 11/19/xx

---

1. Divide *dextroscoliosis* into its three word parts and give the meaning of each word part.

Word Part	Meaning
_____	_____
_____	_____
_____	_____

2. The adjective *spinal* refers to the spine or backbone while the adjective *spinous* refers to a bony process. **True**   **False**

3. Divide *orthopedist* into its three word parts and give the meaning of each word part.

Word Part	**Meaning**
_____	_____
_____	_____
_____	_____

4. The patient's leg length was measured using what two anatomical structures? _____

5. The medial malleolus is located on the distal end of what bone? _____

6. Which leg was shorter, the patient's right leg or left leg? _____

7. The spinous processes are located on what bones? _____

8. What is the single-letter designation for the vertebrae in the lumbar region? _____

9. Which way did the patient's spine curve? To the right or to the left?

_____

10. What category of drugs does Motrin belong to? What drug action does it have?

_____

11. What will the orthopedist measure that this physician did not measure during the office visit?

_____

MyMedicalTerminologyLab™

MyMedicalTerminologyLab is a premium online homework management system that includes a host of features to help you study. Registered users will find:

- A multitude of quizzes and activities built within the MyLab platform

- Powerful tools that track and analyze your results—allowing you to create a personalized learning experience

- Videos and audio pronunciations to help enrich your progress

- Streaming lesson presentations (Guided Lectures) and self-paced learning modules

- A space where you and your instructor can check your progress and manage your assignments

Chapter 9
Orthopedics

Muscular System

Orthopedics (OR-thoh-PEE-diks) is the medical specialty that studies the anatomy and physiology of the muscular and skeletal systems and uses laboratory and diagnostic procedures, medical and surgical procedures, and drugs to treat muscular and skeletal diseases. In Chapter 8, you studied orthopedics from the perspective of the skeletal system. In this chapter, you will study the muscular system.

 ## Learning Outcomes

After you study this chapter, you should be able to

9.1 Identify structures of the muscular system.

9.2 Describe the process of muscle contraction and how muscles produce movement.

9.3 Describe common muscular diseases, laboratory and diagnostic procedures, medical and surgical procedures, and drugs.

9.4 Form the plural and adjective forms of nouns related to orthopedics (muscular).

9.5 Give the meanings of word parts and abbreviations related to orthopedics (muscular).

9.6 Divide orthopedics (muscular) words and build orthopedics (muscular) words.

9.7 Spell and pronounce orthopedic (muscular) words.

9.8 Research sound-alike and other orthopedic (muscular) words.

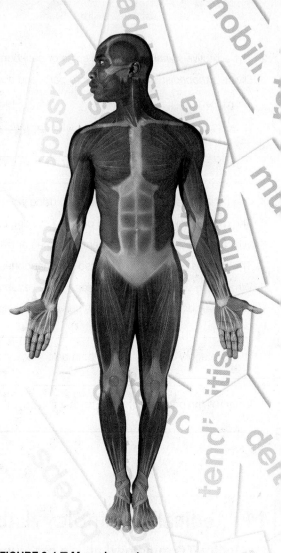

FIGURE 9-1 ■ Muscular system.
The muscular system is a widespread body system that consists of the voluntary skeletal muscles and other structures throughout the body.
Source: Pearson Education

9.9 Analyze the medical content and meaning of orthopedic (muscular) reports.

Medical Language Key

To unlock the definition of a medical word, break it into word parts. Give the meaning of each word part. Put the meanings of the word parts in order, beginning with the meaning of the suffix, then the prefix (if present), then the combining form(s).

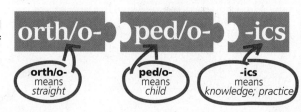

	Word Part	Word Part Meaning
Suffix	**-ics**	*knowledge; practice*
Combining Form	**orth/o-**	*straight*
Combining Form	**ped/o-**	*child*

Orthopedics: ▶ *Knowledge and practice (of producing) straight(ness of the bones and muscles in a) child (or adult).* *Orthopedics* can also be spelled *orthopaedics*. Some hospitals keep this spelling in the title *Department of Orthopaedics.*

Anatomy and Physiology

The **muscular system** is the engine that moves the bony framework of the body (see Figure 9-1 ■). There are approximately 700 skeletal muscles in the body, as well as tendons and other structures of the muscular system. The contours of some skeletal muscles are visible under the skin, particularly when they contract. Others are located more deeply, and their movements may be felt. The purpose of the muscular system is to produce body movement. All of the muscles of the body (or the muscles in a particular part of the body) are referred to as the **musculature**. The muscular system is also known as the **musculoskeletal system** because of the close relationship between the muscles and the bones. Without the muscles, the bones would not be able to move and, without the bones, the muscles would lack support.

Anatomy of the Muscular System

Types of Muscles

There are three types of muscles: skeletal muscles, the cardiac muscle, and smooth muscles (see Figure 9-2 ■).

- **Skeletal muscles**: Skeletal muscles provide the means by which the body can move. Skeletal muscles are **voluntary muscles** that contract and relax in response to conscious thought. They are **striated**, have multiple nuclei, and show bands of color when seen under a microscope.
- **Cardiac muscle**: The cardiac muscle of the heart pumps blood through the circulatory system. It is an involuntary muscle that is not under conscious control. The heart was discussed in "Cardiology," Chapter 5.
- **Smooth muscles**: Smooth muscles are involuntary, nonstriated muscles. They form a continuous, thin layer around many organs and structures (blood vessels, bronchi, intestines, etc.). Smooth muscles are discussed in various chapters.

Of the three types of muscles, only skeletal muscle belongs to the muscular system. In the rest of this chapter, the word *muscle* should be understood to mean *skeletal muscle*.

Pronunciation/Word Parts

muscle (MUS-el)

muscular (MUS-kyoo-lar)
  muscul/o- *muscle*
  -ar *pertaining to*
The combining forms **my/o-** and **myos/o-** also mean *muscle*.

musculature (MUS-kyoo-lah-CHUR)
  muscul/o- *muscle*
  -ature *system composed of*

musculoskeletal
(MUS-kyoo-loh-SKEL-eh-tal)
  muscul/o- *muscle*
  skelet/o- *skeleton*
  -al *pertaining to*

voluntary (VAW-lun-TAIR-ee)
  volunt/o- *person's own free will*
  -ary *pertaining to*

striated (STRY-aa-ted)

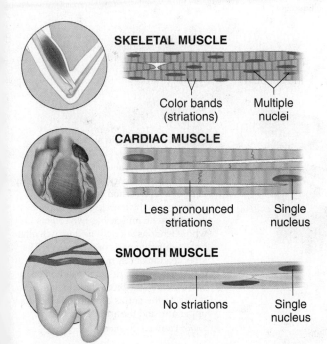

SKELETAL MUSCLE
Color bands (striations)　Multiple nuclei

CARDIAC MUSCLE
Less pronounced striations　Single nucleus

SMOOTH MUSCLE
No striations　Single nucleus

FIGURE 9-2 ■ Types of muscle.
There are three types of muscles—skeletal muscles, the cardiac muscle, and smooth muscles. Each has a different appearance under a microscope. Note the very pronounced color bands (striations) and multiple nuclei in each skeletal muscle cell. Cardiac muscle cells have less pronounced bands, and nonstriated smooth muscle cells have no bands.
Source: Pearson Education

Muscle Origins, Insertions, and Related Structures

A muscle is attached to a bone by a **tendon**, a cordlike, nonelastic, white fibrous band of connective tissue (see Figure 9-3 ■). The **origin** or beginning of a muscle is where its tendon is attached to a stationary or nearly stationary bone (see Figure 9-4 ■). The **insertion** or ending of a muscle is where its tendon is attached to the bone that moves when the muscle contracts and relaxes. The **belly** of a muscle is where its mass is the greatest, usually midway between the origin and insertion. From its origin on a bone, the muscle often travels across a joint; this is the joint that will move when the muscle contracts.

A **bursa**, a thin sac of synovial membrane filled with synovial fluid, acts as a cushion to reduce friction where a tendon rubs against the bone near a synovial joint. Each muscle is wrapped in **fascia**, a thin connective tissue that joins with the tendon (see Figure 9-3). An **aponeurosis** is a wide, white fibrous sheet of connective tissue, sometimes composed of several tendons, that attaches a flat muscle to a bone or to other, deeper muscles (see Figures 9-9, 9-11, and 9-14). A **retinaculum** is a nearly translucent band of fibrous tissue and fascia that holds down tendons that cross the wrist and ankle (see Figures 9-12, 9-13, and 9-15).

Muscle Names

Muscle names can seem complex because they are in Latin, but you will recognize some of the Latin words because they relate to the bones you studied in Chapter 8. Other Latin words become familiar because they consistently describe where the muscle is located, its shape, its size, or what action it performs (see Table 9-1 ■).

Pronunciation/Word Parts

tendon (TEN-dun)

tendinous (TEN-dih-nus)
 tendin/o- *tendon*
 -ous *pertaining to*
The combining form **ten/o-** also means *tendon*.

origin (OR-ih-jin)

insertion (in-SER-shun)
 insert/o- *introduce; put in*
 -ion *action; condition*

bursa (BER-sah)

bursae (BER-see)
Bursa is a Latin singular noun. Form the plural by changing *-a* to *-ae*.

bursal (BER-sal)
 burs/o- *bursa*
 -al *pertaining to*

fascia (FASH-ee-ah)

fascial (FASH-ee-al)
 fasci/o- *fascia*
 -al *pertaining to*

aponeurosis (AP-oh-nyoor-OH-sis)

retinaculum (RET-ih-NAK-yoo-lum)

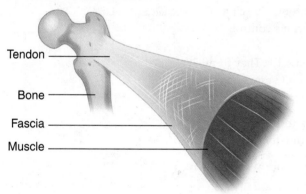

Tendon

Bone

Fascia

Muscle

FIGURE 9-3 ■ Tendon.
At their origins and insertions, most muscles are attached to the bone by a tendon. As the muscle transitions to the tendon, the red color of the muscle is replaced by the white fibrous tissue of the tendon. The fascia that surrounds the muscle also merges with the tendon.
Source: Pearson Education

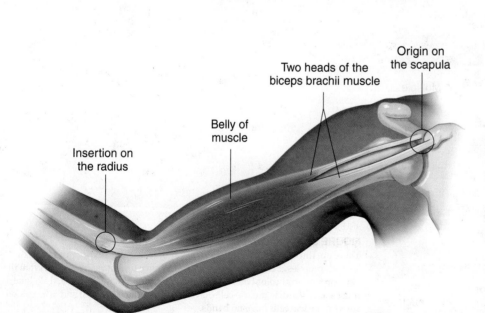

Two heads of the biceps brachii muscle

Origin on the scapula

Belly of muscle

Insertion on the radius

FIGURE 9-4 ■ Origin and insertion of a muscle.
Every muscle has at least one point of origin on a stationary (or nearly stationary) bone and an insertion on a bone that moves when the muscle contracts. The biceps brachii muscle has two origins whose tendons are right next to each other but on different parts of the scapula. The other tendon of this muscle crosses the elbow joint and ends at its insertion on the radius. When the biceps brachii muscle contracts, the radius is pulled toward the upper arm and the arm flexes.
Source: Pearson Education

Table 9-1 Muscle Names and Their Meanings

Muscle Name	What the Muscle Name Tells You	Pronunciation/Word Parts
biceps brachii	Shape: Origin of the muscle has two parts or heads (*biceps*) Location: Arm (*brachii*)	**biceps** (BY-seps) The prefix *bi-* means *two*, and *-ceps* is from the Latin noun *caput* (*head*). **brachii** (BRAY-kee-eye)

brachioradialis	Location: Radial bone (*radi/o-*) in the arm (*brachi/o-*)	**brachioradialis**
		 (BRAY-kee-oh-RAY-dee-AL-is)
		    brachi/o- *arm*
		    radi/o- *forearm bone; radiation; x-rays*
		    -alis *pertaining to*

extensor digitorum	Action: Extends
	 Location: Digits (*digitorum*)
		extensor (eks-TEN-sor)
		    extens/o- *straightening*
		    -or *person who does; person who produces; thing that does; thing that produces*
		
		 digitorum (DIJ-ih-TOR-um)

flexor hallucis brevis	Action: Flexes
	 Location: Big toe (*hallux*)
	 Size: Short (*brevis*)
		flexor (FLEK-sor)
		    flex/o- *bending*
		    -or *person who does; person who produces; thing that does; thing that produces*
		
		 hallucis (HAL-yoo-sis)
		
		 brevis (BREV-is)

gluteus maximus	Location: Buttocks (*gluteus*) Size: Large (*maximus*)	**gluteus** (gloo-TEE-us) **maximus** (MAK-sih-mus)
rectus abdominis	Orientation: Straight up and down (*rectus*) Location: Abdomen (*abdominis*)	**rectus** (REK-tus) **abdominis** (ab-DAW-mih-nis)

temporalis	Location: Temporal bone (*temporalis*) of the cranium	**temporalis** (TEM-poh-RAY-lis)
		    tempor/o- *side of the head; temple*
		    -alis *pertaining to*

triceps brachii	Shape: Origin of the muscle has three parts or heads (*triceps*) Location: Arm (*brachii*)	**triceps** (TRY-seps) The prefix *tri-* means *three*.

Types of Muscle Movement

Muscles function in antagonistic pairs to produce movement. When the first muscle contracts, the second muscle relaxes to allow the movement or it partially contracts to control the movement. Flexion and extension, abduction and adduction, rotation to the right and to the left, supination and pronation, and eversion and inversion are opposite movements that are controlled by muscle pairs (see Figures 9-5 ■ through 9-8 ■ and Table 9-2 ■).

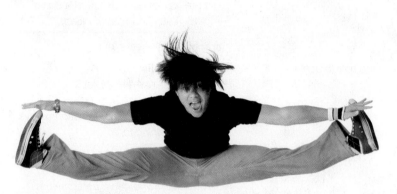

FIGURE 9-5 ■ Extension, abduction, and dorsiflexion.
This dancer has his arms and legs extended and abducted. His feet are in dorsiflexion.
Source: Photodisc/Getty Images

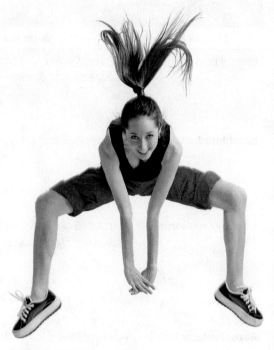

FIGURE 9-6 ■ Extension, adduction, pronation, abduction, flexion, and plantar flexion.
This dancer has her arms extended and adducted, with her hands in pronation. Her thighs are abducted, and her knees flexed. Her feet are in plantar flexion.
Source: Photodisc/Getty Images

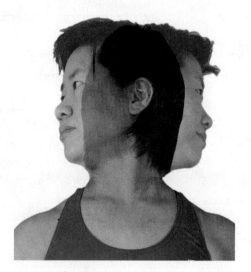

FIGURE 9-7 ■ Rotation.
The head rotates to the right and left around its axis, which is the vertebral column.
Source: Pearson Education

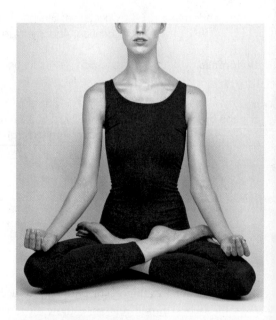

FIGURE 9-8 ■ Extension, supination, abduction, flexion, and inversion.
This person has her arms extended and her hands in supination. Her thighs are abducted, and her knees flexed. Her feet are in inversion.
Source: Anthony Saint James/Photodisc/Getty Images

Table 9-2 Types of Muscle Movement

Movement	Description	Muscle Type	Pronunciation/Word Parts

flexion	Bending a joint to decrease the angle between two bones or two body parts. (*Note*: Plantar flexion of the foot causes the toes to point downward. Dorsiflexion of the foot causes the toes to point upward.)	**flexor**	**flexion** (FLEK-shun)
			  flex/o- *bending*
			  -ion *action; condition*
			
			flexor (FLEK-sor)
			  flex/o- *bending*
			  -or *person who does; person who produces; thing that does; thing that produces*

extension	Straightening and extending a joint to increase the angle between two bones or two body parts	**extensor**	**extension** (eks-TEN-shun)
			  extens/o- *straightening*
			  -ion *action; condition*
			
			extensor (eks-TEN-sor)
			  extens/o- *straightening*
			  -or *person who does; person who produces; thing that does; thing that produces*

abduction	Moving a body part away from the midline of the body	**abductor**	**abduction** (ab-DUK-shun)
			  ab- *away from*
			  duct/o- *bring; duct; move*
			  -ion *action; condition*
			
			abductor (ab-DUK-tor)
			  ab- *away from*
			  duct/o- *bring; duct; move*
			  -or *person who does; person who produces; thing that does; thing that produces*

adduction	Moving a body part toward the midline of the body	**adductor**	**adduction** (ad-DUK-shun)
			  ad- *toward*
			  duct/o- *bring; duct; move*
			  -ion *action; condition*
			
			adductor (ad-DUK-tor)
			  ad- *toward*
			  duct/o- *bring; duct; move*
			  -or *person who does; person who produces; thing that does; thing that produces*

rotation	Moving a body part around its axis	**rotator**	**rotation** (roh-TAY-shun)
			  rotat/o- *rotate*
			  -ion *action; condition*
			
			rotator (ROH-tay-tor)
			  rotat/o- *rotate*
			  -or *person who does; person who produces; thing that does; thing that produces*

supination	Turning the palm of the hand anteriorly or upward. (*Note*: Here, *lying on the back* refers to the back of the hand.)	**supinator**	**supination** (soo-pih-NAY-shun)
			  supinat/o- *lying on the back*
			  -ion *action; condition*
			
			supinator (SOO-pih-NAY-tor)
			  supinat/o- *lying on the back*
			  -or *person who does; person who produces; thing that does; thing that produces*

(continued)

Table 9-2 Types of Muscle Movement (*continued*)

Movement	Description	Muscle Type	Pronunciation/Word Parts

pronation	Turning the palm of the hand posteriorly or downward. (*Note*: Here, *face down* refers to the face of the palm.)	**pronator**	**pronation** (proh-NAY-shun)
			  pronat/o- *face down*
			  -ion *action; condition*

			pronator (proh-NAY-tor)
			  pronat/o- *face down*
			  -or *person who does; person who produces; thing that does; thing that produces*

eversion	Turning a body part outward and toward the side	**evertor**	**eversion** (ee-VER-zhun)
			  e- *out; without*
			  vers/o- *travel; turn*
			  -ion *action; condition*

			evertor (ee-VER-tor)
			  e- *out; without*
			  vert/o- *travel; turn*
			  -or *person who does; person who produces; thing that does; thing that produces*

inversion	Turning a body part inward	**invertor**	**inversion** (in-VER-zhun)
			  in- *in; not; within*
			  vers/o- *travel; turn*
			  -ion *action; condition*

			invertor (in-VER-tor)
			  in- *in; not; within*
			  vert/o- *travel; turn*
			  -or *person who does; person who produces; thing that does; thing that produces*

Muscles of the Head and Neck

These are the most important muscles of the head and neck (see Figure 9-9 ■):

- **Frontalis**: Moves the eyebrows or wrinkles the forehead skin.
- **Temporalis**: Moves the mandible (lower jaw) upward and backward.
- **Orbicularis oculi**: Closes the eyelids or presses them together.
- **Orbicularis oris**: Closes the lips or presses them together.
- **Masseter**: Moves the mandible (lower jaw) upward.

Pronunciation/Word Parts

frontalis (frun-TAY-lis)
  front/o- *front*
  -alis *pertaining to*

temporalis (TEM-poh-RAY-lis)
  tempor/o- *side of the head; temple*
  -alis *pertaining to*

orbicularis (or-BIH-kyoo-LAIR-is)
  orbicul/o- *small circle*
  -aris *pertaining to*

oculi (AW-kyoo-lie)

oris (OR-is)

masseter (MAS-eh-ter)
  masset/o- *chewing*
  -er *person who does; person who produces; thing that does; thing that produces*

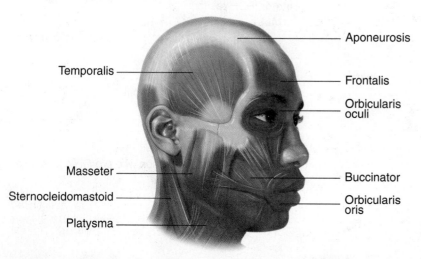

Temporalis — Aponeurosis
Masseter — Frontalis
Sternocleidomastoid — Orbicularis oculi
Platysma — Buccinator
Orbicularis oris

FIGURE 9-9 ■ Muscles of the head and neck.
These muscles contract and relax when you close your eyes, make facial expressions, chew food, or move your head.
Source: Pearson Education

- **Buccinator**: Moves the cheeks.
- **Sternocleidomastoid**: Bends the head toward the sternum (flexion) and turns the head to either side (rotation).
- **Platysma**: Moves the mandible (lower jaw) down.

Muscles of the Shoulders, Chest, and Back

These are the most important muscles of the shoulders, chest, and back (see Figures 9-10 ■ and 9-11 ■):

- **Deltoid**: Raises the arm and moves the arm away from the body (abduction).
- **Pectoralis major**: Moves the arm anteriorly and medially across the chest (adduction).
- **Intercostal muscles**: Muscle pairs between the ribs; one contracts during inspiration to spread the ribs apart; the other contracts during forced expiration, coughing, or sneezing to pull the ribs together.
- **Trapezius**: Raises the shoulder, pulls the shoulder blades together, elevates the clavicle. Turns the head from side to side (rotation). Moves the head posteriorly (extension).
- **Latissimus dorsi**: Moves the arm posteriorly and medially toward the vertebral column (adduction).

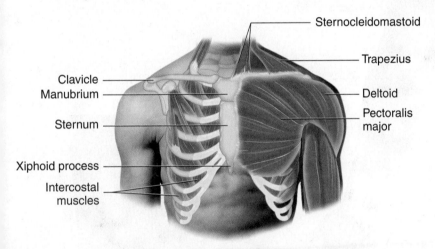

FIGURE 9-10 ■ Muscles of the shoulders and chest.
These muscles contract and relax when you raise your arms, move your arms and shoulders toward the midline to hug someone, or rotate your arms inwardly.
Source: Pearson Education

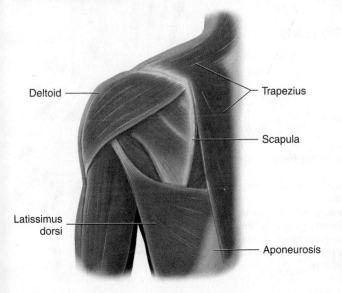

FIGURE 9-11 ■ Muscles of the shoulder and back.
These muscles contract and relax when you shrug your shoulders or pull your shoulder blades together to sit up straight. They also move your head backward and to the side, and turn your trunk to the right or left.
Source: Pearson Education

Pronunciation/Word Parts

buccinator (BUK-sih-NAY-tor)
  buccinat/o- *cheek*
  -or *person who does; person who produces; thing that does; thing that produces*

sternocleidomastoid
(STER-noh-KLY-doh-MAS-toyd)
  stern/o- *breastbone; sternum*
  cleid/o- *clavicle; collar bone*
  mast/o- *breast; mastoid process*
  -oid *resembling*
Note: The origin of this muscle is at two heads, one on the sternum and one on the clavicle. Its insertion is at the mastoid process of the temporal bone behind the ear.

platysma (plah-TIZ-mah)

deltoid (DEL-toyd)
  delt/o- *triangle*
  -oid *resembling*
This muscle is shaped like a triangle. In the Greek alphabet, the capital letter *delta* is in the shape of a triangle.

pectoralis (PEK-toh-RAY-lis)
  pector/o- *chest*
  -alis *pertaining to*

intercostal (IN-ter-KAW-stal)
  inter- *between*
  cost/o- *rib*
  -al *pertaining to*

trapezius (trah-PEE-zee-us)
This muscle is shaped like a trapezoid, a geometric figure that has two parallel sides and two nonparallel sides.

latissimus (lah-TIH-sih-mus)

dorsi (DOR-sigh)

Muscles of the Upper Extremity

These are the most important muscles of the arm and hand (see Figures 9-12 ■ and 9-13 ■):

- **Biceps brachii**: Bends the upper arm toward the shoulder (flexion) and bends the lower arm toward the upper arm (flexion).
- **Triceps brachii**: Straightens the lower arm (extension).
- **Brachioradialis**: Bends the lower arm toward the upper arm (flexion).
- **Thenar muscles**: Bend the thumb (flexion) and move it toward the palm (adduction).

Pronunciation/Word Parts

biceps (BY-seps)
The origin of the biceps muscle is divided into two parts (*bi-*) or heads (*-ceps*).

brachii (BRAY-kee-eye)

triceps (TRY-seps)
The origin of the triceps muscle is divided into three parts (*tri-*) or heads (*-ceps*).

brachioradialis
(BRAY-kee-oh-RAY-dee-AL-is)
   brachi/o- *arm*
   radi/o- *forearm bone; radiation; x-rays*
   -alis *pertaining to*

thenar (THEE-nar)
   then/o- *thumb*
   -ar *pertaining to*

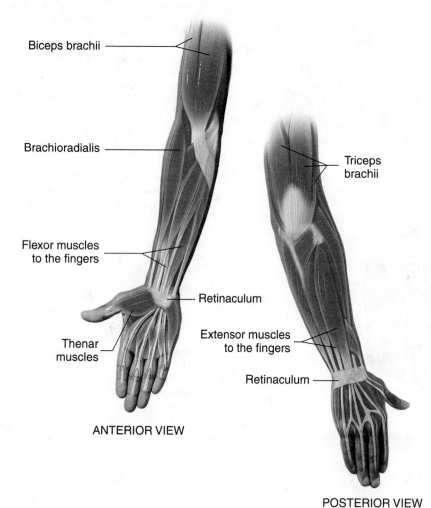

ANTERIOR VIEW

POSTERIOR VIEW

FIGURE 9-12 ■ Muscles of the upper extremity.
These muscles contract and relax when you lift a heavy box, straighten your arms to do a handstand, shake hands, make a fist, or play the piano.
Source: Pearson Education

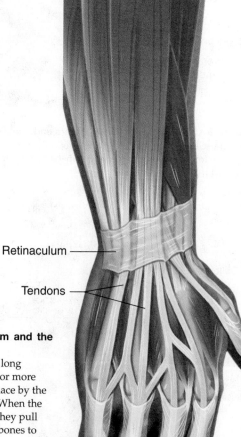

FIGURE 9-13 ■ Muscles of the forearm and the retinaculum.
Each extensor muscle of the forearm has a long tendon that travels across the wrist to one or more of the fingers. These tendons are held in place by the retinaculum, a translucent band of tissue. When the extensor muscles in the forearm contract, they pull the tendons which then pull on the finger bones to straighten and extend the fingers.
Source: Pearson Education

Muscles of the Abdomen

These are the most important muscles of the abdomen (see Figure 9-14 ■):

- **External abdominal oblique**: Bends the upper body forward (flexion), rotates the side of the body medially, and compresses the side of the abdominal wall.
- **Internal abdominal oblique**: Bends the upper body forward (flexion), rotates the side of the body medially, and compresses the side of the abdominal wall.
- **Rectus abdominis**: Bends the upper body forward (flexion) and compresses the anterior abdominal wall.

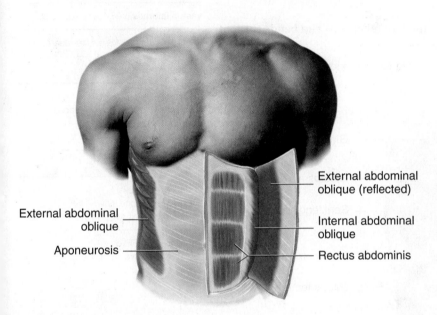

FIGURE 9-14 ■ Muscles of the abdomen.
These muscles contract and relax when you rotate the trunk of your body from side to side, flatten your abdomen, bend forward, do a sit-up, or take a bow for learning medical language!
Source: Pearson Education

Pronunciation/Word Parts

external (eks-TER-nal)
  extern/o- *outside*
  -al *pertaining to*

abdominal (ab-DAW-mih-nal)
  abdomin/o- *abdomen*
  -al *pertaining to*

oblique (oh-BLEEK)

internal (in-TER-nal)
  intern/o- *inside*
  -al *pertaining to*

rectus (REK-tus)

abdominis (ab-DAW-mih-nis)

WORD ALERT
Sound-Alike Words

rectus	(noun)	Latin word meaning *straight*. The segments of the rectus abdominis muscle are in a straight row, top to bottom, on the abdomen.

Example: When the rectus abdominis muscle contracts, it pulls the chest toward the legs.

rectum	(noun)	Straight part of the large intestine that comes after the curving S-shaped sigmoid colon

Example: Digested food travels through the colon, through the rectum, through the anus, and is then expelled from the body.

Muscles of the Lower Extremity

These are the most important muscles of the lower extremity (see Figure 9-15 ■).

Anterior Leg

These muscles are in the anterior leg:

- **Rectus femoris**: Bends the upper leg toward the abdomen (flexion); straightens the lower leg (extension).
- **Sartorius**: Bends the upper leg toward the abdomen (flexion) and rotates it laterally.
- **Vastus lateralis and vastus medialis**: Bend the upper leg toward the abdomen (flexion); straighten the lower leg (extension).
- **Peroneus longus**: Raises the lateral edge of the foot (eversion) and bends the foot downward (plantar flexion).
- **Tibialis anterior**: Bends the foot up toward the leg (dorsiflexion).

Pronunciation/Word Parts

rectus (REK-tus)

femoris (FEM-oh-ris)

sartorius (sar-TOR-ee-us)

vastus lateralis (VAS-tus LAT-er-AL-is)

vastus medialis (VAS-tus MEE-dee-AL-is)

peroneus (PAIR-oh-NEE-us)

peroneal (PAIR-oh-NEE-al)
  perone/o- *fibula; lower leg bone*
  -al *pertaining to*
Peroneal is the adjective form for *fibula*.

longus (LONG-gus)

tibialis (TIB-ee-AL-is)
  tibi/o- *shin bone; tibia*
  -alis *pertaining to*

anterior (an-TEER-ee-or)
  anter/o- *before; front part*
  -ior *pertaining to*

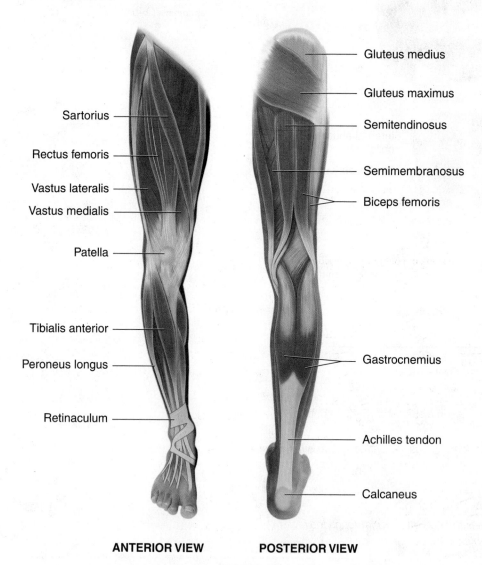

Sartorius

Rectus femoris

Vastus lateralis

Vastus medialis

Patella

Tibialis anterior

Peroneus longus

Retinaculum

Gluteus medius

Gluteus maximus

Semitendinosus

Semimembranosus

Biceps femoris

Gastrocnemius

Achilles tendon

Calcaneus

ANTERIOR VIEW   **POSTERIOR VIEW**

FIGURE 9-15 ■ Muscles of the lower extremity.
The muscles of the legs and buttocks contract and relax when you move your legs in any direction, bend your knees, walk on tiptoe, climb the stairs, or get up from a sitting position.
Source: Pearson Education

Quadriceps femoris is a collective name for the group of four muscles—the rectus femoris, vastus lateralis, vastus intermedius (beneath the vastus lateralis), and vastus medialis—on the anterior and lateral upper leg. The tendons of the four heads of these muscles join together and insert on the tibia. These muscles straighten the lower leg (extension).

Posterior Leg

These muscles are in the posterior leg:

- **Gluteus maximus**: Moves the upper leg posteriorly (extension) and rotates it laterally.
- **Biceps femoris**: Moves the upper leg posteriorly (extension) and bends the lower leg toward the buttocks (flexion).
- **Semitendinosus** and **semimembranosus**: Move the upper leg posteriorly (extension), bend the lower leg toward the buttocks (flexion), and rotate the leg medially.
- **Gastrocnemius**: Bends the foot downward (plantar flexion) and lets you stand on tiptoe.

Hamstrings is a collective name for the group of three muscles—the biceps femoris, semitendinosus, and semimembranosus—on the posterior upper leg. These muscles move the upper leg posteriorly (extension) and bend the lower leg toward the buttocks (flexion).

Pronunciation/Word Parts

quadriceps (KWAD-rih-seps)
The prefix *quadri-* means *four.*

femoris (FEM-oh-ris)

gluteus (gloo-TEE-us)

maximus (MAK-sih-mus)

biceps (BY-seps)

semitendinosus
(SEM-eye-TEN-dih-NOH-sus)

semimembranosus
(SEM-eye-MEM-brah-NOH-sus)

gastrocnemius (GAS-trawk-NEE-mee-us)
  gastr/o- *stomach*
  -cnemius *leg*
The gastrocnemius muscle is shaped somewhat like a stomach filled with food, which may be how it got its name.

DID YOU KNOW?

The gastrocnemius muscle has its insertion on the calcaneus (heel bone). This tendon is known as the *Achilles tendon* in reference to Achilles, the mythical Greek hero of Homer's *Iliad* who was wounded in the heel, his only vulnerable spot.

ACROSS THE LIFE SPAN

Pediatrics. Babies are evaluated by the pediatrician on their ability to attain developmental milestones. A 1-month-old baby can lift its head only briefly. By 3 months of age, a baby has developed the muscular coordination to turn over in bed. One of the next developmental milestones is being able to lift up the head and chest (see Figure 9-16 ■).

Geriatrics. Throughout life, regular exercise is an important part of wellness and physical fitness. Aging and chronic disease can limit mobility and decrease muscle strength. The size and strength of the muscles decrease over time. There is less flexibility because elastic muscle tissue is replaced by fibrous connective tissue, but active exercise helps maintain muscle strength and flexibility.

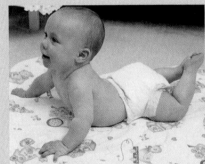

FIGURE 9-16 ■ Growth and development milestones.
This baby is able to lift his head and support his entire upper body with his arms, an activity that requires strength and coordination in the muscles of the neck, shoulders, and arms.
Source: Pearson Education

Physiology of a Muscle Contraction

A **muscle** is composed of several muscle fascicles, each of which is individually wrapped in fascia (see Figure 9-17 ■). Each **muscle fascicle** is a bundle of individual muscle fibers. These run parallel to each other so that, when they contract, they all pull in the same direction. A **muscle fiber** (which is actually one long muscle cell) has hundreds of nuclei along its length to speed up the chemical processes that occur as it contracts. Each muscle fiber is composed of **myofibrils** that contain thin strands of the protein actin and thick strands of the protein myosin that give skeletal muscle its characteristic striated (striped) appearance under a microscope (see Figure 9-2).

A muscle contracts in response to an electrical impulse from a nerve. On a microscopic level, each muscle fiber is connected to a single nerve cell at a **neuromuscular junction**. The nerve cell releases the **neurotransmitter acetylcholine**, a chemical messenger that changes the permeability of the muscle fiber and allows sodium ions to flow into it. This releases calcium ions from their storage site within the muscle fiber. Calcium causes the thin strands (actin) to slide between the thick strands (myosin), which shortens the muscle and produces a muscle **contraction**. The muscle eventually relaxes when acetylcholine is inactivated by an enzyme and the calcium ions are pumped back into their storage site.

Even when not actively moving, your muscles are in a state of mild, partial contraction because of nerve impulses from the brain and spinal cord. This produces muscle tone that keeps the muscles firm and ready to act. This is the only aspect of muscle activity that is not under conscious control.

Pronunciation/Word Parts

fascicle (FAS-ih-kl)
  fasci/o- *fascia*
  -cle *small thing*

myofibril (MY-oh-FY-bril)
  my/o- *muscle*
  fibr/o- *fiber*
  -il *thing*

neuromuscular (NYOOR-oh-MUS-kyoo-lar)
  neur/o- *nerve*
  muscul/o- *muscle*
  -ar *pertaining to*

neurotransmitter
(NYOOR-oh-TRANS-mit-er)
(NYOOR-oh-trans-MIT-er)
  neur/o- *nerve*
  transmitt/o- *send across; send through*
  -er *person who does; person who produces; thing that does; thing that produces*

acetylcholine (AS-eh-til-KOH-leen)

contraction (con-TRAK-shun)
  contract/o- *pull together*
  -ion *action; condition*

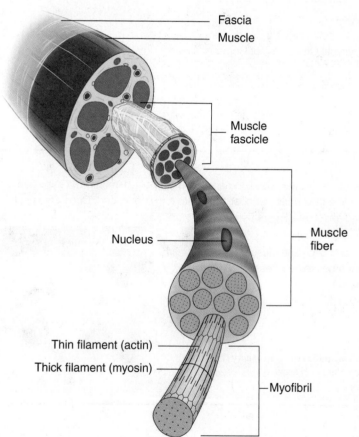

Fascia
Muscle
Muscle fascicle
Nucleus
Muscle fiber
Thin filament (actin)
Thick filament (myosin)
Myofibril

FIGURE 9-17 ■ Parts of a muscle.
A muscle is composed of muscle fascicles. Around each fascicle are arteries, veins, nerves, and fascia. Each fascicle contains several muscle fibers (muscle cells). Within each muscle fiber are myofibrils that contain thin strands of actin and thick strands of myosin.
Source: Pearson Education

CLINICAL CONNECTIONS

Sports Medicine. Professional athletes depend on their muscles to help them win. The muscle fibers of a marathon runner are different from those of a sprinter. Marathon runners have mostly slow-twitch muscle fibers that can contract many times without becoming fatigued. Sprinters have fast-twitch muscle fibers that can contract very quickly and repeatedly, but soon become tired. Because of the effect of the male hormone testosterone, men have larger muscles than women and a bulkier musculature, but vigorous weight training can increase the size of a muscle (**muscle hypertrophy**) in either sex. Bodybuilders work to enlarge, define, and sculpt their muscles (see Figure 9-18 ■). Some athletes try to enhance their performance with the use of illicit drugs, particularly anabolic steroid drugs that add bulk to the muscles.

hypertrophy (hy-PER-troh-fee)
   hyper- *above; more than normal*
   -trophy *process of development*
The ending *-trophy* contains the combining form *troph/o-* and the one-letter suffix *-y*.

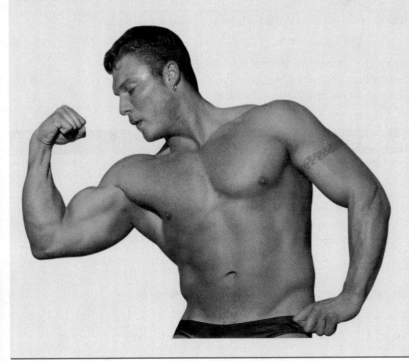

FIGURE 9-18 ■ Muscle strength and size.
This bodybuilder has highly developed muscles: the biceps brachii of the flexed right arm, the deltoid muscle of the shoulder, and the well-defined pectoral muscle of the chest. The individual segments of the rectus abdominis muscles can be seen on either side of the umbilicus.
Source: Pearson Education

Vocabulary Review

Anatomy and Physiology

Word or Phrase	Description	Combining Forms
muscle	Structure that produces movement of the body	**muscul/o-** *muscle* **my/o-** *muscle* **myos/o-** *muscle*
muscular system	Provides movement for the body in conjunction with support from the bones. It is also known as the **musculoskeletal system**.	**muscul/o-** *muscle* **skelet/o-** *skeleton*
musculature	Skeletal muscles in one body part or all of the muscles in the body as a whole	**muscul/o-** *muscle*
skeletal muscle	One of three types of muscles in the body, but the only one that is under **voluntary** control. Skeletal muscles contract and relax in response to conscious thought, and they provide the means by which the body can move.	**skelet/o-** *skeleton* **volunt/o-** *person's own free will*

Muscle Structures

Word or Phrase	Description	Combining Forms
aponeurosis	Wide, white, fibrous sheet of connective tissue that attaches a flat muscle to a bone or other structure	
belly of the muscle	Area of greatest mass, usually the center of the muscle midway between the origin and insertion	
bursa	Sac of synovial membrane that contains synovial fluid. It decreases friction where a tendon rubs against a bone near a synovial joint.	**burs/o-** *bursa*
fascia	Thin connective tissue around each muscle. It joins to become part of the tendon.	**fasci/o-** *fascia*
insertion	Where the tendon of a muscle ends on a bone that moves when the muscle contracts or relaxes	**insert/o-** *introduce; put in*
origin	Where the tendon of a muscle begins and is attached to a stationary (or nearly stationary) bone	
retinaculum	Thin, nearly translucent band of fibrous tissue and fascia that holds down tendons that cross the wrist and ankle	
tendon	Cordlike, nonelastic, white fibrous band of connective tissue that attaches a muscle to a bone	**tendin/o-** *tendon* **ten/o-** *tendon*

Muscle Movements

Word or Phrase	Description	Combining Forms
abduction	Moving a body part away from the midline. It is the opposite of adduction. An **abductor** is a muscle that produces abduction when it contracts.	**duct/o-** *bring; duct; move*
adduction	Moving a body part toward the midline. It is the opposite of abduction. An **adductor** is a muscle that produces adduction when it contracts.	**duct/o-** *bring; duct; move*
eversion	Turning a body part outward and toward the side. It is the opposite of inversion. An **evertor** is a muscle that produces eversion when it contracts.	**vers/o-** *travel; turn* **vert/o-** *travel; turn*
extension	Straightening and extending a joint to increase the angle between two bones or two body parts. It is the opposite of flexion. An **extensor** is a muscle that produces extension when it contracts.	**extens/o-** *straightening*

Word or Phrase	Description	Combining Forms
flexion	Bending a joint to decrease the angle between two bones or two body parts. It is the opposite of extension. A **flexor** is a muscle that produces flexion when it contracts.	**flex/o-** *bending*
inversion	Turning a body part inward. It is the opposite of eversion. An **invertor** is a muscle that produces inversion when it contracts.	**vers/o-** *travel; turn* **vert/o-** *travel; turn*
pronation	Turning the palm of the hand posteriorly or downward. It is the opposite of supination. A **pronator** is a muscle that produces pronation when it contracts.	**pronat/o-** *face down*
rotation	Moving a body part around its axis. A **rotator** is a muscle that produces rotation when it contracts.	**rotat/o-** *rotate*
supination	Turning the palm of the hand anteriorly or upward. It is the opposite of pronation. A **supinator** is a muscle that produces supination when it contracts.	**supinat/o-** *lying on the back*
<td colspan="3" align="center">**Muscles of the Head and Neck**</td>
buccinator muscle	Muscle of the side of the face that moves the cheek	**buccinat/o-** *cheek*
frontalis muscle	Muscle of the forehead that moves the forehead skin and eyebrows	**front/o-** *front*
masseter muscle	Muscle of the side of the jaw that moves the mandible upward	**masset/o-** *chewing*
orbicularis oculi muscle	Muscle around the eye that closes the eyelids	**orbicul/o-** *small circle*
orbicularis oris muscle	Muscle around the mouth that closes the lips	**orbicul/o-** *small circle*
platysma muscle	Muscle of the neck that moves the mandible down	
sternocleido-mastoid muscle	Muscle of the neck that bends the head toward the sternum (flexion) and turns the head to either side (rotation). Its origin is at two muscle heads on the sternum and clavicle. Its insertion is at the mastoid process of the temporal bone behind the ear.	**stern/o-** *breast bone; sternum* **cleid/o-** *clavicle; collar bone* **mast/o-** *breast; mastoid process*
temporalis muscle	Muscle of the side of the head that moves the mandible upward and backward	**tempor/o-** *side of the head; temple*
<td colspan="3" align="center">**Muscles of the Shoulders, Chest, and Back**</td>
deltoid muscle	Muscle of the shoulder that raises the arm and moves the arm away from the body (abduction)	**delt/o-** *triangle*
intercostal muscles	Muscles between the ribs that work in pairs to spread the ribs apart during inspiration and pull the ribs together during forced expiration, coughing, or sneezing	**cost/o-** *rib*
latissimus dorsi muscle	Muscle of the back that moves the arm posteriorly and medially toward the vertebral column (adduction)	

Word or Phrase	Description	Combining Forms
pectoralis major muscle	Muscle of the chest that moves the arm anteriorly and medially across the chest (adduction)	**pector/o-** *chest*
trapezius muscle	Muscle of the shoulder that raises the shoulder, pulls the shoulder blades together, and elevates the clavicle. It turns the head from side to side (rotation) and moves the head posteriorly (extension).	
Muscles of the Upper Extremity		
biceps brachii muscle	Muscle of the anterior upper arm that bends the upper arm toward the shoulder (flexion) and bends the lower arm toward the upper arm (flexion). The origin of this muscle has two heads.	
brachioradialis muscle	Muscle of the anterior lower arm that bends the lower arm toward the upper arm (flexion)	**brachi/o-** *arm* **radi/o-** *forearm bone; radiation; x-rays*
extensor digitorum muscle	Muscle that extends the fingers or toes	**extens/o-** *straightening*
thenar muscles	Group of muscles in the palm side of the hand that bends the thumb (flexion) and moves it toward the palm (adduction)	**then/o-** *thumb*
triceps brachii muscle	Muscle of the posterior upper arm that straightens the lower arm (extension). The origin of this muscle has three heads.	
Muscles of the Abdomen		
external abdominal oblique muscle	Muscle of the side of the abdomen that bends the upper body forward (flexion), rotates the side of the body medially, and compresses the side of the abdominal wall. The **internal abdominal oblique muscle** lies directly beneath it and performs the same movements, but its muscle fibers are oriented in the opposite direction.	**extern/o-** *outside* **abdomin/o-** *abdomen* **intern/o-** *inside*
rectus abdominis muscle	Muscle of the anterior abdomen that bends the upper body forward (flexion) and compresses the anterior abdominal wall	
Muscles of the Lower Extremity		
biceps femoris muscle	Muscle of the posterior upper leg that moves the upper leg posteriorly (extension) and bends the lower leg toward the buttocks (flexion). The origin of this muscle has two heads.	
gastrocnemius muscle	Muscle of the posterior lower leg that bends the foot downward (plantar flexion) and lets you stand on tiptoe	**gastr/o-** *stomach* *Note:* The shape of this muscle is somewhat like a stomach filled with food.
gluteus maximus muscle	Muscle of the buttocks that moves the upper leg posteriorly (extension) and rotates it laterally	
hamstrings	Collective name for three muscles in the posterior upper leg that move the upper leg posteriorly (extension) and bend the lower leg toward the buttocks (flexion). It includes the biceps femoris, semitendinosus, and semimembranosus muscles.	
peroneus longus muscle	Muscle of the lateral lower leg that raises the lateral edge of the foot (eversion) and bends the foot downward (plantar flexion)	**perone/o-** *fibula; lower leg bone*

Build Medical Words

Combining Form and Suffix Exercise

Read the definition of the medical word. Look at the combining form that is given. Select the correct suffix from the Suffix List and write it on the blank line. Then build the medical word and write it on the line. (Remember: You may need to remove the combining vowel. Always remove the hyphens and slash.) Be sure to check your spelling. The first one has been done for you.

SUFFIX LIST

-al (pertaining to)	-ary (pertaining to)	-oid (resembling)
-alis (pertaining to)	-ature (system composed of)	-or (person who does;
-ar (pertaining to)	-er (person who does; thing that produces)	thing that produces)
-aris (pertaining to)	-ion (action; condition)	-ous (pertaining to)

	Definition of the Medical Word	Combining Form	Suffix	Build the Medical Word
1.	Thing that produces (or makes something) rotate	**rotat/o-**	**-or**	rotator

(You think *thing that produces* (-or) + *rotate* (rotat/o-). You change the order of the word parts to put the suffix last. You write *rotator*.)

	Definition of the Medical Word	Combining Form	Suffix	Build the Medical Word
2.	Pertaining to (a) tendon	tendin/o-	_____	_____
3.	Pertaining to (a) muscle	muscul/o-	_____	_____
4.	Action (of) bending	flex/o-	_____	_____
5.	Pertaining to (the) fascia	fasci/o-	_____	_____
6.	System composed of muscle(s)	muscul/o-	_____	_____
7.	(Muscle) resembling (a) triangle	delt/o-	_____	_____
8.	Pertaining to (being done of a) person's own free will	volunt/o-	_____	_____
9.	Thing that produces chewing	masset/o-	_____	_____
10.	Pertaining to (a muscle that is a) small circle	orbicul/o-	_____	_____
11.	(Muscle name that means) pertaining to (the) chest	pector/o-	_____	_____
12.	Action (of) lying on the back (of the hand)	supinat/o-	_____	_____
13.	Action (of a muscle to) pull together	contract/o-	_____	_____

Diseases

Diseases of the Muscles

Word or Phrase	Description	Pronunciation/Word Parts
atrophy	Loss of muscle bulk in one or more muscles. It is caused by a lack of use or by malnutrition, or it can occur in any part of the body that is paralyzed because the muscles receive no electrical impulses from the nerves. The muscle is **atrophic**. It is also known as **muscle wasting**. Treatment: Correct the underlying cause.	**atrophy** (AT-roh-fee) **a-** *away from; without* **-trophy** *process of development* The ending *-trophy* contains the combining form *troph/o-* and the one-letter suffix *-y*. **atrophic** (ah-TROH-fik) **a-** *away from; without* **troph/o-** *development* **-ic** *pertaining to*
avulsion	Condition in which the muscle tears away from the tendon or the tendon tears away from the bone. Treatment: Surgical repair (myorrhaphy or tenorrhaphy).	**avulsion** (ah-VUL-shun) **a-** *away from; without* **vuls/o-** *tear* **-ion** *action; condition*
compartment syndrome	The result of a severe blunt or crushing injury that causes bleeding in the muscles of the leg. The fascia acts as a compartment, holding in the accumulating blood. The increased pressure causes muscle and nerve damage and tissue death. Treatment: Fasciotomy to allow the blood and fluid to drain out.	
contracture	Inactivity or paralysis coupled with continuing nerve impulses can cause an arm or leg muscle to become progressively flexed and drawn into a position where it becomes nearly immovable (see Figure 9-19 ■). Treatment: Range of motion (ROM) exercises and frequent repositioning.	**contracture** (con-TRAK-chur) **contract/o-** *pull together* **-ure** *result of; system*

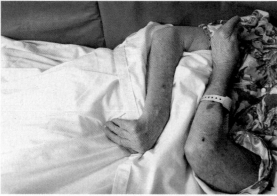

FIGURE 9-19 ■ Muscle contracture.
This elderly woman has severe arthritis and is a patient in a long-term care facility. She has developed contractures of the arms and wrists, which could have been prevented by proper body positioning and regular range of motion exercises.
Source: Michael Heron/Pearson Education

WORD ALERT

Sound-Alike Words

contraction	(noun)	the normal tensing and shortening of a muscle in response to a nerve impulse
		Example: It requires a strong, sustained contraction of the arm muscles to lift a heavy box.
contracture	(noun)	abnormal, fixed position in which the muscle is permanently flexed
		Example: Range of motion exercises help prevent a contracture from occurring.

Word or Phrase	Description	Pronunciation/Word Parts
fibromyalgia	Pain located at specific, hyperirritable trigger points in the muscles of the neck, back, or hips. The trigger points are tender to the touch and feel firm. The cause is not known, but may be related to an overreaction to painful stimuli with a possible history of prior injury or a genetic predisposition. Fibromyalgia is associated with disturbed sleep patterns and sometimes depression. Treatment: Analgesic drug, muscle relaxant drug, massage, and trigger point injections with a local anesthetic drug.	**fibromyalgia** (FY-broh-my-AL-jah) **fibr/o-** *fiber* **my/o-** *muscle* **alg/o-** *pain* **-ia** *condition; state; thing*
hyperextension– hyperflexion injury	Injury that occurs during a car accident as a person's head snaps forward and then backward in response to the car's changing speed. This causes a muscle strain or muscle tear, as well as damage to the nerves. It is also known as **acceleration–deceleration injury** or **whiplash**. Treatment: Soft cervical collar to support the neck, rest, analgesic drug, nonsteroidal anti-inflammatory drug.	**hyperextension** (HY-per-eks-TEN-shun) **hyper-** *above; more than normal* **extens/o-** *straightening* **-ion** *action; condition* **hyperflexion** (HY-per-FLEK-shun) **hyper-** *above; more than normal* **flex/o-** *bending* **-ion** *action; condition*
muscle contusion	Condition in which blunt trauma causes some bleeding in the muscle. It is also known as a **bruise**. Treatment: Analgesic drug.	**contusion** (con-TOO-shun) **contus/o-** *bruising* **-ion** *action; condition*
muscle spasm	Painful but temporary condition with a sudden, severe, involuntary contraction of a muscle, often in the legs. It can be brought on by overexercise. It is also known as a **muscle cramp**. **Torticollis** is a painful spasm of the muscles on one side of the neck. It is also known as **wryneck**. Treatment: Massage, muscle relaxant drug, analgesic drug.	**spasm** (SPAZM) **torticollis** (TOR-tih-KOH-lis) **tort/i-** *twisted position* **-collis** *condition of the neck*
muscle strain	Overstretching of a muscle, often due to physical overexertion. This causes **inflammation**, pain, swelling, and bruising as capillaries in the muscle tear. It is also known as a **pulled muscle**. Treatment: Rest, analgesic drug, nonsteroidal anti-inflammatory drug.	**strain** (STRAYN) **inflammation** (IN-flah-MAY-shun) **inflammat/o-** *redness and warmth* **-ion** *action; condition*
muscular dystrophy	Genetic mutation of the gene that normally makes the muscle protein dystrophin. Without dystrophin, the muscles weaken and then atrophy. It begins in early childhood with weakness in the lower extremities and then the upper extremities (see Figure 9-20 ■). The most common and most severe form is **Duchenne's muscular dystrophy**; Becker's muscular dystrophy is a milder form. Weakness of the diaphragm with an inability to breathe is the most frequent cause of death. Treatment: Supportive care.	**dystrophy** (DIS-troh-fee) **dys-** *abnormal; difficult; painful* **-trophy** *process of development* The ending *-trophy* contains the combining form *troph/o-* and the one-letter suffix *-y*. **Duchenne** (doo-SHAYN)

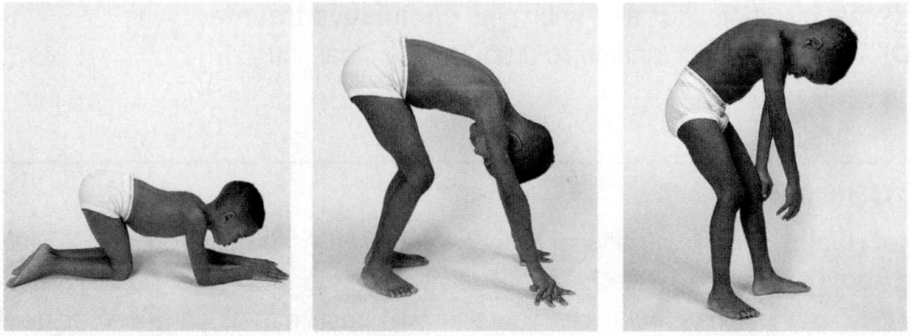

FIGURE 9-20 ■ Muscular dystrophy.
Weakness of the muscles in the legs causes this patient with muscular dystrophy to stand up in a way that is characteristic of this disease. The legs and arms must work together to raise the body. Because muscular dystrophy is a progressive disease, this patient soon may not be able to walk at all.
Source: Pearson Education

Word or Phrase	Description	Pronunciation/Word Parts
myalgia	Pain in a muscle due to injury or muscle disease. **Polymyalgia** is pain in several muscle groups. Treatment: Analgesic drug, massage.	**myalgia** (my-AL-jah) **my/o-** *muscle* **alg/o-** *pain* **-ia** *condition; state; thing* **polymyalgia** (PAW-lee-my-AL-jah) **poly-** *many; much* **my/o-** *muscle* **alg/o-** *pain* **-ia** *condition; state; thing*
myasthenia gravis	Autoimmune disorder with abnormal and rapid fatigue of the muscles, particularly in the muscles of the face, where there is **ptosis** (drooping) of the eyelids. The weakness worsens during the day, but is relieved by rest. The body produces antibodies against its own acetylcholine receptors on the muscle fibers. The antibodies destroy many of the receptors. There are normal levels of acetylcholine, but too few receptors remain to produce a sustained muscle contraction. Treatment: Thymectomy to remove the thymus because it contributes to the abnormal immune response; drug that prolongs the action of acetylcholine. Plasmapheresis to remove antibodies from the blood.	**myasthenia gravis** (MY-as-THEE-nee-ah GRAV-is) **my/o-** *muscle* **asthen/o-** *lack of strength* **-ia** *condition; state; thing* **ptosis** (TOH-sis)
myopathy	Category that includes many different diseases of the muscles. Treatment: Correct the underlying cause.	**myopathy** (my-AW-pah-thee) **my/o-** *muscle* **-pathy** *disease*
myositis	Inflammation of a muscle with localized swelling and tenderness. It can be caused by injury or strain. **Polymyositis** is a chronic, progressive disease that causes widespread inflammation of muscles with weakness and fatigue. The cause is unknown, although it may be an autoimmune disorder. **Dermatomyositis** causes a skin rash as well as muscle weakness and inflammation. Treatment: Analgesic drug, nonsteroidal anti-inflammatory drug, corticosteroid drug.	**myositis** (MY-oh-SY-tis) **myos/o-** *muscle* **-itis** *infection of; inflammation of* **polymyositis** (PAW-lee-MY-oh-SY-tis) **poly-** *many; much* **myos/o-** *muscle* **-itis** *infection of; inflammation of* **dermatomyositis** (DER-mah-toh-MY-oh-SY-tis) **dermat/o-** *skin* **myos/o-** *muscle* **-itis** *infection of; inflammation of*
repetitive strain injury (RSI)	Condition affecting the muscles, tendons, and sometimes the nerves. It occurs as a result of trauma caused by repetitive movements over an extended period of time. It includes tennis elbow, carpal tunnel syndrome, and other disorders. It is also known as **cumulative trauma disorder (CTD)**. Treatment: Rest, analgesic drug, nonsteroidal anti-inflammatory drug.	

CLINICAL CONNECTIONS

Occupational Health. The Occupational Safety and Health Administration (OSHA) educates healthcare professionals about workplace-related injuries. Lifting, carrying, pulling, or pushing something heavy and not using proper body mechanics can cause injury as can repetitive motions done constantly, such as typing on a computer.

Word or Phrase	Description	Pronunciation/Word Parts
rhabdomyoma	**Benign** tumor in a muscle. Treatment: Surgical removal.	**rhabdomyoma** (RAB-doh-my-OH-mah) **rhabd/o-** *rod shaped* **my/o-** *muscle* **-oma** *mass; tumor* *Note:* The immature muscle cells in this tumor are shaped like a rod. **benign** (bee-NINE)
rhabdomyo-sarcoma	Cancerous tumor in a muscle. This **cancer** usually occurs in children and young adults. Treatment: Surgical removal, chemotherapy, and radiation therapy.	**rhabdomyosarcoma** (RAB-doh-MY-oh-sar-KOH-mah) **rhabd/o-** *rod shaped* **my/o-** *muscle* **sarc/o-** *connective tissue* **-oma** *mass; tumor* **cancer** (KAN-ser) **cancerous** (KAN-ser-us) **cancer/o-** *cancer* **-ous** *pertaining to*
rotator cuff tear	Tear in the rotator muscles of the shoulder that surround the head of the humerus. These muscles help to abduct the arm. The tear can be caused by acute trauma or repetitive overuse, particularly motions in which the arm is above the head. Treatment: Surgical repair.	

> ### CLINICAL CONNECTIONS
> **Forensic Science. Rigor mortis** is not a muscle disease of the living, but rather a normal condition of the muscles that occurs several hours after death. As each muscle fiber dies, its stored calcium is released and this causes the muscle fiber—and then each muscle of the body—to contract. The muscle fiber is no longer able to pump calcium ions back into the storage site, and so the muscles remain contracted for about 72 hours until the muscle fibers begin to decompose. This is also known as **postmortem rigidity**. Forensic scientists use the presence or absence of rigor mortis to help determine the time of death.
>
> **rigor mortis** (RIG-or MOR-tis)
>
> **postmortem** (post-MOR-tem)

Movement Disorders

Word or Phrase	Description	Pronunciation/Word Parts
ataxia	Incoordination of the muscles during movement, particularly incoordination of the gait. It is caused by disease of the brain or spinal cord, cerebral palsy, or an adverse reaction to a drug. The patient is **ataxic**. Treatment: Correct the underlying cause. Leg braces or crutches, if needed.	**ataxia** (ah-TAK-see-ah) **a-** *away from; without* **tax/o-** *coordination* **-ia** *condition; state; thing* **ataxic** (ah-TAK-sik) **a-** *away from; without* **tax/o-** *coordination* **-ic** *pertaining to*
bradykinesia	Abnormally slow muscle movements or a decrease in the number of spontaneous muscle movements. It is usually associated with Parkinson's disease, a neurologic disease of the brain. Treatment: Drug for Parkinson's disease.	**bradykinesia** (BRAD-ee-kih-NEE-zha) **brady-** *slow* **kines/o-** *movement* **-ia** *condition; state; thing*

Word or Phrase	Description	Pronunciation/Word Parts
dyskinesia	Abnormal motions that occur because of difficulty controlling the voluntary muscles. Attempts at movement become tics, muscle spasms, muscle jerking (**myoclonus**), or slow, wandering, purposeless writhing of the hand (**athetoid movements**) in which some muscles of the fingers are flexed and others are extended. It is associated with neurologic disorders (Parkinson's disease, Huntington's chorea, cerebral palsy, etc.). Treatment: Correct the underlying cause.	**dyskinesia** (DIS-kih-NEE-zha) **dys-** *abnormal; difficult; painful* **kines/o-** *movement* **-ia** *condition; state; thing* Select the correct prefix meaning to get the definition of *dyskinesia*: *condition of abnormal movement.*
	CLINICAL CONNECTIONS **Neurology (Chapter 10).** Cerebral palsy is caused by a lack of oxygen to parts of a fetus' brain before or during birth. The extent of the symptoms varies, but can include spastic muscles; dyskinesia; lack of coordination in walking, eating, and talking; or even muscle paralysis.	**myoclonus** (MY-oh-KLOH-nus) **my/o-** *muscle* **-clonus** *rapid contracting and relaxing* **athetoid** (ATH-eh-toyd) **athet/o-** *without place; without position* **-oid** *resembling*
hyperkinesis	An abnormally increased amount of muscle movements. Restlessness. It can be a side effect of a drug. Treatment: Correct the underlying cause.	**hyperkinesis** (HY-per-kih-NEE-sis) **hyper-** *above; more than normal* **kin/o-** *movement* **-esis** *condition; process*
restless legs syndrome (RLS)	An uncomfortable restlessness and twitching of the muscles of the legs, particularly the calf muscles, along with an indescribable tingling, aching, or crawling-insect sensation. This usually occurs at night and can interfere with sleep. The exact cause is unknown. Treatment: The drug Requip, which stimulates dopamine receptors in the brain. Tranquilizer drug may be of some help.	
tremor	Small, involuntary, sometimes jerky, back-and-forth movements of the hands, head, jaw, or extremities. These are continuous and cannot be controlled by the patient. These are usually due to essential familial tremor, an inherited condition. Treatment: Beta-blocker drug.	**tremor** (TREM-or)

Diseases of the Bursa, Fascia, or Tendon

Word or Phrase	Description	Pronunciation/Word Parts
bursitis	Inflammation of the bursal sac because of repetitive muscle contractions or pressure on the bone underneath the bursa. It can occur with any joint that has a bursa, but most often occurs in the shoulders and knees. Prolonged periods of kneeling cause bursitis known as **housemaid's knee**. Treatment: Rest, analgesic drug, nonsteroidal anti-inflammatory drug.	**bursitis** (ber-SY-tis) **burs/o-** *bursa* **-itis** *infection of; inflammation of*
Dupuytren's contracture	Progressive disease in which collagen fibers in the fascia in the palm of the hand become thickened and shortened. This causes a contracture and flexion deformity of the fingers. Treatment: Injection of a drug to dissolve the collagen fibers. Surgery to remove the fascia (fasciectomy).	**Dupuytren** (DOO-pyoo-tren) **contracture** (con-TRAK-chur) **contract/o-** *pull together* **-ure** *result of; system*
fasciitis	Inflammation of the fascia around a muscle. Plantar fasciitis is inflammation of the fascia on the bottom of the foot that is caused by excessive running or exercise. There is aching or stabbing pain around the heel. It is the most common cause of heel pain. Treament: Analgesic drug, nonsteroidal anti-inflammatory drug. Injection into the fascia of a corticosteroid drug.	**fasciitis** (FAS-ee-EYE-tis) **fasci/o-** *fascia* **-itis** *infection of; inflammation of*

Word or Phrase	Description	Pronunciation/Word Parts
ganglion	Semisolid or fluid-containing cyst that develops on a tendon, often in the wrist, hand, or foot. A ganglion is a rounded lump under the skin and may or may not be painful (see Figure 9-21 ■). Treatment: Needle aspiration of fluid from the ganglion or surgical removal (ganglionectomy).	**ganglion** (GANG-glee-on)

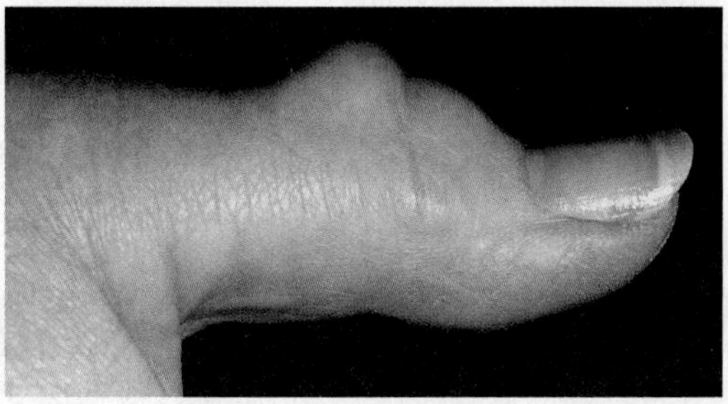

FIGURE 9-21 ■ Ganglion.
This patient has a semisolid ganglion on the extensor tendon of the thumb. Even after a ganglionectomy is done to surgically remove it, it may recur.
Source: Dr. P. Marazzi/Science Source

Word or Phrase	Description	Pronunciation/Word Parts
pitcher's elbow	Inflammation and pain of the flexor and pronator muscles of the forearm where their tendons originate on the medial epicondyle of the humerus (by the elbow joint). This is an overuse injury caused by repeated flexing of the wrist while the fingers tightly grasp. It is also known as **golfer's elbow** or **medial epicondylitis**. Treatment: Rest, analgesic drug, nonsteroidal anti-inflammatory drug.	
shin splints	Pain and inflammation of the tendons of the flexor muscles of the anterior lower leg over the tibia (shin bone). It is an overuse injury common to athletes who run. Treatment: Rest, analgesic drug, nonsteroidal anti-inflammatory drug.	
tendinitis	Inflammation of any tendon from injury or overuse. Treatment: Rest, analgesic drug, nonsteroidal anti-inflammatory drug.	**tendinitis** (TEN-dih-NY-tis) **tendin/o-** *tendon* **-itis** *infection of; inflammation of*
tennis elbow	Inflammation and pain of the extensor and supinator muscles where their tendons originate on the lateral epicondyle of the humerus (by the elbow joint). It is an overuse injury caused by repeated extension and supination of the wrist. It is also known as **lateral epicondylitis**. Treatment: Rest, analgesic drug, nonsteroidal anti-inflammatory drug.	
tenosynovitis	Inflammation and pain due to overuse of a tendon and inability of the synovium to produce enough lubricating fluid. Treatment: Rest, analgesic drug, nonsteroidal anti-inflammatory drug.	**tenosynovitis** (TEN-oh-SIN-oh-VY-tis) **ten/o-** *tendon* **synov/o-** *joint membrane; synovium* **-itis** *infection of; inflammation of*

Laboratory and Diagnostic Procedures

Blood Tests		
Word or Phrase	**Description**	**Pronunciation/Word Parts**
acetylcholine receptor antibody test	Test that detects antibodies that the body produces against its acetylcholine receptors. It is used to diagnose myasthenia gravis.	**antibody** (AN-tee-BAW-dee) (AN-tih-BAW-dee) The prefix *anti-* means *against*.
creatine phosphokinase (CPK-MM)	Test that measures the level of serum CPK-MM, an isoenzyme found in the muscles. A high blood level of CPK-MM is present in various diseases, particularly muscular dystrophy, in which muscle tissue is being destroyed.	**creatine phosphokinase** (KREE-ah-teen FAWS-foh-KY-nays)
Muscle Tests		
electromyography (EMG)	Procedure to diagnose muscle disease or nerve damage. A needle electrode inserted into a muscle records electrical activity as the muscle contracts and relaxes. The electrical activity is displayed as waveforms on a computer screen and recorded as an **electromyogram**.	**electromyography** (ee-LEK-troh-my-AW-grah-fee) **electr/o-** *electricity* **my/o-** *muscle* **-graphy** *process of recording* **electromyogram** (ee-LEK-troh-MY-oh-gram) **electr/o-** *electricity* **my/o-** *muscle* **-gram** *picture; record*
edrophonium test	Procedure in which the drug edrophonium is given to confirm a diagnosis of myasthenia gravis. The drug blocks the enzyme that breaks down acetylcholine, and patients with myasthenia gravis show temporarily increased muscle strength during the test.	**edrophonium** (EH-droh-FOH-nee-um)

Medical and Surgical Procedures

Medical Procedures		
braces and adaptive devices	A brace is an orthopedic device known as an **orthosis** that supports and straightens a body part. It keeps the body part in anatomical alignment while still permitting movement (see Figure 9-22 ■). An adaptive or assistive device increases **mobility** and independence by helping a physically challenged patient perform activities of daily living (ADLs). Examples: A grasper to extend the reach, spoons that can be attached to the wrist, and extra-large pens that can be easily grasped	**orthosis** (or-THOH-sis) **orth/o-** *straight* **-osis** *condition; process* **mobility** (moh-BIL-ih-tee) **mobil/o-** *movement* **-ity** *condition; state*

A CLOSER LOOK

The Americans with Disabilities Act (ADA) of 1990 is a federal law that prohibits discrimination against disabled persons. It provides guidelines and requirements for accommodating persons with disabilities at work and in public buildings and transportation vehicles. Instead of *handicapped*, the correct phrase is *physically challenged*.

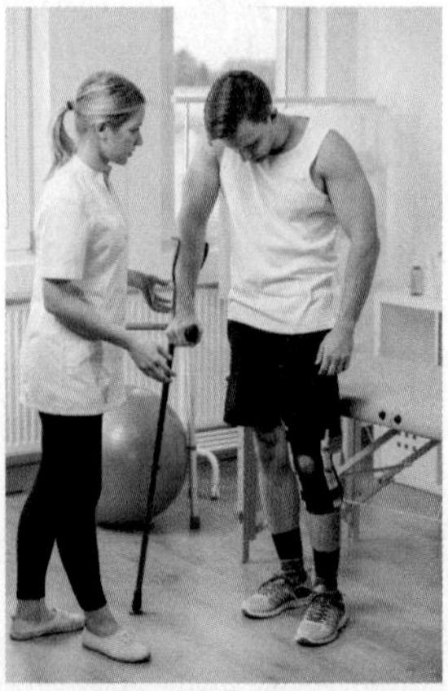

FIGURE 9-22 ■ **Braces.**
Braces provide support and stability. The physical therapist is instructing and assisting this patient in how to safely walk with a crutch and a knee brace.
Source: Photographee.eu/Shutterstock

Word or Phrase	Description	Pronunciation/Word Parts
deep tendon reflexes (DTR)	Procedure that tests whether the muscular–nervous pathway is functioning normally. Tapping briskly on a tendon causes an involuntary, automatic contraction of the muscle connected to that tendon. This test can be done in several places, but the most common site is at the knee (see Figure 9-23 ■). It is also known as the **knee jerk** or **patellar reflex**.	**reflex** (REE-fleks)

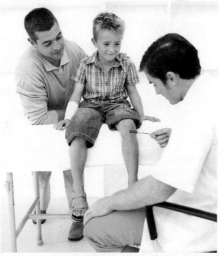

FIGURE 9-23 ■ Deep tendon reflex.
A percussion hammer with a rounded rubber end is used to tap just below the patella on the combined tendons of the quadriceps femoris muscle group. A normal response is a sudden involuntary contraction of the muscles that briskly extends the lower leg. The response in both legs is tested and compared.
Source: WavebreakMediaMicro/Fotolia

WORD ALERT

Sound-Alike Words

reflex   (noun)   involuntary, automatic response of the muscular–nervous pathway
          Example: The patient's knee jerk reflexes were equal bilaterally.

reflux   (noun)   backward flowing of fluid
          Example: Acid reflux from the stomach can cause inflammation and ulcers in the esophagus.

Word or Phrase	Description	Pronunciation/Word Parts
muscle strength test	Procedure used to test the **motor strength** of certain muscle groups. For muscles in the legs and feet, the physician presses against the lower leg or foot and asks the patient to extend the leg or flex the foot upward. For shoulder muscles, the physician presses down and the patient tries to shrug the shoulders. For muscles in the hand, the patient grasps two of the physician's fingers and squeezes them as tightly as possible. Muscle strength is measured on a scale of 0 to 5, with 5 being normal strength and 0 being an inability to move the muscles being tested.	**motor** (MOH-tor) **mot/o-** *movement* **-or** *person who does; person who produces; thing that does; thing that produces*

Word or Phrase	Description	Pronunciation/Word Parts

rehabilitation exercises	Physical therapy that includes exercises to increase muscle strength and improve coordination and balance. It is prescribed as part of a rehabilitation plan. In active exercise, the patient exercises without assistance (see Figure 9-24 ■). In passive exercise, a physical therapist or nurse performs range of motion (ROM) exercises for a patient who is unable to move. This does not build muscle strength, but it does decrease stiffness and spasticity and prevent contractures. 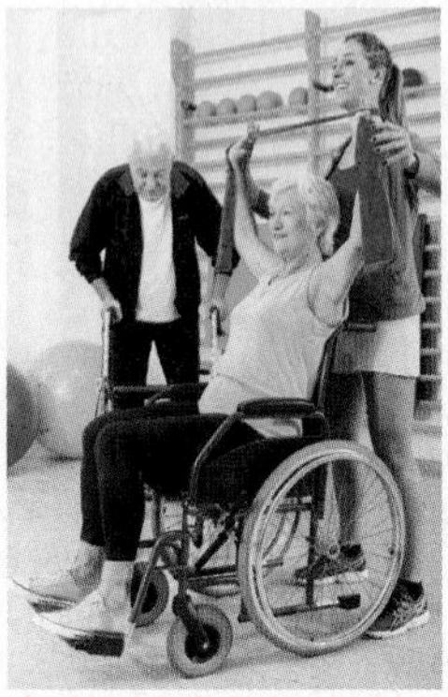
	
	FIGURE 9-24 ■ Active exercise. These patients are part of a physical therapy group. Even patients confined to wheelchairs benefit from regular exercise.
	Source: Kzenon/Fotolia
		rehabilitation (REE-hah-BIL-ih-TAY-shun)
		  re- *again and again; backward; unable to*
		  habilitat/o- *give ability*
		  -ion *action; condition*
		Select the correct prefix meaning to get the definition of *rehabilitation*: *action (of) again and again (exercises) (to) give ability*. During rehabilitation, exercises are repeated again and again.

trigger point injections	Procedure to treat fibromyalgia. A combination of a local anesthetic drug and a corticosteroid drug are injected into each fibromyalgia trigger point to relieve pain and decrease inflammation.	
Surgical Procedures		

fasciectomy	Procedure to partially or totally remove the fascia that is causing Dupuytren's contracture	**fasciectomy** (FASH-ee-EK-toh-mee)
		  fasci/o- *fascia*
		  -ectomy *surgical removal*

fasciotomy	Procedure to cut the fascia and release pressure from built-up blood and tissue fluid in a patient with compartment syndrome	**fasciotomy** (FASH-ee-AW-toh-mee)
		  fasci/o- *fascia*
		  -tomy *process of cutting; process of making an incision*

ganglionectomy	Procedure to remove a ganglion from a tendon	**ganglionectomy** (GANG-glee-oh-NEK-toh-mee)
		  ganglion/o- *ganglion*
		  -ectomy *surgical removal*

muscle biopsy	Procedure to diagnose muscle weakness that could be caused by many different muscular diseases. An incision is made in the muscle and a piece of tissue is removed and sent to the pathology department for examination under a microscope. This is an **incisional biopsy** or open biopsy. Alternatively, a needle is inserted and some muscle tissue is aspirated through the needle; this is a closed biopsy.	**biopsy** (BY-awp-see)
		  bi/o- *life; living organism; living tissue*
		  -opsy *process of viewing*
		incisional (in-SIH-zhun-al)
		  incis/o- *cut into*
		  -ion *action; condition*
		  -al *pertaining to*

myorrhaphy	Procedure to suture together a torn muscle after an injury	**myorrhaphy** (my-OR-ah-fee)
		  my/o- *muscle*
		  -rrhaphy *procedure of suturing*

Word or Phrase	Description	Pronunciation/Word Parts
tenorrhaphy	Procedure to suture together a torn tendon after an injury	**tenorrhaphy** (teh-NOR-ah-fee) **ten/o-** *tendon* **-rrhaphy** *procedure of suturing*
thymectomy	Procedure to remove the thymus gland. It is used to treat patients with myasthenia gravis because, after a thymectomy, the patient produces fewer antibodies against the remaining acetylcholine receptors.	**thymectomy** (thy-MEK-toh-mee) **thym/o-** *rage; thymus* **-ectomy** *surgical removal* Select the correct combining form meaning to get the definition of *thymectomy*: surgical removal (of the) thymus.

Drugs

These drug categories and drugs are used to treat muscular diseases. The most common generic and trade name drugs in each category are listed.

Category	Indication	Examples	Pronunciation/Word Parts
analgesic drugs	Over-the-counter drugs aspirin and acetaminophen decrease mild-to-moderate inflammation and pain. They are used to treat minor injuries, muscle strains, tendinitis, bursitis, and muscle overuse. Prescription narcotic drugs are used to treat chronic, severe pain.	aspirin (Bayer, Ecotrin), acetaminophen (Tylenol). Prescription narcotic drugs: meperidine (Demerol), oxycodone (OxyContin), morphine sulfate (MS Contin)	**analgesic** (AN-al-JEE-zik) **an-** *not; without* **alges/o-** *sensation of pain* **-ic** *pertaining to*
beta-blocker drugs	Block the action of epinephrine to suppress essential familial tremor	propranolol (Inderal)	
corticosteroid drugs	Decrease severe inflammation. They are given orally; some are injected into the fascia.	dexamethasone, hydrocortisone (Cortef, Solu-Cortef), prednisone Injection into the fascia or tendon: betamethasone (Celestone), methylprednisolone (Depo-Medrol), triamcinolone (Kenalog). *Note*: This is often referred to as a "cortisone shot," even though it is not the drug cortisone (which is only available as a tablet).	**corticosteroid** (KOR-tih-koh-STAIR-oyd) **cortic/o-** *cortex; outer region* **-steroid** *steroid*
dopamine stimulant drugs	Stimulate dopamine receptors to treat restless legs syndrome	ropinirole (Requip)	
drugs for fibromyalgia	Include an oral muscle relaxant drug (cyclobenzaprine), injected local anesthetic drugs (lidocaine, procaine), and oral pregabalin	cyclobenzaprine (Flexeril), lidocaine (Xylocaine), pregabalin (Lyrica), procaine (Novocain)	
drugs for myasthenia gravis	Inhibit the enzyme that breaks down acetylcholine	neostigmine (Prostigmin), pyridostigmine (Mestinon)	

Category	Indication	Examples	Pronunciation/Word Parts
muscle relaxant drugs	Relieve muscle spasm and stiffness. They are used to treat muscle injuries. They are also used to treat muscle spasms in patients with neurologic diseases such as multiple sclerosis, cerebral palsy, and stroke.	carisoprodol (Soma), cyclobenzaprine (Flexeril), methocarbamol (Robaxin)	**relaxant** (ree-LAK-sant) **relax/o-** *relax* **-ant** *pertaining to*
neuromuscular blocker drugs	Block acetylcholine receptors to prevent muscle contraction. They are used during surgery to produce muscle relaxation, particularly during abdominal surgery to allow visualization of the organs in the abdominal cavity.	atracurium (Tracrium)	**neuromuscular** (NYOOR-oh-MUS-kyoo-lar) **neur/o-** *nerve* **muscul/o-** *muscle* **-ar** *pertaining to*
nonsteroidal anti-inflammatory drugs (NSAIDs)	Decrease mild-to-moderate inflammation and pain. They are used to treat minor injuries, muscle strains, tendinitis, bursitis, and muscle overuse. Celebrex is a COX-2 inhibitor drug, a type of NSAID that blocks the COX-2 enzyme that produces prostaglandins that cause pain.	celecoxib (Celebrex), diclofenac (Cataflam, Voltaren), ibuprofen (Advil, Motrin), naproxen (Aleve, Naprosyn)	**nonsteroidal** (NON-stair-OYD-al) **non-** *not* **steroid/o-** *steroid* **-al** *pertaining to* **anti-inflammatory** (AN-tee-in-FLAM-ah-TOR-ee) **anti-** *against* **inflammat/o-** *redness and warmth* **-ory** *having the function of*

CLINICAL CONNECTIONS

Pharmacology. Some drugs are administered by **intramuscular (IM) injection**. Intramuscular injections are given in a large muscle that is not near a large artery, vein, or nerve. In adults, these sites include the deltoid muscle (lateral upper arm), the vastus lateralis (anterolateral thigh), the gluteus medius muscle (lateral hip), and the gluteus maximus (upper outer quadrant of the buttocks). In infants, the only suitable site for an intramuscular injection is in the anterolateral thigh (see Figure 9-25 ■).

intramuscular (IN-trah-MUS-kyoo-lar)
  intra- *within*
  muscul/o- *muscle*
  -ar *pertaining to*

injection (in-JEK-shun)
  inject/o- *insert; put in*
  -ion *action; condition*

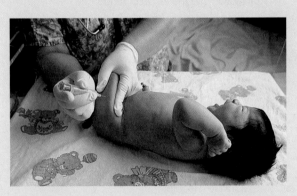

FIGURE 9-25 ■ Intramuscular injection.
The thigh muscles are the largest muscles in a baby's body, and immunizations are injected there.
Source: Pearson Education

Abbreviations

ADA	Americans with Disabilities Act	**OOB**	out of bed
ADLs	activities of daily living	**ortho**	orthopedics (short form)
COTA	certified occupational therapy assistant	**OSHA**	Occupational Safety and Health Administration
CPK-MM	creatine phosphokinase-MM (band)	**OT**	occupational therapist; occupational therapy
CTD	cumulative trauma disorder	**PM&R**	physical medicine and rehabilitation
D.C.	Doctor of Chiropracty or Chiropractic Medicine	**PT**	physical therapist; physical therapy
DTR	deep tendon reflex	**rehab**	rehabilitation (short form)
EMG	electromyogram; electromyography	**RICE**	rest, ice, compression, and elevation
IM	intramuscular	**RLE**	right lower extremity
LLE	left lower extremity	**ROM**	range of motion
LUE	left upper extremity	**RSI**	repetitive strain injury
MD	muscular dystrophy	**RUE**	right upper extremity
NSAID	nonsteroidal anti-inflammatory drug		

WORD ALERT

Abbreviations

Abbreviations are commonly used in all types of medical documents; however, they can mean different things to different people and their meanings can be misinterpreted. Always verify the meaning of an abbreviation.

ADA means *Americans with Disabilities Act*, but it also means *American Diabetes Association*, *American Dental Association*, or *American Dietetic Association*.

MD means *muscular dystrophy*, but it also means *macular degeneration* or *Doctor of Medicine (M.D.)*.

PT means *physical therapist* and *physical therapy*, but it also means *prothrombin time*.

ROM means *range of motion*, but it also means *rupture of membranes* (prior to delivery of a baby).

IT'S GREEK TO ME!

Did you notice that some words have two different combining forms? Combining forms from both Greek and Latin remain a part of medical language today.

Word	Greek	Latin	Medical Word Examples
movement	kines/o-, kin/o-	mobil/o-, mot/o-	dyskinesia, hyperkinesis, mobility, motor strength
muscle	my/o-	muscul/o-, myos/o-	fibromyalgia, muscular, myositis
tendon	ten/o-	tendin/o-	tenorrhaphy, tendinitis

CAREER FOCUS

Meet Iris, a massage therapist

"I became a massage therapist because I wanted to help people. I get to see clients that I can honestly say I enjoy, and to see the progress of them, physically—and emotionally, sometimes—is very rewarding. Massage therapy is basically known for its relaxation qualities, but more and more people are understanding that it increases circulation, increases range of motion, and reduces pain. I personally use a lot of medical terminology. I use the names of muscles—origins and insertions. The education involved with massage therapy begins with intense anatomy and physiology. There's a lot of ethics training, a lot of training in dealing with people."

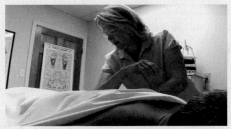

Source: Pearson Education

Massage therapists are allied health professionals who use pressure and manipulation of the muscles and soft tissues to relieve stress and prevent or treat muscular injuries. Massage therapists work in athletic clubs, resorts, chiropractic or orthopedic offices, or in their own private offices.

 Osteopaths, Doctors of **Osteopathy or Osteopathic Medicine** (D.O.), can diagnose and treat any patient that an orthopedist with an M.D. can treat, but they base their treatment on osteopathy, the study of how to prevent and treat diseases by using proper nutrition and keeping the body structures in a normal anatomical relationship.

 Chiropractors, Doctors of **Chiropracty or Chiropractic Medicine** (D.C.), diagnose and treat patients with injuries involving the bones, muscles, and nerves by manipulating the alignment of the vertebral column.

 Podiatrists, Doctors of **Podiatry or Podiatric Medicine** (D.P.M.), diagnose and treat medical and surgical conditions of the foot.

Physiatrists are physicians who specialize in physical medicine and rehabilitation. **Physiatry** is the medical specialty that diagnoses and treats musculoskeletal diseases and acute and chronic pain by using the physical properties of cold, heat, light, and water in conjunction with exercise and some drugs. It is also known as the field of **physical medicine and rehabilitation (PM&R)**. **Sports medicine** encompasses the prevention, treatment, and rehabilitation of musculoskeletal injuries from sports, as well as athletic training and endurance, biomechanics, nutrition, and psychology. A physician (M.D.) or Doctor of Osteopathy can take additional training and become board certified in physical medicine and rehabilitation or in sports medicine.

---

therapist (THAIR-ah-pist)
 therap/o- *treatment*
 -ist *person who specializes in*

---

osteopath (AW-stee-oh-PATH)
 oste/o- *bone*
 -path *person involved with disease*

---

osteopathy (AW-stee-AW-pah-thee)
 oste/o- *bone*
 -pathy *disease*

---

chiropractor (KY-roh-PRAK-tor)
 chir/o- *hand*
 pract/o- *medical practice*
 -or *person who does; person who produces; thing that does; thing that produces*
Add words to make a complete definition of *chiropractor*: *person who does (manipulation and alignment of the body by using the) hands (to perform) medical practice.*

---

chiropractic (KY-roh-PRAK-tik)
 chir/o- *hand*
 pract/o- *medical practice*
 -ic *pertaining to*

---

podiatrist (poh-DY-ah-trist)
 pod/o- *foot*
 iatr/o- *medical treatment; physician*
 -ist *person who specializes in*

---

podiatry (poh-DY-ah-tree)
 pod/o- *foot*
 -iatry *medical treatment*

---

podiatric (POH-dee-AT-rik)
 pod/o- *foot*
 iatr/o- *medical treatment; physician*
 -ic *pertaining to*

---

physiatrist (fih-ZY-ah-trist)
 physi/o- *physical function*
 iatr/o- *medical treatment; physician*
 -ist *person who specializes in*

---

physiatry (fih-ZY-ah-tree)
 physi/o- *physical function*
 -iatry *medical treatment*

MyMedicalTerminologyLab™ To see Iris's complete video profile, log into MyMedicalTerminologyLab and navigate to the Multimedia Library for Chapter 9. Check the Video box, and then click the Career Focus - Massage Therapist link.

PREFIX EXERCISE

Read the definition of the medical word. Look at the medical word or partial word that is given (it already contains a combining form and a suffix). Select the correct prefix from the Prefix List and write it on the blank line. Then build the medical word and write it on the line. Be sure to check your spelling. The first one has been done for you.

PREFIX LIST

a- (away from; without)	dys- (abnormal; difficult; painful)	inter- (between)	re- (again and again;
an- (not; without)	hyper- (above; more than	intra- (within)	backward; unable to)
brady- (slow)	normal)	poly- (many; much)	

Definition of the Medical Word	Prefix	Word or Partial Word	Build the Medical Word
1. Action (to) again and again give ability	re-	habilitation	rehabilitation
2. Pertaining to within (a) muscle	_____	muscular	_____
3. Condition (of) slow movement	_____	kinesia	_____
4. Condition (of being) without coordination	_____	taxia	_____
5. Action (of) more than normal straightening	_____	extension	_____
6. Pertaining to (muscles) between (the) ribs	_____	costal	_____
7. Pertaining to (muscles being) without development	_____	trophic	_____
8. Condition (in) many muscles (of) pain	_____	myalgia	_____
9. Condition (of the muscle or tendon) away from (the bone to) tear	_____	vulsion	_____
10. Condition (of) abnormal movement	_____	kinesia	_____
11. Inflammation of many muscles	_____	myositis	_____
12. Pertaining to (a drug that makes you be) without (the) sensation of pain	_____	algesic	_____

MULTIPLE COMBINING FORMS AND SUFFIX EXERCISE

Read the definition of the medical word. Select the correct suffix and combining forms. Then build the medical word and write it on the line. Be sure to check your spelling. The first one has been done for you.

SUFFIX LIST · COMBINING FORM LIST

SUFFIX LIST	COMBINING FORM LIST	
-al (pertaining to)	alg/o- (pain)	myos/o- (muscle)
-alis (pertaining to)	brachi/o- (arm)	neur/o- (nerve)
-ar (pertaining to)	dermat/o- (skin)	pod/o- (foot)
-ia (condition; state; thing)	electr/o- (electricity)	radi/o- (forearm bone; radiation; x-rays)
-ist (person who specializes in)	fibr/o- (fiber)	rhabd/o- (rod shaped)
-itis (infection of; inflammation of)	iatr/o- (medical treatment; physician)	skelet/o- (skeleton)
-graphy (process of recording)	muscul/o- (muscle)	synov/o- (joint membrane; synovium)
-oma (mass; tumor)	my/o- (muscle)	ten/o- (tendon)

Definition of the Medical Word · Build the Medical Word

Definition of the Medical Word	Build the Medical Word
1. Pertaining to (the) muscle(s) and skeleton	musculoskeletal
2. Pertaining to (a muscle of the) arm (near the) forearm bone (radius)	_____
3. Pertaining to nerve(s and) muscle(s)	_____
4. Infection of (or) inflammation of (the) skin (and) muscle	_____
5. Condition (in which) fibers (in the) muscles (cause) pain	_____
(*Hint*: Use three combining forms.)	

Definition of the Medical Word	**Build the Medical Word**
6. Process of recording electricity (in a) muscle	_____
7. (Benign) tumor (with cells that are) rod shaped (and occur in a) muscle	_____
8. Infection of (or) inflammation of (the) tendon and joint membrane	_____
9. Person who specializes in (the) foot medical treatment	_____

9.7A Spell Medical Words

PROOFREADING AND SPELLING EXERCISE

Read the following paragraph. Identify each misspelled medical word and write the correct spelling of it on the line provided.

Orothopedics is the study of the bones and muscles. A tendin connects the bone to the muscle and the facsia around it. The rectis femoris is in the leg. Fibromialgia has pain at trigger points, while bersitis is inflammation of a fluid-filled sac. A ganglian forms on a tendon. A muscle biopsee is used to diagnose muscular dystrophee. A tenorhaphy sews together a tendon after an injury.

1. _____   6. _____
2. _____   7. _____
3. _____   8. _____
4. _____   9. _____
5. _____   10. _____

ENGLISH AND MEDICAL WORD EQUIVALENTS EXERCISE

For each English word, write its equivalent medical word. Be sure to check your spelling. The first one has been done for you.

English Word	**Medical Word**	**English Word**	**Medical Word**
1. housemaid's knee	*bursitis*	5. whiplash	_____
2. muscle wasting	_____	6. bruise	_____
3. wryneck	_____	7. pitcher's elbow	_____
4. pulled muscle	_____	8. tennis elbow	_____

HEARING MEDICAL WORDS EXERCISE

You hear someone speaking the medical words given below. Read each pronunciation and then write the medical word it represents. Be sure to check your spelling. The first one has been done for you.

1. BER-sah	*bursa*	6. GAS-trawk-NEE-mee-us MUS-el	_____
2. AT-roh-fee	_____	7. my-AL-jah	_____
3. BRAD-ee-kih-NEE-zha	_____	8. poh-DY-ah-trist	_____
4. ee-LEK-troh-my-AW-grah-fee	_____	9. REE-hah-BIL-ih-TAY-shun	_____
5. FASH-ee-ah	_____	10. teh-NOR-ah-fee	_____

9.7B Pronounce Medical Words

PRONUNCIATION EXERCISE

Read the medical word and the syllables in its pronunciation. Circle the primary (main) accented syllable. The first one has been done for you.

1. abduction (ab-**duk**-shun)
2. atrophy (at-roh-fee)
3. chiropractor (ky-roh-prak-tor)
4. fibromyalgia (fy-broh-my-al-jah)
5. hypertrophy (hy-per-troh-fee)
6. intramuscular (in-trah-mus-kyoo-lar)
7. musculoskeletal (mus-kyoo-loh-skel-eh-tal)
8. sternocleidomastoid (ster-noh-kly-doh-mas-toyd)

9.8 Research Medical Words

ON THE JOB CHALLENGE

1. On the job, you will often encounter new medical words. Practice your medical dictionary skills by looking up *muscle* and *musculus* (the Latin word for *muscle*). Which entry has subentries with a full description of each muscle?

   _____

2. Also look up *tendon* and *tendo* (the Latin word for *tendon*). Are these complete lists of all the tendons in the body? Circle the correct answer: **Yes   No**

3. What other anatomical structure might lend its name to a tendon?

   _____

SOUND-ALIKE WORDS

Compare and contrast the medical meanings of these sound-alike orthopedic (muscular) and other words.

1. *rectum* (Chapter 3) and *rectus*
2. *reflex* and *reflux* (Chapter 3)
3. *contraction* and *contracture*

9.9 Analyze Medical Reports

ELECTRONIC PATIENT RECORD #1

This contains two related reports: an Operative Report and a Pathology Report. Read both reports and answer the questions.

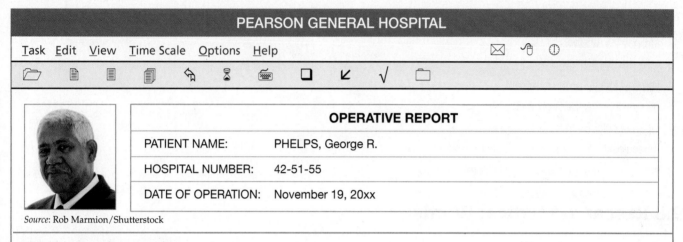

PEARSON GENERAL HOSPITAL

Task   Edit   View   Time Scale   Options   Help

OPERATIVE REPORT

PATIENT NAME:	PHELPS, George R.
HOSPITAL NUMBER:	42-51-55
DATE OF OPERATION:	November 19, 20xx

Source: Rob Marmion/Shutterstock

PREOPERATIVE DIAGNOSIS
Myopathy of undetermined etiology.

POSTOPERATIVE DIAGNOSIS
Myopathy of undetermined etiology.

PROCEDURE
Right quadriceps muscle biopsy.

ANESTHESIA
Xylocaine 1% local anesthetic with I.V. sedation.

SPECIMEN
Muscle biopsy x3.

COMPLICATIONS
None.

CLINICAL HISTORY
The patient is a 68-year-old male who has had progressive lower back and right leg weakness for approximately 6 months. He notes difficulty climbing stairs or getting up from a chair or bed. He moves slowly. There is mild eyelid ptosis noted.

OPERATIVE TECHNIQUE
After the induction of I.V. sedation, the right thigh skin was prepped with Betadine and draped in the usual fashion. After infiltration with local anesthesia, a longitudinal incision was made over the anterolateral aspect of the thigh. The incision was deepened through subcutaneous tissue to the quadriceps fascia, which was incised. Three muscle specimens were obtained for biopsy as per Armed Forces Institute of Pathology (AFIP) protocol. A thin core of muscle, approximately the thickness of a pencil, going deep into the muscle was submitted for the first biopsy. Then two muscle segments were grasped with biopsy clamps and excised. Pressure was held over the muscle for hemostasis. The wound was irrigated with warm saline solution, and the fascia was reapproximated with two interrupted sutures of #2-0 Vicryl. The subcutaneous tissue was approximated with interrupted sutures of #3-0 Vicryl. The skin was approximated with skin staples. A sterile dressing was applied. The patient was transferred to the recovery room in stable condition. Blood loss during the procedure was minimal.

Jamison R. Smith, M.D.

Jamison R. Smith, M.D.

JRS:srd
D: 11/19/xx
T: 11/19/xx

Chapter 10
Neurology

Nervous System

Neurology (nyoor-AW-loh-jee) is the medical specialty that studies the anatomy and physiology of the nervous system and uses laboratory and diagnostic procedures, medical and surgical procedures, and drugs to treat nervous system diseases.

 ## Learning Outcomes

After you study this chapter, you should be able to

10.1 Identify structures of the nervous system.

10.2 Describe the process of nerve transmission.

10.3 Describe common nervous system diseases, laboratory and diagnostic procedures, medical and surgical procedures, and drugs.

10.4 Form the plural and adjective forms of nouns related to neurology.

10.5 Give the meanings of word parts and abbreviations related to neurology.

10.6 Divide neurology words and build neurology words.

10.7 Spell and pronounce neurology words.

10.8 Research sound-alike and other neurology words.

10.9 Analyze the medical content and meaning of neurology reports.

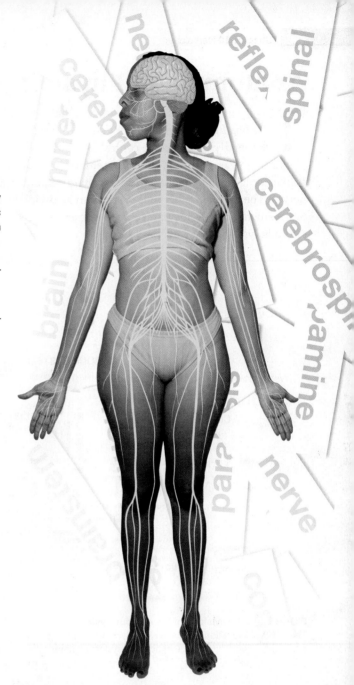

FIGURE 10-1 ■ Nervous system.
The nervous system is a widespread body system that consists of the brain, spinal cord, and nerves that form a connected pathway through which nerve impulses travel throughout the body.
Source: Pearson Education

Medical Language Key

To unlock the definition of a medical word, break it into word parts. Give the meaning of each word part. Put the meanings of the word parts in order, beginning with the meaning of the suffix, then the prefix (if present), then the combining form(s).

	Word Part	Word Part Meaning
Suffix	**-logy**	*study of*
Combining Form	**neur/o-**	*nerve*

Neurology: ▶ *Study of (the) nerves (and related structures).*

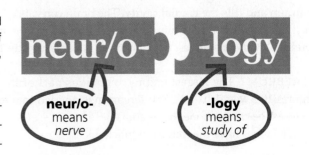

Anatomy and Physiology

The **nervous system** is a body system that is found in every part of the body from the head to the tips of the fingers and toes (see Figure 10-1 ■). The nervous system is divided into the central nervous system (CNS) and the peripheral nervous system (see Figure 10-2 ■). The **central nervous system** contains the brain and the spinal cord. The **peripheral nervous system** contains the cranial nerves and the spinal nerves. The peripheral nervous system can be divided into the autonomic nervous system (which includes the parasympathetic and sympathetic divisions) and the somatic nervous system.

Pronunciation/Word Parts

nervous (NER-vus)
  nerv/o- *nerve*
  -ous *pertaining to*

central (SEN-tral)

peripheral (peh-RIF-eh-ral)
  peripher/o- *outer aspects*
  -al *pertaining to*

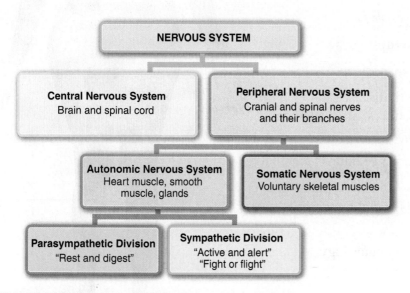

FIGURE 10-2 ■ **Divisions of the nervous system.**
The two main divisions of the nervous system are the central nervous system and the peripheral nervous system. The peripheral nervous system contains other subdivisions.
Source: Pearson Education

Anatomy of the Central Nervous System

Brain

The **brain** is the largest part of the central nervous system. It is located within the bony **cranium** and fills the **cranial cavity**. The brain consists of the cerebrum (and its lobes), the thalamus, hypothalamus, ventricles, brainstem, and cerebellum. The brain is surrounded by the meninges, three layers of membranes (see the section "Meninges.").

CEREBRUM   The largest and most obvious part of the brain is the **cerebrum** (see Figures 10-3 ■ and 10-4 ■). The cerebrum is divided into **lobes**. Each lobe has the same name as the cranial bone that is above it.

The lobes have the following functions.

brain (BRAYN)
The combining form **encephal/o-** means *brain*.

cranium (KRAY-nee-um)

cranial (KRAY-nee-al)
  crani/o- *cranium; skull*
  -al *pertaining to*

cavity (KAV-ih-tee)
  cav/o- *hollow space*
  -ity *condition; state*

cerebrum (seh-REE-brum)
(SAIR-eh-brum)

cerebral (seh-REE-bral) (SAIR-eh-bral)
  cerebr/o- *cerebrum*
  -al *pertaining to*

lobe (LOHB)

Frontal Lobe

- Originates conscious thought and intelligence
- Predicts future events and the benefits or consequences of actions
- Coordinates and analyzes information coming from other lobes of the cerebrum

Pronunciation/Word Parts

frontal (FRUN-tal)
   front/o- *front*
   -al *pertaining to*

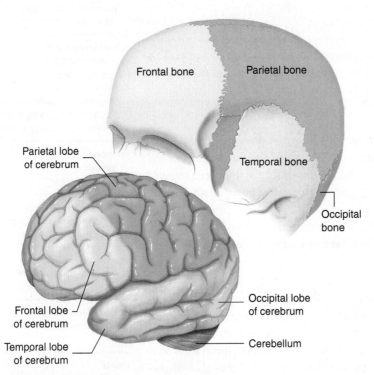

FIGURE 10-3 ■ Lobes of the cerebrum.
Each lobe of the cerebrum takes its name from the bone of the cranium that is above it.
Source: Pearson Education

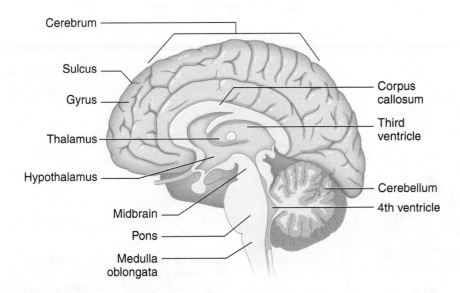

FIGURE 10-4 ■ Midline cut section of the brain.
This cut section shows the right half of the brain. The large size of the cerebrum is seen in comparison to the cerebellum and other structures. Many gyri and sulci are visible on the surface of the cerebrum. The thalamus, hypothalamus, midbrain, pons, medulla oblongata and cerebellum are seen.
Source: Pearson Education

- Exerts conscious, voluntary control over the skeletal muscles
- Coordinates the muscles of the mouth, lips, tongue, pharynx, and larynx to produce speech. This is done in the **speech center**, which is only in the left frontal lobe.
- Analyzes sensory information about taste. This information comes from taste receptors in the tongue and throat and is analyzed by the **gustatory cortex** of the frontal lobe.

Parietal Lobe

- Analyzes sensory information about touch, temperature, vibration, and pain. This information comes from receptors in the skin, joints, and muscles and is analyzed by the **somatosensory** area of the parietal lobe.

Temporal Lobe

- Analyzes sensory information about hearing. This information comes from receptors in the cochlea of the inner ear and is analyzed by the **auditory cortex** of the temporal lobe. (The auditory cortex of the right temporal lobe analyzes sensory information from the left ear, and the auditory cortex of the left temporal lobe analyzes sensory information from the right ear.)
- Analyzes sensory information about smells. This information comes from olfactory receptors in the nose and is analyzed by the **olfactory cortex** of the temporal lobe.

Occipital Lobe

- Analyzes sensory information about vision. This information comes from receptors in the retina of the eye and is analyzed by the **visual cortex** of the occipital lobe. (The visual cortex of the right occipital lobe analyzes sensory information from some parts of both eyes, and the visual cortex of the left occipital lobe analyzes sensory information from the other parts of both eyes, and this gives three-dimensional vision.)

There is a very deep, anterior-to-posterior **fissure** in the superior surface of the cerebrum (see Figure 10-5 ■). It divides the cerebrum into right and left halves. Each half of the cerebrum is a **hemisphere**. The only connection between the right and left hemispheres

Pronunciation/Word Parts

gustatory (GUS-tah-TOR-ee)
  gustat/o- *sense of taste*
  -ory *having the function of*

parietal (pah-RY-eh-tal)
  pariet/o- *wall of a cavity*
  -al *pertaining to*

somatosensory
(soh-MAH-toh-SEN-soh-ree)
  somat/o- *body*
  sens/o- *sensation*
  -ory *having the function of*
The combining forms **esthes/o-** and **esthet/o-** mean *feeling; sensation*

temporal (TEM-poh-ral)
  tempor/o- *side of head; temple*
  -al *pertaining to*

auditory (AW-dih-TOR-ee)
  audit/o- *sense of hearing*
  -ory *having the function of*

olfactory (ol-FAK-toh-ree)
  olfact/o- *sense of smell*
  -ory *having the function of*

occipital (awk-SIP-ih-tal)
  occipit/o- *back of the head; occiput*
  -al *pertaining to*

visual (VIH-shoo-al)
  vis/o- *sight; vision*
  -ual *pertaining to*

fissure (FIH-shur)
  fiss/o- *splitting*
  -ure *result of; system*

hemisphere (HEM-ih-sfeer)
  hemi- *one half*
  -sphere *ball; sphere*
The ending *-sphere* contains the combining form *spher/o-* and the one-letter suffix *-e*.

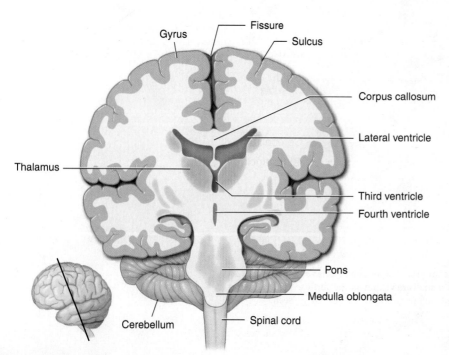

FIGURE 10-5 ■ Posterior half of the brain.
The anterior part of the cerebrum has been removed. The fissure that divides the right and left hemispheres of the cerebrum can be seen at the top. The corpus callosum is the white connecting bridge between the hemispheres. The right and left lateral ventricles and the small, central third ventricle can be seen. The medulla oblongata, the most posterior part of the brainstem, merges with the spinal cord.
Source: Pearson Education

is the **corpus callosum**. This connecting band of neurons deep within the brain allows the two hemispheres to communicate with each other and coordinate their activities. The hemisphere on one side of the brain receives sensory information from the other side of the body and sends motor commands to that side. In general, the right hemisphere of the cerebrum plays an important role in recognizing faces, patterns, and three-dimensional structures. The right hemisphere also analyzes the emotional content of words but not the actual words. The left hemisphere of the cerebrum performs mathematical and logical reasoning, problem-solving (see Figure 10-6 ■), and it coordinates the recall of memories. It is important in language skills and processing language.

The surface of the cerebrum has elevated folds (**gyri**) and narrow grooves (**sulci**) (see Figure 10-4). The **cerebral cortex** or gray matter is the outermost layer of tissue that follows the curves of the gyri and sulci (see Figure 10-5). The gray matter is composed of the cell bodies of neurons. Beneath it, the white matter of the cerebrum is composed of the axons of neurons. Most of these axons are covered by a fatty, white insulating layer of myelin. Myelin increases the speed of an electrical impulse along the neuron and gives the white color to the white matter of the cerebrum.

THALAMUS   The **thalamus** is located near the center of the cerebrum (see Figures 10-4 and 10-5). Its two lobes form the walls of the third ventricle. The thalamus acts as a relay station, receiving sensory information (sight, hearing, taste, smell, and touch) from the cranial nerves and the spinal nerves. The thalamus sends this to (1) the midbrain (that generates motor commands if the sensory information suggests an immediate danger) and (2) the cerebrum (that analyzes sensory information, compares it with memories, and uses it to plan future actions). The thalamus is also part of the limbic system that deals with emotions (discussed in "Psychiatry," Chapter 17).

HYPOTHALAMUS   The **hypothalamus**, as its name indicates, is located below the thalamus (see Figure 10-4). It forms the floor and part of the walls of the third ventricle, and it has a stalk of blood vessels and nerves that connects it to the pituitary gland. The hypothalamus functions as part of both the endocrine system and the nervous system. As part of the endocrine system, the hypothalamus produces hormones that control

Pronunciation/Word Parts

corpus callosum (KOR-pus kah-LOH-sum)

cerebral (seh-REE-bral) (SAIR-eh-bral)
   cerebr/o- *cerebrum*
   -al *pertaining to*

gyri (JY-rye)
Gyrus is a Latin singular noun. Form the plural by changing *-us* to *-i*.

gyrus (JY-rus)

sulci (SUL-sigh)
Sulcus is a Latin singular noun. Form the plural by changing *-us* to *-i*.

sulcus (SUL-kus)

cortex (KOR-teks)

cortical (KOR-tih-kal)
   cortic/o- *cortex; outer region*
   -al *pertaining to*

thalamus (THAL-ah-mus)

thalamic (thah-LAM-ik)
   thalam/o- *thalamus*
   -ic *pertaining to*

hypothalamus (HY-poh-THAL-ah-mus)

hypothalamic (HY-poh-thah-LAM-ik)
   hypo- *below; deficient*
   thalam/o- *thalamus*
   -ic *pertaining to*

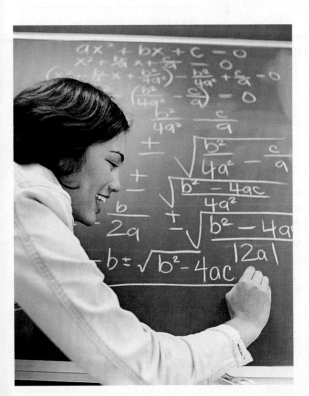

FIGURE 10-6 ■ Left-brain thinking.
Left-brain thinking uses the left hemisphere of the cerebrum, the site of mathematical and logical reasoning.
Source: Pearson Education

the functions of the anterior pituitary gland; it also produces other hormones that are stored in, and released by, the posterior pituitary gland (discussed in "Endocrinology," Chapter 14). As part of the nervous system, the hypothalamus coordinates the activities of the pons and medulla oblongata, which control the heart rate, blood pressure, and respiratory rate. The hypothalamus also regulates body temperature and sensations of hunger and thirst. The hypothalamus also plays a role in emotions and the sexual drive (discussed in "Psychiatry," Chapter 17).

VENTRICLES   The **ventricles** are four interconnected cavities within the brain. The largest of these are the lateral ventricles, two C-shaped cavities, one in each hemisphere in the cerebrum (see Figures 10-4 and 10-5). The third ventricle, a small central cavity, lies between the two lobes of the thalamus. The fourth ventricle is a long, narrow cavity that connects to the spinal cavity. The **ependymal cells** that line the ventricles produce **cerebrospinal fluid (CSF)**, a clear fluid that cushions and protects the brain and contains glucose and other nutrients. Cerebrospinal fluid flows through the ventricles, into the spinal cavity, then back toward the brain, and through the subarachnoid space in the meninges where it is absorbed into the blood of large veins.

BRAINSTEM   The **brainstem** (see Figures 10-4 and 10-5) is a column of tissue that begins in the center of the brain and continues inferiorly until it meets the spinal cord. It is composed of the midbrain, the pons, and the medulla oblongata.

The **midbrain** is the most superior part of the brainstem. It keeps the mind conscious. It coordinates immediate reflex responses to things you see or hear (such as a child suddenly crossing in front of your car or a very loud noise). It maintains muscle tone and the position of the extremities so that you do not have to consciously think about them. It contains the **substantia nigra**, a gray-to-black pigmented area that produces the neuro-transmitter dopamine that regulates muscle tone.

The **pons** is the middle part of the brainstem. It relays nerve impulses from the spinal cord to the midbrain, hypothalamus, thalamus, and cerebrum.

The **medulla oblongata** is the most inferior part of the brainstem. It contains the **respiratory centers** that automatically set the respiratory rate and other centers that control the heart rate. (In the medulla oblongata, nerve tracts cross, and nerve impulses from the right side of the body are relayed to the left side of the cerebrum, and vice versa.)

CEREBELLUM   The **cerebellum** is the separate, rounded section of the brain that is inferior and posterior to the cerebrum (see Figures 10-3, 10-4, and 10-5). The cerebellum receives sensory information about muscle tone and the position of the body and uses this to help maintain balance. It receives information from the cerebrum about motor commands and makes minor adjustments to coordinate those movements, especially intricate movements such as typing or skiing.

MENINGES   The brain is surrounded by the **meninges**, three separate membrane layers (see Figure 10-7 ■). The outermost membrane (beneath the bony cranium) is the **dura mater**, a tough, fibrous layer that protects the brain. The second layer is the **arachnoid**. Beneath the arachnoid is the **subarachnoid space**, which is filled with cerebrospinal fluid and contains large, branching fibers that connect the arachnoid to the pia mater beneath it. The innermost layer is the **pia mater**, a thin, delicate membrane next to the brain; it contains a spider-weblike network of small blood vessels.

Pronunciation/Word Parts

ventricle (VEN-trih-kl)

ventricular (ven-TRIH-kyoo-lar)
 ventricul/o- *chamber that is filled; ventricle*
 -ar *pertaining to*

ependymal (eh-PEN-dih-mal)
 ependym/o- *cellular lining*
 -al *pertaining to*

cerebrospinal (seh-REE-broh-SPY-nal)
(SAIR-eh-broh-SPY-nal)
 cerebr/o- *cerebrum*
 spin/o- *backbone; spine*
 -al *pertaining to*

brainstem (BRAYN-stem)

substantia nigra
(sub-STAN-shee-ah NY-grah)

pons (PAWNZ)

medulla (meh-DUL-ah) (meh-DOOL-ah)

oblongata (AWB-long-GAW-tah)

cerebellum (SAIR-eh-BEL-um)

cerebellar (SAIR-eh-BEL-ar)
 cerebell/o- *cerebellum*
 -ar *pertaining to*

meninges (meh-NIN-jeez)
Meninx, the singular form, is seldom used.

meningeal (meh-NIN-jee-al) (MEN-in-JEE-al)
 mening/o- *meninges*
 -eal *pertaining to*
The combining form **meningi/o-** also
means *meninges.*

dura mater (DOOR-ah MAY-ter)
(DOOR-ah MAH-ter)

dural (DOOR-al)
 dur/o- *dura mater*
 -al *pertaining to*

arachnoid (ah-RAK-noyd)
 arachn/o- *spider; spider web*
 -oid *resembling*

subarachnoid (SUB-ah-RAK-noyd)
 sub- *below; underneath*
 arachn/o- *spider; spider web*
 -oid *resembling*

pia mater (PY-ah MAY-ter)
(PEE-ah MAH-ter)

DID YOU KNOW?

Although the brain contains 100 billion neurons, it cannot feel pain. Only the meninges have sensory receptors for pain.

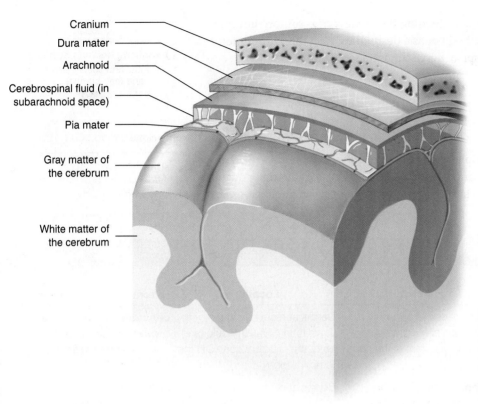

Cranium
Dura mater
Arachnoid
Cerebrospinal fluid (in subarachnoid space)
Pia mater
Gray matter of the cerebrum
White matter of the cerebrum

FIGURE 10-7 ■ Meninges.
The meninges have three membrane layers: the dura mater, arachnoid, and pia mater. Between the arachnoid and the pia mater is the subarachnoid space, which is filled with cerebrospinal fluid.
Source: Pearson Education

Spinal Cord

The **spinal cord** is part of the central nervous system. The spinal cord is a long, narrow column of neural tissue within the **spinal cavity** (or **spinal canal**). At its superior end, the spinal cord joins the medulla oblongata of the brain. The spinal cord extends to the level of the second lumbar vertebra in the vertebral column. There, at its inferior end, the spinal cord becomes a group of nerve roots known as the **cauda equina**. The spinal cord is protected because it is within the central opening (foramen) of each bony vertebra (see Figure 10-8 ■). The spinal cord is also protected and nourished by the meninges, which continue in an uninterrupted fashion from the brain down the spinal cavity. A narrow canal at the center of the spinal cord is lined with ependymal cells that also produce cerebrospinal fluid. There is one difference between the meninges around the brain and those around the spinal cord; between the dura mater and the bony vertebrae is the **epidural space**, an area that is unique to the spinal cord. This space is filled with fatty tissue and blood vessels.

The gray matter of the spinal cord is composed of the cell bodies of neurons in the spinal cord and spinal nerves. The white matter of the spinal cord is composed of the

Pronunciation/Word Parts

spinal (SPY-nal)
  spin/o- *backbone; spine*
  -al *pertaining to*
The combining form **myel/o-** means *bone marrow; myelin; spinal cord*

cavity (KAV-ih-tee)
  cav/o- *hollow space*
  -ity *condition; state*

canal (kah-NAL)

cauda equina (KAW-dah ee-KWY-nah)

epidural (EP-ih-DOOR-al)
  epi- *above; upon*
  dur/o- *dura mater*
  -al *pertaining to*

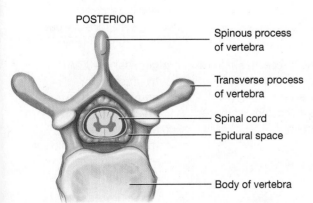

POSTERIOR

Spinous process of vertebra
Transverse process of vertebra
Spinal cord
Epidural space
Body of vertebra

FIGURE 10-8 ■ Spinal cord.
The spinal cord passes through the foramen (opening) within each vertebra. It is protected by the bony vertebra as well as by the dura mater of the meninges.
Source: Pearson Education

axons of neurons bundled together as an ascending tract that carries sensory information from a sensory spinal nerve to the brain or as a descending tract that carries motor commands from the brain to a motor spinal nerve connected to a muscle.

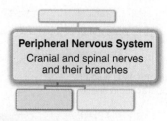

Peripheral Nervous System
Cranial and spinal nerves and their branches

Anatomy of the Peripheral Nervous System
Cranial Nerves

The **cranial nerves** are part of the peripheral nervous system (see Table 10-1 ▦). There are 12 pairs of cranial nerves. Each pair consists of a cranial nerve to the right side of the body and a cranial nerve to the left side of the body. Each pair of cranial nerves has

Pronunciation/Word Parts

cranial (KRAY-nee-al)
  crani/o- *cranium; skull*
  -al *pertaining to*

Table 10-1 Cranial Nerves

Cranial Nerve	Type of Nerve	Function	Location	Pronunciation/Word Parts
I olfactory nerve	sensory	**Smell.** Receives sensory information about smells from olfactory receptors in the nose	Begins at receptors in the nose Goes to the olfactory bulb (and on to the olfactory cortex) in the temporal lobe	**olfactory** (ol-FAK-toh-ree) **olfact/o-** *sense of smell* **-ory** *having the function of*
II optic nerve	sensory	**Vision.** Receives sensory information about light, dark, and color from rods and cones in the retina of the eye	Begins at receptors in the retina Goes to the optic chiasm in the brain	**optic** (AWP-tik) **opt/o-** *eye; vision* **-ic** *pertaining to*
III oculomotor nerve	motor	**Eye movement.** Sends motor commands to the extraocular muscles to move the eye. Sends motor commands to move the eyelid and to muscles of the iris to increase or decrease the diameter of the pupil.	Begins in the midbrain (of the brainstem) Goes to four of the six extraocular muscles around the eye Goes to the eyelid Goes to the iris	**oculomotor** (AW-kyoo-loh-MOH-tor) **ocul/o-** *eye* **mot/o-** *movement* **-or** *person who does; person who produces; thing that does; thing that produces*
IV trochlear nerve	motor	**Eye movement.** Sends motor commands to the extraocular muscles to move the eye	Begins in the midbrain (of the brainstem) Goes to one of the six extraocular muscles around the eye	**trochlear** (TROH-klee-ar) **trochle/o-** *structure shaped like a pulley* **-ar** *pertaining to* In the bony socket of the eye, there is a loop of ligament attached to the bone. When a nerve impulse from the trochlear nerve stimulates the superior oblique muscle, it contracts, pulling its tendon through that loop like the rope of a pulley, and this moves the eye.
V trigeminal nerve	sensory	**Facial and oral sensation.** Receives sensory information about touch, temperature, vibration, and pain from the skin of the face, the nasal cavity, oral cavity, gums, teeth, tongue, and palate	Begins at receptors in the skin and mucous membranes of those areas Goes to the pons (of the brainstem)	**trigeminal** (try-JEM-ih-nal) **tri-** *three* **gemin/o-** *group; set* **-al** *pertaining to* The trigeminal nerve is composed of three different branches: the ophthalmic, maxillary, and mandibular nerves.

Table 10-1 Cranial Nerves   *(continued)*

Cranial Nerve	Type of Nerve	Function	Location	Pronunciation/Word Parts
V trigeminal nerve *(continued)*	motor	**Chewing.** Sends motor commands to move the muscles for chewing	Begins in the pons (of the brainstem) Goes to the lower jaw (mandibular branch of the nerve)	
VI abducens nerve	motor	**Eye movement.** Sends motor commands to the extraocular muscles to move the eye	Begins in the pons (of the brainstem) Goes to one of the six extraocular muscles around the eye	**abducens** (ab-DOO-senz)
VII facial nerve	sensory	**Taste.** Receives sensory information about taste (sweet, sour, bitter, etc.) from taste receptors in the front of the tongue	Begins at receptors in the tongue Goes to the pons (of the brainstem)	**facial** (FAY-shal) **faci/o-** *face* **-al** *pertaining to*
	motor	**Facial movement. Tears and saliva.** Sends motor commands to move the facial muscles. Contracts the lacrimal glands to secrete tears. Contracts the submandibular and sublingual salivary glands to secrete saliva.	Begins in the pons (of the brainstem) Goes to the facial muscles Goes to the muscles in the lacrimal glands Goes to the muscles in the submandibular and sublingual salivary glands	
VIII vestibulo-cochlear nerve	sensory	**Hearing and balance.** Receives sensory information about sounds from the cochlea (in the inner ear). Receives sensory information from the semicircular canals to keep the balance of the body.	Begins at receptors in the vestibule (entrance to the cochlea) and in the semicircular canals in the inner ear Goes to the pons and medulla oblongata (of the brainstem)	**vestibulocochlear** (ves-TIH-byoo-loh-KOH-klee-ar) **vestibul/o-** *entrance; vestibule* **cochle/o-** *cochlea; spiral-shaped structure* **-ar** *pertaining to* It is also known as the **auditory nerve**.
				auditory (AW-dih-TOR-ee) **audit/o-** *sense of hearing* **-ory** *having the function of*
IX glossopharyn-geal nerve	sensory	**Taste.** Receives sensory information about taste (sweet, sour, bitter, etc.) from taste receptors at the back of the tongue, palate, and pharynx. Receives sensory information about the blood pressure and oxygen/carbon dioxide levels in arterial blood from pressure receptors in the carotid artery.	Begins at receptors in the tongue, palate, and pharynx Begins at receptors in the carotid artery Goes to the medulla oblongata (of the brainstem)	**glossopharyngeal** (GLAW-soh-fah-RIN-jee-al) **gloss/o-** *tongue* **pharyng/o-** *pharynx; throat* **-eal** *pertaining to*
	motor	**Swallowing.** Sends motor commands to move the muscles involved in swallowing. **Saliva.** Contracts the parotid gland to secrete saliva.	Begins in the medulla oblongata (of the brainstem) Goes to muscles in the pharynx and parotid gland	

(continued)

Table 10-1 Cranial Nerves *(continued)*

Cranial Nerve	Type of Nerve	Function	Location	Pronunciation/Word Parts
X vagus nerve	sensory	**Taste.** Receives sensory information about taste (sweet, sour, bitter, etc.) from taste receptors in the soft palate and pharynx. **Ear, chest, and abdomen sensation.** Receives sensory information about touch, temperature, vibration, and pain from receptors in the ear, diaphragm, and organs in the thoracic cavity and abdominopelvic cavity.	Begins at receptors in the soft palate and pharynx Begins at receptors in the skin and smooth muscles Goes to the medulla oblongata (of the brainstem)	**vagus** (VAY-gus) **vagal** (VAY-gal) **vag/o-** *vagus nerve; wandering* **-al** *pertaining to* The vagus nerve travels farther into the body than any other cranial nerve.
	motor	**Heart rate.** Sends motor commands to slow the heart rate. **Bronchi.** Contracts smooth muscle around the bronchi. **Peristalsis.** Contracts smooth muscle in the gastrointestinal tract to produce peristalsis.	Begins in the medulla oblongata (of the brainstem) Goes to the heart muscle and involuntary smooth muscles around the bronchi, blood vessels, esophagus, stomach, and intestines	
XI accessory nerve	motor	**Swallowing.** Sends motor commands to move the muscles involved in swallowing. **Vocal cord and neck movement.** Moves the vocal cords. Moves the muscles of the neck and upper back.	Begins in the medulla oblongata (of the brainstem) Goes to muscles in the pharynx, larynx, neck, and upper back	**accessory** (ak-SES-oh-ree) **access/o-** *contributing part; supplemental part* **-ory** *having the function of* The accessory nerve supplements the functions of the vagus nerve.
XII hypoglossal nerve	motor	**Tongue movement.** Sends motor commands to move the tongue	Begins in the medulla oblongata (of the brainstem) Goes to the muscles of the tongue	**hypoglossal** (HY-poh-GLAW-sal) **hypo-** *below; deficient* **gloss/o-** *tongue* **-al** *pertaining to*

a name that reflects its location or function. Some cranial nerves receive **sensory** information from the body (visual images, sounds, smells, tastes, touch, pressure, vibration, temperature, pain, or position). Other cranial nerves send **motor** commands from the brain to voluntary muscles (to move the face, head, and neck) or to involuntary muscles (to slow the heart rate, to cause peristalsis in the digestive tract, to cause the bronchioles to constrict, to cause the lacrimal or salivary glands to secrete tears or saliva). Some cranial nerves carry both sensory and motor nerve impulses.

Spinal Nerves

The **spinal nerves** are part of the peripheral nervous system because they are found in the periphery of the body (those parts away from the center). There are 31 pairs of spinal nerves that originate at regular intervals along the spinal cord. Each pair consists of a spinal nerve to the right side of the body and a spinal nerve to the left side of the body. Each pair of spinal nerves is named according to the vertebra next to it.

Each spinal nerve has two different groups of nerve roots that connect it to the spinal cord: dorsal nerve roots and ventral nerve roots (see Figure 10-9 ■).

Pronunciation/Word Parts

sensory (SEN-soh-ree)
  sens/o- *sensation*
  -ory *having the function of*

motor (MOH-tor)
  mot/o- *movement*
  -or *person who does; person who produces; thing that does; thing that produces*

spinal (SPY-nal)
  spin/o- *backbone; spine*
  -al *pertaining to*

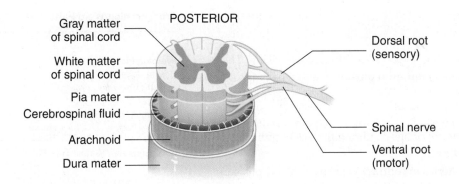

POSTERIOR

Gray matter of spinal cord

White matter of spinal cord

Pia mater

Cerebrospinal fluid

Arachnoid

Dura mater

Dorsal root (sensory)

Spinal nerve

Ventral root (motor)

FIGURE 10-9 ■ Spinal nerves.
The spinal nerves originate at regular intervals along the spinal cord. Each spinal nerve consists of dorsal nerve roots that receive sensory information from the body and ventral nerve roots that carry motor commands to the body.
Source: Pearson Education

The posterior or **dorsal nerve roots** receive sensory information (touch, pressure, vibration, temperature, pain, and body position) from the skin. Each dorsal nerve root receives sensory information from a specific area of the skin known as a *dermatome* (discussed in "Dermatology," Chapter 7) (see Figure 7-3). Dermatomes are important in the diagnosis of nerve injuries because they correlate a specific spinal nerve and its dermatome to an area of the skin where there is loss of sensation or movement. The dorsal nerve roots also receive sensory information from the muscles and joints. Dorsal nerve roots and their spinal nerve are an **afferent nerve** because they carry nerve impulses from the body to the spinal cord.

The anterior or **ventral nerve roots** carry motor commands from the spinal cord to skeletal muscles and involuntary smooth muscles within organs, glands, and other structures. Ventral nerve roots and their spinal nerve are an **efferent nerve** because they carry nerve impulses from the spinal cord to the body.

A **reflex** is a rapid, involuntary muscle reaction that is controlled by the spinal cord. The spinal cord reacts immediately to certain types of sensory information (sudden pain or when a physician uses a percussion hammer to tap on a tendon that stretches a muscle) (see Figure 9-23). For example, accidentally placing your hand on a hot stove causes you to pull your hand away, even before your brain understands what is wrong. Sensory information from a spinal nerve in the hand reached the spinal cord, and the spinal cord immediately sent a motor command to muscles to make you move your hand. This circuit is known as a **reflex arc**. Later, the sensory information is analyzed by the brain, and you say "Ouch."

Autonomic Nervous System

The **autonomic nervous system** controls the contractions of involuntary cardiac muscle in the heart, as well as smooth muscles around organs, glands, and other structures. The autonomic nervous system can be further broken down into two divisions: the parasympathetic division and the sympathetic division.

The **parasympathetic division** is active when the body is sleeping, resting, eating, or doing light activity (so-called "rest and digest" activities). The neurotransmitter of the parasympathetic division is **acetylcholine**. The action of the parasympathetic division and acetylcholine is to

- Decrease the heart rate, blood pressure, and metabolic rate
- Increase or decrease the diameter of the pupils in response to changing levels of light
- Increase peristalsis in the gastrointestinal tract
- Cause the secretion of saliva, digestive enzymes, and insulin

dorsal (DOR-sal)
dors/o- *back; dorsum*
-al *pertaining to*

nerve root (NERV ROOT)
The combining forms **radicul/o-** and **rhiz/o-** mean *spinal nerve root*.

afferent (AF-eh-rent)
affer/o- *toward the center*
-ent *pertaining to*

ventral (VEN-tral)
ventr/o- *abdomen; front*
-al *pertaining to*

efferent (EF-eh-rent)
effer/o- *away from the center*
-ent *pertaining to*

reflex (REE-fleks)

autonomic (AW-toh-NAW-mik)
autonom/o- *independent; self-governing*
-ic *pertaining to*

parasympathetic
(PAIR-ah-SIM-pah-THEH-tik)
para- *abnormal; apart from; beside; two parts of a pair*
sym- *together; with*
pathet/o- *suffering*
-ic *pertaining to*
The parasympathetic division is one of two parts of a pair in the autonomic nervous system. It works together with the sympathetic division.

acetylcholine (AS-eh-til-KOH-leen)

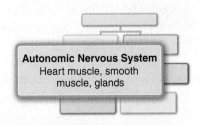

Autonomic Nervous System
Heart muscle, smooth muscle, glands

- Prepare the body for sexual activity
- Contract the bladder for urination.

The **sympathetic division** is active when the body is active or exercising. The neurotransmitter of the sympathetic division is **norepinephrine**. The action of the sympathetic division and norepinephrine is to

- Increase mental alertness
- Dilate the pupils to increase the amount of light entering the eye to optimize vision
- Increase the heart rate and metabolic rate
- Cause the smooth muscles in the arteries to contract to raise the blood pressure
- Cause the smooth muscles in the bronchioles to relax to increase air flow to the lungs
- Increase the respiratory rate
- Cause the skeletal muscles and liver to release glycogen (stored glucose) to meet increased energy needs.

During stress, anxiety, fear, or anger, the hypothalamus sends nerve impulses to the sympathetic division, which then stimulates the medulla of the adrenal gland to secrete the hormone **epinephrine** into the blood to prepare the body for more intense activity as in "fight or flight."

sympathetic (SIM-pah-THEH-tik)
  sym- *together; with*
  pathet/o- *suffering*
  -ic *pertaining to*
The sympathetic nervous system is active when the body is suffering from fear.

norepinephrine (NOR-ep-ih-NEF-rin)

epinephrine (EP-ih-NEF-rin)

Somatic Nervous System

The **somatic nervous system** controls the voluntary movements of skeletal muscles. Cranial nerves and spinal nerves send nerve impulses as motor commands to skeletal muscles and cause them to contract. These motor commands are the result of conscious thoughts in the brain, and the movements produced are voluntary movements. For example, if you decide to open this book and begin studying, your brain sends nerve impulses as motor commands through specific spinal nerves to the skeletal muscles in your arms and hands, and you open the book and find the correct page. Then your brain sends nerve impulses as motor commands through specific cranial nerves to the extraocular muscles of the eyes, and your eyes move across the page as you read.

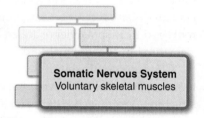

Somatic Nervous System
Voluntary skeletal muscles

somatic (soh-MAT-ik)
  somat/o- *body*
  -ic *pertaining to*

neural (NYOOR-al)
  neur/o- *nerve*
  -al *pertaining to*

Neurons and Neuroglia

All of the structures of the nervous system are composed of neural tissue. **Neural tissue** is made up of two categories of cells: neurons and neuroglia.

A **neuron**, an individual nerve cell, is the functional unit of the nervous system. **Nerves** are bundles of individual nerve cells (neurons).

Neuroglia are the other category of neural tissue. Neuroglia do not generate or conduct electrical impulses like neurons do. However, their role in the function of the nervous system is very important. Neuroglia perform specialized tasks to help neurons do their work (see Table 10-2 ■). Cancers of the nervous system arise from the neuroglia, not from the neurons.

neuron (NYOOR-on)
  neur/o- *nerve*
  -on *structure; substance*

nerve (NERV)
The combining forms **nerv/o-** and **neur/o-** mean *nerve*.

neuroglia (nyoor-OH-glee-ah)
  neur/o- *nerve*
  -glia *cells that provide support*

dendrite (DEN-dryt)
  dendr/o- *branching structure*
  -ite *thing that pertains to*

Physiology of a Neuron and Neurotransmitters

A neuron is the functional unit of the nervous system. It consists of three parts: dendrites, the cell body, and an axon (see Figure 10-10 ■). The **dendrites** are multiple branching structures at the beginning of the neuron. The cell body contains the **nucleus** of the neuron, which directs cellular activities. The cell body also contains **cytoplasm**; structures in the cytoplasm produce neurotransmitters as well as energy for the neuron. The **axon** is an elongated extension of cytoplasm at the end of the neuron. At the tip of

nucleus (NOO-klee-us)

cytoplasm (SY-toh-plazm)
  cyt/o- *cell*
  -plasm *formed substance; growth*

axon (AK-sawn)

Table 10-2 Neuroglia

Cell Name	Cell Description and Function	Pronunciation/Word Parts
astrocytes	Cells with branches that radiate outward like a star. They support the dendrites of neurons and connect them to capillaries. Astrocytes form the blood–brain barrier that keeps certain harmful substances in the blood from getting to the brain.	**astrocyte** (AS-troh-site) **astr/o-** *star-like structure* **-cyte** *cell*
ependymal cells	Cells that line the ventricles of the brain, the spinal cavity, and the narrow, central canal within the spinal cord; they produce cerebrospinal fluid	**ependymal** (eh-PEN-dih-mal) **ependym/o-** *cellular lining* **-al** *pertaining to*
microglia	Cells that move throughout the tissues of the brain and spinal cord. They engulf and destroy dead tissue and pathogens (bacteria, viruses, etc.). Microglia are the smallest of all the neuroglia.	**microglia** (my-KROH-glee-ah) **micr/o-** *one millionth; small* **-glia** *cells that provide support*
oligodendroglia	Cells that provide structural support. They also produce myelin that surrounds the larger axons of neurons in the brain and spinal cord	**oligodendroglia** (OH-lih-GOH-den-DROH-glee-ah) **olig/o-** *few; scanty* **dendr/o-** *branching structure* **-glia** *cells that provide support* Add words to make a complete definition of *oligodendroglia: cells that provide support (to a neuron but have) few branching structures.*
Schwann cells	Cells that produce myelin that surrounds the larger axons of neurons of the cranial nerves and the spinal nerves	**Schwann** (SHVAWN)

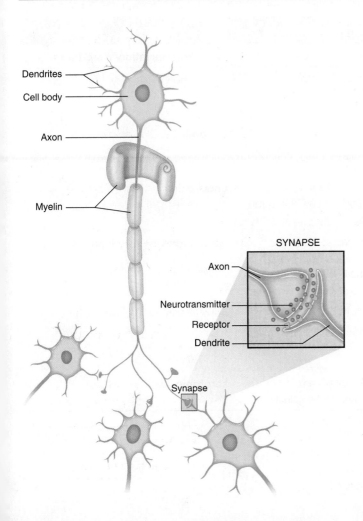

Dendrites

Cell body

Axon

Myelin

SYNAPSE

Axon

Neurotransmitter

Receptor

Dendrite

Synapse

FIGURE 10-10 ■ Neuron.
A neuron consists of several dendrites, a cell body, and an axon. The dendrites receive nerve impulses from other neurons. The cell body contains the nucleus of the neuron. The axon transmits nerve impulses to other neurons (or to a muscle fiber, to a cell in an organ, or to a cell in a gland). Larger axons are covered with myelin to increase the speed of electrical impulses.
Source: Pearson Education

the axon are vesicles (fluid-filled sacs) that store a neurotransmitter. The axon of one neuron does not connect directly to the dendrites of the next neuron. Instead, there is a space or **synapse** between the two neurons. There is also a synapse between a neuron and other structures, such as the cell of a muscle, organ, or gland.

A neuron is able to (1) generate an electrical impulse when stimulated, (2) conduct that electrical impulse throughout its length, and (3) change that electrical impulse into a chemical substance (neurotransmitter). An electrical impulse is relayed from one neuron to the next neuron in the following way. An electrical impulse travels along the dendrite, cell body, and to the end of the axon. The electrical impulse cannot travel across the synapse, and so vesicles at the tip of the axon release a **neurotransmitter** stored inside of them. The neurotransmitter is a chemical messenger that travels across the synapse and binds with a **receptor**, a structure on the cell membrane of a dendrite of the next neuron (or on the cell membrane of a muscle, organ, or gland). This causes a change in the cell membrane of the dendrite that then produces an electrical impulse that travels along that dendrite, etc. All of these events happen in a fraction of a second. The presence of myelin dramatically increases the speed at which an electrical impulse can travel along the axon. Larger axons are covered by a fatty, white insulating layer of **myelin** and are said to be myelinated. Smaller axons do not have myelin.

There are many different neurotransmitters in the nervous system. The most common ones are described in the following table (see Table 10-3 ■).

Pronunciation/Word Parts

synapse (SIN-aps)

neurotransmitter
(NYOOR-oh-TRANS-mit-er)
   neur/o- *nerve*
   transmitt/o- *send across; send through*
   -er *person who does; person who produces; thing that does; thing that produces*

receptor (ree-SEP-tor)
   recept/o- *receive*
   -or *person who does; person who produces; thing that does; thing that produces*

myelin (MY-eh-lin)

myelinated (MY-eh-lih-NAY-ted)
   myelin/o- *myelin*
   -ated *composed of; pertaining to a condition*

Table 10-3 Neurotransmitters, Neuromodulators, and Hormones

Neurotransmitter	Location	Pronunciation/Word Parts
acetylcholine	Neurotransmitter between neurons of the parasympathetic division. It is also in the somatic nervous system in synapses between a motor neuron and a voluntary skeletal muscle.	**acetylcholine** (AS-eh-til-KOH-leen)
dopamine	Neurotransmitter in the brain between neurons in the cerebral cortex, hypothalamus, midbrain, and limbic system. Produced by the substantia nigra of the midbrain.	**dopamine** (DOH-pah-meen)
endorphins	Neuromodulators in the brain between neurons in the hypothalamus, thalamus, and brainstem. They are one of several natural pain relievers produced by the brain.	**endorphins** (en-DOR-finz)
epinephrine	Hormone secreted by the adrenal gland and released into the blood. It stimulates neurons in the sympathetic division during times of anxiety, fear, or anger to prepare the body for "fight or flight."	**epinephrine** (EP-ih-NEF-rin)
norepinephrine	Neurotransmitter of the sympathetic division. It is also found between neurons in the cerebral cortex, hypothalamus, cerebellum, brainstem, and spinal cord. It is also a hormone secreted by the adrenal gland.	**norepinephrine** (NOR-ep-ih-NEF-rin)
serotonin	Neurotransmitter between neurons of the limbic system, hypothalamus, and cerebellum in the brain, and in the spinal cord	**serotonin** (SAIR-oh-TOH-nin)

Vocabulary Review

Anatomy and Physiology

Word or Phrase	Description	Combining Forms
afferent nerves	Nerves that carry sensory nerve impulses from the body to the spinal cord or brain	**affer/o-** *toward the center*
autonomic nervous system	Division of the peripheral nervous system that carries nerve impulses to the heart, involuntary smooth muscles, and glands. It includes the parasympathetic division and the sympathetic division.	**autonom/o-** *independent; self-governing*
central nervous system	Division of the nervous system that includes the brain and the spinal cord	**nerv/o-** *nerve*
efferent nerves	Nerves that carry motor nerve impulses from the spinal cord or brain to the body	**effer/o-** *away from the center*
nervous system	Body system that consists of the brain, spinal cord, cranial nerves, and spinal nerves. It includes the central nervous system and the peripheral nervous system and its divisions. The nervous system is made of **neural tissue**.	**nerv/o-** *nerve* **neur/o-** *nerve*
parasympathetic division	Division of the autonomic nervous system. Its neurotransmitter is acetylcholine. It directs the activity of the heart, involuntary smooth muscles, and glands while the body is at rest.	**pathet/o-** *suffering*
peripheral nervous system	Division of the nervous system that includes the cranial nerves and the spinal nerves	**peripher/o-** *outer aspects*
receptor	Structure on the cell membrane of a dendrite (or on a muscle, organ, or gland) where a neurotransmitter binds	**recept/o-** *receive*
reflex	Rapid, involuntary muscle reaction that is controlled by the spinal cord. In response to sudden pain or muscle stretch, the spinal cord immediately sends a motor command to move. All of this takes place without conscious thought or processing by the brain. The entire circuit that the nerve impulse travels is also known as a **reflex arc**.	
somatic nervous system	Division of the peripheral nervous system that controls the movements of voluntary skeletal muscles	**somat/o-** *body*
sympathetic division	Division of the autonomic nervous system. Its neurotransmitter is norepinephrine. It directs the activity of the heart, involuntary muscles, and glands during times of increased activity. During danger or stress ("fight or flight"), it stimulates the adrenal gland to release the hormone epinephrine into the blood.	**pathet/o-** *suffering*

Brain

Word or Phrase	Description	Combining Forms
arachnoid	Thin, middle layer of the meninges. Beneath it is a spider-weblike network of fibers that goes into the subarachnoid space and connects the arachnoid to the pia mater layer.	**arachn/o-** *spider; spiderweb*
auditory cortex	Area in the temporal lobe of the cerebrum that analyzes sensory information from receptors in the cochlea for the sense of hearing	**audit/o-** *sense of hearing*
brain	Largest organ of the nervous system. It is part of the central nervous system and is located in the cranial cavity.	**encephal/o-** *brain*

Word or Phrase	Description	Combining Forms
brainstem	Column of tissue that begins in the center of the brain and continues inferiorly to join the spinal cord. The brainstem is composed of the midbrain, pons, and medulla oblongata.	
cerebellum	Small, rounded structure that is the most posterior part of the brain. It receives information about muscle tone and body position. It maintains the balance and coordinates muscle movements.	**cerebell/o-** *cerebellum*
cerebral cortex	The outermost surface of the cerebrum. It consists of gray matter that contains the cell bodies of neurons.	**cortic/o-** *cortex; outer region*
cerebrospinal fluid	Clear fluid that is produced by the ependymal cells that line the ventricles in the brain and the canal within the spinal cord. It circulates through the ventricles, into the spinal cavity, back to the brain, and through the subarachnoid space of the meninges. It cushions and protects the brain and contains glucose and other nutrients.	**cerebr/o-** *cerebrum* **spin/o-** *backbone; spine*
cerebrum	The largest and most visible part of the brain. Its surface contains gyri and sulci, and it is divided into two hemispheres. It is also divided into lobes.	**cerebr/o-** *cerebrum*
corpus callosum	Connecting band of neurons between the two hemispheres of the cerebrum that allows them to communicate and coordinate their activities	
cranial cavity	Hollow cavity inside the bony cranium that contains the brain	**crani/o-** *cranium; skull* **cav/o-** *hollow space*
dura mater	Tough, outermost layer of the meninges. The dura mater lies just beneath the bones of the cranium and within the foramen of each vertebra.	**dur/o-** *dura mater*
fissure	Deep division that runs in an anterior-to-posterior direction through the superior surface of the cerebrum and divides it into right and left hemispheres	**fiss/o-** *splitting*
frontal lobe	Lobe of the cerebrum that originates conscious thought and intelligence and predicts future events and consequences. Exerts conscious control over the skeletal muscles. Contains the speech center that coordinates muscles for speaking. Contains the gustatory cortex for the sense of taste.	**front/o-** *front*
gustatory cortex	Area in the frontal lobe of the cerebrum that analyzes sensory information from taste receptors in the tongue for the sense of taste.	**gustat/o-** *sense of taste*
gyrus	One of many elevated folds on the surface of the cerebrum. In between each gyrus is a sulcus (narrow groove).	
hemisphere	One half of the cerebrum. The right hemisphere recognizes faces, patterns, three-dimensional structures and the emotions of words. The left hemisphere deals with mathematical and logical reasoning, problem-solving, and recall of memories. It is active in language skills and processing language.	
hypothalamus	Area in the center of the brain just below the thalamus that coordinates the activities of the pons and medulla oblongata. It controls the heart rate, blood pressure, respiratory rate, body temperature, and sensations of hunger and thirst. It also produces hormones as part of the endocrine system; it has a stalk of tissue that connects it to the pituitary gland of the endocrine system.	**thalam/o-** *thalamus*
lobe	Large area of the cerebrum. Each lobe is named for the bone of the cranium that is above it: frontal lobe, parietal lobe, temporal lobe, and occipital lobe.	

Word or Phrase	Description	Combining Forms
medulla oblongata	Most inferior part of the brainstem that joins to the spinal cord. It contains the respiratory centers. The motor portions of cranial nerves IX through XII begin here. The sensory portions of cranial nerves IX and X end here.	
meninges	Three separate membranes that envelop and protect the entire brain and spinal cord. The meninges include the dura mater, arachnoid, and pia mater.	**meningi/o-** *meninges* **mening/o-** *meninges*
midbrain	Most superior part of the brainstem. It keeps the mind conscious, coordinates immediate responses, and maintains muscle tone and body position. It contains the substantia nigra. Cranial nerves III and IV begin here.	
occipital lobe	Lobe of the cerebrum that receives and analyzes sensory information from the eyes. Contains the visual cortex for the sense of sight.	**occipit/o-** *back of the head; occiput*
olfactory cortex	Area in the temporal lobe of the cerebrum that analyzes sensory information from receptors in the nose for the sense of smell	**olfact/o-** *sense of smell*
parietal lobe	Lobe of the cerebrum that receives and analyzes sensory information about touch, temperature, vibration, and pain from the skin, joints, and muscles.	**pariet/o-** *wall of a cavity*
pia mater	Thin, delicate, innermost layer of the meninges. It covers the surface of the brain and contains many small blood vessels.	
pons	Middle part of the brainstem that relays nerve impulses from the spinal cord to the midbrain, hypothalamus, thalamus, and cerebrum. The motor portions of cranial nerves V through VII begin here. The sensory portions of cranial nerves V and VII end here.	
somatosensory area	Area of the parietal lobe of the cerebrum that analyzes sensory information (touch, temperature, vibration, and pain) from receptors in the skin, joints, and muscles	**somat/o-** *body* **esthes/o-** *feeling; sensation* **esthet/o-** *feeling; sensation*
subarachnoid space	Space beneath the arachnoid layer of the meninges. It is filled with cerebrospinal fluid.	**arachn/o-** *spider; spider web*
substantia nigra	A gray-to-black pigmented area in the midbrain of the brainstem that produces the neurotransmitter dopamine	
sulcus	Groove between two gyri on the surface of the cerebrum	
temporal lobe	Lobe of the cerebrum that receives and analyzes sensory information about hearing and smells. It contains the auditory cortex for the sense of hearing and the olfactory cortex for the sense of smell.	**tempor/o-** *side of the head; temple*
thalamus	Area in the center of the cerebrum that is a relay station. It takes sensory information from the cranial and spinal nerves and sends it to the midbrain and the cerebrum.	**thalam/o-** *thalamus*
ventricle	One of four interconnected cavities in the brain that contains cerebrospinal fluid. The two lateral ventricles are in the right and left hemispheres of the cerebrum. The small third ventricle is between the two lobes of the thalamus. The long, narrow fourth ventricle connects to the spinal cavity.	**ventricul/o-** *chamber that is filled; ventricle*
visual cortex	Area in the occipital lobe of the cerebrum that receives and analyzes sensory information from the retina of each eye for the sense of sight	**vis/o-** *sight; vision*

Spinal Cord

Word or Phrase	Description	Combining Forms
cauda equina	Group of nerve roots that begin where the spinal cord ends and continue inferiorly within the spinal cavity. They look like the tail (cauda) of a horse (equine).	
epidural space	Area between the dura mater and the vertebral body. It is filled with fatty tissue and blood vessels.	dur/o- *dura mater*
spinal cavity	Hollow cavity within each vertebra. It contains the spinal cord. It is also known as the **spinal canal**.	spin/o- *backbone; spine* cav/o- *hollow space*
spinal cord	Part of the central nervous system. It begins at the medulla oblongata of the brain and extends down the back within the spinal cavity. It ends at lumbar vertebra L2 where it separates into nerve roots (cauda equina).	spin/o- *backbone; spine* myel/o- *bone marrow; myelin;* *spinal cord*

Cranial Nerves

Word or Phrase	Description	Combining Forms
abducens nerve	Cranial nerve VI. Motor nerve. Movement of the eye.	
accessory nerve	Cranial nerve XI. Motor nerve. Movement of the muscles for swallowing, the vocal cords, and muscles of the neck and upper back. Two of its nerve branches also assist the vagus nerve.	access/o- *contributing part;* *supplemental part*
cranial nerves (I–XII)	Twelve pairs of nerves that originate in the brain. They carry **sensory** nerve impulses to the brain and/or **motor** nerve impulses from the brain.	crani/o- *cranium; skull* sens/o- *sensation* mot/o- *movement*
facial nerve	Cranial nerve VII. Sensory and motor nerve. Sense of taste for the front of the tongue. Movement of the facial muscles and salivary and lacrimal glands.	faci/o- *face*
glossopharyngeal nerve	Cranial nerve IX. Sensory and motor nerve. Sense of taste for the back of the tongue. Receives information about blood pressure and oxygen/carbon dioxide levels. Movement of the muscles for swallowing and the parotid salivary glands.	gloss/o- *tongue* pharyng/o- *pharynx; throat*
hypoglossal nerve	Cranial nerve XII. Motor nerve. Movement of the tongue.	gloss/o- *tongue*
oculomotor nerve	Cranial nerve III. Motor nerve. Movement of the eye, eyelids, and iris (to change the diameter of the pupil).	ocul/o- *eye* mot/o- *movement*
olfactory nerve	Cranial nerve I. Sensory nerve. Sense of smell.	olfact/o- *sense of smell*
optic nerve	Cranial nerve II. Sensory nerve. Sense of vision.	opt/o- *eye; vision*
trigeminal nerve	Cranial nerve V. Sensory and motor nerve. Sensation in the face and mouth. Movement of the muscles for chewing. It consists of three branches: ophthalmic nerve, maxillary nerve, mandibular nerve.	gemin/o- *group; set*
trochlear nerve	Cranial nerve IV. Motor nerve. Movement of the eye.	trochle/o- *structure shaped like* *a pulley*
vagus nerve	Cranial nerve X. Sensory and motor nerve. Sensation of taste from the soft palate and throat. Sensation in the ears, diaphragm, and the internal organs. It controls the heart rate and the smooth muscles in the bronchi and GI tract.	vag/o- *vagus nerve; wandering*

Build Medical Words

Combining Form and Suffix Exercise

Read the definition of the medical word. Look at the combining form that is given. Select the correct suffix from the Suffix List and write it on the blank line. Then build the medical word and write it on the line. (Remember: You may need to remove the combining vowel. Always remove the hyphens and slash.) Be sure to check your spelling. The first one has been done for you.

SUFFIX LIST

-al (pertaining to)
-ar (pertaining to)
-ated (composed of; pertaining to a condition)
-cyte (cell)
-eal (pertaining to)

-ent (pertaining to)
-glia (cells that provide support)
-ic (pertaining to)
-ite (thing that pertains to)
-oid (resembling)
-on (structure; substance)

-or (person who does; person who produces; thing that does; thing that produces)
-ory (having the function of)
-ous (pertaining to)
-ure (result of; system)

Definition of the Medical Word	Combining Form	Suffix	Build the Medical Word
1. (Division of the nervous system) pertaining to (the) body	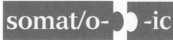 somat/o- -ic		somatic

(You think *pertaining to* (-ic) + *body* (somat/o-). You change the order of the word parts to put the suffix last. You write *somatic*.)

Definition of the Medical Word	Combining Form	Suffix	Build the Medical Word
2. Pertaining to (the) cerebrum	cerebr/o-		
3. Pertaining to (the top of the) skull	crani/o-		
4. Pertaining to (the) nerves	nerv/o-		
5. Having the function of (the) sense of hearing	audit/o-		
6. Pertaining to (the) ventricles (in the brain)	ventricul/o-		
7. Resembling (a) spider web	arachn/o-		
8. Pertaining to (the) meninges	mening/o-		
9. Cell (that is a) star-like structure	astr/o-		
10. Pertaining to (the) spine	spin/o-		
11. Thing that pertains to (a) branching structure	dendr/o-		
12. Pertaining to away from the center	effer/o-		
13. (Structure that is the) result of splitting	fiss/o-		
14. Pertaining to (the) outer aspects (of the body)	peripher/o-		
15. Pertaining to (the) thalamus	thalam/o-		
16. Having the function of sensation	sens/o-		
17. Thing that does receive	recept/o-		
18. Composed of myelin	myelin/o-		
19. Pertaining to independent or self-governing	autonom/o-		
20. Structure (of a single) nerve (cell)	neur/o-		
21. Pertaining to (the) temple (of the cranium)	tempor/o-		
22. Having the function of (the) sense of smell	olfact/o-		
23. Pertaining to (the) cerebellum	cerebell/o-		
24. Cells that provide support (for) nerves	neur/o-		
25. Pertaining to (the) dura mater	dur/o-		
26. Pertaining to (the) back of the head	occipit/o-		

Prefix Exercise

Read the definition of the medical word. Look at the medical word or partial word that is given (it already contains a combining form and a suffix). Select the correct prefix from the Prefix List and write it on the blank line. Then build the medical word and write it on the line. Be sure to check your spelling. The first one has been done for you.

PREFIX LIST

epi- (above; upon)	hypo- (below; deficient)	sym- (together; with)
hemi- (one half)	sub- (below; underneath)	tri- (three)

Definition of the Medical Word	Prefix	Word or Partial Word	Build the Medical Word
1. Pertaining to with suffering	**sym-**	**pathetic**	sympathetic
2. (Structure) below (the) thalamus	_____	thalamus	_____
3. Pertaining to above (the) dura mater	_____	dural	_____
4. (Cranial nerve) pertaining to three (in a) group or set	_____	geminal	_____
5. Resembling (an) underneath (layer like a) spider web	_____	arachnoid	_____
6. Sphere (divided into a shape like) one half	_____	sphere	_____
7. (Cranial nerve) pertaining to below (the) tongue	_____	glossal	_____

Diseases

Brain		
Word or Phrase	**Description**	**Pronunciation/Word Parts**
amnesia	Partial or total (global) loss of memory of recent or remote (past) experiences. It is often a consequence of brain injury or a stroke that damages the hippocampus where short-term memories are converted to long-term memories. Treatment: None.	**amnesia** (am-NEE-zha) **amnes/o-** *forgetfulness* **-ia** *condition; state; thing*
anencephaly	Rare congenital condition in which some or all of the cranium and cerebrum are missing. The newborn breathes because the respiratory centers in the medulla oblongata are present, but only survives a few hours or days. Treatment: None.	**anencephaly** (AN-en-SEF-ah-lee) **an-** *not; without* **-encephaly** *condition of the brain* The ending *-encephaly* contains the combining form *encephal/o-* and the one-letter suffix *-y*.
aphasia	Loss of the ability to communicate verbally or in writing. Aphasia can occur with head trauma, a stroke, or Alzheimer's disease when there is injury to the areas of the brain that deal with language and the interpretation of sounds and symbols. Patients with aphasia are said to be **aphasic**. **Expressive aphasia** is the inability to verbally express thoughts. **Receptive aphasia** is the inability to understand the spoken or written word. Patients with both types are said to have **global aphasia**. Limited impairment that involves some difficulty speaking or understanding words is known as **dysphasia**. Treatment: Correct the underlying cause.	**aphasia** (ah-FAY-zha) **a-** *away from; without* **phas/o-** *speech* **-ia** *condition; state; thing* **aphasic** (ah-FAY-sik) **a-** *away from; without* **phas/o-** *speech* **-ic** *pertaining to* **expressive** (eks-PREH-siv) **express/o-** *communicate* **-ive** *pertaining to* **receptive** (ree-SEP-tiv) **recept/o-** *receive* **-ive** *pertaining to* **global** (GLOH-bal) **glob/o-** *comprehensive; shaped like a globe* **-al** *pertaining to* **dysphasia** (dis-FAY-zha) **dys-** *abnormal; difficult; painful* **phas/o-** *speech* **-ia** *condition; state; thing*
arteriovenous malformation (AVM)	Abnormality in which arteries in the brain connect directly to veins (rather than to capillaries), forming an abnormal twisted nest of blood vessels. An AVM can rupture and cause a stroke. Treatment: Focused beam radiation to destroy the AVM or embolization to block blood flow to the AVM; surgical removal, if needed.	**arteriovenous** (ar-TEER-ee-oh-VEE-nus) **arteri/o-** *artery* **ven/o-** *vein* **-ous** *pertaining to* **malformation** (MAL-for-MAY-shun) **mal-** *bad; inadequate* **format/o-** *arrangement; structure* **-ion** *action; condition*

Word or Phrase	Description	Pronunciation/Word Parts

brain tumor	**Benign** or **malignant** tumor of any area of the brain. Brain tumors arise from the neuroglia or meninges, rather than from neurons themselves. They are named according to the type of cell from which they originated (see Table 10-4 ■). Malignant brain tumors can also be secondary tumors that metastasized from a primary malignant tumor elsewhere in the body. Because the cranium is rigid, the enlarging benign or malignant tumor causes increased **intracranial pressure (ICP)**, cerebral edema, and sometimes seizures. The pressure compresses and destroys brain tissue (see Figure 10-11 ■). Treatment: Surgery to remove or debulk the tumor; chemotherapy drugs or radiation therapy for malignant tumors. 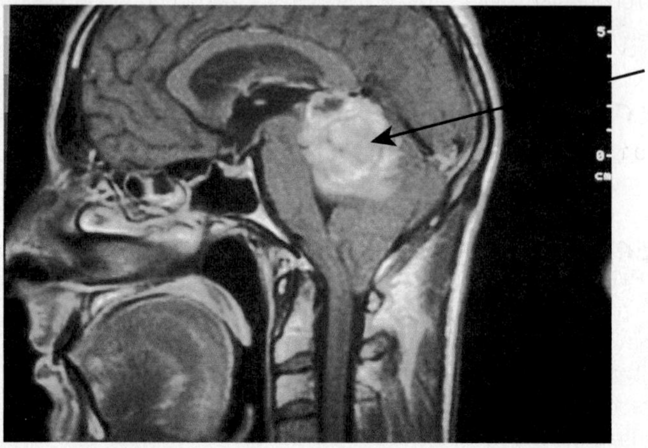
	
	FIGURE 10-11 ■ Glioma.
	This patient's MRI scan of the brain shows a large glioma that is pressing on the cerebellum. This tumor would affect the patient's ability to keep his balance and coordinate movements.
	Source: Simon Fraser/Science Source
		benign (bee-NINE)
		Note: A benign tumor is one that is not malignant (cancerous).
		
		malignant (mah-LIG-nant)
		  malign/o- *cancer; intentionally causing harm*
		  -ant *pertaining to*
		
		intracranial (IN-trah-KRAY-nee-al)
		  intra- *within*
		  crani/o- *cranium; skull*
		  -al *pertaining to*

cephalalgia	Pain in the head. It is commonly known as a **headache**. It can be caused by eyestrain, muscle tension in the face or neck, generalized infections such as the flu, migraine headaches, sinus infections, hypertension, or by more serious conditions such as head trauma, meningitis, or brain tumors. Treatment: Correct the underlying cause.	**cephalalgia** (SEF-al-AL-jah)
		  cephal/o- *head*
		  alg/o- *pain*
		  -ia *condition; state; thing*

cerebral palsy (CP)	Cerebral palsy is caused by a lack of oxygen to parts of the fetus' brain during birth. The result can include spastic muscles; lack of coordination in walking, eating, and talking; muscle paralysis; seizures; or mental retardation. Treatment: Braces, muscle relaxant drug, physical therapy, speech therapy.	**cerebral**
		(seh-REE-bral) (SAIR-eh-bral)
		  cerebr/o- *cerebrum*
		  -al *pertaining to*
		
		palsy (PAWL-zee)

Table 10-4   Types of Brain Tumors

Brain Tumor	Characteristic	Originating Cell or Structure	Pronunciation/Word Parts
astrocytoma	malignant	astrocyte in the cerebrum	**astrocytoma** (AS-troh-sy-TOH-mah) **astr/o-** *star-like structure* **cyt/o-** *cell* **-oma** *mass; tumor*
ependymoma	benign	ependymal cells that line the ventricles	**ependymoma** (eh-PEN-dih-MOH-mah) **ependym/o-** *cellular lining* **-oma** *mass; tumor*
glioblastoma multiforme	malignant	immature astrocyte in the cerebrum	**glioblastoma multiforme** (GLY-oh-blas-TOH-mah MUL-tih-FOR-may) **gli/o-** *supporting cells* **blast/o-** *embryonic; immature* **-oma** *mass; tumor*
glioma (see Figure 10-11)	benign or malignant	any neuroglial cell	**glioma** (gly-OH-mah) **gli/o-** *supporting cells* **-oma** *mass; tumor*
lymphoma	malignant	microglia in the cerebrum	**lymphoma** (lim-FOH-mah) **lymph/o-** *lymph; lymphatic system* **-oma** *mass; tumor*
meningioma	benign	meninges around the brain or spinal cord	**meningioma** (meh-NIN-jee-OH-mah) **meningi/o-** *meninges* **-oma** *mass; tumor*
oligodendroglioma	malignant	oligodendroglia in the cerebrum	**oligodendroglioma** (OH-lih-GOH-den-DROH-gly-OH-mah) **olig/o-** *few; scanty* **dendr/o-** *branching structure* **gli/o-** *supporting cells* **-oma** *mass; tumor*
schwannoma	benign	Schwann cells near the cranial or spinal nerves	**schwannoma** (shwah-NOH-mah)

Word or Phrase	Description	Pronunciation/Word Parts
cerebrovascular accident (CVA)	Disruption or blockage of blood flow to the brain, which causes tissue death and an area of necrosis known as an **infarct**. This can be caused by an embolus, arteriosclerosis, or hemorrhage. An embolus is a thrombus (blood clot) that forms in the heart or aorta because of arteriosclerosis, breaks free, travels through the blood, and becomes lodged in a small artery to the brain. Hemorrhage occurs when high blood pressure causes an artery to rupture or when an aneurysm or AVM ruptures. A CVA is also known as a **stroke** or **brain attack**. A **transient ischemic attack (TIA)**, a temporary lack of oxygenated blood to an area of the brain, is like a CVA, but its effects last only 24 hours. A **reversible ischemic neurologic deficit (RIND)** is a TIA whose effects last several days. TIAs and RINDs are precursors to an impending CVA. A cerebrovascular accident on the left side of the brain affects the right side of the body and vice versa (see Figure 10-12 ■).	**cerebrovascular** (seh-REE-broh-VAS-kyoo-lar) (SAIR-eh-broh-VAS-kyoo-lar) **cerebr/o-** *cerebrum* **vascul/o-** *blood vessel* **-ar** *pertaining to* **infarct** (IN-farkt) **infarction** (in-FARK-shun) **infarct/o-** *small area of dead tissue* **-ion** *action; condition* **ischemia** (is-KEE-mee-ah) **isch/o-** *block; keep back* **-emia** *condition of the blood; substance in the blood* **ischemic** (is-KEE-mik) **isch/o-** *block; keep back* **-emic** *pertaining to a condition of the blood; pertaining to a substance in the blood* **neurologic** (NYOOR-oh-LAW-jik) **neur/o-** *nerve* **log/o-** *study of; word* **-ic** *pertaining to* **hemiparesis** (HEM-ee-pah-REE-sis) (HEM-ee-PAIR-eh-sis) The prefix *hemi-* means *one half. Paresis* is a Greek word that means *condition of weakness.* **hemiplegia** (HEM-ee-PLEE-jah) **hemi-** *one half* **pleg/o-** *paralysis* **-ia** *condition; state; thing* **hemiplegic** (HEM-ee-PLEE-jik) **hemi-** *one half* **pleg/o-** *paralysis* **-ic** *pertaining to*

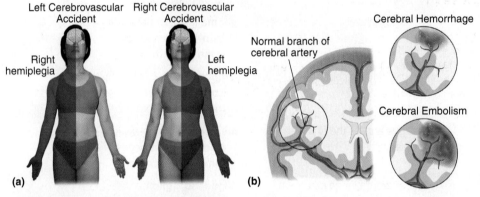

FIGURE 10-12 ■ **Cerebrovascular accident.**
(a) A cerebrovascular accident on the left side of the brain affects the right side of the body and vice versa. (b) Hemorrhage of an aneurysm disrupts blood flow to the brain and causes a cerebrovascular accident. An embolus blocks blood flow to the brain and causes a cerebrovascular accident.
Source: Pearson Education

The severity and symptoms of the CVA depend on how much brain tissue dies. **Hemiparesis** is muscle weakness on one side of the body. **Hemiplegia** is paralysis on one side of the body, and the patient is said to be **hemiplegic** (see Figure 10-13 ■). A CVA can also cause amnesia, aphasia, dysphasia, or dysphagia (difficulty swallowing). Prevention: Carotid endarterectomy, aneurysm clipping, or aneurysmectomy to prevent a CVA. Treatment: Thrombolytic drug to break up an embolus that is occluding the artery. Physical therapy, speech therapy.

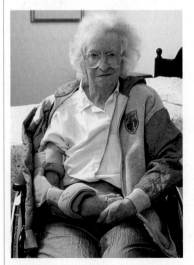

FIGURE 10-13 ■ **Patient with a cerebrovascular accident.**
This patient had a cerebrovascular accident on the left side of her brain that has paralyzed the right side of her body. Notice the drooping of the right side of her mouth and her right shoulder. The elbow and wrist of her right arm are covered with protective padding. She is using her functioning left hand to hold her paralyzed right hand in her lap and move her right arm from time to time.
Source: Pearson Education

Word or Phrase	Description	Pronunciation/Word Parts

coma	Deep state of unconsciousness and unresponsiveness caused by trauma or disease in the brain, by metabolic imbalance with accumulation of waste products in the blood (hepatic coma), or by too little glucose in the blood (hypoglycemia). A coma may be temporary or permanent. The patient is said to be **comatose**. Treatment: Correct the underlying cause.
	
	    Brain death is a condition in which there is irreversible loss of all brain function as confirmed by an electroencephalogram (EEG) that is flat, showing no brain wave activity of any kind for 30 minutes. The patient is said to be "brain dead."
		coma (KOH-mah)
		
		comatose (KOH-mah-tohs)
		    comat/o- *unconsciousness*
		    -ose *full of*

concussion	Traumatic injury to the brain that results in an immediate loss of consciousness (LOC) for a brief or prolonged period of time (see Figure 10-14 ■). Even after consciousness returns, the patient must be watched closely for signs of a slowly enlarging hemorrhage in the brain. These signs include sleepiness or irritability, a vacant stare, slowness in answering questions, inability to follow commands, disorientation to time and place, slurred speech, or a lack of coordination. A **contusion** is a traumatic injury to the brain or spinal cord. There is no loss of consciousness, but there is bruising with some bleeding in the tissues. **Shaken baby syndrome** is caused by an adult vigorously shaking an infant in anger or to discipline. Because the infant's head is large and the neck muscles are weak, severe shaking causes the head to whip back and forth. This can cause a contusion, concussion, hemorrhaging, mental retardation, coma, or even death.	**concussion** (con-KUH-shun)
		    concuss/o- *violent impact*
		    -ion *action; condition*
		
		contusion (con-TOO-shun)
		    contus/o- *bruising*
		    -ion *action; condition*

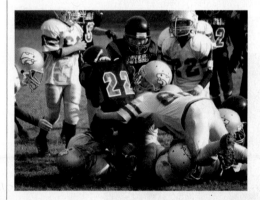

FIGURE 10-14 ■ Concussion.
Although football helmets are padded and constructed to protect the head, this player sustained a concussion with loss of consciousness. Repeated concussions can result in developing Alzheimer's disease in middle age. Former National Football League players have sued the NFL in class-action lawsuits for financial reimbursement because of concussions and brain damage.
Source: cfarmer/Fotolia

CLINICAL CONNECTIONS

Public Health. New variant **Creutzfeldt-Jakob disease**, a fatal neurologic disorder, is caused by a prion (a small infectious protein particle). This disease is contracted from cows infected with mad cow disease (bovine spongiform encephalopathy). It was first discovered in Great Britain. It is transmitted to cows when they eat animal feed contaminated with the processed spinal cords and brains of infected cows. All such animal feed has been banned in the United States. The disease can be transmitted to humans who eat meat from the infected cows. People who have lived or traveled extensively in England are even prohibited from donating blood to prevent possible transmission of this disease.

Creutzfeldt-Jakob
(KROITS-felt YAH-kohp)

Word or Phrase	Description	Pronunciation/Word Parts

dementia	Disease of the brain in which many neurons in the cerebrum die, the cerebral cortex shrinks in size, and there is progressive deterioration in mental function (see Figure 10-15 ■). At first, there is a gradual decline in mental abilities, with forgetfulness, inability to learn new things, inability to perform daily activities, and difficulty making decisions. The patient uses the wrong words and is unable to comprehend what others say. This becomes progressively more severe over time and includes inability to care for personal needs, inability to recognize friends and family, and complete memory loss. The more neurons that are destroyed, the greater the cognitive impairment. Psychiatric symptoms of depression, anxiety, impulsiveness, and combativeness can also occur. Dementia is most often associated with old age (**senile-onset dementia**) and the cumulative effect of multiple small cerebrovascular accidents (**multi-infarct dementia**). Dementia can also be caused by brain trauma, chronic alcoholism or drug abuse, or chronic neurodegenerative diseases such as multiple sclerosis, Parkinson's disease, and Huntington's chorea. However, the most common cause of dementia is Alzheimer's disease. **Alzheimer's disease** is a hereditary dementia that is known to run in families with inherited mutations on chromosomes 1, 14, and 21. At autopsy, the neurons show characteristic **neurofibrillary tangles** that distort the cells. There are also microscopic beta amyloid **senile plaques**. The brain also has a decreased level of the neurotransmitter acetylcholine. Alzheimer's disease that occurs in early middle age is known as early-onset Alzheimer's disease or **presenile dementia**. Treatment: Drug to inhibit the enzyme that breaks down acetylcholine.	**dementia** (deh-MEN-sha)
		  de- *reversal of; without*
		  ment/o- *chin; mind*
		  -ia *condition; state; thing*
		Select the correct prefix and combining form meanings to get the definition of *dementia*: *condition (of being) without (the) mind.*
		
		senile (SEE-nile)
		  sen/o- *old age*
		  -ile *pertaining to*
		
		Alzheimer (AWLZ-hy-mer)
		
		neurofibrillary (NYOOR-oh-FIB-rih-LAIR-ee)
		  neur/o- *nerve*
		  fibrill/o- *muscle fiber; nerve fiber*
		  -ary *pertaining to*
		
		plaque (PLAK)
		
		presenile (pree-SEE-nile)
		  pre- *before; in front of*
		  sen/o- *old age*
		  -ile *pertaining to*

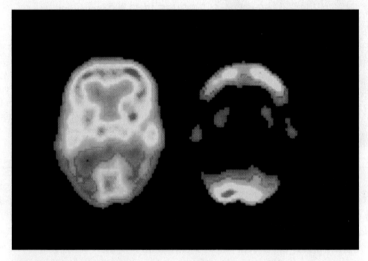

FIGURE 10-15 ■ PET scan of a normal brain and the brain of a patient with Alzheimer's disease.
The PET scan on the left shows the metabolic activity of a normal brain. This patient's scan shows large, symmetrical areas of metabolism and brain activity. Areas with the highest metabolic activity appear yellow to red. The PET scan on the right shows the metabolic activity of the brain in a patient with Alzheimer's disease. Notice the large, central area that is without any evidence of metabolism or brain activity.
Source: Science Source

Word or Phrase	Description	Pronunciation/Word Parts

Down syndrome	Naturally occurring, random error in cell division that creates a genetic defect in which there are three of chromosome 21, instead of the normal two. This defect affects every cell in the body, but is most obvious as mild-to-severe **mental retardation** and characteristic physical features of a large, protruding tongue, short fingers, and a single transverse crease on the palm of the hand (see Figure 10-16 ■). Prenatal test: Amniocentesis of fluid around the developing fetus.
	
	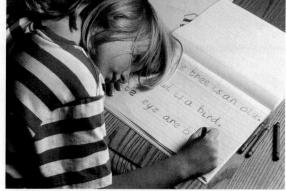
	
	FIGURE 10-16 ■ Down syndrome.
	This patient with Down syndrome shows the characteristic facial features that accompany mental retardation.
	Source: Hattie Young/Science Source
		mental (MEN-tal)
		  ment/o- *chin; mind*
		  -al *pertaining to*
		
		retardation (REE-tar-DAY-shun)
		  retard/o- *delay; slow down*
		  -ation *being; having; process*

dyslexia	Difficulty reading and writing words even though visual acuity and intelligence are normal (see Figure 10-17 ■). Dyslexia tends to run in families and is more prevalent in left-handed persons and in males. It is caused by an abnormality in the occipital lobe of the cerebrum that interprets moving visual images (as the eye moves quickly across the page). A person with dyslexia is said to be **dyslexic**. Treatment: Educational techniques that help a child learn to compensate or overcome this difficulty.
	
	FIGURE 10-17 ■ Dyslexia.
	A child with dyslexia may write certain alphabet letters backward or may change the order of the letters in a word.
	Source: Will & Deni McIntyre/Science Source
		dyslexia (dis-LEK-see-ah)
		  dys- *abnormal; difficult; painful*
		  lex/o- *word*
		  -ia *condition; state; thing*
		
		dyslexic (dis-LEK-sik)
		  dys- *abnormal; difficult; painful*
		  lex/o- *word*
		  -ic *pertaining to*

encephalitis	Inflammation and infection of the brain caused by a virus. Herpes simplex virus is the most common cause of encephalitis, but others include herpes zoster virus, West Nile virus, and cytomegalovirus. There is fever, headache, stiff neck, lethargy, vomiting, irritability, and **photophobia**. Treatment: Corticosteroid drug to decrease inflammation of the brain. Only encephalitis caused by the herpes virus responds to an antiviral drug. Antibiotic drugs are not effective against viruses.	**encephalitis** (en-SEF-ah-LY-tis)
		  encephal/o- *brain*
		  -itis *infection of; inflammation of*
		
		photophobia
		(FOH-toh-FOH-bee-ah)
		  phot/o- *light*
		  phob/o- *avoidance; fear*
		  -ia *condition; state; thing*

Word or Phrase	Description	Pronunciation/Word Parts
epilepsy	Recurring condition in which a group of neurons in the brain spontaneously sends out electrical impulses in an abnormal, uncontrolled way. These impulses spread from neuron to neuron. The type and extent of the seizures depend on the number and location of the affected neurons. A patient with epilepsy is said to be **epileptic**. It is also known as **seizures** or **convulsions**. There are four common types of epilepsy (see Table 10-5 ■). With each type of epilepsy, the patient displays a specific EEG pattern during a seizure (see Figure 10-18 ■). A seizure can be triggered by a flashing light, stress, lack of sleep, alcohol or drugs, or the cause can be unknown. Before the onset of a seizure, some epileptic patients experience an **aura**—a visual, olfactory, sensory, or auditory sign (flashing lights, strange odor, tingling, or buzzing sound)—that warns them of an impending seizure. After a tonic-clonic seizure, the patient experiences sleepiness and confusion. This is known as the **postictal state**. Over time, seizures can cause memory loss and personality changes. **Status epilepticus** is a prolonged, continuous seizure or repeated seizures that occur without the patient regaining consciousness. Treatment: Antiepileptic drug. Sometimes surgery, if a tumor or a specific area of the brain is causing the seizures.	**epilepsy** (EP-ih-LEP-see)
		seizure (SEE-zher)

		convulsion (con-VUL-shun)
		    convuls/o- *seizure*
		    -ion *action; condition*

		epileptic (EP-ih-LEP-tik)
		    epilept/o- *seizure*
		    -ic *pertaining to*

		aura (AW-rah)

		postictal (post-IK-tal)
		    post- *after; behind*
		    ict/o- *seizure*
		    -al *pertaining to*

		status epilepticus (STAT-us EP-ih-LEP-tih-kus)

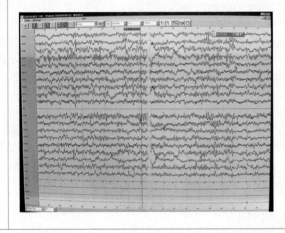

FIGURE 10-18 ■ Epilepsy.
A neurologist will read this record of a patient's brain-wave patterns. The characteristic body movements of the patient recorded during a seizure plus the specific EEG pattern will lead to a diagnosis of the type of seizure disorder that the patient has.

Source: Burger Phanie/Phanie Sarl/CanopyCorbis

Table 10-5 Seizures

Type of Seizure	Description	Pronunciation/Word Parts

tonic-clonic (grand mal)	Unconsciousness with excessive motor activity. The body alternates between excessive muscle tone with rigidity (tonic) and jerking muscle contractions (clonic) in the extremities, with tongue biting and sometimes incontinence. This lasts 1–2 minutes.	**tonic** (TAW-nik)
		  ton/o- *pressure; tone*
		  -ic *pertaining to*
		
		clonic (KLAW-nik)
		  clon/o- *identical group derived from one; rapid contracting and relaxing*
		  -ic *pertaining to*
		
		grand mal (GRAN MAWL)

absence (petit mal)	Impaired consciousness with slight or no muscle activity. Muscle tone is retained and the patient does not fall down, but is unable to respond to external stimuli. There is vacant staring, repetitive blinking, or facial tics. This lasts 5–15 seconds, after which the patient resumes activities and is unaware of the seizure. A patient can have many absence seizures during the course of a day.	**absence** (AB-sens) **petit mal** (peh-TEE MAWL)

complex partial (psychomotor)	Some degree of impairment of consciousness. Involuntary contractions of one or several muscle groups. There can be **automatisms**, such as lip smacking or repetitive muscle movements. This lasts 1–2 minutes.	**psychomotor** (SY-koh-MOH-tor)
		  psych/o- *mind*
		  mot/o- *movement*
		  -or *person who does; person who produces; thing that does; thing that produces*
		
		automatism (aw-TAW-mah-tizm)

simple partial (focal motor)	No impairment of consciousness. The patient is aware of the seizure but is unable to stop the involuntary motor activity, such as jerking of one hand or turning of the head. There can also be sensory hallucinations. This lasts 1–2 minutes.	**focal** (FOH-kal)
		  foc/o- *point of activity*
		  -al *pertaining to*

Word or Phrase	Description	Pronunciation/Word Parts

hematoma	Localized collection of blood that forms in the brain because of trauma to the cranium or the rupture of an intracranial aneurysm or an AVM. An **intraventricular hematoma** occurs within one of the ventricles. A **subdural hematoma** forms under the dura mater (see Figure 10-19 ■). Treatment: Surgery to remove the hematoma.	**hematoma** (HEE-mah-TOH-mah)
		  hemat/o- *blood*
		  -oma *mass; tumor*
		
		intraventricular (IN-trah-ven-TRIH-kyoo-lar)
		  intra- *within*
		  ventricul/o- *chamber that is filled; ventricle*
		  -ar *pertaining to*
		
		subdural (sub-DOOR-al)
		  sub- *below; underneath*
		  dur/o- *dura mater*
		  -al *pertaining to*

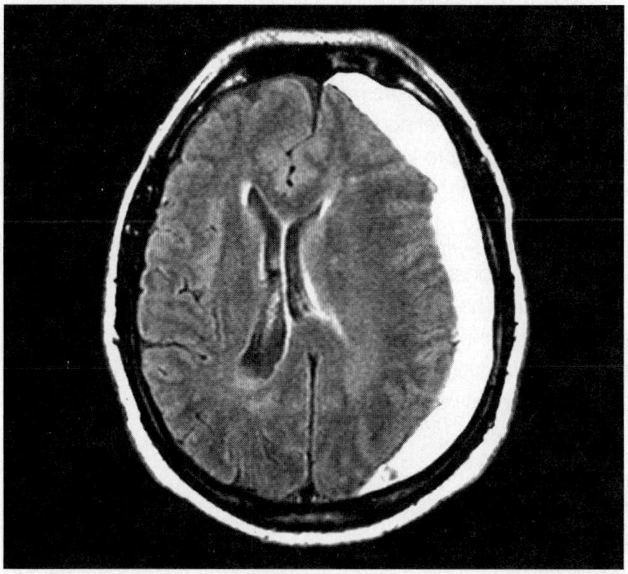

FIGURE 10-19 ■ Subdural hematoma.
This patient developed a subdural hematoma after trauma to the side of the head. An MRI scan shows how the hematoma has compressed the brain on that side.
Source: Science Source/Getty Images

Word or Phrase	Description	Pronunciation/Word Parts
Huntington's chorea	Progressive inherited degenerative disease of the brain that begins in middle age. It is characterized by dementia with spasms of the extremities and face (chorea), alternating with slow writhing movements of the hands and feet (athetosis). Treatment: None.	**Huntington** (HUN-ting-ton) **chorea** (kor-EE-ah)

hydrocephalus	Condition in which an excessive amount of cerebrospinal fluid is produced or the flow of cerebrospinal fluid is blocked. Intracranial pressure increases, distends the ventricles in the brain, and compresses the brain tissue (see Figure 10-20 ■). Hydrocephalus is most often associated with the congenital conditions of meningocele or myelomeningocele (see Figure 10-22), although it can occur in adults (normal pressure hydrocephalus) when the cerebrospinal fluid is not absorbed back into the blood. Untreated hydrocephalus causes a grossly enlarged head and mental retardation. The patient is said to be **hydrocephalic**. A layman's phrase for this condition is "water on the brain." Treatment: Placement of a ventriculoperitoneal shunt to move excess cerebrospinal fluid from the ventricles in the cerebrum to the peritoneal cavity.	**hydrocephalus** (HY-droh-SEF-ah-lus)
		  hydr/o- *fluid; water*
		  -cephalus *head*
		
		hydrocephalic (HY-droh-sih-FAL-ik)
		  hydr/o- *fluid; water*
		  cephal/o- *head*
		  -ic *pertaining to*

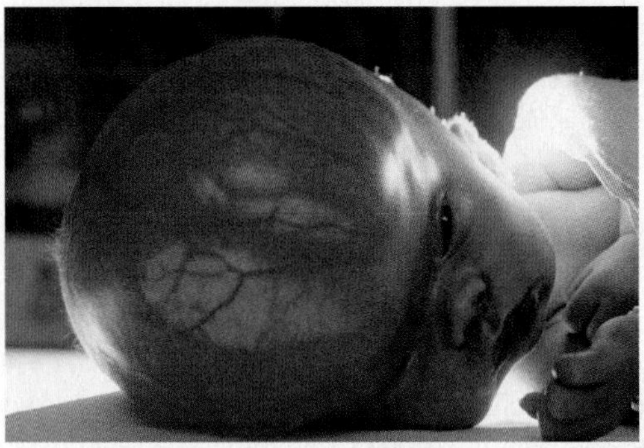

FIGURE 10-20 ■ Hydrocephalus.
This infant has pronounced hydrocephalus. A light shown on the cranium reveals large areas of illumination where the enlarged ventricles are filled with cerebrospinal fluid and the more dense brain tissue has been pushed aside.
Source: Southern Illinois University/Science Source

Word or Phrase	Description	Pronunciation/Word Parts

meningitis	Inflammation and infection of the meninges of the brain or spinal cord caused by a bacterium or virus. There is fever, headache, **nuchal rigidity** (stiff neck with pain and inability to touch the chin to the chest), lethargy, vomiting, irritability, and sensitivity to light (photophobia). Treatment: Vaccination to prevent bacterial meningitis in susceptible groups (particularly college students); antibiotic drug to treat bacterial meningitis. Corticosteroid drug to decrease inflammation.	**meningitis** (MEN-in-JY-tis)
		  mening/o- *meninges*
		  -itis *infection of; inflammation of*
		
		nuchal (NOO-kal)
		  nuch/o- *neck*
		  -al *pertaining to*

migraine headache	Specific type of recurring headache that has a sudden onset with severe, throbbing pain, often on just one side of the head. This is often accompanied by nausea and vomiting and sensitivity to light (photophobia). Migraines are caused by a constriction of the arteries in the brain followed by a sudden dilation (which causes pain), accompanied by the release of neuropeptides by the trigeminal nerve (cranial nerve V) (which causes inflammation). Treatment: Drug to keep the blood vessels from dilating to prevent or treat a migraine.	**migraine** (MY-grayn)

narcolepsy	Brief, involuntary episodes of falling asleep during the daytime while engaged in activity. The patient is not unconscious and can be aroused, but is unable to keep from falling asleep. There is a hereditary component to narcolepsy, and it may be an autoimmune disorder. There is also an underlying abnormality of the rapid eye movement (REM) sleep that is needed to feel refreshed. Treatment: Central nervous system stimulant drug.	**narcolepsy** (NAR-koh-LEP-see)
		  narc/o- *sleep; stupor*
		  -lepsy *seizure*

Word or Phrase	Description	Pronunciation/Word Parts
Parkinson's disease	Chronic, degenerative disease due to an imbalance in the levels of the neurotransmitters dopamine and acetylcholine in the brain. There is muscle rigidity and tremors. In the later stages, it is difficult for the patient to initiate voluntary movements except with effort and concentration (see Figure 10-21 ■). There is also a mask-like facial expression, shuffling gait, or inability to ambulate. It is also known as **parkinsonism**. Treatment: Drug that balances the neurotransmitters by increasing the amount of dopamine or inhibiting the action of acetylcholine in the brain.	**Parkinson** (PAR-kin-son) **parkinsonism** (PAR-kin-son-IZM) The suffix *-ism* means *disease from a specific cause; process*

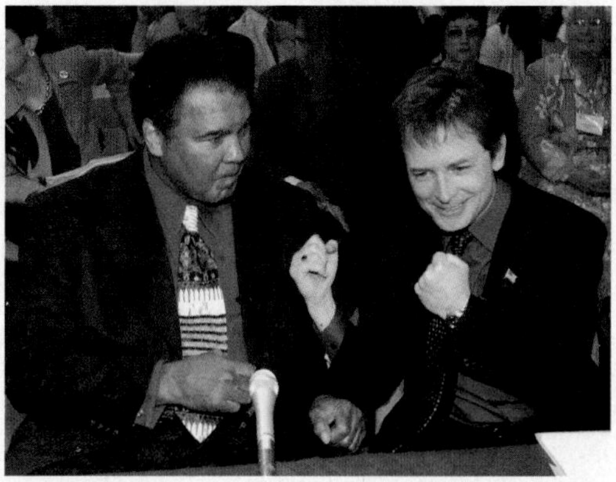

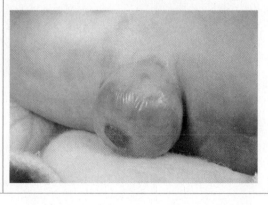

FIGURE 10-21 ■ Parkinson's disease.
Parkinson's patients boxing legend Mohammad Ali and actor Michael J. Fox talk with each other before testifying at a Senate hearing on Parkinson's disease research. Muhammad Ali has had Parkinson's disease for many years, as evidenced by his advanced symptoms of an expressionless face and difficulty initiating movement of his hands.
Source: Kenneth Lambert/AP Images

Word or Phrase	Description	Pronunciation/Word Parts
syncope	Temporary loss of consciousness. A **syncopal episode** is one in which the patient becomes lightheaded and then faints and remains unconscious briefly. It is most often caused by carotid artery stenosis and plaque that block blood flow or by cardiac arrhythmias that decrease blood flow to the brain. Treatment: Correct the underlying cause.	**syncope** (SIN-koh-pee) **syncopal** (SIN-koh-pal) **syncop/o-** *fainting* **-al** *pertaining to*

Spinal Cord

Word or Phrase	Description	Pronunciation/Word Parts
neural tube defect	Congenital abnormality of the neural tube (embryonic structure that becomes the fetal brain and spinal cord). The fetus' vertebrae form incompletely (**spina bifida**), and there is an abnormal opening in the vertebral column that is only covered by meninges and skin. A **meningocele** is a protrusion of the meninges through the skin. A meningomyelocele is a protrusion of the meninges and the spinal cord through the skin (see Figure 10-22 ■).	**neural** (NYOOR-al) **neur/o-** *nerve* **-al** *pertaining to* **spina bifida** (SPY-nah BIF-ih-dah) **meningocele** (meh-NING-goh-seel) **mening/o-** *meninges* **-cele** *hernia*

FIGURE 10-22 ■ Meningomyelocele.
This newborn has a meningomyelocele with part of the meninges and spinal cord in a sac outside the body. These delicate tissues are easily traumatized, allowing infection to enter and affect the brain, so surgery is done shortly after birth to close the defect.
Source: Biophoto Associates/Science Source

Word or Phrase	Description	Pronunciation/Word Parts

neural tube defect (*continued*)	This is also known as **myelomeningocele**. Children with meningocele or **meningomyelocele** may also have hydrocephalus. The amount of spinal cord involvement determines the degree of impairment of muscle control of the legs and bladder and bowel function. A sample of amniotic fluid taken during the pregnancy shows an elevated level of alpha fetoprotein. Treatment: Surgery to close the defect immediately after birth because of the risk of infection. The surgery is not able to restore impaired function to the muscles. The hydrocephalus is treated separately.
	
	CLINICAL CONNECTIONS
	Dietetics. A folic acid supplement taken during pregnancy greatly reduces the risk of neural tube defects. Folic acid is present in prenatal vitamins and in enriched cereals and breads.
		myelomeningocele
		(MY-eh-LOH-meh-NING-goh-seel)
		  myel/o- *bone marrow; myelin; spinal cord*
		  mening/o- *meninges*
		  -cele *hernia*
		
		meningomyelocele
		(meh-NING-goh-MY-eh-loh-SEEL)
		  mening/o- *meninges*
		  myel/o- *bone marrow; myelin; spinal cord*
		  -cele *hernia*
		Select the correct combining form meaning to get the definition of *meningomyelocele: hernia (of the) meninges (and) spinal cord.*

radiculopathy	Acute or chronic condition that occurs because of a tumor, arthritis, or a **herniated nucleus pulposus (HNP)** (when the contents of an intervertebral disk are forced out through a weak area in the disk wall). Any of these press on nearby spinal nerve roots (see Figure 10-23 ■). An HNP usually involves a lumbar disk and is often caused by heavy lifting and poor body mechanics. It is also known as a **slipped disk**. It is also known as **sciatica** because the disk presses on branches of the sciatic nerve whose nerve roots come from between the L4 and L5 vertebrae. The sciatic nerve is a combined sensory and motor nerve; depending on where it is compressed, there is pain and tingling (paresthesias) or numbness and muscle weakness. Treatment: Anti-inflammatory drug, bed rest, traction to the spine, physical therapy; injection into the nerve root of a corticosteroid drug to decrease inflammation. Surgery: Rhizotomy, diskectomy, or laminectomy.	**radiculopathy**
		(rah-DIH-kyoo-LAW-pah-thee)
		  radicul/o- *spinal nerve root*
		  -pathy *disease*
		
		herniated (HER-nee-AA-ted)
		  herni/o- *hernia*
		  -ated *composed of; pertaining to a condition*
		
		nucleus pulposus
		(NOO-klee-us pul-POH-sus)
		
		sciatica (sy-AT-ih-kah)

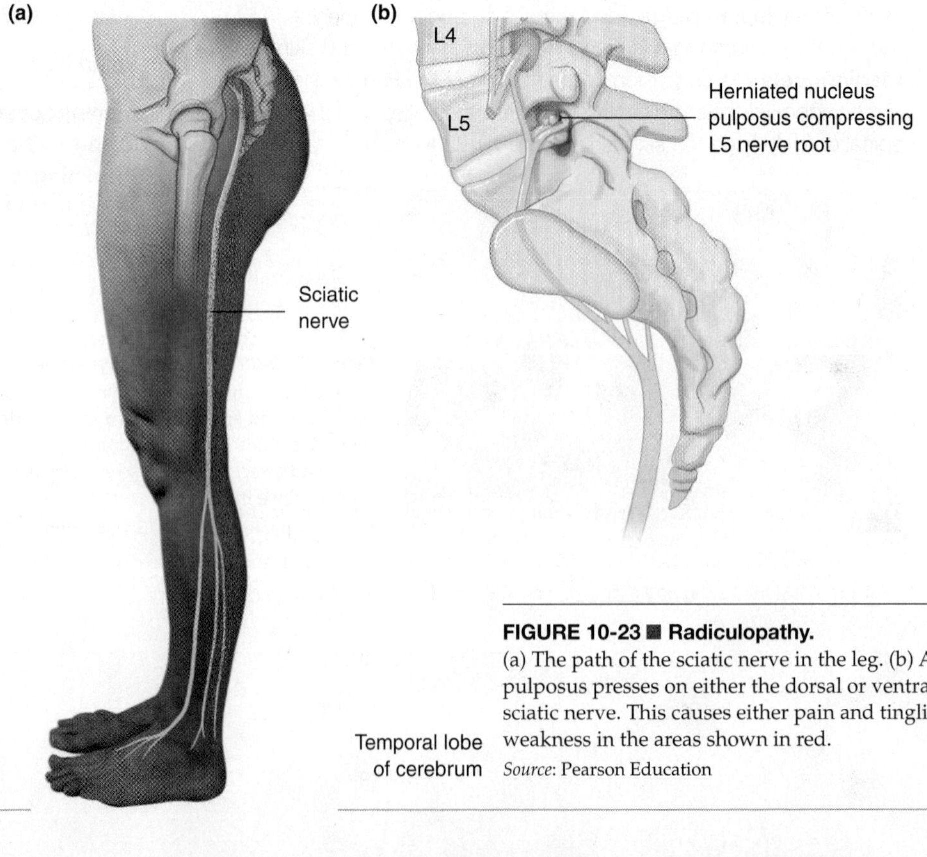

(a)

(b)

L4

L5

Sciatic nerve

Herniated nucleus pulposus compressing L5 nerve root

Temporal lobe of cerebrum

FIGURE 10-23 ■ Radiculopathy.
(a) The path of the sciatic nerve in the leg. (b) A herniated nucleus pulposus presses on either the dorsal or ventral nerve roots of the sciatic nerve. This causes either pain and tingling or numbness and weakness in the areas shown in red. *Source*: Pearson Education

Word or Phrase	Description	Pronunciation/Word Parts
spinal cord injury (SCI)	Trauma to the spinal cord with a partial or complete **transection** of the cord. This interrupts nerve impulses to particular dermatomes, causing partial or complete anesthesia (loss of sensation) and **paralysis** (an inability to voluntarily move the muscles). An injury to the lower spinal cord causes **paraplegia** with paralysis of the legs (see Figure 10-24 ■). A patient with paraplegia is known as a **paraplegic**. An injury to the upper spinal cord causes **quadriplegia** with paralysis of all four extremities. A patient with quadriplegia is known as a **quadriplegic**. Without nerve impulses, the muscles lose their tone and firmness and eventually atrophy. This is known as **flaccid paralysis**. However, the reflex arc of the lower spinal cord often remains intact and, in response to pain or a full bladder, the spinal cord below the injury will send nerve impulses that cause the muscles to spasm. This is known as **spastic paralysis**. The bladder may also contract spontaneously, causing incontinence. Treatment: After a suspected spinal cord injury, the patient is carefully transported to the hospital on a rigid spinal board, with a cervical collar in place, and with the head taped to the board to prevent any movement of the head, neck, or back that might further injure the spinal cord; traction to the skull to align the vertebrae; surgery may be needed to fuse damaged vertebrae; corticosteroid drug to decrease spinal cord inflammation; passive range-of-motion exercises, splints, muscle relaxant drug.	**transection** (tran-SEK-shun) **trans-** *across; through* **sect/o-** *cut* **-ion** *action; condition* The duplicate "s" is omitted. **paralysis** (pah-RAL-ih-sis) **para-** *abnormal; apart from; beside; two parts of a pair* **ly/o-** *break down; destroy* **-sis** *condition; process* Select the correct prefix and suffix meanings to get the definition of *paralysis*: *condition (of) two parts of a pair (arms or legs) break down (being paralyzed).* **paraplegia** (PAIR-ah-PLEE-jah) **para-** *abnormal; apart from; beside; two parts of a pair* **pleg/o-** *paralysis* **-ia** *condition; state; thing* **paraplegic** (PAIR-ah-PLEE-jik) **para-** *abnormal; apart from; beside; two parts of a pair* **pleg/o-** *paralysis* **-ic** *pertaining to* **quadriplegia** (KWAH-drih-PLEE-jah) **quadri-** *four* **pleg/o-** *paralysis* **-ia** *condition; state; thing* Add words to make a complete definition of *quadriplegia*: *condition (in which all) four (extremities have) paralysis.* **quadriplegic** (KWAH-drih-PLEE-jik) **quadri-** *four* **pleg/o-** *paralysis* **-ic** *pertaining to* **flaccid** (FLAS-id) (FLAK-sid) **spastic** (SPAS-tik) **spast/o-** *spasm* **-ic** *pertaining to*

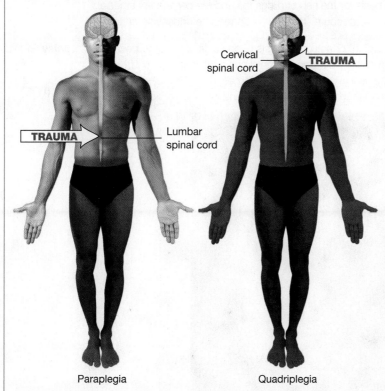

Cervical spinal cord

TRAUMA

Lumbar spinal cord

TRAUMA

Paraplegia   Quadriplegia

FIGURE 10-24 ■ Spinal cord injury.
The level of the spinal cord where an injury occurs and whether the spinal cord was partially or completely transected determines how much of the body is affected and to what extent. Paraplegia affects the lower body and the legs. Quadriplegia affects the body from the neck down and all four extremities.
Source: Pearson Education

Nerves		
Word or Phrase	**Description**	**Pronunciation/Word Parts**
amyotrophic lateral sclerosis (ALS)	Chronic, progressive disease of the motor nerves coming from the spinal cord. There is muscle wasting and spasms, with eventual paralysis of all the muscles, including the swallowing and respiratory muscles. There is no damage to the sensory nerves and so sensation remains intact and thinking is not affected. Some cases of ALS are caused by the lack of an enzyme, which is an inherited defect; but in most cases the cause is not known. It is also known as *Lou Gehrig's disease* after the famous baseball player who developed the disease in the late 1930s. Treatment: Supportive care.	**amyotrophic** (ah-MY-oh-TROH-fik) **a-** *away from; without* **my/o-** *muscle* **troph/o-** *development* **-ic** *pertaining to* **sclerosis** (skleh-ROH-sis) **scler/o-** *hard; white of the eye* **-osis** *condition; process*
anesthesia	Condition in which sensation of any type, including touch, pressure, proprioception, or pain, has been lost. Local areas of anesthesia can occur temporarily when your hand goes numb from pressing on a nerve in your arm as you sleep. Third-degree burns cause permanent anesthesia of the damaged skin.s Permanent anesthesia along a dermatome can occur after a spinal cord injury. Temporary therapeutic anesthesia to relieve pain can be produced in specific regions by injecting an **anesthetic drug** under the skin, near a nerve root, or into the epidural space in the spinal cavity. Unconsciousness is accompanied by an inability to perceive any sensation, and this is the basis for the use of drugs that induce general anesthesia prior to a surgical procedure. Treatment: Correct the underlying cause.	**anesthesia** (AN-es-THEE-zha) **an-** *not; without* **esthes/o-** *feeling; sensation* **-ia** *condition; state; thing* **anesthetic** (AN-es-THEH-tik) **an-** *not; without* **esthet/o-** *feeling; sensation* **-ic** *pertaining to*
Bell's palsy	Weakness, drooping, or actual paralysis of one side of the face because of inflammation of the facial nerve (cranial nerve VII) (see Figure 10-25 ■). It is caused by a viral infection, possibly herpes virus. The condition usually lasts a month and then disappears. Treatment: Corticosteroid drug.	**palsy** (PAWL-zee)

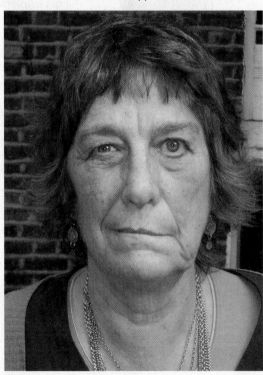

FIGURE 10-25 ■ Bell's palsy.
This patient with Bell's palsy has paralysis of the facial nerve on the left side of her face, as shown by the drooping of her left lower eyelid, cheek, and the corner of her mouth.
Source: Sally Greenhill/Alamy

Word or Phrase	Description	Pronunciation/Word Parts

carpal tunnel syndrome (CTS)	Chronic condition caused by repetitive motions of the hand and wrist, often from constant typing or data entry. There is tingling in the hand because of inflammation and swelling of the tendons from the forearm muscles that go through the carpal tunnel of the wrist bones to reach the hand. This swelling compresses the median nerve. Bending or extending the wrist for 60 seconds (Phalen's maneuver) aggravates the pain and is a positive diagnostic test. Treatment: Rest, splinting the wrist, using a split keyboard to position the wrists, physical therapy; injection of a corticosteroid drug; surgery, if needed.	**carpal** (KAR-pal)
		  carp/o- *wrist*
		  -al *pertaining to*

Guillain-Barré syndrome	Autoimmune disorder in which the body makes antibodies against myelin. There is acute inflammation of the peripheral nerves, loss of myelin with interruption of nerve conduction, muscle weakness, and changes in sensation (paresthesias). This disease is caused by a triggering event such as an infection (often a viral respiratory illness), stress, or trauma. The muscle weakness begins in the legs and then rapidly involves the entire body. The patient may even temporarily require respiratory support until the inflammation subsides. Guillain-Barré does not recur, and the patient recovers some or all neurologic function over a period of days to months. Treatment: Corticosteroid drug to treat inflammation.	**Guillain-Barré** (GEE-yah bah-RAY)

hyperesthesia	Condition in which there is a heightened awareness and sensitivity to touch and increased response to painful stimuli. Treatment: Antidepressant drug or tranquilizer drug.	**hyperesthesia**
		(HY-per-es-THEE-zha)
		  hyper- *above; more than normal*
		  esthes/o- *feeling; sensation*
		  -ia *condition; state; thing*

multiple sclerosis (MS)	Chronic, progressive, degenerative autoimmune disorder in which the body makes antibodies against myelin. There is acute inflammation of the nerves and loss of myelin (**demyelination**) with interruption of nerve conduction in the brain and spinal cord. The areas of demyelination eventually become scar tissue that is hard (sclerosis). These areas are known as *plaque* and can be seen on MRI scans of the brain. This disease can be caused by a triggering event such as a viral infection. Patients are typically in their 20s to early middle age. There is double vision, nystagmus, large muscle weakness, uncoordinated gait, spasticity, early fatigue after repeated muscle contractions, tremors, paresthesias, inability to walk, and sometimes dementia. Heat, stress, and fatigue temporarily worsen the symptoms. There can be periodic remissions in which there is some improvement, followed by exacerbations or flare-ups, but always with worsening of the condition over time. Treatment: Corticosteroid drug, muscle relaxant drug.	**sclerosis** (skleh-ROH-sis)
		  scler/o- *hard; white of the eye*
		  -osis *condition; process*
		Select the correct combining form and suffix meanings to get the definition of *sclerosis*: *condition (of) hard(ness)*.
		
		demyelination
		(dee-MY-eh-lih-NAY-shun)
		  de- *reversal of; without*
		  myelin/o- *myelin*
		  -ation *being; having; process*

neuralgia	Pain along the path of a nerve and its branches that is caused by an injury. Neuralgia can cause mild-to-severe pain. **Trigeminal neuralgia**, also known as **tic douloureux**, is characterized by episodes of brief but severe, stabbing pain (like an electrical shock) on one or both sides of the face or jaw along the distribution of the trigeminal nerve (cranial nerve V). **Causalgia** is severe, burning pain along a nerve and its branches. **Complex regional pain syndrome (CRPS)** consists of causalgia with hyperesthesia, changes in skin color and temperature, and swelling. Treatment: Anti-inflammatory drug, topical anesthetic drug, corticosteroid drug, antidepressant drug, anticonvulsant drug, skeletal muscle relaxant drug, nerve block, TENS unit, and physical therapy.	**neuralgia** (nyoor-AL-jah)
		  neur/o- *nerve*
		  alg/o- *pain*
		  -ia *condition; state; thing*
		
		trigeminal (try-JEM-ih-nal)
		  tri- *three*
		  gemin/o- *group; set*
		  -al *pertaining to*
		
		tic douloureux (TIK doo-loo-ROO)
		
		causalgia (kawz-AL-jah)
		  caus/o- *burning*
		  alg/o- *pain*
		  -ia *condition; state; thing*

Word or Phrase	Description	Pronunciation/Word Parts
neuralgia (*continued*)	**CLINICAL CONNECTIONS** **Dermatology (Chapter 7).** Shingles is a painful skin condition caused by the herpes zoster virus, the virus that causes chickenpox in children. The virus remains dormant in the body until later in life when a stress triggers it to erupt. It affects nerves and the skin of the dermatomes, causing redness, pain, and vesicles. Lingering, chronic pain from shingles is known as *postherpetic neuralgia.* Treatment: Antiviral drug.	

neuritis	Inflammation or infection of a nerve. **Polyneuritis** is a generalized inflammation of many nerves in one part of the body or all the nerves in the body. Treatment: Correct the underlying cause; analgesic drug, anti-inflammatory drug, corticosteroid drug, or antibiotic drug.	**neuritis** (nyoor-EYE-tis)
		   neur/o- *nerve*
		   -itis *infection of;*
		      inflammation of
		
		polyneuritis
		(PAW-lee-nyoor-EYE-tis)
		   poly- *many; much*
		   neur/o- *nerve*
		   -itis *infection of;*
		      inflammation of

neurofibromatosis	Hereditary disease with multiple benign fibrous tumors (**neurofibromata**) that grow on the peripheral nerves. These are most noticeable on the skin, but they can be anywhere in the body—on the internal organs and even in the eye. They range in size from small nodules to large tumors. It is also known as **von Recklinghausen's disease**. Treatment: Surgical removal of large tumors that cause pain or disability.	**neurofibromatosis**
		(NYOOR-oh-fy-BROH-mah-TOH-sis)
		   neur/o- *nerve*
		   fibr/o- *fiber*
		   -omatosis *condition of*
		      masses; condition of tumors
		
		neurofibroma
		(NYOOR-oh-fy-BROH-mah)
		   neur/o- *nerve*
		   fibr/o- *fiber*
		   -oma *mass; tumor*
		Neurofibroma is a Greek singular noun. Form the plural by changing *-oma* to *-omata*.
		
		von Recklinghausen
		(vawn REK-ling-HOW-sen)

neuroma	Benign tumor of a nerve or any of the specialized cells of the nervous system. A **Morton's neuroma** specifically forms from repetitive damage to the nerve that is near the metatarsophalangeal joints between the ball of the foot and the toes. Treatment: Surgical removal.	**neuroma** (nyoor-OH-mah)
		   neur/o- *nerve*
		   -oma *mass; tumor*

neuropathy	General category for any type of disease or injury to a nerve. Treatment: Correct the underlying cause.	**neuropathy**
		(nyoor-AW-pah-thee)
		   neur/o- *nerve*
		   -pathy *disease*

	CLINICAL CONNECTIONS
	Endocrinology (Chapter 14). Diabetic neuropathy is a chronic, slowly progressive condition that affects the peripheral nerves in diabetic patients. It is caused by a lack of blood flow (arteriosclerosis) to the nerves. There is severe pain and a loss of sensation and sense of position. Treatment: Treat the diabetes mellitus.
		diabetic (DY-ah-BET-ik)
		   diabet/o- *diabetes*
		   -ic *pertaining to*
		
		neuropathy (nyoor-AW-pah-thee)
		   neur/o- *nerve*
		   -pathy *disease*

Word or Phrase	Description	Pronunciation/Word Parts
paresthesia	Condition in which abnormal sensations, such as tingling, burning, or pinpricks, are felt on the skin (see Figure 10-26 ■). Paresthesias are often the result of chronic nerve damage from a pinched nerve or diabetic neuropathy. Treatment: Correct the underlying cause. Anticonvulsant drug, antianxiety drug, or antidepressant drug. 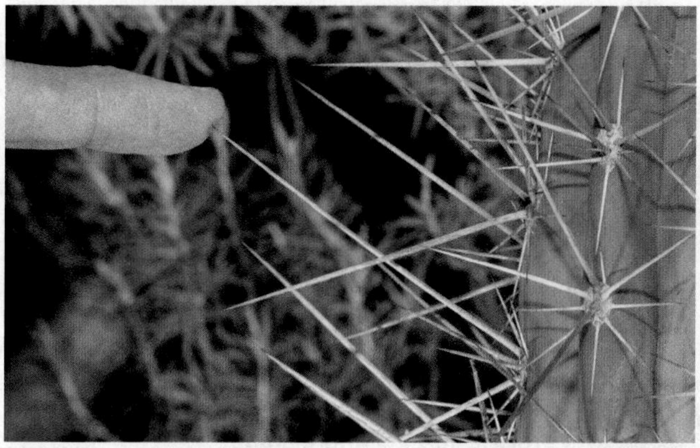	**paresthesia** (PAIR-es-THEE-zha) **para-** *abnormal; apart from; beside; two parts of a pair* **esthes/o-** *feeling; sensation* **-ia** *condition; state; thing* The final "a" in the prefix *para-* is omitted when the word *paresthesia* is formed. Select the correct prefix meaning to get the definition of *paresthesia*: *condition (of) abnormal feeling or sensation.*

FIGURE 10-26 ■ Paresthesias.
This shows the sensation that some patients have with paresthesias: shooting or stabbing pain. Other sensations include burning, tingling, or numbness. Other paresthesias feel like ants crawling on the feet or thumbtacks pricking the feet.
Source: F.C.G./Fotolia

Laboratory and Diagnostic Procedures

Laboratory Tests		
Word or Phrase	**Description**	**Pronunciation/Word Parts**
alpha fetoprotein (AFP)	Test of a sample of amniotic fluid taken from the uterus by amniocentesis (see Figure 13-27) during pregnancy. It is used to diagnose a neural tube defect in the fetus before birth. The fetal liver makes alpha fetoprotein, and small amounts are normally present in the amniotic fluid. However, an increased level indicates that alpha fetoprotein is leaking into the amniotic fluid through a meningocele or meningomyelocele.	**alpha fetoprotein** (AL-fah FEE-toh-PROH-teen)
cerebrospinal fluid (CFS) examination	Test that visually examines the CSF for clarity and color, microscopically for cells, and chemically for proteins and other substances. Normal CSF is clear and colorless. CSF with a pink or reddish tint contains a large number of red blood cells, and this indicates bleeding in the brain from a stroke or trauma. Cloudy CSF contains a large number of white blood cells because of a bacterial infection such as encephalitis or meningitis. An elevated level of protein indicates infection or the presence of a tumor. The presence of oligoclonal bands points to multiple sclerosis. Myelin-basic protein is elevated in multiple sclerosis and amyotrophic lateral sclerosis.	

Radiologic and Nuclear Medicine Procedures

Word or Phrase	Description	Pronunciation/Word Parts

cerebral angiography	Procedure in which a radiopaque contrast dye is injected into the carotid artery, and an x-ray is taken to visualize the arterial circulation in the brain (see Figure 10-27 ■). This is done to show an aneurysm, stenosis, plaque in the arteries, or a tumor. A tumor is seen as an interwoven collection of new blood vessels, or it can be seen indirectly when it forces the arteries into abnormal positions. It is also known as **arteriography**. The x-ray image is an **angiogram** or an **arteriogram**.
	
	FIGURE 10-27 ■ Arteriogram. The injected dye clearly outlines the patient's left carotid artery and its many smaller branches within the cranial cavity. There is no evidence of carotid artery plaques or cerebral aneurysm.
	Source: Larry Mulvehill/Keepsake/Corbis
		angiography (AN-jee-AW-grah-fee)
		  angi/o- *blood vessel; lymphatic vessel*
		  -graphy *process of recording*
		
		angiogram (AN-jee-oh-GRAM)
		  angi/o- *blood vessel; lymphatic vessel*
		  -gram *picture; record*
		
		arteriography (ar-TEER-ee-AW-grah-fee)
		  arteri/o- *artery*
		  -graphy *process of recording*
		
		arteriogram (ar-TEER-ee-oh-GRAM)
		  arteri/o- *artery*
		  -gram *picture; record*

computed axial tomography (CAT, CT)	Procedure that uses x-rays to create many individual, closely spaced images ("slices"). CT scans are used to view the cranium, brain, vertebral column, and spinal cord. Radiopaque contrast dye can be injected to provide more detail.	**axial** (AK-see-al)
		  axi/o- *axis*
		  -al *pertaining to*
		
		tomography (toh-MAW-grah-fee)
		  tom/o- *cut; layer; slice*
		  -graphy *process of recording*

Doppler ultrasonography	Procedure that uses ultra high-frequency sound waves to produce a two-dimensional image to visualize areas of stenosis and plaque and turbulence in the blood flow in the carotid arteries (see Figure 5-25). This is also known as a **carotid duplex scan**.	**carotid** (kah-RAW-tid) **duplex** (DOO-pleks)

magnetic resonance imaging (MRI)	Procedure that uses a magnetic field and radiowaves to align the protons in the body and cause them to emit signals that create an image. Magnetic resonance imaging is a type of tomography that creates images as many individual "slices." MRI scans are used to view the cranium, brain, vertebral column, and spinal cord (see Figure 10-11). Radiopaque contrast dye can be injected to provide more detail.	**magnetic** (mag-NET-ik)
		  magnet/o- *magnet*
		  -ic *pertaining to*
		
		resonance (REZ-oh-nans)

myelography	Procedure in which a radiopaque contrast dye is injected into the subarachnoid space at the level of the L3 and L4 vertebrae. The contrast dye outlines the spinal cavity and shows spinal nerves, nerve roots, and intervertebral disks, as well as tumors, herniated disks, or obstructions within the cavity. The x-ray image is a **myelogram**. Because a myelogram can cause the side effect of a severe headache, an MRI scan of the spine is more often done.	**myelography** (MY-eh-LAW-grah-fee)
		  myel/o- *bone marrow; myelin; spinal cord*
		  -graphy *process of recording*
		
		myelogram (MY-eh-loh-GRAM)
		  myel/o- *bone marrow; myelin; spinal cord*
		  -gram *picture; record*

Word or Phrase	Description	Pronunciation/Word Parts
positron emission tomography (PET) scan	Procedure that uses a radioactive substance that is combined with glucose molecules and injected intravenously. As the glucose is metabolized, the radioactive substance emits positrons, and these form gamma rays that are detected by a gamma camera. The camera produces an image that reflects the amount of metabolism in that area (see Figure 10-15). An area of increased metabolism can be due to a cancerous tumor. Areas of decreased metabolism can be due to Alzheimer's disease, Parkinson's disease, or epilepsy (see Figure 10-16).	**positron** (PAW-zih-trawn) **emission** (ee-MIH-shun) **emiss/o-** *send out* **-ion** *action; condition* **tomography** (toh-MAW-grah-fee) **tom/o-** *cut; layer; slice* **-graphy** *process of recording*
skull x-ray	Procedure in which a plain film (without contrast dye) is taken of the skull. An x-ray can show fractures of the bones of the skull but cannot clearly show the soft tissues of the brain or the blood vessels.	

Other Diagnostic Tests

Word or Phrase	Description	Pronunciation/Word Parts
electroencephalo-graphy (EEG)	Procedure to record the electrical activity of the brain (see Figure 10-28 ■). Multiple electrodes are placed on the scalp overlying specific lobes of the brain. The electrodes are attached by lead wires to an **electroencephalograph**, a machine that records brain waves. The computerized recording of the brain waves is an **electroencephalogram**. There are four types of normal brain waves (named for letters of the Greek alphabet): alpha, beta, delta, and theta. The patterns of brain waves in the lobes of the right and left hemispheres of the cerebrum should be the same. A difference between the two hemispheres suggests a tumor or injury. The presence of abnormal waves suggests encephalopathy or dementia. Brain waves during an epileptic seizure show specific patterns that are used to diagnose the particular type of epilepsy (see Figure 10-19). In order to induce an epileptic seizure during the EEG, the patient may look at flashing lights or have a sleep-deprived EEG recording. An EEG is also done as part of a polysomnography to diagnose sleep disorders and also as part of evoked potential testing.	**electroencephalography** (ee-LEK-troh-en-SEF-ah-LAW-grah-fee) **electr/o-** *electricity* **encephal/o-** *brain* **-graphy** *process of recording* **electroencephalograph** (ee-LEK-troh-en-SEF-ah-loh-GRAF) **electr/o-** *electricity* **encephal/o-** *brain* **-graph** *instrument used to record* **electroencephalogram** (ee-LEK-troh-en-SEF-ah-loh-GRAM) **electr/o-** *electricity* **encephal/o-** *brain* **-gram** *picture; record*

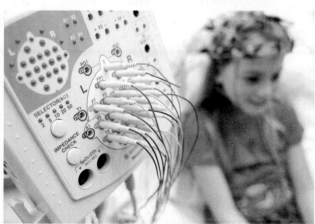

FIGURE 10-28 ■ Electroencephalography (EEG).
This girl is having an EEG done to diagnose what type of epileptic seizures she is having. The electrodes are placed on her scalp in a specific pattern, as shown in the upper left of the EEG machine. The electrodes pick up the electrical impulses of brain waves and display them on a computer screen.
Source: Science Photo LibraryBrand X Pictures/Getty Images

Word or Phrase	Description	Pronunciation/Word Parts
evoked potential testing	Procedure in which an EEG is used to record changes in brain waves that occur following various stimuli. It is used to evaluate the potential ability of a particular nervous pathway to conduct nerve impulses. A stimulus is presented to evoke (stimulate) a response, and this procedure is also called *evoked response testing.* For a **visual evoked potential (VEP)** or **visual evoked response (VER)**, the patient watches a computer monitor that displays rapidly alternating checkerboard patterns. This evaluates nerve pathways from the eye to the cerebrum. For a **brainstem auditory evoked potential (BAEP)** or **brainstem auditory evoked response (BAER)**, the patient has on headphones and listens to a series of clicks in one ear and then the other. This evaluates nerve pathways from the ears to the cerebrum. For a **somatosensory evoked potential (SSEP)** or **somatosensory evoked response (SSER)**, a small electrical impulse is administered to the arm or leg. This evaluates nerve pathways from the extremities to the cerebrum. These tests are particularly helpful with patients who are very young or are unable to respond to standard vision and hearing tests. These tests are also used to detect subtle abnormalities in patients with multiple sclerosis, head trauma, or spinal cord injury. The patient cannot voluntarily alter the results of these tests.	**evoked** (ee-VOKED) **potential** (poh-TEN-shal) **potent/o-** *capable of doing* **-al** *pertaining to* **somatosensory** (soh-MAH-toh-SEN-soh-ree) **somat/o-** *body* **sens/o-** *sensation* **-ory** *having the function of*
nerve conduction study	Procedure to measure the speed at which an electrical impulse travels along a nerve. An electrical impulse through an electrode applied to the skin is used to stimulate a peripheral nerve. Another electrode a measured distance away records how long it takes for the electrical impulse to reach it. This test is usually performed in conjunction with electromyography to help differentiate between weakness due to nerve disorders versus weakness due to muscle disorders.	**conduction** (con-DUK-shun) **conduct/o-** *carrying; conveying* **-ion** *action; condition*
polysomnography	Procedure to diagnose the underlying conditions that can cause insomnia, sleep disruption, sleep apnea, or narcolepsy. Electrodes on the face and head and various other monitors are used to record the patient's EEG, eye movements, muscle activity, heartbeat, and respirations during sleep. It is also known as a **sleep study**.	**polysomnography** (PAW-lee-sawm-NAW-grah-fee) **poly-** *many; much* **somn/o-** *sleep* **-graphy** *process of recording* Add words to make a complete definition of *polysomnography*: *process of recording many (of the body's activities that occur during) sleep.*

Medical and Surgical Procedures

Medical Procedures		
Word or Phrase	**Description**	**Pronunciation/Word Parts**
Babinski's sign	Neurologic test in which the end of the metal handle of a percussion hammer is used to firmly stroke the lateral sole of the foot from the heel to the toes. A normal test (negative Babinski) produces a downward curling of the toes. An abnormal test (positive Babinski) produces extension of the great toe and fanning out of the other toes (see Figure 10-29 ■). A positive Babinski indicates injury to the parietal lobe of the cerebrum or to the spinal nerves. **FIGURE 10-29 ■ Positive Babinski's sign.** This patient has a positive (abnormal) Babinski's sign with extension of the great toe and fanning out of the other toes laterally. *Source*: Pearson Education	**Babinski** (bah-BIN-skee)
Glasgow Coma Scale (GCS)	Numerical scale that measures the depth of a coma. The total score ranges from 1 to 15 and is the sum of individual scores for eye opening, motor response, and verbal response following a painful stimulus (such as pressure on the nailbed or on the bony ridge over the eye). For example, if a patient opens his eyes to a verbal command, has confused answers, and withdraws from the painful stimulus, his GCS would be Eyes (3) + Verbal (4) + Motor (4) = 11.	**Glasgow** (GLAS-goh)
lumbar puncture (LP)	Procedure to obtain cerebrospinal fluid (CSF) for testing. It is also known as a **spinal tap**. The patient is positioned with the upper legs flexed toward the chest. This curves the spine and widens the space between the spinous processes of two vertebrae, allowing accurate positioning of the spinal needle (see Figure 10-30 ■). A needle is inserted in the space between the L3–4 or L4–5 vertebrae and into the subarachnoid space. Cerebrospinal fluid flows through the needle and is collected and sent to a laboratory. Before the spinal needle is removed, a calibrated **manometer** (a thin tube) can be attached to measure the intracranial pressure as the CSF rises in the manometer.	**lumbar** (LUM-bar) **lumb/o-** *area between the ribs and pelvis; lower back* **-ar** *pertaining to* **puncture** (PUNGK-chur) **punct/o-** *hole; perforation* **-ure** *result of; system* **manometer** (mah-NAW-meh-ter) **man/o-** *frenzy; thin* **-meter** *instrument used to measure*

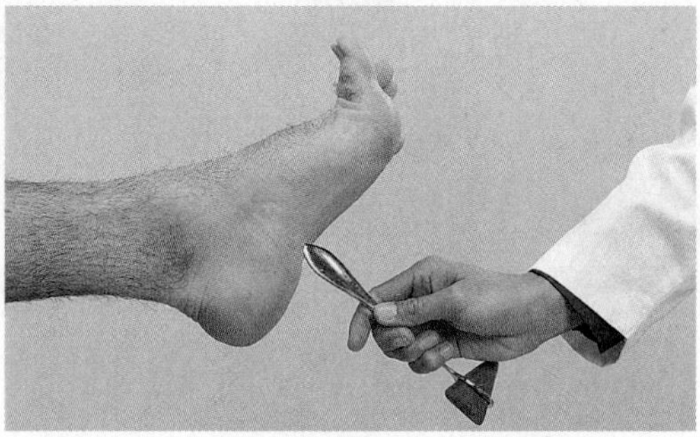

Word or Phrase	Description	Pronunciation/Word Parts

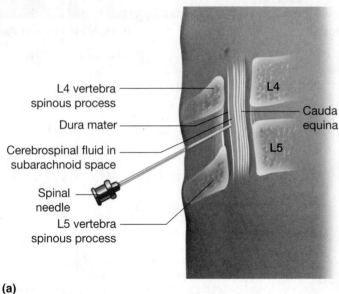

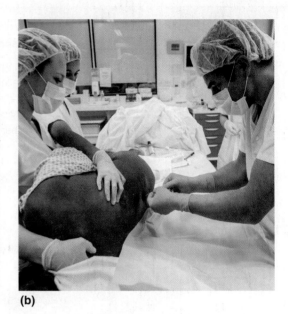

(a)

(b)

FIGURE 10-30 ■ Lumbar puncture.
(a) For a lumbar puncture, the needle is inserted into the subarachnoid space where there is cerebrospinal fluid. (b) This patient is having a lumbar puncture. He does not have much flexibility of the spine and is only able to flex the head and shoulders forward. A nurse is helping the patient to maintain this position while the physician inserts the spinal needle.

Source: Pearson Education; Voisin Phanie/Phanie Sarl/Canopy/Corbis

Word or Phrase	Description	Pronunciation/Word Parts
mini mental status examination (MMSE)	Tests the patient's concrete and abstract thought processes and long- and short-term memory. The patient is asked to state his/her name, the date, and where he/she is. If the answers are all correct, the patient is said to be oriented to person, time, and place (oriented x3). The patient is asked to perform simple mental arithmetic, recall objects or words, name the current president and recent past presidents, spell a word backwards, and give the meaning of a proverb. A full mental status examination is done during a psychiatric evaluation (discussed in "Psychiatry," Chapter 17).	**mental** (MEN-tal) **ment/o-** *chin; mind* **-al** *pertaining to*
neurologic examination	Tests coordination, sensation, balance, and gait. Coordination tests: (1) Rapid alternating movements. The patient taps the tip of the index finger against the thumb as rapidly as possible. (2) Finger-to-nose test. With eyes closed, the patient touches the tip of the index finger to the nose. (3) The patient touches the nose, then touches the physician's finger as it moves to various locations, then touches the nose again. (4) Heel-to-shin test: The patient puts the heel of one foot onto the opposite leg and then runs it from the knee down the shin to the toes. Sensation tests: (1) With the patient's eyes closed, the skin is touched in various places with a cotton swab (to test light touch), a vibrating tuning fork (to test vibration), and the point of a pin (pinprick to test pain). One or two pins are used to see if the patient can distinguish the number of things touching the skin (two-point discrimination). (2) The patient's toe or finger is moved up and down and the patient is asked to identify the direction (to test body position and **proprioception**). Balance tests: (1) **Romberg test**. The patient stands with the feet together and the eyes closed. In a normal test, the patient does not sway excessively or lose balance. The Romberg test is also known as the **station test**. Gait tests: (1) The manner of walking is assessed for a normal arm swing and stride. (2) The patient is asked to walk across the room in a heel-to-toe fashion. The patient is asked to walk on the toes, on the heels, and then hop in place on each foot.	**proprioception** (PROH-pree-oh-SEP-shun) *Proprioception* comes from the combining form *propri/o- (one's own self)*, part of the word *receptor*, and the suffix *-tion (being; having; process)*. **Romberg** (RAWM-berg)

Word or Phrase	Description	Pronunciation/Word Parts
spinal traction	Procedure in which a fracture of the vertebra is immobilized while it heals. Two metal pins are surgically inserted into the cranium and attached to a set of tongs with a rope and pulley and 7–10 pounds of weight. A patient with a partially healed fracture of the vertebra can be fitted for a halo vest with pins in the cranium attached to a metal ring (halo). This allows the patient to walk around.	**traction** (TRAK-shun) 　**tract/o-** *pulling* 　**-ion** *action; condition*
transcutaneous electrical nerve stimulation (TENS) unit	Procedure that uses an electrical device to control chronic pain (see Figure 10-31 ■). A battery produces regular, preset electrical impulses that travel through wires to electrodes on the skin. These impulses block the transmission of pain sensations to the brain. The impulses also stimulate the body to produce its own natural pain-relieving endorphins.	**transcutaneous** (TRANS-kyoo-TAY-nee-us) 　**trans-** *across; through* 　**cutane/o-** *skin* 　**-ous** *pertaining to*

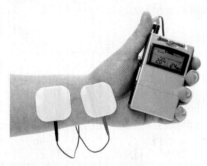

FIGURE 10-31 ■ Transcutaneous electrical nerve stimulation (TENS) unit.
Electrode patches placed on the skin transmit electrical impulses at regular, preset intervals from a battery pack to a painful area.
Source: Rob Byron/Fotolia LLC

Surgical Procedures

Word or Phrase	Description	Pronunciation/Word Parts
biopsy	Procedure to remove a tumor or mass from the brain or other part of the nervous system. In an **excisional biopsy**, the entire tumor or mass is removed and sent to a laboratory for microscopic examination to determine if it is benign or malignant. Even a benign brain tumor must be totally removed because it causes increasing intracranial pressure within the inflexible bony cranium.	**biopsy** (BY-awp-see) 　**bi/o-** *life; living organism; living tissue* 　**-opsy** *process of viewing* **excisional** (ek-SIH-zhun-al) 　**excis/o-** *cut out* 　**-ion** *action; condition* 　**-al** *pertaining to*
carotid endarterectomy	Procedure to remove plaque from the carotid artery. This opens up the lumen of the artery, restores blood flow to the brain, and decreases the possibility of a stroke.	**endarterectomy** (END-ar-ter-EK-toh-mee) 　**endo-** *innermost; within* 　**arter/o-** *artery* 　**-ectomy** *surgical removal*
craniotomy	Incision into the cranium to expose the brain tissue. A craniotomy is the first phase of any type of brain surgery, such as removal of a subdural hematoma or excising a brain tumor.	**craniotomy** (KRAY-nee-AW-toh-mee) 　**crani/o-** *cranium; skull* 　**-tomy** *process of cutting; process of making an incision*
diskectomy	Procedure to remove part or all of a herniated nucleus pulposus from an intervertebral disk. This relieves pressure on the adjacent dorsal nerve roots and relieves the pain.	**diskectomy** (dis-KEK-toh-mee) 　**disk/o-** *disk* 　**-ectomy** *surgical removal*

Word or Phrase	Description	Pronunciation/Word Parts
laminectomy	Procedure to remove the lamina (the flat area of the arch of the vertebra). Removal of this bony segment relieves pressure on the dorsal nerve roots and relieves pain from a herniated nucleus pulposus.	**laminectomy** (LAM-ih-NEK-toh-mee) **lamin/o-** *flat area on a vertebra; lamina* **-ectomy** *surgical removal*
	CLINICAL CONNECTIONS **Pain Management.** This subspecialty for treating chronic or severe pain is shared by both neurology and anesthesiology. Pain management procedures include a dorsal nerve root injection into an area where a nerve is compressed. Surgical treatment includes a **rhizotomy**, an incision to cut spinal nerve roots. The dorsal (sensory) nerve roots can be cut to relieve severe pain. The ventral (motor) nerve roots can be cut to relieve severe muscle spasticity and spasm.	**rhizotomy** (ry-ZAW-toh-mee) **rhiz/o-** *spinal nerve root* **-tomy** *process of cutting; process of making an incision*
stereotactic neurosurgery	Procedure to remove a tumor deep within the cerebrum. A CT or MRI scan is used to show the tumor in three dimensions and give its precise coordinates. The patient's head is fixed in a stereotactic apparatus that guides the position of a probe as it is inserted into the brain. Then heat, cold, or high-energy gamma rays are used to destroy the tumor.	**stereotactic** (STAIR-ee-oh-TAK-tik) **stere/o-** *three dimensions* **tact/o-** *touch* **-ic** *pertaining to* **neurosurgery** (NYOOR-oh-SER-jer-ee) **neur/o-** *nerve* **surg/o-** *operative procedure* **-ery** *process*
ventriculo-peritoneal shunt	Procedure to insert a plastic tube to connect the ventricles of the brain to the peritoneal cavity. The shunt continuously removes excess cerebrospinal fluid associated with hydrocephalus.	**ventriculoperitoneal** (ven-TRIH-kyoo-loh-PAIR-ih-toh-NEE-al) **ventricul/o-** *chamber that is filled; ventricle* **peritone/o-** *peritoneum* **-al** *pertaining to* **shunt** (SHUNT)

Drugs

These drug categories and drugs are used to treat neurologic diseases. The most common generic and trade name drugs in each category are listed.

Category	Indication	Examples	Pronunciation/Word Parts
analgesic drugs	Aspirin, nonsalicylate drugs, such as acetaminophen, and nonsteroidal anti-inflammatory drugs, are used to treat mild-to-moderate pain. **Narcotic** drugs are used to treat severe, chronic pain.	acetaminophen (Tylenol), aspirin (Bayer, Empirin), ibuprofen (Advil, Motrin), naproxen (Aleve, Naprosyn). Narcotic drugs: fentanyl (Actiq, Duragesic), meperidine (Demerol), morphine (MS Contin), oxycodone (OxyContin)	**analgesic** (AN-al-JEE-zik) **an-** *not; without* **alges/o-** *sensation of pain* **-ic** *pertaining to* **narcotic** (nar-KAW-tik) **narc/o-** *sleep; stupor* **-tic** *pertaining to*
antiepileptic drugs	Prevent the seizures of epilepsy. They are also known as **anticonvulsant drugs**.	ethosuximide (Zarontin), phenytoin (Dilantin), topiramate (Topamax), valproic acid (Depakene, Depakote)	**antiepileptic** (AN-tee-EP-ih-LEP-tik) (AN-tih-EP-ih-LEP-tik) **anti-** *against* **epilept/o-** *seizure* **-ic** *pertaining to* **anticonvulsant** (AN-tee-con-VUL-sant) (AN-tih-con-VUL-sant) **anti-** *against* **convuls/o-** *seizure* **-ant** *pertaining to*
corticosteroid drugs	Suppress inflammation in chronic pain conditions and multiple sclerosis. They are used to treat swelling and edema in the brain or spinal cord following traumatic injury or stroke.	dexamethasone, prednisone	**corticosteroid** (KOR-tih-koh-STAIR-oyd) **cortic/o-** *cortex; outer region* **-steroid** *steroid*
drugs for Alzheimer's disease	Inhibit an enzyme that breaks down acetylcholine	donepezil (Aricept), rivastigmine (Exelon), tacrine (Cognex)	
drugs for neuralgia and neuropathy	Work in various ways to treat the many different causes of neuralgia and neuropathy. These drugs are classified as anticonvulsant drugs. Antianxiety and antidepressant drugs are also used.	gabapentin (Neurontin), pregabalin (Lyrica)	
drugs for Parkinson's disease	Stimulate dopamine receptors, inhibit the action of acetylcholine, or inhibit the enzyme that metabolizes the drug levodopa (this allows more levodopa to reach the brain)	amantadine (Symmetrel), benztropine (Cogentin), entacapone (Comtan), ropinirole (Requip), Sinemet (combination of carbidopa and levodopa)	

CLINICAL CONNECTIONS

Pharmacology. Patients who take drugs to treat Parkinson's disease can develop a tolerance to the drug and require higher and higher doses. However, the higher doses produce more side effects. When the drug dose can no longer be increased, or the side effects of a high dose become intolerable, the physician will place the patient on a **drug holiday**. When the drug is restarted at a lower dose, it is effective.

Abbreviations

AFP	alpha fetoprotein		**ICP**	intracranial pressure
ALS	amyotrophic lateral sclerosis		**LOC**	loss of consciousness
AVM	arteriovenous malformation		**LP**	lumbar puncture
BAEP	brainstem auditory evoked potential		**MMSE**	mini mental status examination
BAER	brainstem auditory evoked response		**MRI**	magnetic resonance imaging
CAT	computerized axial tomography		**MS* ■**	multiple sclerosis
CNS	central nervous system		**NICU**	neurologic intensive care unit (pronounced
CP	cerebral palsy			"NIK-yoo")
CRPS	chronic regional pain syndrome; complex		**PET**	positron emission tomography
	regional pain syndrome		**REM**	rapid eye movement
CSF	cerebrospinal fluid		**RIND**	reversible ischemic neurologic deficit
CT	computerized tomography		**SCI**	spinal cord injury
CTS	carpal tunnel syndrome		**SSEP**	somatosensory evoked potential
CVA	cerebrovascular accident		**SSER**	somatosensory evoked response
EEG	electroencephalogram; electroencephalography		**TENS**	transcutaneous electrical nerve stimulation (unit)
END	electroneurodiagnostic (technician)		**TIA**	transient ischemic attack
GCS	Glasgow Coma Scale (or Score)		**VEP**	visual evoked potential
HNP	herniated nucleus pulposus		**VER**	visual evoked response

*According to The Joint Commission and ■ the Institute for Safe Medication Practices (ISMP), this abbreviation should not be used. However, because it is still used by some healthcare professionals, it is included here.

WORD ALERT
Abbreviations

Abbreviations are commonly used in all types of medical documents; however, they can mean different things to different people and their meanings can be misinterpreted. Always verify the meaning of an abbreviation.

CP means *cerebral palsy,* but it also means *cardiopulmonary.*

CNS means *central nervous system*, but it can be confused with the sound-alike abbreviation *C&S,* which means *culture and sensitivity.*

HNP means *herniated nucleus pulposus,* but it can be confused with the sound-alike abbreviation *H&P,* which means *history and physical (examination).*

MS means *multiple sclerosis,* but it also means the drugs *morphine sulfate* or *magnesium sulfate.*

NICU means *neurologic intensive care unit,* but it also means *neonatal intensive care unit.*

Word Part	Meaning	Word Part	Meaning
27. dys-		72. my/o-	
28. -ectomy		73. myelin/o-	
29. effer/o-		74. myel/o-	
30. electr/o-		75. narc/o-	
31. encephal/o-		76. neur/o-	
32. endo-		77. nuch/o-	
33. ependym/o-		78. olig/o-	
34. epilept/o-		79. -oma	
35. esthes/o-		80. -omatosis	
36. esthet/o-		81. -ory	
37. express/o-		82. -ose	
38. fibr/o-		83. para-	
39. format/o-		84. -pathy	
40. gemin/o-		85. phas/o-	
41. gli/o-		86. phob/o-	
42. glob/o-		87. phot/o-	
43. -gram		88. pleg/o-	
44. -graph		89. poly-	
45. -graphy		90. post-	
46. hemat/o-		91. pre-	
47. hemi-		92. propri/o-	
48. herni/o-		93. psych/o-	
49. hydr/o-		94. punct/o-	
50. hyper-		95. quadri-	
51. -ia		96. radicul/o-	
52. ict/o-		97. recept/o-	
53. -ile		98. retard/o-	
54. infarct/o-		99. rhiz/o-	
55. intra-		100. sen/o-	
56. -ion		101. sens/o-	
57. isch/o-		102. -sis	
58. -itis		103. somat/o-	
59. lamin/o-		104. somn/o-	
60. -lepsy		105. sub-	
61. lex/o-		106. surg/o-	
62. log/o-		107. syncop/o-	
63. lymph/o-		108. tom/o-	
64. ly/o-		109. -tomy	
65. mal-		110. ton/o-	
66. man/o-		111. tract/o-	
67. meningi/o-		112. tri-	
68. mening/o-		113. troph/o-	
69. ment/o-		114. -ure	
70. -meter		115. vascul/o-	
71. mot/o-		116. ventricul/o-	

RELATED COMBINING FORMS EXERCISE

Write the combining forms on the line provided. (Hint: See the It's Greek to Me feature box.)

1. Two combining forms that mean *mind.* _____

2. Two combining forms that mean *nerve.* _____

3. Two combining forms that mean *spinal nerve root.* _____

4. Three combining forms that mean *sensation.* _____

5. Three combining forms that mean *seizure.* _____

10.5B Define Abbreviations

MATCHING EXERCISE

Match each abbreviation to its description

1. ALS	_____	Presses on spinal nerve roots
2. CP	_____	Congenital disorder from lack of oxygen to the fetal brain
3. CSF	_____	Lou Gehrig's disease
4. CVA	_____	Trauma that can result in paraplegia or quadriplegia
5. EEG	_____	Also known as a *spinal tap*
6. HNP	_____	Circulates through the subarachnoid space
7. LP	_____	Test that records brain-wave patterns
8. SCI	_____	A stroke

10.6A Divide Medical Words

DIVIDING WORDS EXERCISE

Separate these words into their component parts (prefix, combining form, suffix). Note: Some words do not contain all three word parts. The first one has been done for you.

Medical Word	Prefix	Combining Form	Suffix	Medical Word	Prefix	Combining Form	Suffix
1. aphasia	a-	phas/o-	-ia	6. meningioma	_____	_____	_____
2. dementia	_____	_____	_____	7. narcolepsy	_____	_____	_____
3. epidural	_____	_____	_____	8. neuroglia	_____	_____	_____
4. hypothalamic	_____	_____	_____	9. postictal	_____	_____	_____
5. intracranial	_____	_____	_____	10. subdural	_____	_____	_____

10.6B Build Medical Words

COMBINING FORM AND SUFFIX EXERCISE

Read the definition of the medical word. Select the correct suffix from the Suffix List. Select the correct combining form from the Combining Form List. Build the medical word and write it on the line. Be sure to check your spelling. The first one has been done for you.

SUFFIX LIST	COMBINING FORM LIST	
-al (pertaining to)	bi/o- (life; living organism; living tissue)	hemat/o- (blood)
-cele (hernia)	clon/o- (rapid contracting and relaxing)	hydr/o- (fluid; water)
-cephalus (head)	comat/o- (unconsciousness)	infarct/o- (small area of dead tissue)
-ectomy (surgical removal)	concuss/o- (violent impact)	mening/o- (meninges)
-graphy (process of recording)	convuls/o- (seizure)	ment/o- (chin; mind)
-ic (pertaining to)	crani/o- (cranium; skull)	myel/o- (bone marrow; myelin;
-ion (action; condition)	disk/o- (disk)	spinal cord)
-itis (infection of; inflammation of)	encephal/o- (brain)	narc/o- (sleep; stupor)
-lepsy (seizure)	ependym/o- (cellular lining)	neur/o- (nerve)
-oma (mass; tumor)	epilept/o- (seizure)	radicul/o- (spinal nerve root)
-opsy (process of viewing)	gli/o- (supporting cells)	rhiz/o- (spinal nerve root)
-ose (full of)		syncop/o- (fainting)
-pathy (disease)		
-tomy (process of cutting; process of making an incision)		

Definition of the Medical Word

1. Pertaining to (the) mind
2. Pertaining to (a person with) seizures
3. Mass (localized collection of) blood (within the cranium)
4. Inflammation of (a) nerve
5. Process of (removing and) viewing living tissue (with a microscope)
6. Process of making an incision (into the) cranium
7. Infection of (or) inflammation of (the) meninges
8. Seizure(-like state of being unable to keep from going to) sleep
9. (Condition of the) head (of having too much cerebrospinal) fluid
10. Pertaining to rapid contracting and relaxing (during a seizure)
11. Condition (caused by) violent impact (of the head)
12. Tumor (of the) cellular lining (in the ventricle of the cerebrum)
13. Condition (that results in a) small area of dead tissue
14. Process of recording (an image of the) spinal cord (using a contrast dye)
15. Disease (of the) nerve(s)
16. Process of cutting (the) spinal nerve root
17. Condition (of having a) seizure
18. Infection of (or) inflammation of (the) brain
19. (Condition of a person being) full of unconsciousness
20. Tumor (in the brain composed of) supporting cells
21. Pertaining to fainting
22. Hernia (of the) meninges (to the outside of the body)
23. Disease (of the) spinal nerve root
24. Tumor (of a) nerve
25. Surgical removal (of an intervertebral) disk

Build the Medical Word

mental

PREFIX EXERCISE

Read the definition of the medical word. Look at the medical word or partial word that is given (it already contains a combining form and a suffix). Select the correct prefix from the Prefix List and write it on the blank line. Then build the medical word and write it on the line. Be sure to check your spelling. The first one has been done for you.

PREFIX LIST

a- (away from; without)	dys- (abnormal; difficult; painful)	poly- (many; much)
an- (not; without)	hemi- (one half)	post- (after; behind)
anti- (against)	hyper- (above; more than normal)	quadri- (four)
de- (reversal of; without)	intra- (within)	sub- (below; underneath)

Definition of the Medical Word	Prefix	Word or Partial Word	Build the Medical Word
1. Pertaining to within (the) ventricle	intra-	ventricular	intraventricular
2. State (of being) without (the) mind	_____	mentia	_____
3. Pertaining to (the time) after (a) seizure	_____	ictal	_____
4. State (of being) without feeling or sensation	_____	esthesia	_____
5. Inflammation of many nerves	_____	neuritis	_____
6. Pertaining to (a drug that is) against seizures	_____	convulsant	_____
7. Pertaining to (having a) difficult (time with) words	_____	lexic	_____
8. Pertaining to within (the) cranium	_____	cranial	_____
9. State (of being) without speech	_____	phasia	_____
10. Pertaining to one half (of the body having) paralysis	_____	plegic	_____
11. Pertaining to underneath (the) dura mater	_____	dural	_____
12. Condition (of) four (extremities having) paralysis	_____	plegia	_____
13. Process of recording many (types of tests during) sleep	_____	somnography	_____
14. State (of) more than normal (response to) feelings or sensations	_____	esthesia	_____
15. Condition (of) difficult speech (after a stroke)	_____	phasia	_____

MULTIPLE COMBINING FORMS AND SUFFIX EXERCISE

Read the definition of the medical word. Select the correct suffix and combining forms. Then build the medical word and write it on the line. Be sure to check your spelling. The first one has been done for you.

SUFFIX LIST	COMBINING FORM LIST	
-ar (pertaining to)	alg/o- (pain)	log/o- (study of; word)
-cele (hernia)	astr/o- (star-like structure)	mening/o- (meninges)
-ery (process)	caus/o- (burning)	myel/o- (bone marrow; myelin; spinal cord)
-gram (picture; record)	cephal/o- (head)	neur/o- (nerve)
-ia (condition; state; thing)	cerebr/o- (cerebrum)	phot/o- (light)
-ic (pertaining to)	cyt/o- (cell)	phob/o- (avoidance; fear)
-oma (mass; tumor)	electr/o- (electricity)	surg/o- (operative procedure)
-omatosis (condition of masses; condition of tumors)	encephal/o- (brain)	vascul/o- (blood vessel)
	fibr/o- (fiber)	

Definition of the Medical Word

1. Pertaining to nerves (and the) study of (them)
2. Condition (in which) light (causes) avoidance or fear
3. Hernia (of the) spinal cord (and the) meninges (to the outside of the body)
4. Condition (of) burning pain
5. Condition of tumors (of the) nerve (that are) fibrous
6. Record (of the) electricity (of brain waves) (in the) brain
7. Condition (of the) nerves (having) pain
8. Process (of a) nerve (or brain) operative procedure
9. Pertaining to (the) cerebrum (and) blood vessels
10. Tumor (composed of) star-like structure cells
11. Condition (of the) head (having) pain

Build the Medical Word

neurologic

_____

_____

_____

_____

_____

_____

_____

_____

_____

_____

10.7A Spell Medical Words

PROOFREADING AND SPELLING EXERCISE

Read the following paragraph. Identify each misspelled medical word and write the correct spelling of it on the line.

A patient might need nurosurgery because of a subdural hematomma or a tumor such as a menengioma. A cerebrohvascular accident is a stroke or brain attack and is from an infarkt. An ordinary headache is cephalalga, while having half of the body paralysed from a stroke is called hemeplegia. A seizure or a convulsion is known as epilepsee. Inflammation of many individual nerves is polyneuritus. The study of the brain, spinal cord, and nerves is neurology.

1. _____
2. _____
3. _____
4. _____
5. _____

6. _____
7. _____
8. _____
9. _____
10. _____

HEARING MEDICAL WORDS EXERCISE

You hear someone speaking the medical words given below. Read each pronunciation and then write the medical word it represents. Be sure to check your spelling. The first one has been done for you.

1. SEE-zher   seizure
2. SEF-al-AL-jah   _____
3. KRAY-nee-AW-toh-mee   _____
4. HEM-ee-PLEE-jik   _____
5. MY-grayn   _____

6. IN-trah-KRAY-nee-al   _____
7. awk-SIP-ih-tal   _____
8. SIN-koh-pee   _____
9. MEN-in-JY-tis   _____
10. KOH-mah-tohs   _____

10.7B Pronounce Medical Words

PRONUNCIATION EXERCISE

Read the medical word and the syllables in its pronunciation. Circle the primary (main) accented syllable. The first one has been done for you.

1. nervous (ner-vus)
2. anesthesia (an-es-thee-zha)
3. aphasic (ah-fay-sik)
4. astrocytoma (as-troh-sy-toh-mah)
5. hydrocephalus (hy-droh-sef-ah-lus)
6. infarct (in-farkt)
7. meninges (meh-nin-jeez)
8. paralysis (pah-ral-ih-sis)
9. sciatica (sy-at-ih-kah)
10. syncope (sin-koh-pee)

10.8 Research Medical Words

SOUND-ALIKE WORDS

Compare and contrast the medical meanings of these sound-alike neurology and other words.

1. *convulsion* and *seizure* and *epilepsy*
2. *convulsion* and *contusion* (Chapter 7)
3. What is the difference between the ventricles in the brain and the ventricles in the heart?

10.9 Analyze Medical Reports

ELECTRONIC PATIENT RECORD #1

This is an office visit in the format of a SOAP note. Read the note and answer the questions.

PEARSON PEDIATRIC ASSOCIATES

Task   Edit   View   Time Scale   Options   Help

OFFICE VISIT SOAP NOTE

PATIENT NAME:	JOHNSON, Clarissa
DATE OF BIRTH:	11/19/20xx
DATE OF VISIT:	11/19/20xx

Source: Michael Gray/123RF

SUBJECTIVE
This is a follow-up visit for this 10-year-old black female who recently presented with an initial seizure that happened during school hours. The patient was reported to have vacant staring, was unresponsive to the teacher's voice, and had facial tics. She was sent for a neurologic consult. An EEG showed that she had absence seizures.

OBJECTIVE
Today, the patient is alert and oriented x3. Her vital signs are all within normal limits. Her mother reports that she has not had any convulsions since beginning her antiseizure medication.

ASSESSMENT
Absence seizures, controlled on medication.

PLAN
Continue taking her ethosuximde (Zarontin) at the dose prescribed by the neurologist. Call this office in the event of any seizure activity.

1. What is the name of the overall disease category for absence seizures?

   _____

2. During this type of seizure, would you expect that the patient would have fallen down at school?

   _____

3. What does the abbreviation *EEG* stand for and how is one performed?

   _____

4. What does the **phrase** *oriented x3* mean?

   _____

ELECTRONIC PATIENT RECORD #2

This is a neurologic consultation. Read the report and answer the questions.

PEARSON NEUROLOGIC ASSOCIATES

Task   Edit   View   Time Scale   Options   Help

CONSULTATION REPORT

PATIENT NAME:	JENCKS, Justine
PATIENT NUMBER:	12798
DATE OF CONSULTATION:	November 19, 20xx

Source: Vgstudio/Fotolia

PEARSON NEUROLOGIC ASSOCIATES
Centennial Medical Building, Suite 312
5005 Frankstown Road
Pittsburgh, PA 15237

November 19, 20xx

Marshall Gibbons, M.D.
Primary Care Associates
19 Walker Avenue
Middletown, PA 15222

Re: JENCKS, Justine

Dear Dr. Gibbons:

I saw your patient, Justine Jencks, in neurologic consultation on November 19, 20xx. She is a 38-year-old, right-handed Caucasian female who has complained of intermittent dizziness and other symptoms for the past year. She reports temporary dizziness with hyperextension of the neck when raising her hands above her head to reach a high shelf or hang drapes. Two months ago, the patient had an acute episode in which she awoke with a sense of doom, headache, profuse perspiration, nausea, paresthesias of the fingers, dizziness, tachycardia, and felt the room was spinning. On the way to the emergency room, her husband commented about their dogs, but she could only remember her older dog and had no recollection of having another dog. In the emergency room, she commented to the nurse that she felt like her "blood pressure was zero." When asked about her last menstrual period, she felt that she might be pregnant but could not explain why she felt this way. On the mini mental status exam, she could not name the current and most recent presidents but was otherwise oriented x3. She was able to count backward by serial 7s. The physical examination in the emergency room was essentially negative. Her blood pressure and blood sugar results were normal.

The patient has a past history that is significant for possible MS. This was tentatively diagnosed 10 years ago. At that time, laboratory test results were inconclusive: visual evoked responses were abnormal, but the CSF showed no oligoclonal bands and an MRI scan of the brain was read as negative. At that time, her symptoms included extreme muscle weakness. She could only walk a short distance by using a wide-based gait for stability. This initial episode lasted 2 months and then the symptoms gradually resolved.

She does not routinely have headaches. She denies ever having had seizures. She denies any smell or taste disturbances. She denies difficulty swallowing. She has no speech difficulties and is able to relate her medical history easily.

Examination of cranial nerves V through XII was normal. Examination of the motor system revealed normal muscle strength. Babinski was negative. Sensory examination to light touch, pinprick, vibration, position, and 2-point discrimination was normal. Cerebellar functions in the form of finger-to-nose and heel-to-shin tests were normal. Gait was normal. Romberg's sign was negative. There was marked muscle spasm of the trapezius muscles bilaterally and limitation of neck motion laterally to the right and rotationally to the left.

Several of the patient's complaints could be due to a vestibular migraine, but the episode with the 2-hour alteration in memory is problematic and may suggest a TIA. She has some typical migraine symptoms, but the dizziness points to a vestibular focus to the migraine. Because of the past history of possible MS, I will have her undergo an MRI scan with contrast to pinpoint any demyelination that has occurred since her last MRI. I have also ordered carotid arteriography to rule out blockage of the carotid arteries.

After these tests are obtained, I will follow up with her in about 3 weeks to review the test results.

Thank you for referring this interesting and delightful patient to me.

Sincerely yours,

Renworth R. Pitman, M.D.

Rentworth R. Pitman, M.D.

RRP: sct
D: 11/19/xx

T: 11/19/xx

1. Divide *neurologic* into its three word parts and give the meaning of each word part.

Word Part   **Meaning**

_____   _____

_____   _____

_____   _____

2. Divide *paresthesia* into its three word parts and give the meaning of each word part.

Word Part   **Meaning**

_____   _____

_____   _____

_____   _____

3. What is the abbreviation for *visual evoked response?* _____

4. Divide *arteriography* into its two word parts and give the meaning of each word part.

Word Part   **Meaning**

_____   _____

_____   _____

5. Two months ago, what symptom did the patient experience in her fingers? _____

6. Define these neurologic abbreviations.

MS _____

TIA _____

CSF _____

7. The sensory examination consisted of five separate tests. Name them.

a. _____

b. _____

c. _____

d. _____

e. _____

8. The mini mental status examination done 2 months ago in the emergency room mentions what three mental status tests?

   a. _____

   b. _____

   c. _____

9. Which test showed that the patient's balance was intact? (**Babinski, Romberg, serial 7s**)

10. Which of the patient's symptoms is directly related to the nervous system? (**nausea, paresthesias, tachycardia**)

11. The carotid arteriography will be done to look for evidence of what disease? (**blockage of the artery, demyelination, muscle weakness**)

12. If present, oligoclonal bands are found in what body fluid? _____

13. When the patient could remember the name of her older dog but not the name of her newest dog, this would be described as which of the following?

   a. Impairment of both remote and recent memory

   b. Impairment of remote memory; recent memory intact

   c. Remote memory intact; impairment of recent memory

14. A specimen of the patient's CSF was tested in the laboratory. What medical procedure was done to obtain that specimen?

   _____

15. The finger-to-nose and heel-to-shin tests for cerebellar function were related to: (**coordination, eye sight, memory**).

16. If the carotid arteriography showed a blockage of those arteries, this would relate to which of the patient's symptoms? (**alteration in memory, multiple sclerosis, wide-based gait**)

17. If the MRI with contrast does show areas of demyelination, what diagnosis would that confirm?

   _____

MyMedicalTerminologyLab™

MyMedicalTerminologyLab is a premium online homework management system that includes a host of features to help you study. Registered users will find:

- A multitude of quizzes and activities built within the MyLab platform

- Powerful tools that track and analyze your results—allowing you to create a personalized learning experience

- Videos and audio pronunciations to help enrich your progress

- Streaming lesson presentations (Guided Lectures) and self-paced learning modules

- A space where you and your instructor can check your progress and manage your assignments

Chapter 11
Urology

Urinary System

Urology (yoor-AW-loh-jee) is the medical specialty that studies the anatomy and physiology of the urinary system and uses laboratory and diagnostic procedures, medical and surgical procedures, and drugs to treat urinary diseases.

Learning Outcomes

After you study this chapter, you should be able to

11.1 Identify structures of the urinary system.

11.2 Describe the process of urine production and excretion.

11.3 Describe common urinary diseases, laboratory and diagnostic procedures, medical and surgical procedures, and drugs.

11.4 Form the plural and adjective forms of nouns related to urology.

11.5 Give the meanings of word parts and abbreviations related to urology.

11.6 Divide urology words and build urology words.

11.7 Spell and pronounce urology words.

11.8 Research sound-alike and other urology words.

11.9 Analyze the medical content and meaning of a urology report.

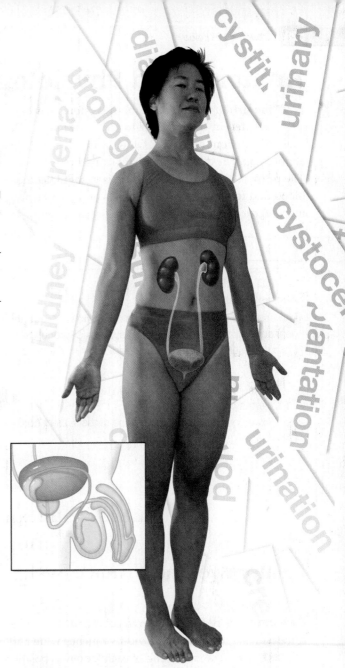

FIGURE 11-1 ■ Urinary system.
The urinary system consists of the kidneys that produce urine, and other structures that transport, store, or excrete urine. In a male, the urinary system continues into the penis (see insert box).

Source: Pearson Education

Medical Language Key

To unlock the definition of a medical word, break it into word parts. Give the meaning of each word part. Put the meanings of the word parts in order, beginning with the meaning of the suffix, then the prefix (if present), then the combining form(s).

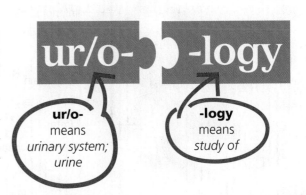

	Word Part	Word Part Meaning
Suffix	**-logy**	*study of*
Combining Form	**ur/o-**	*urinary system; urine*

Urology: ▶ *Study of (the) urinary system, urine, (and related structures).*

Anatomy and Physiology

The **urinary system** is a body system that begins with the kidneys. They are located in the **retroperitoneal space**, a small area behind the peritoneum of the abdominal cavity. Other structures of the urinary system are located in the abdominopelvic cavity, and the male urethra is located in the penis (see Figure 11-1 ■). The purpose of the urinary system is to regulate and maintain the composition of the blood and to remove waste products of metabolism by producing, transporting, storing, and excreting urine.

Pronunciation/Word Parts

urinary (YOOR-ih-NAIR-ee)
  urin/o- *urinary system; urine*
  -ary *pertaining to*

retroperitoneal
(REH-troh-PAIR-ih-toh-NEE-al)
  retro- *backward; behind*
  peritone/o- *peritoneum*
  -al *pertaining to*

WORD ALERT
Alternate Names

The urinary system is also known as the **urinary tract**, the **genitourinary (GU) system** or genitourinary tract, the **urogenital system** or urogenital tract, and the **excretory system**. Each name highlights a different characteristic of this body system.

1. Genitourinary and urogenital: two body systems in close proximity and with shared structures. The reproductive (genital) system is studied in Chapters 12 and 13.
2. Tract: a continuing pathway.
3. Excretory: describes the purpose of the system (to excrete urine).

genitourinary (JEN-ih-toh-YOOR-ih-NAIR-ee)
  genit/o- *genitalia*
  urin/o- *urinary system; urine*
  -ary *pertaining to*

urogenital (YOOR-oh-JEN-ih-tal)
  ur/o- *urinary system; urine*
  genit/o- *genitalia*
  -al *pertaining to*

excretory (EKS-kreh-TOR-ee)
(eks-KREE-tor-ee)
  excret/o- *removing from the body*
  -ory *having the function of*

Anatomy of the Urinary System

Kidneys

Each **kidney** is reddish-brown in color and shaped like (of all things!) a kidney bean. It measures four inches long and two inches wide and weighs less than ½ pound (see Figure 11-2 ■). The upper end of each kidney is positioned under the lower edge of the rib cage in the **flank** area of the back. Each kidney sits in a cushion of fatty tissue in the retroperitoneal space. The **hilum** is an indentation in the medial surface of the kidney. The **renal artery** enters there, and the renal vein and ureter exit there.

kidney (KID-nee)

renal (REE-nal)
  ren/o- *kidney*
  -al *pertaining to*
Renal is the adjective for *kidney*.
The combining form **nephr/o-** means *kidney; nephron*.

flank (FLANK)

hilum (HY-lum)

hila (HY-lah)
Hilum is a Latin singular noun. Form the plural by changing *-um* to *-a*.

hilar (HY-lar)
  hil/o- *indentation*
  -ar *pertaining to*

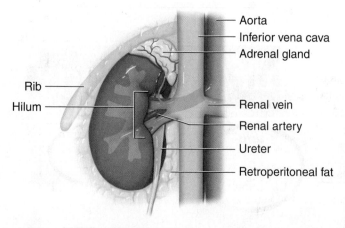

Aorta
Inferior vena cava
Adrenal gland

Rib
Hilum

Renal vein
Renal artery
Ureter
Retroperitoneal fat

FIGURE 11-2 ■ Right kidney.
The kidney is shaped and colored like a kidney bean. The adrenal gland of the endocrine system sits on top of the kidney but is not part of the urinary system. Notice the hilum of the kidney where the renal artery enters and the renal veins and ureter exit.
Source: Pearson Education

The adrenal glands sit on top of the kidneys like caps, but they are not part of the urinary system. The adrenal glands are discussed in "Endocrinology," Chapter 14.

A fibrous capsule surrounds the kidney. Just beneath it is the **cortex** (see Figure 11-3 ■). Beneath that is the **medulla**, an inner layer that contains triangular-shaped **renal pyramids**. The tip of each renal pyramid connects to a **minor calyx**, an area that collects urine. Several minor calices drain into a **major calyx**. Major calices drain into the **renal pelvis**, a large, funnel-shaped area that narrows to become the ureter. Urine flows continuously through minor calices, major calices, the renal pelvis, and into the ureter.

Ureters

Each **ureter** is a 12-inch tube that connects the renal pelvis of the kidney to the bladder (see Figures 11-3, 11-4, 11-5, and 11-6). The ureters enter the bladder on its posterior side. The **ureteral orifices** are the openings into the bladder. The walls of the ureters are smooth muscle that contracts to move urine into the bladder, a process known as **peristalsis**. Valves prevent urine from going back into the ureters.

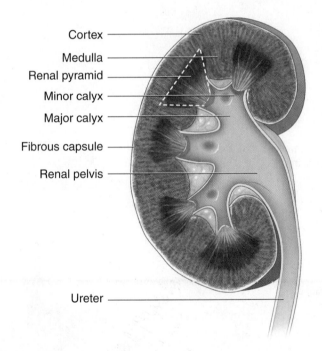

Cortex —
Medulla —
Renal pyramid —
Minor calyx —
Major calyx —
Fibrous capsule —
Renal pelvis —

Ureter —

FIGURE 11-3 ■ Cut section of a kidney.
The internal structures of the kidney include the cortex, medulla, renal pyramids, calices, and renal pelvis. The minor and major calices and the pelvis are known as the *collecting system* because they collect the urine as it is produced. The renal pelvis narrows to become the ureter.
Source: Pearson Education

Bladder

The **bladder** is an expandable reservoir for holding urine (see Figure 11-4 ■). It is located in the pelvic cavity (see Figures 11-5 ■ and 11-6 ■) and it is held in place by ligaments. The rounded top of the bladder is the dome or **fundus**. The bladder is lined with **mucosa**, a mucous membrane. When the bladder is empty, the mucosa collapses into folds or **rugae**. When the bladder is full, smooth muscle in the bladder wall contracts to expel urine. The base of the bladder where it connects to the urethra is the bladder neck. In the bladder neck is the **internal urethral sphincter**, a muscular ring that relaxes when the bladder is full so that urine can flow into the urethra. The opening and closing of this sphincter is an involuntary reflex that cannot be consciously controlled.

Pronunciation/Word Parts

cortex (KOR-teks)

cortices (KOR-tih-seez)
Cortex is a Latin noun. Form the plural by changing -ex to -ices.

cortical (KOR-tih-kal)
  cortic/o- cortex; outer region
  -al pertaining to

medulla (meh-DUL-ah), (meh-DOOL-ah)

medullae (meh-DUL-ee), (meh-DOOL-ee)
Medulla is a Latin singular noun. Form the plural by changing -a to -ae.

calyx (KAY-liks)

calices (KAL-ih-seez)
Calyx is a Latin singular noun. Form the plural by changing -yx to -ices. *Calix* is an alternate spelling.

caliceal (KAL-ih-SEE-al)
  calic/o- calyx
  -eal pertaining to
The combining form **cali/o-** also means calyx.

pelvis (PEL-vis)

pelves (PEL-veez)
Pelvis is a Latin singular noun. Form the plural by changing -is to -es.

pelvic (PEL-vik)
  pelv/o- hip bone; pelvis; renal pelvis
  -ic pertaining to
The combining form **pyel/o-** means renal pelvis.

ureter (YOOR-eh-ter) (yoor-EE-ter)

ureteral (yoor-EE-ter-al)
  ureter/o- ureter
  -al pertaining to

orifice (OR-ih-fis)

peristalsis (PAIR-ih-STAL-sis)
  peri- around
  stal/o- contraction
  -sis condition; process

bladder (BLAD-er)

vesical (VES-ih-kal)
  vesic/o- bladder; fluid-filled sac
  -al pertaining to
Vesical is the adjective form for bladder. The combining form **cyst/o-** means bladder; fluid-filled sac; semisolid cyst

fundus (FUN-dus)

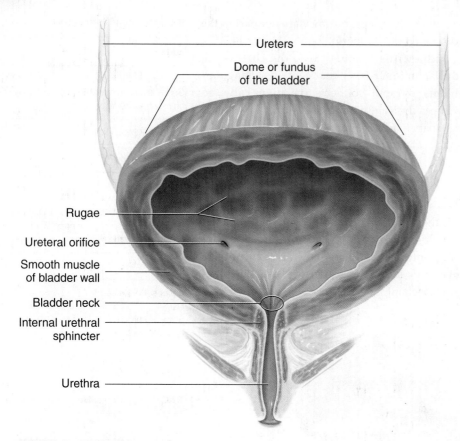

FIGURE 11-4 ■ **Bladder.**
The bladder is a hollow cavity that collects and temporarily stores urine. Rugae are mucous membrane folds in the bladder wall that allow it to expand as it fills.
Source: Pearson Education

Pronunciation/Word Parts

mucosa (myoo-KOH-sah)

mucosal (myoo-KOH-sal)
  mucos/o- *mucous membrane*
  -al *pertaining to*

rugae (ROO-gee)
Ruga is a Latin singular noun. Form the plural by changing *-a* to *-ae*. Because there are so many rugae in the bladder, the singular form is seldom used.

sphincter (SFINK-ter)

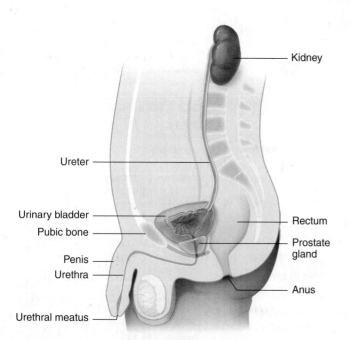

FIGURE 11-5 ■ **Male urinary system.**
The male urethra is long and travels through the prostate gland and the penis before reaching the outside of the body.
Source: Pearson Education

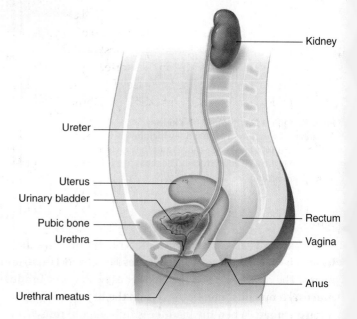

FIGURE 11-6 ■ **Female urinary system.**
The female urethra is short and straight. Notice how the bladder is beneath the uterus. During pregnancy, the bladder is often compressed by the expanding uterus and growing fetus.
Source: Pearson Education

WORD ALERT

Sound-Alike Words

ureter	(noun)	tube that connects the kidney to the bladder
ureteral	(adjective)	descriptive word for the ureter
		Example: The ureteral orifice is the opening of the ureter into the bladder.
urethra	(noun)	tube that connects the bladder to the outside of the body
urethral	(adjective)	descriptive word for the urethra
		Example: The urethral meatus opens to the outside of the body.
vesical	(adjective)	descriptive word for the bladder
		Example: Intravesical chemotherapy drugs are put into the bladder to treat bladder cancer.
vesicle	(noun)	small fluid-filled blister on the skin
		Example: Herpes zoster virus infection causes vesicles on the skin.

Urethra

The **urethra** is a tube that carries urine from the bladder to the outside of the body. The **external urethral sphincter** is a muscular ring that can be consciously controlled to release or hold back urine. The **urethral meatus** is where the urethra opens to the outside of the body.

In men, the urethra is 7–8 inches long. As the urethra leaves the bladder, it travels though the center of the **prostate gland**, a donut-shaped gland at the base of the bladder. This part is known as the **prostatic urethra**. The prostate gland is not part of the urinary system; however, enlargement of the prostate gland can affect the urinary system by pressing on and narrowing the urethra. The prostate gland is discussed in "Male Reproductive Medicine," Chapter 12. The external urethral sphincter is located just distal to the prostate gland. The urethra is part of both the urinary and the male reproductive system because it transports both urine and semen. The urethra travels the length of the **penis** (see Figure 11-5). This part is known as the **penile urethra**. In men, the urethral meatus is located at the tip of the penis. If the male is uncircumcised, the urethral meatus is covered by the foreskin of the penis.

In women, the urethra is much shorter, traveling only 1–2 inches from the bladder to the external surface of the body (see Figure 11-6). The external urethral sphincter is near the distal end of the urethra. The urethral meatus is located just anterior to the external opening of the vagina.

Physiology of the Formation of Urine

The **parenchyma** is the functional or working tissue of an organ (as opposed to its structural framework). The parenchyma of the kidney is made up of the cortex and medulla because these areas contain nephrons. The **nephron**, a microscopic structure, is the functional unit of the kidney and the site of urine production (see Figure 11-7 ■).

The process of urine production begins as the renal artery enters the kidney and divides into smaller arterioles. A single arteriole enters each nephron. The first part of the nephron is the **glomerular capsule**. Within this cup-shaped structure, the arteriole becomes the **glomerulus**, a network of intertwining capillaries.

Blood flowing through these capillaries contains nutritional substances that are needed by the body and waste products that must be excreted. The nutritional substances include electrolytes, glucose, amino acids, vitamins, and so on. **Electrolytes** are chemical elements that have a positive or negative electrical charge and include sodium

urethra (yoor-EE-thrah)

urethral (yoor-EE-thrawl)
  urethr/o- *urethra*
  -al *pertaining to*

sphincter (SFINGK-ter)

meatus (mee-AA-tus)

prostate (PRAW-stayt)

prostatic (praw-STAT-ik)
  prostat/o- *prostate gland*
  -ic *pertaining to*

penis (PEE-nis)

penile (PEE-nIle)
  pen/o- *penis*
  -ile *pertaining to*

parenchyma (pah-RENG-kih-mah)

nephron (NEH-frawn)
The combining form **nephr/o-** means *kidney; nephron.*

glomerular (gloh-MAIR-yoo-lar)
  glomerul/o- *glomerulus*
  -ar *pertaining to*

glomerulus (gloh-MAIR-yoo-lus)

glomeruli (gloh-MAIR-yoo-lie)
Glomerulus is a Latin singular noun. Form the plural by changing *-us* to *-i.*

electrolyte (ee-LEK-troh-lite)
  electr/o- *electricity*
  -lyte *dissolved substance*
Add word parts to make a complete definition of *electrolyte*: *dissolved substance (that can conduct) electricity (through a solution).*

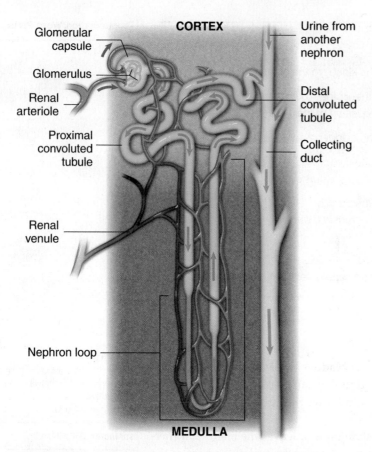

CORTEX

Glomerular capsule

Glomerulus

Renal arteriole

Proximal convoluted tubule

Renal venule

Nephron loop

MEDULLA

Urine from another nephron

Distal convoluted tubule

Collecting duct

FIGURE 11-7 ■ Nephron.
The functional unit of the kidney is the nephron. It filters substances and water out of the blood, helps certain nutritional substances and some water return to the blood, and sends the remaining water and waste substances as urine to the ureter and bladder.
Source: Pearson Education

(Na^+), potassium (K^+), chloride (Cl^-), and bicarbonate (HCO_3^-). Glucose is the simple sugar that the body uses for energy. Amino acids are the building blocks of proteins. These nutritional substances are essential to the health of the body. Waste products include:

- **urea** (from protein metabolism)
- **creatinine** (from muscle contractions)
- **uric acid** (from purine metabolism to construct cellular DNA and RNA)
- drugs and products of drug metabolism.

If these waste products are not excreted in the urine, they would quickly reach toxic levels.

The capillaries in the glomerulus have special pores in their walls that are not in other capillaries in the body. Some things in the blood (red blood cells, white blood cells, platelets, and albumin molecules) are too large to pass through these pores, so they remain in the blood. But other things (nutritional substances, water, and waste products) are pushed by the pressure of the blood through the pores and into the cup-shaped glomerular capsule. This process is known as **filtration**. The capillaries of the glomerulus then combine into a single arteriole that travels along the tubules of the nephron (see Figure 11-7).

The **filtrate** (the solution of nutritional substances, water, and waste products) in the glomerular capsule flows into the **proximal convoluted tubule** of the nephron. There,

Pronunciation/Word Parts

urea (yoor-EE-ah)

creatinine (kree-AT-ih-neen)

uric acid (YOOR-ik AS-id)

filtration (fil-TRAY-shun)
  filtrat/o- *filtering; straining*
  -ion *action; condition*

filtrate (FIL-trayt)
  filtr/o- *filter*
  -ate *composed of; pertaining to*

proximal (PRAWK-sih-mal)
  proxim/o- *near the center; near the point of origin*
  -al *pertaining to*

convoluted (CON-voh-LOO-ted)

tubule (TOO-byool)
  tub/o- *tube*
  -ule *small thing*

tubular (TOO-byoo-lar)
  tubul/o- *small tube*
  -ar *pertaining to*

most of the water and nutritional substances move out of the tubule and return to the blood. This process is known as **reabsorption**. However, if the blood already has a high level of glucose in it (because of just eating a sugary food or because of uncontrolled diabetes mellitus) it cannot reabsorb additional glucose, then that glucose remains in the proximal convoluted tubule and is excreted in the urine.

The proximal convoluted tubule becomes a U-shaped tubule known as the **nephron loop**. There, more water and electrolytes are reabsorbed back into the blood. The nephron loop widens to become the distal convoluted tubule. In the **distal convoluted tubule**, more water and electrolytes as well as amino acids and other nutritional substances are reabsorbed back into the blood. The distal convoluted tubules of many nephrons empty into a common **collecting duct**. Some reabsorption continues to take place in the collecting duct. The fluid that remains is **urine**. Urine is produced continuously by nephrons in the kidneys (see Figure 11-8 ■).

The process of eliminating urine from the body is described in several ways: **urination**, **micturition**, **voiding**, or passing water (a layperson's phrase).

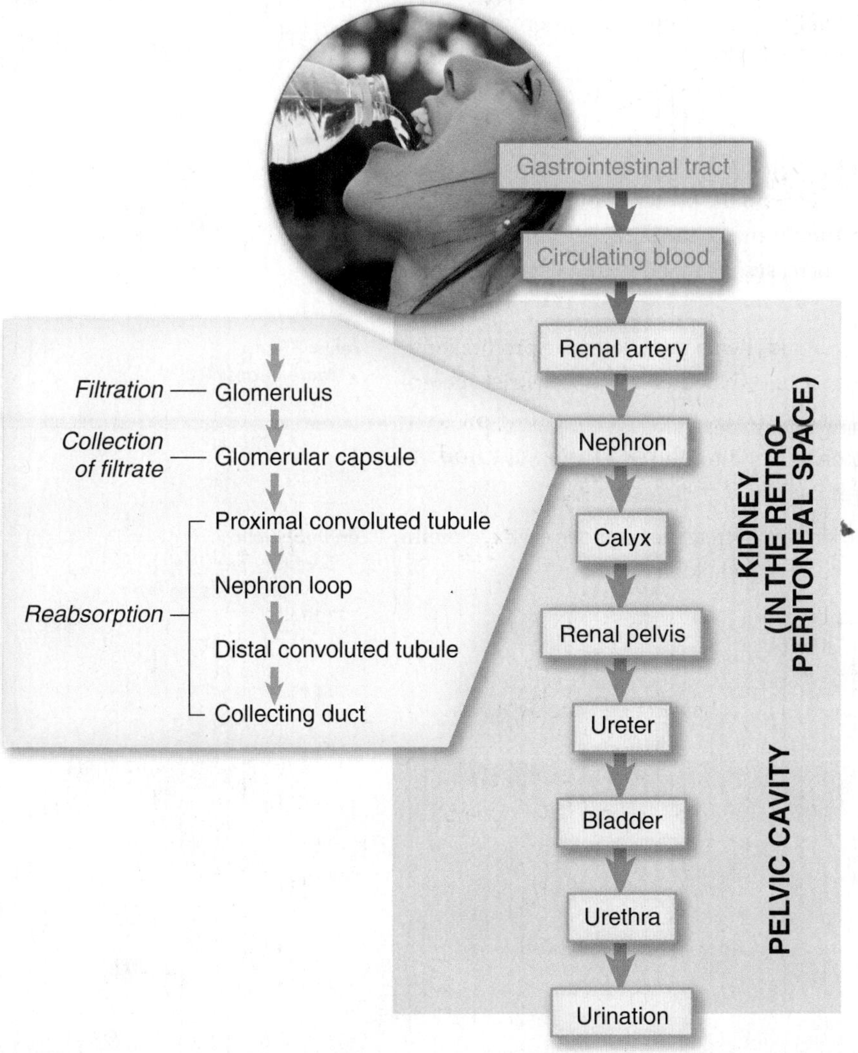

Pronunciation/Word Parts

reabsorption (REE-ab-SORP-shun)
  re- *again and again; backward; unable to*
  absorpt/o- *absorb; take in*
  -ion *action; condition*

nephron loop (NEH-frawn LOOP)

distal (DIS-tal)
  dist/o- *away from the center; away from the point of origin*
  -al *pertaining to*

urine (YOOR-in)
  ur/o- *urinary system; urine*
  -ine *pertaining to; thing pertaining to*

urination (YOOR-ih-NAY-shun)
  urin/o- *urinary system; urine*
  -ation *being; having; process*

micturition (MIK-tyoor-IH-shun)
  micturi/o- *making urine*
  -tion *being; having; process*
The combining form **enur/o-** means *urinate*.

voiding (VOY-ding)

FIGURE 11-8 ■ Pathway of urine production and urination.

Source: Glamy/Fotolia; Pearson Education

ACROSS THE LIFE SPAN

Pediatrics. The kidneys of a fetus begin to produce urine by about the 12th week of life. The urine is excreted and becomes part of the amniotic fluid around the fetus. Children ages 1–3 produce about 400–600 cc (about a pint) of urine each day. Children ages 3–8 produce about 600–1000 cc (about a quart) of urine daily.

Adults produce about 1200–1500 cc (1–3 quarts) of urine each day. Each kidney contains more than 1 million individual nephrons. If laid end to end, these nephrons would be 80 miles in length.

Geriatrics. As a person ages, some nephrons deteriorate and die. Because the body does not repair or replace nephrons, the total number of nephrons in the kidneys continues to decline with age, and kidney function also decreases. Poor renal function can significantly prolong the effects of some drugs. Patients with renal disease and older adults are prescribed lower doses of drugs to prevent toxic symptoms due to decreased excretion of drugs.

Physiology of Other Functions of the Kidneys

The kidneys help the body to maintain a normal and constant internal environment. *Note:* These functions are in addition to urine production.

1. If the blood pressure decreases, the kidneys

   - produce concentrated urine with less water in it. The hormone aldosterone (from the adrenal gland) and antidiuretic hormone (from the posterior pituitary gland in the brain) act on the distal convoluted tubule and collecting duct to cause more sodium and water to be reabsorbed. This increases the blood volume and the blood pressure.

   - secrete the enzyme **renin** directly into the blood. Renin stimulates the production of angiotensin, a powerful vasoconstrictor that causes blood vessels to constrict, increasing blood pressure.

     renin (REE-nin)
     ren/o- *kidney*
     -in *substance*

2. If the pH of the blood decreases, the electrolyte bicarbonate (HCO_3^-) moves from the tubule back into the blood, and this increases the pH.

3. If the number of red blood cells decreases, the kidneys secrete the hormone **erythropoietin**, which stimulates the bone marrow to produce more red blood cells.

   erythropoietin (eh-RITH-roh-POY-eh-tin)
   erythr/o- *red*
   -poietin *substance that forms*

Vocabulary Review

Anatomy and Physiology

Word or Phrase	Description	Combining Forms
urinary system	Body system that includes the kidneys, ureters, bladder, and urethra. Its function is to produce, transport, store, and excrete urine. It also helps regulate the internal environment of the body by secreting the enzyme renin and the hormone erythropoietin. It is also known as the **urinary tract**, **genitourinary system** or tract, **urogenital system** or tract, and the **excretory system**.	**urin/o-** *urinary system; urine* **ur/o-** *urinary system; urine* **genit/o-** *genitalia* **excret/o-** *removing from the body*

Kidney

calyx	Area at the tip of each renal pyramid. The minor calices and then the major calices collect urine.	**calic/o-** *calyx* **cali/o-** *calyx*
cortex	Layer of tissue beneath the fibrous capsule of the kidney	**cortic/o-** *cortex; outer region*
flank	Area on the back (between the ribs and the hip bone) that overlies the kidneys	
hilum	Indentation in the medial side of each kidney where the renal artery enters and the renal vein and ureter exit	**hil/o-** *indentation*
kidney	Organ of the urinary system that produces urine. It is in the **retroperitoneal space**, an area behind the peritoneum of the abdominal cavity.	**ren/o-** *kidney* **nephr/o-** *kidney; nephron* **peritone/o-** *peritoneum*
medulla	Layer of tissue beneath the cortex of the kidney. It contains the renal pyramids.	
parenchyma	Functional area in the cortex and medulla of the kidney that contains the nephrons	
renal pelvis	Large, funnel-shaped area within each kidney. It collects urine from the major calices and then narrows to become the ureter.	**pelv/o-** *hip bone; pelvis; renal pelvis* **pyel/o-** *renal pelvis*
renal pyramids	Triangular-shaped areas in the medulla of the kidney	**ren/o-** *kidney*

Nephron

collecting duct	Large duct that collects fluid from the distal convoluted tubules of many nephrons. The final step of reabsorption takes place there, and the fluid that remains is urine.	
distal convoluted tubule	Tubule of the nephron that begins at the nephron loop and ends at the collecting duct. Reabsorption takes place there.	**dist/o-** *away from the center; away from the point of origin* **tub/o-** *tube* **tubul/o-** *small tube*
glomerular capsule	First part of a nephron. It is a cup-shaped structure that surrounds the glomerulus and collects filtrate.	**glomerul/o-** *glomerulus*
glomerulus	Network of intertwining capillaries within the glomerular capsule. Filtration takes place there.	**glomerul/o-** *glomerulus*

Word or Phrase	Description	Combining Forms
nephron	Microscopic, functional unit of the kidney	**nephr/o-** *kidney; nephron*
nephron loop	Tubule of the nephron that is U-shaped. It begins at the proximal convoluted tubule and ends at the distal convoluted tubule. Reabsorption takes place there.	
proximal convoluted tubule	Tubule of the nephron that begins at the glomerular capsule and ends at the nephron loop. Reabsorption takes place there.	**proxim/o-** *near the center; near the point of origin* **tub/o-** *tube* **tubul/o-** *small tube*
Ureter		
peristalsis	Process of smooth muscle contractions that move urine through the ureter	**stal/o-** *contraction*
ureter	Tube that carries urine from the kidney to the bladder	**ureter/o-** *ureter*
ureteral orifice	Opening at the end of the ureter as it enters the bladder	**ureter/o-** *ureter*
Bladder		
bladder	Expandable reservoir for storing urine. It is located in the pelvic cavity.	**vesic/o-** *bladder; fluid-filled sac* **cyst/o-** *bladder; fluid-filled sac; semisolid cyst*
fundus	Rounded top or dome of the bladder	
mucosa	Mucous membrane lining of the bladder	**mucos/o-** *mucous membrane*
rugae	Folds in the mucosa of the bladder that disappear as the bladder fills with urine	
sphincter	Muscular ring. The sphincter in the bladder neck is not under conscious control.	
Urethra		
external urethral sphincter	Muscular ring in the urethra. It can be consciously controlled to release or hold back urine.	**urethr/o-** *urethra*
penis	Structure that is part of the male reproductive system. In a man, the urethra passes through the length of the penis as the **penile urethra**.	**pen/o-** *penis*
prostate gland	Gland that is part of the male reproductive system. In a man, the urethra passes through the center of the prostate gland as the **prostatic urethra**.	**prostat/o-** *prostate gland*
urethra	Tube that carries urine from the bladder to the outside of the body. In women, it is a short tube; in men, it goes through the prostate gland and the length of the penis.	**urethr/o-** *urethra*
urethral meatus	Opening to the outside of the body at the end of the urethra	**urethr/o-** *urethra*

Diseases

Kidneys and Ureters

Word or Phrase	Description	Pronunciation/Word Parts

glomerulonephritis	Complication that develops following an acute infection with streptococcal bacteria or with viruses. The original infection, which is often a strep throat, causes the immune system to produce antibodies. Antibodies combine with the bacteria or viruses to form antigen–antibody complexes that clog the pores of the capillaries of the glomerulus. The kidneys become inflamed and urine production decreases. Treatment: Antibiotic drug; corticosteroid drug to decrease inflammation; renal dialysis, if necessary.	**glomerulonephritis**
		(gloh-MAIR-yoo-LOH-neh-FRY-tis)
		  glomerul/o- *glomerulus*
		  nephr/o- *kidney; nephron*
		  -itis *infection of; inflammation of*

hydronephrosis	Enlargement of the kidney. This is due to pressure from urine that is backed up in the ureter because of an obstructing stone or stricture. In **caliectasis**, the calices of the kidney are enlarged. In **hydroureter**, only the ureter is enlarged. Treatment: Removal of the stone or stricture.	**hydronephrosis**
		(HY-droh-neh-FROH-sis)
		  hydr/o- *fluid; water*
		  nephr/o- *kidney; nephron*
		  -osis *condition; process*
		
		caliectasis (KAY-lee-EK-tah-sis)
		  cali/o- *calyx*
		  -ectasis *condition of dilation*
		
		hydroureter (HY-droh-YOOR-eh-ter)
		(HY-droh-yoor-EE-ter)
		Hydroureter is a combination of the combining form *hydr/o-* (fluid; water) and the word *ureter*.

nephrolithiasis	Kidney stone or **calculus** formation in the urinary system. Kidney stones can vary in size from microscopic (often referred to as *sand* or *gravel*) (see Figure 11-9 ■) to large enough to block the ureter or fill the renal pelvis (see Figure 11-10 ■). Kidney stones are composed of magnesium, calcium, or uric acid crystals. **Calculogenesis** or **lithogenesis** is the process of forming stones. **Renal colic** is a spasm of smooth muscle of the ureter or bladder as the kidney stone's jagged edges scrape the mucosa. This causes severe pain, nausea and vomiting, and hematuria. Many stones reach the bladder and are eliminated from the body with the urine. Stones that do not pass spontaneously can be destroyed by lithotripsy (see Figure 11-25) or removed surgically. Treatment: Analgesic drug; lithotripsy; surgical procedure of stone basketing or nephrolithotomy, depending on the stone's size and location.	**nephrolithiasis**
		(NEH-froh-lith-EYE-ah-sis)
		  nephr/o- *kidney; nephron*
		  lith/o- *stone*
		  -iasis *process; state*
		
		calculus (KAL-kyoo-lus)
		
		calculi (KAL-kyoo-lie)
		Calculus is a Latin singular noun. Form the plural by changing *-us* to *-i*.
		
		calculogenesis
		(KAL-kyoo-loh-JEN-eh-sis)
		  calcul/o- *stone*
		  gen/o- *arising from; produced by*
		  -esis *condition; process*
		
		lithogenesis (LITH-oh-JEN-eh-sis)
		  lith/o- *stone*
		  gen/o- *arising from; produced by*
		  -esis *condition; process*
		
		colic (KAW-lik)
		  col/o- *colon*
		  -ic *pertaining to*
		Note: Spasm of the smooth muscle of the ureter or bladder with pain is similar to that of colic that occurs in the colon.

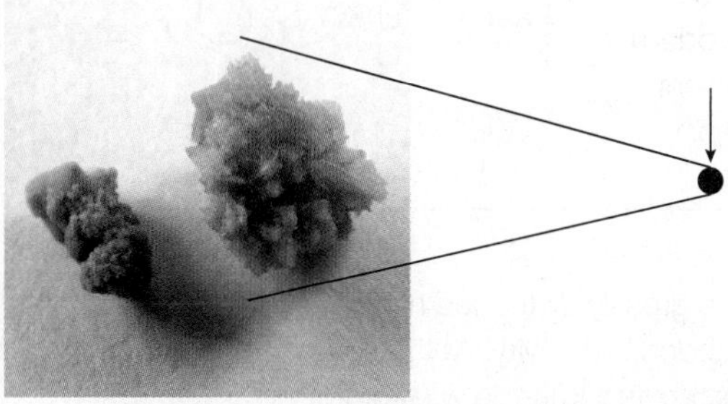

FIGURE 11-9 ■ Kidney stone.
A kidney stone no bigger than this dot caused hematuria, vomiting, renal colic, and severe pain. On close examination, the many sharp, jagged edges of the kidney stone can be seen.
Source: Remik44992/Shutterstock

DID YOU KNOW?
Egyptian mummies have been found to have kidney stones.

Word or Phrase	Description	Pronunciation/Word Parts
nephrolithiasis (*continued*)	**FIGURE 11-10** ■ **Nephrolithiasis.** This x-ray shows multiple kidney stones in the kidney that have become so large that they cannot pass spontaneously. They leave little room in the renal pelvis for urine to collect. *Source*: Dr. E. Walker/Science Source; Tewan Banditrukkanka/Shutterstock	

WORD ALERT
Words with Two Different Meanings
calculus   A kidney stone
It is also the name of an advanced branch of mathematics.
colic   Spasm of the smooth muscle around the ureters and bladder
Spasm of the smooth muscle around the intestines
pelvis   Funnel-shaped area in the kidney that collects urine
Hip bones (as well as the sacrum and coccyx of the vertebral column)

Word or Phrase	Description	Pronunciation/Word Parts
nephropathy	General word for any disease of the kidney. Diabetic nephropathy involves progressive damage to the glomeruli because of diabetes mellitus. The tiny arteries of the glomerulus harden (**glomerulosclerosis**) because of accelerated arteriosclerosis throughout the body. Treatment: Correct the underlying cause; manage the diabetes mellitus.	**nephropathy** (neh-FRAW-pah-thee) **nephr/o-** *kidney; nephron* **-pathy** *disease* **glomerulosclerosis** (gloh-MAIR-yoo-LOH-skleh-ROH-sis) **glomerul/o-** *glomerulus* **scler/o-** *hard; sclera of the eye* **-osis** *condition; process* Select the correct suffix and combining form meanings to get the definition of *glomerulosclerosis*: *condition (of the) glomerulus (becoming) hard*.
nephroptosis	Abnormally low position of a kidney. It sometimes requires surgery, but more often is mentioned as an incidental finding seen on an x-ray.	**nephroptosis** (NEH-frawp-TOH-sis) **nephr/o-** *kidney; nephron* **-ptosis** *state of drooping; state of falling*
nephrotic syndrome	Damage to the pores of the capillaries of the glomerulus. This allows large amounts of albumin (protein) to leak into the urine, decreasing the amount of protein in the blood. This changes the osmotic pressure of the blood and allows fluid to go into the tissues, producing edema in the extremities; fluid also goes into the abdominal cavity, producing **ascites** (a grossly enlarged, fluid-distended abdomen). Treatment: Diuretic drug to decrease edema; correct the underlying cause.	**nephrotic** (neh-FRAW-tik) **nephr/o-** *kidney; nephron* **-tic** *pertaining to* **ascites** (ah-SY-teez)

CLINICAL CONNECTIONS
Dietetics. In the nutritional disease kwashiorkor (protein malnutrition), patients have grossly distended abdomens. The lack of dietary protein causes low blood protein, and fluid moves from the blood into the abdominal cavity. At the same time, muscle tissue is broken down to meet the protein needs of the body. This results in thin extremities (muscle wasting).

Word or Phrase	Description	Pronunciation/Word Parts

polycystic kidney disease	Hereditary disease characterized by cysts in the kidney that eventually destroy the nephrons, causing kidney failure (see Figures 11-11 ■ and 11-12). The early stage of this progressive degenerative disease shows few symptoms or signs; often it is not detected until hypertension and already enlarged kidneys are found during a physical examination. Treatment: Dialysis or kidney transplantation. 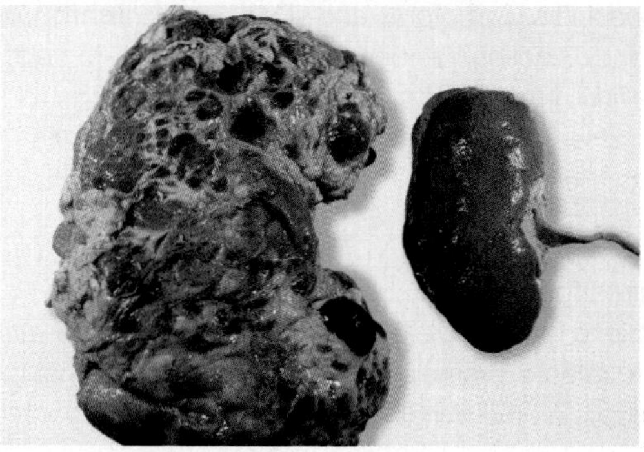
	
	FIGURE 11-11 ■ Polycystic kidney disease.
	(a) As nonfunctioning cysts replace large numbers of nephrons, the patient's kidney function progressively decreases. (b) A normal kidney, for comparison.
	Source: Arthur Glauberman/Science Source
		polycystic (PAW-lee-SIS-tik)
		  poly- *many; much*
		  cyst/o- *bladder; fluid-filled sac; semisolid cyst*
		  -ic *pertaining to*
		Select the correct combining form meaning to get the definition of *polycystic*: *pertaining to many semisolid cysts*.

pyelonephritis	Inflammation and infection of the renal pelvis of the kidney. Infection of the kidney (**nephritis**) also involves the renal pelves. It is caused by a bacterial infection of the bladder that goes up the ureters to the kidneys.	**pyelonephritis**
		(PY-eh-LOH-neh-FRY-tis)
		  pyel/o- *renal pelvis*
		  nephr/o- *kidney; nephron*
		  -itis *infection of; inflammation of*
		
		nephritis (neh-FRY-tis)
		  nephr/o- *kidney; nephron*
		  -itis *infection of; inflammation of*

renal cell cancer	**Cancerous** tumor (**carcinoma**) that arises from tubules in the nephron (see Figure 11-12 ■). **Wilms' tumor** is cancer of the kidney that occurs in children from residual embryonic or fetal tissue; it is also known as a **nephroblastoma**. Treatment: Surgery to remove the kidney (nephrectomy), radiation therapy, chemotherapy drugs. 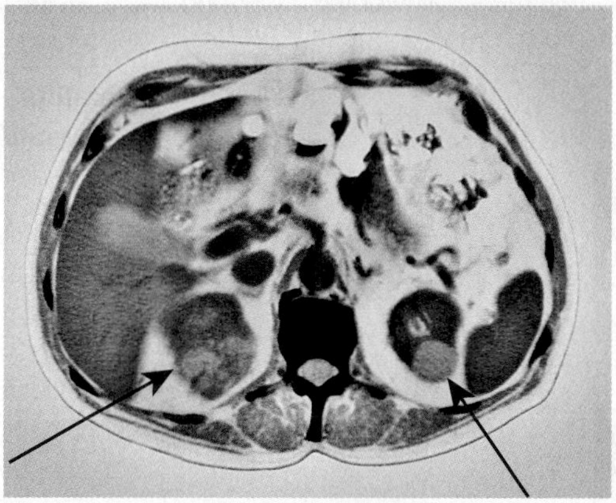	**cancer** (KAN-ser)
		
		cancerous (KAN-ser-us)
		  cancer/o- *cancer*
		  -ous *pertaining to*
		
		carcinoma (KAR-sih-NOH-mah)
		  carcin/o- *cancer*
		  -oma *mass; tumor*
		
		Wilms' (WILMZ)
		
		nephroblastoma
		(NEH-froh-blas-TOH-mah)
		  nephr/o- *kidney; nephron*
		  blast/o- *embryonic; immature*
		  -oma *mass; tumor*

FIGURE 11-12 ■ CT scan of the kidneys.
This colorized computerized tomography (CT) scan shows the abdominal organs and the kidneys. The bottom center of the image shows the patient's vertebral column in black. Small black areas around both sides are the patient's ribs. The top of the image is the patient's abdomen. The abdominal organs will seem to be in an abnormal, reversed position, unless you understand that a CT scan is read as if you were standing at the patient's feet and looking up. Therefore, the patient's liver (light and dark blue) is along the left-hand side of the image. The patient's right kidney (bottom left, see arrow) is enlarged from a cancerous tumor. The patient's left kidney (bottom right, see arrow) has a large cyst.
Source: Simon Fraser/Freeman Hospital, Newcastle upon Tyne/Science Source

Word or Phrase	Description	Pronunciation/Word Parts
renal failure	Disease in which the kidneys decrease urine production, and then stop producing urine. **Acute renal failure (ARF)** occurs suddenly and is usually due to trauma, severe blood loss, or overwhelming infection. It is caused by **acute tubular necrosis**, the sudden destruction of large numbers of nephrons and their tubules. **Chronic renal failure (CRF)** begins with **renal insufficiency**, followed by gradual worsening with progressive damage to the kidneys from chronic, uncontrolled diabetes mellitus, hypertension, or glomerulonephritis. Symptoms and signs do not appear until 80 percent of kidney function has been lost. **End-stage renal disease (ESRD)** is the final, irreversible stage of chronic renal failure in which there is little or no remaining kidney function. Treatment: Treat the underlying cause; treat end-stage failure with dialysis.	**acute** (ah-KYOOT) **necrosis** (neh-KROH-sis) **necr/o-** *dead body; dead cells; dead tissue* **-osis** *condition; process* **chronic** (KRAW-nik) **chron/o-** *time* **-ic** *pertaining to*
uremia	An excessive amount of the waste product urea in the blood because of renal failure. The kidneys are unable to remove urea, and it reaches a toxic level in the blood. It is then excreted to a small degree through the sweat glands, making white deposits on the skin that look like ice (uremic frost). Treatment: Dialysis.	**uremia** (yoor-EE-mee-ah) **ur/o-** *urinary system; urine* **-emia** *condition of the blood; substance in the blood*

Bladder

Word or Phrase	Description	Pronunciation/Word Parts
bladder cancer	Cancerous tumor (carcinoma) of the lining of the bladder, most commonly seen in men over age 60. Hematuria is often the first sign. Treatment: Transurethral resection of the bladder tumor (TURBT), surgery to remove the bladder (cystectomy), radiation therapy, or **intravesical** insertion of a chemotherapy drug through a catheter into the bladder.	**intravesical** (IN-trah-VES-ih-kal) **intra-** *within* **vesic/o-** *bladder; fluid-filled sac* **-al** *pertaining to*
cystitis	Inflammation or infection of the bladder. This is often caused by bacteria in the urethra that ascend into the bladder, particularly in women because of the short length of the urethra. **Interstitial cystitis** is a chronic, progressive infection in which the bladder mucosa becomes extremely irritated and red, with bleeding (see Figure 11-13 ■). **Radiation cystitis** is caused by the irritating effects of radiation therapy given to treat bladder cancer. Treatment: Correct the underlying condition; analgesic drug and antispasmodic drug.	**cystitis** (sis-TY-tis) **cyst/o-** *bladder; fluid-filled sac; semisolid cyst* **-itis** *infection of; inflammation of* Select the correct combining form meaning to get the definition of *cystitis: infection or inflammation of the bladder.* **interstitial** (IN-ter-STIH-shal) **interstiti/o-** *spaces within tissue* **-al** *pertaining to* **radiation** (RAY-dee-AA-shun) **radi/o-** *forearm bone; radiation; x-rays* **-ation** *being; having; process* Select the correct combining form meaning to get the definition of *radiation: being (exposed to) x-rays.*

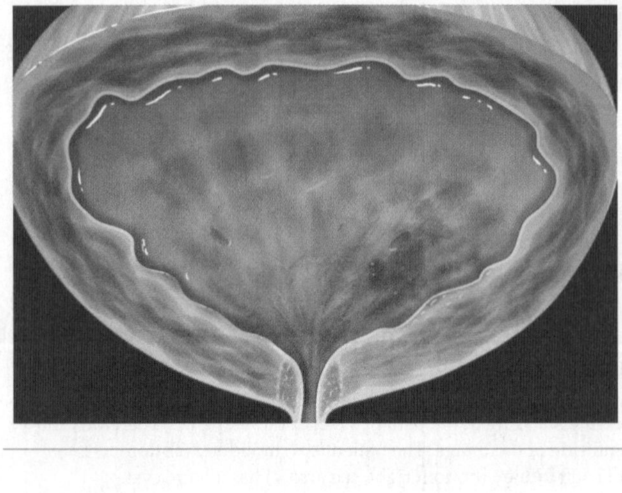

FIGURE 11-13 ■ Acute cystitis.
This bladder shows severe irritation and inflammation of the mucosa with areas of hemorrhage.
Source: Pearson Education

Word or Phrase	Description	Pronunciation/Word Parts
cystocele	Hernia in which the bladder bulges through a weakness in the muscular wall of the vagina or rectum. This causes retention of the urine that is in the bulge of the hernia. This is also known as a **vesicocele**. Treatment: Surgical repair of the vagina or rectum, if severe.	**cystocele** (SIS-toh-seel) **cyst/o-** *bladder; fluid-filled sac; semisolid cyst* **-cele** *hernia* **vesicocele** (VES-ih-koh-SEEL) **vesic/o-** *bladder; fluid-filled sac* **-cele** *hernia*
neurogenic bladder	Urinary retention due to a lack of innervation of the nerves of the bladder. This can be due to a spinal cord injury, spina bifida, multiple sclerosis, or Parkinson's disease. The bladder must be catheterized intermittently because it does not contract to expel urine. Treatment: Catheterization.	**neurogenic** (NYOOR-oh-JEN-ik) **neur/o-** *nerve* **gen/o-** *arising from; produced by* **-ic** *pertaining to*
overactive bladder	Urinary urgency and frequency due to involuntary contractions of the bladder wall as the bladder fills with urine. This sometimes causes incontinence. Treatment: Drug for overactive bladder.	
urinary retention	Inability to empty the bladder because of an obstruction (enlargement of the prostate gland, kidney stone), nerve damage (neurogenic bladder), or as a side effect of certain drugs. Even when the bladder contracts, a large amount of **postvoid residual** urine remains in the bladder. Treatment: Correct the underlying cause.	**retention** (ree-TEN-shun) **retent/o-** *hold back; keep* **-ion** *action; condition* **postvoid** (POST-voyd) *Postvoid* is a combination of the prefix *post-* (after; behind) and the word *void* (urinate).
vesicovaginal fistula	Formation of an abnormal passageway connecting the bladder to the vagina. Urine flows from the bladder into the vagina and leaks continually to the outside of the body. Treatment: Surgical correction.	**vesicovaginal** (VES-ih-koh-VAJ-ih-nal) **vesic/o-** *bladder; fluid-filled sac* **vagin/o-** *vagina* **-al** *pertaining to* **fistula** (FIS-tyoo-lah)

Urethra

Word or Phrase	Description	Pronunciation/Word Parts
epispadias	Congenital condition in which the female urethral meatus is in an abnormal location near the clitoris, or the male urethral meatus is in an abnormal location on the upper surface of the shaft of the penis rather than at the tip of the glans penis. **Hypospadias** is when the male urethral meatus is on the underside of the shaft of the penis. Treatment: Surgery (urethroplasty) to reposition the urethral meatus.	**epispadias** (EP-ih-SPAY-dee-as) **epi-** *above; upon* **spad/o-** *opening; tear* **-ias** *condition* **hypospadias** (HY-poh-SPAY-dee-as) **hypo-** *below; deficient* **spad/o-** *opening; tear* **-ias** *condition*
urethritis	Inflammation or infection of the urethra. Gonococcal urethritis is a symptom of the sexually transmitted disease gonorrhea caused by the bacterium *Neisseria gonorrhoeae*. Nongonococcal urethritis is a sexually transmitted disease caused by the bacterium *Chlamydia trachomatis*. Nonspecific urethritis is an inflammation or infection of the urethra from bacteria, chemicals, or trauma; it is not a sexually transmitted disease. Treatment: Antibiotic drug for an infection.	**urethritis** (YOOR-ee-THRY-tis) **urethr/o-** *urethra* **-itis** *infection of; inflammation of*

Urine and Urination

Word or Phrase	Description	Pronunciation/Word Parts
albuminuria	Presence of albumin in the urine. Albumin is the major protein in the blood, and so this condition is also called **proteinuria**. Normally there is no protein in the urine because albumin molecules are too large to pass through pores in the capillaries of the glomerulus; but when there is kidney disease, albumin passes through the damaged pores and is excreted in the urine. Albuminuria is an important first sign of kidney disease. It is also present in pregnant women who are developing preeclampsia. Treatment: Correct the underlying cause.	**albuminuria** (AL-byoo-mih-NYOOR-ee-ah) **albumin/o-** *albumin* **ur/o-** *urinary system; urine* **-ia** *condition; state; thing*
		proteinuria (PROH-teh-NYOOR-ee-ah) **protein/o-** *protein* **ur/o-** *urinary system; urine* **-ia** *condition; state; thing*
anuria	Absence of urine production by the kidneys because of acute or chronic renal failure. Treatment: Diuretic drug or renal dialysis.	**anuria** (an-YOOR-ee-ah) **an-** *not; without* **ur/o-** *urinary system; urine* **-ia** *condition; state; thing*
bacteriuria	Presence of bacteria in the urine. Normally, urine is sterile. Bacteria indicate an infection somewhere in the urinary tract. *Note*: A urine specimen that is not collected properly can be contaminated with bacteria. Treatment: Antibiotic drug.	**bacteriuria** (BAK-teer-ih-YOOR-ee-ah) **bacteri/o-** *bacterium* **ur/o-** *urinary system; urine* **-ia** *condition; state; thing*
dysuria	Difficult or painful urination. It can be due to many factors (kidney stone, cystitis, etc.). Treatment: Correct the underlying cause.	**dysuria** (dis-YOOR-ee-ah) **dys-** *abnormal; difficult; painful* **ur/o-** *urinary system; urine* **-ia** *condition; state; thing*
enuresis	Involuntary release of urine in an otherwise normal person who should have bladder control. Nocturnal enuresis is involuntary urination during sleep. Laypersons call this *childhood bedwetting*. Treatment: Antidiuretic hormone (ADH), a pituitary gland hormone drug; psychological therapy.	**enuresis** (EN-yoor-EE-sis) **enur/o-** *urinate* **-esis** *condition; process* Add words to make a complete definition of *enuresis*: *process (that causes the patient to) urinate (involuntarily)*.
frequency	Urinating often, usually in small amounts. This can be due to a kidney stone or enlarged prostate gland blocking the urine, a urinary tract infection, or overactive bladder. Treatment: Correct the underlying cause. Frequency is present during pregnancy when the enlarging uterus limits the capacity of the bladder; this is not a disease.	
glycosuria	Glucose in the urine. This is an indication of an elevated blood sugar level, that "spills over" into the urine, as seen in diabetes mellitus. Treatment: Correct the underlying cause.	**glycosuria** (GLY-kohs-YOOR-ee-ah) **glycos/o-** *glucose; sugar* **ur/o-** *urinary system; urine* **-ia** *condition; state; thing*
hematuria	Blood in the urine. This can be gross or frank blood (easily seen with the naked eye), or it can be microscopic hematuria that can only be detected with laboratory testing. Hematuria can be caused by a kidney stone, cystitis, bladder cancer, etc. It can also be due to menstrual blood that contaminates a urine specimen. Treatment: Correct the underlying cause.	**hematuria** (HEE-mah-TYOOR-ee-ah) **hemat/o-** *blood* **ur/o-** *urinary system; urine* **-ia** *condition; state; thing*

Word or Phrase	Description	Pronunciation/Word Parts
hesitancy	Inability to initiate a normal stream of urine. There is dribbling, and the urinary stream has a decreased **caliber**. The volume of urine passed is less, and residual urine may remain in the bladder. It can be caused by blockage of the urethra by a kidney stone, a urinary tract infection, or an enlarged prostate gland. Treatment: Correct the underlying cause.	**caliber** (KAL-ih-ber)
hypokalemia	A decreased amount of potassium in the blood. It is usually due to a diuretic drug that causes the kidneys to excrete an excessive amount of urine (and potassium). Treatment: Adjust the dose of the diuretic drug.	**hypokalemia** (HY-poh-kay-LEE-mee-ah) **hypo-** *below; deficient* **kal/i-** *potassium* **-emia** *condition of the blood; substance in the blood*
incontinence	Inability to voluntarily keep urine in the bladder. It can be due to a spinal cord injury, surgery on the prostate gland, unconsciousness, or a mental condition such as dementia. Treatment: Correct the underlying cause.	**incontinence** (in-CON-tih-nens) **in-** *in; not; within* **contin/o-** *hold together* **-ence** *state* Add words to make a complete definition of *incontinence*: *state (of) not (being able to) hold together (urine in the bladder).*

ACROSS THE LIFE SPAN

Pediatrics. Incontinence of urine is normal in babies because the nerve connections to the external urethral sphincter do not develop until about 2 years of age—about the time that parents begin toilet training.

Geriatrics. Incontinence can begin as early as middle age. There is relaxation of the muscles of the pelvic floor. When the patient laughs, coughs, or sneezes, increased intra-abdominal pressure causes urine to pass. This is known as **stress incontinence**. Muscle tone can be improved by doing Kegel exercises (the perineum is alternatively tensed and relaxed), or surgery may be needed. In older adults, the bladder has a decreased capacity and does not contract as well, which leaves a postvoid residual of urine with frequency of urination. Dementia often results in incontinence.

Word or Phrase	Description	Pronunciation/Word Parts
ketonuria	Ketone bodies in the urine. Ketones are waste products produced when fat is metabolized. Ketonuria is seen in patients with diabetes mellitus who metabolize fat for energy because they cannot metabolize glucose. It is also seen in malnourished patients who do not have enough glucose in the blood and must metabolize their own body fat. Treatment: Correct the underlying cause.	**ketonuria** (KEE-toh-NYOOR-ee-ah) **keton/o-** *ketones* **ur/o-** *urinary system; urine* **-ia** *condition; state; thing*
nocturia	Increased frequency and urgency of urination during the night. It can be due to cystitis, an enlarged prostate gland, or decreased capacity of the bladder in older adults. Nocturia is expressed as the number of times the patient voids each night (for example, nocturia x3). Treatment: Correct the underlying cause.	**nocturia** (nawk-TYOOR-ee-ah) **noct/o-** *night* **ur/o-** *urinary system; urine* **-ia** *condition; state; thing*
oliguria	Decreased production of urine due to kidney failure. Dehydration can cause temporary oliguria. Treatment: Correct the underlying cause.	**oliguria** (OH-lih-GYOOR-ee-ah) **olig/o-** *few; scanty* **ur/o-** *urinary system; urine* **-ia** *condition; state; thing*

Word or Phrase	Description	Pronunciation/Word Parts
polyuria	Excessive production of urine due to diabetes mellitus or diabetes insipidus. Treatment: Correct the underlying cause.	**polyuria** (PAW-lee-YOOR-ee-ah) **poly-** *many; much* **ur/o-** *urinary system; urine* **-ia** *condition; state; thing*
pyuria	White blood cells (WBCs) in the urine, indicating a urinary tract infection. Severe pyuria can cause the urine to be cloudy or milky, or the number of white blood cells may be so few that they can be detected only by microscopic examination during a urinalysis. Treatment: Antibiotic drug.	**pyuria** (py-YOOR-ee-ah) **py/o-** *pus* **ur/o-** *urinary system; urine* **-ia** *condition; state; thing*
urgency	Strong urge to urinate and a sense of pressure in the bladder as the bladder contracts repeatedly. It is caused by obstruction from an enlarged prostate gland, a kidney stone, or inflammation from a urinary tract infection. Treatment: Correct the underlying cause.	
urinary tract infection (UTI)	Bacterial infection somewhere in the urinary tract, most often caused by *Escherichia coli* (*E. coli*), which is normally found in the intestines and rectum. Urethritis is when the infection is only in the urethra. Cystitis is when the infection is in the bladder. Pyelonephritis is when the infection is in the kidney. Because of the short length of the urethra in women and its location close to the anus, women are more prone than men to develop urinary tract infections. Catheterization can also introduce bacteria into the urinary tract. Prevention: Patients with frequent urinary tract infections may be told to drink cranberry juice (see Figure 11-14 ■) to make their urine more acidic, as bacteria prefer to grow in alkaline, not acidic, urine. Treatment: Antibiotic drug.	**infection** (in-FEK-shun) **infect/o-** *disease within* **-ion** *action; condition*

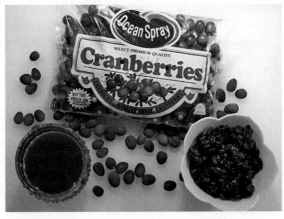

FIGURE 11-14 ■ Cranberry juice.
Patients with urinary tract infections can drink cranberry juice to make their urine more acidic. Bacteria that cause a urinary tract infection multiply rapidly in alkaline urine, but not in acidic urine. Some types of kidney stones form in alkaline urine, but not in acidic urine.
Source: Pearson Education

Laboratory and Diagnostic Procedures

Blood Tests

Word or Phrase	Description	Pronunciation/Word Parts
blood urea nitrogen (BUN)	Test that measures the amount of urea in the blood. It is used to monitor kidney function and the progression of kidney disease or to watch for signs of nephrotoxicity in patients taking aminoglycoside antibiotic drugs.	
creatinine	Test that measures the amount of creatinine in the blood. It is used to monitor kidney function and the progression of kidney disease. Creatinine with the BUN gives a comprehensive picture of kidney function.	

Urine Tests

Word or Phrase	Description	Pronunciation/Word Parts

culture and sensitivity (C&S)	Test that puts urine onto a culture medium in a Petri dish to identify the cause of a urinary tract infection (see Figure 11-15 ■). Microorganisms in the urine grow into colonies. The specific disease-causing microorganism is identified and tested to determine its sensitivity to various antibiotic drugs.	**culture** (KUL-chur)
		
		 sensitivity (SEN-sih-TIV-ih-tee)
		   sensitiv/o- *affected by; sensitive to*
		   -ity *condition; state*

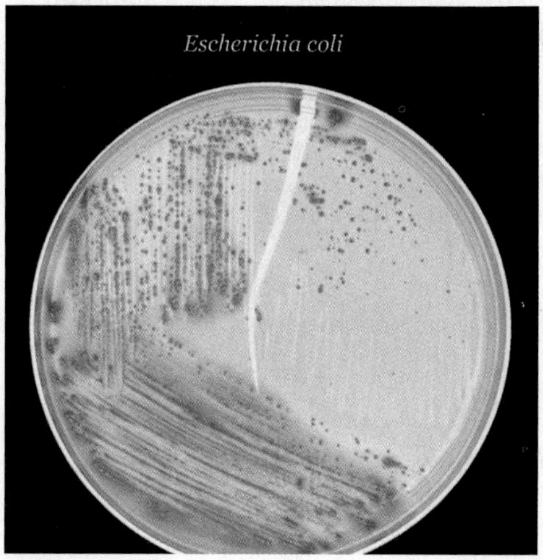

Escherichia coli

FIGURE 11-15 ■ Culture and sensitivity testing.
This Petri dish grew colonies of the bacterium *E. coli*, the most common cause of a urinary tract infection. Now that the bacterium has been identified by culture, the next step will be to do the sensitivity testing. Disks of different antibiotic drugs will be placed in a Petri dish and the bacterium allowed to grow. The antibiotic drugs that are most effective against *E. coli* will show a large zone of inhibition (clear ring) around the disk where the drug kept the bacterium from growing (see Figure 4-18). One of those antibiotic drugs will then be prescribed to treat this patient's urinary tract infection.
Source: Centers for Disease Control and Prevention

Word or Phrase	Description	Pronunciation/Word Parts
drug screening	Test performed on employees' or athletes' urine to detect any individual who is using illegal, addictive, or performance-enhancing drugs	

leukocyte esterase	Test that detects esterase, an enzyme associated with leukocytes (white blood cells) and a urinary tract infection. This urine dipstick test gives a quick result so that an antibiotic drug can be started immediately. At the same time, a urine specimen is sent for C&S.	**leukocyte** (LOO-koh-site)
		   leuk/o- *white*
		   -cyte *cell*
		
		 esterase (ES-ter-ays)

24-hour creatinine clearance	Test that collects all urine for 24 hours to measure the total amount of creatinine "cleared" (excreted) by the kidneys. The result is compared to the level of creatinine in the blood to determine kidney function.	

Word or Phrase	Description	Pronunciation/Word Parts
urinalysis (UA)	Test that describes the urine and detects substances in it. A quick urinalysis can be done with a dipstick test (see Figure 11-16 ■) or the urine specimen can be sent to a laboratory for a full analysis. 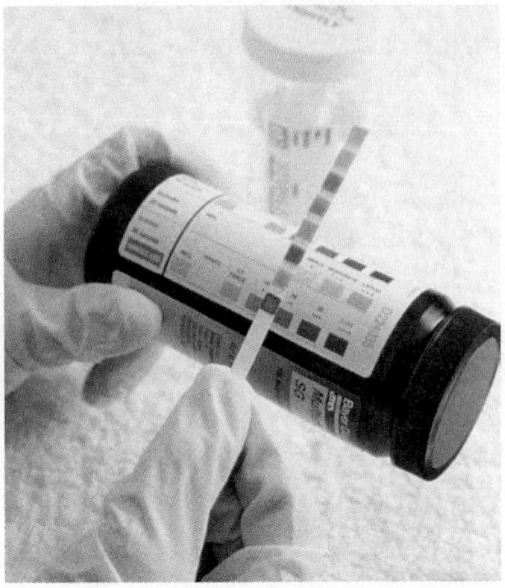 FIGURE 11-16 ■ **Urine dipstick.** This plastic strip with chemical-impregnated pads can perform several different laboratory tests (pH, protein, glucose, blood, and ketones) with a single dip in a urine specimen. The pads change color over time. The final color of each pad is compared to a chart on the back of the container that gives a range of colors and the associated test result numbers. *Source*: Faye Norman/Science Source	**urinalysis** (YOOR-ih-NAL-ih-sis) *Urinalysis* is a combination of the combining form *urin/o-* (urinary system; urine) plus a shortened form of *analysis*.
color	Normal urine is light yellow to amber in color, depending on its concentration. Pink or smoky-colored urine indicates red blood cells from bleeding in the urinary tract. **Turbid** (cloudy or milky) urine indicates white blood cells and a urinary tract infection. The urinary analgesic drug phenazopyridine (Pyridium, Urogesic) turns the urine bright orange.	**turbid** (TUR-bid)
odor	Urine has a faint odor due to the waste products in it. The urine of a patient with uncontrolled diabetes mellitus has a fruity smell because of the glucose in it. When urine stands at room temperature, bacteria from the air grow in it, breaking down the urea into ammonia; this gives old urine its characteristic smell.	
pH	A test of how **acidic** or **alkaline** the urine is. Acidic urine has a pH lower than 7. Alkaline urine has a pH higher than 7. Urine is normally slightly alkaline. Bacteria grow quickly and some types of kidney stones form more readily in alkaline urine.	**pH** (pee-H) **acidic** (ah-SID-ik) **acid/o-** *acid; low pH* **-ic** *pertaining to* **alkaline** (AL-kah-line) **alkal/o-** *base; high pH* **-ine** *pertaining to*
protein	Protein (or albumin) is not normally found in urine. Its presence (proteinuria or albuminuria) indicates damage to the glomerulus.	**protein** (PROH-teen)
glucose	Glucose is not normally found in urine. Its presence (glycosuria) indicates uncontrolled diabetes mellitus, with excess glucose in the blood "spilling" over into the urine.	**glucose** (GLOO-kohs)
red blood cells (RBCs)	Microscopic examination of urine under high-power magnification to count the number of erythrocytes (red blood cells). Even clear urine can contain **occult (hidden) blood**. This microscopic hematuria is reported as the number of RBCs per high-power field (hpf). If the urine has visible blood, the red blood cell count is reported as "TNTC" (too numerous to count). Menstrual blood can give a false-positive result of blood in the urine.	**occult** (oh-KULT)
white blood cells (WBCs)	Microscopic examination of urine under high-power magnification to count the number of leukocytes (white blood cells) to identify a urinary tract infection. If the specimen is milky or cloudy, the white blood cell count is reported as "TNTC."	

Word or Phrase	Description	Pronunciation/Word Parts
ketones	Ketones are not normally found in urine. They are produced when the body cannot use (or does not have enough) glucose and instead metabolizes fat. It is seen in patients with uncontrolled diabetes mellitus, malnutrition, or in marathon runners.	**ketones** (KEE-tohnz)
specific gravity (SG)	Measurement of the concentration of the urine as compared to that of water (specific gravity 1.000). Dilute (not concentrated) urine has a specific gravity of 1.005, while concentrated urine is 1.030. Above 1.030 means the patient is dehydrated. Instruments used to measure specific gravity include a **urinometer** (see Figure 11-17 ■) or a **refractometer**, a handheld instrument that uses light rays that are bent (refracted) by a thin layer of urine spread on glass.	**urinometer** (YOOR-ih-NAW-meh-ter) **urin/o-** *urinary system; urine* **-meter** *instrument used to measure* **refractometer** (REE-frak-TAW-meh-ter) **re-** *again and again; backward; unable to* **fract/o-** *bend; break up* **-meter** *instrument used to measure* Add words to make a complete definition of *refractometer*: *instrument used to measure again and again (the) bend(ing of light rays in urine).*

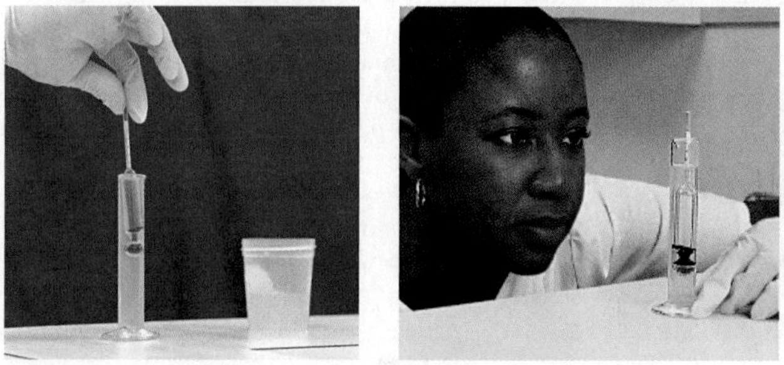

FIGURE 11-17 ■ Urinometer.
This test tube–like container holds the urine. A calibrated glass weight floats higher or lower, depending on the specific gravity of the urine. The specific gravity is the number where the surface of the urine touches the calibrated scale on the narrowed top of the glass float.
Source: Susan M. Turley

Word or Phrase	Description	Pronunciation/Word Parts
sediment	There are several types of sediment in the urine. Crystals (calcium oxalate, uric acid, etc.) can become a kidney stone. Casts are protein molecules (**hyaline casts**) or blood (red cell casts) that is molded by the cylindrical shape of the tubules. Epithelial cells are normal in urine sediment because they are shed continuously from the lining of the urinary tract.	**hyaline** (HY-ah-lin) **hyal/o-** *clear, glass-like substance* **-ine** *pertaining to; thing pertaining to*
other substances	Chemical compounds whose presence helps to diagnose certain disease conditions. Vanillylmandelic acid (VMA) is seen in pheochromocytoma and neuroblastoma, while 5-HIAA is seen in carcinoid syndrome.	
urine protein electrophoresis (UPEP)	Test that uses electricity to move substances in a gel. Detects immunoglobulins and Bence-Jones protein, an abnormal protein in the urine of patients with the cancer multiple myeloma.	**electrophoresis** (ee-LEK-troh-foh-REE-sis) **electr/o-** *electricity* **phor/o-** *bear; carry; range* **-esis** *condition; process* Add words to make a complete definition of *electrophoresis*: *process (of using) electricity (to) carry (immunoglobulins in a gel).*

Radiology and Nuclear Medicine Procedures

Word or Phrase	Description	Pronunciation/Word Parts
intravenous pyelography (IVP)	Procedure that uses x-rays and radiopaque contrast dye (see Figure 11-18 ■). The dye is injected intravenously and flows through the blood and into the kidneys. It outlines the renal pelves, ureters, bladder, and urethra. It shows any obstruction, blockage, kidney stone, or abnormal anatomy in the urinary tract. It is also known as an **excretory urography**. The x-ray image is known as a **pyelogram** or **urogram**. Alternatively, **retrograde pyelography** can be done in which a cystoscopy is performed and a catheter is advanced into the ureter and dye is injected. The dye outlines the ureter, as well as the pelvis and calices of the kidney. **FIGURE 11-18 ■ Intravenous pyelogram.** In this color-enhanced image, contrast dye has outlined the calices and renal pelvis of each kidney and on to the ureters and bladder. This is a normal pyelogram with no evidence of tumor, obstruction, or kidney stone. *Source*: Cnri/Science Source	**intravenous** (IN-trah-VEE-nus) **intra-** *within* **ven/o-** *vein* **-ous** *pertaining to* **pyelography** (PY-eh-LAW-grah-fee) **pyel/o-** *renal pelvis* **-graphy** *process of recording* **excretory** (EKS-kreh-TOR-ee) (eks-KREE-tor-ee) **excret/o-** *removing from the body* **-ory** *having the function of* **urography** (yoor-AW-grah-fee) **ur/o-** *urinary system; urine* **-graphy** *process of recording* **pyelogram** (PY-eh-loh-GRAM) **pyel/o-** *renal pelvis* **-gram** *picture; record* **urogram** (YOOR-oh-gram) **ur/o-** *urinary system; urine* **-gram** *picture; record* **retrograde** (REH-troh-grayd) **retro-** *backward; behind* **-grade** *pertaining to going* The ending *-grade* contains the combining form *grad/o-* and the single-letter suffix *–e*.
kidneys, ureters, bladder (KUB) x-ray	Procedure that uses an x-ray of the kidneys, ureters, and bladder done without contrast dye. It is used to find kidney stones or as a preliminary x-ray (scout film) before performing intravenous pyelography.	
nephrotomography	Procedure that uses a computerized tomography (CT) scan and radiopaque contrast dye injected intravenously. It takes x-ray images as multiple "slices" through the kidneys. The images can be examined layer by layer to show the exact location of tumors.	**nephrotomography** (NEH-froh-toh-MAW-grah-fee) **nephr/o-** *kidney; nephron* **tom/o-** *cut; layer; slice* **-graphy** *process of recording*
renal angiography	Procedure that uses x-rays and radiopaque contrast dye. The dye is injected intravenously and flows through the blood into the renal artery. It outlines the renal artery and shows any obstruction or blockage. It is also known as **renal arteriography**. The x-ray image is known as a **renal angiogram** or **renal arteriogram**.	**angiography** (AN-jee-AW-grah-fee) **angi/o-** *blood vessel; lymphatic vessel* **-graphy** *process of recording* **arteriography** (ar-TEER-ee-AW-grah-fee) **arteri/o-** *artery* **-graphy** *process of recording* **angiogram** (AN-jee-oh-GRAM) **angi/o-** *blood vessel; lymphatic vessel* **-gram** *picture; record* **arteriogram** (ar-TEER-ee-oh-GRAM) **arteri/o-** *artery* **-gram** *picture; record*

Word or Phrase	Description	Pronunciation/Word Parts
renal scan	Procedure that uses a radioactive isotope injected intravenously. It is taken up by the kidney and emits radioactive particles that are captured by a scanner and made into an image. It is performed after a kidney transplantation to look for signs of organ rejection.	
ultrasonography	Procedure that uses ultra high-frequency sound waves emitted by a transducer or probe to produce an image of the kidneys, ureters, or bladder. The ultrasound image is known as a **sonogram** (see Figure 11-19 ■). FIGURE 11-19 ■ Sonogram. The ultrasound image on the left shows a kidney stone, as designated by the arrow. *Source*: Puwadol Jaturawutthichai/Shutterstock	**ultrasonography** (UL-trah-soh-NAW-grah-fee) **ultra-** *beyond; higher* **son/o-** *sound* **-graphy** *process of recording* **sonogram** (SAW-noh-gram) **son/o-** *sound* **-gram** *picture; record*

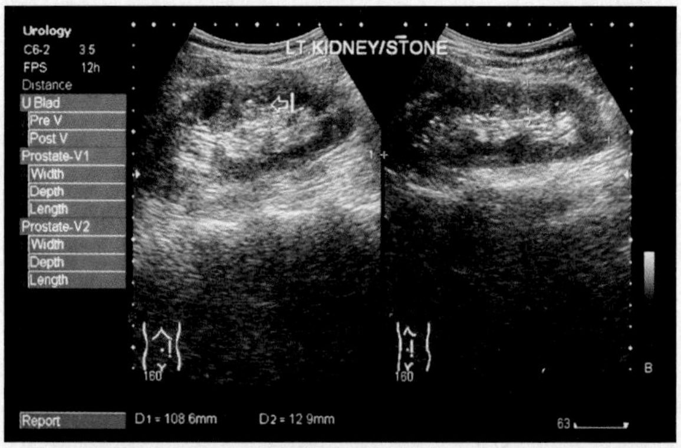

<table>
<tr><th colspan="3" align="center">Other Diagnostic Tests</th></tr>
<tr><td>cystometry</td><td>Procedure that evaluates the function of the nerves to the bladder. A catheter is used to inflate the bladder with liquid (or gas). A cystometer attached to the catheter measures the amount of liquid and the pressure in the bladder. The patient indicates when the first urge to urinate occurs. At that time, the cystometer makes a graphic recording known as a cystometrogram (CMG).</td><td>cystometry (sis-TAW-meh-tree)
cyst/o- bladder; fluid-filled sac; semisolid cyst
-metry process of measuring

cystometer (sis-TAW-meh-ter)
cyst/o- bladder; fluid-filled sac; semisolid cyst
-meter instrument used to measure

cystometrogram
(SIS-toh-MEH-troh-gram)
cyst/o- bladder; fluid-filled sac; semisolid cyst
metr/o- measurement; uterus; womb
-gram picture; record</td></tr>
<tr><td>voiding cystourethrography (VCUG)</td><td>Procedure that uses x-rays and radiopaque contrast dye. The dye, which is inserted into the bladder through a catheter, outlines the bladder and urethra. The x-ray image, taken while the patient is urinating, is known as a voiding cystourethrogram.</td><td>cystourethrography
(SIS-toh-YOOR-eh-THRAW-grah-fee)
cyst/o- bladder; fluid-filled sac; semisolid cyst
urethr/o- urethra
-graphy process of recording

cystourethrogram
(SIS-toh-yoor-EE-throh-gram)
cyst/o- bladder; fluid-filled sac; semisolid cyst
urethr/o- urethra
-gram picture; record</td></tr>
</table>

Medical and Surgical Procedures

Medical Procedures		
Word or Phrase	**Description**	**Pronunciation/Word Parts**
catheterization	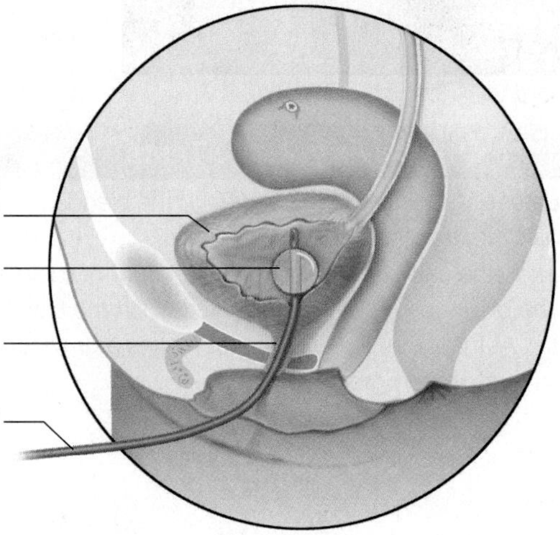 Procedure in which a **catheter** (flexible tube) is inserted through the urethra and into the bladder to drain the urine (see Figure 11-20 ■). A straight catheter is inserted each time the bladder becomes full, or it can also be used to obtain a single urine specimen for testing. A **Foley catheter** is an indwelling tube that drains urine continuously. It has an expandable balloon tip that keeps it positioned in the bladder. A **suprapubic catheter** is inserted through the abdominal wall (just above the pubic bone) and into the bladder. It is sometimes inserted after bladder or prostate gland surgery. A **condom catheter** is shaped like a condom (male contraceptive device). It fits snugly over the penis and collects the urine as it leaves the urethral meatus. Foley, suprapubic, and condom catheters are connected to a urine-collecting bag (see Figure 11-22).	**catheterization** (KATH-eh-TER-ih-ZAY-shun) **catheter/o-** *catheter* **-ization** *process of creating; process of inserting; process of making* **catheter** (KATH-eh-ter) **Foley** (FOH-lee) **suprapubic** (soo-prah-PYOO-bik) **supra-** *above* **pub/o-** *hip bone; pubis* **-ic** *pertaining to* **condom** (CON-dom)

FIGURE 11-20 ■ Foley catheter.
The inflated balloon at the tip of the Foley catheter holds it in place in the bladder. The catheter continuously drains urine from the bladder, and the urine is collected in a drainage bag.
Source: Pearson Education

Labels: Urinary bladder, Inflated balloon, Urethra, Foley catheter

Word or Phrase	Description	Pronunciation/Word Parts

dialysis	Procedure to remove waste products from the blood of a patient in renal failure. Patients undergo dialysis several times a week while waiting for a kidney transplantation. There are two types: hemodialysis and peritoneal dialysis. **Hemodialysis** uses a shunt or a fistula to allow easy and reliable access to the blood (see Figure 11-21 ■). A shunt (surgically implanted internal and external tubing) is used when a patient's blood vessels are small. A fistula is created by surgically joining an artery and vein. After surgery, the fistula enlarges to accommodate two needles, one that removes blood and sends it to the dialysis machine and another that receives purified blood from the dialysis machine and returns it to the body. **Peritoneal dialysis** uses a permanent catheter inserted through the abdominal wall. **Dialysate fluid** flows through the catheter and remains in the abdominal cavity for several hours. During that time, the fluid pulls body wastes from the blood. Then the fluid is removed, carrying waste products with it. In **continuous ambulatory peritoneal dialysis (CAPD)**, the patient is able to walk around between the three or four daily episodes of dialysis. In **continuous cycling peritoneal dialysis (CCPD)**, a machine inserts and removes dialysate fluid several times a night while the patient sleeps.	**dialysis** (dy-AL-ih-sis)
		   dia- *complete; completely through*
		   ly/o- *break down; destroy*
		   -sis *condition; process*
		 Add words to make a complete definition of *dialysis*: *process (of a) complete break(ing) down (of body wastes)*.
		
		 hemodialysis
		 (HEE-moh-dy-AL-ih-sis)
		   hem/o- *blood*
		   dia- *complete; completely through*
		   ly/o- *break down; destroy*
		   -sis *condition; process*
		
		 peritoneal (PAIR-ih-toh-NEE-al)
		   peritone/o- *peritoneum*
		   -al *pertaining to*
		
		 dialysate (dy-AL-ih-sayt)
		   dia- *complete; completely through*
		   lys/o- *break down; destroy*
		   -ate *composed of; pertaining to*
		
		 ambulatory (AM-byoo-lah-TOR-ee)
		   ambulat/o- *walking*
		   -ory *having the function of*

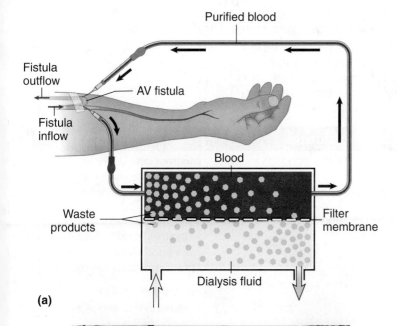

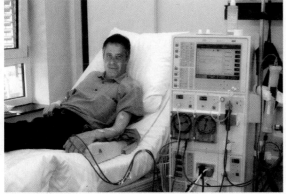

FIGURE 11-21 ■ **Hemodialysis.**
(a) A dialysis machine pumps blood through tubing whose wall is a selectively permeable membrane. Dialysate fluid surrounds the tubing. Wastes and excess amounts of electrolytes and glucose move from an area of higher concentration (the blood) to an area of lower concentration (dialysate fluid). The cleansed blood is pumped back through the shunt or fistula to the patient. (b) This patient is undergoing hemodialysis. He comes to the dialysis center three times a week, and each session takes 3–5 hours to complete.
Source: Pearson Education; Gopixa/Shutterstock

Word or Phrase	Description	Pronunciation/Word Parts
intake and output (I&O)	Nursing procedure that documents the total amount of fluid intake (oral, nasogastric tube, intravenous line, etc.) and the total amount of fluid output (urine, wound drainage, etc.) (see Figure 11-22 ■). It is used to monitor the body's fluid balance in patients with renal failure, burns, congestive heart failure, large draining wounds, dehydration, overdose of diuretic drugs, etc. **FIGURE 11-22 ■ Urine output.** This nurse is measuring the urine output from a patient who has an indwelling Foley catheter that continuously drains urine into a collecting bag. The volume of a liquid (urine) is measured in cubic centimeters (cc) or milliliters (mL). *Source*: Pearson Education	
urine specimen	Procedure to obtain a urine specimen for testing. Urine specimens can be tested in the doctor's office with a dipstick (see Figure 11-16). A clean-caught specimen (the urethral meatus is first cleansed) or a catheterized specimen (obtained directly from a catheter) is placed in a sterile container and sent to a laboratory for culture and sensitivity testing. An improperly obtained urine specimen can be contaminated with bacteria or menstrual blood and give incorrect results.	

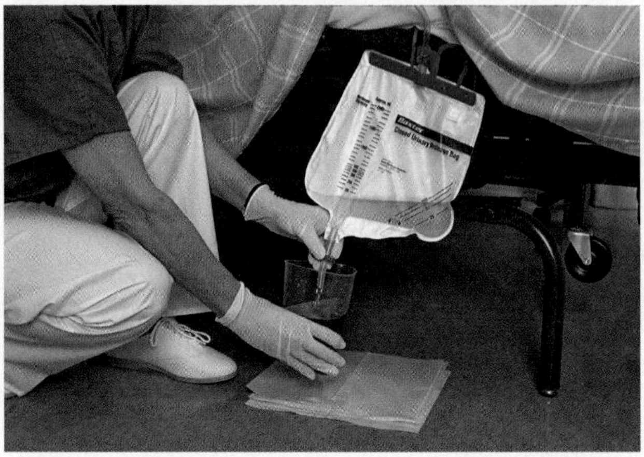

Surgical Procedures

Word or Phrase	Description	Pronunciation/Word Parts
bladder neck suspension	Procedure to correct stress urinary incontinence. A supportive sling of muscle tissue or synthetic material is inserted around the base of the bladder and the urethra to elevate them to a normal position.	**suspension** (sus-PEN-shun) **suspens/o-** *hanging* **-ion** *action; condition*
cystectomy	Procedure to remove the bladder because of bladder cancer. A **radical cystectomy** removes the bladder, surrounding tissues, and lymph nodes.	**cystectomy** (sis-TEK-toh-mee) **cyst/o-** *bladder; fluid-filled sac; semisolid cyst* **-ectomy** *surgical removal* **radical** (RAD-ih-kal) **radic/o-** *root and all parts* **-al** *pertaining to*

Word or Phrase	Description	Pronunciation/Word Parts
cystoscopy	Procedure that uses a rigid or flexible **cystoscope** inserted through the urethra in order to examine the inside of the bladder (see Figure 11-23 ■). A wide-angle lens and a light allow a full view of the bladder. A video attachment can be used to create a permanent visual record.	**cystoscopy** (sis-TAW-skoh-pee) **cyst/o-** *bladder; fluid-filled sac; semisolid cyst* **-scopy** *process of using an instrument to examine* **cystoscope** (SIS-toh-skohp) **cyst/o-** *bladder; fluid-filled sac; semisolid cyst* **-scope** *instrument used to examine*

DID YOU KNOW?
Cystoscopes have been used since the early 1800s. Because this was before the invention of the light bulb, early cystoscopes used a platinum wire that glowed when an electrical current ran through it to illuminate the inside of the bladder.

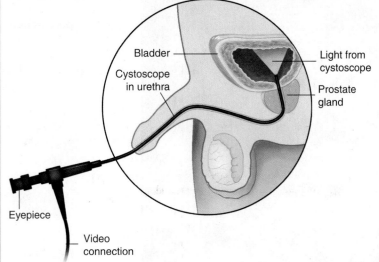

Bladder
Cystoscope in urethra
Light from cystoscope
Prostate gland
Eyepiece
Video connection

FIGURE 11-23 ■ Cystoscopy.
The cystoscope is a flexible tube that is inserted through the urethra and into the bladder. It has a viewing eyepiece and a light to illuminate the inside of the bladder.
Source: Pearson Education

| **kidney transplantation** | Procedure to remove a severely damaged kidney from a patient with end-stage kidney failure and insert a new kidney from a donor. The patient (the recipient) is matched by blood type and tissue type to the **donor**. The patient's diseased kidney is removed and the donor kidney is sutured in place (see Figure 11-24 ■). Kidney transplantation patients must take an immunosuppressant drug for the rest of their lives to keep their bodies from rejecting their new kidney. | **transplantation** (TRANS-plan-TAY-shun) **transplant/o-** *move something across and put in another place* **-ation** *being; having; process*

donor (DOH-nor) |

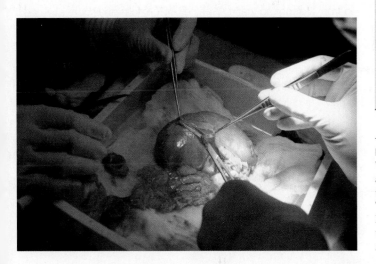

DID YOU KNOW?
The first successful kidney transplant occurred in 1954 in the United States between identical twins. It was not until FDA approval of the antirejection immunosuppressant drug cyclosporine in 1984 that transplantation of kidneys from cadavers or unrelated living donors could be performed successfully. In 2015, there were over 100,000 patients waiting for kidney transplantations.

FIGURE 11-24 ■ Kidney transplantation.
When it was donated, this kidney was flushed with a cold solution and kept on ice to preserve it. Now, it is in a basin, being prepared for transplantation. The patient's diseased kidney was already removed. The surgeons will suture the renal artery and vein of the donor kidney to the patient's iliac artery and vein in the pelvic cavity. The ureter of the donor kidney will be sutured to the patient's bladder.
Source: Owen Franken/Terra/Corbis

Word or Phrase	Description	Pronunciation/Word Parts
lithotripsy	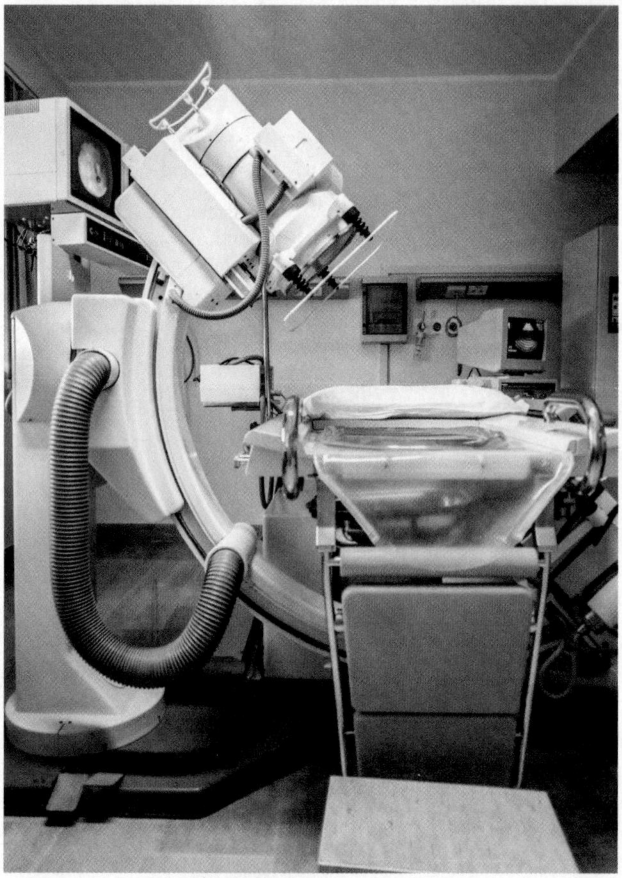 Procedure that uses sound waves to break up a kidney stone (see Figure 11-25 ■). After an x-ray pinpoints the location of the stone, a **lithotriptor** generates sound waves that break up the stone. Because the sound waves are generated by a source outside the body, the procedure is known as **extracorporeal shock wave lithotripsy (ESWL)**. In the surgical procedure **percutaneous ultrasonic lithotripsy**, an endoscope is inserted through the flank skin and into the kidney. A lithotriptor probe is inserted through the endoscope and into the kidney to break up large stones. Sometimes a laser beam is used to break up very hard kidney stones.	**lithotripsy** (LITH-oh-TRIP-see) **lith/o-** *stone* **-tripsy** *process of crushing* **lithotriptor** (LITH-oh-TRIP-tor) **lith/o-** *stone* **-triptor** *thing that crushes* **extracorporeal** (EKS-trah-kor-POOR-ee-al) **extra-** *outside* **corpor/o-** *body* **-eal** *pertaining to* **percutaneous** (PER-kyoo-TAY-nee-us) **per-** *through; throughout* **cutane/o-** *skin* **-ous** *pertaining to* **ultrasonic** (UL-trah-SAW-nik) **ultra-** *beyond; higher* **son/o-** *sound* **-ic** *pertaining to*

FIGURE 11-25 ■ Lithotripsy.
The patient lies on a table or is immersed in a tank of water. The lithotriptor emits ultrasonic frequencies that create shock waves to break up a kidney stone. The urologist watches the process on a computer screen.
Source: Dario Lo Presti/Fotolia

Word or Phrase	Description	Pronunciation/Word Parts
nephrectomy	Procedure to surgically remove a diseased or cancerous kidney. Alternatively, a healthy kidney may be removed from a donor so that it can be transplanted into a patient with renal failure.	**nephrectomy** (neh-FREK-toh-mee) **nephr/o-** *kidney; nephron* **-ectomy** *surgical removal*
nephrolithotomy	Procedure in which a small incision is made in the skin and an endoscope is inserted in a percutaneous approach into the kidney to remove a kidney stone embedded in the renal pelvis or calices.	**nephrolithotomy** (NEH-froh-lith-AW-toh-mee) **nephr/o-** *kidney; nephron* **lith/o-** *stone* **-tomy** *process of cutting; process of making an incision*
nephropexy	Procedure to correct a kidney that is in an abnormally low position (nephroptosis) by suturing it back into anatomical position.	**nephropexy** (NEH-froh-PEK-see) **nephr/o-** *kidney; nephron* **-pexy** *process of surgically fixing in place*

Word or Phrase	Description	Pronunciation/Word Parts
renal biopsy	Procedure in which a small piece of kidney is excised for microscopic analysis. This is done to confirm or exclude a diagnosis of cancer or kidney disease.	**biopsy** (BY-awp-see) **bi/o-** *life; living organism; living tissue* **-opsy** *process of viewing*
stone basketing	Procedure in which a cystoscope is inserted into the bladder. A stone basket (a long-handled instrument with several interwoven wires at its end) is then passed through the cystoscope to snare a kidney stone and remove it.	
transurethral resection of a bladder tumor (TURBT)	Procedure to remove a bladder tumor from inside the bladder. A special cystoscope known as a **resectoscope** is inserted through the urethra into the bladder. It has built-in instruments that resect the bladder tumor, cauterize bleeding blood vessels, and use irrigating fluid to flush pieces of tissue out of the bladder.	**transurethral** (TRANS-yoor-EE-thral) **trans-** *across; through* **urethr/o-** *urethra* **-al** *pertaining to* **resection** (ree-SEK-shun) **resect/o-** *cut out; remove* **-ion** *action; condition* **resectoscope** (ree-SEK-toh-skohp) **resect/o-** *cut out; remove* **-scope** *instrument used to examine*
urethroplasty	Procedure that involves plastic surgery to reposition the urethral meatus. It is used to correct congenital hypospadias or epispadias.	**urethroplasty** (yoor-EE-throh-PLAS-tee) **urethr/o-** *urethra* **-plasty** *process of reshaping by surgery*

Drugs

These drug categories and drugs are used to treat urinary diseases. The most common generic and trade name drugs in each category are listed.

Category	Indication	Examples	Pronunciation/Word Parts
antibiotic drugs	Used to treat urinary tract infections. These urinary antibiotic drugs have a special affinity for the urinary tract, although other categories of antibiotic drugs are also used to treat urinary tract infections.	nitrofurantoin (Macrobid, Macrodantin)	**antibiotic** (AN-tee-by-AW-tik) (AN-tih-by-AW-tik) **anti-** *against* **bi/o-** *life; living organism; living tissue* **-tic** *pertaining to*
	CLINICAL CONNECTIONS **Pharmacology.** Aminoglycoside antibiotic drugs can cause a severe, **nephrotoxic** effect on the kidneys. Patients taking these drugs have their kidney function monitored by periodic BUN and creatinine tests.		**nephrotoxic** (NEH-froh-TAWK-sik) **nephr/o-** *kidney; nephron* **tox/o-** *poison* **-ic** *pertaining to*
antispasmodic drugs	Relax the smooth muscle in the walls of the ureter, bladder, and urethra. Used to treat spasm from cystitis and overactive bladder.	hyoscyamine (Cystospaz)	**antispasmodic** (AN-tee-spaz-MAW-dik) **anti-** *against* **spasmod/o-** *spasm* **-ic** *pertaining to*
diuretic drugs	Block sodium from being reabsorbed from the tubule into the blood. As the sodium is excreted in the urine, it brings water and potassium with it because of osmotic pressure. This process is known as *diuresis*. This decreases the volume of blood and is used to treat hypertension, congestive heart failure, and nephrotic syndrome.	furosemide (Lasix), hydrochlorothiazide (HCTZ)	**diuretic** (DY-yoor-EH-tik) **dia-** *complete; completely through* **ur/o-** *urinary system; urine* **-etic** *pertaining to* The "*a*" in *dia-* is deleted when the word is formed.
drugs for overactive bladder	Block the action of acetylcholine and decrease contractions of the smooth muscle of the bladder	solifenacin (Vesicare), tolterodine (Detrol)	
potassium supplements	Used as a replacement for potassium lost due to diuretic drugs. (Diuretic drugs increase sodium excretion but also potassium excretion because they are both positively charged electrolytes.) The presence of *K* in the drug name refers to the chemical symbol for potassium K^+).	potassium (K-Dur, K-Tab)	
urinary analgesic drugs	Exert a pain-relieving effect on the mucosa of the urinary tract	phenazopyridine (Pyridium, Urogesic)	**analgesic** (AN-al-JEE-zik) **an-** *not; without* **alges/o-** *sensation of pain* **-ic** *pertaining to*

Abbreviations

ADH	antidiuretic hormone	**I&O**	intake and output
ARF	acute renal failure	**IVP**	intravenous pyelogram; intravenous pyelography
BUN	blood urea nitrogen	**K, K⁺**	potassium
C&S	culture and sensitivity	**KUB**	kidneys, ureters, bladder
CAPD	continuous ambulatory peritoneal dialysis	**mL**	milliliter (measure of volume)
cath	catheterize or catheterization (short form)	**Na⁺**	sodium
cc*■	cubic centimeter (measure of volume)	**pH**	potential of hydrogen (acid or alkaline)
CCPD	continuous cycling peritoneal dialysis	**RBC**	red blood cell
Cl⁻	chloride	**SG, sp gr**	specific gravity
CMG	cystometrogram	**TNTC**	too numerous to count
CRF	chronic renal failure	**TURBT**	transurethral resection of bladder tumor
CT	computerized tomography	**UA**	urinalysis
cysto	cystoscopy (short form)	**UPEP**	urine protein electrophoresis (pronounced "U-pep")
epis	epithelial cells (in the urine specimen) (short form)	**UTI**	urinary tract infection
ESRD	end-stage renal disease	**VCUG**	voiding cystourethrogram; voiding cystourethrography
ESWL	extracorporeal shock wave lithotripsy	**VMA**	vanillylmandelic acid
GU	genitourinary gonococcal urethritis	**WBC**	white blood cell
HCO₃⁻	bicarbonate		
HCTZ	hydrochlorothiazide (drug)		
hpf	high-power field		

*According to The Joint Commission or ■ the Institute for Safe Medication Practices (ISMP), this abbreviation should not be used. However, because it is still used by some healthcare professionals, it is included here.

WORD ALERT
Abbreviations

Abbreviations are commonly used in all types of medical documents; however, they can mean different things to different people and their meanings can be misinterpreted. Always verify the meaning of an abbreviation.

ARF means *acute renal failure*, but it also means *acute respiratory failure* or *acute rheumatic fever*.

C&S means *culture and sensitivity*, but the sound-alike word *CNS* means *central nervous system*.

CRF means *chronic renal failure*, but it also means *cardiac risk factors*.

GU means *genitourinary*, but it also means *gonococcal urethritis*.

IT'S GREEK TO ME!

Did you notice that some words have two different combining forms? Combining forms from both Greek and Latin remain a part of medical language today.

Word	Greek	Latin	Medical Word Examples
bladder	cyst/o-	vesic/o-	cystitis, vesicovaginal
kidney	nephr/o-	ren/o-	nephritis, renal
(kidney) stone	lith/o-	calcul/o-	lithotripsy, calculogenesis
urinate, making urine, or urine	enur/o- urin/o- ur/o-	micturi/o-	enuresis, micturition, urination; urology
renal pelvis	pyel/o-	pelv/o-	pyelonephritis, renal pelvis

CAREER FOCUS

Meet Cindy, a dialysis nurse

"I came into dialysis because my brother actually was on dialysis for a very long time, and it was something I thought would be interesting. The dialysis center let me come in and let me observe for a few hours, and I found that was also very fascinating. I had already been a nurse for over eight years. This dialysis center gave me all the on-the-job training. It was just a whole different field. You really get to know your patients. You do have the time to actually sit down and talk to them. The majority of our patients have hypertension or they have diabetes, so we do a lot of diabetic teaching."

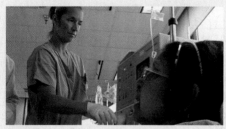

Source: Pearson Education

Dialysis nurses are allied health professionals who work in dialysis centers. They specialize in caring for patients with end-stage kidney disease who are receiving dialysis.

Urologists are physicians who practice in the specialty of urology. They diagnose and treat patients with diseases of the urinary tract. Some urologists further specialize and become **nephrologists** who only treat patients with kidney disease. Physicians can take additional training and become board certified in the subspecialty of pediatric nephrology. Cancerous tumors of the urinary tract are treated medically by an oncologist or surgically by a urologist or a general surgeon.

urologist (yoor-AW-loh-jist)
  ur/o- *urinary system; urine*
  log/o- *study of; word*
  -ist *person who specializes in*

nephrologist (neh-FRAW-loh-jist)
  nephr/o- *kidney; nephron*
  log/o- *study of; word*
  -ist *person who specializes in*

MyMedicalTerminologyLab™ To see Cindy's complete video profile, log into MyMedicalTerminologyLab and navigate to the Multimedia Library for Chapter 11. Check the Video box, and then click the Career Focus - Dialysis Nurse link.

Word Part	Meaning	Word Part	Meaning
11. blast/o-		53. leuk/o-	
12. calcul/o-		54. lith/o-	
13. cancer/o-		55. ly/o-	
14. carcin/o-		56. lys/o-	
15. catheter/o-		57. -meter	
16. -cele		58. -metry	
17. chron/o-		59. necr/o-	
18. col/o-		60. neur/o-	
19. contin/o-		61. noct/o-	
20. cyst/o-		62. olig/o-	
21. -cyte		63. -oma	
22. dia-		64. -ory	
23. dys-		65. -osis	
24. -ectasis		66. -pathy	
25. -ectomy		67. -pexy	
26. -emia		68. -plasty	
27. -ence		69. poly-	
28. enur/o-		70. protein/o-	
29. epi-		71. -ptosis	
30. -esis		72. pub/o-	
31. fract/o-		73. py/o-	
32. gen/o-		74. re-	
33. glycos/o-		75. retent/o-	
34. -gram		76. scler/o-	
35. -graphy		77. -scope	
36. hemat/o-		78. -scopy	
37. hem/o-		79. sensitiv/o-	
38. hyal/o-		80. -sis	
39. hydr/o-		81. son/o-	
40. hypo-		82. spad/o-	
41. -ia		83. spasmod/o-	
42. -iasis		84. super-	
43. in-		85. tom/o-	
44. infect/o-		86. -tomy	
45. interstiti/o-		87. tox/o-	
46. intra-		88. trans-	
47. -ion		89. transplant/o-	
48. -itis		90. -tripsy	
49. -ity		91. -triptor	
50. -ization		92. ultra-	
51. kal/i-		93. vagin/o-	
52. keton/o-			

RELATED COMBINING FORMS EXERCISE

Write the combining forms on the line provided. (Hint: See the It's Greek to Me feature box.)

1. Two combining forms that mean *bladder*. _____

2. Two combining forms that mean *kidney*. _____

3. Two combining forms that mean *(kidney) stone*. _____

4. Two combining forms that mean *renal pelvis*. _____

5. Four combining forms that mean *to urinate, making urine, or urine*. _____

11.5B Define Abbreviations

DEFINE AND MATCH EXERCISE

Give the definition for each abbreviation listed below, then match it to its description.

1. BUN _____ _____ X-ray image of the kidneys after injection of dye

2. cc _____ _____ Test to determine what is causing a UTI and how to treat it

3. CRF _____ _____ Long-term decrease in kidney function

4. C&S _____ _____ Presence of this cell in the urine means infection

5. ESWL _____ _____ X-ray of the kidneys, ureters, and bladder

6. I&O _____ _____ Unit of measurement of volume of urine

7. IVP _____ _____ Used when there are too many cells to count

8. K _____ _____ Blood test that measures kidney function

9. KUB _____ _____ Measures consumption and excretion of fluids

10. TNTC _____ _____ Includes multiple tests done on one urine specimen

11. UA _____ _____ An electrolyte

12. WBC _____ _____ Shock waves that dissolve kidney stones

11.6A Divide Medical Words

DIVIDING WORDS EXERCISE

Separate these words into their component parts (prefix, combining form, suffix). Note: Some words do not contain all three word parts. The first one has been done for you.

Medical Word	Prefix	Combining Form	Suffix	Medical Word	Prefix	Combining Form	Suffix
1. retroperitoneal	retro-	peritone/o-	-al	7. vesicocele	_____	_____	_____
2. excretory	_____	_____	_____	8. epispadias	_____	_____	_____
3. electrolyte	_____	_____	_____	9. dysuria	_____	_____	_____
4. reabsorption	_____	_____	_____	10. cystectomy	_____	_____	_____
5. nephropathy	_____	_____	_____	11. catheterization	_____	_____	_____
6. polycystic	_____	_____	_____	12. transurethral	_____	_____	_____

11.9 Analyze Medical Reports

ELECTRONIC PATIENT RECORD

This is an Emergency Department Report. Read the report and answer the questions.

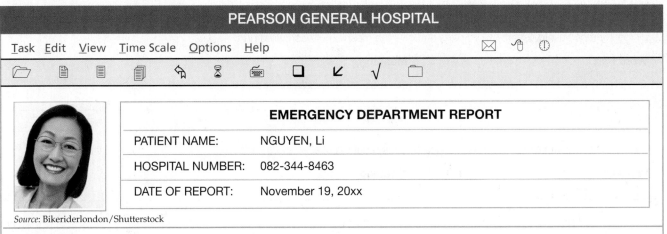

PEARSON GENERAL HOSPITAL

Task Edit View Time Scale Options Help

EMERGENCY DEPARTMENT REPORT

PATIENT NAME:	NGUYEN, Li
HOSPITAL NUMBER:	082-344-8463
DATE OF REPORT:	November 19, 20xx

Source: Bikeriderlondon/Shutterstock

CHIEF COMPLAINT
This 40-year-old female presented to the emergency department with complaints of abdominal pain, nausea, and vomiting.

HISTORY OF PRESENT ILLNESS
The patient had been seen 3 days earlier in the office of her primary care physician for a complaint of pressure and pain in the urethra. She was given a tentative diagnosis of urinary tract infection. The physician ordered a clean-catch urine specimen, and the patient provided this to a nearby laboratory. The patient was given a prescription for the antibiotic drug Bactrim and the urinary analgesic drug Pyridium. She was told to call the office in 3 days for the result of the urine culture.

The patient states that, even though she was on the antibiotic drug, her symptoms worsened over the next 48 hours. She was taking Pyridium regularly, as well as Extra Strength Tylenol, and using a heating pad. She was drinking fluids, including cranberry juice as recommended by her primary care physician to acidify the urine to decrease the growth of bacteria.

This evening, when her pain became acute, with pressure in the bladder area, a sense of urgency to urinate, spasm, renal colic, and nausea and vomiting, she presented to the emergency department.

PAST MEDICAL HISTORY
Appendectomy in the remote past. She has a history of kidney stones x2, the last episode being several years ago.

SOCIAL HISTORY
She is married and sexually active in a monogamous relationship. Her husband had a vasectomy several years ago.

PHYSICAL EXAMINATION
Vital signs: Temperature 98.8, pulse 120, respirations 28, blood pressure 140/100; normal blood pressure for her is 116/90. There is tenderness to palpation over the right lumbar and flank areas. There is tenderness to palpation over the suprapubic area. There is no tenderness to palpation elsewhere in the abdomen. Vaginal examination is normal with no vaginal discharge or tenderness. The patient is not currently menstruating.

LABORATORY DATA
A catheterized urine specimen was obtained. It showed no bacteria, no gross blood, and no white blood cells. There was, however, microscopic hematuria. A KUB x-ray revealed no abnormalities. A pregnancy test was negative. However, a CT scan revealed a moderately sized kidney stone located in the bladder neck.

DIAGNOSIS
Solitary kidney stone at the bladder neck.

TREATMENT
The patient was given a urine strainer and will strain all urine. She will call to schedule an appointment with a urologist next week so that these multiple episodes of kidney stones can be investigated. If she passes the stone, the patient will bring it to the hospital laboratory for analysis.

In the emergency department, the patient was given pain medication and hydrated with I.V. fluids. When her pain had subsided, she was released. She will follow up as described above.

Alfred J. Strawberry, M.D.

Alfred J. Strawberry, M.D.

AJS:ljs
D: 11/19/xx
T: 11/19/xx

1. Divide *urologist* into its three word parts and give the meaning of each word part.

   Word Part   **Meaning**

   _____   _____

   _____   _____

   _____   _____

2. Divide *suprapubic* into its three word parts and give the meaning of each word part.

   Word Part   **Meaning**

   _____   _____

   _____   _____

   _____   _____

3. Divide *hematuria* into its three word parts and give the meaning of each word part.

   Word Part   **Meaning**

   _____   _____

   _____   _____

   _____   _____

4. Divide *antibiotic* into its three word parts and give the meaning of each word part.

   Word Part   **Meaning**

   _____   _____

   _____   _____

   _____   _____

5. Define these abbreviations.

   KUB _____

   I.V. _____

6. The phrase "tentative diagnosis of a urinary tract infection" could be written with an abbreviation as "tentative diagnosis of a _____."

7. What type of urine specimen was obtained by the physician's office lab? _____

8. What was the purpose of drinking cranberry juice? _____

9. Define these phrases.

   renal colic _____

   suprapubic pain _____

10. What type of urine specimen was obtained in the emergency department? _____

11. Why was the patient given a urine strainer? _____

12. Why was it important that the patient has had an appendectomy? _____

13. Why was it important that the patient's husband has had a vasectomy? _____

14. Why were the patient's pulse, respirations, and blood pressure elevated on admission to the emergency department, but not her temperature? _____

15. Why is it important to know that the patient is not menstruating? _____

16. What is the most likely explanation for the microscopic hematuria? _____

MyMedicalTerminologyLab™

MyMedicalTerminologyLab is a premium online homework management system that includes a host of features to help you study. Registered users will find:

- A multitude of quizzes and activities built within the MyLab platform
- Powerful tools that track and analyze your results—allowing you to create a personalized learning experience
- Videos and audio pronunciations to help enrich your progress
- Streaming lesson presentations (Guided Lectures) and self-paced learning modules
- A space where you and your instructor can check your progress and manage your assignments

Chapter 12
Male Reproductive Medicine

Male Genitourinary System

Male reproductive (RE-proh-DUK-tive) medicine is the medical specialty that studies the anatomy and physiology of the male genitourinary system and uses laboratory and diagnostic procedures, medical and surgical procedures, and drugs to treat male reproductive diseases.

 ## Learning Outcomes

After you study this chapter, you should be able to

12.1 Identify structures of the male genitourinary system.

12.2 Describe the processes of spermatogenesis and ejaculation.

12.3 Describe common male genitourinary diseases, laboratory and diagnostic procedures, medical and surgical procedures, and drugs.

12.4 Form the plural and adjective forms of nouns related to male reproductive medicine.

12.5 Give the meanings of word parts and abbreviations related to male reproductive medicine.

12.6 Divide and build male reproductive medicine words.

12.7 Spell and pronounce male reproductive medicine words.

12.8 Research sound-alike and other male reproductive medicine words.

12.9 Analyze the medical content and meaning of male reproductive medicine reports.

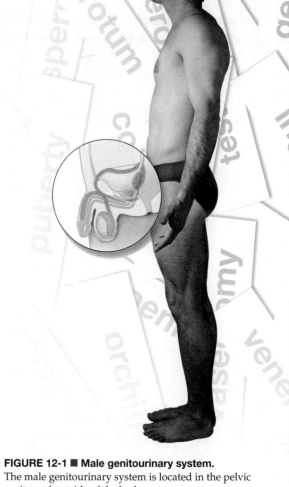

FIGURE 12-1 ■ Male genitourinary system.
The male genitourinary system is located in the pelvic cavity and outside of the body.
Source: Pearson Education

Medical Language Key

To unlock the definition of a medical word, break it into word parts. Give the meaning of each word part. Put the meanings of the word parts in order, beginning with the meaning of the suffix, then the prefix (if present), then the combining form(s).

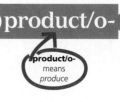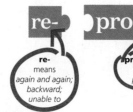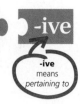

	Word Part	Word Part Meaning
Suffix	**-ive**	*pertaining to*
Prefix	**re-**	*again and again; backward; unable to*
Combining Form	**product/o-**	*produce*

Reproductive Medicine: ▶ *(Medical specialty) pertaining to again and again producing (children).*

Anatomy and Physiology

The **male genitourinary system** includes both the external and internal genitalia or **genital organs** (see Figure 12-1 ■). The **external genitalia** outside of the body include the scrotum, testes, epididymides, penis, and urethra. The **internal genitalia** within the pelvic cavity include the vas deferens, seminal vesicles, ejaculatory ducts, prostate gland, and bulbourethral glands. The male genitourinary system shares the urethra with the urinary system. The genitourinary system is also known as the **urogenital system** because of the close proximity of these two body systems and their shared structures. The function of the male genitourinary system is to secrete the male hormones, develop male secondary sexual characteristics, produce spermatozoa, and release spermatozoa.

Anatomy of the Male Genitourinary System

Scrotum

The **scrotum** is a soft pouch of skin behind the penis and in front of the legs (see Figure 12-2 ■). The scrotum is always a few degrees cooler than the core body temperature. This temperature difference is necessary for the proper development of spermatozoa. Muscles in the wall of the scrotum contract or relax to move the scrotum closer to or farther away from the body to adjust to temperature changes in the environment. The **perineum** is the area on the outside of the body between the anus and the scrotum.

Pronunciation/Word Parts

genitourinary (JEN-ih-toh-YOOR-ih-NAIR-ee)
  genit/o- *genitalia*
  urin/o- *urinary system; urine*
  -ary *pertaining to*

genital (JEN-ih-tal)
  genit/o- *genitalia*
  -al *pertaining to*

genitalia (JEN-ih-TAY-lee-ah)

urogenital (YOOR-oh-JEN-ih-tal)
  ur/o- *urinary system; urine*
  genit/o- *genitalia*
  -al *pertaining to*

scrotum (SKROH-tum)

scrotal (SKROH-tal)
  scrot/o- *bag; scrotum*
  -al *pertaining to*

perineum (PAIR-ih-NEE-um)

perineal (PAIR-ih-NEE-al)
  perine/o- *perineum*
  -al *pertaining to*

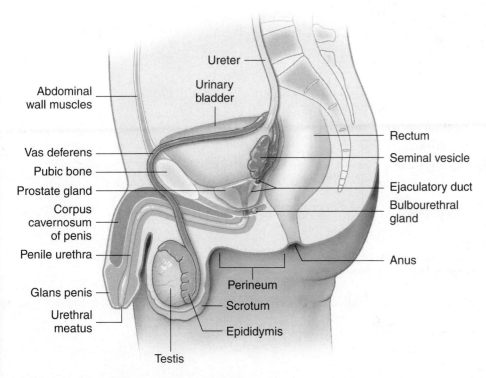

FIGURE 12-2 ■ External and internal male genitalia.
The external male genitalia are interconnected with the internal male genitalia. Structures of the urinary system are also involved: the urinary bladder is located near the internal male genitalia, and the urethra is shared by the male genitourinary system and the urinary system.
Source: Pearson Education

Testis and Epididymis

The scrotum contains the **testes** or **testicles**. Each testis is an egg-shaped gland about 2 inches in length (see Figures 12-2 and 12-3 ■). The testes are the **gonads** or sex glands in a male. They function as part of the male genitourinary system and also as part of the endocrine system (discussed in "Endocrinology," Chapter 14). The word *gonads* also includes the ovaries, the female sex glands that produce ova, (discussed in "Gynecology and Obstetrics," Chapter 13).

Pronunciation/Word Parts

testis (TES-tis)

testes (TES-teez)
Testis is a Latin singular noun. Form the plural by changing *-is* to *-es.*

testicle (TES-tih-kl)
Testicle is a combination of *testis* and the suffix *-cle* (small thing). *Testis* and *testicle* are used interchangeably (like *drop* and *droplet*), without implying any difference in the size.

testicular (tes-TIH-kyoo-lar)
  testicul/o- *testicle; testis*
  -ar *pertaining to*
The combining forms **didym/o-, orchid/o-, orchi/o-, orch/o-,** and **test/o-** also mean *testicle; testis.*

gonad (GOH-nad)
  gon/o- *ovum; seed; spermatozoon*
  -ad *in the direction of; toward*

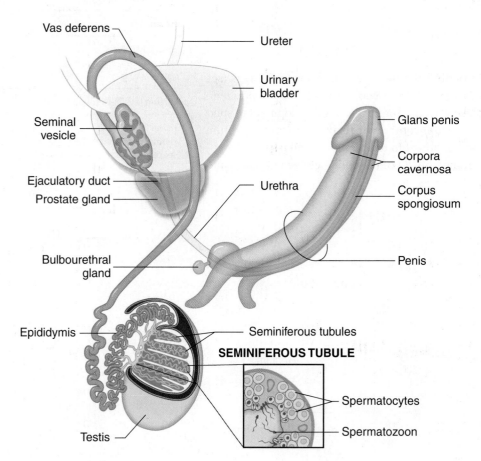

FIGURE 12-3 ■ Structures of the testis and penis.
The tightly coiled seminiferous tubules and epididymis become the long tubule of the vas deferens. It connects the external genitalia to the internal genitalia. The three columns of erectile tissue in the penis can be seen.
Source: Pearson Education

The testes contain the **seminiferous tubules**, tightly coiled tubules that produce **spermatozoa** or **sperm**. Each spermatozoon has a head and a tail or **flagellum** that propels it. The testes are also endocrine glands; their **interstitial cells** (between the seminiferous tubules) secrete the hormone testosterone. **Testosterone** is the most abundant and biologically active of all the male sex hormones; it stimulates spermatozoa to mature. Mature spermatozoa are continuously released into the **lumen** (internal opening) of the seminiferous tubules and carried by fluid into the epididymis. The testes also secrete a small amount of the female hormone estradiol.

The **epididymis** is a long, tightly coiled tube (over 20 feet in length) that is attached to the outer wall of each testis (see Figures 12-2 and 12-3). Within the epididymis, the head of each spermatozoon is given a cap-like layer of enzymes that helps it penetrate and fertilize the ovum of the female. The epididymis also destroys defective spermatozoa. Spermatozoa in the epididymis are mature but not yet moving. The tubules of the epididymis become a larger, uncoiled tube known as the *vas deferens* or *ductus deferens*.

Pronunciation/Word Parts

seminiferous (SEM-ih-NIF-er-us)
   semin/i- *sperm; spermatozoon*
   fer/o- *bear*
   -ous *pertaining to*

tubule (TOO-byool)
   tub/o- *tube*
   -ule *small thing*

spermatozoon (SPER-mah-toh-ZOH-on)
   spermat/o- *sperm; spermatozoon*
   -zoon *animal; living thing*

spermatozoa (SPER-mah-toh-ZOH-ah)
Spermatozoon is a Greek noun. Form the plural by changing *-on* to *-a.*

sperm (SPERM)
The combining form **sperm/o-** also means *sperm; spermatozoon.*

CLINICAL CONNECTIONS

Neonatology. Before birth, the fetal testes develop in the pelvic cavity. Each testis has a **spermatic cord** that contains arteries, veins, nerves, and the vas deferens. Two months before birth, a testis and its spermatic cord enter the **inguinal canal**, a passageway that goes through the abdominal muscles, over the pubic bone, through the groin area, and into one side of the scrotum (see Figure 12-4 ■). At some point between birth and 2 years of age, the inguinal canal closes. If it fails to close, a loop of intestine can slip through the inguinal canal and create a bulge in the groin or in the scrotum. This is known as an *indirect inguinal hernia*.

spermatic (sper-MAT-ik)
   spermat/o- *sperm; spermatozoon*
   -ic *pertaining to*

inguinal (ING-gwih-nal)
   inguin/o- *groin*
   -al *pertaining to*

canal (kah-NAL)

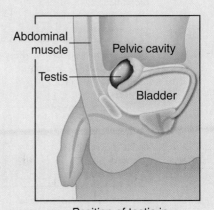 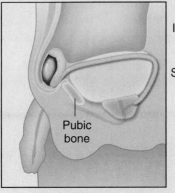 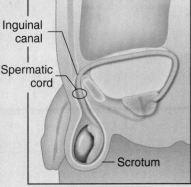

FIGURE 12-4 ■ Descent of the testes.
Before birth, the testes and their spermatic cords move from the pelvic cavity, through the inguinal canals, and into the scrotum.
Source: Pearson Education

Position of testis in 5-month fetus — Abdominal muscle, Pelvic cavity, Testis, Bladder

Position of testis in 7-month fetus — Pubic bone

Position of testis in newborn — Inguinal canal, Spermatic cord, Scrotum

flagellum (flah-JEL-um)

interstitial (IN-ter-STIH-shal)
   interstiti/o- *spaces within tissue*
   -al *pertaining to*

testosterone (tes-TAW-steh-rohn)
Testosterone contains the combining forms *test/o-* (testicle; testis) and *steroid/o-* (steroid) and the suffix *–one* (chemical substance).

Vas Deferens, Seminal Vesicles, and Ejaculatory Duct

The **vas deferens** (or **ductus deferens**) is a long tube (or duct) that receives spermatozoa from the epididymis (see Figures 12-2 and 12-3). Spermatozoa can be stored in the vas deferens for several months in an inactive state. The vas deferens travels superiorly through the inguinal canal inside the spermatic cord. At the superior end of the inguinal canal, however, the vas deferens continues on alone and goes behind the urinary bladder. There, the vas deferens merges with a seminal vesicle. The **seminal vesicles** are two elongated glands that form a *V* along the posterior wall of the urinary bladder. These glands produce **seminal fluid**, which makes up most of the volume of **semen**. The **ejaculatory duct** is a large collecting duct that holds spermatozoa from each vas deferens and seminal fluid from the seminal vesicles. The ejaculatory duct enters the prostate gland and then joins the prostatic urethra within the prostate gland.

Prostate Gland and Bulbourethral Glands

The **prostate gland** is a donut-shaped gland at the base of the bladder (see Figures 12-2 and 12-3). It completely surrounds the first part of the urethra (the prostatic urethra). The prostate gland is not part of the urinary system, however. The prostate gland produces **prostatic fluid**, a milky substance that makes up some of the volume of semen. This fluid contains an antibiotic substance that kills bacteria in the woman's vagina, as well as a substance that activates the enzymes in the head of a spermatozoon so that it can penetrate the woman's ovum to fertilize it. Prostatic fluid also contains acid phosphatase, an enzyme that breaks the deposit of semen apart and releases the spermatozoa in the woman's vagina.

The **bulbourethral glands** are small, bulb-like glands about the size of peas that are located on either side of the urethra at the base of the penis (see Figures 12-2 and 12-3). They produce thick mucus that makes up some of the volume of the semen. This mucus helps the spermatozoa survive by neutralizing the acidity of any urine remaining in the urethra at the time of ejaculation and neutralizing the normally acidic environment of the female vagina.

WORD ALERT

Sound-Alike Words

prostate	(noun)	gland that surrounds the urethra in men
		Example: When the prostate gland is enlarged, it interferes with urination in men.
prostrate	(adjective)	descriptive word for *lying in a face-down position from humility or exhaustion*
		Example: After the marathon race, the exhausted winner lay prostrate on the track.

Penis

The **penis** functions as an organ of the male genitourinary system and the urinary system (see Figures 12-2 and 12-3). The urethra leaves the prostate gland and passes through the length of the penis (penile urethra). The urethral meatus is located at the tip of the **glans penis**. In uncircumcised males, the urethral meatus is covered by the **prepuce** or **foreskin** of the penis. The penis and urethra serve as a passageway for semen (as part of the male genitourinary system) and as a passageway for urine (as part of the urinary system).

Three columns of erectile tissue run the length of the penis. Two of the columns, the **corpora cavernosa**, are located along the upper surface of the penis. The third column, the **corpus spongiosum**, is centered along the underside of the penis. The urethra is located within the corpus spongiosum. These three columns are composed of **erectile tissue** that fills with blood during sexual arousal, causing an **erection** as the penis becomes firm and erect.

Pronunciation/Word Parts

lumen (LOO-men)

epididymis (EP-ih-DID-ih-mis)
  epi- *above; upon*
  -didymis *testicle; testis*

epididymides (EP-ih-dih-DIM-ih-deez)
Epididymis is a Greek singular noun. Form the plural by changing *-is* to *-ides*. The ending *–didymis* contains the combining form *didym/o-* and the two-letter suffix *-is.*

vas deferens (VAS DEF-er-enz)
The combining form **vas/o-** means *blood vessel; vas deferens.*

ductus (DUK-tus)

seminal (SEM-ih-nal)
  semin/o- *sperm; spermatozoon*
  -al *pertaining to*

vesicle (VES-ih-kl)

semen (SEE-men)

ejaculatory (ee-JAH-kyoo-lah-TOR-ee)
  ejaculat/o- *expel suddenly*
  -ory *having the function of*

prostate (PRAW-stayt)

prostatic (praw-STAT-ik)
  prostat/o- *prostate gland*
  -ic *pertaining to*

bulbourethral (BUL-boh-yoor-EE-thral)
  bulb/o- *bulb-like structure*
  urethr/o- *urethra*
  -al *pertaining to*

penis (PEE-nis)

penile (PEE-nile)
  pen/o- *penis*
  -ile *pertaining to*

glans penis (GLANZ PEE-nis)
The combining form **balan/o-** means *glans penis.*

prepuce (PREE-poos)

corpora cavernosa
(KOR-por-ah KAV-er-NOH-sah)
Corpus is a Latin singular noun. Form the plural by changing *-us* to *-ora.*

corpus spongiosum
(KOR-pus SPUN-jee-OH-sum)

erectile (ee-REK-tile)
  erect/o- *stand up*
  -ile *pertaining to*

erection (ee-REK-shun)
  erect/o- *stand up*
  -ion *action; condition*

WORD ALERT

Sound-Alike Words

gland   (noun)   one of the structures of the endocrine system that secretes hormones into the blood

Example: The anterior pituitary gland in the brain secretes hormones that stimulate the testes at the beginning of puberty.

glans   (noun)   rounded area on top of the shaft of the penis

Example: The glans is covered by the foreskin in uncircumcised males.

Physiology of Spermatogenesis, Sexual Maturity, and Ejaculation

Spermatogenesis

At the onset of **puberty** (or **adolescence**), the anterior pituitary gland in the brain (discussed in "Endocrinology," Chapter 14) begins to secrete two hormones to stimulate the testes. **Follicle-stimulating hormone (FSH)** causes the seminiferous tubules to enlarge.

puberty (PYOO-ber-tee)
   puber/o- *growing up*
   -ty *quality; state*

adolescence (AD-oh-LES-sens)
   adolesc/o- *beginning of being an adult*
   -ence *state*

follicle (FAW-lih-kl)

A CLOSER LOOK

Most cells in the body divide by the process of **mitosis**, in which the 46 chromosomes in the nucleus duplicate and then split, creating two identical cells each with 46 chromosomes. However, the production of spermatozoa is different from that of other cells in the body.

During childhood, the seminiferous tubules contain immature **spermatocytes**. These cells are round and each contains 46 chromosomes. First, the 46 chromosomes duplicate by mitosis, and the duplicated chromosomes randomly exchange genetic material. This is how different combinations of genes from the male are passed on to his children. Then the spermatocyte divides two more times and becomes four individual spermatozoon, each with 23 chromosomes; this process is **meiosis**. Spermatozoa (and also ova from the female) are **gametes**, and they have only half of the usual number of chromosomes. Each spermatozoon contains 23 chromosomes. **Spermatogenesis** is the process of producing many mature spermatozoa.

mitosis (my-TOH-sis)
   mit/o- *thread-like strand*
   -osis *condition; process*

spermatocyte (sper-MAT-oh-site)
   spermat/o- *sperm; spermatozoon*
   -cyte *cell*

meiosis (my-OH-sis)

gamete (GAM-eet)

spermatogenesis
(SPER-mah-toh-JEN-eh-sis)
   spermat/o- *sperm; spermatozoon*
   gen/o- *arising from; produced by*
   -esis *condition; process*

Because these tubules make up 80% of each testis, the testes themselves enlarge during puberty. FSH also stimulates spermatocytes in the testes to begin dividing. **Luteinizing hormone (LH)** stimulates the interstitial cells to begin to secrete testosterone.

luteinizing (LOO-tee-ih-NY-zing)

Sexual Maturity

Also during puberty, testosterone causes the development of the male sexual characteristics: enlargement of the external genitalia; development of large body muscles; deepening of the voice (as the larynx grows); growth of body hair on the face, chest, axillae, and genital area; and development of the sexual drive (see Figure 12-5 ■).

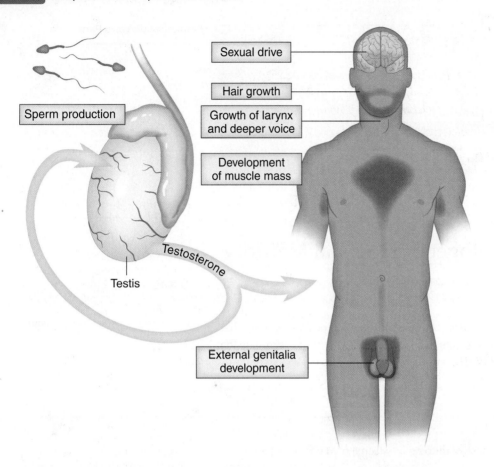

FIGURE 12-5 ■ Testosterone.
Testosterone is secreted by interstitial cells between the seminiferous tubules of the testes. Testosterone causes the development of the male sexual characteristics during puberty. It also causes spermatozoa to develop and mature.
Source: Pearson Education

Ejaculation

The process of ejaculation begins in response to thoughts or sensations that initiate sexual arousal. Smooth muscle relaxes in the wall of arteries in the penis, and vasodilation increases blood flow within the penis. Veins constrict to keep the corpora cavernosa and the corpus spongiosum distended with blood and produce an erection.

   Stimulation from the sympathetic division of the nervous system causes muscles at the base of the penis to contract. Spermatozoa in the vas deferens move into the ejaculatory duct, where they are mixed with fluid from the seminal vesicles. This fluid has a high level of sugar, a source of energy for the spermatozoa. It is at this point that the spermatozoa become active. Then the spermatozoa move into the urethra. The prostate gland contracts, forcing prostatic fluid through ducts into the urethra. As the spermatozoa move through the urethra, they are mixed with mucus from the bulbourethral glands. Semen is a combination of spermatozoa and secretions from the seminal vesicles, prostate gland, and the bulbourethral glands. A series of contractions cause 2–5 mL of semen to be expelled from the penis through the urethral meatus. This process is **ejaculation**. Within this small volume of semen are 100–500 million spermatozoa! Sugar and other nutrients in the semen keep the spermatozoa swimming strongly as they travel through the female cervix, uterus, and uterine tube to fertilize an ovum. The physical union of a male and a female during **sexual intercourse** is known as **coitus**.

ejaculation (ee-JAH-kyoo-LAY-shun)
   ejaculat/o- *expel suddenly*
   -ion *action; condition*

coitus (KOH-ih-tus)
The combining forms **coit/o-**, **pareun/o-**, and **venere/o-** mean *sexual intercourse*.

Vocabulary Review

Anatomy and Physiology		
Word or Phrase	**Description**	**Combining Forms**
external genitalia	Scrotum, testes, epididymides, penis, and urethra	**genit/o-** *genitalia*
genital organs	Male internal and external **genitalia**	**genit/o-** *genitalia*
genitourinary system	Two body systems (male reproductive system, urinary system) that share some structures. It is also known as the **urogenital system**.	**genit/o-** *genitalia* **urin/o-** *urinary system; urine* **ur/o-** *urinary system; urine*
internal genitalia	Vas deferens, seminal vesicles, ejaculatory ducts, prostate gland, and bulbourethral glands in the pelvic cavity	**genit/o-** *genitalia*
Scrotum, Testis, and Epididymis		
epididymis	Long, coiled tube on the outer wall of each testis. It receives spermatozoa from the seminiferous tubules, adds a cap-like layer of enzymes to them, and destroys defective spermatozoa.	**didym/o-** *testicle; testis*
gonads	The male sex glands (i.e., the testes)	**gon/o-** *ovum; seed; spermatozoon*
inguinal canal	Passageway through the abdominal muscles, over the pubic bone, and through the groin area through which the testes travel before birth as they descend from the pelvic cavity to the scrotum. The open inguinal canal should close around the spermatic cord sometime before age 2.	**inguin/o-** *groin*
interstitial cells	Cells between the seminiferous tubules of the testes. They secrete testosterone when stimulated by luteinizing hormone (LH).	**interstiti/o-** *spaces within tissue*
lumen	Central open area throughout the length of a tube or duct (such as the seminiferous tubule, vas deferens, ejaculatory duct, or urethra)	
perineum	Area on the outside of the body between the anus and the scrotum	**perine/o-** *perineum*
scrotum	Pouch of skin behind the penis that holds the two testes	**scrot/o-** *bag; scrotum*
seminiferous tubules	Tubules within each testis that produce spermatozoa	**semin/i-** *sperm; spermatozoon* **fer/o-** *bear* **tub/o-** *tube*
spermatic cord	Tube that, before birth, contains arteries, veins, and nerves for each testis as well as the vas deferens. It passes through the inguinal canal.	**spermat/o-** *sperm; spermatozoon*
spermatozoon	An individual mature **sperm.** Because it contains 23 chromosomes, it is a gamete. The **flagellum** is the long tail on a spermatozoon that makes it move.	**spermat/o-** *sperm; spermatozoon* **sperm/o-** *sperm; spermatozoon*
testes	Egg-shaped gland in each side of the scrotum. It is also known as a **testicle**. It contains interstitial cells that secrete testosterone and seminiferous tubules that produce spermatozoa.	**test/o-** *testicle; testis* **testicul/o-** *testicle; testis* **didym/o-** *testicle; testis* **orchid/o-** *testicle; testis* **orchi/o-** *testicle; testis* **orch/o-** *testicle; testis*
testosterone	Most abundant and most biologically active of the male sex hormones secreted by the interstitial cells of the testes. It causes the male sexual characteristics to develop and spermatozoa to mature.	**test/o-** *testicle; testis*

Penis

Word or Phrase	Description	Combining Forms
erection	During sexual arousal, erectile tissue in the penis fills with blood, causing the penis to become firm and erect.	erect/o- *stand up*
penis	Organ of **erectile tissue** that fills with blood during male sexual arousal. The **glans penis** is the rounded area on top of the shaft of the penis. The **corpora cavernosa** are two columns of tissue along the upper surface of the penis. The **corpus spongiosum** is a column of tissue on the underside of the penis. The urethra of the urinary system travels through the corpus spongiosum.	pen/o- *penis* erect/o- *stand up* balan/o- *glans penis*
prepuce	**Foreskin** of the penis that covers the urethral meatus in an uncircumcised male	

Other Structures

bulbourethral glands	Small, bulb-like glands at the base of the penis that produce mucus that becomes part of the semen	bulb/o- *bulb-like structure* urethr/o- *urethra*
ejaculatory duct	Duct that collects spermatozoa from the vas deferens and fluid from the seminal vesicles and empties into the urethra during ejaculation	ejaculat/o- *expel suddenly*
prostate gland	Donut-shaped gland at the base of the bladder. It surrounds the first part of the urethra and produces **prostatic fluid** that becomes part of semen.	prostat/o- *prostate gland*
semen	Fluid expelled from the penis during ejaculation. Semen contains spermatozoa, seminal fluid, prostatic fluid, and mucus from the bulbourethral glands.	
seminal vesicles	Glands along the posterior wall of the bladder that secrete **seminal fluid**, a source of energy for the spermatozoa and the main fluid of semen	semin/o- *sperm; spermatozoon*
vas deferens	Long tube that receives spermatozoa from the epididymis and carries them to the seminal vesicles. It is also known as the **ductus deferens**.	vas/o- *blood vessel; vas deferens*

Spermatogenesis, Sexual Maturity, and Ejaculation

coitus	The physical union of two people during **sexual intercourse**	coit/o- *sexual intercourse* pareun/o- *sexual intercourse* venere/o- *sexual intercourse*
ejaculation	Sudden expelling of semen from the penis during sexual arousal of the male	ejaculat/o- *expel suddenly*
follicle-stimulating hormone (FSH)	Hormone secreted by the anterior pituitary gland. It causes the seminiferous tubules of the testes to enlarge during puberty and spermatocytes in the testes to begin dividing.	
gamete	A cell (male spermatozoon or female ovum) that has 23 chromosomes instead of the usual 46 chromosomes like other cells	
luteinizing hormone (LH)	Hormone secreted by the anterior pituitary gland. It causes the interstitial cells of the testes to begin secreting testosterone during puberty.	
meiosis	Process by which a spermatocyte reduces the number of chromosomes in its nucleus to 23, or half the normal number, to create gametes	
mitosis	Process by which most body cells reproduce. The 46 chromosomes in the nucleus duplicate, and then split, creating two identical cells, each with 46 chromosomes.	mit/o- *thread-like strand*

Build Medical Words

Combining Form and Suffix Exercise

Read the definition of the medical word. Look at the combining form that is given. Select the correct suffix from the Suffix List and write it on the blank line. Then build the medical word and write it on the line. (Remember: You may need to remove the combining vowel. Always remove the hyphens and slash.) Be sure to check your spelling. The first one has been done for you.

SUFFIX LIST				
-al (pertaining to)	-cyte (cell)	-ic (pertaining to)	-ion (action; condition)	-ty (quality; state)
-ar (pertaining to)	-ence (state)	-ile (pertaining to)	-ory (having the function of)	-ule (small thing)

Definition of the Medical Word	Combining Form	Suffix	Build the Medical Word
1. Pertaining to (the) perineum	**perine/o-**	**-al**	perineal
(You think *pertaining to* (-al) + *perineum* (perine/o-). You change the order of the word parts to put the suffix last. You write *perineal*.)			
2. Pertaining to (the) scrotum	scrot/o-	_____	_____
3. State (of) growing up	puber/o-	_____	_____
4. Cell (that will become) sperm	spermat/o-	_____	_____
5. Small thing (that is a) tube	tub/o-	_____	_____
6. Action (of the penis to) stand up	erect/o-	_____	_____
7. State (of the) beginning of being an adult	adolesc/o-	_____	_____
8. Pertaining to (the) genitalia	genit/o-	_____	_____
9. Pertaining to (the) testis	testicul/o-	_____	_____
10. Pertaining to (the) penis	pen/o-	_____	_____
11. Pertaining to (the) prostate gland	prostat/o-	_____	_____
12. Having the function of expel(ing semen) suddenly	ejaculat/o-	_____	_____
13. Pertaining to (the) groin	inguin/o-	_____	_____

Diseases

Testis and Epididymis

Word or Phrase	Description	Pronunciation/Word Parts
cryptorchidism	Failure of one or both of the testicles to descend through the inguinal canal into the scrotum. This causes a low sperm count and male infertility. It is also known as *cryptorchism.* Treatment: Testosterone drug; orchiopexy.	**cryptorchidism** (krip-TOR-kih-dizm) **crypt/o-** *hidden* **orchid/o-** *testicle; testis* **-ism** *disease from a specific cause; process*
epididymitis	Inflammation and infection of the epididymis. It is caused by a bacterial urinary tract infection or sexually transmitted diseases such as gonorrhea or chlamydia. Treatment: Antibiotic drug.	**epididymitis** (EP-ih-DID-ih-MY-tis) **epi-** *above; upon* **didym/o-** *testicle; testis* **-itis** *infection of; inflammation of*
infertility	Failure of the woman to conceive after at least 1 year of regular sexual intercourse. If the man is infertile, it can be because of a hormone imbalance of FSH or LH, undescended testicles, a varicocele, damage to the testes from mumps, infection in the testes, too few spermatozoa, or abnormal spermatozoa. Treatment: Correct the underlying cause.	**infertility** (IN-fer-TIL-ih-tee) **in-** *in; not; within* **fertil/o-** *conceive; form* **-ity** *condition; state*
oligospermia	Fewer than the normal number of spermatozoa are produced by the testes (see Figure 12-6 ■). This is the most common cause of male infertility. It is caused by a hormone imbalance or an undescended testis. Treatment: Correct the underlying cause.	**oligospermia** (OH-lih-goh-SPER-mee-ah) **olig/o-** *few; scanty* **sperm/o-** *sperm; spermatozoon* **-ia** *condition; state; thing*

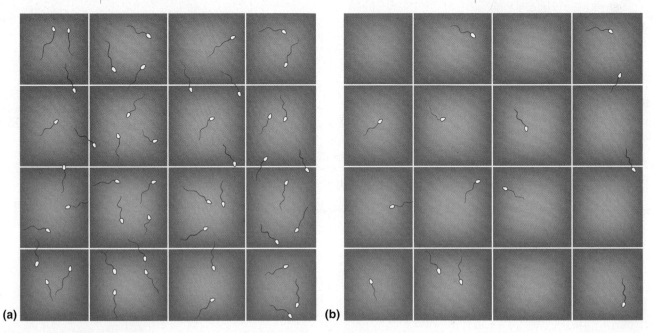

(a)   (b)

FIGURE 12-6 ■ Oligospermia.
(a) This semen specimen shows a normal number of sperm as seen on a counting grid under the microscope. (b) This semen specimen shows a decreased number of sperm in a patient with oligospermia.
Source: Pearson Education

Word or Phrase	Description	Pronunciation/Word Parts
orchitis	Inflammation or infection of the testes. It is caused by bacteria, the mumps virus, or trauma. Treatment: Antibiotic drug for a bacterial infection; an antibiotic drug is not effective against a virus.	**orchitis** (or-KY-tis) **orch/o-** *testicle; testis* **-itis** *infection of; inflammation of*
testicular cancer	Cancerous tumor of one of the testes. It arises from abnormal spermatocytes, not from other parts of the testes. It is also known as a **seminoma**. Treatment: Surgery to remove the testis (orchiectomy); chemotherapy drugs.	**seminoma** (SEM-ih-NOH-mah) **semin/o-** *sperm; spermatozoon* **-oma** *mass; tumor*
varicocele	Varicose vein in the spermatic cord to the testis. The valves in the vein do not close completely. The vein becomes distended with blood and is painful. A varicocele can cause a low sperm count and infertility. Treatment: Surgical removal of the varicocele.	**varicocele** (VAIR-ih-koh-SEEL) **varic/o-** *varicose vein; varix* **-cele** *hernia*

Prostate Gland

Word or Phrase	Description	Pronunciation/Word Parts
benign prostatic hypertrophy (BPH)	Benign, gradual enlargement of the prostate gland that normally occurs as a man ages. The enlarged prostate gland compresses the urethra and causes the bladder to retain urine. There is hesitancy and dribbling on urination and a narrowed caliber of the urine stream. Treatment: Drug to decrease the size of the prostate gland. Surgery: Transurethral resection of the prostate gland (TURP) or an alternate procedure with a laser, microwaves, or radiowaves.	**benign** (bee-NINE) **hypertrophy** (hy-PER-troh-fee) **hyper-** *above; more than normal* **-trophy** *process of development* The ending *-trophy* contains the combining form *troph/o-* and the one-letter suffix *-y*.
cancer of the prostate gland	**Cancerous** tumor of the prostate gland. This **malignancy** is the most common cancer in men. There are few early symptoms or signs because the cancer grows slowly. Later, the cancer makes the prostate feel hard or nodular on digital rectal examination. Treatment: "Watch and wait" approach if the cancer is small and the patient is elderly. Surgery to remove the prostate gland (prostatectomy), radiation therapy, cryosurgery, or female hormone drug therapy, chemotherapy drugs.	**cancerous** (KAN-ser-us) **cancer/o-** *cancer* **-ous** *pertaining to* **malignancy** (mah-LIG-nan-see) **malign/o-** *cancer; intentionally causing harm* **-ancy** *state*
prostatitis	Acute or chronic bacterial infection of the prostate gland. It is caused by a urinary tract infection or a sexually transmitted disease. Treatment: Antibiotic drug.	**prostatitis** (PRAW-stah-TY-tis) **prostat/o-** *prostate gland* **-itis** *infection of; inflammation of*

Penis

Word or Phrase	Description	Pronunciation/Word Parts
balanitis	Inflammation and infection of the glans penis caused by a bacterium, virus, yeast, or fungus. It is often associated with phimosis and inadequate hygiene of the prepuce. Treatment: Antibiotic drug (for a bacterial infection); antifungal drug (for a yeast or fungal infection).	**balanitis** (BAL-ah-NY-tis) **balan/o-** *glans penis* **-itis** *infection of; inflammation of*
chordee	Downward curvature of the penis during an erection. It is caused by a constricting, cordlike band of tissue along the underside of the penis. This is a congenital abnormality that is often associated with hypospadias. Treatment: Surgical correction.	**chordee** (kor-DEE)
dyspareunia	Painful or difficult sexual intercourse or **postcoital** pain. It is caused by infection of the penis or prostate gland, chordee of the penis, or phimosis. Treatment: Correct the underlying cause.	**dyspareunia** (DIS-pah-ROO-nee-ah) **dys-** *abnormal; difficult; painful* **pareun/o-** *sexual intercourse* **-ia** *condition; state; thing* **postcoital** (post-KOH-ih-tal) **post-** *after; behind* **coit/o-** *sexual intercourse* **-al** *pertaining to*

Word or Phrase	Description	Pronunciation/Word Parts
erectile dysfunction (ED)	Inability to achieve or sustain an erection of the penis. It can be caused by hypertension, arteriosclerosis that blocks blood flow into the penis, neurologic disease (such as a spinal cord injury) that impairs sensory stimuli and nerve transmission, diabetes mellitus, a low level of testosterone, smoking, alcoholism, the side effects of certain drugs, or psychological factors. It is also known as **impotence**. Treatment: Drug to stimulate an erection; penile implant.	**erectile** (ee-REK-tile) **erect/o-** *stand up* **-ile** *pertaining to* **dysfunction** (dis-FUNK-shun) *Dysfunction* is a combination of the prefix *dys-* (abnormal; difficult; painful) and the word *function*. **impotence** (IM-poh-tens)
phimosis	Congenital condition in which the opening of the foreskin is too small to allow the foreskin to pull back over the glans penis. This traps **smegma** (a white, cheesy discharge of skin cells and oil) and can cause infection. Treatment: Circumcision.	**phimosis** (fih-MOH-sis) **phim/o-** *closed tight* **-osis** *condition; process* **smegma** (SMEG-mah)
premature ejaculation	Ejaculation of semen that often occurs with minimal stimulation and before the penis becomes fully erect to penetrate the vagina. This lessens the enjoyment of sexual intercourse and decreases the chance of conception. It can be caused by a hormone imbalance but is more often caused by stress or a psychological reason. Treatment: Correct the underlying cause.	
priapism	Abnormal, continuing erection of the penis with pain and tenderness. It is caused by spinal cord injury or a side effect of drugs used to treat erectile dysfunction. Treatment: Correct the underlying cause.	**priapism** (PRY-ah-pizm) **priap/o-** *persistent erection* **-ism** *disease from a specific cause; process*
sexually transmitted disease (STD)	Infectious disease that is contracted during sexual intercourse with an infected individual (see Table 12-1 ■). A positive test for a sexually transmitted disease means that the patient and all sexual partners need to be treated. Sexually transmitted diseases can also be passed to a fetus (in the uterus or as it travels through the birth canal), causing serious illness, blindness, and even death. It is also known as **venereal disease (VD)**. Treatment: Antibiotic drug or antiviral drug.	**venereal** (veh-NEER-ee-al) **venere/o-** *sexual intercourse* **-al** *pertaining to*

Table 12-1 Sexually Transmitted Diseases (STDs)

Physicians are required to report all cases of sexually transmitted diseases to the state health department, which, in turn, reports all cases to the national Centers for Disease Control and Prevention (CDCP). Also known as sexually transmitted infections (STIs).

acquired immunodeficiency syndrome (AIDS)		**immunodeficiency**
Note: This disease, its history, symptoms, diagnosis, and treatment, are discussed in detail in "Hematology and Immunology," Chapter 6.		(IH-myoo-NOH-deh-FIH-shun-see) **immun/o-** *immune response* **defici/o-** *inadequate; lacking* **-ency** *condition of being; condition of having*
Pathogen	Human immunodeficiency virus (HIV), a retrovirus	
Symptoms	Men: Fever, night sweats, weight loss, fatigue Women: Same	
Diagnosis	Blood test (ELISA, Western blot, viral RNA load, p24 antigen, CD4 count) or saliva screening test (OraSure)	
Treatment	Oral antiretroviral drugs taken in combination	
Other	Treatment can only slow the progress of this disease; there is no cure.	

Table 12-1 Sexually Transmitted Diseases (STDs)   *(continued)*

chlamydia		**chlamydia** (klah-MID-ee-ah)
Pathogen	*Chlamydia trachomatis,* a gram-negative coccus (sphere-shaped) bacterium	
Symptoms	Men: Painful urination with burning and itching. Thin, watery discharge from the urethra. Some men have no symptoms.	
	Women: Frequently have no symptoms or a slight vaginal discharge	
Diagnosis	Smear of discharge from urethra (men) or cervix (women) is stained and examined under a microscope	
Treatment	Oral antibiotic drug	
Other	Most common sexually transmitted disease. It is also known as **nongonococcal urethritis**.	

genital herpes		**herpes** (HER-peez)
Pathogen	Herpes simplex virus (HSV), type 2	
Symptoms	Men: Vesicular lesions (blisters) on the penis, scrotum, perineum, or anus. When the blisters break, they become skin ulcers. There may be flu-like symptoms or no symptoms at all.	
	Women: Same, on the vulva, perineum, anus, or vagina	
Diagnosis	Culture grown from swab of a lesion, polymerase chain reaction test	
Treatment	Topical and oral antiviral drugs shorten the duration of each outbreak	

genital warts (condylomata acuminata) (see Figure 12-7 ■)		**condylomata acuminata**
Pathogen	Human papillomavirus (HPV)	(CON-dih-LOH-mah-tah
	Certain strains cause genital warts; other strains cause dysplasia of the cervix, which can lead to cervical cancer in women	ah-KOO-mih-NAH-tah)
Symptoms	Men: Itching, flesh-colored, irregular lesions that are raised and cauliflower-like	
	Women: Same, with vaginal discharge	
Diagnosis	Visual examination of the skin of the genital area. In women, a Pap smear of the cervix is examined under a microscope.	
Treatment	Topical chemicals or cryosurgery, cautery, or laser to remove warts	
Other	It is also known as **venereal warts**.	

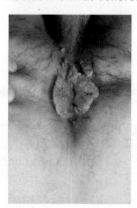

FIGURE 12-7 ■ Genital warts.
These raised, irregular, flesh-colored lesions are caused by the human papillomavirus (HPV). In a male, they occur on the penis, scrotum, or perineum. In a female, they occur on the labia or perineum. Some strains of HPV are associated with cancer of the cervix in women.
Source: Biophoto Associates/Science source

(continued)

Table 12-1 Sexually Transmitted Diseases (STDs)   *(continued)*

gonorrhea		
Pathogen	*Neisseria gonorrhoeae*, a gram-negative diplococcus (double sphere) bacterium. It is also known as **gonococcus (GC)**.	**gonorrhea** (GAW-noh-REE-ah) **gon/o-** *ovum; seed; spermatozoon*
Symptoms	Men: Painful urination. Thick yellow discharge from the urethra (gonococcal urethritis). Some men have no symptoms. Women: Painful urination. Thick yellow vaginal discharge. Half of infected women have no symptoms.	**-rrhea** *discharge; flow*
Diagnosis	Gram stain of a smear of the discharge shows characteristic gram-negative intracellular diplococci under a microscope Culture grown from a swab of discharge from the urethra (men) or cervix (women)	
Treatment	Oral antibiotic drug	
Other	Laypersons call this disease *the clap* because of a similar-sounding French word that means *house of prostitution*.	

syphilis		
Pathogen	*Treponema pallidum,* a spirochete (spiral) bacterium	**syphilis** (SIF-ih-lis)
Symptoms	Men: Single, painless **chancre** (lesion that ulcerates, forms a crust, and then heals) on the penis. Later, there is fever, rash, and various symptoms that mimic other diseases. Women: Same, with chancre on female genitalia	**chancre** (SHANG-ker) **lues** (LOO-ees)
Diagnosis	Fluid from a lesion viewed with special illumination under darkfield microscopy shows the spiral bacterium Blood tests for antibodies (RPR, VDRL, FTA-ABS)	
Treatment	Oral antibiotic drug	
Other	It is also known as **lues**.	

trichomoniasis		
Pathogen	*Trichomonas vaginalis,* a protozoan with a flagellum (tail)	**trichomoniasis** (TRIK-oh-moh-NY-ah-sis)
Symptoms	Men: Almost no symptoms Women: Greenish-yellow frothy or bubbly vaginal discharge with a foul odor. Itching of the vulva and vagina.	
Diagnosis	Wet mount preparation of the vaginal discharge examined under a microscope. Culture of the discharge.	
Treatment	Oral antiprotozoal drug	

Male Breast		
Word or Phrase	**Description**	**Pronunciation/Word Parts**
gynecomastia	Enlargement of the male breast. It is caused by an imbalance of testosterone and estradiol because of puberty, aging, surgical removal of the testes, or female hormone drug treatment for prostate cancer. Treatment: Androgen drug. Plastic surgery to decrease breast size.	**gynecomastia** (GY-neh-koh-MAS-tee-ah) **gynec/o-** *female; woman* **mast/o-** *breast; mastoid process* **-ia** *condition; state; thing* Add words to make a correct definition of *gynecomastia*: *condition (of enlargement in which the male's chest resembles the) female breast.*

Laboratory and Diagnostic Procedures

Blood Tests		
Word or Phrase	**Description**	**Pronunciation/Word Parts**
acid phosphatase	Test for an enzyme found in the prostate gland. Prostatic acid phosphatase (PAP) only measures acid phosphatase from the prostate gland as opposed to the total acid phosphatase level. An increased level in the blood indicates cancer of the prostate that has metastasized to the body.	**acid phosphatase** (AS-id FAWS-fah-tays)
hormone testing	Test that determines the levels of FSH and LH from the anterior pituitary gland and testosterone from the testes. It is used to diagnose infertility problems.	**hormone** (HOR-mohn)
prostate-specific antigen (PSA)	Test that detects a glycoprotein in cells of the prostate gland. PSA is increased in men with prostate cancer. The higher the level, the more advanced the cancer. The PSA level falls after successful treatment of the cancer.	**antigen** (AN-tih-jen) *Antigen* is a combination of part of the word *antibody* and the suffix *-gen* (that which produces).
syphilis testing	Tests that include RPR, VDRL, and FTA-ABS. RPR stands for *rapid plasma reagin.* VDRL stands for *Venereal Disease Research Laboratory.* These tests detect an antibody that is produced with syphilis; however, it is also produced with other diseases. FTA-ABS stands for *fluorescent treponemal antibody absorption.* This test detects the body's specific antibodies against syphilis.	

Semen Tests		
acid phosphatase	Test that detects the presence of acid phosphatase in the vagina and indicates sexual intercourse has occurred because semen contains acid phosphatase. This test is used in rape investigations.	
DNA analysis	DNA analysis of semen from a crime scene or rape victim can be compared to the samples of known DNA in a criminal database. DNA analysis can also be used to prove paternity (that a particular man is the father of the child being tested).	
semen analysis	Microscopic examination of the spermatozoa (see Figure 12-8 ■). A semen analysis is done as part of a workup for infertility. After not ejaculating for 36 hours, the man gives a semen specimen. A normal **sperm count** is greater than 50 million/mL. The **motility** (forward movement) and **morphology** (normal shape) of the spermatozoa are evaluated. A semen analysis is also done after a vasectomy to verify **aspermia** and a successful sterilization.	**motility** (moh-TIL-ih-tee) **motil/o-** *movement* **-ity** *condition; state* **morphology** (mor-FAW-loh-jee) **morph/o-** *shape* **-logy** *study of* **aspermia** (aa-SPER-mee-ah) **a-** *away from; without* **sperm/o-** *sperm; spermatozoon* **-ia** *condition; state; thing*

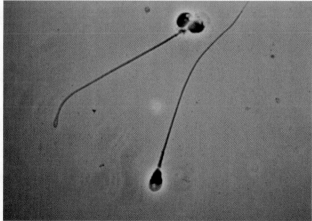

FIGURE 12-8 ■ **Spermatozoa.**
The spermatozoon on the right shows normal morphology. Vigorous movement of its flagellum would indicate normal motility. The spermatozoon on the left has abnormal morphology with a double head and a deformed tail. Abnormal spermatozoa can have enlarged heads, pin heads, or tails that are kinked, doubled, coiled, or missing. All men produce a few abnormal spermatozoa, but exposure to lead, cigarette smoke, pesticides, or chemicals can increase this number. Large numbers of abnormal spermatozoa cause male infertility.
Source: John Walsh/Science Source

Radiologic Tests		
Word or Phrase	**Description**	**Pronunciation/Word Parts**
ProstaScint scan	Procedure that uses ProstaScint to detect areas of metastasis from a primary site of prostate cancer. ProstaScint is a combination of a radioactive tracer (indium-111) and a monoclonal antibody that binds to receptors on cancer cells in the prostate gland and elsewhere in the body. The radioactive tracer emits gamma rays that are detected by a gamma scintillation camera and made into an image.	
ultrasonography	Procedure that uses ultra high-frequency sound waves emitted by a transducer or probe to produce an image. Ultrasonography of the testis is used to detect a varicocele or undescended testes. **Transrectal ultrasonography (TRUS)** uses an ultrasound probe inserted into the rectum to obtain an image of the prostate gland or to help guide a needle biopsy of the prostate gland. The **ultrasound** image is a **sonogram**.	**ultrasonography** (UL-trah-soh-NAW-grah-fee) **ultra-** *beyond; higher* **son/o-** *sound* **-graphy** *process of recording* **transrectal** (trans-REK-tal) **trans-** *across; through* **rect/o-** *rectum* **-al** *pertaining to* **ultrasound** (UL-trah-sound) **sonogram** (SAW-noh-gram) **son/o-** *sound* **-gram** *picture; record*

Medical and Surgical Procedures

Medical Procedures

Word or Phrase	Description	Pronunciation/Word Parts

digital rectal examination (DRE)	Procedure to palpate the prostate gland. A gloved finger inserted into the rectum is used to feel the prostate gland for signs of tenderness, nodules, hardness, or enlargement. This examination should be done yearly in men over age 40.	**digital** (DIJ-ih-tal)
		  digit/o- *digit; finger; toe*
		  -al *pertaining to*

newborn genital examination	Procedure in which the newborn's external male genitalia are examined for any sign of abnormal positioning of the urethral meatus (epispadias, hypospadias), ambiguous genitalia, or undescended testes (see Figure 12-9 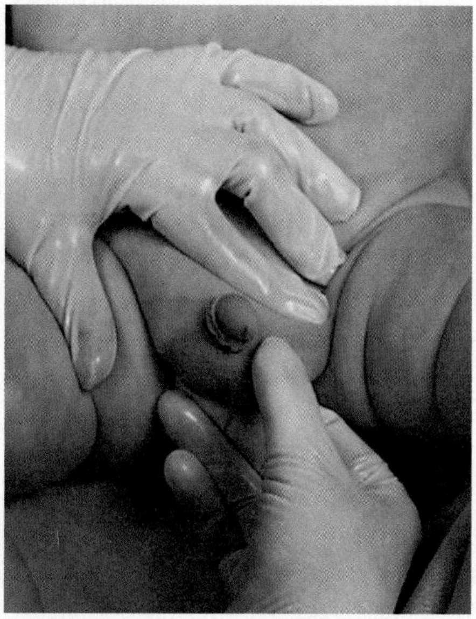 ■).	

FIGURE 12-9 ■ Newborn scrotal examination.
The scrotum is palpated as part of the initial genital examination of a newborn. Both testes should be descended and present in the scrotum at birth.
Source: Susan M. Turley

Word or Phrase	Description	Pronunciation/Word Parts
testicular self-examination (TSE)	Procedure performed by the patient to palpate the testes and scrotum to detect lumps, masses, or enlarged lymph nodes. TSE should be done monthly to detect early signs of testicular cancer.	

Surgical Procedures

Word or Phrase	Description	Pronunciation/Word Parts

biopsy	Procedure to remove tissue from the prostate gland to diagnose prostatic cancer. A large-bore needle is inserted through the rectum or urethra to take a core of prostatic tissue.
	    Fine-needle aspiration biopsy of the testis is performed to investigate a low sperm count. A thin needle is inserted and a syringe is used to aspirate tissue. An **incisional biopsy** (open biopsy) is performed to remove part of a mass in a testis.
		biopsy (BY-awp-see)
		  bi/o- *life; living organism; living tissue*
		  -opsy *process of viewing*
		
		aspiration (AS-pih-RAY-shun)
		  aspir/o- *breathe in; suck in*
		  -ation *being; having; process*
		
		incisional (in-SIH-zhun-al)
		  incis/o- *cut into*
		  -ion *action; condition*
		  -al *pertaining to*

Word or Phrase	Description	Pronunciation/Word Parts
circumcision	Procedure to remove the prepuce (foreskin). This can be done to correct a tight prepuce and allow better hygiene of the glans penis. The foreskin in newborn babies is often removed because of social customs or religious requirements.	**circumcision** (SER-kum-SIH-zhun) **circum-** *around* **cis/o-** *cut* **-ion** *action; condition*
orchiectomy	Procedure to remove a testis because of testicular cancer	**orchiectomy** (OR-kee-EK-toh-mee) **orchi/o-** *testicle; testis* **-ectomy** *surgical removal*
orchiopexy	Procedure to reposition an undescended testis and fix it within the scrotum	**orchiopexy** (OR-kee-oh-PEK-see) **orchi/o-** *testicle; testis* **-pexy** *process of surgically fixing in place*
penile implant	Procedure to implant an inflatable penile **prosthesis** for patients with erectile dysfunction	**prosthesis** (praws-THEE-sis)
prostatectomy	Procedure to remove the entire prostate gland, along with the lymph nodes, seminal vesicles, and vas deferens because of prostate cancer (see Figure 12-10 ■).	**prostatectomy** (PRAW-stah-TEK-toh-mee) **prostat/o-** *prostate gland* **-ectomy** *surgical removal*

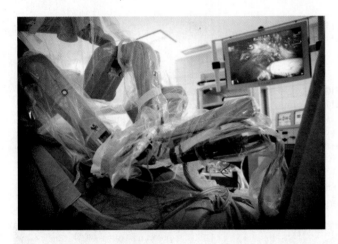

FIGURE 12-10 ■ Robot-assisted prostatectomy.
Procedure to remove a cancerous prostate gland using robot-assisted surgery. Several portals are placed in the patient's abdomen and robotic instruments are inserted. The robotic 3D camera has 10 times the magnification of the human eye. Robotic instruments allow the surgeon to more precisely remove cancerous tissues while preserving nerves that affect sexual function.
Source: Abk/Bsip/Corbis

Word or Phrase	Description	Pronunciation/Word Parts
transurethral resection of the prostate (TURP)	Procedure to reduce the size of the prostate gland in patients with benign prostatic hypertrophy. A special cystoscope (a **resectoscope**) is inserted through the urethra. It has built-in cutting instruments and cautery to resect pieces of the prostate gland and cauterize bleeding blood vessels. Chips of prostatic tissue are then irrigated out (see Figure 12-11 ■). TURP is the most common surgical treatment for a moderately to severely enlarged prostate gland. Other procedures use a laser to vaporize prostatic tissue. These include **photoselective vaporization of the prostate (PVP)** and **holmium laser ablation of the prostate (HoLAP)**. Laser surgery produces the same results as a TURP, but with less bleeding and a shorter recovery time. Minimally invasive procedures for moderate benign prostatic hypertrophy include **transurethral microwave therapy (TUMT)**, which uses a microwave antenna on a catheter inserted through the urethra to destroy prostatic tissue with microwaves and heat, and **transurethral needle ablation (TUNA)**, which uses a resectoscope to place needles in the prostate gland to destroy prostatic tissue with radio waves and heat.	**transurethral** (TRANS-yoor-EE-thral) **trans-** *across; through* **urethr/o-** *urethra* **-al** *pertaining to* **resection** (ree-SEK-shun) **resect/o-** *cut out; remove* **-ion** *action; condition* **resectoscope** (ree-SEK-toh-skohp) **resect/o-** *cut out; remove* **-scope** *instrument used to examine* **ablation** (ah-BLAY-shun) **ablat/o-** *destroy; take away* **-ion** *action; condition*

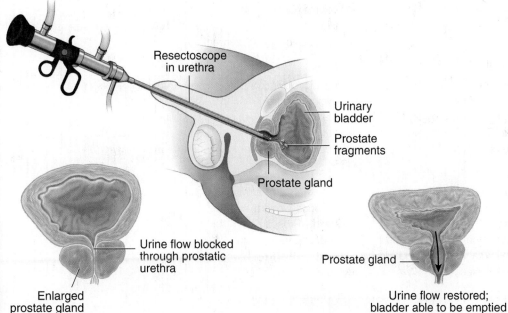

Resectoscope in urethra

Urinary bladder

Prostate fragments

Prostate gland

Urine flow blocked through prostatic urethra

Enlarged prostate gland

Prostate gland

Urine flow restored; bladder able to be emptied

FIGURE 12-11 ■ **Transurethral resection of the prostate (TURP).** This surgical procedure is the "gold standard" of treatment for benign prostatic hypertrophy. *Source*: Pearson Education

Word or Phrase	Description	Pronunciation/Word Parts
vasectomy	Procedure in the male to prevent pregnancy in the female. Through a small incision at the base of the scrotum, both vas deferens are divided, a length of each tube is removed, and the cut ends are sutured and crushed or destroyed with electrocautery. Spermatozoa continue to be produced by the testes, but they are absorbed back into the body. A **vasovasostomy** is a reversal of a vasectomy. The cut ends of the vas deferens are rejoined so that spermatozoa are again present in the ejaculate and the male can cause a woman to become pregnant.	**vasectomy** (vah-SEK-toh-mee) **vas/o-** *blood vessel; vas deferens* **-ectomy** *surgical removal* **vasovasostomy** (VAY-soh-vah-SAW-stoh-mee) **vas/o-** *blood vessel; vas deferens* **vas/o-** *blood vessel; vas deferens* **-stomy** *surgically created opening* Add words to make a complete definition of *vasovasostomy*: *surgically created opening (in one part of the) vas deferens (to join another part of the) vas deferens.*

Drugs

These drug categories and drugs are used to treat male genitourinary diseases. The most common generic and trade name drugs in each category are listed.

Category	Indication	Examples	Pronunciation/Word Parts
androgen drugs	Treat a lack of production of testosterone by the testes because of cryptorchidism, orchiectomy, or a decreased level of LH from the anterior pituitary gland. It is used to treat delayed puberty in boys. *Androgen* refers to testosterone produced by the testes, other testosterone-like hormones, or manufactured testosterone used in drugs.	methyltestosterone (Android, Virilon), testosterone (Androderm, AndroGel)	**androgen** (AN-droh-jen) **andr/o-** *male* **-gen** *that which produces*
antibiotic drugs	Treat bacterial infections that cause chlamydia, gonorrhea, and syphilis	Chlamydia: doxycyline (Vibramycin) Gonorrhea: ampicillin (Principen), cefuroxime (Ceftin), ciprofloxacin (Cipro) Syphilis: penicillin G (Pfizerpen)	**antibiotic** (AN-tee-by-AW-tik), (AN-tih-by-AW-tik) **anti-** *against* **bi/o-** *life; living organism; living tissue* **-tic** *pertaining to*
antiviral drugs, antiretroviral drugs	Treat viral infections that cause genital herpes and condylomata acuminata. These drugs are applied topically to the affected areas. Oral antiretroviral drugs are used to treat HIV and AIDS.	Topical: acyclovir (Zovirax), valacyclovir (Valtrex) Oral: lamivudine (Epivir), tenofovir (Viread), and zidovudine (Retrovir) for HIV or AIDS	**antiviral** (AN-tee-VY-ral) (AN-tih-VY-ral) **anti-** *against* **vir/o-** *virus* **-al** *pertaining to*
drugs for benign prostatic hypertrophy	Androgen inhibitor drugs inhibit the male hormone dihydrotestosterone, which causes the prostate gland to enlarge. Other drugs relax the smooth muscle in the prostate gland and urethra and allow urine to flow more freely.	Androgen inhibitor drugs: dutasteride (Avodart), finasteride (Proscar) Other drugs: tamsulosin (Flomax), terazosin (Hytrin)	

> ### DID YOU KNOW?
> Proscar for benign prostatic hypertrophy is also marketed under the trade name Propecia. Propecia comes in a lower dose and is applied topically to treat male-pattern baldness.

Category	Indication	Examples	Pronunciation/Word Parts
drugs for erectile dysfunction	Promote the release of nitric oxide gas in the tissues and inhibit an enzyme, both of which increases blood flow into the penis to create an erection	sildenafil (Viagra), tadalafil (Cialis), vardenafil (Levitra)	

Abbreviations

AIDS	acquired immunodeficiency syndrome		**LH**	luteinizing hormone
BPH	benign prostatic hypertrophy		**PAP**	prostatic acid phosphatase
CDCP	Centers for Disease Control and Prevention		**PSA**	prostate-specific antigen
	The abbreviation for its older name—Centers for Disease Control (CDC)—is still used.		**PVP**	photoselective vaporization of the prostate
			RPR	rapid plasma reagin (test for syphilis)
DRE	digital rectal examination		**STD**	sexually transmitted disease
ED	erectile dysfunction		**STI**	sexually transmitted infection
FSH	follicle-stimulating hormone		**TRUS**	transrectal ultrasound
GC	gonococcus (*Neisseria gonorrhoeae*)		**TSE**	testicular self-examination
GU	genitourinary; gonococcal urethritis		**TUMT**	transurethral microwave therapy
HIV	human immunodeficiency virus		**TUNA**	transurethral needle ablation
HoLAP	holmium laser ablation of the prostate		**TURP**	transurethral resection of the prostate
HPV	human papillomavirus		**VD**	venereal disease
HSV	herpes simplex virus		**VDRL**	Venereal Disease Research Laboratory (test for syphilis)

WORD ALERT
Abbreviations

Abbreviations are commonly used in all types of medical documents; however, they can mean different things to different people and their meanings can be misinterpreted. Always verify the meaning of an abbreviation.

ED means *erectile dysfunction,* but it also means *emergency department.*

PAP means *prostatic acid phosphatase,* but *Pap* is a short form for *Papanicolaou smear or test.*

IT'S GREEK TO ME!

Did you notice that some words have two different combining forms? Combining forms from both Greek and Latin remain a part of medical language today.

Word	Greek	Latin	Medical Word Examples
glans penis	balan/o-		balanitis
penis		pen/o-	penile
sexual intercourse	pareun/o-	venere/o-	dyspareunia, venereal disease
		coit/o-	postcoital
testicle; testis	didym/o-	test/o-	epididymitis, testosterone
	orchid/o-, orchi/o-	testicul/o-	cryptorchidism, orchiectomy, testicular
	orch/o-		orchitis

CAREER FOCUS

Meet Mindy, a clinical laboratory scientist and blood bank supervisor

"Clinical laboratory scientist is the newer name, but we know ourselves as medical technologists. In college, I took a microbiology class. I enjoyed it so much that I pursued that as my major. A technologist performs the testing, whether it's hematology, chemistry, blood bank, or microbiology. I have to communicate with the doctors and nurses. I have to have an understanding of medical terminology to be able to communicate clearly with them. When we can interact with the nurses and the doctors to give them the answers they need to care for the patients, that's what's rewarding."

Clinical laboratory scientists are allied health professionals who work in a hospital or a large commercial medical laboratory. They perform all types of laboratory tests on blood, urine, and other body fluids and tissues. They work with microscopes and computerized equipment.

Reproductive medicine physicians treat male (and female) patients who have difficulty conceiving a child because of infertility.

Endocrinologists treat patients with disorders of the endocrine system, including hormonal disorders that affect men, such as infertility. Cancerous tumors of the male genitourinary system are treated medically by an oncologist and surgically by a general surgeon.

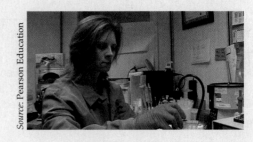

Source: Pearson Education

clinical (KLIN-ih-kal)
   clinic/o- *medicine*
   -al *pertaining to*

laboratory (LAB-oh-rah-TOR-ee)
   laborat/o- *testing place; workplace*
   -ory *having the function of*

scientist (SY-en-tist)
   scient/o- *knowledge; science*
   -ist *person who specializes in; thing that specializes in*

reproductive (REE-proh-DUK-tiv)
   re- *again and again; backward; unable to*
   product/o- *produce*
   -ive *pertaining to*

MyMedicalTerminologyLab™

To see Mindy Langston's complete video profile, log into MyMedicalTerminologyLab and navigate to the Multimedia Library for Chapter 12. Check the Video box, and then click the Career Focus - Medical Technologist link.

12.5B Define Abbreviations

DEFINITION EXERCISE

Write the definition of the following abbreviations.

1. BPH _____
2. ED _____
3. GC _____
4. HSV _____
5. PSA _____
6. STD _____
7. TURP _____
8. VD _____

12.6A Divide Medical Words

DIVIDING WORDS EXERCISE

Separate these words into their component parts (prefix, combining form, suffix). Note: Some words do not contain all three word parts. The first one has been done for you.

Medical Word	Prefix	Combining Form	Suffix	Medical Word	Prefix	Combining Form	Suffix
1. dyspareunia	dys-	pareun/o-	-ia	5. aspermia	_____	_____	_____
2. venereal	_____	_____	_____	6. priapism	_____	_____	_____
3. circumcision	_____	_____	_____	7. reproductive	_____	_____	_____
4. testicular	_____	_____	_____	8. postcoital	_____	_____	_____

12.6B Build Medical Words

PREFIX EXERCISE

Read the definition of the medical word. Look at the medical word or partial word that is given (it already contains a combining form and a suffix). Select the correct prefix from the Prefix List and write it on the blank line. Then build the medical word and write it on the line. Be sure to check your spelling. The first one has been done for you.

PREFIX LIST

a- (away from; without)	in- (in; not; within)	trans- (across; through)
circum- (around)	post- (after; behind)	ultra- (beyond; higher)
dys- (abnormal; difficult; painful)	re- (again and again; backward;	
epi- (above; upon)	unable to)	

Definition of the Medical Word	Prefix	Word or Partial Word	Build the Medical Word
1. Pertaining to through (the) urethra	trans-	urethral	transurethral
2. Condition (of) painful sexual intercourse	_____	pareunia	_____
3. Process of recording higher (frequency) sound (waves)	_____	sonography	_____
4. Condition (of being) without spermatozoa	_____	spermia	_____
5. Action (of going) around (the foreskin to) cut (it off)	_____	cision	_____
6. Pertaining to again and again producing (children)	_____	productive	_____
7. Pertaining to after sexual intercourse	_____	coital	_____
8. Inflammation of (a coiled tube structure) upon (the) testis	_____	didymitis	_____
9. State (of) not (being able to) conceive (a child)	_____	fertility	_____

COMBINING FORM AND SUFFIX EXERCISE

Read the definition of the medical word. Select the correct suffix from the Suffix List. Select the correct combining form from the Combining Form List. Build the medical word and write it on the line. Be sure to check your spelling. The first one has been done for you.

SUFFIX LIST

-al (pertaining to)
-ancy (state)
-cele (hernia)
-ectomy (surgical removal)
-gen (that which produces)
-ism (disease from a specific cause; process)
-itis (infection of; inflammation of)
-ity (condition; state)
-logy (study of)
-oma (mass; tumor)
-opsy (process of viewing)
-osis (condition; process)
-ous (pertaining to)
-pexy (process of surgically fixing in place)
-scope (instrument used to examine)

COMBINING FORM LIST

andr/o- (male)	orch/o- (testicle; testis)
balan/o- (glans penis)	phim/o- (closed tight)
bi/o- (life; living organism; living tissue)	priap/o- (persistent erection)
	prostat/o- (prostate gland)
cancer/o- (cancer)	resect/o- (cut out; remove)
malign/o- (cancer; intentionally causing harm)	semin/o- (sperm; spermatozoon)
	varic/o- (varicose vein; varix)
morph/o- (shape)	vas/o- (blood vessel; vas deferens)
motil/o- (movement)	venere/o- (sexual intercourse)
orchi/o- (testicle; testis)	

Definition of the Medical Word

1. State (of) movement (of spermatozoa)
2. Surgical removal (of part of the) vas deferens
3. Pertaining to cancer
4. Hernia (of a) varicose vein (in the spermatic cord)
5. Tumor (of the structure that produces) sperm
6. Infection of (or) inflammation of (the) testis
7. Study of (the) shape (of spermatozoa)
8. Surgical removal (of the) prostate gland
9. Process of surgically fixing in place (a) testis
10. State (of) intentionally causing harm (cancer)
11. Infection of (or) inflammation of (the) glans penis
12. That (a drug) which produces male (characteristics)
13. Process of viewing living tissue (after it has been removed from the body)
14. Instrument used to examine (and then) cut out and remove (tissue)
15. Pertaining to (a disease transmitted by) sexual intercourse
16. Surgical removal (of a) testis
17. Infection of (or) inflammation of (the) prostate gland
18. Disease from a specific cause (of a) persistent erection
19. Condition (in which the foreskin opening is) closed tight

Build the Medical Word

motility
_____

MULTIPLE COMBINING FORMS AND SUFFIX EXERCISE

Read the definition of the medical word. Select the correct suffix and combining forms. Then build the medical word and write it on the line. Be sure to check your spelling. The first one has been done for you.

SUFFIX LIST	COMBINING FORM LIST	
-ary (pertaining to)	crypt/o- (hidden)	olig/o- (few; scanty)
-ency (condition of being; condition of having)	defici/o- (inadequate; lacking)	orchid/o- (testicle; testis)
	genit/o- (genitalia)	spermat/o- (sperm; spermatozoon)
-esis (condition; process)	gen/o- (arising from; produced by)	sperm/o- (sperm; spermatozoon)
-ia (condition; state; thing)	gynec/o- (female; woman)	urin/o- (urinary system; urine)
-ism (disease from a specific cause; process)	immun/o- (immune response)	vas/o- (blood vessel; vas deferens)
-stomy (surgically created opening)	mast/o- (breast; mastoid process)	

Definition of the Medical Word

1. Condition of having (an) immune response (that is) inadequate
2. Pertaining to (the) genitalia (and) urinary system
3. Surgically created opening (in one part of the) vas deferens (to join another part of the) vas deferens
4. Condition (of enlargement in which the male's chest resembles the) female breast
5. Process (of) spermatozoa produced by (the testis)
6. Disease from a specific cause (of) hidden (undescended) testis
7. Condition (of) few spermatozoa

Build the Medical Word

immunodeficiency
_____

12.7A Spell Medical Words

PROOFREADING AND SPELLING EXERCISE

Read the following paragraph. Identify each misspelled medical word and write the correct spelling of it on the line.

The male anatomy is located in the pelvic area. It shares the urethra with the urinary system, and this exits from the glands penis or tip of the penis. The peroneal area is the skin between the anus and skrotum. The testes produce spermatozon if they have descended through the inguinel canal. The epidydimis holds sperm or gameetes. Then sperm travel through the vas deference and ejaculatory duct. The seminole vesicles add fluid, as does the prostrate gland, to make semen.

1. _____   6. _____

2. _____   7. _____

3. _____   8. _____

4. _____   9. _____

5. _____   10. _____

ENGLISH AND MEDICAL WORD EQUIVALENTS EXERCISE

For each English word or phrase, write its equivalent medical word or phrase. Be sure to check your spelling. The first one has been done for you.

English Word	Medical Word	English Word	Medical Word
1. testicular cancer	seminoma	5. undescended testicle	_____
2. pain during intercourse	_____	6. genital warts	_____
3. impotence	_____	7. enlarged prostate	_____
4. sexually transmitted disease	_____		

HEARING MEDICAL WORDS EXERCISE

You hear someone speaking the medical words given below. Read each pronunciation and then write the medical word it represents. Be sure to check your spelling. The first one has been done for you.

1. PAIR-ih-NEE-um   perineum   6. GAW-noh-REE-ah   _____

2. BAL-ah-NY-tis   _____   7. or-KY-tis   _____

3. SHANG-ker   _____   8. PRAW-stah-TEK-toh-mee   _____

4. DIS-pah-ROO-nee-ah   _____   9. SEM-ih-NOH-mah   _____

5. EP-ih-DID-ih-mis   _____   10. SIF-ih-lis   _____

ELECTRONIC PATIENT RECORD #2

This is a hospital Operative Report. Read the report and answer the questions.

PEARSON GENERAL HOSPITAL

Task   Edit   View   Time Scale   Options   Help

OPERATIVE REPORT

PATIENT NAME:	JENKINS, Daniel
HOSPITAL NUMBER:	206-47-5869
DATE OF OPERATION:	November 19, 20xx

Source: Sirikorn Thamniyom/123 RF

PREOPERATIVE DIAGNOSES

1. Undescended left testis
2. Left indirect inguinal hernia

POSTOPERATIVE DIAGNOSES

1. Undescended left testis, corrected
2. Left indirect inguinal hernia, repaired

PROCEDURES

1. Left orchiopexy
2. Left inguinal herniorrhaphy

DESCRIPTION OF OPERATIVE PROCEDURE

The patient was placed in the dorsal supine position, and general anesthesia was induced via mask anesthesia. The pubic region and external genitalia were prepped and draped with Betadine antibacterial scrub. A transverse incision was made in the suprapubic skin fold on the left side. It was carried down through subcutaneous tissue and fat. Bleeding was controlled with the electrocautery. The left testis was identified in the operative field and was noted to be lying just within the external inguinal ring. The external oblique fascia was incised with a #15 scalpel and Metzenbaum scissors. The left testis was grasped and freed from its surrounding structures up to the level of the internal inguinal ring. This maneuver freed up the cord so that adequate cord length was obtained. The hernia sac was then opened and dissected up to the level of the inguinal ring, where it was closed with 4-0 Vicryl suture. Then we again turned our attention to the undescended left testis. A scrotal incision was made and a subcutaneous pouch created. The left testis was then brought down into the pouch, and a 3-0 silk suture was placed in the lower pole of the testis, brought out through the scrotal skin, and tied over a cotton pledget to secure the testis in place. A careful search detected no bleeding in the scrotal or groin incisions. The scrotal incision was closed with 5-0 Vicryl. The external oblique fascia was closed with a running 4-0 Vicryl suture. The subcutaneous tissue was closed with 4-0 Vicryl. The skin was closed with a running subcuticular 3-0 Prolene suture, and the child was discharged from the operating room in satisfactory condition.

James R. Bentley, M.D.

James R. Bentley, M.D.

JRB:btg
D: 11/19/xx
T: 11/19/xx

1. Divide *orchiopexy* into its two word parts and define each word part.

   Word Part   **Meaning**

   _____   _____

   _____   _____

2. An incision in the suprapubic skin fold would be located _____.

   a. below the pubic bone

   b. around the pubic bone

   c. above the pubic bone

3. In the dorsal supine position, the patient is placed on his (**abdomen**, **back**, **side**).

4. In a male, the external genitalia include what five structures?

   _____   _____

   _____   _____

   _____

5. Incisions were made in what two areas? _____   _____

6. The hernia sac was closed with sutures. **True**   **False**

7. *Subcutaneous* means (**around the testis**, **inside the scrotum**, **under the skin**).

8. The left testis was not descended. What operative procedure was performed to correct this? _____

9. A preoperative diagnosis represents the patient's condition (**before**, **during**, **after**) surgery.

10. "The maneuver freed up the cord . . . " What *cord* does this refer to? **spinal cord**   **spermatic cord**   **umbilical cord**

MyMedicalTerminologyLab™

MyMedicalTerminologyLab is a premium online homework management system that includes a host of features to help you study. Registered users will find:

- A multitude of quizzes and activities built within the MyLab platform

- Powerful tools that track and analyze your results—allowing you to create a personalized learning experience

- Videos and audio pronunciations to help enrich your progress

- Streaming lesson presentations (Guided Lectures) and self-paced learning modules

- A space where you and your instructor can check your progress and manage your assignments

Chapter 13

Gynecology and Obstetrics

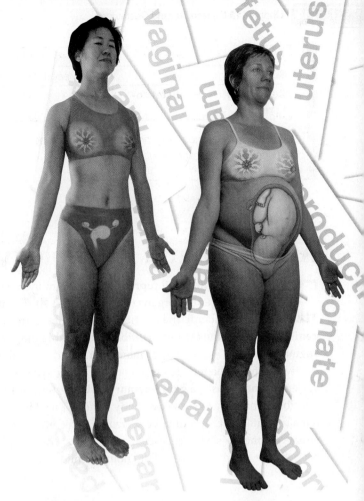

Female Genital and Reproductive System

Gynecology (GY-neh-KAW-loh-jee) is the medical specialty that studies the anatomy and physiology of the female genital system and uses laboratory and diagnostic procedures, medical and surgical procedures, and drugs to treat female genital diseases.

Obstetrics (awb-STEH-triks) is the medical specialty that studies the anatomy and physiology of the female reproductive system and uses laboratory and diagnostic procedures, medical and surgical procedures, and drugs to monitor pregnancy and childbirth and treat diseases.

 ## Learning Outcomes

After you study this chapter, you should be able to

13.1 Identify structures of the female genital and reproductive system.

13.2 Describe the processes of oogenesis, menstruation, conception, labor, and delivery.

13.3 Describe normal and abnormal findings in the neonate.

13.4 Describe common female genital and reproductive, and common neonatal, diseases, laboratory and diagnostic procedures, medical and surgical procedures, and drugs.

13.5 Form the plural and adjective forms of nouns related to gynecology, obstetrics, and neonatology.

13.6 Give the meanings of word parts and abbreviations related to gynecology, obstetrics, and neonatology.

FIGURE 13-1 ■ Female genital and reproductive system. The female genital and reproductive system consists of the ovaries, uterine tubes, uterus, and vagina, as well as the external genitalia on the outside of the body. It also includes the breasts. This body system undergoes significant changes during pregnancy and childbirth.

Source: Pearson Education

13.7 Divide gynecology, obstetrics, and neonatalogy words and build these words.

13.8 Spell and pronounce gynecology, obstetrics, and neonatology words.

13.9 Research sound-alike gynecology and other words.

13.10 Analyze the medical content and meaning of gynecology and neonatal reports.

Medical Language Key

To unlock the definition of a medical word, break it into word parts. Give the meaning of each word part. Put the meanings of the word parts in order, beginning with the meaning of the suffix, then the prefix (if present), then the combining form(s).

	Word Part	Word Part Meaning
Suffix	**-logy**	*study of*
Combining Form	**gynec/o-**	*female; woman*

Gynecology: ▸ *Study of females.*

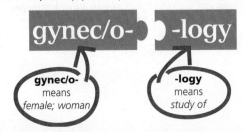

	Word Part	Word Part Meaning
Suffix	-ics	*knowledge; practice*
Combining Form	obstetr/o-	*pregnancy and childbirth*

Obstetrics: ▶ *Knowledge and practice (of treating women during) pregnancy and childbirth.*

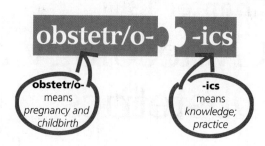

Anatomy and Physiology

The **female genital and reproductive system** includes both internal and external genitalia or **genital organs** (see Figure 13-1 ■). The **internal genitalia** in the pelvic cavity include the ovaries, uterine tubes, uterus, and vagina. The **external genitalia** include the area of the mons pubis, labia majora, labia minora, clitoris, and vaginal introitus. The breasts or mammary glands also play a role in the female reproductive system. The female genital and reproductive system together with the urinary system is known as the **genitourinary (GU) system** or **urogenital system** because of the close proximity of these two body systems (see Figure 13-2 ■). The function of the female genital and reproductive system is to secrete the female hormones, develop the female secondary sexual characteristics, produce ova (eggs), menstruate, conceive and bear children, and produce milk to nourish children.

Pronunciation/Word Parts

genital (JEN-ih-tal)
  genit/o- *genitalia*
  -al *pertaining to*

reproductive (REE-proh-DUK-tiv)
  re- *again and again; backward; unable to*
  product/o- *produce*
  -ive *pertaining to*
Select the correct prefix meaning to get the definition of *reproductive: pertaining to again and again producing (children).*

genitalia (JEN-ih-TAY-lee-ah)

genitourinary (JEN-ih-toh-YOOR-ih-NAIR-ee)
  genit/o- *genitalia*
  urin/o- *urinary system; urine*
  -ary *pertaining to*

urogenital (YOOR-oh-JEN-ih-tal)
  ur/o- *urinary system; urine*
  genit/o- *genitalia*
  -al *pertaining to*

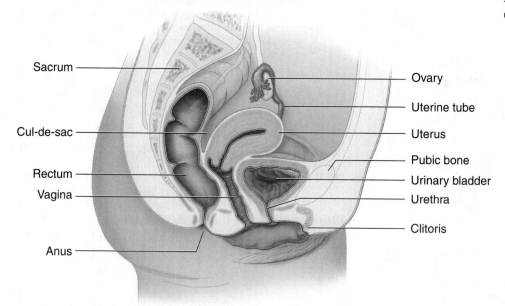

Sacrum — Ovary
Uterine tube
Uterus
Cul-de-sac — Pubic bone
Rectum — Urinary bladder
Vagina — Urethra
Clitoris
Anus —

FIGURE 13-2 ■ Abdominopelvic cavity.
The female genital and reproductive organs in the abdominopelvic cavity lie in close proximity to the organs of the urinary system and gastrointestinal system.
Source: Pearson Education

Anatomy of the Female Genital and Reproductive System

Ovaries

An **ovary** is a small egg-shaped gland about 2 inches in length near the end of a uterine tube (see Figure 13-3 ■). The ovaries are held in place by the **broad ligament**, a folded sheet of peritoneum that extends to the walls of the pelvic cavity, and by other ligaments. The ovaries are the **gonads** or sex glands in a female. They function as part of the female genital and reproductive system and the endocrine system (discussed in "Endocrinology," Chapter 14). The ovaries contain **follicles** that rupture, releasing **ova** (eggs) during the menstrual cycle. The ovaries are glands that secrete three hormones (estradiol, progesterone, and testosterone), and these hormones affect puberty, menstruation, and pregnancy.

Pronunciation/Word Parts

ovary (OH-vah-ree)

ovarian (oh-VAIR-ee-an)
  ovari/o- *ovary*
  -an *pertaining to*
The combining form **oophor/o-** also means *ovary*.

ligament (LIG-ah-ment)

gonad (GOH-nad)
  gon/o- *ovum; seed; spermatozoon*
  -ad *in the direction of; toward*

follicle (FAW-lih-kl)

ovum (OH-vum)

ova (OH-vah)
Form the plural by changing *-um* to *-a*. The combining forms **o/o-**, **ov/i-**, **ov/o-**, and **ovul/o-** mean *egg; ovum*.

DID YOU KNOW?

Before birth, while a female fetus is still in the mother's uterus, the fetal ovary has about 2 million **oocytes** (immature ova). These are all the ova that a female will ever have, as no more are produced after she is born. By puberty only about 25% of these remain and, of those, only about 400 mature ova are released during all the ovulations throughout her lifetime.

oocyte (OH-oh-site)
  o/o- *egg; ovum*
  -cyte *cell*

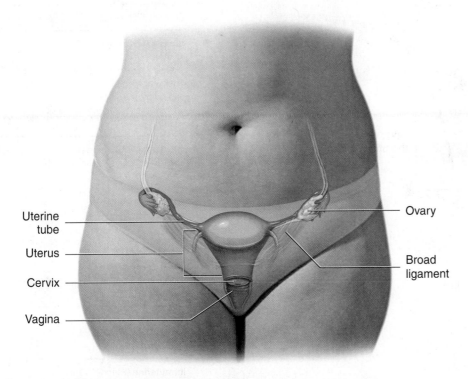

Uterine tube
Uterus
Cervix
Vagina
Ovary
Broad ligament

FIGURE 13-3 ■ Ovaries, uterine tubes, and uterus.
The ovaries and uterine tubes lie on either side of the uterus. They are suspended within the abdominopelvic cavity by ligaments. The cervix of the uterus protrudes downward into the vagina.
Source: Pearson Education

Uterine Tubes

Each **uterine tube** is about 5 inches in length and is held in place by the broad ligament. The function of the uterine tube is to transport an ovum from the ovary to the uterus. The medial end of the uterine tube is connected to the uterus, but its lateral end is not connected to the ovary (see Figure 13-4). There is an open space (part of the abdomino-pelvic cavity) between each ovary and its uterine tube. The ovary releases an ovum into this open space. **Fimbriae**, moving, fingerlike projections at the end of the uterine tube, create currents that carry the ovum into the **lumen** of the tube. Within the uterine tube, **cilia** (tiny hairs) beat in waves while **peristalsis** (coordinated, wavelike contractions of smooth muscle around the tube) propels the ovum toward the uterus. Fluid inside the uterine tube contains nutrients to nourish the ovum on its 3-day journey to the uterus. The uterine tube is also known as the **oviduct**. Together, the ovaries and the uterine tubes are known as the **adnexa**.

Uterus

The **uterus** is an inverted pear-shaped organ about 3 inches in length (see Figure 13-4 ■). The uterus is held in place by the broad ligament and other ligaments that go from the uterus to the sides of the pelvic walls and to the bony sacrum. The broad ligament creates a small pouch, the **cul-de-sac**, between the uterus and the rectum (see Figure 13-2). The **fundus** is the rounded top of the uterus. The body of the uterus is its widest part. The body narrows and becomes the **cervix** (neck of the uterus). Within the uterus is the hollow **intrauterine cavity**, which narrows into the **cervical canal**. The **cervical os** in the center of the cervix is the opening of the cervical canal. The rounded tip of the cervix

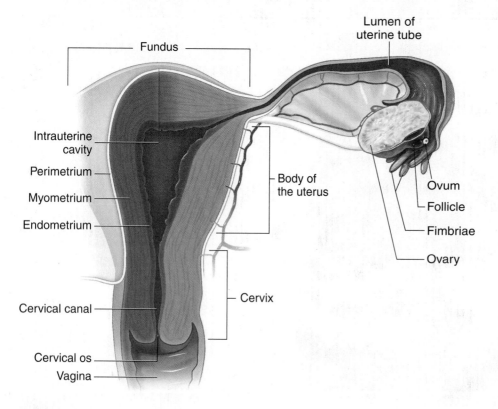

FIGURE 13-4 ■ Uterus.
The fundus, body, and cervix are regions of the uterus. The perimetrium is the outer covering of the uterus. The myometrium is the layer of smooth muscle that makes up the uterine wall. The endometrium is the layer of glands and tissue that lines the intrauterine cavity. The ovary contains a follicle that ruptures and releases an ovum. Movements of the fimbriae draw the ovum into the lumen of the uterine tube that goes to the uterus.
Source: Pearson Education

Pronunciation/Word Parts

uterine (YOO-teh-rin) (YOO-teh-rine)
  uter/o- *uterus; womb*
  -ine *pertaining to; thing pertaining to*
The combining forms **salping/o-** and **fallopi/o-** mean *uterine tube*. The uterine tube was formerly known as the *fallopian tube*.

fimbriae (FIM-bree-ee)
Fimbria is a Latin singular noun. Form the plural by changing *-a* to *-ae*. Because there are so many fimbriae, the singular form is seldom used.

lumen (LOO-men)

cilia (SIL-ee-ah)
Cilium is a Latin singular noun. Form the plural by changing *-um* to *-a*.

peristalsis (PAIR-ih-STAL-sis)
  peri- *around*
  stal/o- *contraction*
  -sis *condition; process*

oviduct (OH-vih-dukt)
  ov/i- *egg; ovum*
  -duct *duct; tube*

adnexa (ad-NEK-sah)

adnexal (ad-NEK-sal)
  adnex/o- *accessory connecting parts*
  -al *pertaining to*

uterus (YOO-ter-us)

uterine (YOO-teh-rin) (YOO-teh-rine)
  uter/o- *uterus; womb*
  -ine *pertaining to; thing pertaining to*
The combining forms **hyster/o-**, **metri/o-**, and **metr/o-** also mean *uterus; womb*. Laypersons refer to the uterus as the *womb*.

cul-de-sac (KUL-deh-sak)
The combining form *culd/o-* means *cul-de-sac*.

fundus (FUN-dus)

fundal (FUN-dal)
  fund/o- *fundus; part farthest from the opening*
  -al *pertaining to*

cervix (SER-viks)

cervical (SER-vih-kal)
  cervic/o- *cervix; neck*
  -al *pertaining to*

intrauterine (IN-trah-YOO-teh-rin) (IN-trah-YOO-teh-rine)
  intra- *within*
  uter/o- *uterus; womb*
  -ine *pertaining to*

os (AWS)

projects about ½ inch into the vagina. The superior portion of the uterus is tipped anteriorly, and part of it rests on the urinary bladder (see Figure 13-2); this normal position is known as **anteflexion**.

The wall of the uterus is composed of three layers: perimetrium, myometrium, and endometrium. The **perimetrium** is the outer layer. It is a serous membrane that is part of the peritoneum that lines the abdominopelvic cavity (discussed in "Gastroenterology," Chapter 3). The **myometrium** or uterine muscle contains smooth muscle fibers that are oriented in different directions. This allows the uterus to contract strongly from all sides during labor and the delivery of a baby. The innermost layer, the **endometrium**, lines the intrauterine cavity. It is a mucous membrane that contains glands, and this layer thickens during the menstrual cycle. If an ovum is not fertilized, this lining is shed during menstruation.

Vagina

The **vagina** is a short, tubelike structure about 3 inches in length (see Figures 13-2 and 13-4). Within the vagina is the open **vaginal canal**. The cervix of the uterus protrudes into the superior end of the vaginal canal. The **fornix** is the area of the vaginal canal that is behind and around the cervix. At the inferior end of the vaginal canal is the **hymen**, an elastic membrane that partially or completely covers the opening, although it is sometimes absent. The hymen, if present, is easily torn by the insertion of a tampon, a vaginal examination, or sexual intercourse.

The vagina has three functions. During menstruation, it transports the shed endometrium to the outside of the body. During sexual intercourse, it holds the penis and collects the ejaculate that contains spermatozoa. During birth, it is part of the birth canal that takes the baby to the outside of the mother's body.

External Genitalia

The external genitalia include the mons pubis, labia majora, labia minora, clitoris, vaginal introitus, and glands that produce lubricating secretions (see Figure 13-5 ■). The **mons pubis** is the rounded, fleshy pad with pubic hair that overlies the pubic bone. The labia

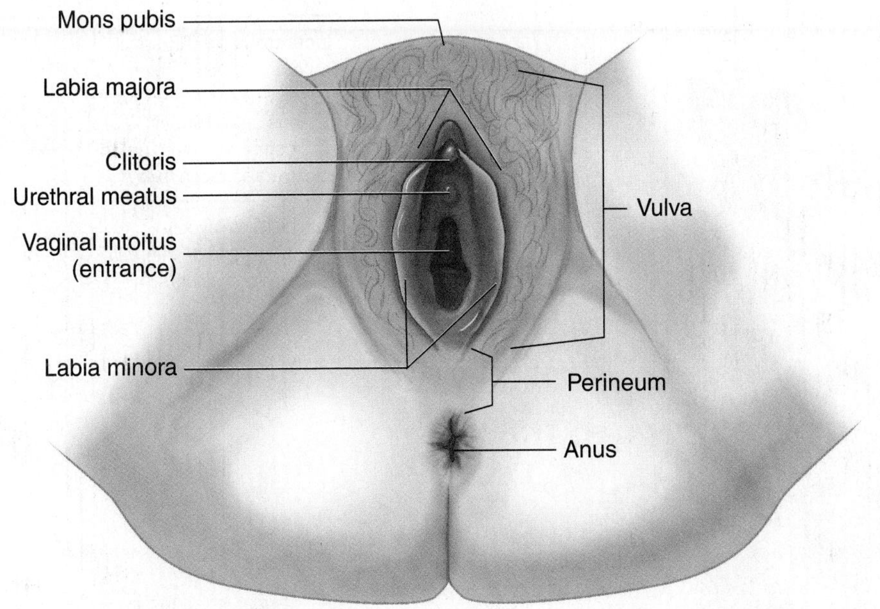

Pronunciation/Word Parts

anteflexion (AN-tee-FLEK-shun)
ante- before; forward
flex/o- bending
-ion action; condition

perimetrium (PAIR-ih-MEE-tree-um)
peri- around
metri/o- uterus; womb
-um period of time; structure

myometrium (MY-oh-MEE-tree-um)
my/o- muscle
metri/o- uterus; womb
-um period of time; structure

endometrium (EN-doh-MEE-tree-um)
endo- innermost; within
metri/o- uterus; womb
-um period of time; structure

endometrial (EN-doh-MEE-tree-al)

vagina (vah-JY-nah)

vaginal (VAJ-ih-nal)
vagin/o- vagina
-al pertaining to
The combining form **colp/o-** also means vagina.

fornix (FOR-niks)
The fornix is also known as the vaginal vault.

hymen (HY-men)

mons pubis (MAWNZ PYOO-bis)

FIGURE 13-5 ■ External female genitalia.
The labia majora and labia minora protect and partially cover the clitoris, vaginal introitus, and the glands that secrete mucus. The vulva includes all these structures but also includes the mons pubis.
Source: Pearson Education

consist of two sets of lip-shaped structures that run anteriorly to posteriorly and partially cover the urethral meatus and vaginal introitus. The thicker, outermost lips, the **labia majora**, are fleshy and covered with pubic hair on their outer surface. The smooth, thin, inner lips, the **labia minora**, lie beneath the labia majora. The **clitoris** is the organ of sexual response in the female. Its tip is located anterior to the urethral meatus. With sexual stimulation, the clitoris enlarges with blood and becomes firm. The **vaginal introitus** is the opening to the outside of the body (see Figure 13-5); it is posterior to the urethral meatus. Three sets of glands near the vaginal introitus—**Bartholin's glands**, the **urethral glands**, and **Skene's glands (BUS)**—secrete mucus during sexual arousal. The **vulva** includes all of these structures. The area between the vulva and the anus is the **perineum**.

Pronunciation/Word Parts

labia majora (LAY-bee-ah mah-JOR-ah)

labia minora (LAY-bee-ah my-NOR-ah)
Labium is a Latin singular noun. Form the plural by changing *-um* to *-a.*

labial (LAY-bee-al)
  labi/o- *labium; lip*
  -al *pertaining to*

clitoris (KLIT-oh-ris)

introitus (in-TROH-ih-tus)

Bartholin (BAR-thoh-lin)

urethral (yoor-EE-thral)
  urethr/o- *urethra*
  -al *pertaining to*

Skene (SKEEN)

vulva (VUL-vah)

vulvar (VUL-var)
  vulv/o- *vulva*
  -ar *pertaining to*
The combining form **episi/o-** also means *vulva.*

perineum (PAIR-ih-NEE-um)
  perine/o- *perineum*
  -um *period of time; structure*

perineal (PAIR-ih-NEE-al)

mammary (MAM-ah-ree)
  mamm/o- *breast*
  -ary *pertaining to*
The combining forms **mamm/a-** and **mast/o-** also mean *breast.*

lactiferous (lak-TIF-er-us)
  lact/i- *milk*
  fer/o- *bear*
  -ous *pertaining to*
The combining forms **galact/o-** and **lact/o-** also mean *milk.*

lobule (LAW-byool)
  lob/o- *lobe of an organ*
  -ule *small thing*

> **WORD ALERT**
> **Sound-Alike Words**
>
> **perineum** (noun) area between the vulva and the anus
> *Example: The perineum is an area of skin on the outside of the body.*
>
> **perimetrium** (noun) serous membrane on the outside of the uterus
> *Example: The perimetrium is the outermost layer of the uterus.*
>
> **peritoneum** (noun) serous membrane that lines the abdominopelvic cavity
> *Example: The peritoneum secretes peritoneal fluid that fills the spaces between the intestines and other organs in the abdominopelvic cavity.*

Breasts

The breasts or **mammary glands** are located on the chest. They contain adipose (fatty) tissue and glands. The breasts develop at puberty in response to estradiol secreted by the ovaries. They are one of the female sexual characteristics, and they also provide milk to nourish the newborn after birth. The breasts contain **lactiferous lobules** that produce milk (see Figure 13-6 ■). Milk flows through the **lactiferous ducts** to

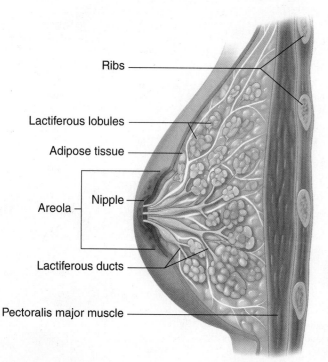

Ribs
Lactiferous lobules
Adipose tissue
Areola
Nipple
Lactiferous ducts
Pectoralis major muscle

FIGURE 13-6 ■ Breast.
The breasts or mammary glands develop during puberty, but the lactiferous lobules do not produce milk until after childbirth.
Source: Pearson Education

the nipple. The **areola** is the pigmented area around the nipple. The surface of the areola is covered with small, elevated areas that secrete oil to protect the nipple when the baby nurses.

Physiology of Sexual Maturity, Oogenesis, Menstruation, and Conception

Sexual Maturity and Oogenesis

At the onset of puberty (adolescence), the anterior pituitary gland in the brain (discussed in "Endocrinology," Chapter 14) begins to secrete two hormones that stimulate the ovaries.

1. **Follicle-stimulating hormone (FSH).** FSH stimulates a follicle in the ovary to enlarge and produce a mature ovum. **Oogenesis** is the process of forming a mature ovum. Like a spermatozoon, the mature ovum is created by mitosis and meiosis. Like a spermatozoon, the mature ovum is known as a **gamete**. However, unlike spermatozoa, only a single ovum is produced. It contains 23 chromosomes, and the remaining chromosomes are discarded in small packets of cytoplasm known as *polar bodies*. FSH also stimulates the follicles to secrete estradiol, which causes the development of the female sexual characteristics during puberty.

2. **Luteinizing hormone (LH).** LH stimulates a single follicle each month to rupture and release its mature ovum. Then it stimulates the ruptured follicle (corpus luteum) to secrete estradiol and progesterone.

The ovary secretes these three hormones:

1. **Estradiol**. The most abundant and most biologically active of the female hormones. It is secreted by each follicle (and also by the ruptured follicle [corpus luteum] after ovulation). Estradiol causes the development of these female sexual characteristics during puberty: enlargement of the external genitalia, development of the breasts, widening of the pelvis, growth of body hair in the axillary and genital areas, and development of the sexual drive (see Figure 13-7 ■). Estradiol also causes the endometrium (lining of the uterus) to thicken during the menstrual cycle. Estradiol is also secreted by the placenta during pregnancy.

2. **Progesterone**. Hormone secreted by a ruptured follicle (corpus luteum) after ovulation. Progesterone also causes the endometrium to thicken during the menstrual cycle. It is also secreted by the placenta during pregnancy.

3. **Testosterone**. A male hormone secreted by cells around the follicle. It plays a role in the female sexual drive.

The Menstrual Cycle

With the onset of puberty, the female begins to ovulate and menstruate. **Menarche** is the beginning of **menstruation**, which occurs with the first **menstrual period** or **menses**.

Each **menstrual cycle**, on average, lasts 28 days and includes four phases: the menstrual phase, the proliferative phase (followed by ovulation), the secretory phase, and the ischemic phase (see Figure 13-8 ■).

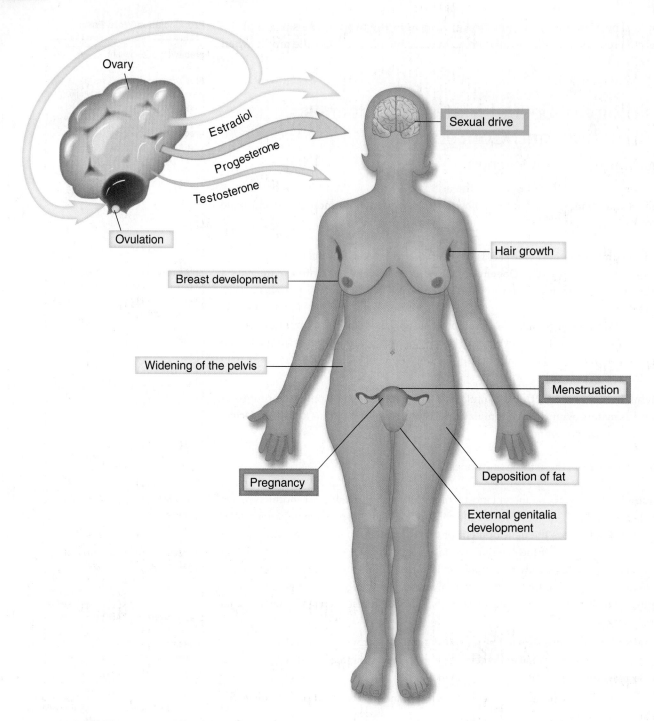

FIGURE 13-7 ■ Hormones secreted by the ovaries.
Estradiol produces the female sexual characteristics that occur during puberty. Estradiol and progesterone stimulate the growth of the endometrium prior to menstruation and also (if an ovum is fertilized) these hormones stimulate the growth of the endometrium during pregnancy when they are secreted by the placenta. Testosterone plays a role in the female sexual drive.
Source: Pearson Education

THE MENSTRUAL CYCLE

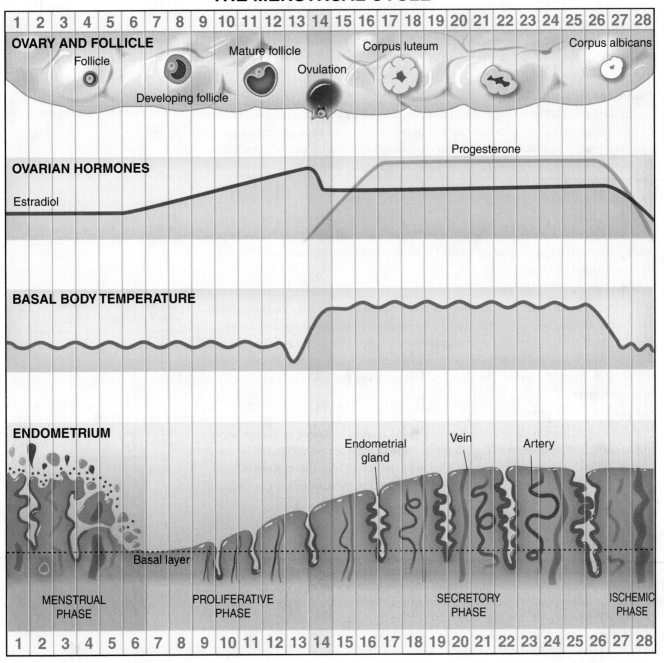

FIGURE 13-8 ■ Menstrual cycle.

Activities in the ovary are related to those in the uterus during the menstrual cycle. Hormones (estradiol and progesterone) produced by the follicle and then by the corpus luteum of the ovary cause the endometrium of the uterus to proliferate and thicken. If the ovum is not fertilized, the declining levels of these hormones cause the endometrium to slough off in menstruation.

Source: Pearson Education

1. **Menstrual phase** (Days 1–6)

    Menstruation begins. Approximately 30 mL of blood, endometrial tissue, and mucus is sloughed off from the uterus and passes through the vagina. All that remains of the endometrium is a thin layer of glands. At the same time, several follicles in the ovary are enlarging and their ova are maturing in preparation for one of them to be released during ovulation on day 14.

2. **Proliferative phase** (Days 7–13)

    Follicle-stimulating hormone (FSH) from the anterior pituitary gland stimulates the ovarian follicles to secrete estradiol. One follicle becomes greatly enlarged and produces a mature ovum. The endometrium in the uterus becomes thicker because of estradiol. At the end of the proliferative phase, mucus in the cervical canal thins to allow spermatozoa to pass through it.

    Ovulation (Day 14)

    Luteinizing hormone (LH) from the anterior pituitary gland causes the enlarged ovarian follicle to rupture, releasing a mature ovum. The **basal (baseline) body temperature** rises about 0.4 degrees at the time of ovulation and stays elevated until the onset of menstruation (see Figure 13-8).

3. **Secretory phase** (Days 15–26)

    The ruptured ovarian follicle fills with yellow fat and becomes the **corpus luteum**. The corpus luteum secretes estradiol and progesterone. Progesterone causes the endometrial glands of the uterus to enlarge, and the endometrium becomes thicker. Small arteries grow to the innermost edge of the endometrium, ready to nourish a fertilized ovum, if one enters the uterus. The basal body temperature continues to be elevated due to progesterone.

4. **Ischemic phase** (Days 27–28)

    The corpus luteum turns into white scar tissue (corpus albicans) and stops secreting estradiol and progesterone. The abrupt decrease in these hormones causes the small arteries in the endometrium to contract. This stops the flow of blood and causes ischemia of the tissue. The endometrium begins to slough off, and menstruation (the first phase of the menstrual cycle) begins again.

Pronunciation/Word Parts

proliferative (proh-LIF-er-ah-TIV)
Proliferate means *to increase in number by producing more of the same.*

ovulation (AW-vyoo-LAY-shun)
ovul/o- *egg; ovum*
-ation *being; having; process*

secretory (SEE-kreh-TOR-ee)
secret/o- *produce; secrete*
-ory *having the function of*

corpus luteum (KOR-pus LOO-tee-um)

ischemic (is-KEE-mik)
isch/o- *block; keep back*
-emic *pertaining to a condition of the blood; pertaining to a substance in the blood*

DID YOU KNOW?

In the 1800s, the average age for menarche (the onset of menstruation) was 18 years old. Now the average age for menarche is 12 years old. Researchers point to better health and nutrition as the reason, but feel that childhood obesity, estrogen in the environment (from discarded birth control pills), and pesticides (which have an estrogen-like effect) are the reason for a decrease in the age.

Conception

Of the 100–500 million spermatozoa deposited in the vagina during sexual intercourse, only some are able to reach the ovum in the uterine tube; this occurs 24–48 hours after sexual intercourse. Chemicals secreted by the ovum attract the spermatozoa. A cap-like layer of enzymes on the head of each spermatozoon begins to dissolve the layer of cells around the ovum (see Figure 13-9 ■). Many spermatozoa attach to the ovum, but only one penetrates its surface. This is the moment of **fertilization** or **conception**. After that, the surface of the ovum changes and actually repels the other spermatozoa. When a spermatozoon unites with an ovum, the resulting cell has 46 chromosomes and is known as a **zygote**. **Pregnancy** begins at the moment of conception.

A zygote immediately begins to divide as it moves through the uterine tube. Within the intrauterine cavity, it sinks into the thickened endometrium. At this point, the zygote is a hollow ball with an inner mass of cells and an outer layer.

fertilization (FER-til-ih-ZAY-shun)
fertil/o- *conceive; form*
-ization *process of creating; process of inserting; process of making*

conception (con-SEP-shun)
concept/o- *conceive; form*
-ion *action; condition*

zygote (ZY-goht)

pregnancy (PREG-nan-see)
pregn/o- *being with child*
-ancy *state*

pregnant (PREG-nant)
pregn/o- *being with child*
-ant *pertaining to*

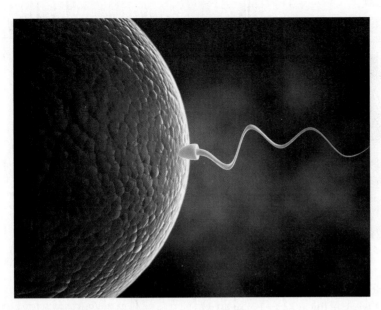

FIGURE 13-9 ■ An ovum and spermatozoon.
An ovum is nearly 100,000 times larger than a spermatozoon. An ovum and a spermatozoon are gametes that each contain only 23 chromosomes. A fertilized ovum contains 46 chromosomes and is known as a *zygote.*
Source: Jezper/Shutterstock

The inner mass of cells becomes the amnion and the embryo. The **amnion** (or bag of waters) is a membrane sac that produces **amniotic fluid**. The developing embryo floats in, and is cushioned by, the amniotic fluid.

The outer layer of the zygote becomes the **chorion**. It sends fingerlike projections (villi) into the endometrium to absorb nutrients and oxygen. The chorion produces the hormone **human chorionic gonadotropin (HCG)**. HCG stimulates the corpus luteum of the ovary to keep producing estradiol and progesterone. This maintains the thickened endometrium to support the developing embryo and prevents menstruation from occurring during the rest of the pregnancy. The chorion becomes the **placenta**, a pancake-like structure about 7 inches in diameter and 1–2 inches thick. By the end of the first trimester of pregnancy, the placenta begins to secrete estradiol and progesterone and takes over the job of the corpus luteum in the ovary. Other structures in the chorion form the rubbery, flexible **umbilical cord** (with its two arteries and one vein) that connects the placenta to the fetus. The umbilical cord and placenta bring oxygen, nutrients, and antibodies from the mother to the fetus and remove carbon dioxide and waste products.

After 4 days of development, the zygote is known as an **embryo**. After 8 weeks, it is known as a **fetus** (see Figure 13-10 ■). The fetus, placenta, and all fluids and tissue in the uterus are known as the **products of conception**.

Pronunciation/Word Parts

amnion (AM-nee-on)

amniotic (AM-nee-AW-tik)
   amni/o- *amnion; membrane around the fetus*
   -tic *pertaining to*

chorion (KOR-ee-awn)

chorionic (KOR-ee-AW-nik)
   chorion/o- *chorion*
   -ic *pertaining to*

gonadotropin (GOH-nah-doh-TROH-pin)
   gonad/o- *gonad; ovary; testis*
   trop/o- *having an affinity for; stimulating; turning*
   -in *substance*

placenta (plah-SEN-tah)

placental (plah-SEN-tal)
   placent/o- *placenta*
   -al *pertaining to*

umbilicus (um-BIL-ih-kus) (UM-bih-LIE-kus)

umbilical (um-BIL-ih-kal)
   umbilic/o- *navel; umbilicus*
   -al *pertaining to*

embryo (EM-bree-oh)

embryonic (EM-bree-AW-nik)
   embryon/o- *embryo; immature form*
   -ic *pertaining to*

fetus (FEE-tus)
Fetus is a Latin singular noun. Its plural form *fetuses* does not follow the regular rule for Latin nouns ending in *-us.*

fetal (FEE-tal)
   fet/o- *fetus*
   -al *pertaining to*

CLINICAL CONNECTIONS

Genetics. The sex chromosomes are one of the chromosome pairs that are in the nucleus of every cell in the body. In a female, every cell contains two X chromosomes. In a male, every cell contains an X chromosome and a Y chromosome.

The ovum always contains an X chromosome. A spermatozoon contains either an X chromosome or a Y chromosome. An X chromosome from the ovum and an X chromosome from the spermatozoon unite to create a female (XX). An X chromosome from the ovum and a Y chromosome from the spermatozoon unite to create a male (XY). **Identical twins** occur when one already developing zygote splits to create two separate but identical zygotes. **Fraternal twins** occur when the ovary releases two ova that are fertilized by different spermatozoa. Multiple zygotes can develop if the ovary releases multiple ova that are all fertilized; this can occur in patients taking ovulation-stimulating drugs for infertility.

fraternal (frah-TER-nal)
   fratern/o- *close association; close relationship*
   -al *pertaining to*

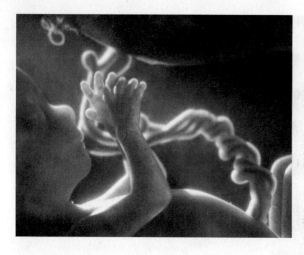

FIGURE 13-10 ■ Fetus at 16 weeks' gestation.
This fetus is 5 inches long from head to buttocks and weighs 3 ½ ounces. It is floating in amniotic fluid. The face, hands, and feet are developed. The eyes are not open, but the face can have expressions of squinting and frowning. The arteries bringing red, oxygenated blood to the fetus are visible in the umbilical cord.
Source: Scanpix Sweden AB

Gestation is from the moment of conception to the moment of birth. The gestational period is approximately 9 months (38–42 weeks), the average being 40 weeks (see Figure 13-11 ■). Gestation can be divided into three time periods, or **trimesters**. Each trimester is 3 months long. For the fetus, the period of time from conception to birth is the **prenatal period**. For the mother, the period of time from conception to birth is known as **antepartum**.

gestation (jes-TAY-shun)
  gestat/o- *conception to birth*
  -ion *action; condition*

trimester (TRY-mes-ter) (try-MES-ter)

prenatal (pree-NAY-tal)
  pre- *before; in front of*
  nat/o- *birth*
  -al *pertaining to*

antepartum (AN-tee-PAR-tum)
  ante- *before; forward*
  part/o- *childbirth; labor*
  -um *period of time; structure*
The combining form **par/o-** means *giving birth.*

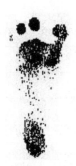

FIGURE 13-11 ■ Fetal footprint.
This is the actual footprint that appeared on the delivery room record of a fetus who was born prematurely at 23 weeks' gestation.
Source: Susan M. Turley

DID YOU KNOW?
The fetus swallows amniotic fluid each day. The fetal kidneys excrete urine into the amniotic fluid. The amniotic fluid contains urea and creatinine (waste products in the urine), skin cells and hair shed by the fetus, and two important substances (lecithin and sphingomyelin) that can be used to determine the maturity of the fetal lungs when the amniotic fluid is tested.

Physiology of Labor and Delivery

As the fetus grows, the uterus expands, taking up space in the mother's abdominal cavity and displacing her abdominal organs. This causes constipation, urinary frequency, and shortness of breath in the mother. During the last trimester of pregnancy, the uterus contracts irregularly to strengthen itself in preparation for childbirth. These are known as **Braxton Hicks contractions** or *false labor*. Progesterone from the placenta keeps these contractions from becoming labor contractions. The cervical os remains closed (not dilated), and the wall of the cervix remains thick (not effaced). A mucus plug in the cervical os keeps out microorganisms. Late in the pregnancy, the head of

Braxton Hicks (BRAK-ston HIKS)

contraction (con-TRAK-shun)
  contract/o- *pull together*
  -ion *action; condition*

the fetus drops into the birth position within the mother's pelvis. This process is known as **engagement**. (It is also known as **lightening** because it eases the mother's shortness of breath.) The fetus usually assumes a head-down position. The head becomes the presenting part (part of the body that will go first through the birth canal). This is a **cephalic presentation**. Any part of the head can be the presenting part, but most commonly it is the top of the head, and this is a **vertex presentation** (see Figure 13-12 ■).

Sometime between 38 and 42 weeks' gestation, labor begins. The weight of the fetus presses on the cervix and vagina. This causes the cervix to begin to dilate and stimulates the release of oxytocin from the posterior pituitary gland. The uterus itself also produces oxytoxin. **Oxytocin** causes the uterus to contract regularly. The cervix softens as collagen fibers in its wall break down. This is known as **cervical ripening**.

Pronunciation/Word Parts

cephalic (seh-FAL-ik)
  cephal/o- *head*
  -ic *pertaining to*

vertex (VER-teks)

oxytocin (AWK-see-TOH-sin)
  ox/y- *oxygen; quick*
  toc/o- *childbirth; labor*
  -in *substance*
Select the correct combining form meaning to get the definition of *oxytoxin*: *substance (that causes) quick childbirth and labor.*

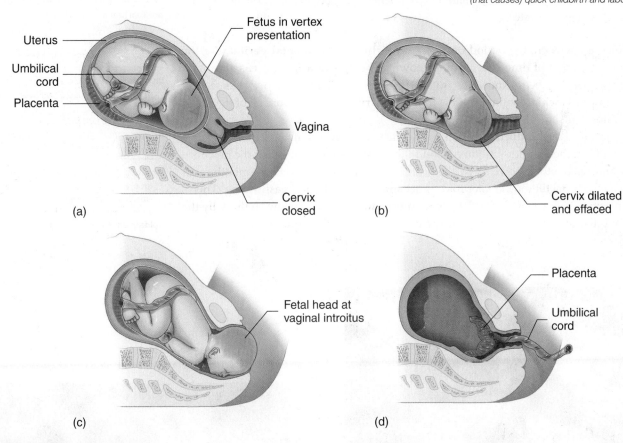

FIGURE 13-12 ■ Labor and delivery.
(a) This fetus is in a vertex presentation with the head as the presenting part. The cervical os is closed at the beginning of labor. (b) Gradually, the cervix dilates to 10 cm, and its wall thins until it is 100% effaced. (c) The head of the fetus moves through the cervical canal and vagina until the top of the head is visible at the vaginal introitus. This is known as *crowning*. (d) After birth, the placenta and umbilical cord are expelled.
Source: Pearson Education

The process of labor and childbirth is known as **parturition**. It is divided into three stages:

1. **First stage of labor.** Uterine contractions occur about every 30 minutes, increasing in intensity and duration. Cervical **dilation** (widening of the cervical os) progresses from 0 cm to 5 cm, and **effacement** (thinning of the cervical wall) progresses from 0 percent to 50 percent. **Rupture of the membranes (ROM)** occurs, and this releases amniotic fluid. As the uterine contractions intensify, the mother may receive epidural anesthesia to help control the pain. After 8 to 20 hours of labor, the cervix is completely dilated at 10 cm and 100% effaced (see Figure 13-12), and the mother is transferred to the delivery room.

parturition (PAR-tyoor-IH-shun)
  parturit/o- *childbirth; labor*
  -ion *action; condition*

dilation (dy-LAY-shun)
  dilat/o- *dilate; widen*
  -ion *action; condition*

effacement (eh-FAYS-ment)
  efface/o- *do away with; obliterate*
  -ment *action; state*

2. **Second stage of labor.** The uterine contractions have brought the head of the fetus into the vagina. The mother is encouraged to push by holding her breath to raise the intra-abdominal pressure. **Crowning** occurs when the top of the head is visible at the vaginal introitus (see Figures 13-12 and 13-13 ■). The head is delivered, and after several more uterine contractions, the shoulders and the rest of the body are delivered. The newborn is placed on the mother's abdomen while the umbilical cord is clamped and cut (see Figure 13-14 ■).

3. **Third stage of labor.** The placenta is delivered about 30 minutes after the birth. The placenta is also known as the *afterbirth* (see Figure 13-12). Oxytocin causes the uterus to contract to stop blood flow from the raw surfaces where the placenta pulled away. The obstetrician sutures up the episiotomy, if one was performed. The placenta and umbilical cord are sent to pathology for examination. Blood in the umbilical cord is rich in stem cells and can be used for stem cell transplantation (discussed in "Hematology and Immunology," Chapter 6).

For the newborn, the period of time after birth is the **postnatal period**. For the mother, the period of time after birth is known as **postpartum**. The uterus gradually shrinks in size, a process known as **involution**. Small amounts of blood, tissue, and fluid, known as **lochia**, continue to flow from the uterus for a week until all of the endometrial lining is shed.

Lactation is the production of milk by the breasts when stimulated by the hormone prolactin from the anterior pituitary gland in the brain. After birth, when the newborn cries or sucks, oxytocin secreted by the posterior pituitary gland causes smooth muscles around the lactiferous lobules to contract and expel milk for breastfeeding. This is known as the *let-down reflex*. The first milk, **colostrum**, is a thick, yellowish fluid. By the third day, the colostrum is replaced by regular breast milk that is thin and white.

Pronunciation/Word Parts

postnatal (post-NAY-tal)
post- *after; behind*
nat/o- *birth*
-al *pertaining to*

postpartum (post-PAR-tum)
post- *after; behind*
part/o- *childbirth; labor*
-um *period of time; structure*

involution (IN-voh-LOO-shun)
involut/o- *enlarged organ returns to normal size*
-ion *action; condition*

lochia (LOH-kee-ah)

lactation (lak-TAY-shun)
lact/o- *milk*
-ation *being; having; process*

colostrum (koh-LAW-strum)

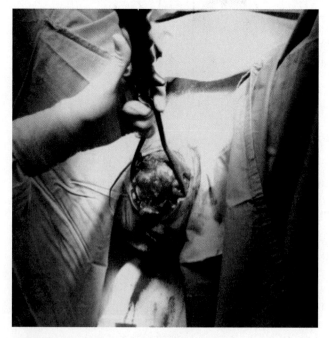

FIGURE 13-13 ■ Crowning of the head.
The hair on the baby's head is visible. The top of the head bulges outwardly with each contraction. The irregular edges of the vagina are from an episiotomy to prevent spontaneous tearing as the baby is born. The obstetrician is using obstetrical forceps to assist in the delivery of the head.
Source: Susan M. Turley

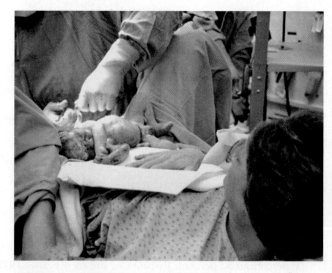

FIGURE 13-14 ■ Cutting the umbilical cord.
The obstetrician uses forceps to clamp the umbilical cord. Notice the length of the umbilical cord from its attachment at the baby's umbilicus, beneath his body, to the obstetrician.
Source: Susan M. Turley

CLINICAL CONNECTIONS

Immunology (Chapter 6). Colostrum is rich in nutrients and contains maternal antibodies. For the first few days of life, the intestinal tract is more permeable and allows these maternal antibodies to be absorbed into the newborn's blood. Maternal antibodies provide passive immunity to common diseases that the mother has already had. This immunity lasts until the newborn begins to make its own antibodies at about 18 months of age.

The Newborn

A newborn who is between 38 and 42 weeks' gestation is a **term neonate**. A newborn between 28 and 37 weeks' gestation is **preterm** or **premature**, a reference to the maturity of the internal organs and their ability to function. Because the date of conception is not always known, the gestational age of a newborn is an estimate.

The skin of the newborn is covered with **vernix caseosa**, a thick, white, cheesy substance that protects the skin from amniotic fluid in the uterus (see Figure 13-15 ■). The head can exhibit **molding**, a temporary elongated reshaping of the cranium that occurs as the head passes through the mother's bony pelvis. On the top of the head, the anterior **fontanel** or soft spot is a soft area that bulges when the newborn cries because it is only covered by a layer of fibrous connective tissue, not by bone (see Figure 8-4). There is also a smaller posterior fontanel at the back of the head. The fontanels allow the brain to grow before the bones fuse together. The newborn's face, hands, and feet are often bluish, a temporary condition known as **acrocyanosis**. The first bowel movement is **meconium**, a thick, greenish-black, tar-like substance. It contains mucus and bile (from the fetal digestive tract) and skin cells (that were in amniotic fluid swallowed by the fetus).

neonate (NEE-oh-nayt)
  ne/o- *new*
  -nate *thing that is born*

neonatal (NEE-oh-NAY-tal)
  ne/o- *new*
  nat/o- *birth*
  -al *pertaining to*

vernix caseosa
(VER-niks KAY-see-OH-sah)

fontanel (FAWN-tah-NEL)

acrocyanosis (AK-roh-SY-ah-NOH-sis)
  acr/o- *extremity; highest point*
  cyan/o- *blue*
  -osis *condition; process*

meconium (meh-KOH-nee-um)

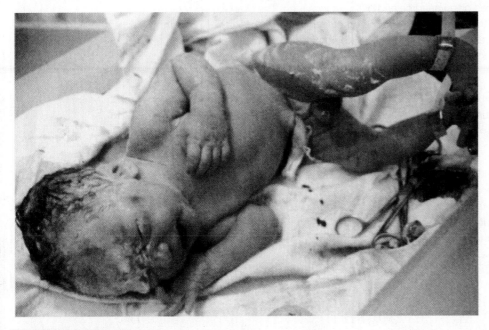

FIGURE 13-15 ■ Term neonate.
This male newborn is on the warming table in the delivery room. The vernix caseosa has been partially cleaned off of his trunk and arms. His eyes are swollen from the pressure of the birth canal. He is crying vigorously, but his distal extremities still show acrocyanosis (note the bluish color of the right hand and both legs). There is a plastic clamp on the stump of the umbilical cord. There are identification bracelets on both legs.
Source: Susan M. Turley

Vocabulary Review

Female Genital and Reproductive System		
Word or Phrase	**Description**	**Combining Forms**
external genitalia	Mons pubis, labia majora, labia minora, clitoris, vaginal introitus, Bartholin's glands, urethral glands, and Skene's glands	genit/o- *genitalia*
genital organs	Internal and external organs and structures of the female genital and reproductive system	genit/o- *genitalia*
genitourinary system	Female genital and reproductive system that is in close proximity to the urinary system. It is also known as the **urogenital system**.	genit/o- *genitalia* urin/o- *urinary system; urine* ur/o- *urinary system; urine*
internal genitalia	Ovaries, uterine tubes, uterus, and vagina	genit/o- *genitalia*
reproductive system	The other role of the female genital system in conceiving, carrying, and giving birth to a child	product/o- *produce*

Ovary and Uterine Tube		
adnexa	Accessory organs (the ovaries and uterine tubes) that are connected to the main organ (the uterus)	adnex/o- *accessory connecting parts*
follicle	Small area in the ovary that holds an oocyte before puberty and a maturing ovum after puberty. A follicle ruptures at the time of ovulation and becomes the corpus luteum.	
gonads	The ovaries or sex glands in a female	gon/o- *ovum; seed; spermatozoon*
oocyte	Immature egg in the follicle of the ovary	o/o- *egg; ovum*
ovary	Small, egg-shaped gland near the end of the uterine tube. The ovary is held in place by the **broad ligament** and other ligaments. The follicles of the ovary secrete estradiol. The corpus luteum of the ovary secretes estradiol and progesterone. The cells around the follicles secrete testosterone.	ovari/o- *ovary* oophor/o- *ovary*
ovum	An egg within a follicle in the ovary. A mature ovum is released during ovulation. An ovum is a gamete because it has only 23 chromosomes.	o/o- *egg; ovum* ov/i- *egg; ovum* ov/o- *egg; ovum* ovul/o- *egg; ovum*
uterine tube	Narrow tube that is connected at one end to the uterus. The other end is not directly connected to the ovary. It has a funnel-shaped end and fingerlike **fimbriae** that draw an ovum into the **lumen** (long central opening of the tube). **Cilia** (tiny hairs) inside the uterine tube beat in waves and **peristalsis** (smooth muscle contractions) move the ovum toward the uterus. It is also known as an **oviduct**. Formerly known as the **fallopian tube**.	uter/o- *uterus; womb* stal/o- *contraction* ov/i- *egg; ovum* salping/o- *uterine tube* fallopi/o- *uterine tube*

Uterus, Cervix, and Vagina

Word or Phrase	Description	Combining Forms
anteflexion	Normal position of the uterus in which the superior portion is tipped anteriorly on top of the bladder	**flex/o-** *bending*
cervix	Narrow, most inferior part of the uterus. It contains the **cervical canal**. Part of the cervix protrudes into the vagina. The **cervical os** is the small central opening in the cervix.	**cervic/o-** *cervix; neck*
cul-de-sac	Small pouch in the broad ligament that is between the uterus and rectum	**culd/o-** *cul-de-sac*
endometrium	Innermost layer of the uterus that lines the intrauterine cavity. It is a mucous membrane that contains many glands. It thickens and then is shed during the menstrual cycle.	**metri/o-** *uterus; womb*
myometrium	Smooth muscle layer of the uterine wall. It contracts during menstruation to expel the endometrial lining. It contracts during labor and delivery of the newborn.	**my/o-** *muscle* **metri/o-** *uterus; womb*
perimetrium	Serous membrane that is the outer layer of the uterus. It is part of the peritoneum that lines the abdominopelvic cavity.	**metri/o-** *uterus; womb*
uterus	Internal female organ of menstruation and pregnancy. It is also known as the *womb*. The uterus is held in place by the **broad ligament** and other ligaments. The **fundus** is the rounded top of the uterus. The cervix is the narrow, most inferior part. The hollow **intrauterine cavity** inside the uterus is lined with endometrium.	**uter/o-** *uterus; womb* **fund/o-** *fundus; part farthest from the opening* **hyster/o-** *uterus; womb* **metri/o-** *uterus; womb* **metr/o-** *measurement; uterus; womb*
vagina	Short tubular structure connected at its superior end to the cervix and at its inferior end to the outside of the body. It contains the **vaginal canal**. The **fornix** is the area of the vaginal canal that is behind and around the cervix. The **hymen** is the elastic membrane that partially or completely covers the inferior end of the vaginal canal. The opening to the outside of the body is the **vaginal introitus**.	**vagin/o-** *vagina* **colp/o-** *vagina*

External Genitalia

Word or Phrase	Description	Combining Forms
BUS	**Bartholin's glands**, **urethral glands**, and **Skene's glands** are located in or near the vaginal introitus. They secrete mucus during sexual arousal.	**urethr/o-** *urethra*
clitoris	Organ of sexual response in the female that enlarges and becomes engorged with blood	
labia	A pair of fleshy lips covered with pubic hair (the **labia majora**) and a small, thin, inner pair of lips (the **labia minora**) that partially cover the clitoris, urethral meatus, and vaginal introitus	**labi/o-** *labium; lip*
mons pubis	Rounded, fatty pad of tissue covered with pubic hair that lies on top of the pubis (anterior hip bone)	
perineum	Area of skin between the vulva and the anus	**perine/o-** *perineum*
vulva	Area between the inner thighs that includes the external genitalia as well as the mons pubis	**vulv/o-** *vulva* **episi/o-** *vulva*

Breasts

Word or Phrase	Description	Combining Forms
areola	Pigmented area around the nipple of the breast.	**areol/o-** *small, circular area*
lactiferous lobules	Site of milk production in the mammary glands. Prolactin from the anterior pituitary gland stimulates milk production during pregnancy. After birth, oxytocin from the posterior pituitary gland is released when the newborn cries or sucks and this causes the release of milk with the let-down reflex. The milk flows through the **lactiferous ducts** to the nipple.	**lact/i-** *milk* **fer/o-** *bear* **lact/o-** *milk* **galact/o-** *milk*
mammary glands	The breasts. A female sexual characteristic that develops during puberty. The breasts contain adipose (fatty) tissue and lactiferous lobules. The breasts provide milk to nourish the baby after birth. The nipple is the projecting point of the breast where the lactiferous ducts converge.	**mamm/o-** *breast* **mamm/a-** *breast* **mast/o-** *breast; mastoid process*

Sexual Maturity and Oogenesis

Word or Phrase	Description	Combining Forms
estradiol	Most abundant and biologically active of the female hormones. It is secreted by the follicles of the ovary. During puberty, it causes the development of the female sexual characteristics. It causes the endometrium to thicken during the menstrual cycle. After ovulation, it is secreted by the corpus luteum of the ovary. During pregnancy, it is secreted by the placenta.	**estr/a-** *female* **estr/o-** *female* **gynec/o-** *female; woman*
follicle-stimulating hormone (FSH)	Hormone secreted by the anterior pituitary gland in the brain. It causes a follicle in the ovary to enlarge and produce a mature ovum. FSH also stimulates the follicles to secrete estradiol, which causes the development of the female sexual characteristics.	
gamete	An ovum or spermatozoon. It has 23 chromosomes instead of the usual 46 chromosomes like other cells in the body.	
luteinizing hormone (LH)	Hormone secreted by the anterior pituitary gland in the brain. It causes a follicle to rupture and release a mature ovum.	
oogenesis	Production of a mature ovum from an oocyte through the processes of mitosis and then meiosis	**o/o-** *egg; ovum* **gen/o-** *arising from; produced by*
progesterone	Hormone secreted by the corpus luteum of the ovary after ovulation. It causes the uterine lining to thicken to prepare for a possible fertilized ovum. During pregnancy, it is secreted by the placenta.	
testosterone	Male hormone secreted by cells around the follicles in the ovary. It plays a role in the female sexual drive.	

Menstruation

Word or Phrase	Description	Combining Forms
corpus luteum	Remnants of a ruptured follicle in the ovary. The corpus luteum is filled with yellow fat and secretes estradiol and progesterone during the menstrual cycle. If the ovum is fertilized, the placenta begins to secrete these hormones, and the corpus luteum becomes white scar tissue.	
ischemic phase	Days 27–28 of the menstrual cycle. The corpus luteum degenerates into white scar tissue (corpus albicans) and stops producing estradiol and progesterone. The endometrium sloughs off, and menstruation begins.	**isch/o-** *block; keep back*
menarche	The first cycle of menstruation at the onset of puberty. This is the first **menstrual period** or **menses**.	**men/o-** *month* **menstru/o-** *monthly discharge of blood*

Word or Phrase	Description	Combining Forms
menstrual cycle	A 28-day cycle that consists of the menstrual phase, proliferative phase, ovulation, secretory phase, and ischemic phase	**menstru/o-** *monthly discharge of blood*
menstrual phase	Days 1–6 of the menstrual cycle. The endometrial lining of the uterus is shed.	**menstru/o-** *monthly discharge of blood*
menstruation	Process in which the endometrium of the uterus is shed each month, causing a flow of blood and tissue through the vagina. Under the influence of estradiol, the endometrium thickens in preparation to receive a fertilized ovum. If the ovum is not fertilized, the endometrium is again shed to begin another menstrual cycle.	**menstru/o-** *monthly discharge of blood*
ovulation	Day 14 of the menstrual cycle. Luteinizing hormone from the anterior pituitary gland causes the ovarian follicle to rupture, releasing the mature ovum. The **basal (baseline) body temperature** rises during ovulation.	**ovul/o-** *egg; ovum*
proliferative phase	Days 7–13 of the menstrual cycle. A follicle matures in the ovary and the thickness of the endometrium increases.	
secretory phase	Days 15–26 of the menstrual cycle. A ruptured follicle becomes the corpus luteum and secretes estradiol and progesterone. The thickness of the endometrium increases.	**secret/o-** *produce; secrete*

Conception

Word or Phrase	Description	Combining Forms
amnion	Membrane sac that produces **amniotic fluid** that surrounds and cushions the developing embryo and fetus. It is also known as the *bag of waters.*	**amni/o-** *amnion; membrane around the fetus*
antepartum	From the mother's standpoint, the period of time from conception until labor and delivery	**part/o-** *childbirth; labor*
chorion	Cells in a zygote that send out fingerlike projections (villi) to penetrate the endometrium to bring nutrients and oxygen to the embryo. It produces human chorionic gonadotropin. It later develops into the placenta.	**chorion/o-** *chorion*
embryo	A fertilized ovum (a zygote) is an embryo from 4 days after fertilization through 8 weeks of gestation. Then it becomes a fetus.	**embryon/o-** *embryo; immature form*
fertilization	The act of a spermatozoon uniting with an ovum. It is also known as **conception**.	**fertil/o-** *conceive; form* **concept/o-** *conceive; form*
fetus	An embryo becomes a fetus beginning at 9 weeks of gestation. It is called a fetus until the moment of birth.	**fet/o-** *fetus*
fraternal twins	The ovary releases two ova that are then fertilized at the same time but by different spermatozoa	**fratern/o-** *close association; close relationship*
gestation	Period of time from the moment of fertilization of the ovum until birth, approximately 9 months (38–42 weeks)	**gestat/o-** *conception to birth*
human chorionic gonadotropin (HCG)	Hormone secreted by the chorion of the zygote. It stimulates the corpus luteum of the ovary to keep producing estradiol and progesterone. This maintains the endometrium to support the developing embryo and prevents menstruation for the duration of the pregnancy.	**chorion/o-** *chorion* **gonad/o-** *gonad; ovary; testis* **trop/o-** *having an affinity for; stimulating; turning*
identical twins	An already developing zygote splits in two. This develops into two separate but identical embryos.	

Word or Phrase	Description	Combining Forms
placenta	Large, pancake-like organ that develops from the chorion. It provides nutrients and oxygen to the developing fetus and removes carbon dioxide and waste products. By the end of the first trimester of pregnancy, it assumes the job of the corpus luteum and secretes estradiol and progesterone to maintain the endometrium during pregnancy. It is also known as the *afterbirth*.	**placent/o-** *placenta*
pregnancy	State of being with child. It begins at the moment of conception and ends with delivery of the newborn.	**pregn/o-** *being with child*
prenatal period	From the fetus' standpoint, the period of time from conception to birth	**nat/o-** *birth*
products of conception	The fetus, placenta, and all fluids and tissue in the pregnant uterus	**concept/o-** *conceive; form*
trimester	A period of 3 months. The time of gestation is divided into three trimesters.	
umbilical cord	Rubbery, flexible cord that connects the placenta to the **umbilicus** (navel) of the fetus. It contains two arteries and one vein.	**umbilic/o-** *navel; umbilicus*
zygote	Cell that is the union of a spermatozoon and an ovum. A zygote has 46 chromosomes.	

Labor, Delivery, and Postpartum

Word or Phrase	Description	Combining Forms
Braxton Hicks contractions	Irregular uterine contractions during the last trimester. These strengthen the uterine muscle in preparation for labor. Also known as *false labor*.	**contract/o-** *pull together*
cephalic presentation	Position of the fetus in which the head is the presenting part that is first to go through the birth canal. **Vertex presentation** is a type of cephalic presentation in which the top of the head is the presenting part.	**cephal/o-** *head*
cervical ripening	Softening of the cervix as collagen fibers in its wall break down prior to the onset of labor	
colostrum	First milk from the breasts. It is a thick, yellowish fluid that is rich in nutrients and contains maternal antibodies to give the newborn passive immunity to common diseases.	
crowning	The top of the fetal head is visible at the vaginal introitus	
dilation	Widening of the cervical os from 0 cm to 10 cm during labor to allow passage of the fetal head	**dilat/o-** *dilate; widen*
effacement	Thinning of the cervical wall, measured as a percentage from 0 percent to 100 percent	**efface/o-** *do away with; obliterate*
engagement	The fetal head drops into position within the mother's pelvis in anticipation of birth. It is also known as **lightening**.	
involution	Process by which the uterus gradually returns to a normal size after childbirth	**involut/o-** *enlarged organ returns to normal size*
lactation	Production of colostrum and then breast milk by the mammary glands after childbirth	**lact/o-** *milk* **lact/i-** *milk* **galact/o-** *milk*

Give Word Part Meanings

Use the Answer Key at the end of the book to check your answers.

Combining Forms Exercise

Next to each combining form, write its meaning. The first one has been done for you.

Combining Form	Meaning	Combining Form	Meaning
1. **gon/o-**	*ovum; seed; spermatozoon*	39. lob/o-	_____
2. acr/o-	_____	40. mamm/a-	_____
3. adnex/o-	_____	41. mamm/o-	_____
4. amni/o-	_____	42. mast/o-	_____
5. areol/o-	_____	43. men/o-	_____
6. cephal/o-	_____	44. menstru/o-	_____
7. cervic/o-	_____	45. metri/o-	_____
8. chorion/o-	_____	46. metr/o-	_____
9. colp/o-	_____	47. my/o-	_____
10. concept/o-	_____	48. nat/o-	_____
11. contract/o-	_____	49. ne/o-	_____
12. culd/o-	_____	50. o/o-	_____
13. cyan/o-	_____	51. oophor/o-	_____
14. dilat/o-	_____	52. ovari/o-	_____
15. efface/o-	_____	53. ov/i-	_____
16. embryon/o-	_____	54. ov/o-	_____
17. episi/o-	_____	55. ovul/o-	_____
18. estr/a-	_____	56. ox/y-	_____
19. estr/o-	_____	57. par/o-	_____
20. fallopi/o-	_____	58. part/o-	_____
21. fer/o-	_____	59. parturit/o	_____
22. fertil/o-	_____	60. perine/o-	_____
23. fet/o-	_____	61. placent/o-	_____
24. flex/o-	_____	62. pregn/o-	_____
25. fratern/o-	_____	63. product/o-	_____
26. fund/o-	_____	64. salping/o-	_____
27. galact/o-	_____	65. secret/o-	_____
28. genit/o-	_____	66. stal/o-	_____
29. gen/o-	_____	67. toc/o-	_____
30. gestat/o-	_____	68. trop/o-	_____
31. gonad/o-	_____	69. umbilic/o-	_____
32. gynec/o-	_____	70. urethr/o-	_____
33. hyster/o-	_____	71. urin/o-	_____
34. involut/o-	_____	72. ur/o-	_____
35. isch/o-	_____	73. uter/o-	_____
36. labi/o-	_____	74. vagin/o-	_____
37. lact/i-	_____	75. vulv/o-	_____
38. lact/o-	_____		

Build Medical Words

Combining Form and Suffix Exercise

Read the definition of the medical word. Look at the combining form that is given. Select the correct suffix from the Suffix List and write it on the blank line. Then build the medical word and write it on the line. (Remember: You may need to remove the combining vowel. Always remove the hyphens and slash.) Be sure to check your spelling. The first one has been done for you.

SUFFIX LIST

-al (pertaining to)	-ary (pertaining to)	-ion (action; condition)
-an (pertaining to)	-ation (being; having; process)	-ization (process of
-ancy (state)	-cyte (cell)	inserting)
-ant (pertaining to)	-duct (duct; tube)	-ment (action; state)
-ar (pertaining to)	-ic (pertaining to)	-nate (thing that is born)
-arche (beginning)	-ine (pertaining to; thing pertaining to)	-tic (pertaining to)

Definition of the Medical Word	Combining Form	Suffix	Build the Medical Word
1. Pertaining to (the) fundus (of the uterus)	fund/o-	-al	fundal
(You think pertaining to (-al) + fundus (fund/o-). You change the order of the word parts to put the suffix last. You write fundal.)			
2. Pertaining to (the) breasts	mamm/o-	_____	_____
3. Pertaining to (the) uterus	uter/o-	_____	_____
4. Cell (that is an immature) ovum	o/o-	_____	_____
5. Pertaining to (the) ovary	ovari/o-	_____	_____
6. Pertaining to (the) areola	areol/o-	_____	_____
7. Process (of having an) ovum (released from the follicle)	ovul/o-	_____	_____
8. Beginning (of) month(ly periods)	men/o-	_____	_____
9. Pertaining to (the) cervix	cervic/o-	_____	_____
10. Process (of having) monthly discharge of blood	menstru/o-	_____	_____
11. Pertaining to (the) amnion	amni/o-	_____	_____
12. Process (of having) milk	lact/o-	_____	_____
13. Pertaining to accessory connecting parts (the ovary and uterine tube)	adnex/o-	_____	_____
14. Pertaining to (the) fetus	fet/o-	_____	_____
15. Action (to) conceive (or) form (a child)	concept/o-	_____	_____
16. Pertaining to being with child	pregn/o-	_____	_____
17. Pertaining to (the) embryo	embryon/o-	_____	_____
18. Duct (tube that transports the) ovum	ov/i-	_____	_____
19. Pertaining to (the) vagina	vagin/o-	_____	_____
20. Pertaining to (a) lip (structure in the vulvar area)	labi/o-	_____	_____
21. State (of) being with child	pregn/o-	_____	_____
22. Process of inserting (sperm into an ovum to) conceive (a child)	fertil/o-	_____	_____
23. Pertaining to (the) perineum	perine/o-	_____	_____
24. Thing (baby) that is born new	ne/o-	_____	_____

Definition of the Medical Word	Combining Form	Suffix	Build the Medical Word
25.　Pertaining to (the) placenta	placent/o-	_____	_____
26.　Action (when an) enlarged organ (the uterus) returns to normal size	involut/o-	_____	_____
27.　Pertaining to (the) vulva	vulv/o-	_____	_____
28.　Action (to) do away with (or) obliterate (the thick wall of the cervix)	efface/o-	_____	_____
29.　Condition (from) conception to birth	gestat/o-	_____	_____

Prefix Exercise

Read the definition of the medical word. Look at the medical word or partial word that is given (it already contains a combining form and a suffix). Select the correct prefix from the Prefix List and write it on the blank line. Then build the medical word and write it on the line. Be sure to check your spelling. The first one has been done for you.

PREFIX LIST

ante- (before; forward)	peri- (around)	re- (again and again;
endo- (innermost; within)	post- (after; behind)	backward; unable to)
intra- (within)	pre- (before; in front of)	tri- (three)

Definition of the Medical Word	Prefix	Word or Partial Word	Build the Medical Word
1.　Pertaining to before birth	pre-	natal	prenatal
2.　Pertaining to within (the) uterus	_____	uterine	_____
3.　Pertaining to again and again producing (children)	_____	productive	_____
4.　Condition (of the uterus of) forward bending	_____	flexion	_____
5.　Structure (that is) around (the) uterus	_____	metrium	_____
6.　Pertaining to after birth	_____	natal	_____
7.　Structure (that is the) innermost (lining of the) uterus	_____	metrium	_____
8.　Thing that produces (months of pregnancy that are) three	_____	mester	_____

Multiple Combining Forms and Suffix Exercise

Read the definition of the medical word. Select the correct suffix and combining forms. Then build the medical word and write it on the line. Be sure to check your spelling. The first one has been done for you.

SUFFIX LIST	COMBINING FORM LIST	
-al (pertaining to)	acr/o- (extremity; highest point)	my/o- (muscle)
-ary (pertaining to)	cyan/o- (blue)	nat/o- (birth)
-esis (condition; process)	fer/o- (bear)	ne/o- (new)
-in (substance)	genit/o- (genitalia)	o/o- (egg; ovum)
-osis (condition; process)	gen/o- (arising from; produced by)	ox/y- (oxygen; quick)
-ous (pertaining to)	lact/i- (milk)	toc/o- (childbirth; labor)
-um (period of time; structure)	metri/o- (uterus; womb)	urin/o- (urinary system; urine)

	Definition of the Medical Word	Combining Form	Combining Form	Suffix	Build the Medical Word
1.	Pertaining to milk bear(ing)	lact/i-	fer/o-	-ous	lactiferous

(You think *pertaining to* (-ous) + *milk* (lact/i-) + *bear* (fer/o-). You change the order of the word parts to put the suffix last. You write *lactiferous*.)

2.	Structure (of the) muscle (in the) uterus				
3.	Process (of an) ovum (being) produced by (the follicle)				
4.	Pertaining to (a) new birth				
5.	Substance (a hormone that causes) quick childbirth				
6.	Condition (of the) extremities (of a newborn being) blue				
7.	Pertaining to (the) genitalia (and) urinary system				

Diseases

Ovaries and Uterine Tubes		
Word or Phrase	**Description**	**Pronunciation/Word Parts**
anovulation	Failure of the ovaries to release a mature ovum at the time of ovulation, although the menstrual cycle is normal. This results in infertility. Anovulation is a normal condition prior to menarche, during pregnancy, and during menopause. Treatment: Hormone drug to stimulate ovulation.	**anovulation** (AN-aw-vyoo-LAY-shun) **an-** *not; without* **ovul/o-** *egg; ovum* **-ation** *being; having; process*
ovarian cancer	**Cancerous** tumor of an ovary. This **malignancy** often does not cause symptoms until it is quite large and has already metastasized. Treatment: Surgery to remove the ovary (oophorectomy), or the uterus (hysterectomy), and chemotherapy drugs.	**cancer** (KAN-ser) **cancerous** (KAN-ser-us) **cancer/o-** *cancer* **-ous** *pertaining to* **malignancy** (mah-LIG-nan-see) **malign/o-** *cancer; intentionally causing harm* **-ancy** *state*
polycystic ovary syndrome	The ovaries contain multiple cysts (see Figure 13-16 ■). A follicle matures and enlarges, but fails to rupture to release an ovum; it then becomes a cyst. With each menstrual cycle, the cysts enlarge, causing pain. This happens month after month until the ovaries are filled with cysts. This syndrome is associated with amenorrhea or menometrorrhagia, infertility, obesity, and insulin resistance syndrome with the development of type 2 diabetes mellitus. Treatment: Oral contraceptive drug (to correct hormone levels), weight control, oral antidiabetic drug. 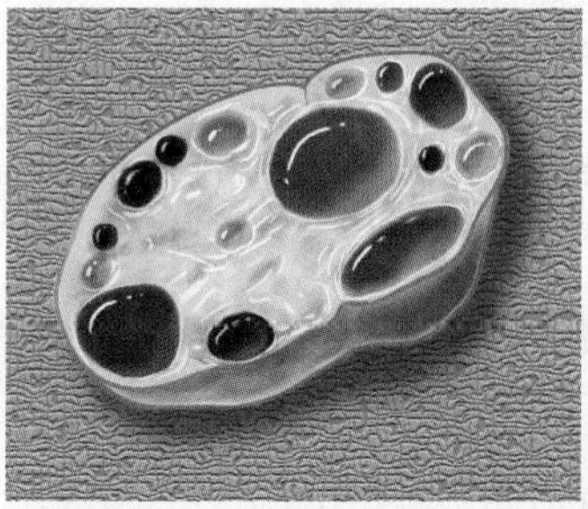 **FIGURE 13-16 ■ Polycystic ovary syndrome.** The ovary is filled with both small and large cysts. Some of the cysts contain blood. *Source*: Pearson Education	**polycystic** (PAW-lee-SIS-tik) **poly-** *many; much* **cyst/o-** *bladder; fluid-filled sac; semisolid cyst* **-ic** *pertaining to*
salpingitis	Inflammation or infection of the uterine tube. It is due to endometriosis or pelvic inflammatory disease. This narrows or blocks the lumen of the tube and can lead to an ectopic pregnancy. With **hydrosalpinx**, inflammation fills the tube with fluid. With **pyosalpinx**, infection fills the tube with pus. Treatment: Treat the underlying cause.	**salpingitis** (SAL-ping-JY-tis) **salping/o-** *uterine tube* **-itis** *infection of; inflammation of* **hydrosalpinx** (HY-droh-SAL-pinks) **hydr/o-** *fluid; water* **-salpinx** *uterine tube* **pyosalpinx** (PY-oh-SAL-pinks) **py/o-** *pus* **-salpinx** *uterine tube*

Uterus		
Word or Phrase	**Description**	**Pronunciation/Word Parts**
endometriosis	Endometrial tissue in abnormal places. The endometrium sloughs off during menstruation but is forced upward through the uterine tubes and out into the pelvic cavity because the uterus is bent backward in an abnormal position. This is known as **retroflexion** or **retroversion**. These endometrial tissues remain alive and sensitive to hormones. Endometrial implants in the uterine tubes cause blockage, scarring, and infertility. The endometrial tissue implants itself on the outside of the ovaries and uterus and on the walls of the abdominopelvic cavity. Endometriosis on the outside of the ovary forms "chocolate cysts" that contain old, dark blood. During each menstrual cycle, the implants in the abdominopelvic cavity thicken and slough off, forming more implants with old blood and tissue debris (see Figure 13-17 ■). They can form adhesions between the internal organs. Endometriosis causes pelvic inflammation, pelvic pain, and pain during sexual intercourse. Treatment: Hormone drug to suppress the menstrual cycle (to make the implants shrivel up) or laparoscopic surgery to destroy the implants. 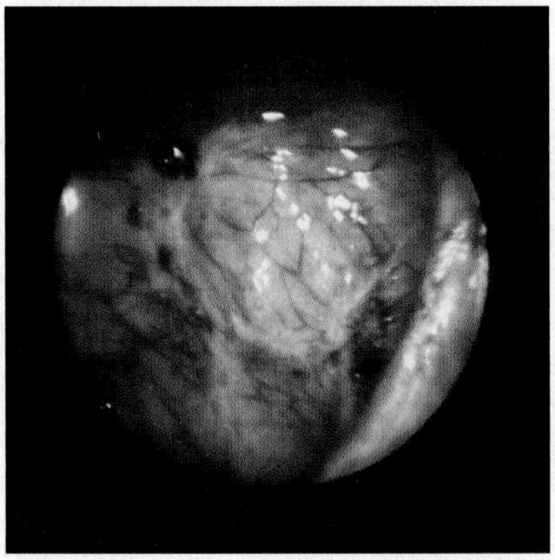	**endometriosis** (EN-doh-MEE-tree-OH-sis) **endo-** *innermost; within* **metri/o-** *uterus; womb* **-osis** *condition; process* **retroflexion** (REH-troh-FLEK-shun) **retro-** *backward; behind* **flex/o-** *bending* **-ion** *action; condition* **retroversion** (REH-troh-VER-shun) **retro-** *backward; behind* **vers/o-** *travel; turn* **-ion** *action; condition*

FIGURE 13-17 ■ Endometriosis.
This area on the outside of the uterus, as seen through a laparoscope inserted through the abdominal wall, shows many endometrial implants with evidence of old blood.
Source: CNRI/Science Source

leiomyoma	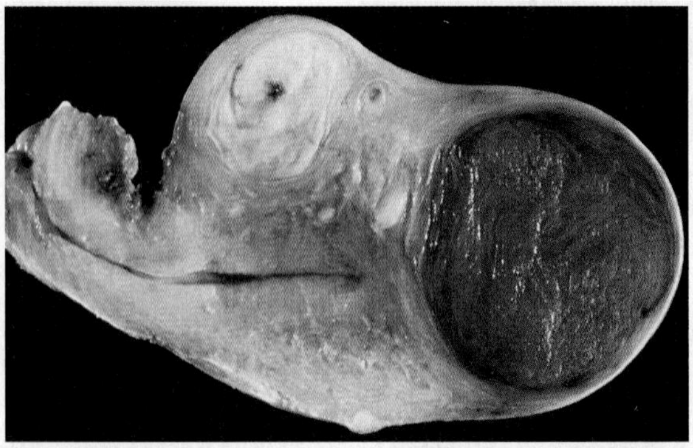 Benign, fibrous tumor in the smooth muscle of the myometrium (see Figure 13-18 ■). It can be small or as large as a soccer ball. Several tumors are **leiomyomata**; they are also known as **uterine fibroids**. There is pelvic pain, excessive uterine bleeding, and painful sexual intercourse. Treatment: Uterine artery embolization. Surgery to remove the tumor (myomectomy) or the uterus (hysterectomy), depending on the size of the tumor.	**leiomyoma** (LIE-oh-my-OH-mah) **lei/o-** *smooth* **my/o-** *muscle* **-oma** *mass; tumor* **leiomyomata** (LIE-oh-my-OH-mah-tah) *Leiomyoma* is a Greek singular noun. Form the plural by changing *-oma* to *-omata*. **fibroid** (FY-broyd) **fibr/o-** *fiber* **-oid** *resembling*

FIGURE 13-18 ■ Leiomyoma.
This pathology specimen of the cut section of a uterus contains a large, benign, red leiomyoma.
Source: CNRI/Science Source

leiomyosarcoma	Cancerous tumor of the smooth muscle of the myometrium. Treatment: Surgery to remove the uterus (hysterectomy), chemotherapy drugs, or radiation therapy.	**leiomyosarcoma** (LIE-oh-MY-oh-sar-KOH-mah) **lei/o-** *smooth* **my/o-** *muscle* **sarc/o-** *connective tissue* **-oma** *mass; tumor*

Word or Phrase	Description	Pronunciation/Word Parts
myometritis	Inflammation or infection of the myometrium. It is associated with pelvic inflammatory disease. **Pyometritis** is an infection of the myometrium that creates pus in the intrauterine cavity. Treatment: Antibiotic drug.	**myometritis** (MY-oh-mee-TRY-tis) **my/o-** *muscle* **metr/o-** *measurement; uterus; womb* **-itis** *infection of; inflammation of* **pyometritis** (PY-oh-mee-TRY-tis) **py/o-** *pus* **metr/o-** *measurement; uterus; womb* **-itis** *infection of; inflammation of*
pelvic inflammatory disease (PID)	Infection of the cervix that ascends to the uterus, uterine tubes, and ovaries. It is often caused by a sexually transmitted disease. There is pelvic pain, fever, and vaginal discharge. If untreated, it can cause scars that block the uterine tubes and infertility. Treatment: Antibiotic drug.	**inflammatory** (in-FLAM-ah-TOR-ee) **inflammat/o-** *redness and warmth* **-ory** *having the function of*
uterine cancer	Cancerous tumor of the endometrium of the uterus. The earliest sign is abnormal bleeding. It is also known as **endometrial cancer**. Treatment: Surgery to remove the uterus (hysterectomy); chemotherapy drugs.	
uterine prolapse	Descent of the uterus from its normal position. This is caused by stretching of ligaments that support the uterus and weakness in the muscles of the floor of the pelvic cavity. It occurs after childbirth or because of age. The uterus can be so prolapsed that the cervix is visible at the vaginal introitus. It is also known as **uterine descensus**. Severe prolapse affects urination and bowel movements. Treatment: Molded plastic form (a pessary) inserted in the vagina to move it upward; hysterectomy or uterine suspension.	**prolapse** (PROH-laps) **descensus** (dee-SEN-sus)

Menstrual Disorders

Word or Phrase	Description	Pronunciation/Word Parts
amenorrhea	Absence of monthly menstrual periods. It is caused by a hormone imbalance, thyroid disease, or a tumor of the uterus or ovary. Poor nutrition, stress, chronic disease, intense exercise, or the psychiatric illness of anorexia nervosa can also cause amenorrhea. (*Note:* Amenorrhea is normal before puberty, during pregnancy, and after menopause.) Treatment: Correct the underlying cause.	**amenorrhea** (AH-men-oh-REE-ah) **a-** *away from; without* **men/o-** *month* **-rrhea** *discharge; flow*
dysfunctional uterine bleeding (DUB)	Sporadic menstrual bleeding without a true menstrual period. It is related to anovulation. The endometrium sloughs off from time to time, but never reaches a full thickness because there is no ovulation and no corpus luteum to secrete progesterone. Treatment: Hormone drug therapy to restore normal ovulation and menstruation.	**dysfunctional** (dis-FUNK-shun-al) *Dysfunctional* is a combination of the prefix *dys-* (abnormal; difficult; painful), the English word *function* (physiologic working), and the suffix *–al* (pertaining to).

Word or Phrase	Description	Pronunciation/Word Parts
dysmenorrhea	Painful menstruation. During menstruation, the uterus releases **prostaglandin** to constrict blood vessels in the uterine wall and prevent excessive bleeding. A very high level of prostaglandin causes cramping and temporary ischemia of the myometrium, both of which cause pain. There is also nausea, dizziness, backache, and diarrhea. Pelvic inflammatory disease, endometriosis, or uterine fibroids can also cause dysmenorrhea. Treatment: Nonsteroidal anti-inflammatory drug to block the production of prostaglandin; correct the underlying cause.	**dysmenorrhea** (DIS-men-oh-REE-ah) **dys-** *abnormal; difficult; painful* **men/o-** *month* **-rrhea** *discharge; flow* **prostaglandin** (PRAW-stah-GLAN-din)
menopause	Normal cessation of menstrual periods, occurring around middle age. The **perimenopausal period** is the time around menopause when menstrual periods first become irregular and menstrual flow is lighter. Menopause is also known as **climacteric** or the change of life. Treatment: Hormone replacement therapy (HRT) on a short-term basis. Natural estrogen supplements from soy and herbs.	**menopause** (MEN-oh-pawz) **men/o-** *month* **-pause** *cessation* **perimenopausal** (PAIR-ee-MEN-oh-PAW-zal) **peri-** *around* **men/o-** *month* **paus/o-** *cessation* **-al** *pertaining to* **climacteric** (kly-MAK-ter-ik) (KLY-mak-TAIR-ik)

A CLOSER LOOK

As a woman ages, the follicles deteriorate and stop secreting estradiol. Ovulation and menstruation cease. Decreased estradiol causes vaginal dryness, vaginal atrophy, and dryness of the skin. The breasts decrease in size. The anterior pituitary gland responds to a low blood level of estradiol by secreting more follicle-stimulating hormone (FSH). This causes occasional ovulation and menstruation during the perimenopausal period. These bursts of FSH (which often occur at night) produce vasodilation, and the patient experiences hot flashes with perspiration and flushing. Frequent hot flashes throughout the night can cause sleeplessness and fatigue.

Word or Phrase	Description	Pronunciation/Word Parts
menorrhagia	A menstrual period with excessively heavy flow or a menstrual period that lasts longer than 7 days. It is caused by a hormone imbalance, uterine fibroids, or endometriosis. **Menometrorrhagia** is excessively heavy menstrual flow during menstruation or at other times of the month. **Metrorrhagia** is excessively heavy bleeding at a time other than menstruation. This can be caused by a tubal pregnancy or uterine cancer. Heavy uterine bleeding of any type can cause anemia. Treatment: Hormone drug therapy or correct the underlying cause.	**menorrhagia** (MEN-oh-RAY-jah) **men/o-** *month* **rrhag/o-** *excessive discharge; excessive flow* **-ia** *condition; state; thing*
oligomenorrhea	A menstrual period with very light flow or infrequent menstrual cycles (longer than 35 days before the next cycle begins) in a woman who previously had normal menstruation. It is caused by a hormone imbalance. Treatment: Hormone drug therapy.	**oligomenorrhea** (OH-lih-goh-MEN-oh-REE-ah) **olig/o-** *few; scanty* **men/o-** *month* **-rrhea** *discharge; flow*
premenstrual syndrome (PMS)	Breast tenderness, fluid retention, bloating, and mild mood changes (irritability, anger, sadness) a few days before the onset of menstruation. It is caused by high levels of estradiol and progesterone just prior to menstruation. Treatment: Over-the-counter drug that relieves pain and fluid retention.	**premenstrual** (pree-MEN-stroo-al) **pre-** *before; in front of* **menstru/o-** *monthly discharge of blood* **-al** *pertaining to*

Word or Phrase	Description	Pronunciation/Word Parts
	CLINICAL CONNECTIONS	
	Psychiatry. Premenstrual dysphoric disorder (PMDD) includes symptoms of PMS plus feelings of depression, anxiety, tearfulness, mood shifts, difficulty concentrating, sleeping and eating disturbances, and breast, joint, and muscle pain. It is a psychiatric mood disorder caused by an alteration in the levels of the neurotransmitters serotonin and norepinephrine in the brain. Treatment: Antianxiety drug, antidepressant drug, and pain reliever drug.	**dysphoric** (dis-FOR-ik) **dys-** *abnormal; difficult; painful* **phor/o-** *bear; carry; range* **-ic** *pertaining to*

Cervix

Word or Phrase	Description	Pronunciation/Word Parts
cervical cancer	Cancerous tumor of the cervix. If the cancer is still localized, it is **carcinoma in situ (CIS)**. There is severe dysplasia of the cells as seen on a Pap smear. Later there is ulceration and bleeding. Infection with human papillomavirus (HPV), also known as *genital warts* (a sexually transmitted disease) predisposes to the development of cervical cancer. Treatment: Conization of the cervix or surgery to remove the uterus (hysterectomy).	**carcinoma** (KAR-sih-NOH-mah) **carcin/o-** *cancer* **-oma** *mass; tumor* **in situ** (IN SY-too)
cervical dysplasia	Abnormal growth of squamous cells in the surface layer of the cervix (see Figure 13-19 ■). Cervical dysplasia is seen on an abnormal Pap smear. Severe dysplasia is a precancerous or cancerous condition. Treatment: Treat the underlying infection or cancer.	**dysplasia** (dis-PLAY-zha) **dys-** *abnormal; difficult; painful* **plas/o-** *formation; growth* **-ia** *condition; state; thing* Select the correct prefix meaning to get the definition of *dysplasia*: *condition of abnormal growth.*

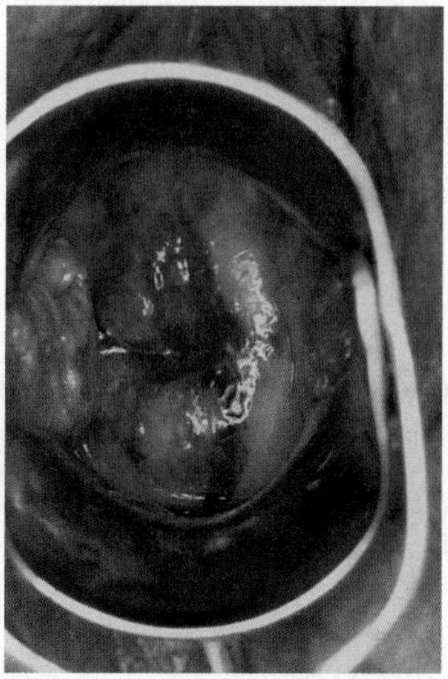

FIGURE 13-19 ■ Cervical dysplasia.
A metal speculum is inserted into the vagina and is used to visualize the cervix. The cervix shows a high degree of cervical dysplasia (classified as CIN II on a Pap smear). These areas of redness are abnormal cells that may develop into cancer.
Source: Spl/Science Source

Vagina

Word or Phrase	Description	Pronunciation/Word Parts
bacterial vaginosis	Bacterial infection of the vagina due to *Gardnerella vaginalis.* There is a white or grayish vaginal discharge that has a fishy odor. This infection is not a sexually transmitted disease. Treatment: Antibiotic drug.	**vaginosis** (VAJ-ih-NOH-sis) **vagin/o-** *vagina* **-osis** *condition; process*
candidiasis	Yeast infection of the vagina due to *Candida albicans.* There is vaginal itching and **leukorrhea**, a cheesy, white discharge. Candidiasis can occur after taking an antibiotic drug for a bacterial infection; the drug kills the disease-causing bacteria but also kills the normal bacterial flora of the vagina. Then yeast, which is not affected by the antibiotic drug, multiplies and causes an infection. Treatment: Antiyeast drug applied topically in the vagina.	**candidiasis** (KAN-dih-DY-ah-sis) **candid/o-** *Candida; yeast* **-iasis** *process; state* **leukorrhea** (LOO-koh-REE-ah) **leuk/o-** *white* **-rrhea** *discharge; flow*
cystocele	Herniation of the bladder into the vagina because of a weakness in the vaginal wall. It is caused by childbirth or age. It can result in urinary retention. Treatment: Colporrhaphy.	**cystocele** (SIS-toh-seel) **cyst/o-** *bladder; fluid-filled sac; semisolid cyst* **-cele** *hernia*
dyspareunia	Painful or difficult sexual intercourse. This can happen when the hymen is across the vaginal introitus or because of infection (of the vagina, cervix, or uterus), pelvic inflammatory disease, endometriosis, or retroflexion of the uterus. Treatment: Correct the underlying cause.	**dyspareunia** (DIS-pah-ROO-nee-ah) **dys-** *abnormal; difficult; painful* **pareun/o-** *sexual intercourse* **-ia** *condition; state; thing*
rectocele	Herniation of the rectum into the vagina because of a weakness in the vaginal wall. It is caused by childbirth or age. It can interfere with bowel movements. Treatment: Colporrhaphy.	**rectocele** (REK-toh-seel) **rect/o-** *rectum* **-cele** *hernia*
vaginitis	Vaginal inflammation or infection. Inflammation can be caused by irritation from chemicals in spermicidal jelly or douches. Infection can be caused by candidiasis (yeast infection) or a sexually transmitted disease. Treatment: Treat the underlying cause.	**vaginitis** (VAJ-ih-NY-tis) **vagin/o-** *vagina* **-itis** *infection of; inflammation of*

CLINICAL CONNECTIONS

Public Health. The first cases of **toxic shock syndrome** were seen in women in 1980. There was a high fever, vomiting, diarrhea, and hypotension (shock). Physicians interviewed patients and family members to discover a common link. All of the patients had used super-absorbent **tampons** during their menstrual period. The super-absorbent tampons held the menstrual blood over an extended period of time until the normally harmless vaginal bacterium *Staphylococcus aureus* multiplied in the old blood and released toxins. Also, the larger size of the tampon caused tears in the vaginal wall that allowed the toxins to enter the blood and cause severe symptoms throughout the body.

toxic (TAWK-sik)
tox/o- *poison*
-ic *pertaining to*

tampon (TAM-pawn)

Breasts		
Word or Phrase	**Description**	**Pronunciation/Word Parts**
breast cancer	Cancerous tumor, usually an **adenocarcinoma** of the lactiferous lobules of the breast (see Figure 13-20 ■). A lump is detected during mammography or breast self-examination. There can be swelling in the area, enlarged lymph nodes, and nipple discharge. Advanced breast cancer has **peau d'orange** (a dimpling of the skin—that looks like the pores in an orange peel—as the tumor pulls on structures inside the breast) and nipple retraction. Long-term hormone replacement therapy with an estrogen drug after menopause increases the risk of breast cancer. Inherited mutations in the BRCA1 or BRCA2 gene increase the risk of developing breast cancer. Treatment: Surgery to remove the tumor (lumpectomy) or remove the breast (mastectomy), chemotherapy drugs, radiation therapy.	**adenocarcinoma** (AD-eh-noh-KAR-sih-NOH-mah) **aden/o-** *gland* **carcin/o-** *cancer* **-oma** *mass; tumor* **peau d'orange** (poh deh-RAHNJ)

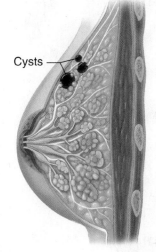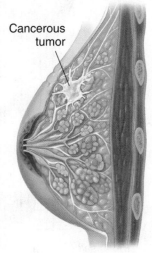

Cysts

Cancerous tumor

FIGURE 13-20 ■ Breast with cysts; breast with cancer.
A lump in the breast can be a benign cyst (fibrocystic disease) or it can be cancer. The presence of many cysts can make it difficult to detect a cancerous tumor on mammography.
Source: Pearson Education

failure of lactation	Lack of production of milk from the breasts after childbirth. It is caused by hyposecretion of prolactin from the anterior pituitary gland. The breasts do not produce milk or produce insufficient milk to breastfeed the baby. Treatment: Switch to bottle feeding.	**lactation** (lak-TAY-shun) **lact/o-** *milk* **-ation** *being; having; process*
fibrocystic disease	Benign condition in which numerous fibrous and fluid-filled cysts form in one or both breasts (see Figure 13-20). The size of the cysts can change in response to hormone levels. The cysts are painful and tender. Severe fibrocystic disease makes it difficult to detect a cancerous tumor on mammography, and so the physician may order an MRI scan instead. Treatment: Hormone therapy. Elimination of certain foods (chocolate, caffeine) from the diet sometimes helps.	**fibrocystic** (FY-broh-SIS-tik) **fibr/o-** *fiber* **cyst/o-** *bladder; fluid-filled sac; semisolid cyst* **-ic** *pertaining to*
galactorrhea	Discharge of milk from the breasts when the patient is not pregnant or breastfeeding. It is caused by an increased level of prolactin from an adenoma (benign tumor) of the anterior pituitary gland. Treatment: Drug to decrease prolactin production or surgery to remove the adenoma from the anterior pituitary gland in the brain.	**galactorrhea** (gah-LAK-toh-REE-ah) **galact/o-** *milk* **-rrhea** *discharge; flow*

Pregnancy and Labor and Delivery

Word or Phrase	Description	Pronunciation/Word Parts
abnormal presentation	Birth position in which the presenting part of the fetus is not the head. In a **breech** presentation, the presenting part is the buttocks, buttocks and feet, or just the feet (see Figure 13-21 ■). If the fetus is in a transverse lie (the fetal vertebral column is perpendicular to the mother's vertebral column), the shoulder or arm is the presenting part. It is also known as **malpresentation** of the fetus (see Figure 13-22 ■). Treatment: Version maneuver to turn the fetus or delivery by cesarean section.	**breech** (BREECH) **malpresentation** (MAL-pree-sen-TAY-shun) The prefix *mal-* means *bad; inadequate.*

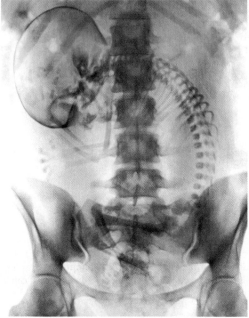

FIGURE 13-21 ■ Breech position.
This colorized three-dimensional CT scan shows a full-term fetus in a breech presentation. The fetal skull is at the top, the spine is along the right side of the image, and the legs are bent.
Source: David Parker/Science Source

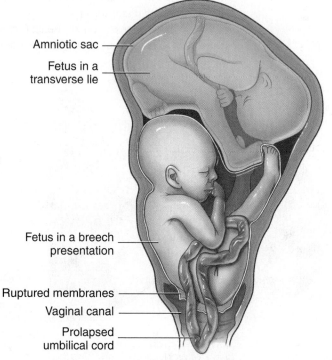

Amniotic sac

Fetus in a transverse lie

Fetus in a breech presentation

Ruptured membranes

Vaginal canal

Prolapsed umbilical cord

FIGURE 13-22 ■ Malpresentation of fraternal twins.
One twin is in the breech position with the buttocks as the presenting part. The amniotic sac around this fetus has already ruptured, and the umbilical cord has prolapsed into the vaginal canal. The second twin, still in its amniotic sac, is in a transverse lie position.
Source: Pearson Education

Word or Phrase	Description	Pronunciation/Word Parts
abruptio placentae	Complete or partial separation of the placenta from the uterine wall before the third stage of labor. This results in uterine hemorrhage that threatens the life of the mother as well as disruption of blood flow and oxygen through the umbilical cord, which threatens the life of the fetus. Treatment: Emergency cesarean section.	**abruptio placentae** (ab-RUP-shee-oh plah-SEN-tee)
cephalopelvic disproportion (CPD)	The size of the fetal head exceeds the size of the opening in the mother's pelvic bones so the fetus cannot be born vaginally. Treatment: Cesarean section.	**cephalopelvic** (SEF-ah-loh-PEL-vik) **cephal/o-** *head* **pelv/o-** *hip bone; pelvis; renal pelvis* **-ic** *pertaining to* **disproportion** (DIS-proh-POR-shun)

DID YOU KNOW?

Skeletons of prehistoric women have been discovered that show cephalopelvic disproportion with the skull of the baby still tightly wedged in the mother's pelvic bones.

Word or Phrase	Description	Pronunciation/Word Parts
dystocia	Any type of difficult or abnormal labor and delivery. Treatment: Correct the underlying cause.	**dystocia** (dis-TOH-sha) **dys-** *abnormal; difficult; painful* **toc/o-** *childbirth; labor* **-ia** *condition; state; thing*
ectopic pregnancy	Implantation of a fertilized ovum somewhere other than in the uterus. It can occur in the cervix, ovary, or abdominal cavity, but most commonly occurs in the uterine tube (a **tubal pregnancy**). This occurs more often if the uterine tube has scar tissue or a blockage in it. The patient has a positive pregnancy test, but there is abdominal tenderness as the uterine tube swells from the developing embryo. The tube can bleed, a condition known as **hemosalpinx**. The tube can suddenly rupture, causing severe blood loss and shock. Treatment: Salpingectomy to remove the embryo and uterine tube.	**ectopic** (ek-TAW-pik) **ectop/o-** *outside* **-ic** *pertaining to* **tubal** (TOO-bal) **tub/o-** *tube* **-al** *pertaining to* **hemosalpinx** (HEE-moh-SAL-pinks) **hem/o-** *blood* **-salpinx** *uterine tube*
gestational diabetes mellitus	Temporary disorder of glucose metabolism that occurs only during pregnancy. Increased levels of estradiol and progesterone during pregnancy block the action of insulin from the pancreas. The function of insulin is to metabolize glucose. A decreased action of insulin leads to a high level of unmetabolized glucose in the mother's blood. Excess glucose crosses the placenta and causes the fetus to grow too rapidly (because its pancreas produces insulin that metabolizes the glucose). Treatment: Dietary management, oral antidiabetic drug during pregnancy. This condition ceases with childbirth, but the mother often develops type 2 diabetes mellitus later in life.	**gestational** (jes-TAY-shun-al) **gestat/o-** *conception to birth* **-ion** *action; condition* **-al** *pertaining to* **diabetes** (DY-ah-BEE-teez) **mellitus** (MEL-ih-tus)
hydatidiform mole	Abnormal union of an ovum and spermatozoon. It produces hundreds of small, fluid-filled sacs but no embryo. The chorion produces HCG, so the patient has early signs of pregnancy. However, the hydatidiform mole grows more rapidly than a normal pregnancy, and the uterus is much larger than expected for the gestational age. Surgery: Removal of the hydatidiform mole or hysterectomy.	**hydatidiform** (HY-dah-TID-ih-form) **hydatidi/o-** *fluid-filled sacs* **-form** *having the form of* **mole** (MOHL)
incompetent cervix	Spontaneous, premature dilation of the cervix during the second trimester of pregnancy. This can result in spontaneous abortion of the fetus. Treatment: Bed rest and placement of a cerclage.	**incompetent** (in-COM-peh-tent)
mastitis	Inflammation or infection of the breast. It is caused by milk engorgement in the breast or by an infection due to the bacterium *Staphylococcus aureus* from the nursing infant's mouth or the mother's skin. The affected breast is red and swollen, and the mother has a fever. Treatment: Pumping of breast milk. Antibiotic drug to treat the infection.	**mastitis** (mas-TY-tis) **mast/o-** *breast; mastoid process* **-itis** *infection of; inflammation of*
morning sickness	Nausea and vomiting during the first trimester of pregnancy. It is thought to be due to elevated estradiol and progesterone levels. **Hyperemesis gravidarum** is excessive vomiting that causes weakness, dehydration, and fluid and electrolyte imbalance. Treatment: Intravenous fluids for severe hyperemesis gravidarum.	**hyperemesis** (HY-per-EM-eh-sis) **hyper-** *above; more than normal* **eme/o-** *vomiting* **-sis** *condition; process* **gravidarum** (GRAV-ih-DAIR-um)
oligohydramnios	Decreased volume of amniotic fluid. The fetus swallows amniotic fluid but does not excrete a similar volume in its urine because of a congenital abnormality of the fetal kidneys. Oligohydramnios is identified during a routine prenatal ultrasound test. Treatment: Surgery to the fetus while *in utero* or after birth.	**oligohydramnios** (OH-lih-GOH-hy-DRAM-nee-ohs) **olig/o-** *few; scanty* **hydr/o-** *fluid; water* **-amnios** *amniotic fluid* ***in utero*** (IN YOO-ter-oh)

Word or Phrase	Description	Pronunciation/Word Parts
placenta previa	Incorrect position of the placenta with its edge partially or completely covering the cervical canal (see Figure 13-23 ■). During labor when the cervix dilates, the connection between the placenta and uterus is disrupted. This causes moderate-to-severe bleeding in the mother and disrupts the flow of blood to the fetus. Treatment: Cesarean section.	**placenta previa** (plah-SEN-tah PREE-vee-ah)

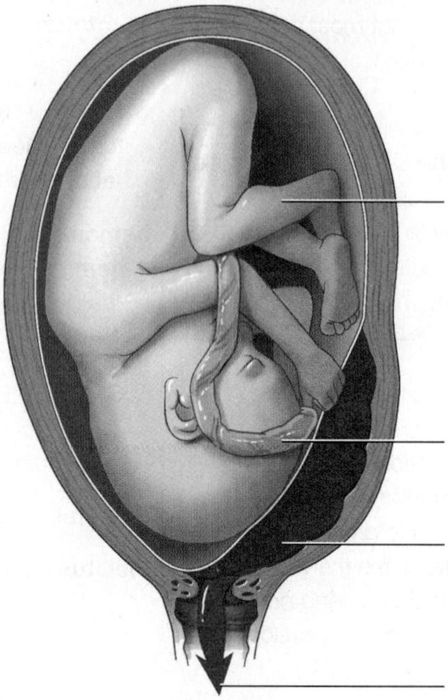

Fetus

Umbilical cord

Placenta previa

Vaginal bleeding

FIGURE 13-23 ■ Placenta previa.
An abnormally low position of the placenta within the uterus can cause bleeding when the cervix dilates during labor and delivery.
Source: Pearson Education

Word or Phrase	Description	Pronunciation/Word Parts
polyhydramnios	Increased volume of amniotic fluid. It is caused by maternal diabetes mellitus, twin gestation, or abnormalities in the fetus. Treatment: Correct the underlying cause.	**polyhydramnios** (PAW-lee-hy-DRAM-nee-ohs) **poly-** *many; much* **hydr/o-** *fluid; water* **-amnios** *amniotic fluid*
postpartum hemorrhage	Continual bleeding from the site where the placenta separated after delivery. The uterus is boggy and does not become firm. It is caused by hyposecretion of oxytocin from the posterior pituitary gland in the brain. Treatment: Manual massage of the uterus. Intravenous oxytocin drug.	**hemorrhage** (HEM-oh-rij) **hem/o-** *blood* **-rrhage** *excessive discharge; excessive flow*
preeclampsia	Hypertensive disorder of pregnancy with increased blood pressure, edema, weight gain, and protein in the urine (proteinuria). The kidneys allow protein from the blood to be lost in the urine. A low level of blood proteins changes the osmotic pressure and allows fluid to move into the tissues and cause edema. Preeclampsia can progress to **eclampsia** in which the woman has seizures and the fetus is endangered. Treatment: Bed rest, antihypertensive and antiseizure drugs.	**preeclampsia** (PREE-ee-KLAMP-see-ah) **pre-** *before; in front of* **eclamps/o-** *seizure* **-ia** *condition; state; thing* **eclampsia** (ee-KLAMP-see-ah)
premature labor	Regular uterine contractions that occur before the fetus is mature. The cervix can dilate and small amounts of blood or amniotic fluid can leak out. Treatment: Bed rest, tocolytic drug to stop labor.	
premature rupture of membranes (PROM)	Spontaneous rupture of the amniotic sac and loss of amniotic fluid before labor begins. The mother must deliver within 24 hours or risk the development of infection. Treatment: Induction of labor.	

Word or Phrase	Description	Pronunciation/Word Parts
prolapsed cord	A loop of umbilical cord becomes caught between the presenting part of the fetus and the birth canal (see Figure 13-22). This occurs if the membranes rupture before the fetal head (or other presenting part) is fully engaged in the mother's pelvis. With each uterine contraction, the umbilical cord is compressed, causing decreased blood flow to the fetus and fetal distress with a decreased heart rate. Treatment: Change the mother's position to move the cord, give oxygen to the mother. Surgery: Cesarean section.	**prolapse** (PROH-laps)
spontaneous abortion (SAB)	Loss of a pregnancy. An early spontaneous abortion usually occurs because of a genetic abnormality or poor implantation of the embryo in the endometrium. A late spontaneous abortion can occur because of preterm labor or an incompetent cervix. In an incomplete abortion, the embryo or fetus is expelled but the placenta and other tissues remain in the uterus. It is also known as a **miscarriage**. The fetus can be born alive or can be a **stillborn**. Treatment: None.	**abortion** (ah-BOR-shun) **abort/o-** *stop prematurely* **-ion** *action; condition*
uterine inertia	Weak or uncoordinated contractions during a long and nonproductive labor. It is caused by (1) a decreased level of oxytocin from the posterior pituitary gland; (2) a uterus that is very distended with multiple fetuses and unable to contract normally; or (3) cephalopelvic disproportion or malpresentation of the fetus. A related condition is **arrest of labor** in which uterine contractions have ceased. It is also known as **failure to progress**, as the cervix does not progressively dilate and efface. Treatment: Intravenous oxytocin drug; cesarean section for cephalopelvic disproportion; version or cesarean section for malpresentation.	**inertia** (in-ER-sha)

CLINICAL CONNECTIONS

Psychiatry (Chapter 17). Postpartum depression is a mood disorder with symptoms of mild-to-moderate depression, anxiousness, irritability, tearfulness, and fatigue. It is caused by hormonal changes after birth and by feelings of overwhelming responsibility and fatigue. It was formerly known as **involutional melancholia** because it occurs at the time of involution of the uterus.

Dietetics. A lack of folic acid during pregnancy can cause a neural tube defect in the fetus. Prenatal vitamins for pregnant women and enrichment of cereals and other grain products with added folic acid have greatly decreased the incidence of neural tube defects.

There are many stories about the food cravings of pregnant women: pickles, ice cream, and so forth. Some pregnant women experience **pica**, an unnatural craving for, and compulsive eating of, substances with no nutritional value, such as clay, chalk, starch, or dirt.

depression (dee-PREH-shun)
 depress/o- *press down*
 -ion *action; condition*

involutional (IN-voh-LOO-shun-al)
 involut/o- *enlarged organ returns to normal size*
 -ion *action; condition*
 -al *pertaining to*

melancholia (MEL-an-KOH-lee-ah)
 melan/o- *black*
 chol/o- *bile; gall*
 -ia *condition; state; thing*

pica (PY-kah) (PEE-kah)

Fetus and Neonate

apnea	Temporary or permanent cessation of breathing in the newborn after birth. The newborn is said to be **apneic**. The immature central nervous system of a newborn fails to maintain a consistent respiratory rate, and there are occasional long pauses between periods of regular breathing. Treatment: Apnea monitor in the hospital and at home that sounds an alarm if the newborn stops breathing.	**apnea** (AP-nee-ah) **a-** *away from; without* **-pnea** *breathing* **apneic** (AP-nee-ik) **a-** *away from; without* **pne/o-** *breathing* **-ic** *pertaining to*

Word or Phrase	Description	Pronunciation/Word Parts
fetal distress	Lack of oxygen to the fetus because of decreased blood flow through the placenta or umbilical cord. The fetus has a decreased heart rate and passes meconium because of the stress of a decreased level of oxygen. Treatment: Mother is given oxygen; possible cesarean section.	
growth abnormalities	Maternal illness, malnutrition, and smoking can make the fetus **small for gestational age (SGA)**. This is known as **intrauterine growth retardation (IUGR)**. Diabetes mellitus in the mother can make the fetus **large for gestational age (LGA)**. A fetus within the normal growth range for weight and length is said to be **appropriate for gestational age (AGA)**. Treatment: Correct the underlying cause.	**intrauterine** (IN-trah-YOO-teh-rin) (IN-trah-YOO-teh-rine) **intra-** *within* **uter/o-** *uterus; womb* **-ine** *pertaining to; thing pertaining to*
jaundice	Yellowish discoloration of the skin in a newborn. During gestation, the fetus has extra red blood cells that are no longer needed after birth. The destruction of those red blood cells releases hemoglobin, which is converted into unconjugated bilirubin. The immature newborn liver is not able to process this much unconjugated bilirubin, and it builds up in the blood (**hyperbilirubinemia**), moves into the tissues, and causes jaundice. The more premature the newborn, the greater the chance of developing jaundice. Treatment: **Phototherapy** with bililights, special fluorescent lights that break down bilirubin in the skin to make it water soluble so it can be excreted by the kidneys.	**jaundice** (JAWN-dis) **hyperbilirubinemia** (HY-per-BIL-ih-ROO-bih-NEE-mee-ah) **hyper-** *above; more than normal* **bilirubin/o-** *bilirubin* **-emia** *condition of the blood; substance in the blood* **phototherapy** (FOH-toh-THAIR-ah-pee) **phot/o-** *light* **-therapy** *treatment*
meconium aspiration	Fetal distress causes the fetus to pass meconium into the amniotic fluid. This can get in the mouth and nose, and, if inhaled with the first breath, it causes severe respiratory distress. Treatment: Suctioning of the newborn's nose and mouth. Use of oxygen and a ventilator after birth.	**aspiration** (AS-pih-RAY-shun) **aspir/o-** *breathe in; suck in* **-ation** *being; having; process*
nuchal cord	Umbilical cord is wrapped around the neck of the fetus. A loose nuchal cord can be present without causing a problem. A tight nuchal cord with one or more loops around the neck can impair blood flow to the brain, causing brain damage or fetal death. Treatment: Emergency cesarean section.	**nuchal** (NOO-kal) **nuch/o-** *neck* **-al** *pertaining to*
respiratory distress syndrome (RDS)	Difficulty inflating the lungs to breathe because of a lack of surfactant. This occurs mainly in premature newborns. It was previously known as *hyaline membrane disease (HMD)*. Treatment: Surfactant drug given through the endotracheal tube; oxygen and a ventilator.	**respiratory** (RES-pih-rah-TOR-ee) (reh-SPY-rah-TOR-ee) **re-** *again and again; backward; unable to* **spir/o-** *breathe; coil* **-atory** *pertaining to*

Laboratory and Diagnostic Procedures

Gynecologic Tests and Procedures		
Word or Phrase	**Description**	**Pronunciation/Word Parts**
acid phosphatase	Test for an enzyme from the prostate gland that is found in the semen. The presence of acid phosphatase in the vagina indicates sexual intercourse and can be used in rape investigations.	**acid phosphatase** (AS-id FAWS-fah-tays)
biopsy	Procedure to remove a small piece of tissue for examination under a microscope to look for abnormal or cancerous cells. A breast biopsy can be done by **fine-needle aspiration** (a very fine needle is inserted into the mass and a syringe is used to aspirate tissue) or by **vacuum-assisted biopsy** (a probe with a cutting device is inserted through the skin and rotated to suck in multiple specimens). For an endometrial biopsy, a speculum is used to visualize the cervix and a dilator expands the cervical os. A pipette or catheter is inserted into the uterus and rotated while suction pulls in tissue. This is used to diagnose abnormal uterine bleeding and uterine cancer. For larger biopsy specimens, a surgical procedure is performed. First, mammography or ultrasound is used to identify the location of the mass, and a needle or wire marker is inserted to pinpoint the site. A **stereotactic biopsy** uses three different angles of mammography to precisely locate the mass. For an **incisional biopsy**, an incision is made in the skin overlying the mass and a large part (but not all) of the mass is removed. For an **excisional biopsy**, the entire mass is removed along with a surrounding margin of normal tissue.	**biopsy** (BY-awp-see) **bi/o-** *life; living organism; living tissue* **-opsy** *process of viewing* **aspiration** (AS-pih-RAY-shun) **aspir/o-** *breathe in; suck in* **-ation** *being; having; process* **stereotactic** (STAIR-ee-oh-TAK-tik) **stere/o-** *three dimensions* **tact/o-** *touch* **-ic** *pertaining to* **incisional** (in-SIH-zhun-al) **incis/o-** *cut into* **-ion** *action; condition* **-al** *pertaining to* **excisional** (ek-SIH-zhun-al) **excis/o-** *cut out* **-ion** *action; condition* **-al** *pertaining to*
BRCA1 or BRCA2 gene	Blood test that shows if a patient has inherited the BRCA1 or BRCA2 gene, **genetic** mutations that significantly increase the risk of developing breast or ovarian cancer. BRCA stands for **br**east **ca**ncer.	**gene** (JEEN) **genetic** (jeh-NET-ik) **gene/o-** *gene* **-tic** *pertaining to*
estrogen receptor assay	**Cytology** test performed on breast tissue that has already been diagnosed as malignant. This test looks for a large number of estrogen receptors on the tumor cell. If present, this means that the tumor requires estrogen (estradiol) in order to grow and that chemotherapy drugs that block estrogen would be effective in treating this cancer.	**receptor** (ree-SEP-tor) **recept/o-** *receive* **-or** *person who does; person who produces; thing that does; thing that produces* **assay** (AS-say) **cytology** (sy-TAW-loh-jee) **cyt/o-** *cell* **-logy** *study of*

Word or Phrase	Description	Pronunciation/Word Parts
Pap smear	Screening cytology test used to detect abnormal cells (dysplasia) or carcinoma *in situ* (CIS) of the cervix. It is also known as a *Pap test*. This is an **exfoliative cytology** test because it examines cells that have been scraped off the cervix. A small plastic or wooden spatula is used to scrape off **ectocervical cells** from the outside wall of the cervix. Then a **cytobrush** is inserted into the cervical os to obtain **endocervical cells** (see Figure 13-24 ■). A cervical broom (Papette®) can obtain both types of cells at the same time and also test for HPV. The cell specimen is transferred to a glass slide and sprayed with a fixative. Alternatively, with **liquid cytology**, the specimen is rinsed in a vial of fixative. This captures all the cells, prevents cell drying, and gives a more accurate result. The slides or vials are sent to the laboratory where the cells are examined under a microscope for abnormalities (see Figure 13-25 ■). The Bethesda System is used to report Pap smear results.	**Pap smear** **exfoliative** (eks-FOH-lee-ah-TIV) **cytology** (sy-TAW-loh-jee) cyt/o- *cell* -logy *study of* **ectocervical** (EK-toh-SER-vih-kal) ecto- *outermost; outside* cervic/o- *cervix; neck* -al *pertaining to* **endocervical** (EN-doh-SER-vih-kal) endo- *innermost; within* cervic/o- *cervix; neck* -al *pertaining to*

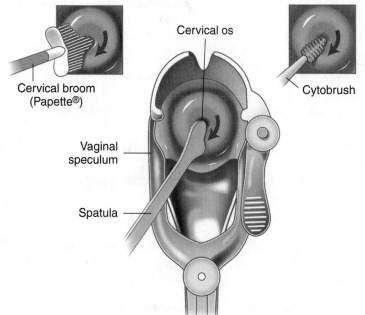

Cervical os

Cervical broom (Papette®)

Cytobrush

Vaginal speculum

Spatula

FIGURE 13-24 ■ Taking a Pap smear.
A metal vaginal speculum is used to spread the vaginal walls apart to reveal the cervix. Cells from the cervix are obtained using a wooden spatula and a cytobrush or a cervical broom (Papette®). A microscope is used to examine the cells and detect cells that are precancerous or cancerous.
Source: Pearson Education

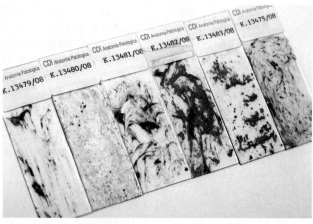

FIGURE 13-25 ■ Pap smears.
These stained slides from Pap smears from different women will be examined under the microscope by a pathologist.
Source: Mauro Fermariello/Science Photo Library/Getty Images

Word or Phrase	Description	Pronunciation/Word Parts

	A CLOSER LOOK
	
	PAP SMEAR TERMINOLOGY
	(Bethesda System Guidelines)
	
	Specimen Adequacy
	• Satisfactory (enough cells were collected; cell quality was sufficient for diagnosis)
	• Unsatisfactory (enough cells were not collected; cell quality was poor)
	
	Normal Pap Smear
	Findings are reported as:
	   Negative for intraepithelial lesion or malignancy. (The presence of infectious organisms [Trichomonas, herpes, HPV] is also reported.)
	
	Abnormal Pap Smear
	Findings are reported as one of the following:
	   ASC-US Atypical squamous cells of unknown significance
	   ASC-H Atypical squamous cells of unknown significance, cannot exclude HSIL
	   LSIL* Low-grade squamous intraepithelial lesion
	   HSIL** High-grade squamous intraepithelial lesion
	   SCC Squamous cell carcinoma
	
	*LSIL includes several levels that are classified as cervical intraepithelial neoplasia (CIN I).
	**HSIL includes several levels that are classified as CIN II through III.	

wet mount	Cytology test for yeasts, parasites, or bacteria. A swab of vaginal discharge is sent to a laboratory. The cells are placed on a slide, mixed with saline solution, and examined under a microscope. It is also known as a **wet prep**.	
Infertility Diagnostic Tests		
antisperm antibody test	Test that detects antibodies against sperm in the woman's cervical mucus. Some antibodies attack the tail of the spermatozoon so that it cannot swim; other antibodies prevent the spermatozoon from penetrating the ovum. Men produce antibodies to their own spermatozoa after a vasectomy when the spermatozoa must be absorbed by the body. These antibodies remain even after reversal of the vasectomy.	**antibody** (AN-tee-BAW-dee) (AN-tih-BAW-dee) The prefix *anti-* means *against.*
hormone testing	Blood test to determine the levels of FSH and LH from the anterior pituitary gland and estradiol and progesterone from the ovaries. It is used to diagnose menstruation and infertility problems.	

Pregnancy and Prenatal Diagnostic Tests

Word or Phrase	Description	Pronunciation/Word Parts

amniocentesis	Procedure to test the amniotic fluid. Using ultrasound guidance, a needle is inserted through the pregnant woman's abdomen and into the uterus to obtain some amniotic fluid (see Figure 13-26 ■). This is done between 15 and 18 weeks' gestation when there is a sufficient amount of amniotic fluid. The following tests are performed:
	
	1. **Chromosome studies** of fetal skin cells can determine the sex of the fetus and identify genetic abnormalities such as Down syndrome.
	2. **Alpha fetoprotein (AFP)**. An increased level indicates a neural tube defect (myelomeningocele).
	3. **L/S ratio** (lecithin/sphingomyelin) test for fetal lung maturity. **Lecithin** is a component of surfactant that keeps the alveoli from collapsing with each exhalation. The **sphingomyelin** level is higher when the fetal lungs are immature; when the lungs are mature the lecithin level is higher.
	
	FIGURE 13-26 ■ Amniocentesis.
	The obstetrician is withdrawing amniotic fluid through a needle inserted into the intrauterine cavity. The position of the needle was verified by ultrasound (the plastic-covered instrument in the background). The sound waves do not injure the developing fetus, and they help the obstetrician locate a pocket of amniotic fluid.
	Source: Astier/Science Source
		amniocentesis
		(AM-nee-OH-sen-TEE-sis)
		  amni/o- *amnion; membrane around the fetus*
		  -centesis *procedure to puncture*
		
		chromosome (KROH-moh-sohm)
		  chrom/o- *color*
		  -some *body*
		Add words to make a complete definition of *chromosome*: *body (within the nucleus that takes on) color (when stained).*
		
		alpha fetoprotein
		(AL-fah FEE-toh-PROH-teen)
		
		lecithin (LES-ih-thin)
		
		sphingomyelin
		(SFING-goh-MY-eh-lin)

chorionic villus sampling (CVS)	Genetic test of the chorionic villi of the placenta. A needle is inserted through the abdomen, or a catheter is inserted through the cervix to aspirate some of the chorionic villi from the placenta. This test is performed when a fetal genetic defect is suspected. It can be performed at 12 weeks, which is earlier than an amniocentesis, but it cannot detect neural tube defects in the fetus.	**chorionic** (KOR-ee-AW-nik)
		  chorion/o- *chorion*
		  -ic *pertaining to*
		
		villus (VIL-us)
		Villus is a Latin singular noun. Form the plural by changing *-us* to *-i*.

pregnancy test	Blood test to detect human chorionic gonadotropin (HCG) secreted by the fertilized ovum. Serum HCG is positive just 9 days after conception. Home pregnancy tests that detect HCG in the urine are easy to use but are not always accurate. Only a positive blood test (serum beta HCG) is diagnostic of pregnancy. The presence of HCG does not indicate that the pregnancy is normal because HCG is also produced when there is an ectopic pregnancy or a hydatidiform mole.	

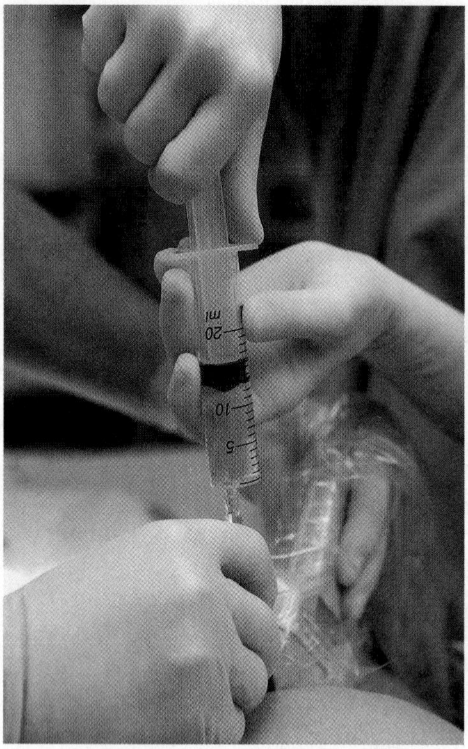

Radiologic Procedures

Word or Phrase	Description	Pronunciation/Word Parts
hystero-salpingography	Procedure in which radiopaque contrast dye is injected through the cervix into the uterus. It coats and outlines the uterus and uterine tubes and shows narrowing, scarring, and blockage. The x-ray image is a **hysterosalpingogram**. This test is done as part of an infertility workup.	**hysterosalpingography** (HIS-ter-oh-SAL-ping-GAW-grah-fee) **hyster/o-** *uterus; womb* **salping/o-** *uterine tube* **-graphy** *process of recording* **hysterosalpingogram** (HIS-ter-OH-sal-PING-goh-gram) **hyster/o-** *uterus; womb* **salping/o-** *uterine tube* **-gram** *picture; record*
mammography	Procedure that uses x-rays to create an image of the breast. The breast is compressed and slightly flattened (see Figure 13-27 ■). Mammography is used to detect areas of microcalcification, infection, cysts, and tumors, many of which cannot be felt on a breast examination. The x-ray image is a **mammogram**. **Xeromammography** uses a special plate instead of an x-ray plate, and the image is developed with dry powder rather than liquid chemicals. The image is printed on paper and is a **xeromammogram**. *Note:* A magnetic resonance image (MRI) scan produces a clearer image than mammography in patients who have multiple cysts in the breasts. 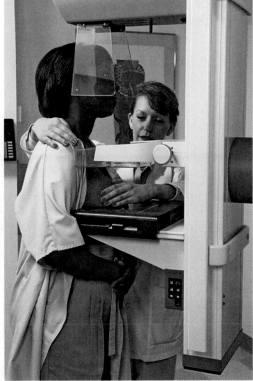 **FIGURE 13-27 ■ Mammography.** A mammogram is the image obtained when an x-ray beam passes through the breast to an x-ray plate. The breast is compressed because, the less distance the x-ray travels, the sharper the image that is obtained. *Source*: Keith Brofsky/Photodisc/Getty Images	**mammography** (mah-MAW-grah-fee) **mamm/o-** *breast* **-graphy** *process of recording* **mammogram** (MAM-oh-gram) **mamm/o-** *breast* **-gram** *picture; record* **xeromammography** (ZEER-oh-mah-MAW-grah-fee) **xer/o-** *dry* **mamm/o-** *breast* **-graphy** *process of recording* **xeromammogram** (ZEER-oh-MAM-oh-gram) **xer/o-** *dry* **mamm/o-** *breast* **-gram** *picture; record*

Word or Phrase	Description	Pronunciation/Word Parts

ultrasonography	Procedure that uses ultra high-frequency sound waves emitted by a transducer or probe to produce an image on a computer screen. Three-dimensional ultrasonography couples the ultrasound with a position sensor to generate a high-resolution image in three dimensions (see Figure 13-28 ■). The **ultrasound** image is a **sonogram**.
	
	Ultrasonography of the breast or uterus can differentiate between benign, fluid-filled tumors (cysts) and solid tumors that need to be biopsied. A pelvic ultrasound can be used to diagnose a normal pregnancy versus a hydatidiform mole or ectopic pregnancy. In early pregnancy, the beating heart is seen. The image can show multiple fetuses and the sex of the fetus. An ultrasound is done routinely at 16–20 weeks in a normal pregnancy to estimate the gestational age. Serial ultrasounds can be done over time if there is a question of intrauterine growth retardation. The length of the femur, the **biparietal diameter (BPD)** (distance between the two parietal bones of the cranium), and the crown-to-rump length are used to calculate the gestational age of the fetus. Ultrasound can show the position of the placenta to diagnose placenta previa. Pelvic ultrasound is used during amniocentesis to locate a large area of amniotic fluid in which to insert the needle (see Figure 13-26). A **transvaginal ultrasound** uses an ultrasound probe inserted into the vagina to determine the thickness of the endometrium in patients with abnormal uterine bleeding. 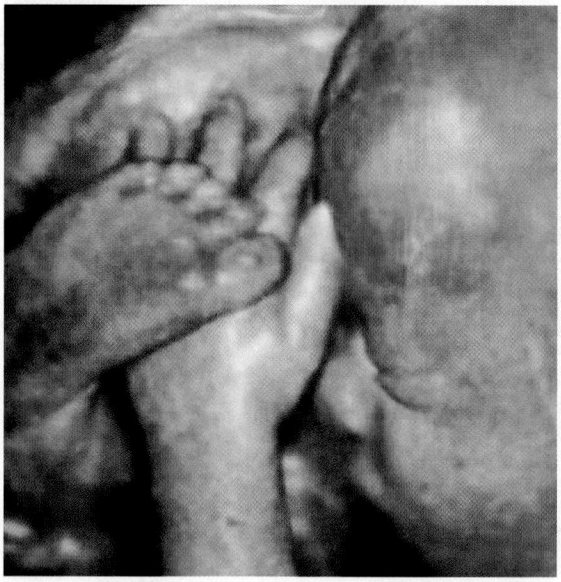
		ultrasonography (UL-trah-soh-NAW-grah-fee)
		  ultra- *beyond; higher*
		  son/o- *sound*
		  -graphy *process of recording*
		
		ultrasound (UL-trah-sound)
		
		sonogram (SAW-noh-gram)
		  son/o- *sound*
		  -gram *picture; record*
		
		biparietal (BY-pah-RY-eh-tal)
		  bi- *two*
		  pariet/o- *wall of a cavity*
		  -al *pertaining to*
		
		transvaginal (trans-VAJ-ih-nal)
		  trans- *across; through*
		  vagin/o- *vagina*
		  -al *pertaining to*

FIGURE 13-28 ■ **Three-dimensional ultrasonography.**
Sound waves generated by a transducer bounce off the fetus and are used to create a computer image. Details of the fetus are clearly visible in this type of ultrasound. Sound waves, rather than x-rays, are used so that the fetus is not exposed to any radiation.
Source: Ge Medical Systems/Science Source

Medical and Surgical Procedures

Medical Procedures of the Internal Genitalia

Word or Phrase	Description	Pronunciation/Word Parts
colposcopy	Procedure that uses a magnifying, lighted scope to visually examine the vagina and cervix	**colposcopy** (kol-PAW-skoh-pee) **colp/o-** *vagina* **-scopy** *process of using an instrument to examine*
cryosurgery	Procedure to destroy small areas of abnormal tissue on the cervix. Colposcopy is used to visualize the cervical lesions. Then a **cryoprobe** containing extremely cold liquid nitrogen is touched to the areas to freeze and destroy the abnormal tissues.	**cryosurgery** (KRY-oh-SER-jer-ee) **cry/o-** *cold* **surg/o-** *operative procedure* **-ery** *process* **cryoprobe** (KRY-oh-prohb) **cry/o-** *cold* **-probe** *rod-like instrument*
gynecologic examination	Procedure to physically examine the external and internal genitalia. This is performed with the patient supine in the **dorsal lithotomy position**. The hips and knees are flexed, and the feet are elevated in stirrups. The external genitalia are examined visually for any skin lesions, rashes, or discharge from the vagina. The internal genitalia are examined using a **bimanual examination** (see Figure 13-29 ■). A mass, cystocele, rectocele, or any enlargement of the uterus can be palpated with the gloved hands. Tenderness to palpation can indicate infection or endometriosis. A **speculum** is inserted into the vagina and a Pap smear is performed (see Figure 13-30 ■). The cervix is examined visually for abnormalities.	**gynecologic** (GY-neh-koh-LAW-jik) **gynec/o-** *female; woman* **log/o-** *study of; word* **-ic** *pertaining to* **dorsal** (DOR-sal) **dors/o-** *back; dorsum* **-al** *pertaining to* **lithotomy** (lith-AW-toh-mee) **lith/o-** *stone* **-tomy** *process of cutting; process of making an incision* *Note*: This is the same body position that was used in the past to treat patients with kidney stones. **bimanual** (by-MAN-yoo-al) **bi-** *two* **manu/o-** *hand* **-al** *pertaining to* **speculum** (SPEH-kyoo-lum)

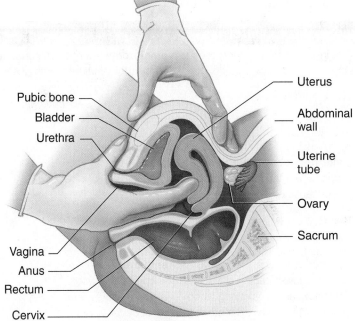

FIGURE 13-29 ■ Bimanual examination.
By using both hands, the gynecologist is able to examine the shape of the nonpregnant uterus and detect tenderness and masses.
Source: Pearson Education

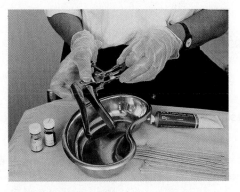

FIGURE 13-30 ■ Vaginal speculum.
A speculum (metal or plastic) has two blades that are closed together as the speculum is inserted into the vagina and then move apart to separate the walls of the vagina so that the cervix can be seen.
Source: Simon Fraser/Science Source

Medical Procedures of the Breast

Word or Phrase	Description	Pronunciation/Word Parts
breast self-examination (BSE)	Procedure to systematically palpate all areas of the breast (starting with the nipple and moving outward in concentric circles) and under the arm to detect lumps, masses, or enlarged lymph nodes (see Figure 13-31 ■). BSE should be done monthly after the menstrual period to detect early signs of breast cancer.	

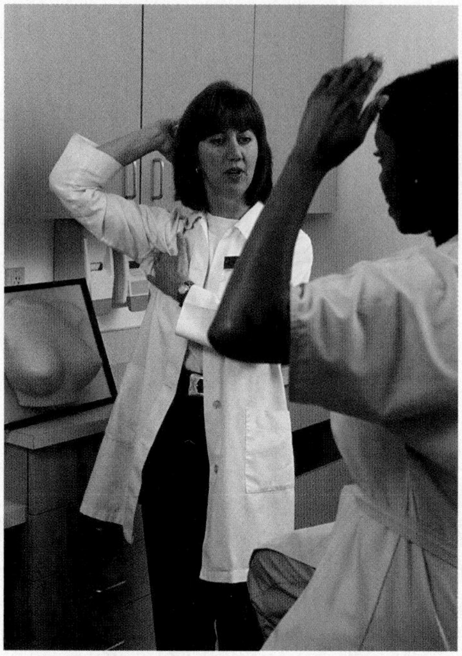

FIGURE 13-31 ■ Breast self-examination.
This nurse is instructing the patient on how to perform self-examination of the breasts to feel for masses or lumps. All areas of the breasts are palpated in a consistent way. The lymph nodes under the arm are also palpated for any sign of enlargement.
Source: Keith Brofsky/Photodisc/Getty Images

Word or Phrase	Description	Pronunciation/Word Parts
Tanner staging	System used to describe the development of the female breasts from childhood through puberty. There are five different stages, from Tanner stage 1 (nipple and areola are flat against the chest wall) to Tanner stage 5 (enlargement of the entire breast). The Tanner system is also used to describe the development of the female external genitalia.	

Medical Procedures for Obstetrics

Word or Phrase	Description	Pronunciation/Word Parts
amniotomy	Procedure in which a hooked instrument is inserted into the cervical os to rupture the amniotic sac and induce labor	**amniotomy** (AM-nee-AW-toh-mee) **amni/o-** *amnion; membrane around the fetus* **-tomy** *process of cutting; process of making an incision*
Apgar score	Procedure that assigns a score to a newborn at 1 and 5 minutes after birth. Points (0–2) are given for the heart rate, respiratory rate, muscle tone, response to stimulation, and skin color, for a total possible score of 10. Normally, one point is always taken off because of acrocyanosis.	**Apgar** (AP-gar)
assisted delivery	Procedure in which obstetrical forceps (see Figure 13-13) or a vacuum extractor is used to facilitate delivery of the head of the fetus	
epidural anesthesia	Procedure to produce local anesthesia by injecting an anesthetic drug into the epidural space between vertebrae in the lower back. This blocks pain and sensation from the abdomen, perineum, and legs during labor and delivery. Epidural anesthesia is not given until the cervix is more than 4 cm dilated; otherwise, it can prolong labor.	**epidural** (EP-ih-DOOR-al) **epi-** *above; upon* **dur/o-** *dura mater* **-al** *pertaining to* **anesthesia** (AN-es-THEE-zha) **an-** *not; without* **esthes/o-** *feeling; sensation* **-ia** *condition; state; thing*

Word or Phrase	Description	Pronunciation/Word Parts
fundal height	Procedure to measure the height of the uterine fundus during each prenatal visit. The fundus of the uterus moves superiorly as pregnancy progresses. The distance in centimeters from the top of the symphysis pubis to the top of the uterine fundus is measured. This is a general indication of fetal growth.	**fundal** (FUN-dal) **fund/o-** *fundus; part farthest from the opening* **-al** *pertaining to*
induction of labor	Procedure that uses an oxytocin drug to induce (cause) labor to begin. This is done when the mother is past her estimated due date or when the health of the mother or fetus necessitates delivery.	**induction** (in-DUK-shun) **induct/o-** *leading in* **-ion** *action; condition*
Nägele's rule	Procedure used to calculate the estimated date of birth (EDB), estimated date of delivery (EDD), or due date. This is done by adding 9 months and 7 days to the date of the first day of the woman's last menstrual period. Often the patient does not remember the first day of her last menstrual period (LMP), and so the EDB is just an approximate date. Estimated date of confinement (EDC) is an older phrase that indicated when a woman was to be confined to her home around her due date.	**Nägele** (NAY-gel)
nonstress test (NST)	Procedure that uses an external monitor on the mother's abdomen to display the fetal heart rate. A normal test (reactive test) will show at least two increases in fetal heart rate associated with fetal movement as felt by the mother. A nonreactive test, which is abnormal, is followed by a **biophysical profile (BPP)** that combines a nonstress test with an ultrasound to show fetal movement, fetal heart rate, and amniotic fluid volume.	**biophysical** (BY-oh-FIZ-ih-kal) **bi/o-** *life; living organism; living tissue* **physic/o-** *body* **-al** *pertaining to*
obstetrical history	Procedure to document past pregnancies and deliveries. This is a standard of good prenatal care. A **nulligravida** is a woman who has never been pregnant and is not pregnant now. A **primigravida** is a woman who is pregnant for the first time. She is primiparous ("primip" for short). A **multigravida** is a woman who has been pregnant more than once. If she has given birth many times, she is said to be **multiparous**. In the past, the obstetrical history was documented as **gravida (G)**, **para (P)**, and **abortion (Ab)**. A woman who was G3, P3, Ab 0 had been pregnant three times and given birth three times. A woman who had had twins would be G1, P2. The G/TPAL system is used more often now because it provides more details. **G** Number of times pregnant **T** Number of term births **P** Number of premature births **A** Number of abortions (spontaneous or therapeutic) **L** Number of living children	**nulligravida** (NUL-ih-GRAV-ih-dah) **null/i-** *none* **-gravida** *pregnancy* **primigravida** (PRY-mih-GRAV-ih-dah) **prim/i-** *first* **-gravida** *pregnancy* **multigravida** (MUL-tih-GRAV-ih-dah) **mult/i-** *many* **-gravida** *pregnancy* **multiparous** (mul-TIP-ah-rus) **mult/i-** *many* **par/o-** *giving birth* **-ous** *pertaining to* **gravida** (GRAV-ih-dah) **para** (PAIR-ah)
therapeutic abortion (TAB)	Procedure for planned termination of a pregnancy at any time during gestation. It is performed because the fetus is abnormal or because the pregnancy is unwanted. All products of conception are removed from the uterus with suction. It is also known as an **elective abortion**.	**therapeutic** (THAIR-ah-PYOO-tik) **therapeut/o-** *therapy; treatment* **-ic** *pertaining to* **abortion** (ah-BOR-shun) **abort/o-** *stop prematurely* **-ion** *action; condition* **elective** (ee-LEK-tiv)
version	Procedure to manually correct a breech or other malpresentation prior to delivery. The obstetrician puts his/her hands on the mother's abdominal wall and manipulates the fetus until it is in a cephalic presentation.	**version** (VER-zhun) **vers/o-** *travel; turn* **-ion** *action; condition*

A CLOSER LOOK

Assisted reproductive technology (ART) uses technology to assist the process of conception. For **in vitro fertilization (IVF)**, the woman receives ovulation-stimulating drugs. Then mature ova are harvested with a needle inserted into the ovary. Some of the ova are combined with spermatozoa and allowed to grow from 2 to 5 days in a culture medium. Then one fertilized ovum (or more) is inserted into the uterus. The newborns born by IVF were known as "test tube babies." For **zygote intrafallopian transfer (ZIFT)**, the same procedure is followed but the fertilized ovum (zygote) is inserted into the uterine (fallopian) tube. For **gamete intrafallopian transfer (GIFT)**, the ova and spermatozoa (gametes) are collected, and both are inserted right away into the uterine (fallopian) tube.

When the man has a low sperm count or the woman's cervical mucus contains antibodies against sperm, the man's semen is collected, concentrated, and inserted into the uterus, a procedure known as **intrauterine insemination**. In men with a very low sperm count, sperm can be taken from the testis or epididymis. Then, under a microscope, a micropipette is used to inject a single sperm into the cytoplasm of one ovum, a procedure known as **intracytoplasmic sperm injection (ICSI)** (see Figure 13-32 ■).

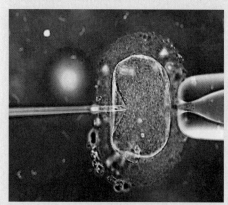

FIGURE 13-32 ■ **Intracytoplasmic sperm injection (ICSI).**
A type of assisted reproductive technology. Under a microscope, a micropipette (on the left) is used to penetrate the cytoplasm of an ovum and insert a single spermatozoon to fertilize it. A glass rod on the right holds the ovum in place during this procedure.
Source: Zephyr/Science Source

in vitro (IN VEE-troh)

intrafallopian
(IN-trah-fah-LOH-pee-an)
  intra- *within*
  fallopi/o- *uterine tube*
  -an *pertaining to*

insemination
(in-SEM-ih-NAY-shun)
  insemin/o- *sow a seed*
  -ation *being; having; process*

intracytoplasmic
(IN-trah-SY-toh-PLAS-mik)
  intra- *within*
  cyt/o- *cell*
  plasm/o- *plasma*
  -ic *pertaining to*

injection (in-JEK-shun)
  inject/o- *insert; put in*
  -ion *action; condition*

Surgical Procedures of the Uterus, Uterine Tubes, and Ovaries

Word or Phrase	Description	Pronunciation/Word Parts

dilation and curettage (D&C)	Procedure to remove abnormal tissue from inside the uterus. The cervix is dilated with progressively larger dilators inserted into the cervical os. A **tenaculum** (long, scissors-like instrument with two curved, pointed ends) is used to grasp and hold the cervix. Then a **curet** (instrument with a sharp-edged circular or oval ring at one end) is inserted to scrape the endometrium. Alternatively, a vacuum aspirator is inserted to suction out pieces of endometrium. This procedure is used to treat abnormal uterine bleeding, to look for uterine cancer, to perform a therapeutic abortion, or remove the products of conception following a spontaneous but incomplete abortion.	**dilation** (dy-LAY-shun)
		  dilat/o- *dilate; widen*
		  -ion *action; condition*
		
		curettage (KYOOR-eh-TAWZH)
		
		tenaculum (teh-NAH-kyoo-lum)
		
		curet (kyoor-ET)

endometrial ablation	Procedure that uses heat or cold to destroy the endometrium. A laser, hot fluid in a balloon, or an electrode with electrical current is inserted into the uterus. Alternatively, a cryoprobe is inserted to freeze the endometrium. It is used to treat dysfunctional uterine bleeding.	**ablation** (ah-BLAY-shun)
		  ablat/o- *destroy; take away*
		  -ion *action; condition*

Word or Phrase	Description	Pronunciation/Word Parts
hysterectomy	Procedure to remove the uterus. An abdominal hysterectomy is performed with a laparoscope through an abdominal incision. A vaginal hysterectomy is performed through the vagina. A total hysterectomy involves removing both the uterus and cervix. A **TAH-BSO** is a total abdominal hysterectomy and bilateral salpingo-oophorectomy (removal of both uterine tubes and ovaries). A hysterectomy is done because of uterine fibroids, endometriosis, uterine prolapse, abnormal uterine bleeding, or uterine or cervical cancer. A radical hysterectomy to treat cancer of the uterus involves removal of the uterus, cervix, upper vagina, and pelvic lymph nodes.	**hysterectomy** (HIS-ter-EK-toh-mee) **hyster/o-** *uterus; womb* **-ectomy** *surgical removal*
laparoscopy	Procedure to visualize the abdominopelvic cavity, uterus, uterine tubes, and ovaries. **Laparoscopic** surgery begins with a small incision near the umbilicus, and carbon dioxide gas is used to inflate the abdominal cavity. Then a **laparoscope**, a fiberoptic **endoscope**, is inserted through the incision (see Figure 13-33 ■). Grasping and cutting instruments are inserted through other abdominal incisions. Pelvic adhesions, pelvic inflammatory disease, and endometriosis can be treated, a biopsy taken, or a hysterectomy performed.	**laparoscopy** (LAP-ar-AW-skoh-pee) **lapar/o-** *abdomen* **-scopy** *process of using an instrument to examine*
		laparoscopic (LAP-ar-oh-SKAW-pik) **lapar/o-** *abdomen* **scop/o-** *examine with an instrument* **-ic** *pertaining to*
		laparoscope (LAP-ar-oh-SKOHP) **lapar/o-** *abdomen* **-scope** *instrument used to examine*
		endoscope (EN-doh-skohp) **endo-** *innermost; within* **-scope** *instrument used to examine*

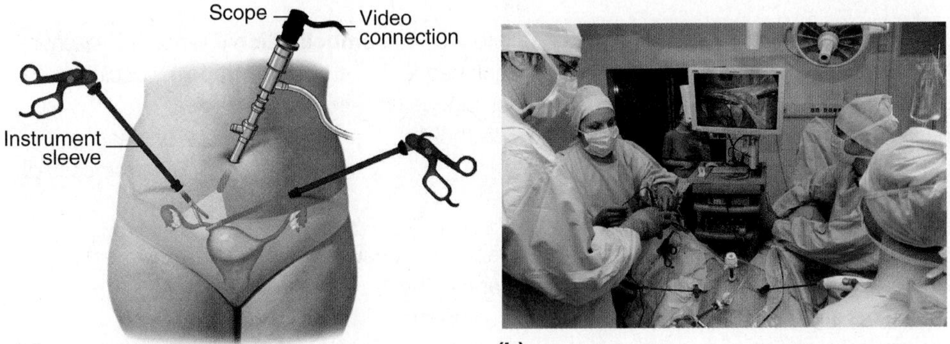

(a)   **(b)**

FIGURE 13-33 ■ Laparoscopic surgery.
(a) Small incisions in the abdomen allow visualization of the uterus, uterine tubes, and ovaries with a lighted scope. (b) The image can be seen on a computer screen in the operating room. The surgeon watches the image on the screen as he manipulates the grasping and cutting instruments.
Source: Pearson Education; Aubert/BSIP SA/Alamy

Word or Phrase	Description	Pronunciation/Word Parts
myomectomy	Procedure to remove leiomyomata (uterine fibroids) from the uterus. This procedure can be done vaginally or through a laparoscope inserted into the abdominal cavity. Large fibroids require a hysterectomy.	**myomectomy** (MY-oh-MEK-toh-mee) **my/o-** *muscle* **om/o-** *mass; tumor* **-ectomy** *surgical removal*
oophorectomy	Procedure to remove an ovary because of large ovarian cysts or ovarian cancer. A **bilateral oophorectomy** removes both ovaries.	**oophorectomy** (OH-of-or-EK-toh-mee) **oophor/o-** *ovary* **-ectomy** *surgical removal*
		bilateral (by-LAT-er-al) **bi-** *two* **later/o-** *side* **-al** *pertaining to*

Word or Phrase	Description	Pronunciation/Word Parts
salpingectomy	Procedure to remove the uterine tube because of ovarian cancer or an ectopic pregnancy in the tube. A bilateral salpingectomy removes both uterine tubes. A **bilateral salpingo-oophoresctomy (BSO)** removes both uterine tubes and both ovaries.	**salpingectomy** (SAL-ping-JEK-toh-mee) **salping/o-** *uterine tube* **-ectomy** *surgical removal* **salpingo-oophorectomy** (sal-PING-goh-OH-of-or-EK-toh-mee) **salping/o-** *uterine tube* **oophor/o-** *ovary* **-ectomy** *surgical removal*
tubal ligation	Procedure to prevent pregnancy. A short segment of each uterine tube is removed. The cut ends are sutured and then crushed or cauterized. The woman continues to ovulate, but the ovum cannot travel to the uterus and sperm cannot reach the ovum. It is also known as "getting your tubes tied." A **tubal anastomosis** is a procedure to rejoin the uterine tube segments so that the woman can get pregnant again.	**tubal** (TOO-bal) **tub/o-** *tube* **-al** *pertaining to* **ligation** (ly-GAY-shun) **ligat/o-** *bind; tie up* **-ion** *action; condition* **anastomosis** (ah-NAS-toh-MOH-sis) **anastom/o-** *create an opening between two structures* **-osis** *condition; process*
uterine artery embolization	Procedure used to treat uterine fibroids. A catheter is inserted into the femoral artery in the groin and threaded to the uterine artery. Radiopaque contrast dye is injected to identify the smaller artery that supplies blood to a large fibroid. Tiny particles are injected to block that artery. Without a blood supply, the fibroid shrinks in size.	**embolization** (EM-bol-ih-ZAY-shun) **embol/o-** *embolus; occluding plug* **-ization** *process of creating; process of inserting; process of making*
uterine suspension	Procedure to suspend and fix the uterus in an anatomically correct position. It is used to correct a retroverted uterus or uterine prolapse. The ligaments holding the uterus are shortened, which pulls the uterus up into a normal position, or surgical mesh (sling) or surgical tape are used to reposition the uterus. It is also known as a **hysteropexy**.	**suspension** (sus-PEN-shun) **suspens/o-** *hanging* **-ion** *action; condition* **hysteropexy** (HIS-ter-oh-PEK-see) **hyster/o-** *uterus; womb* **-pexy** *process of surgically fixing in place*

Surgical Procedures of the Cervix and Vagina

Word or Phrase	Description	Pronunciation/Word Parts
colporrhaphy	Procedure to suture a weakness in the vaginal wall. This procedure is done to correct a cystocele or a rectocele that is bulging into the vaginal canal.	**colporrhaphy** (kol-POR-ah-fee) **colp/o-** *vagina* **-rrhaphy** *procedure of suturing*
conization	Procedure to remove a large, cone-shaped section of tissue that includes the cervical os and part of the cervical canal. It is used to diagnose a lesion or excise an abnormal area identified by a Pap smear. A laser knife or a **loop electrosurgical excision procedure (LEEP)** with a hot wire loop is used to burn and cut away the tissue. Alternately, a scalpel (cold knife conization) can be used so that no cells are damaged by heat.	**conization** (KOH-nih-ZAY-shun) **con/o-** *cone* **-ization** *process of creating; process of inserting; process of making*
culdoscopy	Procedure in which an endoscope is inserted into the vagina and then pushed through the posterior wall of the vagina (in the area of the cul-de-sac behind the cervix) (see Figure 13-2) and into the pelvic cavity. This procedure is performed under local anesthesia and leaves no abdominal scars. It is used to examine the pelvic cavity and the external surfaces of the uterus, uterine tubes, and ovaries for signs of endometriosis or adhesions.	**culdoscopy** (kul-DAW-skoh-pee) **culd/o-** *cul-de-sac* **-scopy** *process of using an instrument to examine*

Surgical Procedures of the Breast

Word or Phrase	Description	Pronunciation/Word Parts
lumpectomy	Procedure to excise a small malignant tumor of the breast. Adjacent normal breast tissue and the axillary lymph nodes are also removed in case any cancerous cells have already spread to them. The rest of the breast is left intact.	**lumpectomy** (lump-EK-toh-mee) *Lumpectomy* is a combination of the English word *lump* and the suffix *-ectomy* (surgical removal).
mammaplasty	Procedure to change the size, shape, or position of the breast. It is also known as a **mammoplasty**. An **augmentation mammaplasty** augments (enlarges) the size of a small breast by inserting a breast **prosthesis** or implant under the skin or chest muscles (see Figure 13-34 ■). A **reduction mammaplasty** reduces the size of a large, **pendulous** breast. The procedure can be performed in conjunction with a **mastopexy** or breast lift to reposition a sagging breast. A **reconstructive mammaplasty** is done to reconstruct a breast after a mastectomy. **FIGURE 13-34 ■ Breast implant.** A breast prosthesis or implant is a soft-walled container filled with silicone gel or saline (salt water). It is placed beneath the skin of the breast or beneath the pectoralis major muscle of the chest during augmentation mammaplasty or reconstructive breast surgery. *Source*: Marko Poplasen/Shutterstock	**mammaplasty** (MAM-ah-PLAS-tee) **mamm/a-** *breast* **-plasty** *process of reshaping by surgery* **mammoplasty** (MAM-oh-PLAS-tee) **mamm/o-** *breast* **-plasty** *process of reshaping by surgery* **augmentation** (AWG-men-TAY-shun) **augment/o-** *increase in degree; increase in size* **-ation** *being; having; process* **prosthesis** (praws-THEE-sis) **reduction** (re-DUK-shun) **reduct/o-** *bring back; decrease* **-ion** *action; condition* **pendulous** (PEN-dyoo-lus) **pendul/o-** *hanging down* **-ous** *pertaining to* **mastopexy** (MAS-toh-PEK-see) **mast/o-** *breast; mastoid process* **-pexy** *process of surgically fixing in place* **reconstructive** (REE-con-STRUK-tiv) **re-** *again and again; backward; unable to* **construct/o-** *build* **-ive** *pertaining to*
mastectomy	Procedure to surgically remove all or part of the breast to excise a malignant tumor. In a **simple** or **total mastectomy**, the entire breast, the overlying skin, and the nipple are removed, but not the chest muscle or axillary (underarm) lymph nodes. In a **modified radical mastectomy**, an **axillary node dissection** is also performed and some of the axillary lymph nodes are removed. In a **radical mastectomy**, the pectoralis major and minor muscles of the chest wall are also removed; this procedure is performed infrequently. A **prophylactic mastectomy** can be performed to prevent breast cancer from occurring in women who have a strong family history of breast cancer or have the BRCA1 or BRCA2 gene.	**mastectomy** (mas-TEK-toh-mee) **mast/o-** *breast; mastoid process* **-ectomy** *surgical removal* **radical** (RAD-ih-kal) **radic/o-** *root and all parts* **-al** *pertaining to* **dissection** (dih-SEK-shun) **dissect/o-** *cut apart* **-ion** *action; condition* **prophylactic** (PROH-fih-LAK-tik) **pro-** *before* **phylact/o-** *guarding; protecting* **-ic** *pertaining to*

Word or Phrase	Description	Pronunciation/Word Parts
reconstructive breast surgery	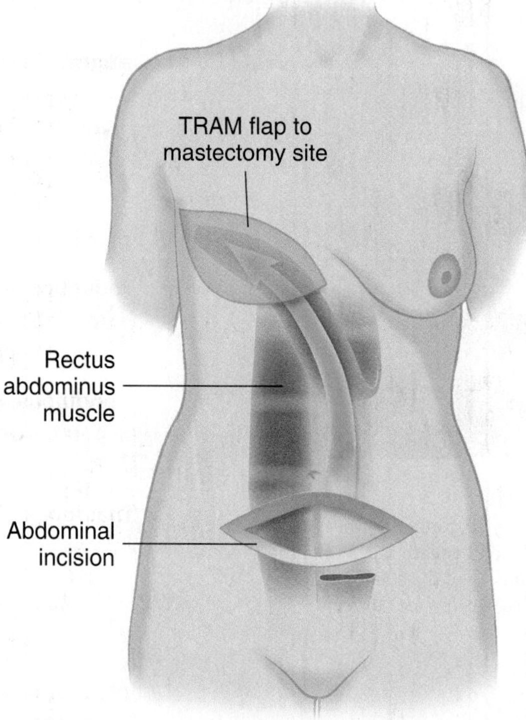 Procedure to rebuild a breast after a mastectomy. This can be done at the same time as the mastectomy or in a later operation. A breast implant or a TRAM flap (see Figure 13-35 ■) is used to recreate the fullness of the breast. With a breast prosthesis procedure, a tissue expander (a saline-filled silicone bag) is first inserted to stretch the skin to accommodate a breast prosthesis, which is inserted later. For a **TRAM (transverse rectus abdominis muscle) flap**, an incision is made around a transverse area of the abdomen. Skin, fat, and muscle are excised, except for one end that is left attached to blood vessels (pedicle graft). Alternatively, the latissimus dorsi muscle of the back can be used. Then the flap is tunneled under the skin of the upper abdomen and positioned at the site of the previous mastectomy. Later, a tattoo is done on the skin to create an areola and nipple.	**reconstructive** (REE-con-STRUK-tiv) **re-** *again and again; backward; unable to* **construct/o-** *build* **-ive** *pertaining to* Select the correct prefix meaning to get the definition of *reconstructive*: *pertaining to again building (the breast).* **transverse** (trans-VERS) **trans-** *across; through* **-verse** *travel; turn* The ending *-verse* contains the suffix *vers/o-* and the one-letter suffix *-e*.

TRAM flap to
mastectomy site

Rectus
abdominus
muscle

Abdominal
incision

FIGURE 13-35 ■ TRAM flap reconstruction.
This reconstructive surgery uses a skin, fat, and muscle flap from the abdomen to reconstruct the breast following a mastectomy. This provides a natural feel to the reconstructed breast and takes the place of a synthetic breast implant.
Source: Pearson Education

Surgical Procedures in Obstetrics

Word or Phrase	Description	Pronunciation/Word Parts
cerclage	Procedure to place a purse-string suture around the cervix to prevent it from dilating prematurely. The suture is removed prior to delivery.	**cerclage** (sir-CLAWJ)
cesarean section	Procedure to deliver a fetus. It is done because of cephalopelvic disproportion, failure to progress during labor, the mother being past the due date, or medical problems in the mother or fetus. The fetus is delivered through an incision in the abdominal wall and uterus. It is also known as a *C section*. A vaginal birth after a previous cesarean section is abbreviated as *VBAC*.	**cesarean** (seh-SAIR-ee-an)
episiotomy	Procedure that makes an incision in the posterior edge of the vagina and into the perineum to prevent a spontaneous tear during delivery of the baby's head (see Figure 13-13). Spontaneous vaginal tears can have ragged tissue edges that are difficult to suture and can extend into the rectum, causing incontinence.	**episiotomy** (eh-PIZ-ee-AW-toh-mee) **episi/o-** *vulva* **-tomy** *process of cutting; process of making an incision*

Drugs

These drug categories and drugs are used to treat female genital and reproductive diseases. The most common generic and trade name drugs in each category are listed.

Category	Indication	Examples	Pronunciation/Word Parts
drugs for amenorrhea and abnormal uterine bleeding	Correct the lack of hormones	medroxyprogesterone (Provera), progesterone (Crinone)	
drugs for contraception to prevent pregnancy	Suppress the release of FSH and LH from the anterior pituitary gland. Other drugs (not listed here) kill sperm or keep them from reaching the uterus.	Oral contraceptive pill (OCP): Cyclessa, Ortho-Novum, Seasonale Intrauterine device: Mirena Transdermal patch: Ortho Evra Vaginal ring: NuvaRing	**contraception** (CON-trah-SEP-shun) *Contraception* is a combination of the prefix *contra-* (against) and a shortened form of the word *conception.*
drugs for dysmenorrhea	Treat the pain associated with dysmenorrhea. These are nonsteroidal anti-inflammatory drugs (NSAIDs).	ibuprofen (Motrin), mefenamic acid (Ponstel), naproxen (Aleve)	
drugs for endometriosis	Suppress the menstrual cycle for several months and cause endometrial implants in the pelvic cavity to atrophy	goserelein (Zoladex), leuprolide (Lupron Depot)	
drugs for premature labor	These are progesterone hormones. They are known as **tocolytic drugs**.	hydroxyprogesterone (Makena)	**tocolytic** (TOH-koh-LIT-ik) **toc/o-** *childbirth; labor* **lyt/o-** *break down; destroy* **-ic** *pertaining to*
drugs for vaginal yeast infections	Topical antifungal drugs used to treat *Candida albicans* infection of the vagina	clotrimazole (Gyne-Lotrimin, Mycelex), miconazole (Monistat 3)	
drugs used to dilate the cervix	Prostaglandin drug applied topically to the cervix to cause dilation and effacement	dinoprostone (Cervidil, Prepidil)	
drugs used to induce labor	Stimulate the uterus and increase the strength and frequency of contractions of the smooth muscle of the uterine wall	oxytocin (Pitocin)	
hormone replacement therapy (HRT) drugs	Treat the symptoms and consequences of menopause (hot flashes, vaginal dryness, osteoporosis) caused by a decreased level of estradiol. Long-term estrogen use has been associated with an increased risk of breast cancer, endometrial cancer, and thrombophlebitis.	conjugated estrogens (Premarin), estradiol (Climara, Estraderm, Vivelle)	**estrogen** (ES-troh-jen) **estr/o-** *female* **-gen** *that which produces* Estrogen is the drug form of the female hormone estradiol.

Category	Indication	Examples	Pronunciation/Word Parts
ovulation-stimulating drugs	Stimulate the anterior pituitary gland to secrete FSH and LH to cause ovulation. Used to treat infertility. These drugs cause several mature ova to be released at the same time for *in vitro* fertilization.	clomiphene (Clomid), human chorionic gonadotropin (Pregnyl, Profasi)	

DID YOU KNOW?

On November 20, 1997, a mother in Iowa gave birth to the world's only surviving set of septuplets. The four boys and three girls were born prematurely at only 30 weeks' gestation. The mother was taking ovulation-stimulating drugs for infertility at the time. On January 26, 2009, a mother in California gave birth to the world's only surviving set of octuplets. With ovulation-stimulating drugs and assisted reproductive technology (ART), the mother had her six previously frozen zygotes implanted in her uterus. Then two zygotes split into identical twins to make a total of eight (six boys and two girls).

Abbreviations

AB, Ab	abortion
AFP	alpha fetoprotein
AGA	appropriate for gestational age
ART	assisted reproductive technology
ASC-H	atypical squamous cells, cannot exclude HSIL
ASC-US	atypical squamous cells of undetermined significance
BBT	basal body temperature
BPD	biparietal diameter (of the fetal head)
BPP	biophysical profile
BRCA	breast cancer (gene)
BSE	breast self-examination
BSO	bilateral salpingo-oophorectomy
BX, Bx	biopsy
Ca	cancer; carcinoma (pronounced "c-a")
CIN	cervical intraepithelial neoplasia
CIS	carcinoma *in situ*
CNM	certified nurse midwife
CPD	cephalopelvic disproportion
CS	cesarean section ("C-section", short form)
CVS	chorionic villus sampling
D&C	dilation and curettage
DUB	dysfunctional uterine bleeding
EDB	estimated date of birth
EDC	estimated date of confinement
EDD	estimated date of delivery
EGA	estimated gestational age
FHR	fetal heart rate
FSH	follicle-stimulating hormone
G	gravida
GIFT	gamete intrafallopian transfer
G/TPAL	see *G* and *TPAL*
GYN	gynecology
HCG, hCG	human chorionic gonadotropin
HPV	human papillomavirus
HRT	hormone replacement therapy
HSG	hysterosalpingogram; hysterosalpingography
HSIL	high-grade squamous intraepithelial lesion

ICSI	intracytoplasmic sperm injection
IUGR	intrauterine growth retardation
IVF	*in vitro* fertilization
L&D	labor and delivery
LEEP	loop electrocautery excision procedure
LGA	large for gestational age
LH	luteinizing hormone
LMP	last menstrual period
L/S	lecithin/sphingomyelin (ratio)
LSIL	low-grade squamous intraepithelial lesion
NB	newborn
NICU	neonatal intensive care unit (pronounced "NIK-yoo")
NST	nonstress test
NSVD	normal spontaneous vaginal delivery
OB	obstetrics
OB/GYN	obstetrics and gynecology
OCP	oral contraceptive pill
P	para
Pap	Papanicolaou (smear or test) (short form)
PID	pelvic inflammatory disease
PMDD	premenstrual dysphoric disorder
PMS	premenstrual syndrome
PROM	premature rupture of membranes
ROM	rupture of membranes
SAB	spontaneous abortion
SCC	squamous cell carcinoma
SGA	small for gestational age
STD	sexually transmitted disease
TAB	therapeutic abortion
TAH-BSO	total abdominal hysterectomy and bilateral salpingo-oophorectomy
TPAL	term newborns, premature newborns, abortions, living children
TRAM	transverse rectus abdominis muscle (flap) (pronounced "tram")
TVH	total vaginal hysterectomy
VBAC	vaginal birth after cesarean section (pronounced "V-back")
ZIFT	zygote intrafallopian transfer

WORD ALERT
Abbreviations

Abbreviations are commonly used in all types of medical documents; however, they can mean different things to different people and their meanings can be misinterpreted. Always verify the meaning of an abbreviation.

AI means *artificial insemination,* but it also means *aortic insufficiency, apical impulse,* and *artificial intelligence.*

Ca means *cancer,* but it also means the mineral *calcium.*

D&C means *dilation and curettage,* but it can be confused with *D/C (discontinue* or *discharge).*

EDC means *estimated date of confinement,* but it also means *extensor digitorum communis* (a muscle).

G means *gravida,* but it also means *gauge (of a needle).*

NICU means *neonatal intensive care unit,* but it also means *neurologic intensive care unit.*

P means *para,* but it also means the mineral *phosphorus* and *pulse (rate).*

ROM means *rupture of membranes,* but it also means *range of motion.*

IT'S GREEK TO ME!

Did *you* notice that some words have two different combining forms? Combining forms from both Greek and Latin remain a part of medical language today.

Word	Greek	Latin	Medical Word Examples
breast	mast/o-	mamm/a-, mamm/o-	mastitis, mammaplasty, mammography
childbirth; labor	toc/o-	part/o-, parturit/o-	oxytocin, postpartum, parturition
egg; ovum	o/o-	ov/i-, ov/o-, ovul/o-	oocyte, oviduct, ovum, ovulation
female; woman	gynec/o-	estr/a-, estr/o-	gynecology, estradiol, estrogen
giving birth or birth	par/o-	nat/o-	multiparous, prenatal
milk	galact/o-	lact/i-, lact/o-	galactorrhea, lactiferous, lactation
ovary	oophor/o-	ovari/o-	oophorectomy, ovarian
sexual intercourse	pareun/o-	coit/o-, venere/o-	dyspareunia, postcoital, venereal
uterus; womb	hyster/o-	uter/o-	hysterectomy, uterine
	metri/o-, metr/o-		endometriosis, metrorrhagia
vagina	colp/o-	vagin/o-	colposcopy, vaginal
vulva	episi/o-	vulv/o-	episiotomy, vulvar

13.8A Spell Medical Words

PROOFREADING AND SPELLING EXERCISE

Read the following paragraph. Identify each misspelled medical word and write the correct spelling of it on the line.

A woman may request a gynicologic exam because of pain and dysparunia. When the gynecologist does an examination, the uteris can be felt, but not the uterin tubes. A pregnant woman's obstetical history notes that she is a primogravida. Her doctor might recommend an amniosentesis and a cecarean section. An older woman might need to have a histerectomy and an ophorectomy.

1. _____   6. _____
2. _____   7. _____
3. _____   8. _____
4. _____   9. _____
5. _____   10. _____

ENGLISH AND MEDICAL WORD EQUIVALENTS EXERCISE

For each English word, write its equivalent medical word or phrase. Be sure to check your spelling.

English Word	Medical Word
1. breasts	_____
2. afterbirth	_____
3. baby, newborn	_____
4. bag of waters	_____
5. false labor	_____
6. getting your tubes tied	_____
7. soft spot (on the newborn's head)	_____
8. womb	_____
9. excessive morning sickness	_____

YOU WRITE THE MEDICAL REPORT

You are a healthcare professional interviewing a patient. Listen to the patient's statements and then enter them in the patient's medical record using medical words and phrases. Be sure to check your spelling. The first one has been done for you.

1. The patient says, "I didn't produce any milk with my last pregnancy."
   You write: The patient has a history of <u>failure of lactation.</u>

2. The patient says, "I had my womb taken out, with all my tubes and my ovaries too. That was last year."
   You write: The patient had a _____ and a bilateral _____ last year.

3. The patient says, "I am having itching and a white, cheesy discharge from my vagina because of a yeast infection. I want an antibiotic drug."
   You write: The patient is complaining of _____ coming from the vagina due to an infection with the yeast _____. She was prescribed the topical _____ drug Monistat.

4. The patient says, "I can finally breathe because the baby's head dropped down yesterday. I am due on January 21."
   You write: Based on my examination and the mother's comments, there is _____ of the fetal head in the maternal pelvis. Her _____ [abbreviation] is January 21.

5. The patient says, "I had a workup done last month because I couldn't get pregnant. They said I had an infection in my tubes and that my ovaries had lots of cysts in them. I also had pain when I had sexual intercourse with my husband. They took a scope and looked into my abdomen to check this out, and they said that was because of pieces of the lining of the uterus being in the wrong places."
   You write: The patient had an _____ workup last month. She was found to have _____ and _____ ovary syndrome. She also complained of _____ during sexual intercourse with her husband. She had a _____ to investigate this and was diagnosed as having _____.

6. The patient says, "I started my periods when I was 16. I always have pain with my periods. Recently, my periods have changed and are very light. But I am too young to be in the change of life."

You write: Patient had _____ at age 16. She reports she has always had _____ with her periods. Recently, she has noticed _____. She is only 30, and so this is probably a hormonal imbalance and not the beginning of _____.

HEARING MEDICAL WORDS EXERCISE

You hear someone speaking the medical words given below. Read each pronunciation and then write the medical word it represents. Be sure to check your spelling. The first one has been done for you.

1. BY-awp-see   *biopsy* _____
2. meh-NAR-kee   _____
3. mah-MAW-grah-fee   _____
4. lak-TAY-shun   _____
5. AM-nee-oh-sen-TEE-sis   _____
6. SIS-toh-seel   _____
7. DIS-pah-ROO-nee-ah   _____
8. eh-PIZ-ee-AW-toh-mee   _____

13.8B Pronounce Medical Words

PRONUNCIATION EXERCISE

Read the medical word and the syllables in its pronunciation. Circle the primary (main) accented syllable. The first one has been done for you.

1. menopause (men-oh-pawz)
2. colostrum (koh-law-strum)
3. mammary (mam-ah-ree)
4. ovarian (oh-vair-ee-an)
5. intrauterine (in-trah-yoo-teh-rin)
6. dysmenorrhea (dis-men-oh-ree-ah)
7. vagina (vah-jy-nah)
8. vaginal (vaj-ih-nal)
9. mastectomy (mas-tek-toh-mee)
10. menstruation (men-stroo-aa-shun)
11. embryonic (em-bree-aw-nik)
12. dyspareunia (dis-pah-roo-nee-ah)
13. episiotomy (eh-piz-ee-aw-toh-mee)
14. endometriosis (en-doh-mee-tree-oh-sis)

13.9 Research Medical Words

SOUND-ALIKE WORDS

Compare and contrast the medical meanings of these sound-alike gynecology and other words.

1. *perineum* and *peritoneum* (Chapter 3)
2. *fundus of the uterus*, *fundus of the stomach* (Chapter 3), and *fundus of the eye* (Chapter 15)
3. *colposcopy* and *colonoscopy* (Chapter 3)
4. *dilation and effacement*, and *dilation and curettage*

13.10 Analyze Medical Reports

ELECTRONIC PATIENT RECORD #1

This is an Office Visit SOAP Note. Read the note and answer the questions.

PEARSON OB/GYN ASSOCIATES

<u>Task</u>   <u>Edit</u>   <u>View</u>   <u>Time Scale</u>   <u>Options</u>   <u>Help</u>

OFFICE VISIT SOAP NOTE

PATIENT NAME:	BRADLEY, Emily
MEDICAL RECORD NUMBER:	16-7934
DATE OF VISIT:	11/19/20xx

Source: Eric Simard/123 RF

SUBJECTIVE: The patient comes in today with complaints of menorrhagia during some months of her menstrual cycle and oligomenorrhea other months. She denies dysmenorrhea or dyspareunia. The patient has a past history of a tubal ligation. She is married and has three children.

OBJECTIVE: With the patient in the dorsal lithotomy position, a colposcopy was performed. There was the presence of old blood in the cervical canal and vagina. Bimanual examination did not show any tenderness or enlargement of the uterus.

ASSESSMENT: Hormone imbalance.

PLAN: The patient will have blood drawn for FSH and LH. Depending on the results, she may need to have an endometrial biopsy done.

---

1. Define these words:

   menorrhagia _____

   oligomenorrhea _____

   dysmenorrhea _____

   dyspareunia _____

2. What surgery did the patient have in the past? _____

3. Could the patient be pregnant? Why not? _____

4. Describe the dorsal lithotomy position. _____

5. What is a colposcopy? _____

6. How is a bimanual examination performed? _____

7. Define FSH and LH. _____

ELECTRONIC PATIENT RECORD #2

This is an Admission History and Physical Examination done in the neonatal intensive care unit. Read the report and answer the questions.

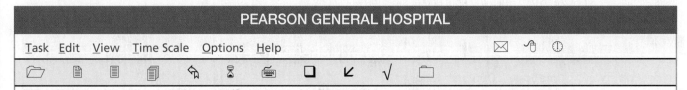

PEARSON GENERAL HOSPITAL

Task   Edit   View   Time Scale   Options   Help

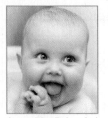

Source: Max Bukovski/ Shutterstock

ADMISSION HISTORY AND PHYSICAL EXAMINATION

PATIENT NAME:	KAISER, Baby Boy
HOSPITAL NUMBER:	03-7843
DATE OF BIRTH:	November 19, 20xx
DATE OF ADMISSION TO NICU:	November 19, 20xx

HISTORY
This is a 3360 g, full-term white male infant, who was transferred from the delivery room to the NICU after birth because of respiratory distress. The infant was born to a 34-year-old mother with an EDB of 11/22/xx, and he had an EGA of 40 weeks.

MATERNAL HISTORY
The mother was G2, TPAL 0-0-1-0 with a SAB 2 years ago. The mother had prenatal care beginning in the first trimester of this pregnancy. She took prenatal vitamins. She denied the use of alcohol, smoking, or drugs. A sonogram on 10/10/xx showed a single fetus in breech presentation at 35 weeks' gestation.

LABOR AND DELIVERY HISTORY
The membranes ruptured spontaneously 14 hours prior to the onset of labor. The mother had a temperature of 103.2 degrees prior to delivery and was started on an antibiotic drug. A version of the breech presentation was performed. Labor was induced and lasted 8 hours.

  The baby was born via a normal spontaneous vaginal delivery. Apgars were 8 and 8 at 1 and 5 minutes, respectively. There was no evidence of meconium aspiration on visualization of the mouth, pharynx, and vocal cords. The infant was tachypneic despite suctioning and the administration of blow-by oxygen and was brought to the neonatal intensive care unit.

PHYSICAL EXAMINATION
Heart rate 200 beats/minute, respiratory rate 70/minute, temperature 101.2, weight 3360 g, length 54 cm, head circumference 33.5 cm. General: Full-term, AGA male. Alert, active, responsive. Head: Moderate molding present. Fontanels soft. Palate intact. Eyes: Pupils equal and reactive to light. Chest symmetrical. Now pink in room air with only mild tachypnea and mild sternal retractions. Breath sounds equal bilaterally. Clavicles intact. Abdomen: Bowel sounds present. No hepatosplenomegaly. There is a three-vessel umbilical cord. Genitalia normal. Anus patent. Neurologic: Strong cry, strong suck, normal muscle tone.

IMPRESSION
Term male infant, estimated gestational age of 38.5 weeks, appropriate for gestational age. Rule out pneumonia.

PLAN
Admit to the neonatal intensive care unit. Vital signs q.1h. until stable. Cardiorespiratory monitor. Intravenous fluids of dextrose 10% in water at 80 cc/kg/day. Hold oral feedings for now. Chest x-ray to rule out pneumonia.

Bonita C. Grant, M.D.

Bonita C. Grant, M.D.

BCG: cgm
D: 11/19/xx
T: 11/19/xx

1. Give the definitions of these abbreviations.

   a. AGA _____

   b. EDB _____

   c. EGA _____

   d. NICU _____

   e. SAB _____

2. A sonogram showed the fetus at 35 weeks' gestation. If you wanted to use the adjective form of *gestation,* you would say, "The fetus had a _____ age of 35 weeks."

3. Divide *gestational* into its three word parts and give the meaning of each word part.

   Word Part   **Meaning**

   _____   _____

   _____   _____

   _____   _____

4. Divide *prenatal* into its three word parts and give the meaning of each word part.

   Word Part   **Meaning**

   _____   _____

   _____   _____

   _____   _____

5. What is the abbreviation for the medical phrase *normal spontaneous vaginal delivery?* _____

6. The sonogram (ultrasound) done on 10/10/xx showed what fetal presentation? _____

7. What procedure was performed to correct this presentation? Circle the correct answer.

   Apgar   repeat sonogram   version   vaginal delivery

8. What does the mother's TPAL score of 0-0-1-0 mean? _____

9. What moderate condition of the head was noted on the physical examination? _____

10. The newborn's estimated gestational age was 38.5 weeks. Is this a term newborn? **Yes No**

11. Where are the fontanels located? _____

12. What test was ordered to rule out pneumonia? _____

13. Rupture of the membranes many hours prior to delivery can cause infection in the mother and in the newborn. What information is given in the record that tells you that the mother and newborn did develop an infection? _____

14. Circle the correct answer. If there had been meconium-stained amniotic fluid, we would know that the fetus had experienced (**apnea**, **fetal distress**, **premature birth**).

MyMedicalTerminologyLab™

MyMedicalTerminologyLab is a premium online homework management system that includes a host of features to help you study. Registered users will find:

- A multitude of quizzes and activities built within the MyLab platform

- Powerful tools that track and analyze your results—allowing you to create a personalized learning experience

- Videos and audio pronunciations to help enrich your progress

- Streaming lesson presentations (Guided Lectures) and self-paced learning modules

- A space where you and your instructor can check your progress and manage your assignments

Chapter 14
Endocrinology

Endocrine System

Endocrinology (EN-doh-krih-NAW-loh-jee) is the medical specialty that studies the anatomy and physiology of the endocrine system and uses laboratory and diagnostic procedures, medical and surgical procedures, and drugs to treat endocrine system diseases.

Learning Outcomes

After you study this chapter, you should be able to

14.1 Identify structures of the endocrine system.

14.2 Describe the process of hormone response and feedback.

14.3 Describe common endocrine diseases, laboratory and diagnostic procedures, medical and surgical procedures, and drugs.

14.4 Form the plural and adjective forms of nouns related to endocrinology.

14.5 Give the meanings of word parts and abbreviations related to endocrinology.

14.6 Divide endocrinology words and build endocrinology words.

14.7 Spell and pronounce endocrinology words.

14.8 Research sound-alike and other endocrinology words.

14.9 Analyze the medical content and meaning of an endocrinology report.

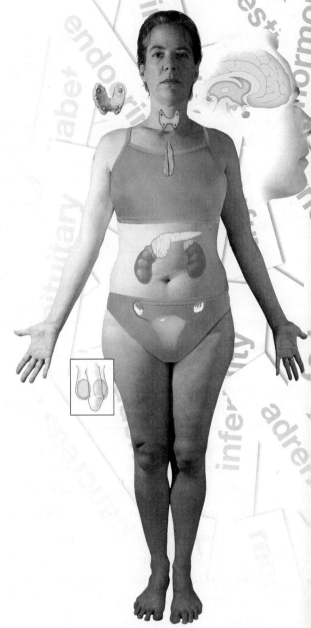

FIGURE 14-1 ■ Endocrine System.
The endocrine system consists of glands that perform very different functions. They are related to each other because they all secrete hormones into the blood.
Source: Pearson Education

Medical Language Key

To unlock the definition of a medical word, break it into word parts. Give the meaning of each word part. Put the meanings of the word parts in order, beginning with the meaning of the suffix, then the prefix (if present), then the combining form(s).

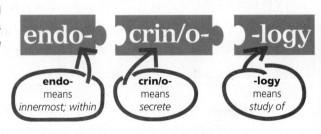

	Word Part	Word Part Meaning
Suffix	**-logy**	*study of*
Prefix	**endo-**	*innermost; within*
Combining Form	**crin/o-**	*secrete*

Endocrinology: ▶ *Study of (glands) within (the body that) secrete (hormones).*

Anatomy and Physiology

The **endocrine system** is different from other body systems in that it is made up of **glands** that are in various parts of the body (see Figure 14-1 ■). Endocrine glands produce and secrete hormones into the blood. These glands include the hypothalamus, pituitary gland, pineal gland, thyroid gland, parathyroid glands, thymus, pancreas, adrenal glands, ovaries, and testes. Some, but not all, of these glands are influenced by hormones from the pituitary gland.

However, all endocrine glands are alike in these ways:

1. They secrete substances known as **hormones**.
2. They secrete their hormones directly into the blood and not through ducts.
3. Their hormones regulate specific body functions.

One of the functions of the endocrine system is to keep the body in **homeostasis**. This is a state of equilibrium of the internal environment so that all body systems can function optimally. The endocrine system plays a role in homeostasis by regulating body fluids, electrolytes, glucose, cell metabolism, growth, and the wake–sleep cycle.

Some endocrine glands do "double duty" as part of another body system, such as the hypothalamus (nervous system), thymus (immune system), pancreas (digestive system), or ovaries and testes (genital and reproductive system).

Pronunciation/Word Parts

endocrine (EN-doh-krin) (EN-doh-krine)
  endo- *innermost; within*
  crin/o- *secrete*
  -ine *pertaining to; thing pertaining to*
The duplicated letters *in* in the combining form and suffix are deleted when the word parts are joined.

gland (GLAND)

glandular (GLAN-dyoo-lar)
  glandul/o- *gland*
  -ar *pertaining to*
The combining form **aden/o-** also means *gland*.

hormone (HOR-mohn)

hormonal (hor-MOH-nal)
  hormon/o- *hormone*
  -al *pertaining to*

homeostasis (HOH-mee-oh-STAY-sis)
  home/o- *same*
  -stasis *standing still; staying in one place*

WORD ALERT
Sound-Alike Words

endocrine	(adjective)	descriptive word for glands that secrete hormones directly into the blood
		Example: The thyroid gland is one of the glands of the endocrine system.
exocrine	(adjective)	descriptive word for glands that release substances through ducts (not directly into the blood)
		Example: The sebaceous glands in the skin are exocrine glands that produce oil.

Anatomy of the Endocrine System

Hypothalamus

The **hypothalamus** is in the center of the brain, on top of the brainstem, and (as its name implies) just below the thalamus. The hypothalamus forms the floor and part of the walls of the third ventricle in the brain, and it has a stalk of blood vessels and nerves that connects it to the pituitary gland (see Figure 14-2 ■). The hypothalamus functions as part of both the nervous system (discussed in "Neurology," Chapter 10) and the endocrine system. As an endocrine gland, the hypothalamus secretes hormones that stimulate or inhibit the secretion of hormones from the anterior pituitary gland. The hypothalamus also produces two hormones of its own—antidiuretic hormone (ADH) and oxytocin—and these are stored in the posterior pituitary gland. These hormones are secreted when the hypothalamus sends a nerve impulse through the stalk to the posterior pituitary gland.

hypothalamus (HY-poh-THAL-ah-mus)

hypothalamic (HY-poh-thah-LAM-ik)
  hypo- *below; deficient*
  thalam/o- *thalamus*
  -ic *pertaining to*

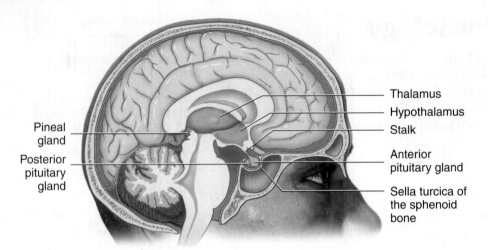

Thalamus
Hypothalamus
Stalk
Anterior pituitary gland
Sella turcica of the sphenoid bone

Pineal gland
Posterior pituitary gland

FIGURE 14-2 ■ Endocrine glands in the brain.
The hypothalamus has a stalk of tissue that goes to the pituitary gland. The pituitary gland sits in a bony cup (the sella turcica) in the sphenoid bone. The pineal gland is located between the two lobes of the thalamus.
Source: Pearson Education

Because the hypothalamus belongs to the nervous system and the endocrine system and the posterior pituitary gland contains the axons of neurons from the hypothalamus, their shared functions and structures are reflected in the word **neuroendocrine**.

Pituitary Gland

The **pituitary gland** (hypophysis) is within the brain, just above the sphenoid sinus, and it sits in a bony cup (the **sella turcica**) of the sphenoid bone (see Figure 14-2). The pituitary gland is a bulb-shaped gland at the end of the stalk from the hypothalamus. Even though it is about the size of a pea and weighs only a fraction of an ounce, the pituitary gland is known as the *master gland of the body* because the effects of its hormones are felt throughout the body. It has two lobes: the **anterior pituitary gland** (or **adenohypophysis**) and the **posterior pituitary gland** (or **neurohypophysis**).

ANTERIOR PITUITARY GLAND   The anterior pituitary gland secretes seven hormones (see Figure 14-3 ■).

1. **Thyroid-stimulating hormone (TSH).**   This hormone causes the thyroid gland to grow, and stimulates it to secrete the thyroid hormones T_3 and T_4.

2. **Follicle-stimulating hormone (FSH).**   In females, this hormone stimulates follicles in the ovaries to produce mature ova and to secrete the hormone estradiol. In males, FSH stimulates the seminiferous tubules of the testes to produce spermatozoa.

DID YOU KNOW?

FSH and LH stimulate the female and male sex glands (ovaries and testes), which are known as *gonads*. So, FSH and LH are known as **gonadotropins**.

3. **Luteinizing hormone (LH).**   In females, this hormone stimulates a follicle each month to release a mature ovum. It stimulates the corpus luteum (ruptured ovarian follicle) to secrete estradiol and progesterone. In males, LH stimulates the interstitial cells of the testes to secrete testosterone.

Pronunciation/Word Parts

neuroendocrine (NYOOR-oh-EN-doh-krin)
  neur/o- *nerve*
  endo- *innermost; within*
  crin/o- *secrete*
  -ine *pertaining to; thing pertaining to*

pituitary (pih-TOO-eh-TAIR-ee)
  pituit/o- *pituitary gland*
  -ary *pertaining to*
The combining forms **hypophys/o-** and **pituitar/o-** also mean *pituitary gland*.

sella turcica (SEL-ah TUR-sih-kah)

adenohypophysis
(AD-eh-NOH-hy-PAW-fih-sis)
  aden/o- *gland*
  hypo- *below; deficient*
  -physis *state of growing*
The adenohypophysis is a true gland (aden/o- means *gland*) because it makes and secretes its own hormones.

neurohypophysis
(NYOOR-oh-hy-PAW-fih-sis)
  neur/o- *nerve*
  hypo- *below; deficient*
  -physis *state of growing*
The neurohypophysis only releases stored hormones when stimulated by a nerve impulse from the hypothalamus.

thyroid (THY-royd)

follicle (FAW-lih-kl)

gonadotropin (GOH-nah-doh-TROH-pin)
  gonad/o- *gonad; ovary; testis*
  trop/o- *having an affinity for; stimulating; turning*
  -in *substance*

luteinizing (LOO-tee-ih-NY-zing)

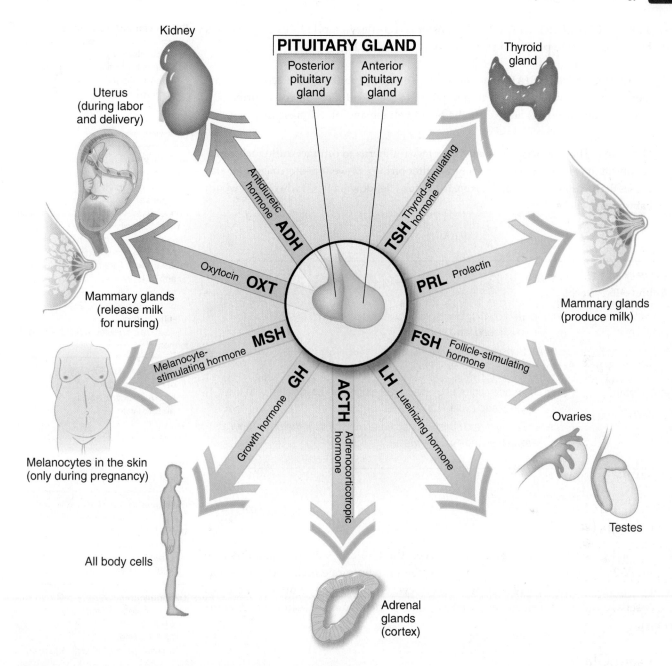

FIGURE 14-3 ■ Hormones of the anterior and posterior pituitary gland.
The anterior pituitary gland produces and secretes seven different hormones. The posterior pituitary gland stores and secretes two hormones that are actually produced by the hypothalamus.
Source: Pearson Education

4. **Prolactin.** This hormone stimulates the development of the breasts during puberty and stimulates the mammary glands to produce milk during pregnancy.

5. **Adrenocorticotropic hormone (ACTH).** This hormone stimulates the cortex of the adrenal gland to secrete its hormones (aldosterone, cortisol, and androgens).

6. **Growth hormone (GH).** This hormone stimulates growth and protein synthesis in all cells. It increases height and weight during childhood and puberty.

7. **Melanocyte-stimulating hormone (MSH).** This hormone does not have any significant function and is not normally present in adults. In pregnant women, however, it is secreted and it stimulates melanocytes in the skin to produce the pigment melanin. This causes a distinctive skin pigmentation on the face (chloasma) and along the midline of the abdomen (linea nigra) (discussed in "Dermatology," Chapter 7).

Pronunciation/Word Parts

prolactin (proh-LAK-tin)
  pro- *before*
  lact/o- *milk*
  -in *substance*
Add words to make a complete definition of *prolactin: substance (that must be secreted) before milk (can be produced).* The combining form **galact/o-** also means *milk.*

POSTERIOR PITUITARY GLAND   The posterior pituitary gland stores and releases two hormones that are produced in the hypothalamus (see Figure 14-3).

1. **Antidiuretic hormone (ADH).**   This hormone affects tubules in the nephron of the kidney, moving water from the tubule back into the blood. This decreases urine output (antidiuretic effect) and keeps the blood volume and blood pressure at normal levels.

2. **Oxytocin.**   This hormone stimulates the pregnant uterus to contract during labor and childbirth. It causes the uterus to contract after birth to prevent hemorrhaging. It also causes the breasts to release milk for breastfeeding ("let-down reflex") when the newborn baby cries or sucks.

WORD ALERT
Sound-Alike Words

melanin	(noun)	dark brown or black pigment produced by melanocytes in the skin in response to sunlight.
		Example: Sunshine increases the level of melanin in the skin, causing it to tan.
melatonin	(noun)	hormone secreted by the pineal gland; it is associated with the wake–sleep cycle.
		Example: Daylight and sunshine decrease melatonin in the brain, helping us to be awake during the daytime.

Pineal Gland

The **pineal gland** (or **pineal body**) is between the two lobes of the thalamus (see Figure 14-2). It is a small, round gland that secretes the hormone **melatonin**. This hormone maintains the body's 24-hour wake–sleep cycle (circadian rhythm) and regulates the onset and duration of sleep. Increased amounts of melatonin are secreted during the winter.

Thyroid Gland

The **thyroid gland** has two lobes connected by a band of tissue. It lies across the anterior surface of the trachea (see Figure 14-4 ■). The thyroid gland secretes three hormones.

1. **T_3 (triiodothyronine).**   This hormone increases the rate of cell metabolism.
2. **T_4 (thyroxine).**   This hormone is secreted, but then most of it is changed by the liver into T_3. The thyroid gland secretes T_3 and T_4 when stimulated by TSH from the anterior pituitary gland.
3. **Calcitonin.**   This hormone regulates the amount of calcium in the blood. If the calcium level is too high, calcitonin moves calcium from the blood and deposits it in the bones. Calcitonin has an opposite effect from that of parathyroid hormone secreted by the parathyroid glands.

When the thyroid gland is functioning properly, producing neither too much nor too little of its hormones, this steady state is known as **euthyroidism**.

Pronunciation/Word Parts

adrenocorticotropic
(ah-DREE-noh-KOR-tih-koh-TROH-pik)
   adren/o- *adrenal gland*
   cortic/o- *cortex; outer region*
   trop/o- *having an affinity for; stimulating; turning*
   -ic *pertaining to*

melanocyte (meh-LAN-oh-site)
(MEL-ah-noh-SITE)
   melan/o- *black*
   -cyte *cell*
Add words to make a complete definition of *melanocyte: cell (in the skin that produces the dark brown or) black (pigment melanin).*

antidiuretic (AN-tee-DY-yoor-EH-tik)
   anti- *against*
   dia- *complete; completely through*
   ur/o- *urinary system; urine*
   -etic *pertaining to*
The *a* in *dia-* is deleted when the word is formed.

oxytocin (AWK-see-TOH-sin)
   ox/y- *oxygen; quick*
   toc/o- *childbirth; labor*
   -in *substance*

pineal (PIN-ee-al)

melatonin (MEL-ah-TOH-nin)

thyroid (THY-royd)
   thyr/o- *shield-shaped structure; thyroid gland*
   -oid *resembling*

triiodothyronine
(try-EYE-oh-doh-THY-roh-neen)
   tri- *three*
   iod/o- *iodine*
   thyr/o- *shield-shaped structure; thyroid gland*
   -nine *pertaining to a single chemical substance*
Each molecule of T_3 contains three iodine atoms.

thyroxine (thy-RAWK-seen) (thy-RAWK-sin)

calcitonin (KAL-sih-TOH-nin)
   calc/i- *calcium*
   ton/o- *pressure; tone*
   -in *substance*
The combining form **calc/o-** also means *calcium.*

euthyroidism (yoo-THY-royd-izm)
   eu- *good; normal*
   thyroid/o- *thyroid gland*
   -ism *disease from a specific cause; process*

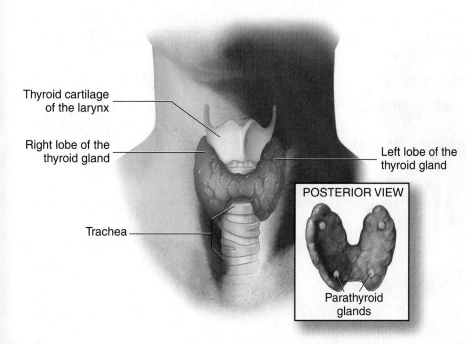

Thyroid cartilage of the larynx

Right lobe of the thyroid gland

Left lobe of the thyroid gland

Trachea

POSTERIOR VIEW

Parathyroid glands

FIGURE 14-4 ■ Thyroid gland and parathyroid glands.
This anterior view of the thyroid gland shows its two lobes. The thyroid cartilage of the larynx sounds and looks like it is related to the thyroid gland, but it is part of the respiratory system, not the endocrine system. The parathyroid glands are located on the posterior surface of the thyroid gland.
Source: Pearson Education; Southern Illinois University/Science Source

Pronunciation/Word Parts

Parathyroid Glands

The four **parathyroid glands** are on the posterior surface of the thyroid gland (see Figure 14-4). Each gland is about the size of a grain of rice. The parathyroid glands secrete **parathyroid hormone**, which regulates the amount of calcium in the blood. If the calcium level is too low, parathyroid hormone moves calcium from the bones into the blood. Parathyroid hormone has an opposite effect from that of calcitonin secreted by the thyroid gland.

parathyroid (PAIR-ah-THY-royd)
para- abnormal; apart from; beside; two parts of a pair
thyr/o- shield-shaped structure; thyroid gland
-oid resembling
Select the correct prefix meaning to get the definition of *parathyroid*: (structures) resembling two parts of a pair (on the) thyroid gland.

Thymus Gland

The **thymus gland** is a pink gland with two lobes. It is posterior to the sternum, within the mediastinum of the thoracic cavity. During childhood and puberty, the thymus gland is large, but it shrinks during adulthood. The thymus gland functions as part of both the body's immune response (discussed in "Hematology and Immunology," Chapter 6) and the endocrine system. As an endocrine gland, the thymus secretes **thymosins**, which cause immature T lymphocytes in the thymus gland to develop and mature.

thymus (THY-mus)

thymic (THY-mik)
thym/o- rage; thymus
-ic pertaining to

thymosin (thy-MOH-sin)

pancreas (PAN-kree-as)

Pancreas

The **pancreas** is a yellow, elongated, triangular gland that is posterior to the stomach (see Figure 14-5 ■). The pancreas functions as part of both the digestive system (discussed in "Gastroenterology," Chapter 3) and the endocrine system. As an endocrine gland, the pancreas secretes three hormones from groups of cells known as the **islets of Langerhans**.

1. **Glucagon.** This hormone is secreted by **alpha cells** in the islets of Langerhans. When the blood glucose level is too low, glucagon breaks down **glycogen** (glucose stored in the liver and skeletal muscles) to release more **glucose** into the blood.

pancreatic (PAN-kree-AT-ik)
pancreat/o- pancreas
-ic pertaining to

islets of Langerhans (EYE-lets of LANG-ger-hanz)

glucagon (GLOO-kah-gawn)
gluc/o- glucose; sugar
ag/o- lead to
-on structure; substance

glycogen (GLY-koh-jen)
glyc/o- glucose; sugar
-gen that which produces

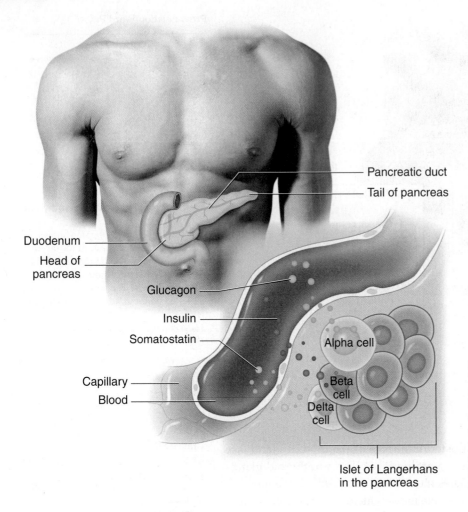

Pancreatic duct
Tail of pancreas
Duodenum
Head of pancreas
Glucagon
Insulin
Somatostatin
Alpha cell
Beta cell
Delta cell
Capillary
Blood
Islet of Langerhans
in the pancreas

FIGURE 14-5 ■ Pancreas.
The pancreas is composed of small groups (islands) of cells known as the *islets of Langerhans*. Each islet is next to a capillary so that the secreted hormones (glucagon, insulin, and somatostatin) go directly into the blood. The pancreas also produces digestive enzymes (amylase, lipase, etc.), and these flow through the pancreatic duct that empties into the duodenum.
Source: Pearson Education

2. **Insulin.**   This hormone is secreted by **beta cells** in the islets of Langerhans. Insulin transports glucose to a body cell, binds to an insulin receptor on the cell membrane, and transports glucose into the cell. Within the cell, glucose is metabolized to produce energy. Insulin decreases the level of glucose in the blood.

3. **Somatostatin.**   This hormone is secreted by **delta cells** in the islets of Langerhans. Somatostatin prevents glucagon and insulin from being secreted. It also prevents growth hormone (from the anterior pituitary gland) from being secreted.

Adrenal Glands

The **adrenal gland** is draped over the superior end of each kidney (see Figure 14-6 ■). The adrenal gland contains two different glands: an outer layer (cortex) and an inner layer (medulla). Each of these layers functions independently of the other and secretes its own hormones.

glucose (GLOO-kohs)
  gluc/o- *glucose; sugar*
  -ose *full of; thing full of*
The combining form **glycos/o-** also means *glucose; sugar.*

insulin (IN-soo-lin)
  insul/o- *island*
  -in *substance*
The combining form **insulin/o-** means *insulin.*

somatostatin (SOH-mah-toh-STAT-in)
  somat/o- *body*
  stat/o- *standing still; staying in one place*
  -in *substance*
Add words to make a complete definition of *somatostatin*: substance (that makes the) body (to be) standing still (without growth).

adrenal (ah-DREE-nal)
  ad- *toward*
  ren/o- *kidney*
  -al *pertaining to*
The combining forms **adrenal/o-** and **adren/o-** mean *adrenal gland.*

WORD ALERT
Sound-Alike Words

aden/o-   (combining form) gland
       Example: An adenoma is a benign tumor of a gland.

adren/o-   (combining form) adrenal gland
       Example: Each adrenal gland sits on top of a kidney.

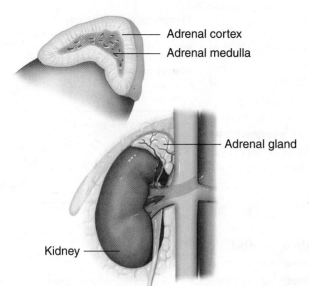

Adrenal cortex
Adrenal medulla
Adrenal gland
Kidney

FIGURE 14-6 ▪ Adrenal gland.
The adrenal gland is on top of the kidney but is part of the endocrine system, while the kidney belongs to the urinary system. The two parts of the adrenal gland—the cortex and the medulla—function as two separate endocrine glands.
Source: Pearson Education

ADRENAL CORTEX   The **adrenal cortex** secretes three groups of hormones: mineralocorticoids, glucocorticoids, and androgens. The adrenal cortex secretes these hormones when stimulated by ACTH from the anterior pituitary gland.

1. **Aldosterone**.   This hormone is the most abundant and biologically active of the **mineralocorticoid** hormones. The adrenal cortex secretes aldosterone when the blood pressure is low. Aldosterone moves sodium and water from tubules in the nephron of the kidney into the blood while allowing potassium to be excreted in the urine. This increases the blood volume and blood pressure.

2. **Cortisol**.   This hormone is the most abundant and biologically active of the **glucocorticoid** hormones. It breaks down stored glycogen to increase the level of glucose in the blood. It decreases the formation of proteins and new tissue, and it also exerts a strong anti-inflammatory effect.

3. **Androgens**.   This group of hormones are male sex hormones. The adrenal cortex secretes androgens, but the testes secrete testosterone, the most abundant and biologically active of the androgens. In the blood, some of the androgens are changed to **estrogens** (female sex hormones). (The ovaries secrete estradiol, the most abundant and biologically active of the estrogens.)

ADRENAL MEDULLA   The **adrenal medulla** secretes the hormones **norepinephrine**, **epinephrine**, and **dopamine** into the blood.

CLINICAL CONNECTIONS

Neurology (Chapter 10). As a hormone, norepinephrine from the adrenal medulla raises the blood pressure during exercise. But, during times of danger or anger, the hypothalamus uses the sympathetic division of the nervous system to trigger the release of epinephrine from the adrenal medulla. Epinephrine prepares the body to either fight or run away from the danger, the "fight-or-flight" response. Norepinephrine and dopamine are also neurotransmitters in the brain.

Pronunciation/Word Parts

cortex (KOR-teks)

cortices (KOR-tih-seez)
Cortex is a Latin singular noun. Form the plural by changing *-ex* to *-ices*.

cortical (KOR-tih-kal)
   cortic/o- *cortex; outer region*
   -al *pertaining to*

aldosterone (al-DAW-steh-rohn)

mineralocorticoid
(MIN-er-AL-oh-KOR-tih-koyd)
   mineral/o- *electrolyte; mineral*
   cortic/o- *cortex; outer region*
   -oid *resembling*

cortisol (KOR-tih-sawl)

glucocorticoid (GLOO-koh-KOR-tih-koyd)
   gluc/o- *glucose; sugar*
   cortic/o- *cortex; outer region*
   -oid *resembling*

androgen (AN-droh-jen)
   andr/o- *male*
   -gen *that which produces*
The combining form **viril/o-** means *masculine*.

estrogen (ES-troh-jen)
   estr/o- *female*
   -gen *that which produces*

medulla (meh-DUL-ah)

medullae (meh-DUL-ee)
Medulla is a Latin singular noun. Form the plural by changing *-a* to *-ae*.

epinephrine (EP-ih-NEF-rin)

norepinephrine (NOR-ep-ih-NEF-rin)

dopamine (DOH-pah-meen)

Ovaries

The **ovaries** are small, egg-shaped glands in the pelvic cavity. The ovaries function as part of both the female reproductive system (discussed in "Gynecology and Obstetrics," Chapter 13) and the endocrine system. As an endocrine gland, the follicles of the ovary secrete **estradiol** when stimulated by FSH from the anterior pituitary gland. Estradiol is the most abundant and biologically active of the female sex hormones. The corpus luteum (ruptured ovarian follicle) secretes estradiol and **progesterone** when stimulated by LH from the anterior pituitary gland. The cells around the follicle secrete testosterone (a male sex hormone) when stimulated by LH from the anterior pituitary gland.

Testes

The **testes** or **testicles** are egg-shaped glands in the scrotum, a pouch of skin behind the penis. The testes function as part of both the male genitourinary system (discussed in "Male Reproductive Medicine," Chapter 12) and the endocrine system. As an endocrine gland, the seminiferous tubules of the testes produce spermatozoa when stimulated by FSH from the anterior pituitary gland. Interstitial cells of the testes secrete testosterone when stimulated by LH from the anterior pituitary gland. **Testosterone** is the most abundant and biologically active of the androgens (male sex hormones).

Physiology of Hormone Response and Feedback

While the nervous system uses neurotransmitters as chemical messengers that travel between two neurons (or a neuron and an organ), the endocrine system uses hormones as chemical messengers. Hormones are secreted into the blood and travel throughout the body. Some neurotransmitters (epinephrine and norepinephrine) are also hormones because they are secreted by a gland and travel in the blood.

In the blood, hormones come in contact with all tissues, but they only exert an effect on glands or organs that have **receptors** to which they can bind. A hormone is like a key that unlocks receptors on a gland or organ and produces an effect. Other hormones cannot unlock those receptors.

A unique feature of the endocrine system is the "chain reaction" sequence of effects: A hormone secreted by an endocrine gland can stimulate another endocrine gland to release its hormones and then those hormones stimulate receptors on an organ to produce an effect.

The action of hormones involves **stimulation** or **inhibition**. Some hormones, such as the releasing hormones of the hypothalamus, stimulate an endocrine gland to secrete its hormones. Other hormones, such as the inhibiting hormones of the hypothalamus, keep an endocrine gland from secreting its hormones.

When two hormones, such as T_3 and T_4, work in conjunction with one another to accomplish an enhanced effect, this is known as **synergism**. When two hormones, such as calcitonin and parathyroid hormone, exert an opposite effect, this is known as **antagonism** (see Figure 14-7 ■).

The endocrine system maintains body homeostasis through the use of hormones and a negative feedback mechanism. For example, after the anterior pituitary gland secretes thyroid-stimulating hormone, it then monitors the blood levels of thyroid hormones. If the levels are still low (negative feedback), the anterior pituitary gland secretes more thyroid-stimulating hormone.

Pronunciation/Word Parts

ovary (OH-vah-ree)

ovarian (oh-VAIR-ee-an)
ovari/o- ovary
-an pertaining to

estradiol (ES-trah-DY-awl)
estr/a- female
di- two
-ol chemical substance

progesterone (proh-JEH-steh-rohn)

testis (TES-tis)

testes (TES-teez)
Testis is a Latin singular noun. Form the plural by changing -is to -es.

testicle (TES-tih-kl)
Testicle is a combination of testis and the suffix -cle (small thing).

testicular (tes-TIH-kyoo-lar)
testicul/o- testicle; testis
-ar pertaining to

testosterone (tes-TAW-steh-rohn)
Testosterone contains the combining forms test/o- (testicle; testis) and steroid/o- (steroid) and the suffix -one (chemical substance).

receptor (ree-SEP-ter)
recept/o- receive
-or person who does; person who produces; thing that does; thing that produces

stimulation (STIM-yoo-LAY-shun)
stimul/o- exciting; strengthening
-ation being; having; process

inhibition (IN-hih-BIH-shun)
inhibit/o- block; hold back
-ion action; condition

synergism (SIN-er-jizm)
syn- together
erg/o- activity; work
-ism disease from a specific cause; process

antagonism (an-TAG-on-izm)
antagon/o- oppose; work against
-ism disease from a specific cause; process

	HORMONE		ACTION	SOURCE	
BODY METABOLISM	T_3 and T_4	↑	Increases metabolism	Thyroid	
BLOOD GLUCOSE	Cortisol	↑	Increases blood glucose	Adrenal cortex	
	Epinephrine	↑	Increases blood glucose	Adrenal medulla	
	Glucagon	↑	Increases blood glucose	Pancreas	
	Insulin	↓	Decreases blood glucose (glucose transported into cells to be metabolized)	Pancreas	
BLOOD CALCIUM	Parathyroid hormone	↑	Increases blood calcium	Parathyroid	
	Calcitonin	↓	Decreases blood calcium	Thyroid	
BLOOD SODIUM	Aldosterone	↑	Increases blood sodium	Adrenal cortex	

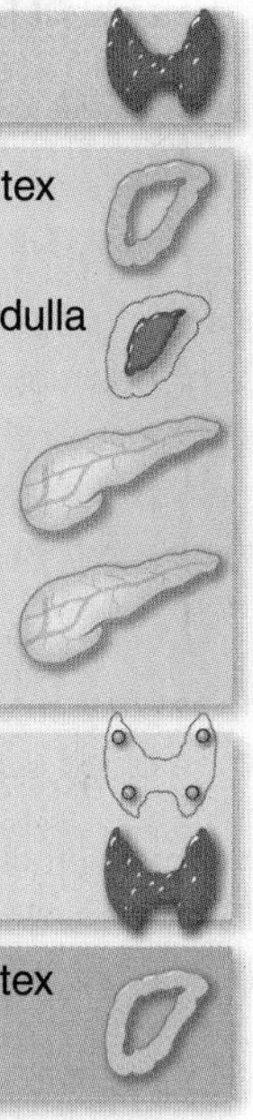

FIGURE 14-7 ■ Effects of hormones. Hormones from various endocrine glands affect cell metabolism, blood glucose, blood calcium, and blood sodium in similar (synergism) or opposite (antagonism) ways.

Source: Pearson Education

Vocabulary Review

Anatomy and Physiology

Word or Phrase	Description	Combining Forms
endocrine system	Body system that includes glands that produce and secrete hormones into the blood. These glands include the hypothalamus, pituitary gland, pineal gland, thyroid gland, parathyroid glands, thymus, pancreas, adrenal glands, ovaries, and testes. The endocrine system is also known as the **neuroendocrine system** because of the connection between it and the nervous system.	crin/o- *secrete* neur/o- *nerve*
gland	Structure of the endocrine system that produces and secretes one or more hormones into the blood	glandul/o- *gland*
homeostasis	State of equilibrium of the internal environment of the body. The endocrine system plays a role in homeostasis by regulating body fluids, electrolytes, glucose, cell metabolism, growth, and the wake–sleep cycle.	home/o- *same*
hormone	Chemical messenger of the endocrine system that is produced by a gland and secreted into the blood	hormon/o- *hormone*

Hypothalamus

hypothalamus	Endocrine gland within the brain just below the thalamus. The hypothalamus secretes hormones that stimulate or inhibit the secretion of hormones from the anterior pituitary gland. It also produces antidiuretic hormone (ADH) and oxytocin. These two hormones are stored in the posterior pituitary gland.	thalam/o- *thalamus*

Pituitary Gland

adrenocortico-tropic hormone (ACTH)	Hormone produced and secreted by the anterior pituitary gland. It stimulates the cortex of the adrenal gland to secrete its hormones.	adren/o- *adrenal gland* cortic/o- *cortex; outer region* trop/o- *having an affinity for; stimulating; turning*
anterior pituitary gland	Part of the pituitary gland that produces and secretes seven hormones: thyroid-stimulating hormone (TSH), follicle-stimulating hormone (FSH), luteinizing hormone (LH), prolactin, adrenocorticotropic hormone (ACTH), growth hormone (GH), and melanocyte-stimulating hormone (MSH). It is also known as the **adenohypophysis**.	pituit/o- *pituitary gland* aden/o- *gland* hypophys/o- *pituitary gland*
antidiuretic hormone (ADH)	Hormone produced by the hypothalamus but stored in and released by the posterior pituitary gland. ADH moves sodium and water from tubules in the nephron of the kidney into the blood. This decreases urine output and keeps the blood volume and blood pressure normal.	ur/o- *urinary system; urine*
follicle-stimulating hormone (FSH)	Hormone produced and secreted by the anterior pituitary gland. In females, it stimulates follicles in the ovary to produce mature ova and to secrete the hormone estradiol. In males, it stimulates the seminiferous tubules of the testes to produce spermatozoa.	stimul/o- *exciting; strengthening*
gonadotropins	Category of hormones that stimulates the male and female sex glands (gonads). It includes FSH and LH.	gonad/o- *gonad; ovary; testis* trop/o- *having an affinity for; stimulating; turning*

Word or Phrase	Description	Combining Forms
growth hormone (GH)	Hormone produced and secreted by the anterior pituitary gland. It stimulates growth and protein synthesis in all cells. It increases height and weight during childhood and puberty.	
luteinizing hormone (LH)	Hormone produced and secreted by the anterior pituitary gland. In females, it stimulates a follicle in the ovary to release a mature ovum. It stimulates the corpus luteum (ruptured ovarian follicle) to secrete estradiol and progesterone. In males, it stimulates the interstitial cells of the testes to secrete testosterone.	
melanocyte-stimulating hormone (MSH)	Hormone produced and secreted by the anterior pituitary gland. It is secreted in pregnant women and stimulates melanocytes in the skin to produce melanin. This causes skin pigmentation on the face and abdomen.	melan/o- *black*
oxytocin	Hormone produced by the hypothalamus but stored in and released by the posterior pituitary gland. It stimulates the pregnant uterus to contract during labor and childbirth. It causes the uterus to contract after birth to prevent hemorrhaging. It causes the breasts to release milk for breastfeeding ("let-down reflex") when the baby cries or sucks.	ox/y- *oxygen; quick* toc/o- *childbirth; labor*
pituitary gland	Endocrine gland in the brain that is connected by a stalk of tissue to the hypothalamus. It sits in the bony cup of the **sella turcica** of the sphenoid bone. It is also known as the **hypophysis**. It is the *master gland of the body.* It consists of two separate glands: the anterior pituitary gland and the posterior pituitary gland.	pituit/o- *pituitary gland* hypophys/o- *pituitary gland* pituitar/o- *pituitary gland*
posterior pituitary gland	Part of the pituitary gland that stores and releases antidiuretic hormone (ADH) and oxytocin produced by the hypothalamus; it releases these hormones in response to a nerve impulse from the hypothalamus. It is also known as the **neurohypophysis**.	pituit/o- *pituitary gland* neur/o- *nerve* hypophys/o- *pituitary gland*
prolactin	Hormone produced and secreted by the anterior pituitary gland. It stimulates the development of the breasts during puberty and stimulates the mammary glands to release milk for breastfeeding.	lact/o- *milk* galact/o- *milk*
thyroid-stimulating hormone (TSH)	Hormone produced and secreted by the anterior pituitary gland. It causes the thyroid gland to grow and stimulates it to secrete the thyroid hormones T_3 and T_4.	thyr/o- *shield-shaped structure;* *thyroid gland* stimul/o- *exciting; strengthening*
Pineal Gland		
melatonin	Hormone secreted by the pineal gland. It maintains the 24-hour wake–sleep cycle.	
pineal gland	Endocrine gland between the two lobes of the thalamus. It secretes the hormone melatonin. It is also known as the **pineal body**.	
Thyroid Gland		
calcitonin	Hormone secreted by the thyroid gland. It regulates the amount of calcium in the blood. If the calcium level is too high, calcitonin moves calcium from the blood and deposits it in the bones.	calc/i- *calcium* ton/o- *pressure; tone* calc/o- *calcium*
euthyroidism	State of normal functioning of the hormones of the thyroid gland	thyroid/o- *thyroid gland*
T_3	Hormone secreted by the thyroid gland. It increases the rate of cell metabolism. It is also known as **triiodothyronine**.	iod/o- *iodine* thyr/o- *shield-shaped structure;* *thyroid gland*

Word or Phrase	Description	Combining Forms
T_4	Hormone secreted by the thyroid gland. Most of it is changed into T_3 by the liver. It is also known as **thyroxine**.	
thyroid gland	Endocrine gland in the neck that secretes the hormones T_3, T_4, and calcitonin. Its two lobes have a shield-like shape with a band of tissue across the trachea.	**thyr/o-** *shield-shaped structure; thyroid gland*

Parathyroid Glands		
parathyroid glands	Four endocrine glands on the posterior surface of the thyroid gland. They secrete parathyroid hormone.	**thyr/o-** *shield-shaped structure; thyroid gland*
parathyroid hormone	Hormone secreted by the parathyroid glands. It regulates the amount of calcium in the blood. If the calcium level is too low, parathyroid hormone moves calcium from the bones to the blood.	**thyr/o-** *shield-shaped structure; thyroid gland*

Thymus Gland		
thymus	Endocrine gland posterior to the sternum and within the mediastinum. It secretes a group of hormones known as **thymosins**. They cause immature T lymphocytes in the thymus to mature.	**thym/o-** *rage; thymus*

Pancreas		
glucagon	Hormone secreted by alpha cells in the islets of Langerhans. It breaks down stored glycogen to increase the glucose in the blood.	**gluc/o-** *glucose; sugar* **ag/o-** *lead to*
glucose	A simple sugar in foods and also the sugar in the blood (produced when the hormones glucagon or cortisol break down stored glycogen)	**gluc/o-** *glucose; sugar* **glycos/o-** *glucose; sugar*
glycogen	Glucose stored in the liver and skeletal muscles. Glycogen is broken down into glucose by the hormone glucagon from the pancreas and by the hormone cortisol from the adrenal cortex.	**glyc/o-** *glucose; sugar*
insulin	Hormone secreted by beta cells in the islets of Langerhans. It transports glucose into the cells where it is metabolized for energy.	**insul/o-** *island* **insulin/o-** *insulin*
pancreas	Endocrine gland posterior to the stomach. It contains the **islets of Langerhans** (alpha, beta, and delta cells) that secrete the hormones glucagon, insulin, and somatostatin.	**pancreat/o-** *pancreas*
somatostatin	Hormone secreted by delta cells in the islets of Langerhans. It prevents the hormones glucagon and insulin from being secreted by the pancreas. It prevents growth hormone from being secreted by the anterior pituitary gland.	**somat/o-** *body* **stat/o-** *standing still; staying in one place*

Adrenal Glands		
adrenal cortex	Outer layer of the adrenal gland. It secretes three groups of hormones: mineralocorticoids (aldosterone), glucocorticoids (cortisol), and androgens (male sex hormones).	**adren/o-** *adrenal gland* **cortic/o-** *cortex; outer region*
adrenal glands	Endocrine glands on top of the kidneys. An adrenal gland contains a cortex and a medulla, each of which is a gland that secretes its own hormones.	**adrenal/o-** *adrenal gland* **adren/o-** *adrenal gland* **ren/o-** *kidney*
adrenal medulla	Inner layer of the adrenal gland. It secretes the hormones norepinephrine, epinephrine, and dopamine.	**adren/o-** *adrenal gland*

Build Medical Words

Combining Form and Suffix Exercise

Read the definition of the medical word. Look at the combining form that is given. Select the correct suffix from the Suffix List and write it on the blank line. Then build the medical word and write it on the line. (Remember: You may need to remove the combining vowel. Always remove the hyphens and slash.) Be sure to check your spelling. The first one has been done for you.

SUFFIX LIST

-al (pertaining to)
-an (pertaining to)
-ar (pertaining to)
-ation (being; having; process)

-gen (that which produces)
-ic (pertaining to)
-ism (disease from a specific
  cause; process)

-oid (resembling)
-or (person who produces; thing that
  produces)
-stasis (standing still; staying in one place)

Definition of the Medical Word	Combining Form	Suffix	Build the Medical Word
1. Pertaining to (the) thymus	**thym/o-**	**-ic**	thymic
(You think *pertaining to* (-ic) + *thymus* (thym/o-). You change the order of the word parts to put the suffix last. You write *thymic*.)			
2. Pertaining to (a) hormone	hormon/o-	_____	_____
3. That which produces male (characteristics)	andr/o-	_____	_____
4. Pertaining to (the) ovary	ovari/o-	_____	_____
5. Staying in one place (and being the) same	home/o-	_____	_____
6. Process (of) exciting	stimul/o-	_____	_____
7. (A gland) resembling (a) shield-shaped structure	thyr/o-	_____	_____
8. Pertaining to (the) pancreas	pancreat/o-	_____	_____
9. Pertaining to (the) testicle	testicul/o-	_____	_____
10. Thing (structure on a cell membrane) that produces (an action to) receive	recept/o-	_____	_____
11. Process (to) oppose or work against	antagon/o-	_____	_____

Prefix Exercise

Read the definition of the medical word. Look at the medical word or partial word that is given (it already contains a combining form and a suffix). Select the correct prefix from the Prefix List and write it on the blank line. Then build the medical word and write it on the line. Be sure to check your spelling. The first one has been done for you.

PREFIX LIST

ad- (toward)
eu- (good; normal)

hypo- (below; deficient)
para- (abnormal; apart from; beside; two parts of a pair)

pro- (before)
syn- (together)

Definition of the Medical Word	Prefix	Word or Partial Word	Build the Medical Word
1. Pertaining to (a gland) toward (the) kidney	**ad-**	**renal**	adrenal
2. Process (of a) normal (level of) thyroid gland (hormones)	_____	thyroidism	_____
3. (Structures) resembling two parts of a pair (on the) thyroid gland	_____	thyroid	_____
4. Pertaining to (a gland) below (the) thalamus	_____	thalamic	_____
5. Substance (that must be secreted) before milk (can be produced)	_____	lactin	_____
6. Process (of two hormones being) together (to) work	_____	ergism	_____

Diseases

Anterior Pituitary Gland: All Hormones

Word or Phase	Description	Pronunciation/Word Parts
hyperpituitarism	Hypersecretion of one or all of the hormones of the anterior pituitary gland. It is caused by a benign tumor (**adenoma**) in the anterior pituitary gland. Treatment: Drug therapy to suppress secretion of the hormones, or surgery to remove the adenoma, with radiation therapy to destroy the remaining adenoma.	**hyperpituitarism** (HY-per-pih-TOO-ih-tair-IZM) **hyper-** *above; more than normal* **pituitar/o-** *pituitary gland* **-ism** *disease from a specific cause; process* **adenoma** (AD-eh-NOH-mah) **aden/o-** *gland* **-oma** *mass; tumor* **adenomata** (AD-eh-NOH-mah-tah) *Adenoma is a Greek noun. Form the plural by changing -oma to -omata.*
hypopituitarism	Hyposecretion of one or more of the hormones of the anterior pituitary gland. It is caused by an injury or a defect in the anterior pituitary gland. **Panhypopituitarism** is hyposecretion of all of the hormones. Treatment: Drug therapy to replace the hormone(s).	**hypopituitarism** (HY-poh-pih-TOO-ih-tair-IZM) **hypo-** *below; deficient* **pituitar/o-** *pituitary gland* **-ism** *disease from a specific cause; process* **panhypopituitarism** (pan-HY-poh-pih-TOO-ih-tair-IZM) *The prefix pan- means all.*

Anterior Pituitary Gland: Prolactin

Word or Phase	Description	Pronunciation/Word Parts
galactorrhea	Hypersecretion of prolactin. It is caused by an adenoma in the anterior pituitary gland. The high level of prolactin causes the mammary glands in the breasts to produce milk, even though the patient is not pregnant. It also inhibits the secretion of FSH and LH and this stops menstruation. Treatment: Drug therapy to suppress secretion of prolactin or surgery to remove the adenoma, with radiation therapy to destroy the remaining adenoma.	**galactorrhea** (gah-LAK-toh-REE-ah) **galact/o-** *milk* **-rrhea** *discharge; flow*
failure of lactation	Hyposecretion of prolactin. It is caused by a defect in the anterior pituitary gland. The low level of prolactin causes the lactiferous lobules (milk glands) in the breasts not to develop during puberty, and the breasts do not make enough milk for breastfeeding after the baby is born. Treatment: None.	**lactation** (lak-TAY-shun) **lact/o-** *milk* **-ation** *being; having; process*

> **CLINICAL CONNECTIONS**
>
> **Pathology.** In 99% of patients with an endocrine gland tumor, the tumor is a benign (not cancerous) adenoma. A microadenoma is a very small tumor.
>
> **Nuclear Medicine.** Radiation therapy uses x-rays delivered in small (fractionated) doses every day for several weeks to destroy any adenoma remaining after surgery.

Anterior Pituitary Gland: Growth Hormone

Word or Phase	Description	Pronunciation/W
gigantism	Hypersecretion of growth hormone during childhood and puberty (see Figure 14-8 ■). It is caused by an adenoma in the anterior pituitary gland. The high level of growth hormone causes the bones and tissues to grow excessively. Treatment: Drug therapy to suppress secretion of growth hormone or surgery to remove the adenoma, with radiation therapy to destroy the remaining adenoma.	**gigantism** (jy-GAN-tizm) (JY-gan-tizm) **gigant/o-** *giant* **-ism** *disease from a specific cause; process*

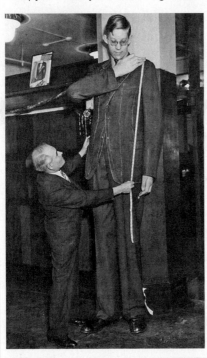

FIGURE 14-8 ■ Gigantism.
The tallest man who ever lived suffered from gigantism. His name was Robert Wadlow. He was born in 1918 in Illinois and was of average weight and length at birth. By the time he was 18 years old, he was 8'11" and weighed 491 pounds. He wore size 37AA shoes that were over 18" in length. He died in 1940, at the age of 22. The tallest living man now is Sultan Kosen of Turkey, who was born in 1982 and is 8'2" tall.
Source: Bettmann/Corbis

Word or Phase	Description	Pronunciation/W
acromegaly	Hypersecretion of growth hormone during adulthood. It is caused by an adenoma in the anterior pituitary gland. Because the growth plates at the ends of the long bones have already fused, the patient cannot grow taller. So, the high level of growth hormone causes the facial features, jaw, hands, and feet to widen and enlarge (see Figure 14-9 ■). Treatment: Drug therapy to suppress secretion of growth hormone or surgery to remove the adenoma, with radiation therapy to destroy the remaining adenoma.	**acromegaly** (AK-roh-MEG-ah-lee) **acr/o-** *extremity; highest point* **-megaly** *enlargement*

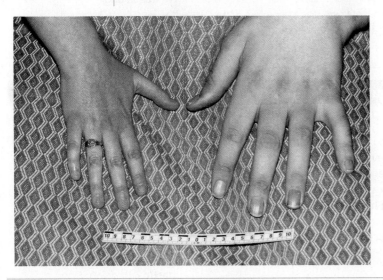

FIGURE 14-9 ■ Acromegaly.
An increased level of growth hormone in adulthood causes the face and extremities to widen. The hand on the left is normal. The hand on the right shows acromegaly with enlargement and widening.
Source: Biophoto Associates/Science Source

Word or Phase	Description	Pronunciation/Word Parts
dwarfism	Hyposecretion of growth hormone during childhood and puberty. It is caused by a defect in the anterior pituitary gland. The low level of growth hormone causes a lack of growth and short stature, but with normal body proportions. Treatment: Drug therapy with growth hormone.	**dwarfism** (DWORF-izm) *Dwarfism* is a combination of the word *dwarf* and the suffix *-ism* (disease from a specific cause; process).

CLINICAL CONNECTIONS

Genetics. Dwarfism has many causes. Achondroplasia is a genetic mutation in which cartilage does not convert to bone. This results in a dwarf with small extremities but a normal-sized trunk. Short stature in an otherwise normal person can also be caused by severe malnutrition, very short parents (heredity), or severe kidney or heart disease as a child.

Posterior Pituitary Gland: Antidiuretic Hormone

Word or Phase	Description	Pronunciation/Word Parts
syndrome of inappropriate ADH (SIADH)	Hypersecretion of ADH. It is caused by an adenoma in the posterior pituitary gland. (It can also be caused by brain infections, multiple sclerosis, or a stroke.) The high level of ADH causes excessive amounts of water to move into the blood. This dilutes the blood, creates a low level of sodium, and causes headache, weakness, confusion, and eventually coma. Treatment: Restriction of water intake. Surgery to remove the adenoma, with radiation therapy to destroy the remaining adenoma.	
diabetes insipidus (DI)	Hyposecretion of ADH. It is caused by a defect in the posterior pituitary gland, a brain infection, head trauma, or heredity. The low level of ADH causes excessive amounts of water to be excreted in the urine (**polyuria**). There is also weakness (due to water loss and dehydration) and thirst, which causes an increased intake of fluids (**polydipsia**). Treatment: Drug therapy with antidiuretic hormone.	**diabetes** (DY-ah-BEE-teez) **insipidus** (in-SIP-ih-dus) **polyuria** (PAW-lee-YOOR-ee-ah) **poly-** *many; much* **ur/o-** *urinary system; urine* **-ia** *condition; state; thing* **polydipsia** (PAW-lee-DIP-see-ah) **poly-** *many; much* **dips/o-** *thirst* **-ia** *condition; state; thing*

DID YOU KNOW?

The Latin word *insipidus* and the English word *insipid* mean *lacking a distinctive appearance or taste.* Patients with diabetes insipidus have tasteless, dilute urine, like water, while the urine of patients with diabetes mellitus is sweet. Before there were laboratories, physicians used to taste the patient's urine to make a diagnosis.

Posterior Pituitary Gland: Oxytocin

Word or Phase	Description	Pronunciation/Word Parts
	There is no specific disease associated with hypersecretion of oxytocin.	
uterine inertia	Hyposecretion of oxytocin. It is caused by a defect in the posterior pituitary gland. Before birth, the low level of oxytocin causes weak and uncoordinated contractions of the pregnant uterus. This prolongs labor and delays the birth of the baby. After the birth of the baby, the low level of oxytocin causes **postpartum hemorrhage** (the uterus does not contract, and there is hemorrhaging at the site where the placenta separated from the uterus). Treatment: Drug therapy with oxytocin hormone.	**uterine** (YOO-teh-rin) (YOO-teh-rine) **uter/o-** *uterus; womb* **-ine** *pertaining to; thing pertaining to* **inertia** (in-ER-sha) **postpartum** (post-PAR-tum) **post-** *after; behind* **part/o-** *childbirth; labor* **-um** *period of time; structure*

Pineal Gland: Melatonin

Word or Phase	Description	Pronunciation/Word Parts
seasonal affective disorder (SAD)	Hypersecretion of melatonin. It is caused by a defect in the pineal gland. The high level of melatonin causes depression, weight gain, and an increased desire for food and sleep. This occurs most often during the winter months when there are fewer hours of bright sunlight. Treatment: Exposure to sunlight or to bright light from a light box (phototherapy) to suppress melatonin secretion. Drug therapy with melatonin and/or an antidepressant drug.	**affective** (ah-FEK-tiv) **affect/o-** *have an influence on; mood; state of mind* **-ive** *pertaining to*
	There is no specific disease associated with hyposecretion of melatonin.	

Thyroid Gland: T₃ and T₄ Thyroid Hormones

hyperthyroidism	Hypersecretion of T_3 and T_4 thyroid hormones. It is caused by an adenoma (also known as a **nodule**) in the thyroid gland. (It can also be caused by hypersecretion of TSH from an adenoma in the anterior pituitary gland.) The high levels of T_3 and T_4 cause tremors of the hands, tachycardia, palpitations, restlessness, nervousness, diarrhea, insomnia, fatigue, and generalized weight loss. The thyroid gland is enlarged (a goiter) and can be felt on palpation of the neck. The eyes are dry and irritated with slow eyelid closing (lid lag). Hyperthyroidism is also known as **thyrotoxicosis** because of the toxic effect of the high levels of thyroid hormones. The sudden onset of severe hyperthyroidism is known as a **thyroid storm**. The most common type of hyperthyroidism is **Graves' disease**. This is an autoimmune disease in which the body produces antibodies that stimulate TSH receptors on the thyroid gland, and this increases the production of thyroid hormones. The entire thyroid gland becomes enlarged (diffuse toxic goiter), and there is **exophthalmos** (see Figure 14-10 ■). Treatment: Antithyroid drug to suppress the secretion of T_3 and T_4 or surgery to remove the thyroid gland (thyroidectomy), with radiation therapy with radioactive iodine to destroy the remaining thyroid gland.	**hyperthyroidism** (HY-per-THY-royd-izm) **hyper-** *above; more than normal* **thyroid/o-** *thyroid gland* **-ism** *disease from a specific cause; process* **thyrotoxicosis** (THY-roh-TAWK-sih-KOH-sis) **thyr/o-** *shield-shaped structure; thyroid gland* **toxic/o-** *poison; toxin* **-osis** *condition; process* Add words to make a complete definition of *thyrotoxicosis*: *condition (in which too much) thyroid gland (hormone acts as a) poison.* **Graves' disease** (GRAYVZ) **exophthalmos** (EKS-off-THAL-mohs) *Exophthalmos* is a combination of the prefix *ex-* (away from; out) and the Greek word *ophthalmos* (eye).

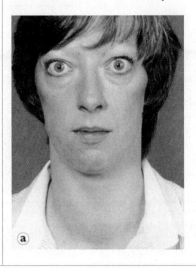

FIGURE 14-10 ■ Exophthalmos.
Exophthalmos is a well-known sign of hyperthyroidism. Edema behind the eyeballs causes them to protrude. This creates a staring expression that shows a large amount of white sclerae. This patient also has swelling of the neck from her enlarged thyroid gland.
Source: Biophoto Associates/Science Source/Getty Images

Word or Phase	Description	Pronunciation/Word Parts
hyperthyroidism (*continued*)		

hyperthyroidism (*continued*)

A CLOSER LOOK

A **goiter** is a chronic and progressive enlargement of the thyroid gland. It is also known as **thyromegaly**. A physician can feel this enlargement during a physical examination (see Figure 14-11 ■) even before it becomes visible. The causes of goiter include the following:

1. An **adenoma** or nodule growing in the thyroid gland. This is known as an **adenomatous goiter** or **nodular goiter**. If there are many nodules, it is a **multinodular goiter**. An adenoma or nodule usually is benign, but can be cancerous.

2. A cancerous tumor growing in the thyroid gland.

3. Chronic inflammation of the thyroid gland as seen in thyroiditis.

4. A lack of iodine in the soil, water, and diet. This causes the thyroid gland to enlarge to help it capture more iodine. This is known as a **simple goiter**, a **nontoxic goiter**, or an **endemic goiter** (because it occurs in people who live in an area where the soil is poor in iodine). The widespread use of iodized salt has decreased the incidence of this type of goiter.

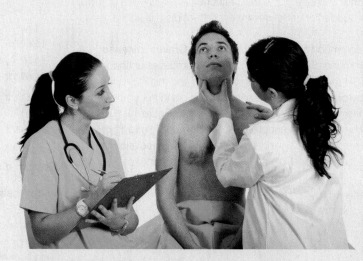

FIGURE 14-11 ■ Physical examination of the thyroid gland.
The anterior location of the thyroid gland means that even mild enlargement can be detected. This physician is palpating the edges of the patient's thyroid gland to determine its size.
Source: Blaj Gabriel/Shutterstock

goiter (GOY-ter)

thyromegaly
(THY-roh-MEG-ah-lee)
  thyr/o- *shield-shaped structure; thyroid gland*
  -megaly *enlargement*

adenoma (AD-eh-NOH-mah)
  aden/o- *gland*
  -oma *mass; tumor*

adenomatous
(AD-eh-NOH-mah-tus)
  aden/o- *gland*
  -oma *mass; tumor*
  -tous *pertaining to*

nodular (NAW-dyoo-lar)
  nodul/o- *small, knobby mass*
  -ar *pertaining to*

multinodular
(MUL-tee-NAW-dyoo-lar)
The combining form *mult/i-* means *many*.

nontoxic (non-TAWK-sik)
  non- *not*
  tox/o- *poison*
  -ic *pertaining to*

endemic (en-DEM-ik)
  en- *in; inward; within*
  dem/o- *people; population*
  -ic *pertaining to*

CLINICAL CONNECTIONS

Dietetics. The production of T_3 is dependent on adequate amounts of the trace mineral iodine in the diet. The ancient Chinese used seaweed to treat goiter because seaweed contains iodine. Iodine can be obtained from eating seafood, from vegetables grown in soil that contains iodine, and from drinking water that contains iodine. In the areas of the Great Lakes and Midwest of the United States, the soil and water are deficient in iodine. This is known as the "goiter belt" because persons living there tend to develop goiters from having too little iodine. Iodine was first added to table salt in 1924, and iodized salt was sold everywhere by 1940.

Word or Phase	Description	Pronunciation/Word Parts
hypothyroidism	Hyposecretion of T_3 and T_4 thyroid hormones. It is usually caused by an inadequate amount of iodine in the diet. It can also be caused by Hashimoto's thyroiditis, by treatments for hyperthyroidism that remove the thyroid gland, or by hyposecretion of TSH from the anterior pituitary gland. Another possible cause is a defect in the thyroid gland at birth that causes **congenital hypothyroidism**. Untreated congenital hypothyroidism results in mental retardation (**cretinism**). The low levels of T_3 and T_4 cause goiter, fatigue, decreased body temperature, dry hair and skin, constipation, and weight gain. Severe hypothyroidism in adults causes **myxedema** with swelling of the subcutaneous and connective tissues, tingling in the hands and feet because of nerve compression, lack of menstruation, hair loss, an enlarged heart, bradycardia, an enlarged tongue, slow speech, and mental impairment. Treatment: Thyroid hormone supplement drug.	**hypothyroidism** (HY-poh-THY-royd-izm) **hypo-** *below; deficient* **thyroid/o-** *thyroid gland* **-ism** *disease from a specific cause; process* **congenital** (con-JEN-ih-tal) **congenit/o-** *present at birth* **-al** *pertaining to* **cretinism** (KREE-tin-izm) **myxedema** (MIKS-eh-DEE-mah) **myx/o-** *mucus-like substance* **-edema** *swelling*
thyroid carcinoma	Malignant tumor of the thyroid gland. There is hoarseness, neck pain, and enlargement of thyroid gland and nearby cancerous lymph nodes. Treatment: Surgery to remove the thyroid gland (thyroidectomy), with radiation therapy to destroy the remaining thyroid gland.	**carcinoma** (KAR-sih-NOH-mah) **carcin/o-** *cancer* **-oma** *mass; tumor*
thyroiditis	Chronic inflammation and progressive destruction of the thyroid gland. The most common type is **Hashimoto's thyroiditis**, an autoimmune disorder in which the body forms antibodies against the thyroid gland. The thyroid becomes inflamed and enlarged (goiter). Over time, the patient develops hypothyroidism as thyroid tissue is destroyed and replaced by fibrous tissue. Treatment: Thyroid hormone supplement drug.	**thyroiditis** (THY-royd-EYE-tis) **thyroid/o-** *thyroid gland* **-itis** *infection of; inflammation of* **Hashimoto** (HAH-shee-MOH-toh)

Parathyroid Glands: Parathyroid Hormone

Word or Phase	Description	Pronunciation/Word Parts
hyperpara-thyroidism	Hypersecretion of parathyroid hormone. It is caused by an adenoma in the parathyroid gland. The high level of parathyroid hormone moves too much calcium from the bones to the blood, and the calcium level in the blood is too high (**hypercalcemia**). The bones become demineralized and prone to fracture. There is also muscle weakness, fatigue, and depression. Excess calcium is excreted in the urine, and this can form kidney stones. Treatment: Surgery to remove the parathyroid glands.	**hyperparathyroidism** (HY-per-PAIR-ah-THY-royd-izm) **hyper-** *above; more than normal* **para-** *abnormal; apart from; beside; two parts of a pair* **thyroid/o-** *thyroid gland* **-ism** *disease from a specific cause; process* **hypercalcemia** (HY-per-kal-SEE-mee-ah) **hyper-** *above; more than normal* **calc/o-** *calcium* **-emia** *condition of the blood; substance in the blood*

Word or Phase	Description	Pronunciation/Word Parts
hypopara-thyroidism	Hyposecretion of parathyroid hormone. It is caused by the accidental removal of the parathyroid glands during surgery to remove the thyroid gland (thyroidectomy). The low level of parathyroid hormone causes the calcium level in the blood to become very low (**hypocalcemia**). This causes irritability of the nerves, skeletal muscle cramps, or sustained muscle spasm (tetany). Treatment: Parathyroid hormone supplement drug.	**hypoparathyroidism** (HY-poh-PAIR-ah-THY-royd-izm) **hypo-** *below; deficient* **para-** *abnormal; apart from; beside; two parts of a pair* **thyroid/o-** *thyroid gland* **-ism** *disease from a specific cause; process* **hypocalcemia** (HY-poh-kal-SEE-mee-ah) **hypo-** *below; deficient* **calc/o-** *calcium* **-emia** *condition of the blood; substance in the blood*

Pancreas: Insulin

Word or Phase	Description	Pronunciation/Word Parts
hyperinsulinism	Hypersecretion of insulin. It is caused by an adenoma in the pancreas. The high level of insulin causes **hypoglycemia** (a low level of glucose in the blood). There is shakiness, headache, sweating, dizziness, and even fainting. If left untreated, hypoglycemia can progress to insulin shock and then coma as the blood glucose level becomes too low to support brain activity. Treatment: Supplemental sugar or sugar drink or dextrose intravenous fluids. Surgery to remove the adenoma.	**hyperinsulinism** (HY-per-IN-soo-lin-IZM) **hyper-** *above; more than normal* **insulin/o-** *insulin* **-ism** *disease from a specific cause; process* **hypoglycemia** (HY-poh-gly-SEE-mee-ah) **hypo-** *below; deficient* **glyc/o-** *glucose; sugar* **-emia** *condition of the blood; substance in the blood*

DID YOU KNOW?

Persons with a normal level of insulin can also become hypoglycemic when they are dieting or fasting. Diabetic patients can become hypoglycemic when they take an oral antidiabetic drug or inject insulin but then skip a meal.

CLINICAL CONNECTIONS

Neonatology. In a mother with uncontrolled gestational diabetes, the fetus is constantly exposed to a high level of glucose in its blood (from the mother via the umbilical cord), and its pancreas constantly secretes large amounts of insulin before birth. After birth, the baby is not drinking much milk at first, but its pancreas continues to produce large amounts of insulin. Then the baby can suddenly become hypoglycemic with seizures or a coma. Treatment: Intravenous fluids with dextrose (sugar).

Word or Phase	Description	Pronunciation/Word Parts
insulin resistance syndrome	Hypersecretion of insulin. This is not caused by an adenoma. It occurs when receptors on body cells resist and do not allow insulin to transport glucose into the cell. There is a high level of glucose remaining in the blood (hyperglycemia), and there is a high level of insulin as the pancreas continues to secrete insulin to try to lower the blood glucose level. Eventually, the pancreas is unable to produce more insulin, and the patient develops diabetes mellitus. Treatment: Appropriate treatment for diabetes mellitus. *Your chart says you have IRS . . . It's either a problem with insulin resistance syndrome or the Internal Revenue Service.*	**resistance** (ree-ZIS-tans) **resist/o-** *withstand the effect of* **-ance** *state*
diabetes mellitus (DM)	Hyposecretion of insulin. It is caused by an inability of the beta cells of the pancreas to secrete enough insulin. A person who has diabetes mellitus is a **diabetic**. The low level of insulin in the blood results in an increased level of glucose in the blood (**hyperglycemia**). Excess glucose in the blood is excreted in the urine (**glycosuria**). As it is excreted, it holds water to it by osmosis, and this increases the amount of urine (**polyuria**). With excessive urination, the patient becomes thirsty and drinks often (**polydipsia**). The patient also feels hungry and eats often (**polyphagia**) because the glucose in the blood cannot be metabolized by the cells. There are three main types of diabetes mellitus: type 1, type 1.5, and type 2 (see Table 14-1 ■). A brittle diabetic has difficulty controlling the blood glucose level, with frequent swings from hyperglycemia to hypoglycemia. "Sugar diabetes" is a layperson's phrase for diabetes mellitus. Treatment: Drug therapy with injections of insulin or an oral -antidiabetic drug (depending on the type of diabetes mellitus). Diet management, weight control, and exercise.	**diabetes** (DY-ah-BEE-teez) **mellitus** (MEL-ih-tus) **diabetic** (DY-ah-BET-ik) **diabet/o-** *diabetes* **-ic** *pertaining to* **hyperglycemia** (HY-per-gly-SEE-mee-ah) **hyper-** *above; more than normal* **glyc/o-** *glucose; sugar* **-emia** *condition of the blood; substance in the blood* **glycosuria** (GLY-kohs-YOOR-ee-ah) **glycos/o-** *glucose; sugar* **ur/o-** *urinary system; urine* **-ia** *condition; state; thing* **polyuria** (PAW-lee-YOOR-ee-ah) **poly-** *many; much* **ur/o-** *urinary system; urine* **-ia** *condition; state; thing* **polydipsia** (PAW-lee-DIP-see-ah) **poly-** *many; much* **dips/o-** *thirst* **-ia** *condition; state; thing* **polyphagia** (PAW-lee-FAY-jah) **poly-** *many; much* **phag/o-** *eating; swallowing* **-ia** *condition; state; thing*

A CLOSER LOOK

Gestational diabetes mellitus occurs only during pregnancy, when increased levels of estradiol and progesterone during pregnancy block the action of insulin. The mother's pancreas is temporarily unable to secrete enough insulin to meet the increased demands from the growing fetus. This type of diabetes mellitus resolves once the baby is delivered. However, many women develop type 2 diabetes later in life.

gestational (jes-TAY-shun-al)
 gestat/o- *conception to birth*
 -ion *action; condition*
 -al *pertaining to*

Table 14-1 Diabetes Mellitus

	Type 1	Type 1.5	Type 2
Other Names	Insulin-dependent diabetes mellitus (IDDM) Juvenile-onset diabetes mellitus	Slow-onset Type I Latent autoimmune diabetes in adults (LADA)	Non-insulin-dependent diabetes mellitus (NIDDM) Adult-onset diabetes mellitus (AODM)
Onset	Child, adolescent, young adult	Adult	Adult
Percentage of all diabetics	10%	15%	75%
Amount of insulin secreted	None	Too little	Too little
Autoimmune disorder	Yes	Yes	No
Antibodies present	Yes	Yes	No
Insulin resistance	No	No	Yes
Body weight	Normal	Normal	Obese
Associated diseases	None	None	Increased cholesterol and triglyceride blood levels, hypertension, gout
Contributing factors	Heredity, triggered by viral illness	Heredity	Heredity, obesity
Drug therapy	Insulin	Insulin and oral antidiabetic drugs	Oral antidiabetic drugs, occasionally insulin

WORD ALERT

Sound-Alike Words

diabetes insipidus   Caused by hyposecretion of antidiuretic hormone (ADH) from the posterior pituitary gland

diabetes mellitus   Caused by hyposecretion of insulin or resistance to the insulin that is secreted

A CLOSER LOOK

Excessive urination (polyuria) is a symptom of both diabetes insipidus and diabetes mellitus, but for different reasons. In diabetes insipidus, a lack of ADH causes excessive amounts of water to be excreted in the urine. In diabetes mellitus, excess glucose excreted in the urine holds water to it by osmotic pressure, increasing the volume of urine.

Word or Phase	Description	Pronunciation/Word Parts
ketoacidosis	A high level of **ketones** in the blood. This occurs in untreated or uncontrolled diabetes mellitus when there is no insulin to metabolize glucose and the body turns to other sources of energy such as fat or protein. Body fat contains the most calories per gram, but fat does not metabolize cleanly and leaves ketones, an acidic by-product. The patient's breath has a unique "fruity" or "nail polish" odor from the high level of glucose and ketones in the blood. A diabetic coma occurs when a very high level of ketones (which are acidic) lowers the pH of the blood to the point that chemical reactions in the body cannot occur and the patient becomes unconscious. Treatment: Drug therapy with insulin.	**ketoacidosis** (KEE-toh-AS-ih-DOH-sis) **ket/o-** *ketones* **acid/o-** *acid; low pH* **-osis** *condition; process* **ketones** (KEE-tohnz)

A CLOSER LOOK

Complications of untreated or uncontrolled diabetes mellitus affect various organs of the body.

1. **Diabetic neuropathy.** Decreased or abnormal sensation in the extremities because of nerve damage due to demyelination of the nerves.

2. **Diabetic nephropathy.** Degenerative changes in the nephrons of the kidneys because of the high levels of glucose and ketones. This causes kidney failure that is treated with dialysis.

3. **Diabetic retinopathy.** Degenerative changes of the retina of the eye because of the local effect of high levels of glucose and ketones. There is formation of new, fragile blood vessels that hemorrhage; this causes blindness.

4. **Atherosclerosis.** Fatty deposits and plaque formation with hardening of the arteries, which is accelerated in diabetes mellitus because of abnormalities in fat metabolism.

5. **Impotence.** Nerve damage and atherosclerosis of the arteries to the penis result in difficulty having an erection.

neuropathy (nyoor-AW-pah-thee)
  neur/o- *nerve*
  -pathy *disease*
nephropathy (neh-FRAW-pah-thee)
  nephr/o- *kidney; nephron*
  -pathy *disease*
retinopathy (RET-ih-NAW-pah-thee)
  retin/o- *retina of the eye*
  -pathy *disease*

CLINICAL CONNECTIONS

Podiatry. Diabetic patients are at high risk for developing gangrene of the feet because of atherosclerosis and poor circulation, coupled with decreased sensation in the extremities (diabetic neuropathy). They are advised to see a podiatrist or physician to have their toenails trimmed. Poor eyesight (from age and diabetic retinopathy) coupled with decreased sensation in the lower extremities (diabetic neuropathy) makes it easy for diabetic patients to cut themselves when trimming their toenails. Small cuts do not heal because of poor blood flow from atherosclerosis. A continuously high level of glucose in the blood suppresses white blood cells that fight infection, and so a small cut can form an ulcer and then gangrene, requiring amputation.

Adrenal Cortex: Aldosterone

Word or Phase	Description	Pronunciation/Word Parts
hyperaldo-steronism	Hypersecretion of aldosterone. It is caused by an adenoma in the adrenal cortex. (It can also be caused by hypersecretion of ACTH from an adenoma in the anterior pituitary gland.) A high level of aldosterone (1) moves large amounts of sodium and water in the nephron of the kidney back to the blood (this causes hypertension) and (2) sends large amounts of potassium to be excreted in the urine (this causes electrolyte imbalance and weakness). Treatment: Surgery to remove the adenoma.	**hyperaldosteronism** (HY-per-al-DAW-steh-rohn-IZM) *Hyperaldosteronism* is a combination of the prefix *hyper-* (above; more than normal), *aldosterone* (with the *-e* deleted), and the suffix *-ism* (disease from a specific cause; process).

Word or Phrase	Description	Pronunciation/Word Parts
hypoaldosteronism	Hyposecretion of aldosterone. It is caused by a defect in the adrenal cortex. There is dizziness, a low level of sodium in the blood, weakness, and decreased blood pressure. Treatment: Drug therapy with an aldosterone hormone drug.	**hypoaldosteronism** (HY-poh-al-DAW-steh-rohn-IZM)

Adrenal Cortex: Cortisol

Word or Phrase	Description	Pronunciation/Word Parts
Cushing's syndrome	Hypersecretion of cortisol. It is caused by an adenoma in the adrenal cortex. (It can also occur in a patient who takes corticosteroid drugs on a long-term basis.) The high level of cortisol breaks down too much glycogen, causing a high level of glucose in the blood. This results in rapid weight gain, with deposits of fat in the face (moon face) (see Figure 14-12 ■), upper back (buffalo hump), and abdomen. There is a thinning of connective tissue in the skin of the face that allows the blood vessels to show through, giving a reddened appearance to the cheeks. The thinned connective tissue in the skin across the obese abdomen is stretched, causing small hemorrhages and red and purple striae. There is also a wasted appearance of the muscles in the extremities and muscle weakness because of the lack of protein synthesis (see Figure 14-12). Note: When there is hypersecretion of ACTH because of an adenoma in the anterior pituitary gland, this causes the adrenal cortex to secrete an excess of all of its hormones, including androgens, which produces dark facial hair (hirsutism) and amenorrhea in women. This condition is then known as *Cushing's disease*. Treatment: Surgery to remove the adenoma. Discontinue corticosteroid drugs.	**Cushing** (KOOSH-ing) **syndrome** (SIN-drohm) **syn-** *together* **-drome** *running* The ending *-drome* contains the combining form *drom/o-* and the one-letter suffix *-e*.

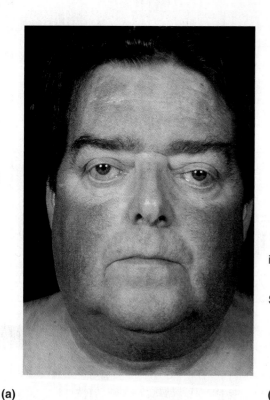

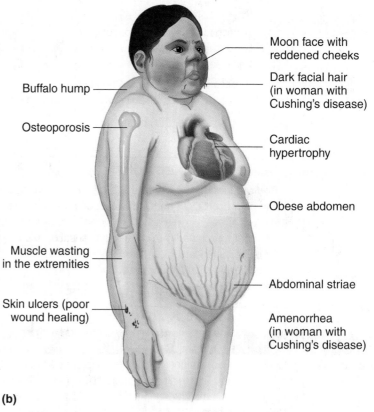

Moon face with reddened cheeks

Dark facial hair (in woman with Cushing's disease)

Buffalo hump

Osteoporosis

Cardiac hypertrophy

Obese abdomen

Muscle wasting in the extremities

Abdominal striae

Skin ulcers (poor wound healing)

Amenorrhea (in woman with Cushing's disease)

(a)

(b)

FIGURE 14-12 ■ Cushing's syndrome.
(a) This patient shows the characteristic signs of Cushing's syndrome. Deposits of fat in the cheeks give a moon face appearance. Breakdown of protein in the connective tissues thins the skin, allowing blood vessels to show through and give the cheeks a reddened appearance. (b) The abdomen is obese, while the extremities are thin and there is muscle wasting and weakness. In female patients with Cushing's disease, there is also dark facial hair and amenorrhea.
Source: Biophoto Associates/Science Source/Getty Images; Pearson Education

Word or Phase	Description	Pronunciation/Word Parts
Addison's disease	Hyposecretion of cortisol. This is an autoimmune disorder in which the body produces antibodies that destroy the adrenal cortex. (It can also be caused by hyposecretion of ACTH from the anterior pituitary gland.) There is a low level of blood glucose, fatigue, weight loss, and decreased ability to tolerate stress, disease, or surgery. Patients have an unusual bronzed color to the skin, even in areas not exposed to the sun. Treatment: Corticosteroid drug.	**Addison** (AD-ih-son)

Adrenal Cortex: Androgens		
adrenogenital syndrome	Hypersecretion of androgens. It is caused by an adenoma in the adrenal gland. In girls, the clitorus and labia enlarge and resemble a penis and scrotum. In boys, it causes precocious puberty. In adult females, it causes **virilism** with masculine facial features and body build, **hirsutism** (excessive, dark hair on the forearms and face), and amenorrhea. Treatment: Surgery to remove the adenoma.	**adrenogenital** (ah-DREE-noh-JEN-ih-tal) **adren/o-** *adrenal gland* **genit/o-** *genitalia* **-al** *pertaining to* **virilism** (VIR-ih-lizm) **viril/o-** *masculine* **-ism** *disease from a specific cause; process* **hirsutism** (HER-soo-tizm) **hirsut/o-** *hairy* **-ism** *disease from a specific cause; process*
	There is no specific disease associated with hyposecretion of androgens.	

Adrenal Medulla: Epinephrine and Norepinephrine		
pheochromo-cytoma	Hypersecretion of norepinephrine and epinephrine because of an adenoma in the adrenal medulla. This adenoma is known as a *pheochromocytoma* because of the appearance of its cells under a microscope. The high levels of norepinephrine and epinephrine cause heart palpitations, severe sweating, and headaches with severe hypertension that can cause a stroke. Treatment: Surgery to remove the pheochromocytoma.	**pheochromocytoma** (FEE-oh-KROH-moh-sy-TOH-mah) **phe/o-** *gray* **chrom/o-** *color* **cyt/o-** *cell* **-oma** *mass; tumor* Add words to make a complete definition of *pheochromocytoma*: *tumor (with a) gray color (to the) cells (when viewed under a microscope).*
	There is no specific disease associated with hyposecretion of epinephrine and norepinephrine.	

Ovaries: Estradiol and Progesterone		
precocious puberty	Hypersecretion of estradiol in a female child. It is caused by an adenoma in the ovary. (It can also be caused by hypersecretion of FSH from an adenoma in the anterior pituitary gland.) The high level of estradiol causes premature development of the breasts and female sexual characteristics, with menstruation and ovulation. Treatment: Surgery to remove the adenoma.	**precocious** (prih-KOH-shus) **puberty** (PYOO-ber-tee) **puber/o-** *growing up* **-ty** *quality; state*
infertility	Hyposecretion of estradiol in an adult female or an imbalance in the amount of estradiol and progesterone. (It can also be caused by a lack of FSH and LH from the anterior pituitary gland.) There is a lack of ovulation, abnormal menstruation, or a history of miscarriages. Treatment: Female hormone drug.	**infertility** (IN-fer-TIL-ih-tee) **in-** *in; not; within* **fertil/o-** *conceive; form* **-ity** *condition; state*

Word or Phase	Description	Pronunciation/Word Parts
menopause	Hyposecretion of estradiol in an adult female. This is a normal result of the aging process in which the ovaries secrete less and less estradiol. It can also be caused by surgical removal of the ovaries (oophorectomy) due to cancer. The resulting low level of estradiol causes vaginal dryness, thinning of the hair, and lack of sexual drive. As the hypothalamus senses a low estradiol level, it stimulates the anterior pituitary gland to secrete FSH to stimulate the ovary. These bursts of FSH cause hot flashes. Treatment: Female hormone replacement therapy, but only for a limited time because these drugs cause an increased risk of breast and endometrial cancer, blood clots, stroke, heart attack, and dementia.	**menopause** (MEN-oh-pawz) **men/o-** *month* **-pause** *cessation*

Testes: Testosterone

Word or Phase	Description	Pronunciation/Word Parts
precocious puberty	Hypersecretion of testosterone in a male child. It is caused by an adenoma in the testis. (It can also be caused by hypersecretion of LH from an adenoma in the anterior pituitary gland.) The high level of testosterone causes the premature development of the male sexual characteristics, with development of a beard, deepening of the voice, and sperm production. Treatment: Surgery to remove the adenoma.	**precocious** (prih-KOH-shus) **puberty** (PYOO-ber-tee) **puber/o-** *growing up* **-ty** *quality; state*
gynecomastia	Hyposecretion of testosterone in an adult male. This is a normal result of the aging process in which the testes secrete less testosterone. (It can also be caused by surgical removal of the testes due to cancer, by estrogen drug treatment for prostate cancer, by excessive alcohol consumption, or as a side effect of some drugs.) However, androgens continue to be secreted by the adrenal cortex and converted to estrogens in the blood. The low level of testosterone now is in an imbalance with the level of estrogens, and this causes enlargement of the male breasts. Treatment: Androgen drug. Plastic surgery to decrease the breast size.	**gynecomastia** (GY-neh-koh-MAS-tee-ah) **gynec/o-** *female; woman* **mast/o-** *breast; mastoid process* **-ia** *condition; state; thing*
infertility	Hyposecretion of testosterone in an adult male. It is caused by failure of one or both of the testes to descend into the scrotum before birth. (It can also be caused by surgical removal of the testes due to cancer, or it can be caused by lack of LH from the anterior pituitary gland.) The low level of testosterone causes too few spermatozoa to be produced. Treatment: Surgery as a child to bring the testes into the scrotum to prevent infertility as an adult. Drug therapy with an androgen drug for an adult.	**infertility** (IN-fer-TIL-ih-tee) **in-** *in; not; within* **fertil/o-** *conceive; form* **-ity** *condition; state*

Laboratory and Diagnostic Procedures

Blood Tests

Word or Phase	Description	Pronunciation/Word Parts
antithyroglobulin antibodies	Test that detects antibodies against thyroglobulin (precursor hormone to T_3 and T_4) in the thyroid gland. A positive test result indicates Hashimoto's thyroiditis.	**antithyroglobulin** (AN-tee-THY-roh-GLAW-byoo-lin) **anti-** *against* **thyr/o-** *shield-shaped structure; thyroid gland* **globul/o-** *shaped like a globe* **-in** *substance*
calcium	Test that measures the level of calcium to determine if the parathyroid gland is secreting a normal amount of parathyroid hormone.	**calcium** (KAL-see-um)

Word or Phase	Description	Pronunciation/Word Parts
cortisol level	Test that measures the level of cortisol to determine if the adrenal cortex is secreting a normal amount of cortisol. (It also determines if the anterior pituitary gland is secreting ACTH to stimulate the adrenal cortex.) A metabolite of cortisol, **17-hydroxycorticosteroids**, can also be measured in the urine to indirectly measure the level of cortisol in the blood.	**cortisol** (KOR-tih-sawl) **hydroxycorticosteroids** (hy-DRAWK-see-KOR-tih-koh-STAIR-oydz)
fasting blood sugar (FBS)	Test that measures the level of glucose after the patient has fasted (not eaten) for at least 12 hours. This shows if the pancreas is secreting a normal amount of insulin. It is the initial screening test for diabetes mellitus. If the result is abnormal, the patient will have a glucose tolerance test. A fasting blood sugar is also known as a **fasting blood glucose (FBG)**.	
FSH assay and LH assay	Test that measures the levels of FSH and LH to determine if the anterior pituitary gland is secreting a normal amount of FSH and LH. It is part of an infertility workup for men and women.	**assay** (AS-say)
glucose self-testing	Self-test that measures the level of glucose (blood sugar). Diabetic patients test their own blood glucose level one or more times each day (see Figure 14-13 ■).	**glucose** (GLOO-kohs) **gluc/o-** *glucose; sugar* **-ose** *full of; thing full of*

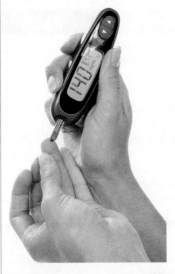

FIGURE 14-13 ■ Blood glucose monitor.
The patient pricks the fingertip and the drop of blood is placed on a test strip. It is inserted into the blood glucose monitor and the monitor displays the numerical value of the patient's blood glucose level. The normal range for blood glucose is between 70 and 150 mg/dL in a healthy person or in a patient whose diabetes mellitus is under control.
Source: Dmitry Lobanov/Fotolia

TECHNOLOGY IN MEDICINE
Now personal medical devices can capture blood glucose readings and transmit them electronically or wirelessly to the patient's physician. This type of remote monitoring dramatically decreases the number of office visits needed by diabetic patients.

Word or Phase	Description	Pronunciation/Word Parts
glucose tolerance test (GTT)	Blood and urine tests that measure the level of glucose to determine if the pancreas is secreting a normal amount of insulin. After the patient has fasted for 12 hours, blood and urine specimens are obtained. Then the patient drinks glucose (in a sugary drink known as **Glucola**) or is given **dextrose** intravenously. Blood and urine specimens are obtained every hour for 4 hours. Normally, the blood glucose returns to normal within 1 to 2 hours. High blood and urine levels of glucose indicate diabetes mellitus. It is also known as an **oral glucose tolerance test (OGTT)**.	**Glucola** (gloo-KOH-lah) **dextrose** (DEKS-trohs) **dextr/o-** *right; sugar* **-ose** *full of; thing full of*
growth hormone (GH)	Test that measures the level of GH to determine if the anterior pituitary gland is secreting a normal amount of growth hormone.	

Word or Phase	Description	Pronunciation/Word Parts
hemoglobin A$_{1C}$ (HbA$_{1C}$)	Test that measures the A$_{1C}$ fraction of hemoglobin in red blood cells. Hemoglobin A$_{1C}$ binds with glucose that is circulating in the blood. Because red blood cells only live about 12 weeks, the hemoglobin A$_{1C}$ result indicates the average level of blood glucose during the previous 12 weeks. It is used to monitor how well a diabetic patient is controlling the blood glucose level with diet and drugs. It is also known as **glycohemoglobin** or **glycosylated hemoglobin**.	**hemoglobin A$_{1C}$** (HEE-moh-GLOH-bin AA-one-see) **glycohemoglobin** (GLY-koh-HEE-moh-GLOH-bin) **glycosylated** (gly-KOH-sih-LAY-ted)
testosterone	Test that measures the levels of total testosterone and free testosterone to determine if the testes are secreting a normal amount of testosterone. (It also indirectly determines if the anterior pituitary gland is secreting luteinizing hormone to stimulate the testes.) This is part of an infertility workup.	
thyroid function tests (TFTs)	Test that measures the levels of T$_3$, T$_4$, and TSH to determine if the thyroid gland is secreting normal amounts of thyroid hormones. (It also determines if the anterior pituitary gland is secreting enough TSH to stimulate the thyroid.) The test uses a radioimmunoassay (RIA) technique in which antibodies labeled with radioactive isotopes combine with thyroid hormones and the amount of radioactivity is measured. Another test value, the **free thyroxine index (FTI)** or **T$_7$**, can be calculated from this.	

Urine Tests		
ADH stimulation test	Test that measures the concentration of urine to determine if the posterior pituitary gland is releasing a normal amount of antidiuretic hormone (ADH). The patient does not drink water for 12 hours; then a urine specimen is obtained. Then ADH is given (as the drug vasopressin), the patient drinks water, and another urine specimen is obtained. In a patient with diabetes insipidus, the second urine specimen will be more concentrated because of the ADH (vasopressin). It is also known as the **water deprivation test**.	
estradiol	Test that measures the level of estradiol to determine if the ovaries are secreting a normal amount of estradiol. (It also determines if the anterior pituitary gland is secreting FSH to stimulate the ovaries.) This is part of an infertility workup.	
urine dipstick	Test that measures glucose, ketones, and other substances in the urine. This is a rapid screening test used to evaluate diabetic patients.	
vanillylmandelic acid (VMA)	A 24-hour urine test that measures the levels of epinephrine and norepinephrine to determine if the adrenal medulla is secreting a normal amount of these hormones. VMA, a by-product of these hormones, is measured.	**vanillylmandelic acid** (VAN-ih-LIL-man-DEL-ik AS-id)

Radiology Tests

Word or Phase	Description	Pronunciation/Word Parts

radioactive iodine uptake (RAIU) and thyroid scan	Procedure that combines a thyroid scan with a radioactive iodine uptake procedure. The thyroid scan shows the size and shape of the thyroid gland. The radioactive iodine uptake shows how well the thyroid gland is able to absorb radioactive iodine from the blood. A normal scan will show uniform distribution of radioactive iodine throughout the thyroid gland. An adenoma appears as a bright ("hot") spot because of its increased uptake of radioactive iodine. A darker area (a "cold" spot) can be a benign cyst or a cancerous tumor of the thyroid gland (neither of which take up iodine) (see Figure 14-14 ■).
	
	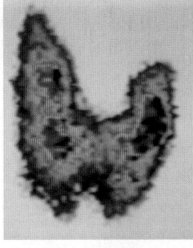
	
	FIGURE 14-14 ■ Thyroid scan.
	This patient's thyroid scan shows two dark blue "cold spots" in the right lobe of the thyroid gland and one large dark blue "cold spot" in the left lobe. These are areas of decreased uptake of radioactive iodine. They could be benign cysts or cancerous tumors. (Remember, when you view the image, your right side corresponds to the patient's left side.)
		radioactive (RAY-dee-oh-AK-tiv)
		  radi/o- *forearm bone; radiation; x-rays*
		  act/o- *action*
		  -ive *pertaining to*
		
		iodine
		(EYE-oh-dine) (EYE-oh-deen)

thyroid ultrasound	Procedure that uses sound waves generated by a transducer that is placed on the neck. It shows thyroid enlargement and thyroid nodules. Also known as **thyroid ultrasonography** (see Figure 14-15 ■).	**ultrasonography**
		(UL-trah-soh-NAW-grah-fee)
		  ultra- *beyond; higher*
		  son/o- *sound*
		  -graphy *process of recording*

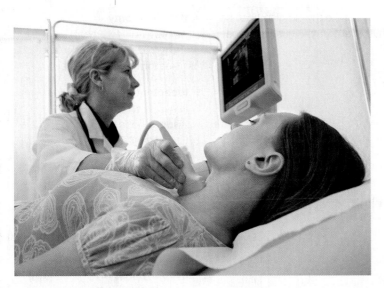

FIGURE 14-15 ■ Thyroid ultrasound.
Ultrasonography uses sound waves rather than radiation to create an image of the thyroid gland.
Source: Alexander Raths/Shutterstock

Medical and Surgical Procedures

Medical Procedures		
Word or Phase	**Description**	**Pronunciation/Word Parts**
ADA diet	Special physician-prescribed diet for diabetic patients that follows the guidelines of the American Diabetes Association (ADA). The amounts of carbohydrate and fat are limited. The physician orders the upper limit for the total daily number of calories for a diabetic patient in the hospital. Example: 1200-calorie ADA diet. Rather than using the ADA diet, diabetic patients can just count calories. A dietitian or diabetes educator helps the patient plan a menu that fits lifestyle and food preferences.	

Surgical Procedures		
adrenalectomy	Procedure to remove the adrenal gland because of an adenoma or cancerous tumor.	**adrenalectomy** (ah-DREE-nal-EK-toh-mee) **adrenal/o-** *adrenal gland* **-ectomy** *surgical removal*
fine-needle biopsy	Procedure that uses a fine needle to take a small sample of tissue from a thyroid nodule seen on a thyroid scan. The tissue is sent to the pathology department to determine if the nodule is benign or cancerous.	**biopsy** (BY-awp-see) **bi/o-** *life; living organism; living tissue* **-opsy** *process of viewing*
parathyroidectomy	Procedure to remove one or more of the parathyroid glands to treat hyperparathyroidism. Also, a parathyroidectomy can occur accidentally when the thyroid gland is surgically removed.	**parathyroidectomy** (PAIR-ah-THY-royd-EK-toh-mee) **para-** *abnormal; apart from; beside; two parts of a pair* **thyroid/o-** *thyroid gland* **-ectomy** *surgical removal*
thymectomy	Procedure to remove the thymus in patients with myasthenia gravis	**thymectomy** (thy-MEK-toh-mee) **thym/o-** *rage; thymus* **-ectomy** *surgical removal*
thyroidectomy	Procedure to remove the thyroid gland. All of the thyroid gland can be removed or just one part (**subtotal thyroidectomy**) or just one lobe (**thyroid lobectomy**).	**thyroidectomy** (THY-royd-EK-toh-mee) **thyroid/o-** *thyroid gland* **-ectomy** *surgical removal* **lobectomy** (loh-BEK-toh-mee) **lob/o-** *lobe of an organ* **-ectomy** *surgical removal*
transsphenoidal hypophysectomy	Procedure to remove an adenoma from the pituitary gland (hypophysis). The pituitary gland is difficult to visualize through an incision in the cranium, so the surgical instruments are inserted in the nose and an incision is made through the sphenoid sinus (transsphenoidal).	**transsphenoidal** (TRANS-sfee-NOY-dal) **trans-** *across; through* **sphenoid/o-** *sphenoid bone; sphenoid sinus* **-al** *pertaining to* **hypophysectomy** (HY-paw-fih-SEK-toh-mee) **hypophys/o-** *pituitary gland* **-ectomy** *surgical removal*

Drugs

These drug categories and drugs are used to treat endocrine diseases. The most common generic and trade name drugs in each category are listed.

Category	Indication	Examples	Pronunciation/Word Parts
antidiabetic drugs	Treat type 2 diabetes mellitus by stimulating the pancreas to secrete more insulin or by increasing the number of insulin receptors on cells. These drugs are given orally. They are not insulin and they are not used to treat patients with type 1 diabetes mellitus.	albiglutide (Tanzeum), dapagliflozin (Farxiga), dulaglutide (Trulicity), glyburide (DiaBeta), metformin (Glucophage), rosiglitazone (Avandia), sitagliptin (Januvia)	**antidiabetic** (AN-tee-DY-ah-BET-ik) **anti-** *against* **diabet/o-** *diabetes* **-ic** *pertaining to*
antithyroid drugs	Treat hyperthyroidism by inhibiting the production of T_3 and T_4. Alternatively, radioactive sodium iodide 131 (I-131) is given orally. It is taken up by the thyroid gland and emits low-level radiation that destroys thyroid cells. It has a short half-life and is excreted in the urine, limiting the number of cells that are destroyed. Some functioning thyroid gland tissue still remains.	methimazole (Tapazole), radioactive sodium iodide 131 (I-131)	**antithyroid** (AN-tee-THY-royd) **anti-** *against* **thyr/o-** *shield-shaped structure; thyroid gland* **-oid** *resembling*
corticosteroid drugs	Mimic the action of cortisol from the adrenal cortex. They are used to treat severe inflammation and as hormone replacement therapy for Addison's disease.	dexamethasone, hydrocortisone (Cortef, Solu-Cortef), prednisone	**corticosteroid** (KOR-tih-koh-STAIR-oyd) **cortic/o-** *cortex; outer region* **-steroid** *steroid*
growth hormone supplement drugs	Provide growth hormone.	somatropin (Humatrope, Nutropin)	

Category	Indication	Examples	Pronunciation/Word Parts
insulin	Treats type 1 and type 1.5 diabetes mellitus. It can also be used to treat type 2 diabetes mellitus that cannot be controlled with oral antidiabetic drugs. Insulin must be injected from one to several times each day to control the blood glucose level (see Figure 14-16 ■). Insulin is classified according to how quickly it acts (which depends on the size of the insulin crystal) and how many hours its therapeutic effect continues.	Rapid-acting (regular) insulins: Humulin R, Novolin R, insulin aspart (NovoLog), insulin lispro (Humalog) Intermediate-acting (NPH) insulins: Humulin N, Novolin N Long-acting insulins: insulin detemir (Levemir), insulin glargine (Lantus)	**insulin** (IN-soo-lin)
thyroid supplement drugs	Treat a lack of thyroid hormones and hypothyroidism	levothyroxine (Levothroid, Synthroid), liothyronine (Cytomel), liotrix (Thyrolar)	

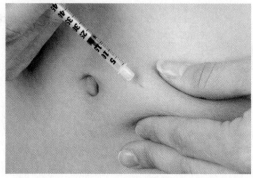

FIGURE 14-16 ■ Insulin injection.
This diabetic patient is injecting insulin using an insulin syringe that is calibrated in units. Insulin as a liquid drug must be injected subcutaneously into the fat layer beneath the skin. The skin is pinched up, and the needle is inserted at an angle so that it does not go into the muscle beneath. The back of the arms, abdomen, and many other sites can be used for insulin injections. A new site must be selected for each injection.
Source: Dmitry Lobanov/Fotolia

Abbreviations

ACTH	adrenocorticotropic hormone		**K, K⁺**	potassium
ADA	American Diabetes Association, American Dietetic Association		**LADA**	latent autoimmune diabetes in adults
			LH	luteinizing hormone
ADH	antidiuretic hormone		**MSH**	melanocyte-stimulating hormone
AODM	adult-onset diabetes mellitus		**Na, Na⁺**	sodium
Ca, Ca⁺⁺	calcium		**NIDDM**	non-insulin-dependent diabetes mellitus
CDE	certified diabetes educator		**NPH**	neutral protamine Hagedorn (insulin)
DI	diabetes insipidus		**OGTT**	oral glucose tolerance test
DKA	diabetic ketoacidosis		**RAIU**	radioactive iodine uptake
DM	diabetes mellitus		**RIA**	radioimmunoassay
FBG	fasting blood glucose		**SAD**	seasonal affective disorder
FBS	fasting blood sugar		**SIADH**	syndrome of inappropriate ADH
FSH	follicle-stimulating hormone		**T₃**	triiodothyronine
FTI	free thyroxine index		**T₄**	thyroxine
GH	growth hormone		**T₇**	free thyroxine index (FTI)
GTT	glucose tolerance test		**TFTs**	thyroid function tests
HbA₁C	hemoglobin A₁C		**TSH**	thyroid-stimulating hormone
IDDM	insulin-dependent diabetes mellitus		**VMA**	vanillylmandelic acid
IRS	insulin resistance syndrome			

WORD ALERT
Abbreviations

Abbreviations are commonly used in all types of medical documents; however, they can mean different things to different people and their meanings can be misinterpreted. Always verify the meaning of an abbreviation.

ADA means *American Diabetes Association,* but it also means *American Dietetic Association*, *American Dental Association,* and *Americans with Disabilities Act*.

Ca means *calcium,* but it also means *cancer.*

GTT means *glucose tolerance test,* but *gtt.* means *drops.*

NPH means *neutral protamine Hagedorn* (insulin), but it also means *normal pressure hydrocephalus.*

IT'S GREEK TO ME!

Did you notice that some words have two different combining forms? Combining forms from both Greek and Latin remain a part of medical language today.

Word	Greek	Latin	Medical Word Examples
female	gynec/o-	estr/a-, estr/o-	gynecomastia, estradiol, estrogens
male, masculine	andr/o-	viril/o-	androgens, virilism
milk	galact/o-	lact/o-	galactorrhea, prolactin
pituitary gland	hypophys/o-	pituitar/o-, pituit/o-	adenohypophysis, hypopituitarism, pituitary

CAREER FOCUS

Meet Maureen, a diabetes educator

"I worked in a large city hospital that had a very large diabetic population, and that's how I got interested in the disease. On a typical day we see patients who have had diabetes anywhere from just a few weeks to years. Diabetic education has really changed a lot because we're really trying to empower the patient. The person lives with diabetes every day, so they should have the tools to take care of their diabetes. The more information they have, the better choices that they're going to make. What we try and do is teach them how—about their food, how to monitor their blood glucose, what their medications are, how to take them properly and consistently, and what to do if their blood glucose is either too high or too low."

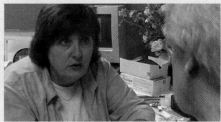

Source: Dan Frank for Pearson Education/PH College/Pearson Education

Diabetes educators are allied health professionals who counsel and educate patients with diabetes mellitus and their families. They work in hospitals, clinics, and some physicians' offices.

Endocrinologists are physicians who practice in the specialty of endocrinology. They diagnose and treat patients with diseases of the endocrine system. Some endocrinologists specialize and become **diabetologists** who only treat patients with diabetes mellitus. Physicians can take additional training and become board certified in the subspecialties of reproductive endocrinology or pediatric endocrinology. Surgery on the endocrine system is performed by a general surgeon or a neurosurgeon. Cancerous tumors of the endocrine system are treated medically by an oncologist or surgically by a general surgeon or neurosurgeon.

---

endocrinologist (EN-doh-krih-NAW-loh-jist)
  endo- *innermost; within*
  crin/o- *secrete*
  log/o- *study of; word*
  -ist *person who specializes in; thing that specializes in*

---

diabetologist (DY-ah-beh-TAW-loh-jist)
  diabet/o- *diabetes*
  log/o- *study of; word*
  -ist *person who specializes in; thing that specializes in*

MyMedicalTerminologyLab™

To see Maureen's complete video profile, log into MyMedicalTerminologyLab and navigate to the Multimedia Library for Chapter 14. Check the Video box, and then click the Career Focus - Diabetic Educator link.

MULTIPLE COMBINING FORMS AND SUFFIX EXERCISE

Read the definition of the medical word. Select the correct suffix and combining forms. Then build the medical word and write it on the line. Be sure to check your spelling. The first one has been done for you.

SUFFIX LIST	COMBINING FORM LIST	
-al (pertaining to)	acid/o- (acid; low pH)	ket/o- (ketones)
-ar (pertaining to)	adren/o- (adrenal gland)	mast/o- (breast; mastoid process)
-ia (condition; state; thing)	chrom/o- (color)	mult/i- (many)
-oma (mass; tumor)	cyt/o- (cell)	nodul/o- (small, knobby mass)
-osis (condition; process)	genit/o- (genitalia)	phe/o- (gray)
	glycos/o- (glucose; sugar)	ur/o- (urinary system; urine)
	gynec/o- (female; woman)	

Definition of the Medical Word

1. Pertaining to many small, knobby mass(es)
2. Condition (in which) ketones (cause the blood to become) acid (with a) low pH
3. Pertaining to (the) adrenal gland (hormones affecting the) genitalia
4. Tumor (with a) gray color (to the) cells (when viewed under the microscope) (*Hint*: Use 3 combining forms.)
5. Condition (of enlargement in which the male's chest resembles the) female breast.
6. Condition (of) glucose (in the) urine

Build the Medical Word

multinodular

_____

_____

_____

_____

_____

14.7A Spell Medical Words

PROOFREADING AND SPELLING EXERCISE

Read the following paragraph. Identify each misspelled medical word and write the correct spelling of it on the line.

Endocrineology is the study of glands and hormones. The pituatary gland is the master gland. In diabetes mellitus, there is too much glukose and not enough insulin. A tumor in the adrenal medula is a feochromocytoma. If there is an adenoma in the thyroid gland, then a thyroectomy would be done. Graves' disease is known for exofthalmos and a goiter. An enlarged thyroid gland is thyromegalee. Galactorhea is milk production in a woman who is not pregnant.

1. _____	6. _____
2. _____	7. _____
3. _____	8. _____
4. _____	9. _____
5. _____	10. _____

HEARING MEDICAL WORDS EXERCISE

You hear someone speaking the medical words given below. Read each pronunciation and then write the medical word it represents. Be sure to check your spelling. The first one has been done for you.

1. DY-ah-BEE-teez	*diabetes*	5. IN-fer-TIL-ih-tee	_____
2. AD-eh-NOH-mah	_____	6. SIN-er-jizm	_____
3. GLAN-dyoo-lar	_____	7. THY-royd-EK-toh-mee	_____
4. HY-per-gly-SEE-mee-ah	_____		

14.7B Pronounce Medical Words

PRONUNCIATION EXERCISE

Read the medical word and the syllables in its pronunciation. Circle the primary (main) accented syllable. The first one has been done for you.

1. hormone (hor-mohn)
2. ovarian (oh-vair-ee-an)
3. cortisol (kor-tih-sawl)
4. diabetic (dy-ah-bet-ik)
5. endocrinology (en-doh-krih-naw-loh-jee)
6. homeostasis (hoh-mee-oh-stay-sis)
7. pituitary (pih-too-eh-tair-ee)

14.8 Research Medical Words

SOUND-ALIKE WORDS

Compare and contrast the medical meanings of these sound-alike endocrinology and other words.

1. *endocrine gland* and *exocrine gland* (Chapter 7)
2. *melatonin* and *melanin* (Chapter 7)
3. *diabetes insipidus* and *diabetes mellitus*

14.9 Analyze Medical Report

ELECTRONIC PATIENT RECORD

This is an Office Visit Note. Read the Note and answer the questions.

PEARSON PRIMARY CARE ASSOCIATES

Task   Edit   View   Time Scale   Options   Help

OFFICE VISIT NOTE

PATIENT NAME:	BAKER, Randolph
PATIENT NUMBER:	86-7943
DATE OF VISIT:	November 19, 20xx

Source: Mat Hayward/Fotolia

HISTORY: This is a 54-year-old male who presents with fatigue. He also has headaches. Because of a history of some visual field defects during his headaches, his ophthalmologist ordered an MRI of the brain. I reviewed the scans and did not see anything but the expected postsurgical changes of the brain. Lab tests show that he does have some residual function of the pituitary gland, so his endocrinologist only placed him on testosterone transdermal patches and thyroid hormone replacement (Synthroid). He also has a history of depression, which could explain the fatigue and headache, or they could be due to low thyroid hormone replacement levels.

PHYSICAL EXAMINATION: HEENT: Normal. Lungs: Clear to auscultation. Cardiovascular: Regular rate and rhythm, without murmurs, rubs, or gallops. Abdomen: Nondistended, nontender. Extremities: No edema.

ASSESSMENT:

1. Fatigue. Possibly hypothyroidism. Will check T_3, T_4, and TSH levels.

2. Headache, possibly within the context of depression. He is on a rather low dose of an antidepressant drug at this time.

3. Hypopituitarism, after surgical removal of an adenoma.

PLAN:

1. Will obtain an FSH, LH, free and total testosterone, and baseline ACTH.

2. Follow up in 1 week.

Edward Allen Selcher, M.D.
_____

Edward Allen Selcher, M.D.

EAS:blg
D: 11/19/xx
T: 11/19/xx

1. Divide *endocrinologist* into its four word parts and give the meaning of each word part.

   Word Part   **Meaning**

   _____   _____

   _____   _____

   _____   _____

   _____   _____

2. Divide *hypopituitarism* into its three word parts and give the meaning of each word part.

   Word Part   **Meaning**

   _____   _____

   _____   _____

   _____   _____

3. What is the abbreviation for *thyroid-stimulating hormone?* _____

4. Besides the physician who dictated this report, what two physician specialists have also recently seen the patient?

   _____   _____

5. What two hormones does the patient already take as drugs for hormone replacement therapy?

   _____   _____

6. What do these abbreviations mean?

   ADH: _____

   FSH: _____

   LH: _____

7. The patient is taking Synthroid for his (**headaches**, **hypothyroidism**, **lungs**). Circle the correct answer.

8. The patient's fatigue, headache, and visual field defects could be signs of a recurring tumor in the brain. What test has already been done to look for a tumor?

   _____

9. The patient's MRI of the brain showed postsurgical changes, meaning changes that are present because of a surgery that was done. Which endocrine gland was operated on in the past?

   _____

10. Which of the patient's drugs correlates with doing the lab tests for T_3, T_4, and TSH?

   _____

MyMedicalTerminologyLab™

MyMedicalTerminologyLab is a premium online homework management system that includes a host of features to help you study. Registered users will find:

- A multitude of quizzes and activities built within the MyLab platform

- Powerful tools that track and analyze your results—allowing you to create a personalized learning experience

- Videos and audio pronunciations to help enrich your progress

- Streaming lesson presentations (Guided Lectures) and self-paced learning modules

- A space where you and your instructor can check your progress and manage your assignments

Chapter 15
Ophthalmology

Eye

Ophthalmology (OFF-thal-MAW-loh-jee) is the medical specialty that studies the anatomy and physiology of the eye and uses laboratory and diagnostic procedures, medical and surgical procedures, and drugs to treat eye diseases.

Learning Outcomes

After you study this chapter, you should be able to

15.1 Identify structures of the eye.

15.2 Describe the process of vision.

15.3 Describe common eye diseases, laboratory and diagnostic procedures, medical and surgical procedures, and drugs.

15.4 Form the plural and adjective forms of nouns related to ophthalmology.

15.5 Give the meanings of word parts and abbreviations related to ophthalmology.

15.6 Divide ophthalmology words and build ophthalmology words.

15.7 Spell and pronounce ophthalmology words.

15.8 Research sound-alike and other ophthalmology words.

15.9 Analyze the medical content and meaning of an ophthalmology report.

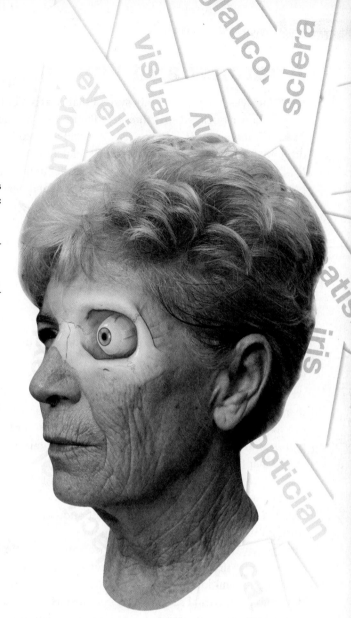

FIGURE 15-1 ■ Eye.
The eyes consist of two identical but individual organs that sit in bony sockets of the cranium. Nerves connect the eyes to the visual cortex in the brain to provide the special sense of sight.
Source: Pearson Education

Medical Language Key

To unlock the definition of a medical word, break it into word parts. Give the meaning of each word part. Put the meanings of the word parts in order, beginning with the meaning of the suffix, then the prefix (if present), then the combining form(s).

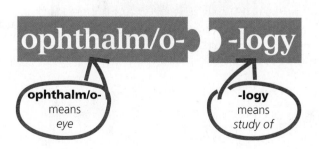

	Word Part	**Word Part Meaning**
Suffix	**-logy**	*study of*
Combining Form	**ophthalm/o-**	*eye*

Ophthalmology: ▶ *Study of (the) eye (and related structures).*

Anatomy and Physiology

The eyes belong to a body system that consists of two identical main organs and many associated structures (see Figure 15-1 ■). Each eye or **optic globe** is located within an **orbit**, a hollow bony socket in the anterior cranium. The walls of the orbit are made up of several different cranial and facial bones (discussed in "Orthopedics," Chapter 8). The bony orbit surrounds all but the anterior surface of the eye. In the posterior wall of the orbit, the optic nerve (cranial nerve II), arteries, and veins come through openings in the bone to reach the eye. Within the bony orbit, a layer of fat cushions and protects the eye. The purpose of the eyes is to provide sensory information that can be interpreted by the visual cortex in the brain to become the sense of sight.

Anatomy of the Eye
Eyelid and Lacrimal Gland

The upper and lower **eyelids** protect the delicate tissues of the eye. The eyelids blink involuntarily to prevent foreign substances from entering the eye. The eyelids also blink many times a minute to spread a layer of tears that keeps the surface of the eye moist. At the edges of the eyelids, sebaceous glands secrete oil that acts as a barrier to keep tears in the eye. The **eyelashes** form a protective barrier that extends outward from the eye to prevent foreign substances from coming in contact with the eye. The sebaceous glands and eyelashes are part of the integumentary system (discussed in "Dermatology," Chapter 7).

The **caruncle** is the red, triangular tissue at the medial corner where the eyelids meet. The **lacrimal gland** is located in the superior-lateral aspect of each eye (see Figure 15-2 ■). The lacrimal glands continuously produce and release tears that travel through the **lacrimal ducts**. Large amounts of tears are produced when the eye is irritated or invaded by a foreign substance and during times of emotional distress. Tears contain an antibacterial enzyme to prevent bacterial infections. At the medial aspects of the upper and lower eyelids, two tiny openings drain away excess tears. Those tears flow into the **lacrimal sac** and then into the **nasolacrimal duct** to the inside of the nose. That is why, when your eyes water, your nose also runs!

Pronunciation/Word Parts

optic (AWP-tik)
   opt/o- *eye; vision*
   -ic *pertaining to*
The combining forms **ocul/o-** and **ophthalm/o-** also mean *eye*.

orbit (OR-bit)

eyelid (EYE-lid)
The combining form **blephar/o-** means *eyelid*.

caruncle (KAR-ung-kl)

lacrimal (LAK-rih-mal)
   lacrim/o- *tears*
   -al *pertaining to*
The combining form **dacry/o-** means *lacrimal sac; tears*.

nasolacrimal (NAY-soh-LAK-rih-mal)
   nas/o- *nose*
   lacrim/o- *tears*
   -al *pertaining to*

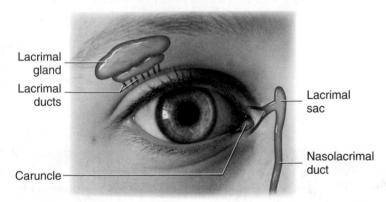

Lacrimal gland
Lacrimal ducts
Caruncle
Lacrimal sac
Nasolacrimal duct

FIGURE 15-2 ■ Lacrimal glands.
The lacrimal glands release tears to lubricate the anterior surface of the eye. Excess tears flow into the lacrimal sac, drain into the nasolacrimal duct, and eventually enter the nose.
Source: Pearson Education

Conjunctiva, Sclera, and Cornea

The **conjunctiva** is a delicate, transparent mucous membrane that covers the insides of the eyelids and the anterior surface of the eye (see Figure 15-4). The conjunctiva produces watery, clear mucus that traps any foreign substances on the surface of the eye.

Beneath that, the **sclera** is a tough, fibrous, connective tissue that forms a continuous outer layer around the eye. This tissue is white and opaque and is known as the *white of the eye* (see Figures 15-3 ■ and 15-4 ■). The sclera protects the internal structures of the eye and helps maintain the shape of the eye. The sclera is the site of attachment for all of the muscles that move the eye (see Figure 15-9).

Pronunciation/Word Parts

conjunctiva (CON-junk-TY-vah)
(con-JUNK-tih-vah)

conjunctivae (CON-junk-TY-vee)
(con-JUNK-tih-vee)
Conjunctiva is a Latin singular noun. Form the plural by changing *-a* to *-ae*.

conjunctival (CON-junk-TY-val)
(con-JUNK-tih-val)
    conjunctiv/o- *conjunctiva of the eye*
    -al *pertaining to*

sclera (SKLEER-ah)

sclerae (SKLEER-ee)
Sclera is a Latin singular noun. Form the plural by changing *-a* to *-ae*.

scleral (SKLEER-al)
    scler/o- *hard; sclera of the eye*
    -al *pertaining to*

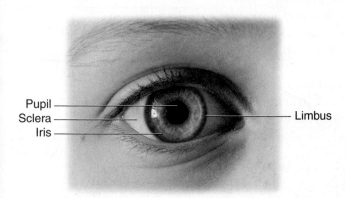

Pupil —
Sclera —
Iris —
— Limbus

FIGURE 15-3 ■ Anterior surface of the eye.
The anterior surface is the only part of the eye that is visible on the surface of the body. The sclera (white of the eye), iris, pupil, and limbus are part of this area. The cornea is the transparent layer over the iris and pupil.
Source: Pearson Education

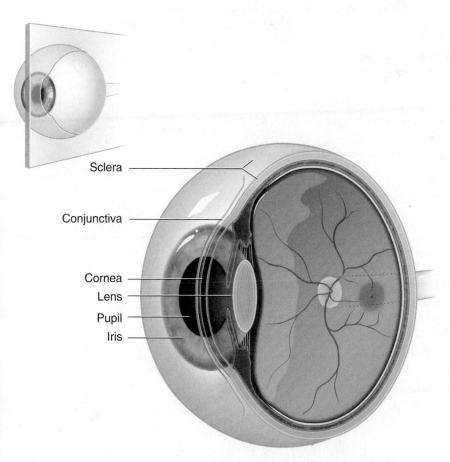

Sclera —

Conjunctiva —

Cornea —
Lens —
Pupil —
Iris —

FIGURE 15-4 ■ External and internal structures at the front of the eye.
The transparent conjunctiva covers the anterior surface of the eye and the inner eyelids. The white sclera surrounds the entire eye. On the anterior surface of the eye, the sclera changes into the transparent cornea. The colored iris and the central pupil can be seen through the cornea. The lens of the eye is behind the iris.
Source: Pearson Education

Across the anterior surface of the eye, the white sclera changes into a transparent layer known as the **cornea** (see Figure 15-4). The transitional line between the white sclera and the clear cornea is known as the **limbus** (see Figure 15-3). The cornea allows light to enter the eye. It also bends (refracts) the rays of light. The cornea itself contains no blood vessels. It receives oxygen and nutrients from tears that flow across its surface and from aqueous humor that flows beneath it in the anterior chamber. The cornea does have nerves, however, and it is the most sensitive area on the anterior surface of the eye.

Iris and Pupil

The iris and pupil can be seen behind the transparent cornea. The **iris** is a circular structure whose color is determined by genetics. At the center of the iris is the **pupil**, a round opening that allows light rays to enter the eye (see Figure 15-4). The pupil itself appears black because very little light is reflected from the back of the eye. However, if you take a picture with flash photography, this intense light does reflect from the back of the eye, and the photograph shows an eye with a red pupil because of blood vessels in the back of the eye.

In bright light, muscles in the iris contract to constrict and decrease the diameter of the pupil. This process, which is known as **miosis**, keeps too much light from entering the eye. In dim light, muscles in the iris relax to dilate and increase the diameter of the pupil. This process, which is known as **mydriasis**, allows more light to enter the eye.

CLINICAL CONNECTIONS

Genetics. Eye color is a genetically determined trait. In each cell, chromosome 15 contains genes for brown/blue and brown/brown eye colors. Chromosome 19 contains a gene for blue/green eye colors. Each parent contributes combinations of these genes to their baby.

At birth, all babies' eyes appear slate gray to blue in color because of the lack of the brown pigment melanin in the iris. Exposure to light triggers the production of melanin by melanocytes in the iris. Babies who inherit a brown/brown or brown/blue gene have a large number of melanocytes in their iris, and they develop dark brown or light brown eyes. Babies who inherit a blue/blue or blue/green gene have no melanocytes in the iris, and their eyes are blue, hazel, or green.

Choroid and Ciliary Body

The **choroid** is a spongy membrane of blood vessels that is part of the internal structure of the eye (see Figure 15-5 ■). It begins at the outer edge of the iris. It cannot be seen on the anterior surface of the eye because it lies beneath the white sclera. In the posterior cavity, the choroid is the middle layer between the sclera and the retina. The blood vessels of the choroid supply blood to the eye.

The **ciliary body** is an extension of the choroid (see Figure 15-5). It attaches to suspensory ligaments that hold the lens in place behind the iris. The ciliary body contains muscles that contract and relax to change the shape of the lens to focus light rays coming through the pupil. The ciliary body also produces aqueous humor.

Pronunciation/Word Parts

cornea (KOR-nee-ah)

corneae (KOR-nee-ee)
Cornea is a Latin singular noun. Form the plural by changing *-a* to *-ae*.

corneal (KOR-nee-al)
    corne/o- *cornea of the eye*
    -al *pertaining to*
The combining form **kerat/o-** means *cornea of the eye; hard, fibrous protein.*

limbus (LIM-bus)

iris (EYE-ris)

irides (IH-rih-deez)
Iris is a Greek singular noun. Form the plural by changing *-is* to *-ides.*

iridal (IH-rih-dal) (EYE-rih-dal)
    irid/o- *iris of the eye*
    -al *pertaining to*
The combining form **ir/o-** also means *iris of the eye.*

pupil (PYOO-pil)

pupillary (PYOO-pih-LAIR-ee)
    pupill/o- *pupil of the eye*
    -ary *pertaining to*
The combining form **cor/o-** also means *pupil of the eye.*

miosis (my-OH-sis)
    mi/o- *narrowing*
    -osis *condition; process*
Add words to make a complete definition of *miosis: process (of) narrowing (the size of the pupil).*

mydriasis (mih-DRY-eh-sis)
    mydr/o- *widening*
    -iasis *process ; state*

choroid (KOH-royd)

choroidal (koh-ROY-dal)
    choroid/o- *choroid of the eye*
    -al *pertaining to*

ciliary (SIL-ee-AIR-ee)
    cili/o- *hair-like structure*
    -ary *pertaining to*
The combining form **cycl/o-** means *ciliary body of the eye; circle; cycle.*

The **uvea** or **uveal tract** is a collective word for the iris, choroid, and ciliary body.

Pronunciation/Word Parts

uvea (YOO-vee-ah)

uveal (YOO-vee-al)
  uve/o- *uvea of the eye*
  -al *pertaining to*

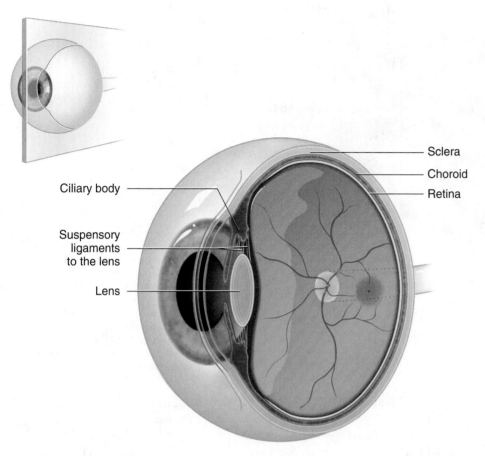

FIGURE 15-5 ■ Tissue layers of the eye.
The sclera (white of the eye) continues around the entire eye except in the area of the transparent cornea. Its tough, fibrous connective tissue helps to maintain the shape of the eye. The choroid layer beneath the sclera contains blood vessels. The ciliary body is an extension of the choroid. The retina lines the curved wall of the posterior cavity.
Source: Pearson Education

lens (LENZ)

lenses (LEN-sez)

capsule (KAP-sool)

lenticular (len-TIH-kyoo-lar)
  lenticul/o- *lens of the eye*
  -ar *pertaining to*
The combining forms **lent/o-**, **phac/o-**, and **phak/o-** also mean *lens of the eye*.

capsular (KAP-soo-lar)
  capsul/o- *capsule; enveloping structure*
  -ar *pertaining to*

accommodation (ah-KAW-moh-DAY-shun)
  accommod/o- *adapt*
  -ation *being; having; process*

anterior (an-TEER-ee-or)
  anter/o- *before; front part*
  -ior *pertaining to*

posterior (pos-TEER-ee-or)
  poster/o- *back part*
  -ior *pertaining to*

Lens

The **lens** is a clear, flexible disk behind the pupil. It contains protein molecules arranged in a crystalline structure that makes the lens transparent (see Figure 15-5). The lens is surrounded by the **lens capsule**, a clear membrane. Through the process of **accommodation**, the lens changes shape. The muscles of the ciliary body contract or relax to move the suspensory ligaments that are attached to the lens. The lens becomes thicker and more rounded to allow you to see objects close by (near vision) or thinner and flatter to see objects at a distance (far vision).

Anterior and Posterior Chambers

The **anterior chamber** is a small space between the cornea and the iris (see Figure 15-6 ■). The **posterior chamber** is a very narrow space posterior to the iris. The iris forms a dividing wall between the anterior and posterior chambers of the anterior

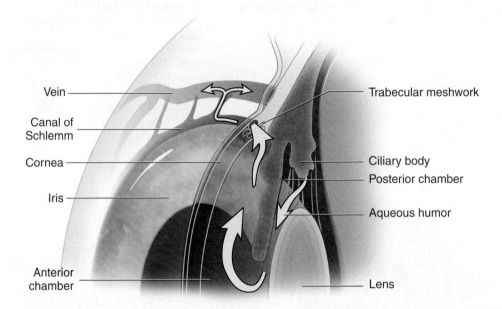

Vein

Canal of Schlemm

Cornea

Iris

Anterior chamber

Trabecular meshwork

Ciliary body

Posterior chamber

Aqueous humor

Lens

FIGURE 15-6 ■ Aqueous humor.
Aqueous humor produced by the ciliary body circulates through the posterior chamber, pupil, and anterior chamber. It drains out through the trabecular meshwork.

Source: Pearson Education

eye. The only opening in this wall is the pupil. The anterior and posterior chambers are both filled with aqueous humor.

Aqueous humor is a clear, watery fluid that is produced continuously by the ciliary body. Aqueous humor carries nutrients and oxygen to the cornea and lens. Aqueous humor circulates through the posterior chamber, through the pupil, and into the anterior chamber. It then drains through the **trabecular meshwork**, interlacing fibers all around the edge of the iris where it meets the cornea and forms an angle. The aqueous humor then drains into the canal of Schlemm, a circular canal around the iris. From there, the aqueous humor is absorbed into the blood. The rate of production of aqueous humor normally equals the rate of drainage.

Posterior Cavity

The **posterior cavity** is the largest space in the eye. It lies between the lens and the retina (see Figure 15-7 ■). It is filled with **vitreous humor**, a clear, gel-like substance that helps maintain the shape of the eye.

Retina

The **retina** is a thin layer of tissue that lines the curved wall of the posterior cavity (see Figures 15-5, 15-7, and 15-8 ■). The choroid layer lies beneath the retina and provides blood to the retina. **Fundus** is a general word for *retina* because the retina is the area that is farthest from the opening to the eye (the pupil).

There are two distinct landmarks on the retina. The **optic disk** is a bright, yellow-white circle with distinct edges in the area of the retina closest to the nose. This is where the **optic nerve** (cranial nerve II) enters the eye. The retinal arteries also enter through

aqueous humor (AA-kwee-us HYOO-mor)
   aque/o- *watery substance*
   -ous *pertaining to*

trabecular (trah-BEH-kyoo-lar)
   trabecul/o- *mesh*
   -ar *pertaining to*

cavity (KAV-ih-tee)
   cav/o- *hollow space*
   -ity *condition; state*

vitreous humor (VIT-ree-us HYOO-mor)
   vitre/o- *transparent substance; vitreous humor*
   -ous *pertaining to*

retina (RET-ih-nah)

retinae (RET-ih-nee)
Retina is a Latin singular noun. Form the plural by changing *-a* to *-ae*.

retinal (RET-ih-nal)
   retin/o- *retina of the eye*
   -al *pertaining to*

fundus (FUN-dus)

fundi (FUN-die)
Fundus is a Latin singular noun. Form the plural by changing *-us* to *-i*.

fundal (FUN-dal)
   fund/o- *fundus; part farthest from the opening*
   -al *pertaining to*
The combining form **fundu/o-** has the same meaning.

optic (AWP-tik)
   opt/o- *eye; vision*
   -ic *pertaining to*

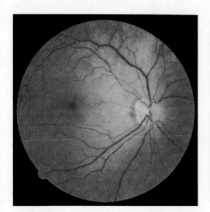

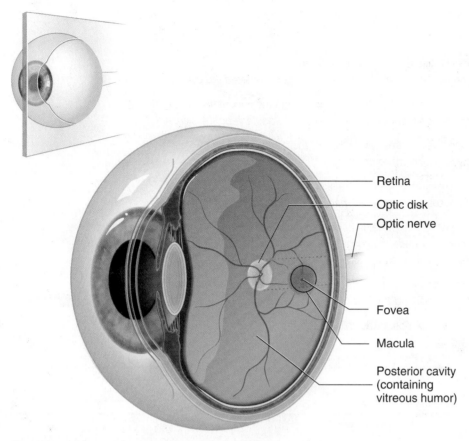

Retina
Optic disk
Optic nerve
Fovea
Macula
Posterior cavity
(containing
vitreous humor)

FIGURE 15-7 ■ Internal structures at the back of the eye.
The posterior cavity is filled with vitreous humor. The retina contains the macula (area of sharpest
vision) and the optic disk (area where the optic nerve enters).
Source: Pearson Education

the optic disk and spread across the retina, and the retinal veins leave the eye at the
optic disk. The optic disk is not stimulated by light or color and cannot receive sensory
information. It is known as the **blind spot**. The second landmark is the **macula**, a dark
yellow-orange area. The **fovea** is a small depression in the center of the macula. The
fovea lies directly opposite the pupil. Light rays entering the pupil fall on the macula,
specifically the fovea, which is the area of sharpest vision.

macula (MAK-yoo-lah)

maculae (MAK-yoo-lee)
Macula is a Latin singular noun. Form the
plural by changing *-a* to *-ae.*

macular (MAK-yoo-lar)
  macul/o- *small area; spot*
  -ar *pertaining to*

fovea (FOH-vee-ah)

foveae (FOH-vee-ee)
Fovea is a Latin singular noun. Form the
plural by changing *-a* to *-ae.*

foveal (FOH-vee-al)
  fove/o- *small, depressed area*
  -al *pertaining to*

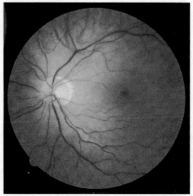

FIGURE 15-8 ■ Retinae of both eyes.
Dilation of the pupil permits visualization of the retina. The structures of the optic
disk, retinal blood vessels, and macula can clearly be seen. Note that the size and
shape of these structures are not identical in each eye.
Source: Susan M. Turley

WORD ALERT
Sound-Alike Words

caruncle (noun) red, triangular tissue at the medial corner of the eye
Example: The caruncle became irritated when a foreign substance entered the eye.

carbuncle (noun) large abscess on the skin that tunnels through the subcutaneous tissue
Example: A carbuncle contains pus from an infection caused by bacteria on the skin.

macula (noun) dark, orange-yellow area with indistinct margins located on the retina
Example: The macula showed degenerative changes.

macule (noun) small, flat, pigmented spot on the skin
Example: Sun exposure increases the number of macules (freckles) on the skin.

macular (adjective) descriptive word that pertains to both the macula of the eye and a macule on the skin
Examples: The patient has macular degeneration of the eye.
The patient has a macular-papular rash on the skin.

miosis (noun) decreasing diameter of the pupil when the muscles of the iris contract
Example: Bright light causes miosis, and the size of the pupil decreases.

mitosis (noun) process by which most body cells reproduce
Example: In mitosis, the dividing cell duplicates and then splits into two cells.

A CLOSER LOOK

The optic nerve (cranial nerve II) is a sensory nerve that carries sensory information from the retina to the optic chiasm (see Figure 15-11). The **oculomotor nerve** (cranial nerve III) is a motor nerve that carries motor commands from the brain to four of the six extraocular muscles to move the eye, to the eyelids to produce movement, and to the muscles of the iris to contract or relax (to decrease or increase the diameter of the pupil). The trochlear nerve (cranial nerve IV) is a motor nerve that carries motor commands from the brain to one extraocular muscle (the superior oblique muscle) to produce movements of the eye. The trigeminal nerve (cranial nerve V) is a sensory nerve that carries sensory information from the skin of the eyelids and eyebrows to the brain. The abducens nerve (cranial nerve VI) is a motor nerve that carries motor commands from the brain to one extraocular muscle (the lateral rectus muscle) to produce movements of the eye. The facial nerve (cranial nerve VII) is a motor nerve that carries motor commands from the brain to the lacrimal glands to produce tears.

oculomotor (AW-kyoo-loh-MOH-tor)
ocul/o- eye
mot/o- movement
-or person who does; person who produces; thing that does; thing that produces

Extraocular Muscles

The **extraocular muscles** control the movements of the eye. Four of these are straight muscles (and have *rectus* in their names). The other two wrap around the eye in a slanted manner (and have *oblique* in their names) (see Figure 15-9 ■). The extraocular muscles are attached to the sclera by tendons. The movement of the extraocular muscles is under voluntary control.

Pronunciation/Word Parts

extraocular (EKS-trah-AW-kyoo-lar)
extra- outside
ocul/o- eye
-ar pertaining to

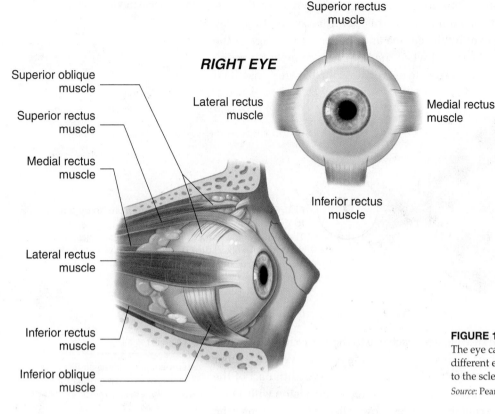

FIGURE 15-9 ■ Extraocular muscles.
The eye can move in all directions because of six different extraocular muscles attached by tendons to the sclera.
Source: Pearson Education

Extraocular Muscles

- **Superior rectus muscle**: Turns the eye superiorly
- **Inferior rectus muscle**: Turns the eye inferiorly
- **Medial rectus muscle**: Turns the eye medially (toward the midline)
- **Lateral rectus muscle**: Turns the eye laterally (away from the midline)
- **Superior oblique muscle**: Turns the eye inferiorly and medially
- **Inferior oblique muscle**: Turns the eye superiorly and laterally

Physiology of Vision

The process of sight or **vision** begins as light rays from an object pass through the cornea, which bends the rays (the process of **refraction**) to begin to focus them. The light rays then enter the pupil and pass through the lens. Muscles in the ciliary body contract or relax to change the shape of the lens to bend and focus the light rays. Light rays from objects directly in the line of vision fall on the macula (specifically the fovea), and these objects produce the clearest, sharpest image. Other parts of the retina pick up light rays from objects at the edges of the visual field.

The retina contains special light-sensitive cells known as *rods* and *cones*. **Rods** are sensitive in all levels of light and detect black and white, but not color. Rods function in daytime and nighttime vision. It only takes one photon (light particle) to activate a rod, so rods can detect objects in very low light, but they only produce a somewhat grainy black-and-white image of that object.

Cones are only sensitive to color. There are three different types of cones that respond to either red light, green light, or blue light. The cones are concentrated in the macula. It takes many photons to activate a cone, which is why it is difficult to see colors in dim light. Cones produce a sharp color image that is superimposed on the black-and-white image created by the rods.

superior (soo-PEER-ee-or)
  super/o- *above*
  -ior *pertaining to*

inferior (in-FEER-ee-or)
  infer/o- *below*
  -ior *pertaining to*

rectus (REK-tus)
Rectus is a Latin word that means *straight*.

medial (MEE-dee-al)
  medi/o- *middle*
  -al *pertaining to*

lateral (LAT-er-al)
  later/o- *side*
  -al *pertaining to*

oblique (oh-BLEEK)
Oblique is an English word that means *on a slant*.

vision (VIH-shun)
  vis/o- *sight; vision*
  -ion *action; condition*

refraction (re-FRAK-shun)
  re- *again and again; backward; unable to*
  fract/o- *bend; break up*
  -ion *action; condition*
Select the correct prefix meaning to get the definition of *refraction*: *action (to) again and again bend (light rays)*.

When a person looks at an object, the rods and cones everywhere in the retina respond to the light rays to create an image. At this point, because of the way in which the light rays have been bent by the cornea and the lens, the image of the object is actually upside down and backward when the light rays come to the retina (see Figure 15-10 ■). The image is then converted to nerve impulses that are transmitted to the optic nerve.

Pronunciation/Word Parts

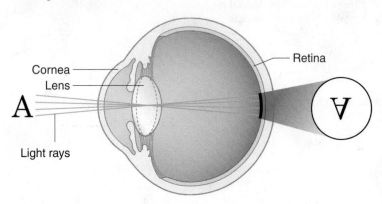

Cornea
Lens
A
Light rays
Retina

FIGURE 15-10 ■ Light rays coming from an object to the retina.
The cornea and lens focus light rays from an object onto the retina. An object directly in the line of vision produces an image on the macula. This image is sharp and clear, but upside down and backward.
Source: Pearson Education

The optic nerve (cranial nerve II) travels from each eye to the **optic chiasm**, a crossing point where parts of one optic nerve cross over to join the optic nerve on the other side, and vice versa. This merges part of the visual field of one eye with part of the visual field of the other eye to create three-dimensional, **stereoscopic vision** with a perception of depth and distance. These combined nerves (now called *optic tracts*) enter the **thalamus** in the brain. There the sensory information they carry is interpreted so that, if needed, there can be a motor command reflex sent out to blink or move away from something coming toward the eye. The sensory information is also sent to the **visual cortex** in the right and left occipital lobes of the brain (see Figure 15-11 ■). The visual cortex merges the image from each eye to create a single, three-dimensional image and turns that image so that it is right side up and facing in the direction of the original object. Another area in the occipital lobe associates this visual image with long-term visual memories and communicates with the frontal lobe of the brain where decisions are made about the meaning of what was seen and what to do about it.

chiasm (KY-azm)

stereoscopic (STAIR-ee-oh-SKAW-pik)
  stere/o- *three dimensions*
  scop/o- *examine with an instrument*
  -ic *pertaining to*

thalamus (THAL-ah-mus)

visual (VIH-shoo-al)
  vis/o- *sight; vision*
  -ual *pertaining to*
The combining from **op/o-** means *vision*.

cortex (KOR-teks)

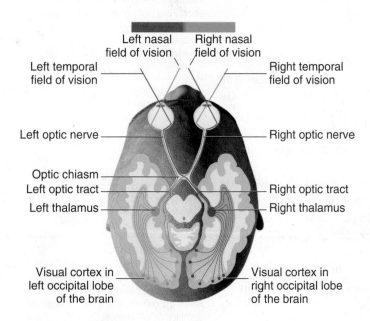

Left nasal field of vision
Right nasal field of vision
Left temporal field of vision
Right temporal field of vision
Left optic nerve
Right optic nerve
Optic chiasm
Left optic tract
Right optic tract
Left thalamus
Right thalamus
Visual cortex in left occipital lobe of the brain
Visual cortex in right occipital lobe of the brain

FIGURE 15-11 ■ Optic nerve, optic chiasm, thalamus, and visual cortex.
The image of an object travels as sensory information through the optic nerve (cranial nerve II) to the optic chiasm, through the optic tracts to the thalamus, and then to the visual cortex in each occipital lobe of the brain where it is interpreted.
Source: Pearson Education

Vocabulary Review

Anatomy and Physiology		
Word or Phrase	**Description**	**Combining Forms**
accommodation	Change in the shape of the lens as the muscles of the ciliary body contract or relax to move the suspensory ligaments to the lens. The lens becomes thicker and more rounded to see objects close by or thinner and flatter to see objects at a distance.	**accommod/o-** *adapt*
anterior chamber	Small space between the cornea and the iris. Aqueous humor circulates through it.	**anter/o-** *before; front part*
aqueous humor	Clear, watery fluid produced continuously by the ciliary body. It circulates through the posterior chamber, pupil, and then the anterior chamber; it takes nutrients and oxygen to the cornea and lens. It drains through the trabecular meshwork, the canal of Schlemm, and then is absorbed into the blood.	**aque/o-** *watery substance*
caruncle	Red, triangular tissue at the medial corner of the eye	
choroid	Spongy membrane of blood vessels that begins at the iris and continues around the eye. In the posterior cavity, it is the middle layer between the sclera and the retina.	**choroid/o-** *choroid of the eye*
ciliary body	Extension of the choroid layer that lies posterior to the iris. It has suspensory ligaments that hold the lens in place. When the ciliary body contracts and relaxes it changes the shape of the lens. It also produces aqueous humor.	**cili/o-** *hair-like structure* **cycl/o-** *ciliary body of the eye; circle; cycle*
cones	Light-sensitive cells in the retina that detect color. There are three different types of cones that respond to either red, green, or blue light.	
conjunctiva	Delicate, transparent mucous membrane that covers the inside of the eyelids and the anterior surface of the eye. It produces clear, watery mucus.	**conjunctiv/o-** *conjunctiva of the eye*
cornea	Transparent layer over the anterior part of the eye. This is the same layer that was previously the white sclera. The transitional area where the change occurs is the limbus.	**corne/o-** *cornea of the eye* **kerat/o-** *cornea of the eye; hard, fibrous protein*
extraocular muscles	Six muscles that are attached to the sclera by tendons: **superior rectus muscle**, **inferior rectus muscle**, **medial rectus muscle**, **lateral rectus muscle**, **superior oblique muscle**, and **inferior oblique muscle**. *Rectus* means *straight,* and *oblique* means *slanted.* They move the eye in all directions. These movements are under voluntary control by the brain through the oculomotor nerve (cranial nerve III), trochlear nerve (cranial nerve IV), and the abducens nerve (cranial nerve VI).	**ocul/o-** *eye* **super/o-** *above* **infer/o-** *below* **medi/o-** *middle* **later/o-** *side*
eye	Organ that provides sensory information that is interpreted by the brain to become the sense of sight. The eye is also known as the **optic globe**.	**opt/o-** *eye; vision* **ocul/o-** *eye* **ophthalm/o-** *eye*
eyelashes	Hairs that form a protective barrier that extends out from the eye to keep foreign substances from coming in contact with the eye	
eyelids	Pair of fleshy structures above and below the eye to protect the eye. They blink to keep the surface of the eye moist with tears and prevent foreign substances from entering the eye. They contain the eyelashes and sebaceous glands.	**blephar/o-** *eyelid*

Word or Phrase	Description	Combining Forms
fovea	Small depression in the center of the macula. It is the area of sharpest vision and lies directly opposite the pupil.	**fove/o-** *small, depressed area*
fundus	General word for the retina because it is the area that is farthest from the opening (the pupil)	**fund/o-** *fundus; part farthest from the opening* **fundu/o-** *fundus; part farthest from the opening*
iris	Circular, colored structure around the pupil. The muscles of the iris contract to decrease or relax to increase the diameter of the pupil. This is controlled by the oculomotor nerve (cranial nerve III). The color of the iris is determined by genetics.	**irid/o-** *iris of the eye* **ir/o-** *iris of the eye*
lacrimal gland	Gland in the superior-lateral aspect of the eye. It continuously produces and releases tears through the **lacrimal ducts**. The lacrimal gland produces tears when stimulated by the facial nerve (cranial nerve VII).	**lacrim/o-** *tears* **dacry/o-** *lacrimal sac; tears*
lacrimal sac	Structure that collects tears as they drain from the medial aspect of the eye. It empties into the nasolacrimal duct.	**lacrim/o-** *tears* **dacry/o-** *lacrimal sac; tears*
lens	Clear, flexible disk behind the pupil. It is surrounded by the lens capsule. The muscles of the ciliary body change the lens shape (accommodation) to focus light rays on the retina.	**lenticul/o-** *lens of the eye* **lent/o-** *lens of the eye* **phac/o-** *lens of the eye* **phak/o-** *lens of the eye*
lens capsule	Clear membrane that surrounds the lens	**capsul/o-** *capsule; enveloping structure*
limbus	Border where the white, opaque sclera becomes the transparent cornea over the anterior aspect of the eye	
macula	Dark yellow-orange area with indistinct edges on the retina. It contains the fovea.	**macul/o-** *small area; spot*
miosis	Contraction of the iris muscle to constrict (reduce the size of) the pupil and limit the amount of light entering the eye	**mi/o-** *narrowing*
mydriasis	Relaxation of the iris muscle to dilate (enlarge the size of) the pupil and increase the amount of light entering the eye	**mydr/o-** *widening*
nasolacrimal duct	Structure that carries tears from the lacrimal sac to the inside of the nose	**nas/o-** *nose* **lacrim/o-** *tears*
oculomotor nerve	Cranial nerve III. A motor nerve that carries motor commands to four of the extraocular muscles to move the eye, to the eyelids to move, and to the muscles of the iris to contract or relax.	**ocul/o-** *eye* **mot/o-** *movement*
optic disk	Bright yellow-white circle in the retina where the optic nerve and retinal arteries enter and the retinal veins leave the posterior cavity. It cannot receive sensory information and is known as the **blind spot**.	**opt/o-** *eye; vision*
optic nerve	Cranial nerve II. It enters the posterior eye at the optic disk. It is a sensory nerve that carries sensory information of visual images from the rods and cones of the retina. At the **optic chiasm** in the brain, parts of each optic nerve cross over to join the optic nerve on the other side. These recombined nerves become the optic tracts that go to the thalamus.	**opt/o-** *eye; vision*
orbit	Bony socket in the cranium that surrounds all but the anterior part of the eye	

Give Word Part Meanings

Use the Answer Key at the end of the book to check your answers.

Combining Forms Exercise

Next to each combining form, write its meaning. The first one has been done for you.

Combining Form	Meaning	Combining Form	Meaning
1. **accommod/o-**	adapt	25. lent/o-	_____
2. anter/o-	_____	26. macul/o-	_____
3. aque/o-	_____	27. medi/o-	_____
4. blephar/o-	_____	28. mi/o-	_____
5. capsul/o-	_____	29. mot/o-	_____
6. cav/o-	_____	30. mydr/o-	_____
7. choroid/o-	_____	31. nas/o-	_____
8. cili/o-	_____	32. ocul/o-	_____
9. conjunctiv/o-	_____	33. ophthalm/o-	_____
10. corne/o-	_____	34. op/o-	_____
11. cor/o-	_____	35. opt/o-	_____
12. cycl/o-	_____	36. phac/o-	_____
13. dacry/o-	_____	37. phak/o-	_____
14. fove/o-	_____	38. poster/o-	_____
15. fract/o-	_____	39. pupill/o-	_____
16. fund/o-	_____	40. retin/o-	_____
17. fundu/o-	_____	41. scler/o-	_____
18. infer/o-	_____	42. scop/o-	_____
19. irid/o-	_____	43. stere/o-	_____
20. ir/o-	_____	44. super/o-	_____
21. kerat/o-	_____	45. trabecul/o-	_____
22. lacrim/o-	_____	46. uve/o-	_____
23. later/o-	_____	47. vis/o-	_____
24. lenticul/o-	_____	48. vitre/o-	_____

Build Medical Words

Combining Form and Suffix Exercise

Read the definition of the medical word. Look at the combining form that is given. Select the correct suffix from the Suffix List and write it on the blank line. Then build the medical word and write it on the line. (Remember: You may need to remove the combining vowel. Always remove the hyphens and slash.) Be sure to check your spelling. The first one has been done for you.

SUFFIX LIST

-al (pertaining to)	-ation (being;	-ic (pertaining to)	-ous (pertaining to)
-ar (pertaining to)	having; process)	-ion (action; condition)	-ual (pertaining to)
-ary (pertaining to)	-iasis (process; state)	-osis (condition; process)	

Definition of the Medical Word	Combining Form	Suffix	Build the Medical Word
1. Pertaining to (the) cornea	**corne/o-**	**-al**	*corneal*
(You think *pertaining to* (-al) + *cornea* (corne/o-). You change the order of the word parts to put the suffix last. You write *corneal*.)			
2. Pertaining to (the) retina	retin/o-	_____	_____
3. Pertaining to sight and vision	vis/o-	_____	_____
4. Pertaining to (the) pupil	pupill/o-	_____	_____
5. Pertaining to (the white part or) sclera of the eye	scler/o-	_____	_____
6. Process (of) widening (of the pupil)	mydr/o-	_____	_____
7. Pertaining to (the) eye or vision	opt/o-	_____	_____
8. Pertaining to (a) watery substance (in the posterior cavity of the eye)	aque/o-	_____	_____
9. Pertaining to (a) small area or spot (on the retina)	macul/o-	_____	_____
10. Pertaining to tears	lacrim/o-	_____	_____
11. Condition (of having) sight	vis/o-	_____	_____
12. Process (of having to) adapt (the lens of the eye)	accommod/o-	_____	_____
13. Pertaining to (the) conjunctiva	conjunctiv/o-	_____	_____
14. Process (of) narrowing (of the pupil)	mi/o-	_____	_____

Diseases

Eyelid		
Word or Phrase	**Description**	**Pronunciation/Word Parts**
blepharitis	Inflammation or infection of the eyelid with redness, crusts, and scales at the bases of the eyelashes. Acute blepharitis is caused by an allergy or infection. Chronic blepharitis is caused by acne rosacea, seborrheic dermatitis, or microscopic mites that live in the sebaceous glands. Treatment: Topical antibiotic or corticosteroid ophthalmic ointment.	**blepharitis** (BLEF-ah-RY-tis) **blephar/o-** *eyelid* **-itis** *infection of; inflammation of*
blepharoptosis	Drooping of the upper eyelid from excessive fat or sagging of the tissues due to age. It can also be from a disease that affects the muscles or nerves (such as myasthenia gravis or stroke). Treatment: Blepharoplasty or treat the underlying cause.	**blepharoptosis** (BLEF-ah-rawp-TOH-sis) **blephar/o-** *eyelid* **-ptosis** *state of drooping; state of falling*
ectropion	Weakening of connective tissue in the lower eyelid. The lower eyelid turns outward (see Figure 15-12 ■), exposing the conjunctiva and causing dryness and chronic conjunctivitis. Treatment: Artificial tears eye drops or surgical correction.	**ectropion** (ek-TROH-pee-on) **ec-** *out; outward* **trop/o-** *having an affinity for; stimulating; turning* **-ion** *action; condition* Select the correct combining form meaning to get the definition of *ectropion*: *condition (of) outward turning (of the eyelid)*.

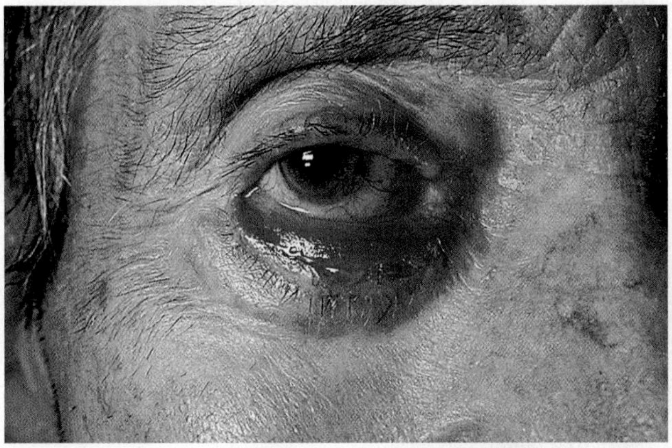

FIGURE 15-12 ■ Ectropion.
With the eyelid turned outward, the exposed conjunctiva becomes inflamed. Tears spill out, and the surface of the eye is dry and irritated.
Source: Pearson Education

entropion	Weakening of the muscle in the lower eyelid. The lower eyelid turns inward, causing the eyelashes to touch the eye, which results in chronic conjunctivitis and pain. Treatment: Artificial tears eye drops or surgical correction.	**entropion** (en-TROH-pee-on) **en-** *in; inward; within* **trop/o-** *having an affinity for; stimulating; turning* **-ion** *action; condition*
hordeolum	Red, painful swelling or a pimple containing pus on the eyelid. It is caused by a bacterial infection (staphylococcus) in a sebaceous (oil) gland. It is also known as a **stye**. Sometimes, when the acute infection subsides, the hordeolum becomes a **chalazion**, a chronically inflamed and granular lump or semisolid cyst. Treatment: Antibiotic drug for a hordeolum; warm compresses or surgical removal for a chalazion.	**hordeolum** (hor-DEE-oh-lum) **chalazion** (kah-LAY-zee-on)

Lacrimal Gland

Word or Phrase	Description	Pronunciation/Word Parts
dacryocystitis	Bacterial infection of the lacrimal sac. The lacrimal sac is tender and contains pus. Treatment: Oral antibiotic drug.	**dacryocystitis** (DAK-ree-OH-sis-TY-tis) **dacry/o-** *lacrimal sac; tears* **cyst/o-** *bladder; fluid-filled sac; semisolid cyst* **-itis** *infection of; inflammation of*
xerophthalmia	Insufficient production of tears resulting in eye irritation. It is associated with the aging process, an ectropion, or a side effect of certain drugs. It is also known as **dry eyes syndrome**. Treatment: Artificial tears eye drops (such as Restasis.) Surgery: Insertion of silicone plugs into the opening in the medial aspect of the lower eyelid to keep tears in the eye.	**xerophthalmia** (ZEER-off-THAL-mee-ah) **xer/o-** *dry* **ophthalm/o-** *eye* **-ia** *condition; state; thing*

Conjunctiva, Sclera, and Cornea

conjunctivitis	Inflamed, reddened, and swollen conjunctiva with dilated blood vessels in the sclera (see Figure 15-13 ■). It is caused by a foreign substance in the eye, a chemical splashed in the eye, allergens or pollution in the air, chlorinated water in swimming pools, mechanical irritation from eyelashes (entropion), or dryness due to a lack of tears. It is also caused by a bacterial or viral infection. Acute contagious bacterial conjunctivitis with mucus discharge is known as **pinkeye**. Treatment: Corticosteroid eye drops for inflammation; topical or oral antibiotic drug for a bacterial infection.	**conjunctivitis** (con-JUNK-tih-VY-tis) **conjunctiv/o-** *conjunctiva of the eye* **-itis** *infection of; inflammation of*

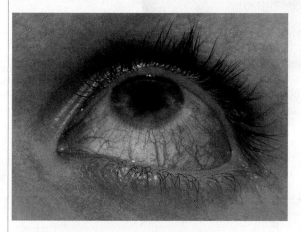

FIGURE 15-13 ■ **Conjunctivitis.**
A viral infection has caused the blood vessels in the conjunctiva to become dilated, giving it a reddened, streaky appearance.
Source: Sergii Chepulskyi/Shutterstock

CLINICAL CONNECTIONS
Neonatology. When a woman with the sexually transmitted disease of gonorrhea gives birth, the eyes of the newborn may become infected from the birth canal. A gonorrheal infection of the eye causes conjunctivitis and can cause blindness. By state law, all newborns are given antibiotic eye drops or eye ointment after birth to prevent blindness caused by gonorrhea. Chlamydia, another organism that causes a sexually transmitted disease of the genital tract, can also cause conjunctivitis in the newborn.

Word or Phrase	Description	Pronunciation/Word Parts
corneal abrasion	Damage to the cornea due to trauma or repetitive irritation, such as a foreign particle under a contact lens. A chronic bacterial infection in a corneal abrasion can become a **corneal ulcer** with sloughing off of necrotic tissue. This is also known as **ulcerative keratitis**. Treatment: Corticosteroid drug for inflammation; antibiotic drug for infection. Surgery: Corneal transplant.	**abrasion** (ah-BRAY-shun) 　**abras/o-** *scrape off* 　**-ion** *action; condition* **ulcer** (UL-ser) **ulcerative** (UL-ser-ah-TIV) 　**ulcerat/o-** *ulcer* 　**-ive** *pertaining to* **keratitis** (KAIR-ah-TY-tis) 　**kerat/o-** *cornea of the eye;* 　　*hard, fibrous protein* 　**-itis** *infection of; inflammation of*
exophthalmos	Pronounced outward bulging of the anterior surface of the eye with a startled, staring expression. If just one eye is affected, it often has a tumor behind it. If both eyes are affected, the patient usually has hyperthyroidism (see Figure 14-10). Treatment: Correct the underlying cause.	**exophthalmos** (EKS-off-THAL-mos) *Exophthalmos* is a combination of the prefix *ex-* (away from; out) and the Greek word *ophthalmos* (eye).
scleral icterus	Yellow discoloration of the conjunctivae, which makes the sclerae also appear yellow. It is caused by **jaundice** due to liver disease (see Figure 15-14 ■). In a patient without jaundice, the normal, white sclerae are said to be **anicteric**. Treatment: Correct the underlying cause. **FIGURE 15-14 ■ Scleral icterus.** This patient's eye has a yellow discoloration. This is due to a high level of bilirubin in the blood that his diseased liver is unable to conjugate. *Source*: James Stevenson/Science Source	**icterus** (IK-ter-us) **icteric** (ik-TAIR-ik) 　**icter/o-** *jaundice* 　**-ic** *pertaining to* **jaundice** (JAWN-dis) **anicteric** (AN-ik-TAIR-ik) 　**an-** *not; without* 　**icter/o-** *jaundice* 　**-ic** *pertaining to*

Iris, Pupil, and Anterior Chamber

Word or Phrase	Description	Pronunciation/Word Parts
anisocoria	Unequal sizes of the pupils. It is caused by glaucoma, head trauma, stroke, or a tumor that damages the cranial nerve that controls the muscle of the iris (and the size of the pupil). Treatment: Correct the underlying cause.	**anisocoria** (an-EYE-soh-KOR-ee-ah) 　**anis/o-** *unequal* 　**cor/o-** *pupil of the eye* 　**-ia** *condition; state; thing*
glaucoma	Increased **intraocular pressure (IOP)** because aqueous humor cannot circulate freely. In open-angle glaucoma, the angle where the edges of the iris and cornea meet is normal and open, but the trabecular meshwork is blocked. Open-angle glaucoma is painless but destroys peripheral vision, leaving the patient with tunnel vision. In closed-angle glaucoma, the angle itself is too narrow and blocks the flow of aqueous humor. Closed-angle glaucoma causes severe pain, blurred vision, and photophobia. Glaucoma can progress to blindness. Treatment: Glaucoma drug to lower intraocular pressure. Surgery: Laser trabeculoplasty.	**glaucoma** (glaw-KOH-mah) 　**glauc/o-** *silver gray* 　**-oma** *mass; tumor* **intraocular** (IN-trah-AW-kyoo-lar) 　**intra-** *within* 　**ocul/o-** *eye* 　**-ar** *pertaining to*

Word or Phrase	Description	Pronunciation/Word Parts
hyphema	Blood in the anterior chamber. It is caused by trauma or increased intraocular pressure. Treatment: Topical corticosteroid eye drops or oral corticosteroid drug; treat underlying glaucoma.	**hyphema** (hy-FEE-mah)
photophobia	Abnormal sensitivity to bright light. It can be associated with inflammation from diseases of the eye or it can be due to increased intracranial pressure or meningitis in the brain. Treatment: Correct the underlying cause.	**photophobia** (FOH-toh-FOH-bee-ah) **phot/o-** *light* **phob/o-** *avoidance; fear* **-ia** *condition; state; thing*
uveitis	Inflammation or infection of the uveal tract. It can be caused by infection in the eye, infection in another part of the body, an allergy, trauma, or an autoimmune disorder. **Iritis** affects the iris. **Choroiditis** affects the choroid membrane. Treatment: Oral corticosteroid or antibiotic drug.	**uveitis** (YOO-vee-EYE-tis) **uve/o-** *uvea of the eye* **-itis** *infection of; inflammation of* **iritis** (eye-RY-tis) **ir/o-** *iris of the eye* **-itis** *infection of; inflammation of* **choroiditis** (KOH-royd-EYE-tis) **choroid/o-** *choroid of the eye* **-itis** *infection of; inflammation of*

Lens

Word or Phrase	Description	Pronunciation/Word Parts
aphakia	Condition in which the lens of the eye has been surgically removed because of a cataract. Treatment: In most patients, an artificial intraocular lens is put into the eye during the cataract surgery. Some cataract patients are not good candidates for an artificial intraocular lens. Their cataract is removed, but they wear special cataract eyeglasses, and they remain aphakic.	**aphakia** (ah-FAY-kee-ah) **a-** *away from; without* **phak/o-** *lens of the eye* **-ia** *condition; state; thing*
cataract	Clouding of the lens (see Figure 15-15 ■). Protein molecules in the lens begin to clump together. It is caused by aging, sun exposure, eye trauma, smoking, and some drugs. The vision is dull and blurry with faded colors and a yellowish tint around lights. Congenital cataracts are present at birth. Treatment: Cataract surgery (see Figure 15-26).	**cataract** (KAT-ah-rakt)

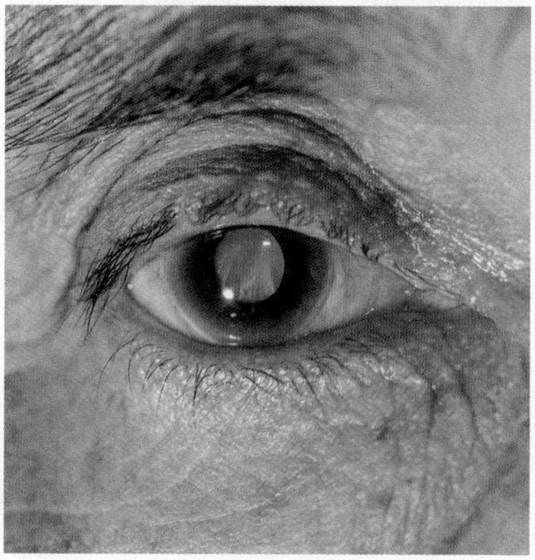

FIGURE 15-15 ■ Cataract.
As a cataract develops, the lens gradually becomes cloudy and opaque. The vision is blurred and colors appear faded and yellowed.
Source: Arztsamui/Shutterstock

Word or Phrase	Description	Pronunciation/Word Parts
presbyopia	Loss of flexibility of the lens with blurry near vision and loss of accommodation. It is caused by aging. Treatment: Corrective eyeglasses.	**presbyopia** (PREZ-bee-OH-pee-ah) **presby/o-** *old age* **op/o-** *vision* **-ia** *condition; state; thing*

Posterior Cavity and Retina

Word or Phrase	Description	Pronunciation/Word Parts
color blindness	Genetic condition in which the cones (usually the green or red cones) are absent or do not contain enough visual pigment to respond to the light from colored objects. Treatment: None.	

diabetic retinopathy	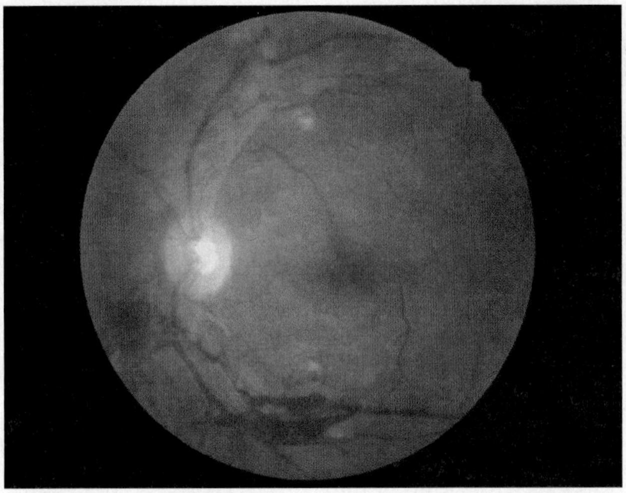 Chronic, progressive condition of the retina in which a large number of new, fragile blood vessels form (**neovascularization**) in patients with uncontrolled diabetes mellitus (see Figure 15-16 ■). These vessels leak, forming exudates (dried fluid deposits) on the retina. They also rupture easily, causing intraocular hemorrhage. Treatment: Management of diabetes mellitus; surgery with laser photocoagulation (see Figure 15-29).	**diabetic** (DY-ah-BET-ik)
		    diabet/o- *diabetes*
		    -ic *pertaining to*
		
		retinopathy
		(RET-ih-NAW-pah-thee)
		    retin/o- *retina of the eye*
		    -pathy *disease*
		
		neovascularization
		(NEE-oh-VAS-kyoo-LAR-ih-ZAY-shun)
		    ne/o- *new*
		    vascul/o- *blood vessel*
		    -ar *pertaining to*
		    -ization *process of creating; process of inserting; process of making*

FIGURE 15-16 ■ Diabetic retinopathy.
This patient's retina shows advanced diabetic retinopathy with neovascularization, the formation of many new, fragile blood vessels in a central cluster, as well as some small areas of hemorrhage.
Source: Satit Umong/123RF

Word or Phrase	Description	Pronunciation/Word Parts
floaters and flashers	Floaters are clumps, dots, or strings of collagen molecules that form in the vitreous humor because of aging. Flashers are brief bursts of bright light that occur when the vitreous humor pulls on the retina. Treatment: None. However, a sudden increase in the number of floaters and flashers can mean a retinal detachment.	

macular degeneration	Chronic, progressive loss of central vision as the macula degenerates. In older patients, this is known as age-related macular degeneration (AMD, ARMD). In dry macular degeneration (the most common type), the macula deteriorates. In wet macular degeneration, abnormal blood vessels grow under the macula. They are fragile and leak, causing the macula to lift away from the retina. Treatment for wet macular degeneration: Photodynamic therapy (PDT) to destroy abnormal blood vessels. Drugs that keep new blood vessels from forming in the retina. There is no treatment for dry macular degeneration.	**macular** (MAK-yoo-lar)
		    macul/o- *small area; spot*
		    -ar *pertaining to*
		
		degeneration
		(DEE-jen-er-AA-shun)
		    de- *reversal of; without*
		    gener/o- *creation; production*
		    -ation *being; having; process*

night blindness	Marked decrease in visual acuity at night or in dim light. This occurs with aging or when the diet does not contain enough vitamin A. Treatment: Dietary supplement, if needed.	

papilledema	Inflammation and edema of the optic disk. It is caused by increased intracranial pressure from a brain tumor or head trauma. It is also known as a **choked optic disk**. Treatment: Correct the underlying cause.	**papilledema** (PAP-il-eh-DEE-mah)
		    papill/o- *elevated structure*
		    -edema *swelling*

Word or Phrase	Description	Pronunciation/Word Parts
retinal detachment	Separation of the retina from the choroid layer beneath it (see Figure 15-17 ■). This can be caused by head trauma. It can occur gradually during aging as the vitreous humor changes from a gel to a watery consistency that flows into small tears in the retina and separates the two layers. In diabetic patients, hemorrhage of the fragile retinal blood vessels can separate the layers. Treatment: Retinopexy with cryotherapy or laser photocoagulation.	**detachment** (dee-TACH-ment)

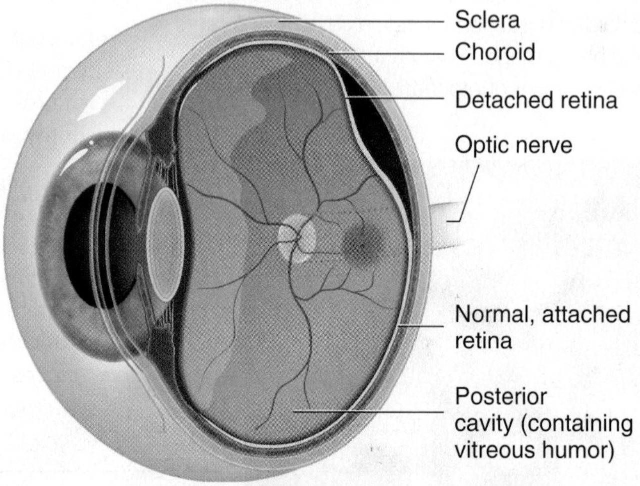

Sclera
Choroid
Detached retina
Optic nerve

Normal, attached retina

Posterior cavity (containing vitreous humor)

FIGURE 15-17 ■ Retinal detachment.
A gradual partial detachment of the retina is painless. The only symptoms are a sudden increase in the number of floaters and brief flashes of light in the visual field. If untreated, however, it can lead to a complete detachment of the retina.
Source: Pearson Education

Word or Phrase	Description	Pronunciation/Word Parts
retinitis pigmentosa (RP)	Hereditary condition linked to 70 different genes. The retina has abnormal deposits of pigmentation behind the rods and cones, causing loss of night vision or color vision and loss of central or peripheral vision. It can progress to blindness. Treatment: None.	**retinitis pigmentosa** (RET-ih-NY-tis PIG-men-TOH-sah) **retin/o-** *retina of the eye* **-itis** *infection of; inflammation of*
retinoblastoma	Cancerous tumor of the retina in children, arising from abnormal embryonic retinal cells. Treatment: Chemotherapy drugs, radiation therapy, and surgical removal.	**retinoblastoma** (RET-ih-NOH-blas-TOH-mah) **retin/o-** *retina of the eye* **blast/o-** *embryonic; immature* **-oma** *mass; tumor*
retinopathy of prematurity	Developing retinal tissue is replaced with fibrous tissue because of using a high level of oxygen to treat premature babies with immature lungs. It is also known as **retrolental fibroplasia**. Treatment: Laser photocoagulation.	**retinopathy** (RET-ih-NAW-pah-thee) **retin/o-** *retina of the eye* **-pathy** *disease* **prematurity** (PREE-mah-TYOOR-ih-tee) **pre-** *before; in front of* **matur/o-** *mature* **-ity** *condition; state* **retrolental** (REH-troh-LEN-tal) **retro-** *backward; behind* **lent/o-** *lens of the eye* **-al** *pertaining to* **fibroplasia** (FY-broh-PLAY-zha) **fibr/o-** *fiber* **plas/o-** *formation; growth* **-ia** *condition; state; thing*

Extraocular Muscles

Word or Phrase	Description	Pronunciation/Word Parts
nystagmus	Involuntary rhythmic motions of the eye, particularly when looking to the side. Each back-and-forth motion is known as a "beat." Nystagmus can be caused by multiple sclerosis or Meniere's disease. Treatment: Correct the underlying cause.	**nystagmus** (nih-STAG-mus)
strabismus	Deviation of one or both eyes medially or laterally. Medial deviation is **esotropia** or **cross-eye** (see Figure 15-18 ■). It is also known as *convergent strabismus*. Lateral deviation is **exotropia** or **wall-eye**. Treatment: Surgical repositioning of the extraocular muscles, which is done during early childhood. **FIGURE 15-18 ■ Esotropia.** In this type of strabismus, one or both eyes deviate medially toward the nose. *Source*: Pearson Education	**strabismus** (strah-BIZ-mus) **esotropia** (ES-oh-TROH-pee-ah) **es/o-** *inward* **trop/o-** *having an affinity for; stimulating; turning* **-ia** *condition; state; thing* **exotropia** (EKS-oh-TROH-pee-ah) **ex/o-** *away from; external; outward* **trop/o-** *having an affinity for; stimulating; turning* **-ia** *condition; state; thing*

Refractive Disorders of the Eyes

Word or Phrase	Description	Pronunciation/Word Parts
astigmatism	Surface of the cornea is curved more steeply in one area, so there is no single point of focus. The patient's vision is blurry both near and at a distance. Treatment: Corrective lenses or surgery.	**astigmatism** (ah-STIG-mah-tizm) **a-** *away from; without* **stigmat/o-** *mark; point* **-ism** *disease from a specific cause; process*
hyperopia	**Farsightedness.** Light rays from a distant object focus correctly on the retina, creating a sharp image. However, light rays from a near object come into focus posterior to the retina, creating a blurred image (see Figure 15-19 ■). Treatment: Corrective lenses or surgery.	**hyperopia** (HY-per-OH-pee-ah) **hyper-** *above; more than normal* **op/o-** *vision* **-ia** *condition; state; thing* Add words to make a complete definition of *hyperopia: condition (at a distance that is) more than normal vision.*

HYPEROPIA (Farsightedness)

Cornea
Lens
A
Far object
Light rays
A

A
Near object

Position of retina in normal eye

FIGURE 15-19 ■ Hyperopia. There is an abnormally short distance between the cornea and the retina. The patient can see objects clearly in the distance (farsightedness), but close objects are blurry. *Source*: Pearson Education

Word or Phrase	Description	Pronunciation/Word Parts
myopia	**Nearsightedness.** Light rays from a near object focus correctly on the retina, creating a sharp image. However, light rays from a distant object come into focus anterior to the retina, creating a blurred image (see Figure 15-20 ■). Treatment: Corrective lenses or surgery.	**myopia** (my-OH-pee-ah) **myop/o-** *near vision* **-ia** *condition; state; thing*

MYOPIA
(Nearsightedness)

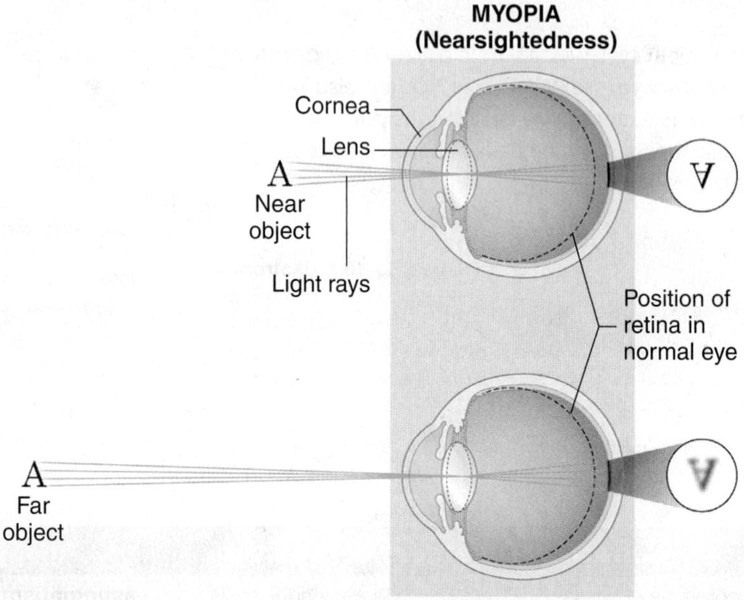

FIGURE 15-20 ■ Myopia.
There is an abnormally long distance between the cornea and the retina. The patient can see objects clearly that are close (nearsightedness), but objects in the distance are blurry.
Source: Pearson Education

Conditions of the Visual Cortex in the Brain

Word or Phrase	Description	Pronunciation/Word Parts
amblyopia	To prevent double vision, the brain ignores the visual image from an eye with strabismus (the most common cause) or from an eye in which the vision is unfocused or cloudy. This is also known as **lazy eye**. Amblyopia may continue even after the strabismus or other defect is surgically corrected. Treatment: The normal eye is patched until the brain accepts the visual image from the other eye.	**amblyopia** (AM-blee-OH-pee-ah) **ambly/o-** *dimness* **op/o-** *vision* **-ia** *condition; state; thing* Add words to make a complete definition of *amblyopia: condition (of) dimness (because of suppression of) vision (in one eye).*
blindness	Condition of complete or partial loss of vision. It is caused by trauma, eye diseases, or defects in the structure of the eye, optic nerve, or visual cortex in the brain. A patient whose best visual acuity is 20/200 even with corrective lenses is legally blind. Treatment: Correct the underlying cause.	
diplopia	Two visual fields are seen rather than one fused image. It can be caused by amblyopia, by a tumor or trauma that increases intracranial pressure, or by multiple sclerosis that affects nerve conduction to the visual cortex. Treatment: Correct the underlying cause.	**diplopia** (dih-PLOH-pee-ah) **dipl/o-** *double* **op/o-** *vision* **-ia** *condition; state; thing*
scotoma	Temporary or permanent visual field defect in one or both eyes. This is seen as a gray spot, area, or curtain in the field of vision. The defect varies in size and can be patchy or solid, stationary or moving. This is caused by glaucoma, diabetic retinopathy, or macular degeneration when various parts of the retina or optic nerve are destroyed. Also, hemorrhage (from a cerebrovascular accident or stroke), a tumor, or trauma in the occipital lobe on one side of the brain can cause a scotoma in the opposite visual field. **Hemianopia** is loss of one half of the visual field (right or left, top or bottom). Prior to a migraine headache, a patient may see a scintillating scotoma, a temporary moving line of brilliantly flashing bars of light in the visual field. This is also known as *hemianopsia.* Treatment: Correct the underlying cause.	**scotoma** (skoh-TOH-mah) **scot/o-** *darkness* **-oma** *mass; tumor* **scotomata** (skoh-TOH-mah-tah) **hemianopia** (HEM-ee-ah-NOH-pee-ah) **hemi-** *one half* **an-** *not; without* **op/o-** *vision* **-ia** *condition; state; thing*

Laboratory and Diagnostic Procedures

Diagnostic Procedures		
Word or Phrase	**Description**	**Pronunciation/Word Parts**

fluorescein angiography	Procedure in which fluorescein (a fluorescent dye) is injected intravenously. The dye travels to the retinal artery in the eye. It glows fluorescent yellow-green on flash photography of the retina. It reveals retinal leaking and hemorrhages common in diabetic patients. The photographic image is an **angiogram**.	**fluorescein** (FLOOR-eh-seen)
		
		angiography (AN-jee-AW-grah-fee)
		  angi/o- *blood vessel; lymphatic vessel*
		  -graphy *process of recording*
		
		angiogram (AN-jee-oh-GRAM)
		  angi/o- *blood vessel; lymphatic vessel*
		  -gram *picture; record*

Radiologic Tests		

ultrasonography	Procedure that uses ultra high-frequency sound waves to create an image of the eye. A-scan ultrasound measures the eye prior to intraocular lens insertion. B-scan creates a two-dimensional image of the inside of the eye to show tumors or hemorrhages. The ultrasound image is a **sonogram**.	**ultrasonography**
		(UL-trah-soh-NAW-grah-fee)
		  ultra- *beyond; higher*
		  son/o- *sound*
		  -graphy *process of recording*
		
		sonogram (SAW-noh-gram)
		  son/o- *sound*
		  -gram *picture; record*

Medical and Surgical Procedures

Medical Procedures		
Word or Phrase	**Description**	**Pronunciation/Word Parts**

accommodation	Procedure to test the ability of the muscles in the ciliary body to contract and flex the lens as demonstrated on near and distance visual acuity tests	**accommodation**
		(ah-KAW-moh-DAY-shun)
		  accommod/o- *adapt*
		  -ation *being; having; process*

color blindness testing	Procedure to determine if a patient has a defect in the red, green, or blue cones in the retina. Each successive color plate requires a higher discrimination of color perception. Color plates that contain numbers are used to test adults (see Figure 15-21 ■), while color plates that contain circles, squares, or animals are used to test children.	

Word or Phrase	Description	Pronunciation/Word Parts

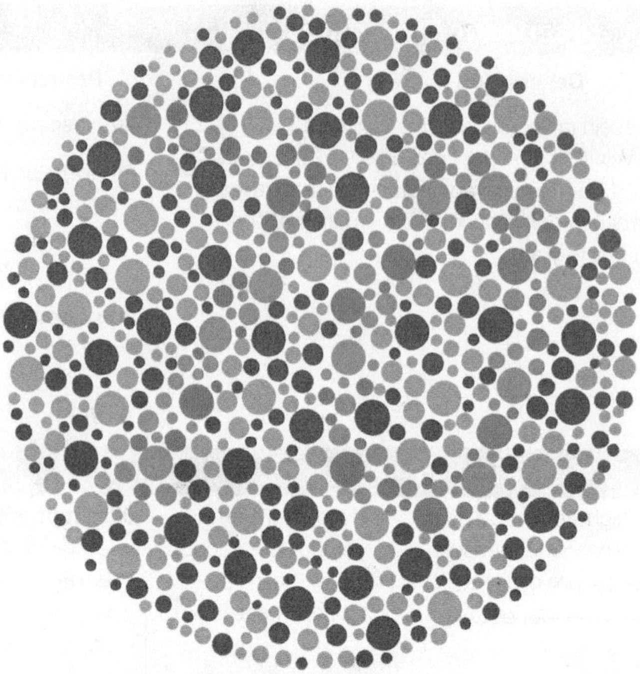

FIGURE 15-21 ■ Ishihara color plate for testing color blindness.
A patient with red-green color blindness would not be able to distinguish the 70 printed in green.
Source: Pearson Education

Word or Phrase	Description	Pronunciation/Word Parts
dilated funduscopy	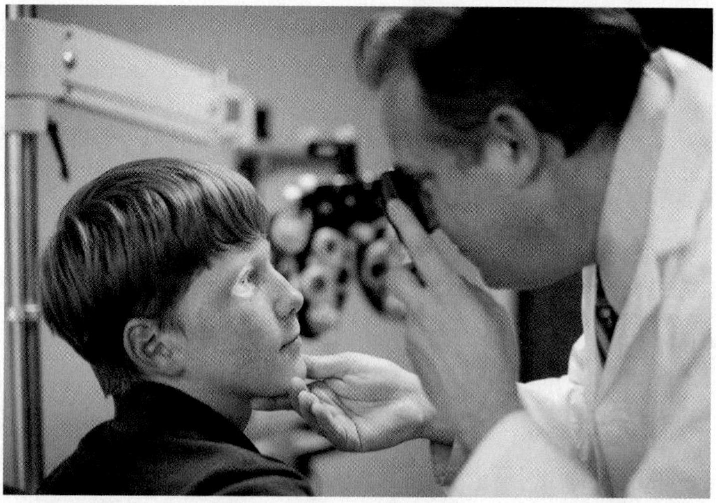 Procedure to examine the posterior cavity. Eye drops are used to dilate the pupil (mydriasis) and to temporarily keep the pupil in a dilated position (**cycloplegia**). An **ophthalmoscope**, a handheld instrument with a light and changeable lenses of different strengths, is used to examine the retina from all angles (see Figure 15-22 ■). Alternatively, the patient can be placed in a darkened room to dilate the pupils. A strobe light creates a sudden flash to illuminate the retina while a photograph is taken. This method is able to show about 30% of the retina. Any abnormalities of the retina must be further examined with a dilated funduscopic exam.	**funduscopy** (fun-DAW-skoh-pee) **fundu/o-** *fundus; part farthest from the opening* **-scopy** *process of using an instrument to examine* **cycloplegia** (SY-kloh-PLEE-jee-ah) **cycl/o-** *ciliary body of the eye; circle; cycle* **pleg/o-** *paralysis* **-ia** *condition; state; thing* **ophthalmoscope** (off-THAL-moh-skohp) **ophthalm/o-** *eye* **-scope** *instrument used to examine*

FIGURE 15-22 ■ Ophthalmoscope.
The ophthalmologist selects and dials in a lens on the ophthalmoscope to see a sharp image of the inside of the patient's eye. The lens that he selects corrects for the visual defects of his own eyes as well as those of the patient.
Source: Erproductions Ltd/Blend Images/Getty Images

Word or Phrase	Description	Pronunciation/Word Parts
eye patching	Procedure in which the eye is covered with a soft bandage and a hard outer shield after eye trauma or eye surgery. Also, a normal eye can be patched to treat amblyopia.	
fluorescein staining	Procedure in which a fluorescein (a fluorescent dye) strip or drops are applied topically to the cornea to detect corneal abrasions and ulcers. As a light is used to examine the eye, any corneal abrasions or ulcers glow fluorescent yellow-green.	**fluorescein** (FLOOR-eh-seen)

Word or Phrase	Description	Pronunciation/Word Parts
gaze testing	Procedure to test the extraocular muscles. The patient's eyes follow the physician's finger from side to side and up and down. **Conjugate gaze** is when both eyes move together as a unit. This is documented in the patient's record as *EOMI (extraocular muscles intact)*. **Dysconjugate gaze** is when the eyes do not move together. **Convergence** tests the medial rectus muscles. The physician's finger moves from far away to close to the patient's nose (the "near point"), and the patient's eyes should both move medially to follow the finger.	**conjugate** (CON-joo-gayt) **conjug/o-** *joined together* **-ate** *composed of; pertaining to* **dysconjugate** (dis-CON-joo-gayt) **dys-** *abnormal; difficult; painful* **conjug/o-** *joined together* **-ate** *composed of; pertaining to* **convergence** (con-VER-jens) **converg/o-** *coming together* **-ence** *state*
gonioscopy	Procedure to look for blockage of the trabecular meshwork in open-angle glaucoma. It uses a slit lamp (see Figure 15-25) with a special lens to illuminate and magnify the tiny trabecular meshwork.	**gonioscopy** (GOH-nee-AW-skoh-pee) **goni/o-** *angle* **-scopy** *process of using an instrument to examine*
peripheral vision	Procedure to test visual acuity at the edges of the visual field. The patient looks straight ahead while the physician moves an object toward the edge of the visual field (from the top, bottom, and both sides). The patient indicates when the object is first seen. Alternatively, a computer projects dots onto a screen with a grid and the patient looks straight ahead and indicates when a dot is seen off to the side.	**peripheral** (peh-RIF-eh-ral) **peripher/o-** *outer aspects* **-al** *pertaining to*
phorometry	Procedure to select from many different lenses to find the strength of lens that corrects the patient's refractive error and produces 20/20 vision. A **phorometer** (see Figure 15-23 ■) holds lenses of successive strengths that are dialed into place as the patient looks through the lens at a Snellen chart. Each eye is tested separately. The specifications of that lens are written as a prescription that is duplicated in eyeglasses or contact lenses.	**phorometry** (foh-RAW-meh-tree) **phor/o-** *bear; carry; range* **-metry** *process of measuring* **phorometer** (foh-RAW-meh-ter) **phor/o-** *bear; carry; range* **-meter** *instrument used to measure*

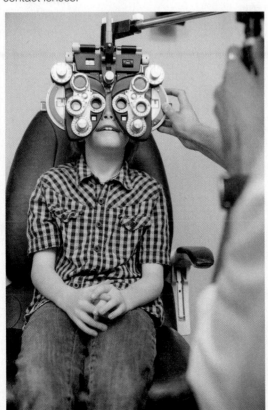

FIGURE 15-23 ■ Phorometer.
This instrument helps the ophthalmologist select the most accurate corrective lens for the patient.
Source: Tyler Olson/123RF

Word or Phrase	Description	Pronunciation/Word Parts
pupillary response	Procedure to test that the pupils constrict briskly and equally in response to a bright light. This is documented in the patient's record as *PERRL* (pupils equal, round, and reactive to light).	
slit-lamp examination	Procedure to look for abnormalities of the cornea, anterior chamber, trabecular meshwork, iris, or lens. The slit lamp combines a low-power microscope with a high-intensity vertical beam of blue light whose width can be adjusted down to a slit (see Figure 15-24 ■). It is used with fluorescein dye to see a corneal abrasion. 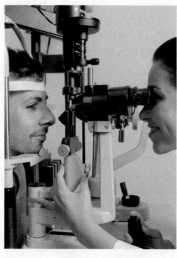 **FIGURE 15-24 ■ Slit lamp examination.** The patient's chin and forehead are in a fixed position as the slit lamp moves around the head to magnify, illuminate, and view the external and internal eye from different angles. *Source*: maxreisgo/Shutterstock	
tonometry	Procedure to detect increased intraocular pressure and glaucoma. The small, flat disk of the **tonometer** is pressed against the cornea to record intraocular pressure. Alternatively, **air-puff tonometry** emits a short burst of air and measures the pressure of the air rebounding from the cornea without touching the patient's eye.	**tonometry** (toh-NAW-meh-tree) **ton/o-** *pressure; tone* **-metry** *process of measuring* **tonometer** (toh-NAW-meh-ter) **ton/o-** *pressure; tone* **-meter** *instrument used to measure*

Word or Phrase	Description	Pronunciation/Word Parts
visual acuity testing	Procedure to test near and distance visual acuity. Each eye is tested separately. A card with typed sentences of decreasing print size is held at a preset distance of 16 inches to test the near vision. The Snellen chart is used to test distance vision from 20 feet away. As an alternative, the Tumbling E chart has capital *E*s facing in various directions, and the patient indicates which way the legs of the *E* are pointing (see Figure 15-25 ■). Children or patients who are illiterate are tested with charts that use pictures. For a patient with severe vision problems, visual acuity can be measured as the ability to count how many fingers the ophthalmologist holds up or by the ability to perceive light.	**visual** (VIH-shoo-al) **vis/o-** *sight; vision* **-ual** *pertaining to* **acuity** (ah-KYOO-ih-tee) **acu/o-** *needle; sharpness* **-ity** *condition; state*

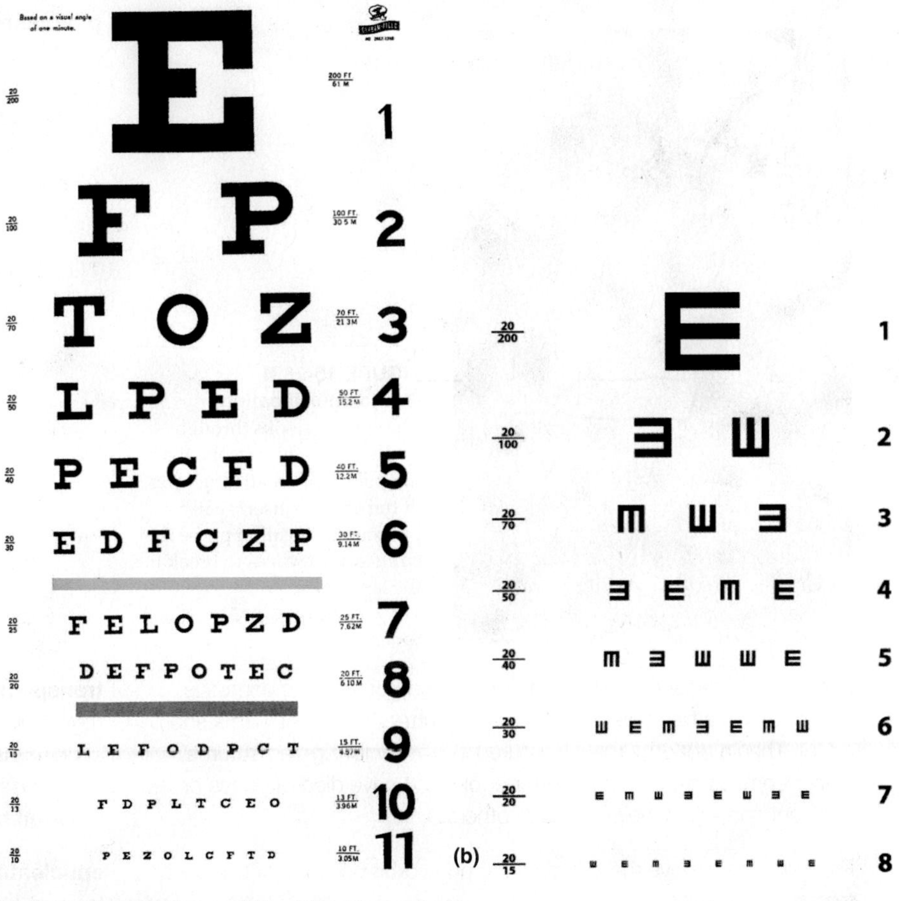

FIGURE 15-25 ■ Snellen and Tumbling E eye charts.
(a) Each line on the Snellen chart corresponds to a visual acuity rating. A normal result for this test is 20/20. The first number stands for 20 feet, the distance between the patient and the chart. The second number stands for 20 feet, the distance at which a person with normal vision could see that line. If a patient stands 20 feet from the chart but can only see the top large *E* (a visual acuity of 20/200), that means he/she can only see at 20 feet what a person with normal vision could see from 200 feet away. (b) Patients who are illiterate are shown the Tumbling E chart and are asked to say which way the legs of the *E* are pointing.
Source: Radu Bercan/Shutterstock; Roman Sotola/Shutterstock

Surgical Procedures

Word or Phrase	Description	Pronunciation/Word Parts
blepharoplasty	Plastic surgery procedure on the eyelids to remove fat and sagging skin. It is often done in conjunction with a facelift. It is also done to correct an ectropion or entropion.	**blepharoplasty** (BLEF-ah-roh-PLAS-tee) **blephar/o-** *eyelid* **-plasty** *process of reshaping by surgery*
capsulotomy	Procedure that is only done during cataract extraction when the remaining posterior part of the lens capsule is cloudy or wrinkled. A laser is used to make an opening in the posterior capsule to restore normal vision.	**capsulotomy** (KAP-soo-LAW-toh-mee) **capsul/o-** *capsule; enveloping structure* **-tomy** *process of cutting; process of making an incision*

Word or Phrase	Description	Pronunciation/Word Parts
cataract extraction	Procedure to remove a lens affected by a cataract. Preoperatively, a laser is used to measure the length of the eye and the curvature of the cornea so that a customized intraocular lens (IOL) can be created before the surgery. During an **extracapsular cataract extraction (ECCE)**, an incision is made in the sclera, the central part of the lens is removed, the posterior part of the lens capsule is left in place, and the IOL is inserted. During **phacoemulsification**, a much smaller, self-sealing (stitchless) incision is made in the cornea. An ultrasonic probe is inserted and sound waves are used to break up the lens (see Figure 15-26 ■). The pieces are removed with irrigation and suction, and the IOL is inserted. The IOL folds to pass through the incision and then unfolds inside the capsule. **FIGURE 15-26 ■ Phacoemulsification.** The surgeon looks through an operating microscope that magnifies the small structures of the eye. He inserts a phacoemulsification probe that emits sound waves to break up the lens. *Source*: Geoff Tompkinson / Science Source	**extracapsular** (EKS-trah-KAP-soo-lar) **extra-** *outside* **capsul/o-** *capsule; enveloping structure* **-ar** *pertaining to* **extraction** (ek-STRAK-shun) **ex-** *away from; out* **tract/o-** *pulling* **-ion** *action; condition* **phacoemulsification** (FAY-koh-ee-MUL-sih-fih-KAY-shun) **phac/o-** *lens of the eye* **emulsific/o-** *liquid with suspended particles* **-ation** *being; having; process*
corneal transplantation	Procedure to replace a damaged or diseased cornea. The cornea is removed with a trephine (a round cookie-cutter instrument with a sharp edge). Then a donor cornea is sutured in place with zig-zag sutures. Donor corneas are obtained from people who have died of illness or accident and willed their organs to others.	**transplantation** (TRANS-plan-TAY-shun) **transplant/o-** *move something across and put in another place* **-ation** *being; having; process*
enucleation	Procedure to remove the eye from the bony orbit because of trauma or a tumor.	**enucleation** (ee-NOO-klee-AA-shun) **enucle/o-** *remove the main part* **-ation** *being; having; process*
hyperopia surgery	Procedure to correct farsightedness. It uses heat to shrink tissues around the edge of the cornea to produce a greater curvature in the cornea that corrects the refractive error. **Conductive keratoplasty (CK)** uses radiowaves delivered by a probe as thin as a hair to spots around the edge of the cornea. **Laser thermal keratoplasty (LTK)** uses a laser to simultaneously place spots in two concentric circles around the cornea.	**conductive** (con-DUK-tiv) **conduct/o-** *carrying; conveying* **-ive** *pertaining to* **keratoplasty** (KAIR-ah-toh-PLAS-tee) **kerat/o-** *cornea of the eye; hard, fibrous protein* **-plasty** *process of reshaping by surgery* **laser** (LAY-zer)

Word or Phrase	Description	Pronunciation/Word Parts
myopia surgery	Procedure to correct nearsightedness. A three-dimensional corneal map is created preoperatively and programmed into the laser. In **laser-assisted *in situ* keratomileusis (LASIK)**, a **microkeratome** creates a very thin flap on the surface of the cornea (see Figure 15-27 ■). The flap is peeled back, and a cold laser that cuts tissue without heating it is used to reshape the underlying cornea. The surface flap is then positioned back in place. In **photorefractive keratectomy (PRK)**, the cold laser reshapes the curvature of the cornea without the creation of a corneal surface flap. 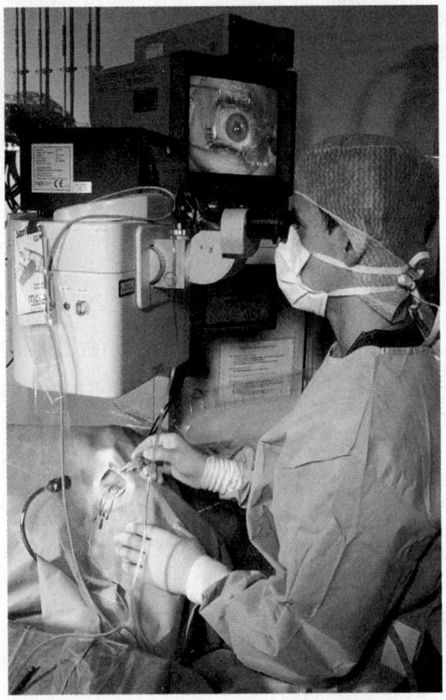 **FIGURE 15-27 ■ Keratomileusis.** During LASIK surgery, a keratomileusis is done in which a thin flap of cornea is lifted up. Then the laser is used to reshape the cornea, and the corneal flap is positioned back in place. The surgeon looks through an operating microscope, while the image is also shown on the computer monitor above. *Source:* Pascal Goetgheluck/Science Source	***in situ*** (IN SY-too) **keratomileusis** (KAIR-ah-TOH-my-LOO-sis) **kerat/o-** *cornea of the eye; hard, fibrous protein* **-mileusis** *process of carving* **microkeratome** (MY-kroh-KAIR-ah-tohm) **micr/o-** *one millionth; small* **kerat/o-** *cornea of the eye; hard, fibrous protein* **-tome** *area with distinct edges; instrument used to cut* **photorefractive** (FOH-toh-ree-FRAK-tiv) **phot/o-** *light* **refract/o-** *bend; deflect* **-ive** *pertaining to* **keratectomy** (KAIR-ah-TEK-toh-mee) **kerat/o-** *cornea of the eye; hard, fibrous protein* **-ectomy** *surgical removal*
photodynamic therapy (PDT)	Procedure to treat wet age-related macular degeneration. A light-sensitive drug is injected into the blood. The drug collects in abnormal vessels under the macula. Laser light then activates the drug and causes it to block blood flow through the abnormal blood vessels.	**photodynamic** (FOH-toh-dy-NAM-ik) **phot/o-** *light* **dynam/o-** *movement; power* **-ic** *pertaining to*
retinopexy	Procedure to reattach a detached retina. **Cryotherapy** is used to freeze the tissue and fix all three layers (sclera, choroid, retina) together. Alternatively, laser photocoagulation can be done to heat spots on the retina to coagulate and seal the detached part to the layers beneath. **Laser photocoagulation** is also done to seal leaking blood vessels in patients with diabetic retinopathy. Light from the laser creates heat that coagulates the tissues (see Figure 15-28 ■). If the vitreous humor contains blood, the laser light cannot reach the retina, and a **vitrectomy** must be done first to remove the vitreous and replace it with clear, man-made fluid. 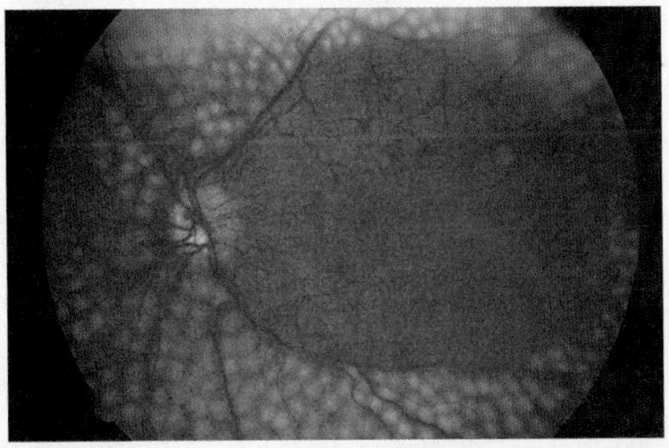 	**retinopexy** (RET-ih-noh-PEK-see) **retin/o-** *retina of the eye* **-pexy** *process of surgically fixing in place* **cryotherapy** (KRY-oh-THAIR-ah-pee) **cry/o-** *cold* **-therapy** *treatment* **photocoagulation** (FOH-toh-koh-AG-yoo-LAY-shun) **phot/o-** *light* **coagul/o-** *clotting* **-ation** *being; having; process* **vitrectomy** (vih-TREK-toh-mee) **vitre/o-** *transparent substance; vitreous humor* **-ectomy** *surgical removal*

FIGURE 15-28 ■ Laser photocoagulation.
This procedure treats leaking or hemorrhaging blood vessels associated with diabetic retinopathy. Here, the laser has been used in multiple small spots around the optic disk to coagulate the tissues.
Source: National Eye Institute

Word or Phrase	Description	Pronunciation/Word Parts
strabismus surgery	Procedure to correct esotropia or exotropia. During a **resection**, the extraocular muscle on one side is shortened. During a **recession**, the extraocular muscle on the other side is lengthened and reattached.	**resection** (ree-SEK-shun) **resect/o-** *cut out; remove* **-ion** *action; condition* **recession** (ree-SEH-shun) **recess/o-** *move back* **-ion** *action; condition*
trabeculoplasty	Procedure to treat open-angle glaucoma. A laser is used to create small holes in half of the trabecular meshwork to increase the flow of aqueous humor. The procedure is usually effective for 5 years, at which time another trabeculoplasty can be performed on the untreated half of the trabecular meshwork.	**trabeculoplasty** (trah-BEH-kyoo-loh-PLAS-tee) **trabecul/o-** *mesh* **-plasty** *process of reshaping by surgery*

Drugs

These drug categories and drugs are used to treat eye diseases. The most common generic and trade name drugs in each category are listed. Note: All drugs used topically in the eye are specially formulated to be physiologically similar to the fluids of the eye so as not to damage the delicate tissues of the eye.

Category	Indication	Examples	Pronunciation/Word Parts
antibiotic drugs	Treat bacterial infections of the eye. Antibiotic drugs are not effective against viral infections of the eye.	erythromycin, gentamicin (Gentak), ofloxacin (Ocuflox)	**antibiotic** (AN-tee-by-AW-tik) (AN-tih-by-AW-tik) **anti-** *against* **bi/o-** *life; living organism; living tissue* **-tic** *pertaining to*
antiviral drugs	Treat viral infections of the eye, specifically herpes simplex virus	trifluridine (Viroptic)	**antiviral** (AN-tee-VY-ral) (AN-tih-VY-ral) **anti-** *against* **vir/o-** *virus* **-al** *pertaining to*
corticosteroid drugs	Treat severe inflammation in the eye	dexamethasone (Maxidex), prednisolone (Pred Forte)	**corticosteroid** (KOR-tih-koh-STAIR-oyd) **cortic/o-** *cortex; outer region* **-steroid** *steroid*
drugs for glaucoma	Lower the intraocular pressure by decreasing the amount of aqueous humor or by constricting the pupil to open the angle between the iris and the cornea	betaxolol (Betoptic), dorzolamide (Trusopt), pilocarpine (Pilopine), timolol (Timoptic)	
mydriatic drugs	Dilate the pupil to prepare the eye for an internal examination	cyclopentolate (Cyclogyl), tropicamide (Mydriacyl)	**mydriatic** (MIH-dree-AT-ik) **mydr/o-** *widening* **-iatic** *pertaining to a process; pertaining to a state*

Abbreviations

AMD, ARMD	age-related macular degeneration	**O.D.**	Doctor of Optometry
CK	conductive keratoplasty	**OS, O.S.*■**	left eye (Latin, *oculus sinister*)
ECCE	extracapsular cataract extraction	**OU, O.U.*■**	both eyes (Latin, *oculus unitas*)
EOM	extraocular movements; extraocular muscles		each eye (Latin, *oculus uterque*)
EOMI	extraocular muscles intact	**PD**	prism diopter
HEENT	head, eyes, ears, nose, and throat	**PDT**	photodynamic therapy
IOL	intraocular lens	**PERRL**	pupils equal, round, and reactive to light
IOP	intraocular pressure	**PERRLA**	pupils equal, round, reactive to light and accommodation
LASIK	laser-assisted *in situ* keratomileusis (pronounced "LAY-sik")	**PRK**	photorefractive keratectomy
LTK	laser thermal keratoplasty	**ROP**	retinopathy of prematurity
OD, O.D.*■	right eye (Latin, *oculus dexter*)	**RP**	retinitis pigmentosa
		VF	visual field

*According to The Joint Commission and ■ the Institute for Safe Medication Practices (ISMP), these abbreviations should not be used. However, because they are still used by some healthcare professionals, they are included here.

WORD ALERT
Abbreviations

Abbreviations are commonly used in all types of medical documents; however, they can mean different things to different people and their meanings can be misinterpreted. Always verify the meaning of an abbreviation.

O.D. means *right eye* or *Doctor of Optometry,* but it also means *overdose.*

LASIK means *laser assisted* in situ *keratomileusis,* but it can be mistaken for *Lasix,* the trade name of a diuretic drug.

IT'S GREEK TO ME!

Did you notice that some words have two different combining forms? Combining forms from both Greek and Latin remain a part of medical language today.

Word	Greek	Latin	Medical Word Examples
cornea	kerat/o-	corne/o-	keratoplasty, corneal
eye	ophthalm/o-	ocul/o-	ophthalmology, ocular
lens	phac/o-, phak/o-	lent/o-	phacoemulsification, aphakia, retrolental
		lenticul/o-	lenticular
pupil	cor/o-	pupill/o-	anisocoria, pupillary
sight, vision	op/o-, opt/o-	vis/o-	hyperopia, optic, visual

CAREER FOCUS

Meet Paul, an optician

"I pick up where the optometrist or ophthalmologist leaves off, by looking at the prescription and suggesting to the patient the selection of frame styles or lens styles. Either we have the lenses here in stock, or we'll order them from a servicing lab that actually manufactures the lens. We use a lensometer to read the prescription of the lens, and we have to make sure we place the optical center of the lens in front of the patient's pupil. This is a fairly busy practice. From 8:00 A.M. to closing, patients come in to purchase new eyewear or have their old eyewear repaired. I've been dealing with the public all my life. When you dispense a pair of glasses to someone and it puts a new light on everything, it's gratifying; it really is."

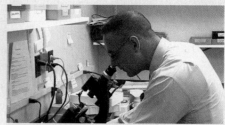

Source: Dan Frank/Ph College/Pearson Education

Opticians are allied health professionals who use automated equipment to cut, grind, and finish lenses to exact specifications based on a written prescription from an optometrist or ophthalmologist. They also prepare contact lenses and instruct the patient in their care and handling. Opticians work in optical stores or in the office of an optometrist or ophthalmologist.

Optometrists are doctors of **optometry** (O.D.) who have graduated from a school of optometry. They diagnose and treat patients with vision problems and diseases of the eyes. They write prescriptions for eyeglasses and contact lenses. They can administer and prescribe ophthalmic drugs. Optometrists do not perform eye surgery.

Ophthalmologists are physicians (M.D.) who practice in the medical specialty of ophthalmology. They do all of the things an optometrist does, but they are also able to perform surgery on the eye. Cancerous tumors of the eye are treated medically by an oncologist or surgically by an ophthalmologist.

---

optician (awp-TIH-shun)
  opt/o- *eye; vision*
  -ician *skilled expert; skilled professional*

---

optometrist (awp-TAW-meh-trist)
  opt/o- *eye; vision*
  metr/o- *measurement; uterus; womb*
  -ist *person who specializes in; thing that specializes in*

---

optometry (awp-TAW-meh-tree)
  opt/o- *eye; vision*
  -metry *process of measuring*

---

ophthalmologist (OFF-thal-MAW-loh-jist)
  ophthalm/o- *eye*
  log/o- *study of; word*
  -ist *person who specializes in; thing that specializes in*

MyMedicalTerminologyLab™   To see Paul's complete video profile, log into MyMedicalTerminologyLab and navigate to the Multimedia Library for Chapter 15. Check the Video box, and then click the Career Focus - Optician link.

MULTIPLE COMBINING FORMS AND SUFFIX EXERCISE

Read the definition of the medical word. Select the correct suffix and combining forms. Then build the medical word and write it on the line. Be sure to check your spelling. The first one has been done for you.

SUFFIX LIST

-ation (being; having; process)
-ia (condition; state; thing)
-ist (person who specializes in)
-itis (infection of; inflammation of)
-oma (mass; tumor)
-tome (instrument used to cut)

COMBINING FORM LIST

anis/o- (unequal)
blast/o- (embryonic; immature)
coagul/o- (clotting)
cor/o- (pupil of the eye)
cycl/o- (ciliary body of the eye)
cyst/o- (fluid-filled sac; semisolid cyst)
dacry/o- (lacrimal sac; tears)
dipl/o- (double)
emulsific/o- (liquid with suspended particles)
es/o- (inward)
kerat/o- (cornea of the eye)

metr/o- (measurement; uterus; womb)
micr/o- (one millionth; small)
ophthalm/o- (eye)
op/o- (vision)
opt/o- (eye; vision)
phac/o- (lens of the eye)
phob/o- (avoidance; fear)
phot/o- (light)
pleg/o- (paralysis)
presby/o- (old age)
retin/o- (retina of the eye)
trop/o- (having an affinity for; stimulating; turning)
xer/o- (dry)

Definition of the Medical Word

1. Condition (of one of the eyes being) inward turning
2. Condition (of) unequal pupils of the eyes
3. Instrument used to cut (a) small (area on the) cornea of the eye
4. Condition (of) light avoidance
5. Tumor (of the) retina (composed of) embryonic (cells)
6. Process (that uses) light (to cause) clotting
7. State (in which the) ciliary body of the eye (has) paralysis (and is kept dilated)
8. Infection of (or) inflammation of (the structure of) tears (that is a) fluid-filled sac
9. Process (in which the) lens (is turned into) liquid with suspended particles
10. Condition (of) dry eyes
11. Person who specializes in vision measurement
12. Condition (of) double vision
13. Condition (of) old age vision

Build the Medical Word

1. *esotropia* _____
2. _____
3. _____
4. _____
5. _____
6. _____
7. _____
8. _____
9. _____
10. _____
11. _____
12. _____
13. _____

15.7A Spell Medical Words

PROOFREADING AND SPELLING EXERCISE

Read the following paragraph. Identify each misspelled medical word and write the correct spelling of it on the line.

The eye works with the vizual cortex of the brain for the sense of sight. The aquous humor is clear in the anterior chamber. The layers of the eye are the conjuntiva, cornea, and sklera. The retina has the macular where the best vision is. Drops in the eyes cause midriasis so the eyes can be examined. It is not good to have a cataract or an entropion or blepharotosis. To diagnose eye diseases, a dilated fundoscopic exam is done. The study of the eye is known as ofthalmology.

1. _____ 6. _____
2. _____ 7. _____
3. _____ 8. _____
4. _____ 9. _____
5. _____ 10. _____

HEARING MEDICAL WORDS EXERCISE

You hear someone speaking the medical words given below. Read each pronunciation and then write the medical word it represents. Be sure to check your spelling. The first one has been done for you.

1. AM-blee-OH-pee-ah   *amblyopia* _____
2. KAT-ah-rakt   _____
3. SY-kloh-PLEE-jee-ah   _____
4. my-OH-pee-ah   _____
5. OFF-thal-MAW-loh-jist _____
6. awp-TIH-shun   _____
7. PREZ-bee-OH-pee-ah   _____
8. strah-BIZ-mus   _____
9. toh-NAW-meh-ter   _____
10. VIT-ree-us HYOO-mor   _____

15.7B Pronounce Medical Words

PRONUNCIATION EXERCISE

Read the medical word and the syllables in its pronunciation. Circle the primary (main) accented syllable. The first one has been done for you.

1. conjunctiva (con-junk-ty-vah)
2. aphakia (ah-fay-kee-ah)
3. conjunctivitis (con-junk-tih-vy-tis)
4. diplopia (dih-ploh-pee-ah)
5. glaucoma (glaw-koh-mah)
6. macular (mak-yoo-lar)
7. optometrist (awp-taw-meh-trist)
8. phacoemulsification (fay-koh-ee-mul-sih-fih-kay-shun)
9. retinopexy (ret-ih-noh-pek-see)
10. strabismus (strah-biz-mus)

15.8 Research Medical Words

SOUND-ALIKE WORDS

Compare and contrast the medical meanings of these sound-alike ophthalmology and other words.

1. *fundus of the eye*, *fundus of the stomach* (Chapter 3), and *fundus of the uterus* (Chapter 13)
2. *miosis* and *mitosis* (Chapter 2)
3. *macula* and *macule* (Chapter 7)
4. *choroid* and *chorion* (Chapter 13)

15.9 Analyze Medical Report

ELECTRONIC PATIENT RECORD

This is a Consultation Report by a specialist physician. Read the report and answer the questions.

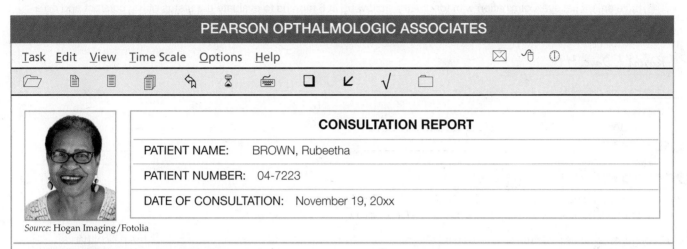

PEARSON OPTHALMOLOGIC ASSOCIATES

Task Edit View Time Scale Options Help

CONSULTATION REPORT

PATIENT NAME: BROWN, Rubeetha

PATIENT NUMBER: 04-7223

DATE OF CONSULTATION: November 19, 20xx

Source: Hogan Imaging/Fotolia

HISTORY OF PRESENT ILLNESS
This 64-year-old, African-American female comes in today as a referral from her primary care physician. She is complaining of bloodshot eyes, headaches, large floaters in her visual field, and blurred vision at close range.

PAST HISTORY
She has had myopia since childhood (onset at age 12). She was diagnosed by a neurologist as having migraines with an aura of scintillating scotomata followed by a temporary visual field defect of hemianopia, "like a gray curtain" coming down. She denies a history of hyperthyroidism, although she has been tested for this on several occasions. She denies hypertension, heart disease, or diabetes. She has some mild osteoarthritis, particularly in her right knee. Past surgeries include a tonsillectomy and an appendectomy in the remote past.

SOCIAL HISTORY
She is married and has two children, both living away from home. She works in the member services department of an HMO and does paperwork and computer work all day.

PHYSICAL EXAMINATION
The conjunctivae are infected, and the sclerae are anicteric. There is a soft, movable mass in the margin of the right upper eyelid. The patient states that this was from a trauma and has remained unchanged for many years. This is not a chalazion, just scar tissue. There is a moderate amount of crusted exudate on the eyelids. There is mild exophthalmos bilaterally. PERRL. Extraocular movements intact. Dilating drops were instilled in each eye, and a funduscopy was performed. There is evidence of a developing cataract in the right eye. The retinae bilaterally were normal. There was no suggestion of macular degeneration. There were no microaneurysms or hemorrhages. There were small clumps of vitreous humor visible in the posterior cavity.

VISUAL TESTING
Distance vision without glasses was 20/200 in both eyes. Peripheral vision was normal. Depth perception was normal. Tonometry showed normal intraocular pressures in both eyes.

DIAGNOSES
1. Eye strain and new-onset presbyopia.
2. Severe myopia. Wears corrective lenses for distance vision.
3. Stage I cataract, O.D.
4. Blepharitis.
5. Vitreous floaters. The patient was advised that although these are annoying and appear large, they are actually small and benign and are the result of the aging process.

(continued)

PLAN
1. The patient has been given a prescription for new eyeglasses. These will be bifocal lenses to correct her myopia and her new-onset presbyopia.
2. The patient was asked to gently cleanse the eyelids and apply bacitracin ophthalmic ointment b.i.d.
3. The patient has been advised of her increased risk of developing glaucoma given her age and race and was advised to have an annual eye examination with tonometry. Follow up in 6 months to evaluate the status of her cataract and do a glaucoma check.

Robert J. Dove, M.D.
_____
Robert J. Dove, M.D.

RJD: smt
D: 11/19/xx
T: 11/19/xx

---

1. A funduscopy was performed. If you wanted to use the adjective form of funduscopy, you would say, "The patient had a _____ examination performed."

2. Divide *intraocular* into its three word parts and give the meaning of each word part.

Word Part	**Meaning**
_____	_____
_____	_____
_____	_____

3. Divide *anicteric* into its three word parts and give the meaning of each word part.

Word Part	**Meaning**
_____	_____
_____	_____
_____	_____

4. What part of the eye does a funduscopy examine? _____

5. What eye condition has the patient had since childhood? _____

6. What two visual symptoms does the patient have before the onset of a migraine? _____ _____

7. The mass on the patient's eyelid is a chalazion.   True   False

8. What is the meaning of PERRL? _____

9. What abbreviation tells you that the patient's cataract was in the right eye? _____

10. The physical finding of crusted exudates on the eyelids corresponds to which diagnosis?

_____

11. Which phrase in the examination of the eye tells you that the patient does not have liver disease?

_____

12. A normal tonometry test shows that the patient does not have what disease?

_____

13. Why have physicians in the past tested the patient for hyperthyroidism?

_____

MyMedicalTerminologyLab™

MyMedicalTerminologyLab is a premium online homework management system that includes a host of features to help you study. Registered users will find:

- A multitude of quizzes and activities built within the MyLab platform

- Powerful tools that track and analyze your results—allowing you to create a personalized learning experience

- Videos and audio pronunciations to help enrich your progress

- Streaming lesson presentations (Guided Lectures) and self-paced learning modules

- A space where you and your instructor can check your progress and manage your assignments

Chapter 16
Otolaryngology

Ears, Nose, and Throat

Otolaryngology (OH-toh-LAIR-ing-GAW-loh-jee) is the medical specialty that studies the anatomy and physiology of the ears, nose, mouth, and throat (ENT) and uses laboratory and diagnostic procedures, medical and surgical procedures, and drugs to treat ENT diseases.

 Learning Outcomes

After you study this chapter, you should be able to

16.1 Identify structures of the ears, nose, and throat (ENT) system.

16.2 Describe the process of hearing.

16.3 Describe common ENT diseases, laboratory and diagnostic procedures, medical and surgical procedures, and drugs.

16.4 Form the plural and adjective forms of nouns related to otolaryngology.

16.5 Give the meanings of word parts and abbreviations related to otolaryngology.

16.6 Divide otolaryngology words and build otolaryngology words.

16.7 Spell and pronounce otolaryngology words.

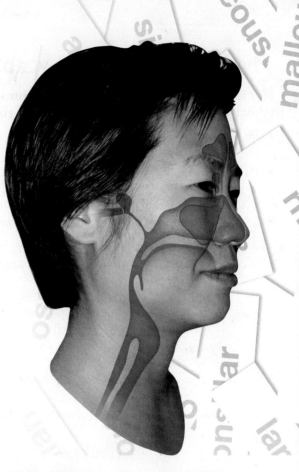

FIGURE 16-1 ■ Ears, nose, and throat (ENT) system.
The ENT system consists of many different structures located in the head and neck. Each of these individual structures is interrelated and connected to one another.
Source: Pearson Education

16.8 Research sound-alike and other otolaryngology words.

16.9 Analyze the medical content and meaning of otolaryngology reports.

Medical Language Key

To unlock the definition of a medical word, break it into word parts. Give the meaning of each word part. Put the meanings of the word parts in order, beginning with the meaning of the suffix, then the prefix (if present), then the combining form(s).

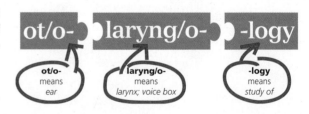

ot/o- means ear
laryng/o- means larynx; voice box
-logy means study of

	Word Part	Word Part Meaning
Suffix	**-logy**	*study of*
Combining Form	**ot/o-**	*ear*
Combining Form	**laryng/o-**	*larynx; voice box*

Otolaryngology ▶ *Study of (the) ears, (nose, throat), larynx, (and related structures).*

Although the word otolaryngology does not contain combining forms for the nose, mouth, throat, or neck, it is understood that these structures are included in this medical specialty. The word otorhinolaryngology does include the combining form rhin/o- for nose.

Anatomy and Physiology

The **ears, nose, and throat (ENT) system** is a compact body system that is contained entirely in the head and neck (see Figure 16-1 ■). The head contains the external and internal structures of the ears, nose, and mouth, and the internal structures of the sinuses. The neck contains the internal structures of the pharynx and larynx. The ENT system has several functions. It shares some structures with the gastrointestinal system and the respiratory system, and it serves as a passageway for both food and air. The ENT system also contains lymphoid tissue that functions as part of the immune response. The body's senses of hearing and smell are also part of the ENT system. The structures of the ENT system (along with those of the respiratory system) are used to generate speech.

Anatomy of the ENT System

External Ear

The external ear is the **auricle** or **pinna** (see Figure 16-2 ■). The **helix** is the outer rim of tissue and cartilage that forms a *C* and ends at the earlobe. The **external auditory meatus** is the opening that leads into the **external auditory canal (EAC)**. The **tragus** is the triangular cartilage anterior to the meatus. The canal has glands that secrete **cerumen**, a waxy, sticky substance that traps dirt and has an antibiotic action against microorganisms that enter the canal. At the end of the canal is the **tympanic membrane (TM)** or **eardrum**, a thin membrane that divides the external ear from the middle ear (see Figure 16-3 ■).

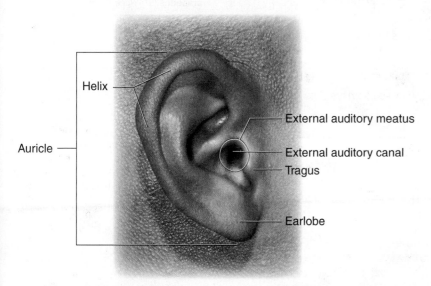

FIGURE 16-2 ■ External ear.
The external ear is composed of several types and shapes of tissue and cartilage. The external ear also includes the external auditory canal that travels into the temporal bone of the cranium.
Source: Pearson Education

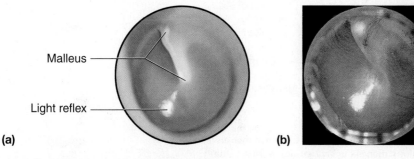

(a) (b)

FIGURE 16-3 ■ Tympanic membrane.
A normal tympanic membrane has a gray, pearly color and is so thin that the malleus can be seen behind it. A shiny strip (reflected light from an otoscope) is seen, which is known as the *light reflex*.
Source: Pearson Education; Ph College/Pearson Education

Pronunciation/Word Parts

auricle (AW-rih-kl)
  aur/i- *ear*
  -cle *small thing*

auricular (aw-RIH-kyoo-lar)
  auricul/o- *ear*
  -ar *pertaining to*

otic (OH-tik)
  ot/o- *ear*
  -ic *pertaining to*
Both *auricular* and *otic* are adjectives that mean *ear*.

pinna (PIN-ah)

pinnae (PIN-ee)
Pinna is a Latin singular noun. Form the plural by changing *-a* to *-ae*.

helix (HEE-liks)

external (eks-TER-nal)
  extern/o- *outside*
  -al *pertaining to*

auditory (AW-dih-TOR-ee)
  audit/o- *sense of hearing*
  -ory *having the function of*
The combining form **acous/o-** means *hearing; sound* and **audi/o-** means *hearing*.

meatus (mee-AA-tus)

meati (mee-AA-tie)
Meatus is a Latin singular noun. Form the plural by changing *-us* to *-i*.

tragus (TRAY-gus)

tragi (TRAY-jeye)
Tragus is a Latin singular noun. Form the plural by changing *-us* to *-i*.

cerumen (seh-ROO-men)

tympanic (tim-PAN-ik)
  tympan/o- *eardrum; tympanic membrane*
  -ic *pertaining to*
The combining form **myring/o-** also means *eardrum; tympanic membrane*.

Just behind the external ear is the **mastoid process**, a bony projection of the temporal bone of the cranium. The mastoid process is not a solid bone; it contains tiny cavities filled with air.

Middle Ear

The middle ear is a hollow area inside the temporal bone of the cranium (see Figure 16-4 ■). The middle ear contains three tiny bones: the **malleus**, **incus**, and **stapes**, collectively known as the **ossicles**. These bones are connected to each other by tiny ligaments to form the **ossicular chain**. The first bone, the malleus, is shaped like and is known as the **hammer**. It is connected to the tympanic membrane. Because the tympanic membrane is nearly transparent, the malleus can be seen through it. The second bone, the incus, is shaped like and is known as the **anvil**. The third bone, the stapes, is shaped like and is known as the **stirrup**. The stapes fits into an opening in the temporal bone known as the oval window. The middle ear is connected to the nasopharynx by the **eustachian tube**. The eustachian tube allows air pressure in the middle ear to equalize with air pressure in the nose and throat and outside the body.

Pronunciation/Word Parts

mastoid (MAS-toyd)
  mast/o- *breast; mastoid process*
  -oid *resembling*
The combining form **mastoid/o-** means *mastoid process.*

malleus (MAL-ee-us)

mallei (MAL-ee-eye)
Malleus is a Latin singular noun. Form the plural by changing *-us* to *-i.*

mallear (MAL-ee-ar)
  malle/o- *hammer-shaped bone; malleus*
  -ar *pertaining to*

incus (ING-kus)

incudes (in-KYOO-deez)

incudal (IN-kyoo-dal)
  incud/o- *anvil-shaped bone; incus*
  -al *pertaining to*

stapes (STAY-peez)

stapedes (STAY-pee-deez)

stapedial (stay-PEE-dee-al)
  staped/o- *stapes; stirrup-shaped bone*
  -ial *pertaining to*

ossicle (AW-sih-kl)
  ossic/o- *bone*
  -cle *small thing*

ossicular (aw-SIH-kyoo-lar)
  ossicul/o- *ossicle; small bone*
  -ar *pertaining to*

eustachian (yoo-STAY-shun)

WORD ALERT		
Sound-Alike Words		
malleus	(noun)	first bone of the middle ear
	Example: An infection in the middle ear caused scar tissue around the malleus and affected the patient's hearing.	
malleolus	(noun)	bony projections on the tibia and fibula of the lower leg near the ankle
	Example: The lateral malleolus is a bony projection from the distal end of the fibula.	

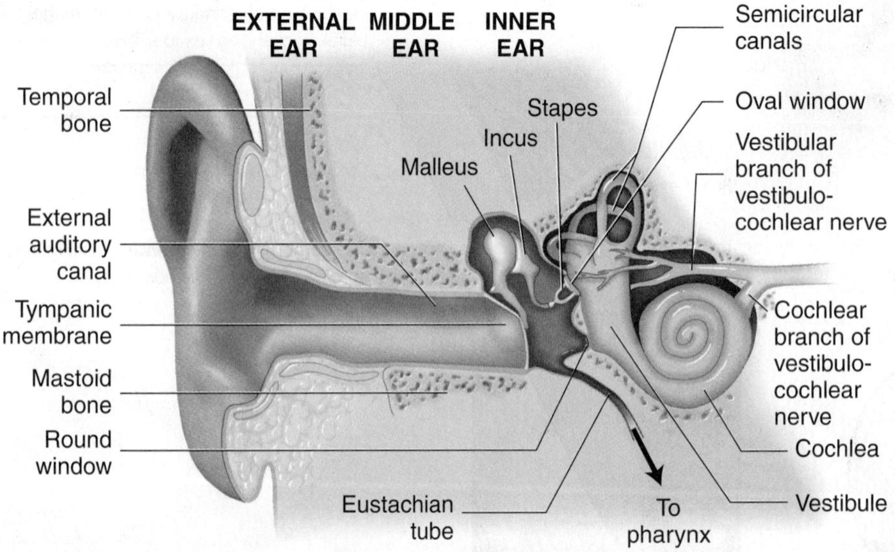

FIGURE 16-4 ■ Structures of the middle ear and inner ear.
Notice the shapes of the malleus, incus, and stapes in the middle ear. Do they look like a hammer, anvil, and stirrup to you? The structures of the inner ear send information about balance and hearing to the brain via the vestibulocochlear nerve.
Source: Pearson Education

Inner Ear

The temporal bone of the cranium divides the middle ear from the inner ear, with openings of the oval window (to the stirrup) and the round window (to the vestibule) connecting the two cavities. The inner ear cavity contains three fluid-filled structures: the vestibule, the semicircular canals, and the cochlea (see Figure 16-4). The **vestibule** is the entrance to the inner ear. The superior part of the vestibule becomes the three **semicircular canals**. Each of these canals is oriented in a different plane: horizontally, vertically, and obliquely. When you move your head, the semicircular canals send information to the brain about the position of your head and this helps you keep your balance. The inferior part of the vestibule becomes the coiled **cochlea**. The cochlea sends sensory information to the brain about the frequency (pitch) and intensity (loudness) of the sound waves entering the ear. Together, all of the structures of the inner ear are known as the **labyrinth**.

External Nose and Mouth

The external nose is supported by the nasal bone, which forms the bridge of the nose and the **dorsum** (see Figure 16-5 ■). At the nasal tip, the nasal bone becomes cartilage. The **nares** are the external openings or nostrils. The flared cartilage on each side of the nostril is a nasal **ala**.

The lips, cheeks, and chin are supported by the maxilla (upper jawbone) and mandible (lower jawbone). The **nasolabial fold** is the crease in the cheek that goes from the nose to the lip at the corner of the mouth. The **philtrum** is the vertical groove in the skin of the upper lip. The chin is also known as the **mentum**.

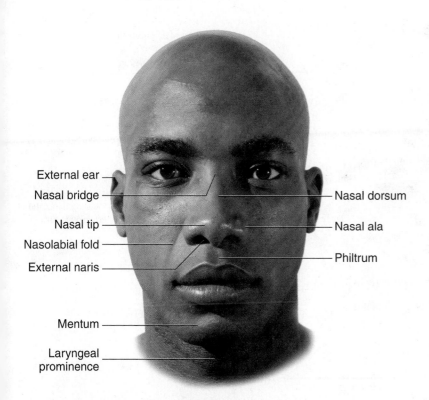

Labels: External ear, Nasal bridge, Nasal tip, Nasolabial fold, External naris, Mentum, Laryngeal prominence, Nasal dorsum, Nasal ala, Philtrum

FIGURE 16-5 ■ External nose, mouth, and neck.
The external nose is supported by the nasal bone, which transitions to cartilage at the tip of the nose. The tissues of the lips, mouth, and chin are supported by the maxilla and mandible bones. The laryngeal prominence in the neck is composed of cartilage around the larynx (voice box).
Source: Pearson Education

Pronunciation/Word Parts

vestibule (VES-tih-byool)

vestibular (ves-TIH-byoo-lar)
 vestibul/o- *entrance; vestibule*
 -ar *pertaining to*

semicircular (SEM-ee-SIR-kyoo-lar)
 semi- *half; partly*
 circul/o- *circle*
 -ar *pertaining to*

cochlea (KOH-klee-ah)

cochleae (KOH-klee-ee)
Cochlea is a Latin singular noun. Form the plural by changing *-a* to *-ae*.

cochlear (KOH-klee-ar)
 cochle/o- *cochlea; spiral-shaped structure*
 -ar *pertaining to*

labyrinth (LAB-ih-rinth)
The combining form **labyrinth/o-** means *labyrinth of the inner ear*.

dorsum (DOR-sum)

dorsal (DOR-sal)
 dors/o- *back; dorsum*
 -al *pertaining to*

naris (NAY-ris)

nares (NAY-reez)
Naris is a Latin singular noun. Form the plural by changing *-is* to *-es*.

ala (AA-lah)

alae (AA-lee)
Ala is a Latin singular noun. Form the plural by changing *-a* to *-ae*.

nasolabial (NAY-zoh-LAY-bee-al)
 nas/o- *nose*
 labi/o- *labium; lip*
 -al *pertaining to*
The combining form **cheil/o-** means *lip*.

philtrum (FIL-trum)

mentum (MEN-tum)
The combining form **ment/o-** means *chin; mind*.

Pronunciation/Word Parts

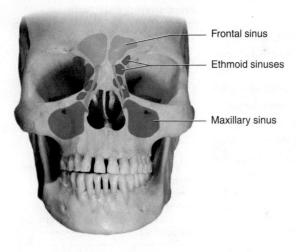

FIGURE 16-6 ■ Sinuses.
The sinuses are hollow cavities or small areas lined with mucosa within the frontal, maxillary, ethmoid, and sphenoid bones of the cranium and face. (The sphenoid sinuses are not seen on this view.)
Source: Alexander Potapov/Fotolia

Sinuses

A **sinus** is a hollow cavity within a bone that is lined with a mucous membrane. There are four pairs of sinuses, each located within the skull bone for which they are named (see Figures 16-6 ■ and 16-7 ■). The **frontal sinuses** are within the frontal bone, just above each eyebrow. The **maxillary sinuses**, the largest of the sinuses, are within each maxilla on either side of the nose. The **ethmoid sinuses**, which are groups of small air cells rather than a hollow cavity, are within the ethmoid bone, between the nose and the eyes. The **sphenoid sinuses** are within the sphenoid bone, posterior to the nasal cavity and near the pituitary gland of the brain (see Figure 16-7). Together, these sinuses are known as the **paranasal sinuses**.

sinus (SY-nus)
The Latin singular and plural forms of *sinus* are the same. An English plural can be formed by adding -*es* (sinuses). The combining form **sinus/o-** means *sinus*.

frontal (FRUN-tal)
   front/o- *front*
   -**al** *pertaining to*

maxillary (MAK-sih-LAIR-ee)
   maxill/o- *maxilla; upper jaw*
   -**ary** *pertaining to*

ethmoid (ETH-moyd)
   ethm/o- *sieve*
   -**oid** *resembling*

sphenoid (SFEE-noyd)
   sphen/o- *wedge shape*
   -**oid** *resembling*

paranasal (PAIR-ah-NAY-zal)
   para- *abnormal; apart from; beside; two parts of a pair*
   nas/o- *nose*
   -**al** *pertaining to*
Select the correct prefix meaning to get the definition of *paranasal*: pertaining to beside the nose.

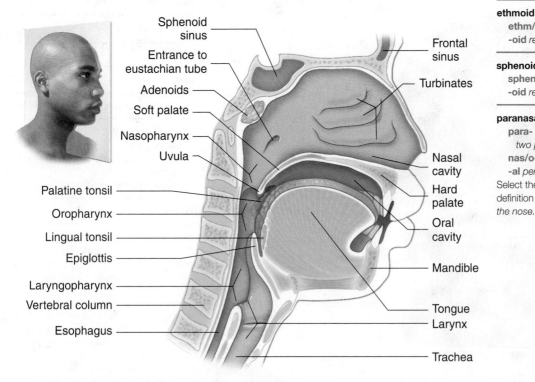

FIGURE 16-7 ■ Structures of the internal nose, mouth, and throat.
This midsagittal section of the head and neck shows the turbinates in the nasal cavity, the structures of the oral cavity, the tonsils and adenoids, and the three parts of the pharynx—the nasopharynx, oropharynx, and laryngopharynx. Note how anatomically close the area of the pharynx is to the bones of the vertebral column.
Source: Pearson Education

Nasal Cavity

The **nasal septum** is a vertical wall of cartilage that divides the nasal cavity into right and left sides. In the posterior nasal cavity, this cartilage becomes the ethmoid bone of the cranium. The walls of the **nasal cavity** are formed by the ethmoid bone of the cranium and maxilla of the upper jaw. Along the walls are three long, bony projections—the **superior**, **middle**, and **inferior turbinates**. These are also known as the **nasal conchae**. They are covered with **mucosa**, a mucous membrane that continuously produces **mucus**. They divide and slow down inhaled air and give it warmth and moisture.

Oral Cavity

The **oral cavity** or mouth contains the tongue, hard palate, soft palate, uvula, and teeth (see Figure 16-7). The oral cavity is lined with oral mucosa; it is known as **buccal mucosa** in the cheek area. The **hard palate** or roof of the mouth divides the oral cavity from the nasal cavity. The hard palate is made up of the maxilla at the front of the mouth, then the palatine bone, and the vomer bone at the back. The hard palate transitions to the tissue of the **soft palate** and the **uvula**, which is the fleshy hanging part of the soft palate. The mandible forms the floor of the mouth, and the base of the **tongue** is attached to it. Each end of the mandible is attached to the temporal bone of the cranium at the moveable **temporomandibular joint (TMJ)**. The salivary glands secrete saliva into the oral cavity (discussed in "Gastroenterology," Chapter 3).

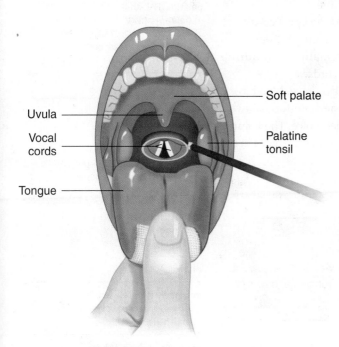

FIGURE 16-8 ■ Pharynx.
The pharynx can be examined by holding the tongue with a piece of gauze and pulling it forward. The palatine tonsils can be seen on either side of the soft palate. A laryngeal mirror can visualize the vocal cords in the larynx, and the mirror can be turned upward to examine the nasopharynx.
Source: Pearson Education

Pronunciation/Word Parts

nasal (NAY-zal)
  nas/o- *nose*
  -al *pertaining to*
Nasal is the adjective form for *nose*. The combining form **rhin/o-** also means *nose*.

septum (SEP-tum)

septal (SEP-tal)
  sept/o- *dividing wall; septum*
  -al *pertaining to*

cavity (KAV-ih-tee)
  cav/o- *hollow space*
  -ity *condition; state*

superior (soo-PEER-ee-or)
  super/o- *above*
  -ior *pertaining to*

inferior (in-FEER-ee-or)
  infer/o- *below*
  -ior *pertaining to*

turbinate (TER-bih-nayt)
  turbin/o- *scroll-like structure; turbinate*
  -ate *composed of; pertaining to*

concha (CON-kah)

conchae (CON-kee)
Concha is a Latin singular noun. Form the plural by changing *-a* to *-ae*.

mucosa (myoo-KOH-sah)

mucosal (myoo-KOH-sal)
  mucos/o- *mucous membrane*
  -al *pertaining to*

mucus (MYOO-kus)

oral (OR-al)
  or/o- *mouth*
  -al *pertaining to*
Oral is the adjective form for *mouth*.

buccal (BUK-al)
  bucc/o- *cheek*
  -al *pertaining to*

palate (PAL-at)

uvula (YOO-vyoo-lah)

glossal (GLAW-sal)
  gloss/o- *tongue*
  -al *pertaining to*
Glossal is the adjective form for *tongue*. The combining form **lingu/o-** also means *tongue*.

temporomandibular
(TEM-poh-ROH-man-DIH-byoo-lar)
  tempor/o- *side of the head; temple*
  mandibul/o- *lower jaw; mandible*
  -ar *pertaining to*

Submental lymph nodes under the chin contain lymphocytes and macrophages that attack bacteria and viruses in the oral cavity.

Pharynx

The **pharynx** or throat is divided into three areas: the nasopharynx, the oropharynx, and the laryngopharynx (see Figure 16-7). As the nasal cavity continues posteriorly, it becomes the **nasopharynx**. The eustachian tubes from the middle ears connect with the nasopharynx. The roof and walls of the nasopharynx contain a collection of lymphoid tissue known as the **adenoids**. The **oropharynx** is the middle portion of the throat. It contains the **palatine tonsils**, which are lymphoid tissue on either side of the soft palate (see Figure 16-8 ■). The **laryngopharynx** extends from the base of the tongue to the entrances to the esophagus and larynx. The laryngopharynx contains the **lingual tonsils** on either side of the base of the tongue. The adenoids and tonsils are part of the lymphatic system, and they function in the immune response. They contain lymphocytes and macrophages that attack bacteria and viruses in the oral cavity and throat.

Larynx

At its inferior end, the pharynx divides into the larynx that leads to the trachea and the esophagus that leads to the stomach. The **larynx**, or voice box, is a short, triangular structure. It is surrounded by cartilage that can be clearly seen at the front of the neck as the **laryngeal prominence** (Adam's apple) (see Figure 16-5). At the superior end of the larynx is the **epiglottis**, a lid-like structure (see Figure 16-7). In the middle of the larynx is the **glottis**, a V-shaped structure of cartilage, ligaments, and the **vocal cords** (see Figure 16-8). When you swallow, the larynx moves up and closes against the epiglottis to keep food from entering the lungs. Otherwise, the larynx remains open during breathing, speaking, or singing to allow air to pass over the vocal cords.

The vocal cords relax or tighten to lower or raise the pitch of the voice. Men have a large larynx and long vocal cords that vibrate at a slow frequency and produce a lower-pitched voice. Women have shorter vocal cords and a higher-pitched voice. The volume of air from the lungs affects how loud or soft the voice is. The voice also resonates in the sinuses, adding fullness to the sound.

DID YOU KNOW?

During speech, exhaled air from the lungs causes the vocal cords to vibrate in a wavelike fashion up to 100 times per second. These vibrations produce sound waves. As the sound waves travel from the vocal cords, they are shaped by the soft palate, tongue, and lips into spoken words.

Physiology of the Sense of Hearing

The external ear captures sound waves. They travel through the external auditory canal to the tympanic membrane (see Figure 16-9 ■). There, the sound waves are converted to mechanical motion as they cause the tympanic membrane to move. As the tympanic membrane moves, it moves the malleus, the incus, and then the stapes of the middle ear. The stapes transmits this mechanical motion to the oval window. This causes the fluid-filled vestibule of the inner ear to vibrate. This vibration is transmitted to the cochlea. Down the length of the cochlea, tiny hair cells detect the loudness (intensity) and pitch (frequency) of the sound. The loudness of the sound correlates to the degree

Pronunciation/Word Parts

submental (sub-MEN-tal)
  sub- *below; underneath*
  ment/o- *chin; mind*
  -al *pertaining to*
Select the correct prefix and combining form meanings to get the definition of *submental*: *pertaining to underneath the chin.*

pharynx (FAIR-ingks)

pharyngeal (fah-RIN-jee-al)
  pharyng/o- *pharynx; throat*
  -eal *pertaining to*

nasopharynx (NAY-zoh-FAIR-ingks)
  nas/o- *nose*
  -pharynx *pharynx; throat*

adenoids (AD-eh-noydz)
  aden/o- *gland*
  -oid *resembling*
The combining form **adenoid/o-** means *structure resembling a gland.*

oropharynx (OR-oh-FAIR-ingks)
  or/o- *mouth*
  -pharynx *pharynx; throat*

palatine (PAL-ah-teen)
  palat/o- *palate*
  -ine *pertaining to; thing pertaining to*
Palatine and *palatal* are both adjectives for *palate.*

tonsil (TAWN-sil)

tonsillar (TAWN-sih-lar)
  tonsill/o- *tonsil*
  -ar *pertaining to*

laryngopharynx (lah-RING-goh-FAIR-ingks)
  laryng/o- *larynx; voice box*
  -pharynx *pharynx; throat*

lingual (LING-gwal)
  lingu/o- *tongue*
  -al *pertaining to*

larynx (LAIR-ingks)

laryngeal (lah-RIN-jee-al)
  laryng/o- *larynx; voice box*
  -eal *pertaining to*

epiglottis (EP-ih-GLAW-tis)

epiglottic (EP-ih-GLAW-tik)
  epi- *above; upon*
  glott/o- *glottis of the larynx*
  -ic *pertaining to*

glottis (GLAW-tis)

vocal (VOH-kal)
  voc/o- *voice*
  -al *pertaining to*

to which the hair cells are distorted. The various frequencies in the sound correlate to the location in the cochlea of the stimulated hairs. (When the vibration has traveled through the cochlea, it comes back to the vestibule where it causes the round window to bulge. The round window acts as a safety valve in the otherwise rigid bony walls of the inner ear.) Then the loudness of the sound and its pitch (as detected by the tiny hair cells of the cochlea) travel as nerve impulses through the cochlear branch of the **vestibulocochlear nerve** (cranial nerve VIII) to the medulla oblongata in the brainstem. From there, the impulses travel to the **auditory cortex** in each temporal lobe of the brain to be interpreted for the sense of hearing.

Pronunciation/Word Parts

vestibulocochlear
(ves-TIH-byoo-loh-KOH-klee-ar)
  vestibul/o- entrance; vestibule
  cochle/o- cochlea; spiral-shaped
    structure
  -ar pertaining to

auditory (AW-dih-TOR-ee)
  audit/o- sense of hearing
  -ory having the function of
The combining form **audi/o-** means
hearing. The combining form **acous/o-**
means hearing; sound.

cortex (KOR-teks)

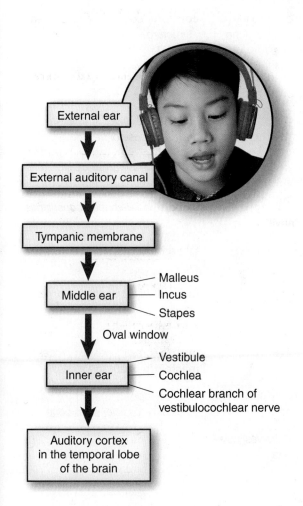

FIGURE 16-9 ■ **The sense of hearing.**
Sound travels as sound waves through the external auditory canal. Then it is converted to mechanical motion in the middle ear. In the inner ear, it is converted to nerve impulses that travel through the cochlear branch of the vestibulocochlear nerve (cranial nerve VIII) to the brain to be interpreted.
Source: Pearson Education; Sirikorn_t/Fotolia

Vocabulary Review

	Ears	
Word or Phrase	**Description**	**Combining Forms**
auditory cortex	Area in each temporal lobe of the brain where sensory information from the ears is interpreted for the sense of hearing	**audit/o-** *sense of hearing* **audi/o-** *hearing* **acous/o-** *hearing; sound*
auricle	The visible external ear. It is also known as the **pinna**.	**aur/i-** *ear* **auricul/o-** *ear* **ot/o-** *ear*
cerumen	Sticky wax secreted by glands in the external auditory canal. It traps dirt.	
cochlea	Coiled structure of the inner ear associated with the sense of hearing. It relays sensory information to the brain via the cochlear branch of the vestibulocochlear nerve.	**cochle/o-** *cochlea; spiral-shaped structure*
eustachian tube	Tube that connects the middle ear to the nasopharynx and equalizes the air pressure between the middle ear, throat, and outside of the body	
external auditory canal	Passageway from the external ear to the middle ear. It contains glands that secrete cerumen. The **external auditory meatus** is the opening to the external auditory canal.	**extern/o-** *outside* **audit/o-** *sense of hearing*
helix	Rim of tissue and cartilage that forms the *C* shape of the external ear	
incus	Second bone of the middle ear. It is attached to the malleus on one end and the stapes on the other end. It is also known as the **anvil**.	**incud/o-** *anvil-shaped bone; incus*
labyrinth	All of the structures of the inner ear	**labyrinth/o-** *labyrinth of the inner ear*
malleus	First bone of the middle ear. It is attached to the tympanic membrane on one end and to the incus on the other end. It is also known as the **hammer**.	**malle/o-** *hammer-shaped bone; malleus*
mastoid process	Bony projection of the temporal bone behind the ear	**mast/o-** *breast; mastoid process* **mastoid/o-** *mastoid process*
ossicles	The three tiny bones of the middle ear: malleus, incus, and stapes. They are also known as the **ossicular chain**.	**ossic/o-** *bone* **ossicul/o-** *ossicle; small bone*
oval window	Opening in the temporal bone between the middle ear and the vestibule of the inner ear. The opening is covered by the end of the stapes.	
round window	Opening in the temporal bone between the middle ear and the vestibule of the inner ear. The opening is covered with a membrane.	
semicircular canals	Three separate but intertwined canals in the inner ear that are oriented in different planes (horizontally, vertically, obliquely). They help the body keep its balance. They relay sensory information to the brain via the vestibular branch of the vestibulocochlear nerve.	**circul/o-** *circle*
stapes	Third bone of the middle ear. It is attached to the incus on one end and to the oval window on the other end. It is also known as the **stirrup**.	**staped/o-** *stapes; stirrup-shaped bone*

Word or Phrase	Description	Combining Forms
tragus	Triangular cartilage anterior to the external auditory meatus of the ear	
tympanic membrane	Membrane that divides the external ear from the middle ear. It is also known as the **eardrum**.	**tympan/o-** *eardrum; tympanic membrane* **myring/o-** *eardrum; tympanic membrane*
vestibule	Structure at the entrance to the inner ear. It is filled with fluid and has two small openings in its wall: the oval window and round window. The ends of the vestibule become the semicircular canals and the cochlea.	**vestibul/o-** *entrance; vestibule*
vestibulocochlear nerve	Cranial nerve VIII whose branches carry impulses from both the semicircular canals and the cochlea to the medulla oblongata of the brainstem	**vestibul/o-** *entrance; vestibule* **cochle/o-** *cochlea; spiral-shaped structure*
Sinuses		
ethmoid sinuses	Groups of small air cells in the ethmoid bone between the nose and the eyes	**ethm/o-** *sieve*
frontal sinuses	Sinuses above each eyebrow in the frontal bone of the cranium	**front/o-** *front*
maxillary sinuses	Largest of the sinuses. They are on either side of the nose in the maxilla (upper jaw bone)	**maxill/o-** *maxilla; upper jaw*
sinus	Hollow cavity within a cranial or facial bone. It is lined with mucosa. The **paranasal sinuses** include all of the sinuses.	**sinus/o-** *sinus* **nas/o-** *nose*
sphenoid sinuses	Sinuses in the sphenoid bone posterior to the nasal cavity and near the pituitary gland of the brain	**sphen/o-** *wedge shape*
Nose and Nasal Cavity		
ala	Flared cartilage on each side of the nostril	
mucosa	Mucous membrane lining the nasal cavity that warms and moistens the incoming air. It also produces **mucus** to trap foreign particles.	**mucos/o-** *mucous membrane*
naris	One nostril, the opening into the nasal cavity	
nasal cavity	Hollow area inside the nose that is formed by the ethmoid and maxillary bones. It is lined with mucosa.	**nas/o-** *nose* **cav/o-** *hollow space* **rhin/o-** *nose*
nasal dorsum	Vertical ridge in the middle of the external nose. It is supported by the nasal bone.	**dors/o-** *back; dorsum*
nasal septum	Vertical wall of cartilage and bone that divides the nasal cavity into right and left sides	**sept/o-** *dividing wall; septum*
turbinates	Three long projections of bone (**superior**, **middle**, and **inferior turbinates**) covered with mucosa that jut into the nasal cavity. They break up and give moisture to the air as it enters the nose. They are also known as the **nasal conchae**.	**turbin/o-** *scroll-like structure; turbinate* **super/o-** *above* **infer/o-** *below*

Mouth and Oral Cavity		
Word or Phrase	**Description**	**Combining Forms**
hard palate	Bone that divides the nasal cavity from the oral cavity. It is made up of the maxilla, palatine, and vomer bones. It is also known as the *roof of the mouth.*	**palat/o-** *palate*
mentum	The chin. The most anterior part of the mandible (lower jaw).	**ment/o-** *chin; mind*
mucosa	Mucous membrane that produces **mucus**. The **oral mucosa** lines the oral cavity. The **buccal mucosa** lines the cheek area of the oral cavity.	**mucos/o-** *mucous membrane* **or/o-** *mouth* **bucc/o-** *cheek*
nasolabial fold	Skin crease in the cheek that goes from the nose to the lip at the corner of the mouth	**nas/o-** *nose* **labi/o-** *labium; lip* **cheil/o-** *lip*
oral cavity	Hollow area inside the mouth that contains the tongue, teeth, hard and soft palates, and uvula. It is lined with mucosa.	**or/o-** *mouth*
philtrum	Vertical groove in the skin of the upper lip	
soft palate	Soft tissue extension of the hard palate at the back of the throat. It ends with the **uvula**.	**palat/o-** *palate*
submental lymph nodes	Lymph nodes beneath the chin	**ment/o-** *chin; mind*
temporo-mandibular joint	Moveable joint where ligaments attach each end of the mandible (lower jaw) to the temporal bones of the cranium	**tempor/o-** *side of the head; temple* **mandibul/o-** *lower jaw; mandible*
tongue	Large muscle in the oral cavity that is attached to the mandible	**gloss/o-** *tongue* **lingu/o-** *tongue*
Pharynx		
adenoids	Lymphoid tissue in the nasopharynx	**aden/o-** *gland* **adenoid/o-** *structure resembling a gland*
laryngopharynx	Most inferior part of the throat. It extends from the base of the tongue to the larynx and the entrance to the esophagus.	**laryng/o-** *larynx; voice box* **pharyng/o-** *pharynx; throat*
lingual tonsils	Lymphoid tissue located on both sides of the base of the tongue in the laryngopharynx	**lingu/o-** *tongue* **tonsill/o-** *tonsil*
nasopharynx	Most superior part of the throat. The nasopharynx contains the adenoids and openings for the eustachian tubes.	**nas/o-** *nose* **pharyng/o-** *pharynx; throat*
oropharynx	Middle part of the throat that lies posterior to the oral cavity. It extends from the soft palate to the epiglottis. It contains the palatine tonsils.	**or/o-** *mouth* **pharyng/o-** *pharynx; throat*
palatine tonsils	Lymphoid tissue in the oropharynx on either side of the soft palate	**palat/o-** *palate* **tonsill/o-** *tonsil*
pharynx	The throat. It is composed of the nasopharynx, oropharynx, and laryngopharynx.	**pharyng/o-** *pharynx; throat*

Give Word Part Meanings

Use the Answer Key at the end of the book to check your answers.

Combining Forms Exercise

Next to each combining form, write its meaning. The first one has been done for you.

Combining Form	Meaning	Combining Form	Meaning
1. **acous/o-**	hearing; sound	27. mast/o-	
2. aden/o-		28. mastoid/o-	
3. adenoid/o-		29. maxill/o-	
4. audi/o-		30. ment/o-	
5. audit/o-		31. mucos/o-	
6. aur/i-		32. myring/o-	
7. auricul/o-		33. nas/o-	
8. bucc/o-		34. or/o-	
9. cav/o-		35. ossic/o-	
10. cheil/o-		36. ossicul/o-	
11. circul/o-		37. ot/o-	
12. cochle/o-		38. palat/o-	
13. dors/o-		39. pharyng/o-	
14. ethm/o-		40. rhin/o-	
15. extern/o-		41. sept/o-	
16. front/o-		42. sinus/o-	
17. gloss/o-		43. sphen/o-	
18. glott/o-		44. staped/o-	
19. incud/o-		45. super/o-	
20. infer/o-		46. tempor/o-	
21. labi/o-		47. tonsill/o-	
22. labyrinth/o-		48. turbin/o-	
23. laryng/o-		49. tympan/o-	
24. lingu/o-		50. vestibul/o-	
25. malle/o-		51. voc/o-	
26. mandibul/o-			

Build Medical Words

Combining Form and Suffix Exercise

Read the definition of the medical word. Look at the combining form that is given. Select the correct suffix from the Suffix List and write it on the blank line. Then build the medical word and write it on the line. (Remember: You may need to remove the combining vowel. Always remove the hyphens and slash.) Be sure to check your spelling. The first one has been done for you.

SUFFIX LIST

-al (pertaining to)	-eal (pertaining to)	-oid (resembling)
-ar (pertaining to)	-ial (pertaining to)	-ory (having the function of)
-ate (composed of; pertaining to)	-ic (pertaining to)	-pharynx (pharynx; throat)
-cle (small thing)		

Definition of the Medical Word	Combining Form	Suffix	Build the Medical Word
1. Pertaining to (the) palate	**palat/o-**	**-al**	palatal

(You think *pertaining to* (-al) + *palate* (palat/o-). You change the order of the word parts to put the suffix last. You write *palatal*.)

2. Pertaining to (the) nose	nas/o-	_____	_____
3. Having the function of (the) sense of hearing	audit/o-	_____	_____
4. Pertaining to (the) eardrum	tympan/o-	_____	_____
5. Pertaining to (the) septum	sept/o-	_____	_____
6. Composed of (a) scroll-like structure	turbin/o-	_____	_____
7. Pertaining to (a) tonsil	tonsill/o-	_____	_____
8. Pertaining to (the) cheek	bucc/o-	_____	_____
9. Pertaining to (the) stirrup-shaped bone (in the middle ear)	staped/o-	_____	_____
10. (Sinus that is) resembling (a) sieve	ethm/o-	_____	_____
11. Pertaining to (the) throat	pharyng/o-	_____	_____
12. Pertaining to (the) tongue	gloss/o-	_____	_____
13. (The part of the) throat (posterior to the) nose	nas/o-	_____	_____
14. (Lymphoid tissue that is) resembling (a) gland	aden/o-	_____	_____
15. Pertaining to (the) mucous membrane	mucos/o-	_____	_____
16. Pertaining to (the) ear	auricul/o-	_____	_____
17. Pertaining to (the) mouth	or/o-	_____	_____
18. Pertaining to (a chain of) small bone(s) (in the middle ear)	ossicul/o-	_____	_____
19. Small thing (that is the) ear	aur/i-	_____	_____
20. (Bony process behind the ear) resembling (a) breast	mast/o-	_____	_____
21. Pertaining to (the) voice box	laryng/o-	_____	_____

Diseases

	Ears	
Word or Phrase	**Description**	**Pronunciation/Word Parts**
acoustic neuroma	Benign (not cancerous) tumor of the vestibulocochlear nerve. Depending on the location of the tumor, it can cause pain, dizziness, or hearing loss. Treatment: Surgical removal.	**acoustic** (ah-KOOS-tik) **acous/o-** *hearing; sound* **-tic** *pertaining to* **neuroma** (nyoor-OH-mah) **neur/o-** *nerve* **-oma** *mass; tumor*
cerumen impaction`	Cerumen (earwax), epithelial cells, and hair form a mass that occludes the external auditory canal. It occurs most commonly in older adults because of dry skin, thick cerumen, growth of hair in the external auditory canal and/or the presence of a hearing aid. Treatment: Ear drops to soften the cerumen and irrigation with a saline solution and bulb syringe to wash it out; removal with forceps (see Figure 16-10 ■).	**impaction** (im-PAK-shun) **impact/o-** *wedged in* **-ion** *action; condition*

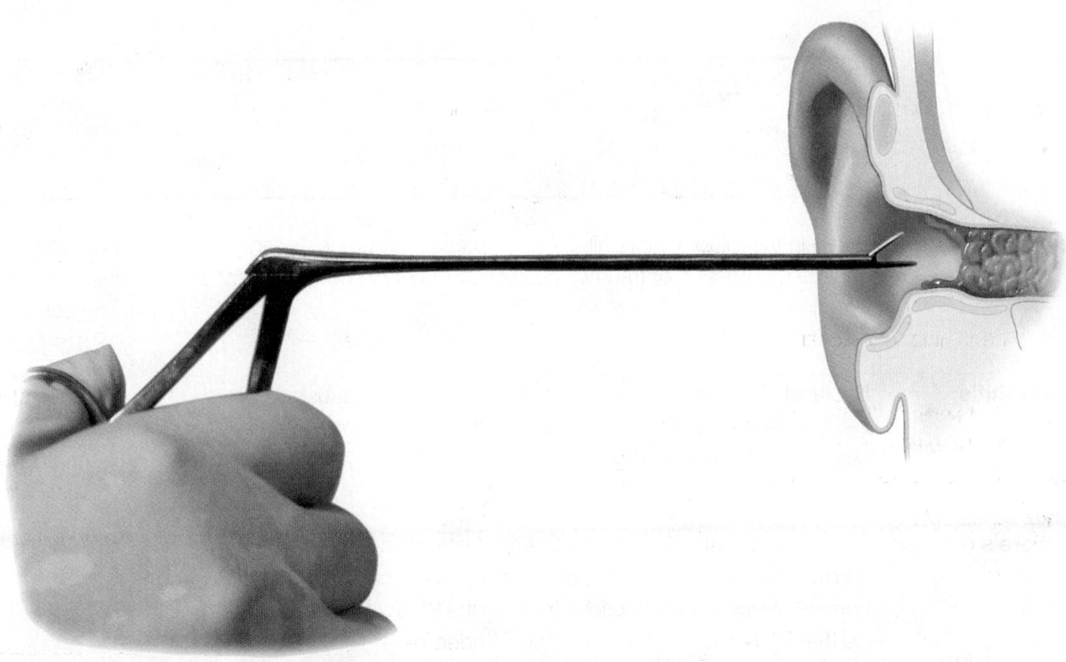

FIGURE 16-10 ■ Cerumen impaction.
Alligator forceps are used to enter the external auditory canal and remove impacted cerumen or a foreign body. Alligator forceps are so-named because their shape resembles the long nose and open, biting jaws of an alligator.
Source: Pearson Education

cholesteatoma	Benign, slow-growing tumor in the middle ear. It contains cholesterol deposits and epithelial cells. It can eventually destroy the bones of the middle ear and extend into the air cells within the mastoid process. The underlying cause usually is chronic otitis media. Treatment: Treat the underlying otitis media. Surgical removal of the cholesteatoma.	**cholesteatoma** (koh-LES-tee-ah-TOH-mah) *Cholesteatoma* is a combination of the word *cholesterol,* the Greek word *stear* (animal fat), and the suffix *-oma* (mass; tumor).

Word or Phrase	Description	Pronunciation/Word Parts
hearing loss	Progressive, permanent decline in the ability to hear sounds in one or both ears. A foreign body or infection in the external auditory canal, perforation of the tympanic membrane, fluid behind the tympanic membrane, degeneration of the ossicles, or otosclerosis (see description on page 796) of the middle ear keep sound waves from reaching the inner ear. These are types of **conductive hearing loss**. Other causes of hearing loss include disease of the cochlea, damage to the inner ear from excessive noise, or changes due to aging that hinder the production or sending of sensory impulses to the vestibulocochlear nerve. These are types of **sensorineural hearing loss**. A combination of both conductive and sensorineural hearing loss is a **mixed hearing loss**. **Low-frequency hearing loss** is the inability to hear low-pitched sounds. **High-frequency hearing loss** is the inability to hear high-pitched sounds. **Presbycusis** is bilateral hearing loss due to aging. Patients with a hearing loss are said to be **hearing impaired** or hard of hearing. Total deafness is known as **anakusis**. Deaf-mutism is deafness coupled with the inability to speak. Treatment: Correct the underlying cause; hearing aid; in some cases a cochlear implant may be needed.	**conductive** (con-DUK-tiv) conduct/o- *carrying; conveying* -ive *pertaining to* **sensorineural** (SEN-soh-ree-NYOOR-al) sensor/i- *sensory* neur/o- *nerve* -al *pertaining to* **presbycusis** (PREZ-bee-KOO-sis) presby/o- *old age* acous/o- *hearing; sound* -sis *condition; process* Delete several letters before joining the word parts. **anakusis** (AN-ah-KOO-sis)

> **DID YOU KNOW?**
> Tone deafness is not a type of hearing loss. It is the inability to identify musical notes and sing in tune with them.

Word or Phrase	Description	Pronunciation/Word Parts
hemotympanum	Blood in the middle ear behind the tympanic membrane. It can be caused by infection or trauma. Treatment: Antibiotic drugs to treat an infection.	**hemotympanum** (HEE-moh-TIM-pah-num) The combining form **hem/o-** means *blood*.
labyrinthitis	Bacterial or viral infection of the semicircular canals, causing severe vertigo. Treatment: Antibiotic drug for a bacterial infection. Viruses are not sensitive to antibiotic drugs.	**labyrinthitis** (LAB-ih-rin-THY-tis) labyrinth/o- *labyrinth of the inner ear* -itis *infection of; inflammation of*
Meniere's disease	Edema of the semicircular canals with destruction of the cochlea, causing tinnitus, vertigo, hearing loss, and nystagmus. It can be caused by head trauma or middle ear infection. Treatment: Correct the underlying cause.	**Meniere's** (MEN-eh-AIRZ)
motion sickness	There is **dysequilibrium** with headache, dizziness, nausea, and vomiting. It is caused by riding in a car, boat, or airplane. Treatment: Drug to treat motion sickness.	**dysequilibrium** (DIS-ee-kwih-LIB-ree-um)
otitis externa	Bacterial infection of the external auditory canal. There is throbbing earache pain (**otalgia**) with a swollen, red canal and serous or purulent drainage. It is caused by a foreign body in the ear or by the patient scratching or probing inside the ear. In swimmers whose ear canals are rubbed by ear plugs or softened by exposure to water, it is known as **swimmer's ear**. Treatment: Correct the underlying cause; topical or oral antibiotic drug.	**otitis externa** (oh-TY-tis eks-TER-nah) ot/o- *ear* -itis *infection of; inflammation of* **otalgia** (oh-TAL-jah) ot/o- *ear* alg/o- *pain* -ia *condition; state; thing*

Word or Phrase	Description	Pronunciation/Word Parts
otitis media	Acute or chronic bacterial infection of the middle ear. There is **myringitis** (redness and inflammation of the tympanic membrane), otalgia, a feeling of pressure, and bulging of the tympanic membrane. There can be an **effusion** (a collection of fluid behind the tympanic membrane that creates an air-fluid level) (see Figure 16-11 ■). This fluid can be **serous** (clear) or **suppurative** (with pus). In children, the effusion can be so thick that it is called **glue ear**. Chronic otitis media can cause a perforation of the tympanic membrane (see Figure 16-12 ■). The mastoid process of the temporal bone can also become infected (**mastoiditis**). Otitis media is common in young children because the short eustachian tube is in a nearly horizontal position that allows bacteria to enter from the nasopharynx. If otitis media is left untreated, the tympanic membrane can rupture or the bones of the middle ear can degenerate, resulting in permanent hearing loss. Treatment: Antibiotic drug; surgery to insert tubes to drain the middle ear.	**otitis media** (oh-TY-tis MEE-dee-ah) **ot/o-** ear **-itis** infection of; inflammation of **myringitis** (MEER-in-JY-tis) **myring/o-** eardrum; tympanic membrane **-itis** infection of; inflammation of **effusion** (ee-FYOO-zhun) **effus/o-** pouring out **-ion** action; condition **serous** (SEER-us) **ser/o-** serum-like fluid; serum of the blood **-ous** pertaining to **suppurative** (SUH-poor-ah-TIV) **suppur/o-** pus formation **-ative** pertaining to **mastoiditis** (MAS-toyd-EYE-tis) **mastoid/o-** mastoid process **-itis** infection of; inflammation of

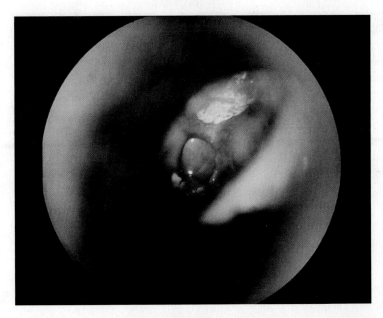

Air-fluid level

Inflammation

Bulging

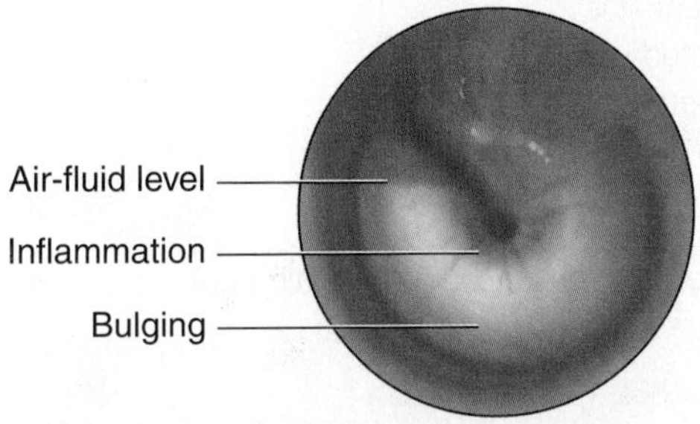

FIGURE 16-11 ■ Myringitis.
The tympanic membrane is red and inflamed. There is dullness with no light reflex. There is a loss of normal landmarks (visibility of the malleus), and the entire tympanic membrane bulges out into the external auditory canal. Fluid from an effusion in the middle ear creates an air-fluid level that can be seen through the tympanic membrane.
Source: Pearson Education

FIGURE 16-12 ■ Perforated tympanic membrane.
A perforated eardrum can be caused by chronic otitis media in the middle ear.
Source: Biophoto Associates/Science Source/Getty Images

WORD ALERT

Sound-Alike Words

mastoiditis	(noun)	infection of the air cells in the bone of the mastoid process
		Example: The middle ear infection progressed to become mastoiditis.
mastitis	(noun)	infection of the mammary glands of the breast
		Example: Mastitis can develop in nursing mothers.

Word or Phrase	Description	Pronunciation/Word Parts
otorrhea	Drainage of serous fluid or pus from the ear. It can be caused by otitis externa or otitis media (with a ruptured tympanic membrane). It can also be caused by a fracture of the temporal bone of the cranium with leakage of cerebrospinal fluid into the ear. Treatment: Correct the underlying cause.	**otorrhea** (OH-toh-REE-ah) **ot/o-** *ear* **-rrhea** *discharge; flow*
otosclerosis	Abnormal deposits of bone in the middle ear, particularly between the stapes and the oval window. The stapes becomes immoveable, causing conductive hearing loss. Certain families have a genetic predisposition to develop otosclerosis. Treatment: Hearing aid, stapedectomy.	**otosclerosis** (OH-toh-skleh-ROH-sis) **ot/o-** *ear* **scler/o-** *hard; sclera of the eye* **-osis** *condition; process*
ruptured tympanic membrane	Tear in the tympanic membrane due to excessive pressure or infection. In pilots and deep sea divers, unequal air pressure in the middle ear compared to the surrounding air or water pressure can rupture the tympanic membrane. Treatment: Tympanoplasty.	
tinnitus	Sounds (buzzing, ringing, hissing, or roaring) that are heard constantly or intermittently in one or both ears, especially in a quiet environment. It is caused by repeated exposure to excessive noise and is associated with hearing loss. It can also be related to the overuse of aspirin. Treatment: Soft background noise (hum of a fan or a device that generates "white noise") to mask tinnitus and allow the patient to sleep.	**tinnitus** (TIN-ih-tus) (tih-NY-tus)
vertigo	Sensation of motion and dizziness when the body is not moving. It is caused by a head cold, middle ear or inner ear infection, head trauma, degenerative changes of the semicircular canals, labyrinthitis, or Meniere's disease. Treatment: Correct the underlying cause.	**vertigo** (VER-tih-goh)

Sinuses, Nose, and Nasal Cavity

Word or Phrase	Description	Pronunciation/Word Parts
allergic rhinitis	Allergic symptoms in the nose. In response to an inhaled antigen (pollen, dust, animal dander, mold), the immune system produces histamine. This causes nasal stuffiness, sneezing, **rhinorrhea** (clear mucus discharge from the nose), hypertrophy (enlargement) of the turbinates in the nose with red, edematous, and boggy mucous membranes, and **postnasal drip (PND)**. When this occurs in spring or fall and coincides with the blooming of certain trees and plants (grasses, maple trees, roses, goldenrod), it is known as **seasonal allergy** or **hay fever**. Treatment: Antihistamine drug, decongestant drug, corticosteroid drug.	**allergic** (ah-LER-jik) **allerg/o-** *allergy* **-ic** *pertaining to* **rhinitis** (ry-NY-tis) **rhin/o-** *nose* **-itis** *infection of; inflammation of* **rhinorrhea** (RY-noh-REE-ah) **rhin/o-** *nose* **-rrhea** *discharge; flow* **postnasal** (post-NAY-zal) **post-** *after; behind* **nas/o-** *nose* **-al** *pertaining to*
anosmia	The temporary or permanent loss of the sense of smell. It is most often caused by head trauma. Treatment: Correct the underlying cause.	**anosmia** (an-AWZ-mee-ah) **an-** *not; without* **osm/o-** *sense of smell* **-ia** *condition; state; thing*
epistaxis	Sudden, sometimes severe bleeding from the nose. It is due to irritation or dryness of the nasal mucosa and the rupture of a small artery, or it can be caused by trauma to the nose. It is known as a **nosebleed**. Treatment: Pack the nostril with gauze or use cautery to stop the bleeding.	**epistaxis** (EP-ih-STAK-sis)
polyp	Benign growth of the mucous membrane in the nose or sinuses. A single polyp may grow large enough to limit the flow of air, or there may be several polyps. Treatment: Polypectomy.	**polyp** (PAW-lip)

Word or Phrase	Description	Pronunciation/Word Parts
rhinophyma	Redness and hypertrophy (enlargement) of the nose with small-to-large, irregular lumps, usually in men. It is caused by the increased number of sebaceous glands associated with acne rosacea of the skin (discussed in "Dermatology," Chapter 7). Treatment: Topical drug for acne rosacea.	**rhinophyma** (RY-noh-FY-mah) **rhin/o-** *nose* **-phyma** *growth; tumor*
septal deviation	Lateral displacement of the nasal septum, significantly narrowing one nasal airway. This can be a congenital condition or it can be caused by trauma to the nose. Treatment: Surgical correction (septoplasty).	
sinusitis	Acute or chronic bacterial infection in one or more of the sinus cavities (see Figure 16-13 ■). There is headache, pain in the forehead or cheekbones over the sinus, postnasal drainage, fatigue, and fever. **Pansinusitis** involves all the sinuses or all of the sinuses on one side of the face. Treatment: Antibiotic drug; endoscopic sinus surgery. ─ Right maxillary sinus **FIGURE 16-13 ■ Sinusitis.** This CT scan of the head shows the nose at the top of the image with the long nasal septum positioned vertically inside the nasal cavity. The right maxillary sinus shows severe swelling of the mucous membrane with no open sinus cavity. The left maxillary sinus shows minimal mucosal swelling with a relatively open sinus cavity (in black). *Source: Maria Zhuravleva/123RF*	**sinusitis** (SY-nyoo-SY-tis) **sinus/o-** *sinus* **-itis** *infection of; inflammation of* **pansinusitis** (PAN-sy-nyoo-SY-tis) **pan-** *all* **sinus/o-** *sinus* **-itis** *infection of; inflammation of*
upper respiratory infection (URI)	Bacterial or viral infection of the nose that can spread to the throat and ears. The nose is a part of the respiratory system as well as the ENT system. This is also known as a **common cold** or **head cold**. Treatment: Antibiotic drug for a bacterial infection.	

Mouth, Oral Cavity, Pharynx, and Neck

Word or Phrase	Description	Pronunciation/Word Parts
cancer of the mouth and neck	**Malignant** tumor (**carcinoma**) of squamous epithelial cells in the oral cavity (lips, tongue, gums, cheeks), throat, or larynx. Smoking and using smokeless chewing tobacco can cause this. Treatment: Surgery to remove the tongue (glossectomy) or larynx (laryngectomy), or jaw bone and neck muscles (radical neck dissection).	**cancer** (KAN-ser) **malignant** (mah-LIG-nant) **malign/o-** *cancer; intentionally causing harm* **-ant** *pertaining to* **carcinoma** (KAR-sih-NOH-mah) **carcin/o-** *cancer* **-oma** *mass; tumor*
cervical lymphadenopathy	Enlargement of the lymph nodes in the neck. It is caused by infection, cancer, or the spread of a cancerous tumor from another site. Treatment: Correct the underlying cause.	**cervical** (SER-vih-kal) **cervic/o-** *cervix; neck* **-al** *pertaining to* **lymphadenopathy** (lim-FAD-eh-NAW-pah-thee) **lymph/o-** *lymph; lymphatic system* **aden/o-** *gland* **-pathy** *disease*

Word or Phrase	Description	Pronunciation/Word Parts
cleft lip and palate	Congenital deformity in which the lip or the bones of the right and left maxilla fail to join in the center before birth. The resulting cleft in the skin and bone can be **unilateral** or **bilateral** (see Figure 16-14 ■). The cleft can also extend into the soft palate. The child has difficulty speaking and eating. Treatment: Surgical correction.	**cleft** (KLEFT) **unilateral** (YOO-nih-LAT-eh-ral) **uni-** *not paired; single* **later/o-** *side* **-al** *pertaining to* **bilateral** (by-LAT-eh-ral) **bi-** *two* **later/o-** *side* **-al** *pertaining to*

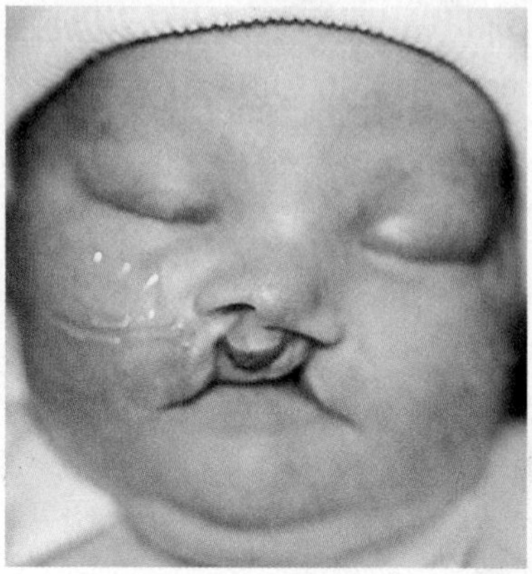

FIGURE 16-14 ■ Cleft lip and palate.
This infant has a bilateral cleft lip and palate. He has difficulty feeding from the breast or bottle because milk flows into the nasal cavity where it could be inhaled into the lungs. Note the feeding tube inserted in the right nostril and taped to the cheek; the tube goes to the stomach.
Source: Ph College/Pearson Education

Word or Phrase	Description	Pronunciation/Word Parts
cold sores	Recurring, painful clusters of blisters on the lips or nose. They are caused by infection with **herpes simplex virus** type 1. After the initial infection, the virus remains dormant in a nerve until triggers of stress, sunlight, illness, or menstruation cause it to erupt again. These are also known as **fever blisters**. Treatment: Topical antiviral drug. *Note:* Herpes simplex type 2 causes genital herpes, a sexually transmitted disease (discussed in "Male Reproductive Medicine," Chapter 12).	**herpes simplex** (HER-peez SIM-pleks)
glossitis	Inflammation or infection of the tongue. It is caused by irritation from spicy or hot food, a food allergy, an infection, or vitamin B deficiency. Treatment: Correct the underlying cause.	**glossitis** (glaw-SY-tis) **gloss/o-** *tongue* **-itis** *infection of; inflammation of*
leukoplakia	Thickened white patch on the mucous membrane of the mouth (see Figure 16-15 ■). If it is caused by chronic irritation from tobacco use, it can become cancerous. It is also caused by irritation from an infection with the Epstein-Barr virus, seen in AIDS patients. Treatment: Correct the underlying cause.	**leukoplakia** (LOO-koh-PLAY-kee-ah) **leuk/o-** *white* **plak/o-** *plaque* **-ia** *condition; state; thing*

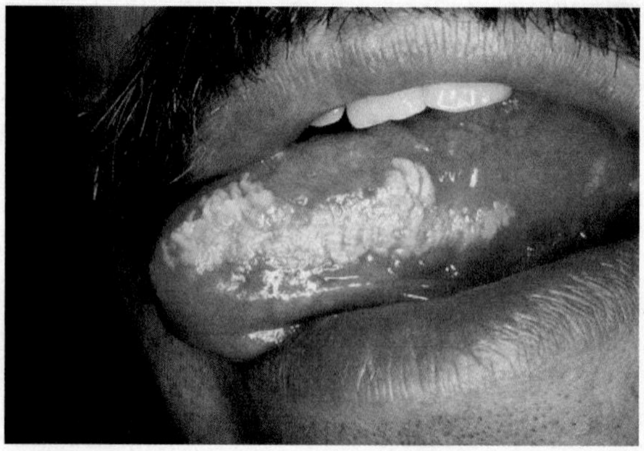

FIGURE 16-15 ■ Leukoplakia.
This white patch of leukoplakia on the tongue is in the mouth of a patient with AIDS. This is under the tongue, but leukoplakia can occur anywhere in the mouth.
Source: Centers for Disease Control and Prevention

Word or Phrase	Description	Pronunciation/Word Parts

pharyngitis	Bacterial or viral infection of the throat. When it is caused by the bacterium group A beta-hemolytic **streptococcus**, it is known as **strep throat**. It is important to diagnose strep throat and treat it with an antibiotic drug so that it does not cause the complication of rheumatic heart disease. Treatment: Antibiotic drug.	**pharyngitis** (FAIR-in-JY-tis)
		  pharyng/o- *pharynx; throat*
		  -itis *infection of; inflammation of*
		
		streptococcus
		(STREP-toh-KAW-kus)
		  strept/o- *curved*
		  -coccus *spherical bacterium*
		Streptococcus is a bacterium shaped as spheres in a long curved chain.

temporo-mandibular joint (TMJ) syndrome	Dysfunction of the movement of the temporomandibular joint. There is clicking of the joint, pain, muscle spasm, and difficulty opening the jaw. It is caused by clenching or grinding the teeth (often during sleep) or by misalignment of the teeth. Treatment: Dental bite guard worn at night, correction of misaligned teeth.	**temporomandibular**
		(TEM-poh-ROH-man-DIH-byoo-lar)
		  tempor/o- *side of the head; temple*
		  mandibul/o- *lower jaw; mandible*
		  -ar *pertaining to*

thrush	Oral infection caused by the yeast *Candida albicans*. It coats the tongue and oral mucosa (see Figure 16-16 ■). Thrush is common in infants, but is also seen in immunocompromised patients with AIDS because their immune system cannot control its growth. It also occurs after an antibiotic drug kills bacteria in the mouth, allowing overgrowth of *Candida albicans*. It is also known as **oral candidiasis**. Treatment: Oral antiyeast drug.	**candidiasis** (KAN-dih-DY-ah-sis)
		  candid/o- *Candida; yeast*
		  -iasis *process; state*

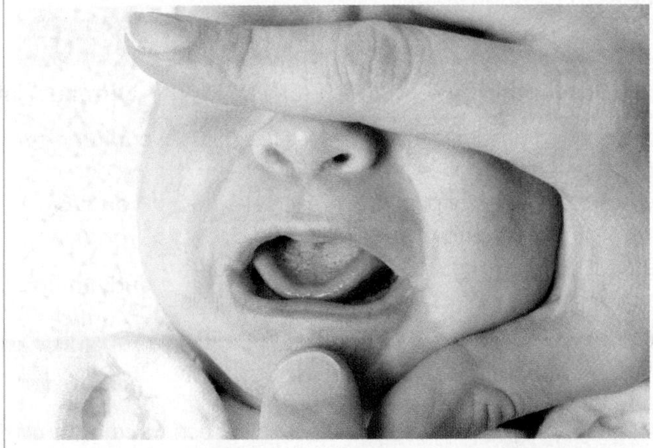

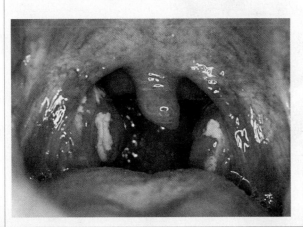

FIGURE 16-16 ■ Thrush.
The warm, moist environment of the mouth encourages the growth of this yeast-like fungus. It forms a thick white coating that resembles milk, but cannot be wiped off.
Source: Rioblanco/123RF

Word or Phrase	Description	Pronunciation/Word Parts

tonsillitis	Acute or chronic bacterial infection of the pharynx and palatine tonsils (see Figure 16-17 ■). There is a sore throat and difficulty swallowing, with mouth breathing and snoring. The tonsils hypertrophy (enlarge) and contain pus and debris. The adenoids may also hypertrophy and block the eustachian tubes. Treatment: Antibiotic drug, tonsillectomy.	**tonsillitis** (TAWN-sil-EYE-tis)
		  tonsill/o- *tonsil*
		  -itis *infection of; inflammation of*

FIGURE 16-17 ■ Tonsillitis.
This patient has acute inflammation, infection, and hypertrophy of the palatine tonsils. There are also some areas of white pus, which indicate a bacterial infection. The uvula and posterior oropharynx are also inflamed.
Source: Dr. P. Marazzi/Science Source

Word or Phrase	Description	Pronunciation/Word Parts

Larynx

Word or Phrase	Description	Pronunciation/Word Parts
laryngitis	Hoarseness or complete loss of the voice, difficulty swallowing, and a cough due to swelling and inflammation of the larynx. It is caused by a bacterial or viral infection. Treatment: Antibiotic drug for a bacterial infection.	**laryngitis** (LAIR-in-JY-tis) **laryng/o-** *larynx; voice box* **-itis** *infection of; inflammation of*
vocal cord nodule or polyp	A nodule is a small, benign, fibrous growth on the surface of the vocal cord. A polyp is a larger, soft growth that contains blood vessels. A nodule or polyp is caused by strain from constant talking or singing or by chronic irritation from smoking or allergies. There is hoarseness and a change in the quality of the voice. Treatment: Voice rest, surgical removal.	**nodule** (NAW-dyool) **polyp** (PAW-lip)

Laboratory and Diagnostic Procedures

Hearing Tests

Word or Phrase	Description	Pronunciation/Word Parts
audiometry	Test that measures hearing acuity and documents hearing loss (see Figure 16-18 ■). The patient puts on headphones that are connected to an **audiometer**, which produces a series of pure tones, each at a different frequency (high or low pitch) and varying in intensity (loud or soft). The frequency is measured in **hertz (Hz)**. The intensity is measured in **decibels (dB)**. The patient presses a button to signal when the tone is heard. The result, printed on graph paper, is an **audiogram**. In **speech audiometry**, the patient hears spoken words and sentences. If he/she can repeat 50% of the words correctly, then this is the threshold of hearing ability for speech sounds. Both pure tone audiometry and speech audiometry are used to determine whether a patient needs a hearing aid.	**audiometry** (AW-dee-AW-meh-tree) **audi/o-** *hearing* **-metry** *process of measuring* **audiometer** (AW-dee-AW-meh-ter) **audi/o-** *hearing* **-meter** *instrument used to measure* **audiogram** (AW-dee-oh-GRAM) **audi/o-** *hearing* **-gram** *picture; record*

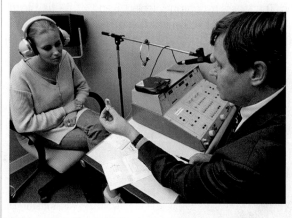

FIGURE 16-18 ■ Audiometry.
This patient is undergoing audiometry. The headphones cover both ears to keep out outside noises. The hearing in each ear is tested separately, and the patient raises her hand when she hears a sound.
Source: Phanie/Science Source

Word or Phrase	Description	Pronunciation/Word Parts
brainstem auditory evoked response (BAER)	Test that analyzes the brain's response to sounds. The patient listens as an audiometer produces a series of clicks. An electroencephalography (EEG) is performed at the same time. A lesion or tumor in the auditory cortex of the brain or on the vestibulocochlear nerve will produce an abnormal EEG. This test is also known as an **auditory brainstem response (ABR)**.	
Rinne and Weber hearing tests	The Rinne tuning fork test evaluates bone conduction versus air conduction of sound in one ear at a time (see Figure 16-19 ■). A vibrating tuning fork is placed against the mastoid process behind one ear to test the bone conduction of sound. Then it is placed next to (but not touching) the same ear. If the sound is louder when the tuning fork is next to the ear, this is normal (because air conduction normally is greater than bone conduction); the test is said to be positive. If the sound is louder when the tuning fork touches the mastoid process, then the patient has a conductive hearing loss.	**Rinne** (RIN-eh) **Weber** (VAH-ber)

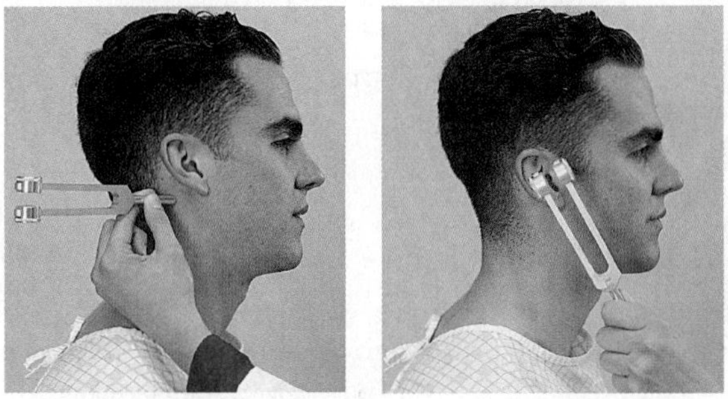

FIGURE 16-19 ■ Rinne test.
This hearing test uses a vibrating tuning fork to compare bone conduction of sound to air conduction of sound in the same ear.
Source: Pearson Education

	The Weber tuning fork test evaluates bone conduction of sound in both ears at the same time. The vibrating tuning fork is placed against the center of the forehead or on top of the head. In a normal test, the sound is heard equally in both ears.	
tympanometry	Test that measures the ability of the tympanic membrane and the bones of the middle ear to move. Air pressure (rather than sound vibration) is used in the external auditory canal. If infection or disease has fixed the middle ear bones, then the tympanic membrane will move very little. This resistance to movement is called **impedance**. The result, printed on graph paper, is called a **tympanogram**.	**tympanometry** (TIM-pah-NAW-meh-tree) **tympan/o-** *eardrum; tympanic membrane* **-metry** *process of measuring* **impedance** (im-PEE-dans) **tympanogram** (tim-PAN-oh-gram) **tympan/o-** *eardrum; tympanic membrane* **-gram** *picture; record*

> **DID YOU KNOW?**
>
> The ear can hear sounds with a frequency as low as 20 Hz or as high as 20,000 Hz. In contrast, a dog can hear from 20 Hz to 45,000 Hz, and a porpoise can hear from 75 Hz to 150,000 Hz. A tuning fork of 256 Hz is used to test the hearing. This frequency corresponds to middle C on the piano.

Laboratory and Radiologic Tests

culture and sensitivity (C&S)	Test in which a swab of mucus or pus from the nose, tonsils, or throat (see Figure 16-20 ■) is placed onto culture medium in a Petri dish to identify the cause of an infection. Microorganisms grow into colonies, and the specific disease-causing microorganism is identified and tested to determine its sensitivity to various antibiotic drugs.	**culture** (KUL-chur)
		
		sensitivity (SEN-sih-TIV-ih-tee)
		  sensitiv/o- *affected by; sensitive to*
		  -ity *condition; state*

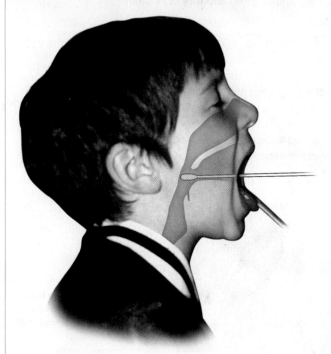

FIGURE 16-20 ■ Throat swab.
This child is having a swab taken of the oropharynx. The material on the swab will be sent to a laboratory for a culture and sensitivity test.
Source: Pearson Education

rapid strep test	Test kit for strep throat. If it detects beta-hemolytic group A streptococcus, a purplish-pink line appears. Unlike a standard culture and sensitivity test, the result of a rapid strep test is available within the hour so that the physician can immediately prescribe an antibiotic drug.
RAST	Blood test that measures the amount of IgE produced when the blood is mixed with a specific antigen. It shows which of many allergens the patient is allergic to and how severe the allergy is. RAST stands for *radioallergosorbent test*.
sinus series	X-rays are taken from various angles to show all of the sinuses and confirm or rule out a diagnosis of sinusitis. Sinusitis shows as cloudy, opacified sinuses or thickened mucous membranes. Sometimes an air-fluid level can be seen within the sinus. If needed, a CT scan is done instead to show additional detail (see Figure 16-13).

Medical and Surgical Procedures

Medical Procedures		
Word or Phrase	**Description**	**Pronunciation/Word Parts**
nose, sinus, mouth, and throat examinations	Procedure in which a nasal **speculum** is used to widen the nostril, while a penlight lights the nasal cavity. The frontal and maxillary sinuses are examined for tenderness by pressing with the fingertips on the forehead and cheekbones. A tongue depressor, penlight, and a laryngeal mirror are used to examine the oral cavity, pharynx, and larynx (see Figure 16-21 ■).	**speculum** (SPEH-kyoo-lum)

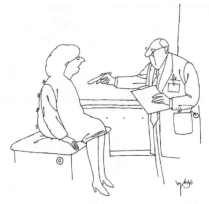

That's all you want me to say . . . Ah?

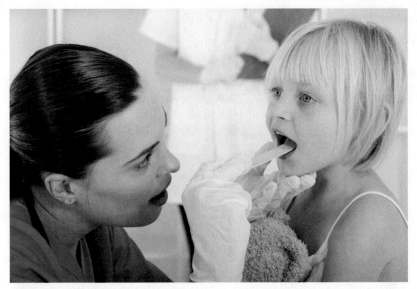

FIGURE 16-21 ■ Throat examination.
This pediatrician is examining this little girl's oropharynx by using a tongue depressor and having the child say "Ah."
Source: Hongqi Zhang/123RF

otoscopy	Procedure to examine the external auditory canal and tympanic membrane (see Figure 16-22 ■). An **otoscope** provides light and magnification. To assess the mobility of the tympanic membrane, some otoscopes have a rubber bulb that is squeezed to force air into the external auditory canal. The otoscope is pressed against the external auditory meatus to form an air-tight seal, and then the bulb is squeezed. A normal tympanic membrane moves in and out in response to this procedure.	**otoscopy** (oh-TAW-skoh-pee) **ot/o-** *ear* **-scopy** *process of using an instrument to examine* **otoscope** (OH-toh-skohp) **ot/o-** *ear* **-scope** *instrument used to examine*

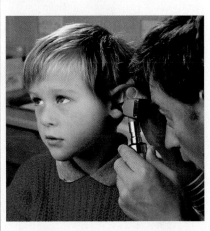

FIGURE 16-22 ■ Otoscopy.
The physician is using an otoscope to examine this child's left external auditory canal and tympanic membrane. Before each use, a disposable black plastic tip (speculum) is placed over the part of the otoscope that enters the ear. For patients from 3 years old to adult, the physician gently pulls the helix backward and upward to straighten the external auditory canal and visualize the tympanic membrane. In infants younger than 3, the helix is pulled backward and downward to straighten the external auditory canal.
Source: Saturn Stills/Science Source

Word or Phrase	Description	Pronunciation/Word Parts
Romberg's sign	Procedure to assess equilibrium. The patient stands with the feet together and the eyes closed. Swaying or falling to one side indicates a loss of balance and an inner ear disorder.	**Romberg** (RAWM-berg)
Surgical Procedures		
cheiloplasty	Procedure to repair the lip, usually because of a laceration. A cheiloplasty can be part of a larger surgical procedure to repair a cleft lip and palate.	**cheiloplasty** (KY-loh-PLAS-tee) **cheil/o-** *lip* **-plasty** *process of reshaping by surgery*
cochlear implant	Procedure to insert a small, battery-powered implant beneath the skin behind the ear. Wires from the implant are placed through the round window and into the cochlea of the inner ear. When the implant "hears" a sound, the implant sends an electrical impulse to stimulate the cochlear portion of the vestibulocochlear nerve.	
endoscopic sinus surgery	Procedure that uses an **endoscope** (a flexible, fiberoptic scope with a magnifying lens and a light source) inserted through the nostril to examine the sinuses. **Endoscopy** is used to remove a polyp, treat sinusitis, or perform a biopsy.	**endoscopic** (EN-doh-SKAW-pik) **endo-** *innermost; within* **scop/o-** *examine with an instrument* **-ic** *pertaining to* **endoscope** (EN-doh-skohp) **endo-** *innermost; within* **-scope** *instrument used to examine* **endoscopy** (en-DAW-skoh-pee) **endo-** *innermost; within* **-scopy** *process of using an instrument to examine*
mastoidectomy	Procedure to remove part of the mastoid process of the temporal bone because of infection	**mastoidectomy** (MAS-toyd-EK-toh-mee) **mastoid/o-** *mastoid process* **-ectomy** *surgical removal*

Word or Phrase	Description	Pronunciation/Word Parts

myringotomy	Procedure that uses a **myringotome** to make an incision in the tympanic membrane to drain fluid from the middle ear. For chronic middle ear infections, a ventilating (or pressure-equalizing [PE]) tube can also be inserted through the incision to form a permanent opening into the middle ear (see Figure 16-23 ■). This procedure is a **tympanostomy**. 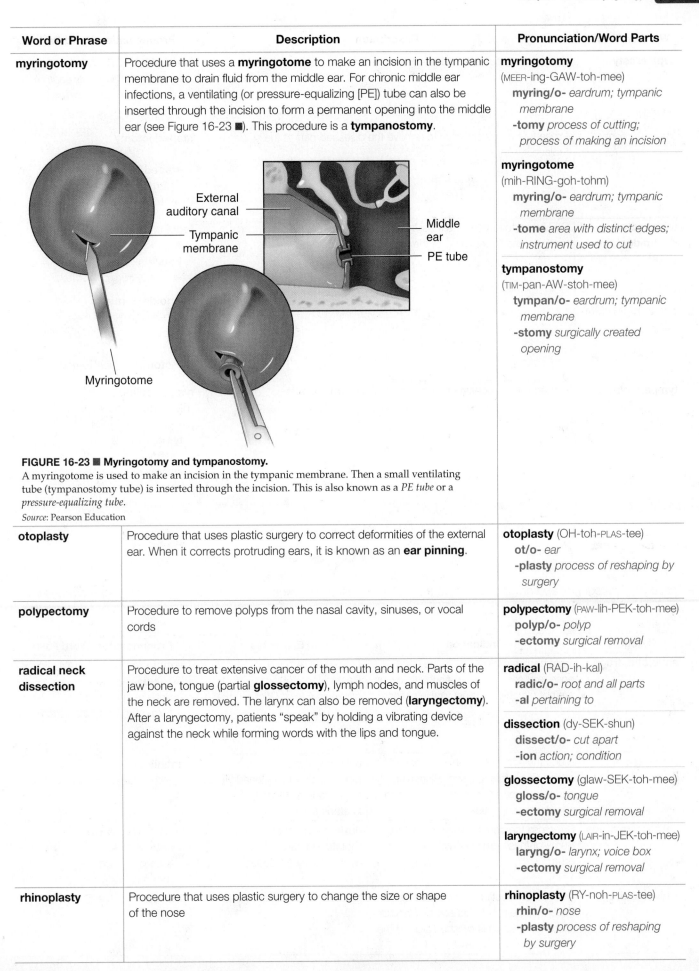
	
	FIGURE 16-23 ■ Myringotomy and tympanostomy.
	A myringotome is used to make an incision in the tympanic membrane. Then a small ventilating tube (tympanostomy tube) is inserted through the incision. This is also known as a *PE tube* or a *pressure-equalizing tube.*
	Source: Pearson Education
		myringotomy
		(MEER-ing-GAW-toh-mee)
		  myring/o- *eardrum; tympanic membrane*
		  -tomy *process of cutting; process of making an incision*
		
		myringotome
		(mih-RING-goh-tohm)
		  myring/o- *eardrum; tympanic membrane*
		  -tome *area with distinct edges; instrument used to cut*
		
		tympanostomy
		(TIM-pan-AW-stoh-mee)
		  tympan/o- *eardrum; tympanic membrane*
		  -stomy *surgically created opening*

otoplasty	Procedure that uses plastic surgery to correct deformities of the external ear. When it corrects protruding ears, it is known as an **ear pinning**.	**otoplasty** (OH-toh-PLAS-tee)
		  ot/o- *ear*
		  -plasty *process of reshaping by surgery*

polypectomy	Procedure to remove polyps from the nasal cavity, sinuses, or vocal cords	**polypectomy** (PAW-lih-PEK-toh-mee)
		  polyp/o- *polyp*
		  -ectomy *surgical removal*

radical neck dissection	Procedure to treat extensive cancer of the mouth and neck. Parts of the jaw bone, tongue (partial **glossectomy**), lymph nodes, and muscles of the neck are removed. The larynx can also be removed (**laryngectomy**). After a laryngectomy, patients "speak" by holding a vibrating device against the neck while forming words with the lips and tongue.	**radical** (RAD-ih-kal)
		  radic/o- *root and all parts*
		  -al *pertaining to*
		
		dissection (dy-SEK-shun)
		  dissect/o- *cut apart*
		  -ion *action; condition*
		
		glossectomy (glaw-SEK-toh-mee)
		  gloss/o- *tongue*
		  -ectomy *surgical removal*
		
		laryngectomy (LAIR-in-JEK-toh-mee)
		  laryng/o- *larynx; voice box*
		  -ectomy *surgical removal*

rhinoplasty	Procedure that uses plastic surgery to change the size or shape of the nose	**rhinoplasty** (RY-noh-PLAS-tee)
		  rhin/o- *nose*
		  -plasty *process of reshaping by surgery*

Figure labels (16-23): External auditory canal; Tympanic membrane; Myringotome; Middle ear; PE tube

Word or Phrase	Description	Pronunciation/Word Parts
septoplasty	Procedure to correct a deviated nasal septum	**septoplasty** (SEP-toh-PLAS-tee) **sept/o-** *dividing wall; septum* **-plasty** *process of reshaping by surgery*
stapedectomy	Procedure for otosclerosis to remove the diseased part of the stapes and replace it with a prosthetic device	**stapedectomy** (STAY-peh-DEK-toh-mee) **staped/o-** *stapes; stirrup-shaped bone* **-ectomy** *surgical removal*
tonsillectomy and adenoidectomy (T&A)	Procedure to remove the tonsils and adenoids in a patient with chronic tonsillitis and hypertrophy of the tonsils and adenoids	**tonsillectomy** (TAWN-sil-EK-toh-mee) **tonsill/o-** *tonsil* **-ectomy** *surgical removal* **adenoidectomy** (AD-eh-noyd-EK-toh-mee) **adenoid/o-** *structure resembling a gland* **-ectomy** *surgical removal*
tympanoplasty	Procedure to reconstruct a ruptured tympanic membrane	**tympanoplasty** (TIM-pah-noh-PLAS-tee) (TIM-pah-noh-PLAS-tee) **tympan/o-** *eardrum; tympanic membrane* **-plasty** *process of reshaping by surgery*

Drugs

These drug categories and drugs are used to treat ENT diseases. The most common generic and trade name drugs in each category are listed.

Category	Indication	Examples	Pronunciation/Word Parts
antibiotic drugs	Treat bacterial infections of the ears, nose, sinuses, or throat. Antibiotic drugs are not effecttive against viral infections.	amoxicillin (Amoxil), Bactrim, ofloxacin (Floxin Otic), Septra	**antibiotic** (AN-tee-by-AW-tik) (AN-tih-by-AW-tik) **anti-** *against* **bi/o-** *life; living organism; living tissue* **-tic** *pertaining to*
antihistamine drugs	Block the effect of histamine released during an allergic reaction. Histamine causes symptoms of runny, itchy nose and nasal congestion.	cetirizine (Zyrtec), diphenhydramine (Benadryl), fexofenadine (Allegra), loratadine (Claritin)	**antihistamine** (AN-tee-HIS-tah-meen)
antitussive drugs	Suppress the cough center in the brain. Some of these drugs contain a narcotic drug.	dextromethorphan (Robitussin, Vicks 44), hydrocodone (Hycodan)	**antitussive** (AN-tee-TUS-iv) **anti-** *against* **tuss/o-** *cough* **-ive** *pertaining to*
antiyeast drugs	Treat yeast infections (oral candidiasis, thrush) of the mouth caused by *Candida albicans*. Solution is swished around the oral cavity and then swallowed.	nystatin (Mycostatin, Nilstat)	**antiyeast** (AN-tee-YEEST)

Category	Indication	Examples	Pronunciation/Word Parts
corticosteroid drugs	Treat severe inflammation of the ears, nose, or mouth. Topical nasal spray, ear drops, or an oral drug that works throughout the body.	beclomethasone (Beconase), fluticasone (Flonase)	**corticosteroid** (KOR-tih-koh-STAIR-oyd) **cortic/o-** *cortex; outer region* **-steroid** *steroid*
decongestant drugs	Constrict blood vessels and decrease swelling of the mucous membranes of the nose and sinuses due to colds and allergies. Topical nasal sprays or oral drugs.	oxymetazoline (Afrin 12-hour, Duration), pseudoephedrine (Dimetapp, Sudafed)	**decongestant** (DEE-con-JES-tant) **de-** *reversal of; without* **congest/o-** *accumulation of fluid* **-ant** *pertaining to*
drugs used to treat vertigo and motion sickness	Decrease the sensitivity of the inner ear to motion and keep nerve impulses from the inner ear from reaching the vomiting center in the brain	dimenhydrinate (Dramamine), meclizine (Antivert), scopolamine (Transderm-Scop)	

CLINICAL CONNECTIONS

Pharmacology. Aminoglycoside antibiotic drugs are known to damage the cochlea of the inner ear. This adverse drug effect is known as **ototoxicity**. Patients taking aminoglycoside drugs need to have audiometry done periodically to monitor their hearing.

    A number of drugs are given by the **sublingual** route. The tablet is placed under the tongue and allowed to dissolve, and then the liquid drug is swallowed.

ototoxicity (OH-toh-tawk-SIS-ih-tee)
ot/o- *ear*
toxic/o- *poison; toxin*
-ity *condition; state*

sublingual (sub-LING-gwal)
sub- *below; underneath*
lingu/o- *tongue*
-al *pertaining to*

Abbreviations

ABR	auditory brainstem response		**HEENT**	head, eyes, ears, nose, and throat
AD, A.D.*■	right ear (Latin, *auris dextra*)		**Hz**	hertz
AS, A.S.*■	left ear (Latin, *auris sinister*)		**PE**	pressure-equalizing (tube)
AU, A.U.*■	both ears (Latin, *auris unitas*); each ear (Latin, *auris uterque*)		**PND**	postnasal drainage; postnasal drip
			RAST	radioallergosorbent test
BAER	brainstem auditory evoked response		**SOM**	serous otitis media
BOM	bilateral otitis media		**T&A**	tonsillectomy and adenoidectomy
C&S	culture and sensitivity		**TM**	tympanic membrane
dB, db	decibel		**TMJ**	temporomandibular joint
EAC	external auditory canal		**URI**	upper respiratory infection
ENT	ears, nose, and throat			

*According to The Joint Commission and ■ the Institute for Safe Medication Practices (ISMP), these abbreviations should not be used. However, because they are still used by some healthcare providers, they are included here.

WORD ALERT
Abbreviations

Abbreviations are commonly used in all types of medical documents; however, they can mean different things to different people and their meanings can be misinterpreted. Always verify the meaning of an abbreviation.

C&S means *culture and sensitivity,* but the sound-alike abbreviation *CNS* means *central nervous system.*

PE means *pressure-equalizing (tube)*, but it also means *physical examination* and *pulmonary embolus.*

PND means *postnasal drainage* or *postnasal drip*, but it also means *paroxysmal nocturnal dyspnea.*

TM means *tympanic membrane*, but *TMJ* means *temporomandibular joint.*

IT'S GREEK TO ME!

Did you notice that some words have two different combining forms? Combining forms from both Greek and Latin remain a part of medical language today.

Word	Greek	Latin	Medical Word Examples
ear	ot/o-	aur/i-, auricul/o-	otic, auricle, auricular
eardrum	tympan/o-	myring/o-	tympanic membrane, myringotomy
hearing	acous/o-	audi/o-, audit/o-	acoustic neuroma, audiogram, auditory canal
lip	cheil/o-	labi/o-	cheiloplasty, nasolabial
nose	rhin/o-	nas/o-	rhinoplasty, nasal
tongue	gloss/o-	lingu/o-	glossectomy, sublingual

Definition of the Medical Word

21. Surgical removal (of the) tongue
22. Record (of the) hearing
23. Infection of (or) inflammation of (the) larynx
24. Process of using an instrument to examine (the) ear
25. Process of reshaping by surgery (on the) nose
26. Surgical removal (of the) tonsils
27. Infection of (or) inflammation of (the) nose
28. Surgically created opening (in the) tympanic membrane
29. Pertaining to (an) allergy
30. Process of reshaping by surgery (on the) ear

Build the Medical Word

_____

_____

_____

_____

_____

_____

_____

_____

_____

_____

PREFIX EXERCISE

Read the definition of the medical word. Look at the medical word or partial word that is given (it already contains a combining form and a suffix). Select the correct prefix from the Prefix List and write it on the blank line. Then build the medical word and write it on the line. Be sure to check your spelling. The first one has been done for you.

<table>
<tr><td colspan="3" align="center">**PREFIX LIST**</td></tr>
<tr><td>an- (not; without)</td><td>de- (reversal of; without)</td><td>pan- (all)</td></tr>
<tr><td>anti- (against)</td><td>endo- (innermost; within)</td><td>post- (after; behind)</td></tr>
<tr><td>bi- (two)</td><td></td><td></td></tr>
</table>

Definition of the Medical Word	Prefix	Word or Partial Word	Build the Medical Word
1. Pertaining to two sides	bi-	lateral	bilateral
2. Pertaining to (a drug that is) against (a) cough	_____	tussive	_____
3. Pertaining to (drainage that is) behind (the) nose	_____	nasal	_____
4. Condition (of being) without (the) sense of smell	_____	osmia	_____
5. Pertaining to (a drug that does a) reversal of accumulation of fluid	_____	congestant	_____
6. Pertaining to (the) innermost (parts to) examine with an instrument	_____	scopic	_____
7. Infection of (or) inflammation of all (of the) sinus(es)	_____	sinusitis	_____

MULTIPLE COMBINING FORMS AND SUFFIX EXERCISE

Read the definition of the medical word. Select the correct suffix and combining forms. Then build the medical word and write it on the line. Be sure to check your spelling. The first one has been done for you.

SUFFIX LIST	COMBINING FORM LIST
-al (pertaining to)	aden/o- (gland)
-ar (pertaining to)	alg/o- (pain)
-ia (condition; state; thing)	audi/o- (hearing)
-ist (person who specializes in; thing that specializes in)	laryng/o- (larynx; voice box)
	leuk/o- (white)
-osis (condition; process)	log/o- (study of; word)
-pathy (disease)	lymph/o- (lymph; lymphatic system)
	mandibul/o- (lower jaw; mandible)
	neur/o- (nerve)
	ot/o- (ear)
	plak/o- (plaque)
	rhin/o- (nose)
	scler/o- (hard; sclera of the eye)
	sensor/i- (sensory)
	tempor/o- (side of the head; temple)

Definition of the Medical Word

1. Pertaining to (a) sensory nerve
2. Condition (of) ear pain
3. Disease (of the) lymph gland
4. Condition (of) white plaque (in the mouth)
5. Condition (in the) ear (of) hard(ness of the bones)
6. Pertaining to (the) temple (and the) mandible (joint)
7. Person who specializes in (the) ear, nose, and larynx study of
8. Person who specializes in (the) hearing study of

Build the Medical Word

1. sensorineural
2. _____
3. _____
4. _____
5. _____
6. _____
7. _____
8. _____

16.7A Spell Medical Words

ENGLISH AND MEDICAL WORD EQUIVALENTS EXERCISE

For each English word, write its equivalent medical word. Be sure to check your spelling. The first one has been done for you.

English Word	Medical Word	English Word	Medical Word
1. ear canal	external auditory canal	9. voice box, Adam's apple	_____
2. eardrum	_____	10. hay fever, seasonal allergies	_____
3. earwax	_____	11. common cold, head cold	_____
4. hammer-shaped bone	_____	12. total deafness	_____
5. anvil-shaped bone	_____	13. nosebleed	_____
6. stirrup-shaped bone	_____	14. earache	_____
7. nostril	_____	15. sore throat	_____
8. throat	_____	16. ringing in the ears	_____

HEARING MEDICAL WORDS EXERCISE

You hear someone speaking the medical words given below. Read each pronunciation and then write the medical word it represents. Be sure to check your spelling. The first one has been done for you.

1. AD-eh-noydz　　　　　adenoids
2. AW-dee-AW-loh-jist　　　_____
3. KY-loh-PLAS-tee　　　_____
4. koh-LES-tee-ah-TOH-mah　_____
5. EP-ih-STAK-sis　　　_____

6. yoo-STAY-shun TOOB　_____
7. LAIR-in-JY-tis　　　_____
8. MEER-ing-GAW-toh-mee　_____
9. SY-nyoo-SY-tis　　　_____
10. TAWN-sih-lar　　　_____

16.7B Pronounce Medical Words

PRONUNCIATION EXERCISE

Read the medical word and the syllables in its pronunciation. Circle the primary (main) accented syllable. The first one has been done for you.

1. mucosa (myoo-(koh)-sah)
2. audiogram (aw-dee-oh-gram)
3. auricular (aw-rih-kyoo-lar)
4. cerumen (seh-roo-men)
5. hemotympanum (hee-moh-tim-pah-num)
6. laryngeal (lah-rin-jee-al)
7. otalgia (oh-tal-jah)
8. postnasal (post-nay-zal)
9. temporomandibular (tem-poh-roh-man-dih-byoo-lar)
10. tonsillar (tawn-sih-lar)

16.8 Research Medical Words

SOUND-ALIKE WORDS

Compare and contrast the medical meanings of these sound-alike otolaryngology and other words.

1. *epistaxis* and *rhinorrhea*
2. *malleus* and *malleolus* (Chapter 8)
3. *mastoiditis* and *mastitis* (Chapter 13)

16.9 Analyze Medical Reports

ELECTRONIC PATIENT RECORD #1

This is an excerpt from an Office Visit Note. Read the Note and answer the questions.

PEARSON PRIMARY CARE ASSOCIATES

Task   Edit   View   Time Scale   Options   Help

OFFICE VISIT NOTE

PATIENT NAME:	STANSBURY, Leona
DATE OF VISIT:	November 19, 20xx

Source: Studio Kwadrat/Fotolia

DIAGNOSIS
Rhinitis medicamentosa, secondary to constant use of Afrin decongestant nasal spray.

PLAN
The patient is to take an oral corticosteroid drug 20 mg every day for 5 days to decrease the chronic inflammation. She will refrain from using Afrin spray. She will return in 3 weeks for a full evaluation of her allergies.

1. Use a medical dictionary or the Internet to look up the definition of *rhinitis medicamentosa*: _____

2. What caused this condition? _____

3. Why did the patient originally begin using a decongestant nasal spray?

4. What does a decongestant nasal spray do?

Chapter 17
Psychiatry

Psychiatry (sy-KY-ah-tree) is the medical specialty that studies the anatomy and physiology of the brain and the functioning of the mind and uses laboratory and diagnostic procedures, medical and psychiatric procedures, and drugs to treat psychiatric diseases.

Learning Outcomes

After you study this chapter, you should be able to

17.1 Identify structures of the brain that are related to psychiatry.

17.2 Describe the process of an emotional response.

17.3 Describe common psychiatric mental disorders, laboratory and diagnostic procedures, medical and psychiatric procedures and therapies, and drugs.

17.4 Form the plural and adjective forms of nouns related to psychiatry.

17.5 Give the meanings of word parts and abbreviations related to psychiatry.

17.6 Divide psychiatric words and build psychiatric words.

17.7 Spell and pronounce psychiatric words.

17.8 Research sound-alike and other psychiatric words.

17.9 Analyze the medical content and meaning of a psychiatric report.

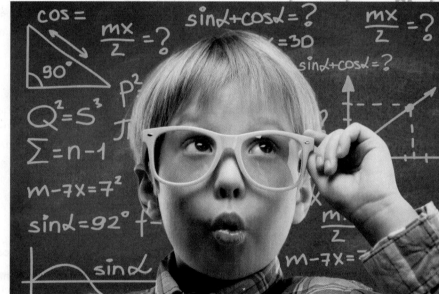

FIGURE 17-1 ■ The mind.
Curiosity for learning, mathematical ability, and short- and long-term memory are only some of the wonderful functions of the mind. The mind is a complex interaction between specific anatomical structures of the brain, the mental functions of reasoning, learning, memory, and conscious and subconscious emotions, drives, and desires.
Source: BillionPhotos/Fotolia

Medical Language Key

To unlock the definition of a medical word, break it into word parts. Give the meaning of each word part. Put the meanings of the word parts in order, beginning with the meaning of the suffix, then the prefix (if present), then the combining form(s).

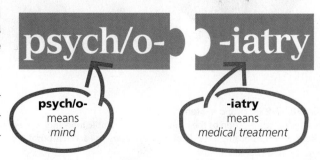

	Word Part	Word Part Meaning
Suffix	-iatry	*medical treatment*
Combining Form	psych/o-	*mind*

Psychiatry ▶ *Medical treatment (of the) mind.*

Anatomy and Physiology

Pronunciation/Word Parts

The structures that pertain to psychiatry are located in the brain (see Figure 17-1 ■). Psychiatry is concerned with physical symptoms and signs as well as behaviors that are the result of thoughts and emotions (for example, a rapid heart rate and agitated behavior due to anger; crying and suicide attempts due to depression; hyperventilation, chest pains, and an anxious facial expression due to fear).

Anatomy Related to Psychiatry

Limbic Lobe and Limbic System

The **limbic lobe** in the brain is along the medial edges of the right and left cerebral hemispheres (just superior to the corpus callosum that is a bridge between the two hemispheres). The limbic lobe includes some of each lobe in the cerebrum, plus a long extension of tissue into the temporal lobe. The limbic lobe is also known as the **cingulate gyrus** because it is in the form of a curved, encircling layer.

The **limbic system** consists of the limbic lobe, thalamus, hypothalamus, hippocampus, amygdaloid bodies, and fornix (see Figure 17-2 ■). The limbic system links the unconscious mind to the conscious mind. The limbic system processes memories and controls emotion, mood, memory, motivation, and behavior.

Thalamus

The **thalamus** is in the center of the cerebrum and forms the walls of the third ventricle (see Figure 17-2). The thalamus is part of the nervous system (discussed in "Neurology," Chapter 10). It acts as a relay station, receiving sensory information from the

limbic (LIM-bik)
  limb/o- *border; edge*
  -ic *pertaining to*

cingulate (SIN-gyoo-layt)
  cingul/o- *structure that surrounds*
  -ate *composed of; pertaining to*

gyrus (JY-rus)

thalamus (THAL-ah-mus)

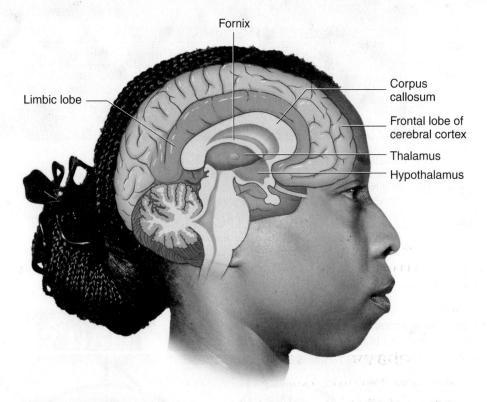

FIGURE 17-2 ■ Limbic system.
This midsagittal section of the brain shows the limbic lobe and some of the structures of the limbic system. The hippocampus and amygdaloid body in each temporal lobe are not visible on this view.
Source: Pearson Education

five senses (sight, hearing, taste, smell, and touch) and relaying it to the midbrain (which sends out a motor command if immediate action is needed). The thalamus also relays sensory information to the cerebrum where it is analyzed and compared with memories.

Hypothalamus

The **hypothalamus**, located below the thalamus, forms the floor and part of the walls of the third ventricle of the brain (see Figure 17-2). The hypothalamus is part of the nervous system and the endocrine system (discussed in "Neurology," Chapter 10 and "Endocrinology," Chapter 14). The hypothalamus controls emotions of pleasure, excitement, fear, anger, and bodily responses to these emotions. The hypothalamus also contains the feeding center and satiety center and regulates the sex drive, sexual arousal, and sexual behavior. (This behavior is also regulated by the male and female sex hormones and by conscious thought processes in the frontal lobe.) During times of fear or anger, the hypothalamus sends nerve impulses to the sympathetic division of the nervous system to trigger the medulla of the adrenal gland to secrete epinephrine for the "fight-or-flight" response to danger.

hypothalamus (HY-poh-THAL-ah-mus)

Hippocampus

The **hippocampus** is an elongated, curving structure with two heads, one of which is located in each temporal lobe. The two tails of the hippocampus join as the fornix in the center of the brain. The hippocampus is active in the learning process. It helps short-term memories become permanent long-term memories, stores long-term memories, and compares past and present emotions and experiences.

hippocampus (HIP-oh-KAM-pus)

Fornix

The **fornix** is along the floor of each lateral ventricle (see Figure 17-2). It connects the hippocampus in each temporal lobe to the thalamus and to amygdaloid bodies.

fornix (FOR-niks)

Amygdaloid Bodies

The **amygdaloid body** is an almond-shaped area within each temporal lobe. The amygdaloid bodies are involved in interpreting facial expressions and new social situations and identifying situations that could be dangerous. They combine visual images and long-term memories and are most active during the intense emotions of fear, anger, and rage.

amygdaloid (ah-MIG-dah-loyd)
  amygdal/o- *almond shape*
  -oid *resembling*

Frontal Lobe

The frontal lobe of the brain is the site of reasoning, judgment, planning, organizing, personality, creativity, and recent memories of all of those things. The frontal lobe exerts conscious control over alertness, concentration, and emotions. The frontal lobe also analyzes situations, predicts future events, and weighs the benefits or consequences of actions.

Physiology of Emotion and Behavior

A current thought, sensory information from one of the five senses, a recalled memory, or a combination of all three can trigger an emotion. An **emotion** is an intense state of feelings. An intense emotion connected with a particular situation causes that situation

emotion (ee-MOH-shun)
  emot/o- *moving; stirring up*
  -ion *action; condition*

to imprint deeply in long-term memory. That situation, when later called to mind, brings with it those same intense emotions.

An emotional thought produces an outward display on the face (the person's **affect**) (see Figure 17-3 ■), changes in behavior, and physical symptoms and signs in the body. A person's emotional state of mind may reflect many emotions at the same time (fear, guilt, and anger), but the prevailing, predominant emotion is known as the person's **mood**.

Pronunciation/Word Parts

affect (AF-ekt)

affective (ah-FEK-tiv)
  affect/o- *have an influence on; mood; state of mind*
  -ive *pertaining to*

mood (MOOD)

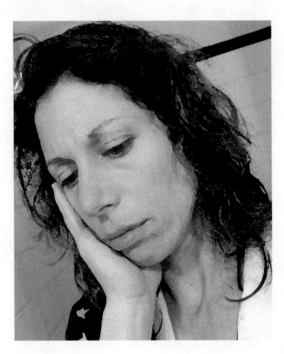

FIGURE 17-3 ■ Affect.
This woman's affect or facial expression reflects sadness and depression. Emotions are inward thoughts that produce an outward display through facial expressions, body position, and behavior.
Source: Pearson Education

Emotions are normal forms of expression, but extremely intense, long-lasting, inappropriate, or absent emotions are signs of a mental disorder. Abnormal emotions and behaviors can be produced by injury to the brain or changes in the levels of neurotransmitters in the brain.

Injury to the hypothalamus can cause overeating and obesity, disinterest in eating, insomnia, or excessive sleepiness.

Injury to, or degeneration of, the hippocampus in the temporal lobe can cause the loss of all long-term memory. A patient with Alzheimer's disease with degeneration of that area may be unable to recognize his/her own face in the mirror.

Hyperstimulation of the amygdaloid bodies can cause violent, aggressive behavior. Injury to, or degeneration of, the amygdaloid bodies can cause a loss of the emotions of anger and fear. The patient may recognize a person's face but cannot say if that person is a friend or an enemy. The patient is also unaware of dangerous situations.

Injury to the frontal lobe can produce these psychiatric symptoms: flat (unchanging) affect, disinterest in life, inability to concentrate, inappropriate laughing or crying, inappropriate social or sexual behavior, indifference to the consequences of behavior, inability to plan or modify behavior, inability to abide by or create rules to govern behavior, inability to keep commitments, impulsiveness, or an absence of goal-directed behavior.

Neurotransmitters are chemicals that relay messages from one neuron to the next. Neurotransmitters play an important role in emotion and behavior. Increased,

neurotransmitter
(NYOOR-oh-TRANS-mih-ter)
  neur/o- *nerve*
  transmitt/o- *send across; send through*
  -er *person who does; person who produces; thing that does; thing that produces*

decreased, or unbalanced levels of neurotransmitters can cause abnormal emotions and behaviors. Here are some of the most common neurotransmitters:

1. **Norepinephrine**. Neurotransmitter of the sympathetic division of the nervous system. It is also a hormone secreted by the medulla of the adrenal gland when stimulated by the sympathetic division of the nervous system. It controls involuntary processes such as the heart rate, respiratory rate, and blood pressure when the body is active or exercising. An increased level of norepinephrine may cause aggression, infatuation, and mania. A decreased level may cause depression.

norepinephrine (NOR-ep-ih-NEF-rin)

2. **Epinephrine**. Neurotransmitter of the sympathetic division of the nervous system. It is also a hormone secreted by the medulla of the adrenal gland when stimulated by the sympathetic division of the nervous system. During stress, anxiety, fear, or anger, epinephrine from the adrenal medulla prepares the body for "fight or flight." An increased level of epinephrine may cause anxiety, social phobia, performance phobia, and panic attacks.

epinephrine (EP-ih-NEF-rin)

3. **Dopamine**. Neurotransmitter in the brain. Cocaine, narcotic drugs, and alcohol increase the amount of dopamine, and this causes the euphoria and excitement ("high") craved by addicts. An increased level of dopamine may also cause infatuation. A decreased level may cause schizophrenia and depression. The combination of an increased level of dopamine in the limbic system and a decreased level of dopamine in the frontal lobe may cause paranoia.

dopamine (DOH-pah-meen)

4. **Serotonin**. Neurotransmitter in the brain and spinal cord. A decreased level of serotonin may cause depression. The combination of a decreased level of serotonin and an increased level of norepinephrine may cause violent behavior.

serotonin (SAIR-oh-TOH-nin)

5. **GABA**. Inhibitory neurotransmitter in the brain. A decreased level may cause anxiety. GABA stands for *gamma-aminobutyric acid*.

Vocabulary Review

Anatomy and Physiology		
Word or Phrase	**Description**	**Combining Forms**
affect	Outward display on the face of inward thoughts and emotions	**affect/o-** *have an influence on; mood; state of mind*
amygdaloid body	Almond-shaped area within each temporal lobe. It interprets facial expressions and new social situations to identify danger. It combines visual images with long-term memory and is active in the emotions of fear, anger, and rage.	**amygdal/o-** *almond shape*
dopamine	Neurotransmitter in the brain	
emotion	Intense state of feelings	**emot/o-** *moving; stirring up*
epinephrine	Neurotransmitter of the sympathetic division of the nervous system. It is also a hormone secreted into the blood by the medulla of the adrenal gland to prepare the body for "fight or flight."	
fornix	Connects the hippocampus to the thalamus and amygdaloid bodies	
GABA	Inhibitory neurotransmitter in the brain	
hippocampus	Elongated, curving structure within each temporal lobe. It helps short-term memories become long-term memories, stores long-term memories, and compares past and present emotions and experiences.	
hypothalamus	Controls emotions (pleasure, excitement, fear, anger) and bodily responses to emotions. It regulates sexual arousal and the sex drive. It contains the feeding and satiety centers. It functions as part of the "fight-or-flight" response of the sympathetic division of the nervous system.	
limbic lobe	Curved, encircling area of the brain that includes the medial edges of the two cerebral hemispheres and extends into the temporal lobes. It is also known as the **cingulate gyrus**.	**limb/o-** *border; edge* **cingul/o-** *structure that surrounds*
limbic system	Related structures in the brain that control emotion, mood, memory, motivation, and behavior and link the conscious to the unconscious mind. The limbic system consists of the limbic lobe, thalamus, hypothalamus, hippocampus, amygdaloid bodies, and fornix.	**limb/o-** *border; edge*
mood	Prevailing, predominant emotion affecting a person's state of mind	
neurotransmitter	Chemicals that relay messages from one neuron to another	**neur/o-** *nerve* **transmitt/o-** *send across; send through*
norepinephrine	Neurotransmitter of the sympathetic division of the nervous system and in the brain. It is also a hormone secreted into the blood by the medulla of the adrenal gland. It controls involuntary processes such as the heart rate, respiratory rate, and blood pressure when the body is active or exercising.	
serotonin	Neurotransmitter in the brain and spinal cord	
thalamus	Relay station that receives sensory information from the five senses and relays it to the midbrain (for immediate action in the face of danger) and to the cerebrum (for analysis and comparison with memories)	

Give Word Part Meanings

Use the Answer Key at the end of the book to check your answers.

Combining Forms Exercise

Next to each combining form, write its meaning. The first one has been done for you.

Combining Form	Meaning	Combining Form	Meaning
1. **amygdal/o-**	almond shape	5. limb/o-	
2. affect/o-		6. neur/o-	
3. cingul/o-		7. transmitt/o-	
4. emot/o-			

Build Medical Words

Combining Form and Suffix Exercise

Read the definition of the medical word. Look at the combining form that is given. Select the correct suffix from the Suffix List and write it on the blank line. Then build the medical word and write it on the line. (Remember: You may need to remove the combining vowel. Always remove the hyphens and slash.) Be sure to check your spelling. The first one has been done for you.

SUFFIX LIST			
-ic (pertaining to)	-ion (action; condition)	-ive (pertaining to)	-oid (resembling)

Definition of the Medical Word	Combining Form	Suffix	Build the Medical Word
1. (Structure) resembling (an) almond shape	**amygdal/o-**	**-oid**	amygdaloid
(You think *resembling* (-oid) + *almond shape* (amygdal/o-). You change the order of the word parts to put the suffix last. You write *amygdaloid*.)			
2. Pertaining to (the) border or edge	limb/o-		
3. Condition (of) stirring up (feelings)	emot/o-		
4. Pertaining to mood or state of mind	affect/o-		

Mental Disorders

Neurosis and Anxiety Disorders

Word or Phrase	Description	Pronunciation/Word Parts
Neurosis is a condition of nervousness and anxiety. **Anxiety disorders** are characterized by the predominant emotion of anxiety, with uneasiness, uncertainty, dread, worry, apprehension, or fear. Bodily symptoms and signs include inability to think clearly, dizziness, dry mouth, chest tightness, palpitations, upset stomach, diarrhea, fine tremor, sweaty palms, inability to relax, heightened startle reflex, fatigue, and irritability. Anxiety itself is an appropriate response to danger, but a neurosis or an anxiety disorder is not associated with a specific dangerous situation, person, or thing. Treatment: Antianxiety drug, antidepressant drug, psychotherapy, group therapy.		**neurosis** (nyoor-OH-sis) **neur/o-** *nerve* **-osis** *condition; process*
generalized anxiety disorder	Dwelling on issues that involve "What if . . . " and predicting or fearing that the worst will happen to self, family, or friends	**anxiety** (ang-ZY-eh-tee) **anxi/o-** *fear; worry* **-ety** *condition; state*
obsessive–compulsive disorder	Constant, persistent, uncontrollable thoughts (**obsessions**) that occupy the mind, cause anxiety, and compel the patient to perform excessive, repetitive, or meaningless activities (**compulsions**) for fear of what might happen if these are not done (see Figure 17-4 ■). These activities include washing and cleaning; checking work again and again; checking doors and locks; ordering, labeling, and arranging belongings in a particular sequence; hoarding useless collections of things with an inability to discard things; or repetitive thinking, counting, praying, or making mental lists. These activities consume a significant portion of each day.	**obsession** (awb-SEH-shun) **obsess/o-** *besieged by thoughts* **-ion** *action; condition* **obsessive** (awb-SEH-siv) **obsess/o-** *besieged by thoughts* **-ive** *pertaining to* **compulsion** (com-PAWL-shun) **compuls/o-** *compel; drive* **-ion** *action; condition* **compulsive** (com-PAWL-siv) **compuls/o-** *compel; drive* **-ive** *pertaining to*

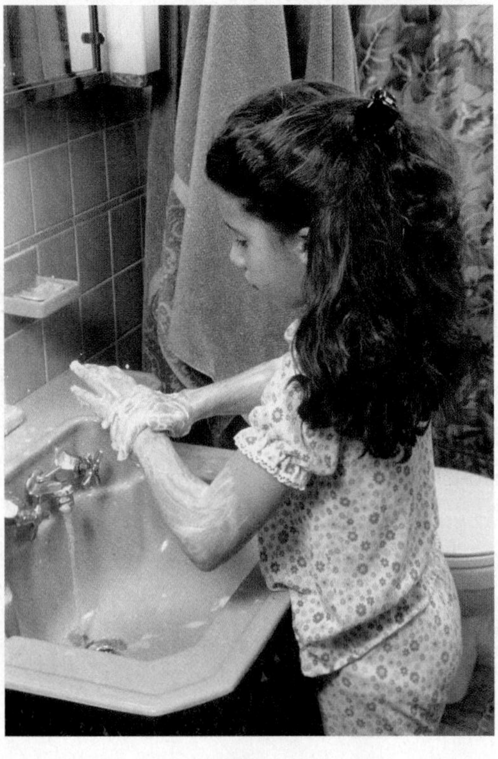

FIGURE 17-4 ■ Obsessive–compulsive disorder.
Washing the hands is a good habit of personal cleanliness. However, when handwashing is excessive and constant to the point that the hands become reddened and raw, and yet the patient cannot stop, then it becomes obsessive–compulsive disorder.
Source: John Greim/Science Source

Word or Phrase	Description	Pronunciation/Word Parts
panic disorder	Sudden attack of severe, overwhelming anxiety without an identifiable cause. Patients often feel that they are choking or dying of a heart attack.	**panic** (PAN-ik)

Word or Phrase	Description	Pronunciation/Word Parts
phobia	Intense, unreasonable fear of a specific thing or situation or even the thought of it (see Table 17-1 ■ and Figure 17-5 ■). Phobias occur when the unconscious mind avoids a real, ongoing conflict by projecting the anxiety onto an unrelated situation or object. While the anxiety exhibited is out of proportion to the actual danger or threat, the patient cannot recognize this. Avoidance of the phobia can severely restrict the normal activities of daily life.	**phobia** (FOH-bee-ah) **phob/o-** *avoidance; fear* **-ia** *condition; state; thing* **phobic** (FOH-bik) **phob/o-** *avoidance; fear* **-ic** *pertaining to*

Table 17-1   Common Phobias

Phobia	Description	Pronunciation/Word Parts
acrophobia	Fear of heights	**acrophobia** (AK-roh-FOH-bee-ah) **acr/o-** *extremity; highest point* **phob/o-** *avoidance; fear* **-ia** *condition; state; thing*
agoraphobia	Fear of crowds or public places	**agoraphobia** (AH-gor-ah-FOH-bee-ah) **agor/a-** *open area; open space* **phob/o-** *avoidance; fear* **-ia** *condition; state; thing*
arachnophobia	Fear of spiders	**arachnophobia** (ah-RAK-noh-FOH-bee-ah) **arachn/o-** *spider; spider web* **phob/o-** *avoidance; fear* **-ia** *condition; state; thing*
claustrophobia	Fear of closed-in spaces	**claustrophobia** (KLAW-stroh-FOH-bee-ah) **claustr/o-** *enclosed space* **phob/o-** *avoidance; fear* **-ia** *condition; state; thing*
microphobia	Fear of germs	**microphobia** (MY-kroh-FOH-bee-ah) **micr/o-** *one millionth; small* **phob/o-** *avoidance; fear* **-ia** *condition; state; thing*
ophidiophobia	Fear of snakes	**ophidiophobia** (oh-FID-ee-oh-FOH-bee-ah) **ophidi/o-** *snake* **phob/o-** *avoidance; fear* **-ia** *condition; state; thing*
social phobia	Fear of being embarrassed or humiliated in front of others, fear of being in a public place, or fear of being the center of attention. This is also known as **social anxiety disorder**.	**social** (SOH-shal) **soci/o-** *community; human beings* **-al** *pertaining to*
thanatophobia	Fear of death	**thanatophobia** (THAN-ah-toh-FOH-bee-ah) **thanat/o-** *death* **phob/o-** *avoidance; fear* **-ia** *condition; state; thing*
xenophobia	Fear of strangers	**xenophobia** (ZEN-oh-FOH-bee-ah) **xen/o-** *foreign* **phob/o-** *avoidance; fear* **-ia** *condition; state; thing*

Word or Phrase	Description	Pronunciation/Word Parts

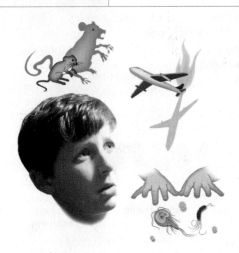

FIGURE 17-5 ■ Phobias.
Phobias are intense, exaggerated fears of a specific thing or situation.
Source: Pearson Education

| posttraumatic stress disorder (PTSD) | Continuing, disabling reaction to an excessively traumatic situation or event, such as a war, terrorist attack, torture, rape, kidnapping, natural disaster (e.g., earthquake, flood), explosion, or fire. The patient feels helpless, has a numbed emotional response with disinterest in people and current events, and relives the trauma of the event over and over. Also, there may be chronic anxiety, insomnia, irritability, or occasional violent outbursts. In the past, this was known as *combat fatigue* or *shell shock*. | **posttraumatic** (POST-trah-MAT-ik) **post-** *after; behind* **traumat/o-** *injury* **-ic** *pertaining to* |

Eating Disorders

Eating disorders are characterized by abnormal eating patterns, distorted body image, fear, guilt, and depression. The majority of patients are young women. Treatment: Antidepressant drugs, psychotherapy, family therapy.

| anorexia nervosa | Extreme, chronic fear of being fat and an obsession with becoming thinner (see Figure 17-6 ■). The patient decreases food intake to the point of starvation. In a patient with long-standing anorexia nervosa, all of the subcutaneous fat on the body is gone and the bones are clearly visible. The patient denies being too thin, denies abnormal eating habits, and tries to keep this a secret from family and friends by making excuses for not eating and wearing clothes that conceal the extreme weight loss. | **anorexia nervosa** (AN-oh-REK-see-ah ner-VOH-sah) **an-** *not; without* **orex/o-** *appetite* **-ia** *condition; state; thing* Anorexia (discussed in "Gastroenterology," Chapter 3) is a simple loss of appetite due to illness. It is not a psychiatric disorder. |

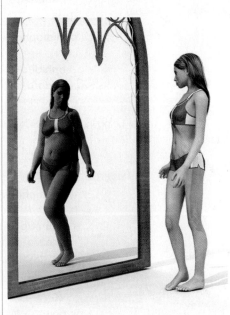

FIGURE 17-6 ■ Anorexia nervosa.
A patient with anorexia nervosa denies being too thin and would, in fact, appear to herself as being fat if she looked in a mirror.
Source: Heywoody/Fotolia

Word or Phrase	Description	Pronunciation/Word Parts
bulimia	Patients gorge themselves on excessive amounts of food (**binge eating**) and then, for fear of gaining weight, they rid (**purge**) themselves of food by using laxative drugs or self-induced vomiting. Long-term vomiting wears away tooth enamel, causes inflammation and ulcers in the esophagus, and can lead to death from a low level of potassium in the blood.	**bulimia** (buh-LEE-ee-ah)

Substance-Related Disorders

Substance-related disorders are characterized by the frequent or constant use and abuse of drugs or chemicals to achieve a desired physical or emotional effect (a "high," sedation, or hallucinations). The drugs may be prescription drugs, over-the-counter drugs, tobacco, alcohol, chemicals, or illegal street drugs. After a brief period of use, patients experience **dependence** (the need for the substance in order to prevent withdrawal symptoms). Later, patients exhibit **tolerance** (decreasing effect even with increasing amounts of the substance). Much of the patient's life may center on drug-seeking behavior. Patients are aware of the serious medical conditions related to the use of the substance, but they choose to ignore this and continue to use the substance. **Addiction** is a state of complete physical and psychological dependence on a substance. Treatment: Psychotherapy, group therapy, family therapy, support groups, aversion therapy, medical support for withdrawal symptoms.

The following substances and drugs are often abused:

- Alcohol (beer, wine, liquor, ETOH, rubbing alcohol, wood alcohol)
- Amphetamines (central nervous system stimulant drugs, diet pills, speed)
- Cannabis (marijuana, hashish)
- Cocaine
- **Hallucinogens** (LSD, PCP)
- Inhalants (fumes from paint, paint thinner, cleaning fluid, lighter fluid, liquid glue, correction fluid, felt-tipped markers, or gasoline; aerosol propellant from spray cans)
- Nicotine (cigarettes, cigars, chewing tobacco)
- Opioids (narcotic drugs such as morphine, codeine, Demerol, OxyContin; the street drug heroin)
- Sedatives and antianxiety drugs (barbiturate drugs, sleeping pills, Valium)

dependence (dee-PEN-dens)
  depend/o- *hang onto*
  -ence *state*

tolerance (TAW-ler-ans)
  toler/o- *become accustomed to*
  -ance *state*

addiction (ah-DIK-shun)
  addict/o- *controlled by; surrender to*
  -ion *action; condition*

hallucinogen
(hah-LOO-sih-noh-JEN)
  hallucin/o- *imagined perception*
  -gen *that which produces*

Affective or Mood Disorders

Word or Phrase	Description	Pronunciation/Word Parts
Mood disorders are characterized by chronic, persistent (longer than 6 months) depression or mood swings alternating between depression and mania. Normal feelings of sadness that diminish over time are considered appropriate and not categorized as a mood disorder. Mood disorders are also known as **affective disorders** because the mood can be seen in the patient's affect (facial expression and body movements). Treatment: Psychotherapy, antidepressant drug, drug for mania.		**affective** (ah-FEK-tiv) **affect/o-** *have an influence on; mood; state of mind* **-ive** *pertaining to*
bipolar disorder	Chronic mood swings between the two opposite emotional poles of **mania** and depression (see Figure 17-7 ■). Patients with mania are hyperactive, with limitless energy and extreme happiness (**euphoria**). They have feelings of power and mastery, need little sleep, and are intensely interested in and talk about one thing after another (flight of ideas), making and then quickly discarding plans. Gradually, their thoughts get out of control; they are unable to concentrate and show increasingly poor judgment and recklessness. After an episode of mania, the patient swings abruptly into severe depression. This is also known as **manic-depressive disorder** because of the cycle between mania and depression.	**bipolar** (by-POH-lar) **bi-** *two* **pol/o-** *pole* **-ar** *pertaining to* **mania** (MAY-nee-ah) **man/o-** *frenzy; thin* **-ia** *condition; state; thing* **euphoria** (yoo-FOR-ee-ah) **eu-** *good; normal* **phor/o-** *bear; carry; range* **-ia** *condition; state; thing* **manic** (MAN-ik) **depressive** (dee-PREH-siv) **depress/o-** *press down* **-ive** *pertaining to*

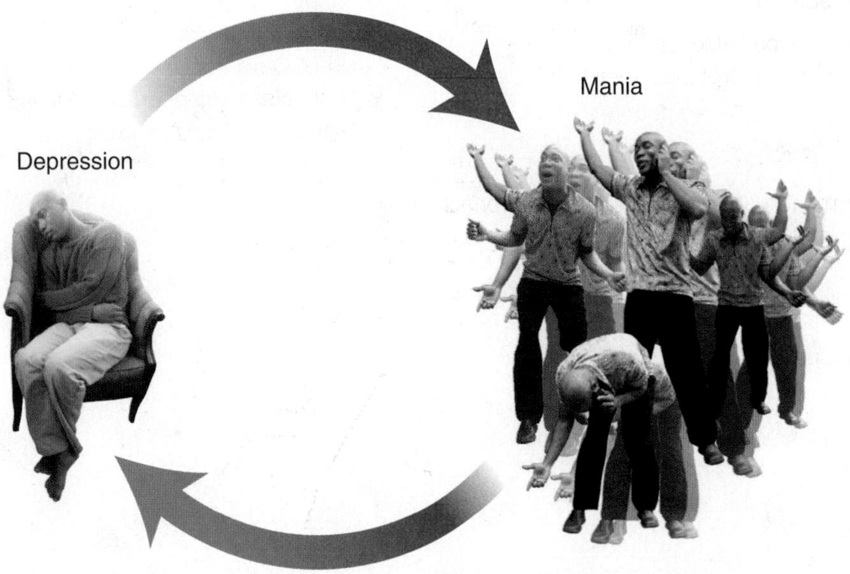

Mania

Depression

FIGURE 17-7 ■ Bipolar disorder.
Depression and mania are characterized by emotions and behaviors that are at opposite poles from each other.
Source: Pearson Education

Word or Phrase	Description	Pronunciation/Word Parts
cyclothymia	Chronic, mild bipolar disorder. In between mood swings, the patient is free of signs and symptoms for several months.	**cyclothymia** (sy-kloh-THY-mee-ah) **cycl/o-** *ciliary body of the eye; circle; cycle* **thym/o-** *rage; thymus* **-ia** *condition; state; thing* Select the correct combining form meanings to get the definition of *cyclothymia*: *condition (of a) cycle (of) rage.*
dysthymia	Chronic, mild-to-moderate depression	**dysthymia** (dis-THY-mee-ah) **dys-** *abnormal; difficult; painful* **thym/o-** *rage; thymus* **-ia** *condition; state; thing*

Word or Phrase	Description	Pronunciation/Word Parts
major depression	Chronic, severe symptoms of depression with **apathy** (indifference), hopelessness, helplessness, worthlessness, crying, insomnia, lack of pleasure in any activity (**anhedonia**), increased or decreased appetite, inability to make decisions or concentrate, fatigue, and slowed movements (see Figure 17-8 ■). During psychiatric interviews, depressed patients are asked if they have current **suicidal ideation** or past suicide attempts. Depression may be caused by decreased levels of norepinephrine, dopamine, and serotonin in the brain. Depression can also occur after a personal loss or traumatic event or as a side effect of certain drugs. 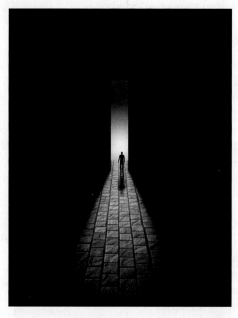 **FIGURE 17-8 ■ Depression.** Psychiatry helps a patient move from a place of darkness toward a normal life. *Source*: Rolffimages/Fotolia	**depression** (dee-PREH-shun) **depress/o-** *press down* **-ion** *action; condition* **apathy** (AP-ah-thee) **a-** *away from; without* **-pathy** *disease* The ending *-pathy* contains the combining form *path/o-* and the one-letter suffix *-y*. **anhedonia** (AN-hee-DOH-nee-ah) **an-** *not; without* **hedon/o-** *pleasure* **-ia** *condition; state; thing* **suicidal** (soo-ih-SY-dal) **su/i-** *self* **cid/o-** *killing* **-al** *pertaining to*

DID YOU KNOW?

Depression was previously known as *melancholia*. This word comes from *melan/o-* (black) and *chol/e-* (bile; gall). The ancient Greeks thought that the body contained four "humors" (blood, yellow bile, black bile, and phlegm) that caused different moods. Depression after childbirth is still known as *involutional melancholia* (see "Gynecology and Obstetrics," Chapter 13).

Word or Phrase	Description	Pronunciation/Word Parts
premenstrual dysphoric disorder (PMDD)	Occurs before the onset of menstruation during each menstrual cycle and combines the symptoms of premenstrual syndrome (PMS) (breast, joint, and muscle pains) with depression, anxiety, tearfulness, difficulty concentrating, and sleeping and eating disturbances.	**premenstrual** (pree-MEN-stroo-al) **pre-** *before; in front of* **menstru/o-** *monthly discharge of blood* **-al** *pertaining to* **dysphoric** (dis-FOR-ik) **dys-** *abnormal; difficult; painful* **phor/o-** *bear; carry; range* **-ic** *pertaining to*
seasonal affective disorder (SAD)	Caused by hypersecretion of melatonin from the pineal gland in the brain. Melatonin is normally produced during the night. The longer nights and decreased hours of sunshine during the winter months increase the production of melatonin, and this causes symptoms of depression, weight gain, and altered sleeping habits. Treatment: Exposure to sunlight or the use of a light box for several hours each day.	**affective** (ah-FEK-tiv) **affect/o-** *have an influence on; mood; state of mind* **-ive** *pertaining to*

Psychosis		
Word or Phrase	**Description**	**Pronunciation/Word Parts**

Psychosis is characterized by a loss of touch with reality and a disintegration of the thought processes. There is a change in affect and behavior, with inability to communicate effectively or maintain life activities. Schizophrenia is the most common form of psychosis. Treatment: Antipsychotic drug, psychotherapy.		**psychosis** (sy-KOH-sis)
		  psych/o- *mind*
		  -osis *condition; process*

delusional disorder	Continued false beliefs (delusions) concerning events of everyday life. These beliefs are fixed and unchanging despite the efforts of others to persuade or evidence showing otherwise. Common delusions: other people or even strangers are in love with you, your husband or wife is unfaithful, or you have the powers of a god or are a famous person (delusions of grandeur). A patient with **paranoia** or delusions of persecution believes that other people are trying to hurt him/her; the patient is **paranoid**.	**delusional** (dee-LOO-shun-al)
		  delus/o- *false belief*
		  -ion *action; condition*
		  -al *pertaining to*
		
		paranoia (PAIR-ah-NOY-ah)

schizophrenia	The most common type of psychosis. There is a chronic loss of touch with reality in most or all aspects of life with bizarre behavior and breakdown of thought processes. The patient is **schizophrenic**. Patients have **hallucinations** (false impressions of vision, smell, sound, taste, or touch). The most common is an auditory hallucination of a voice telling them to do certain things. Patients with paranoid schizophrenia have delusions of persecution or delusions that others are controlling their thoughts. Other schizophrenic patients feel that they can use their own thoughts to control events. Some patients' thoughts are so chaotic that their spoken words are completely meaningless, and they may use **neologisms** (new or made-up words that have no meaning). Patients' emotions and affect are inappropriate and do not correspond to what they are saying. Some patients are rigid and in a stupor (**catatonia**) or their extremities stay fixed in whatever position they are placed (**catalepsy**) (see Figure 17-9 ■), while others have childish, silly behavior (**hebephrenia**). Many patients have their first episode as young adults following a stressful event. Others develop symptoms more slowly over time.
	
	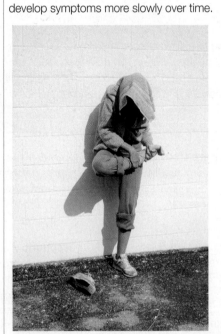
	
	FIGURE 17-9 ■ Catalepsy. This patient is showing the unusual fixed position of the extremities that is a common feature of catalepsy. It is associated with catatonic schizophrenia, Parkinson's disease, epilepsy, or can be caused by antipsychotic drugs used to treat schizophrenia.
	Source: Grunnitus Studio/Science Source/Getty Images
		schizophrenia
		(SKIZ-oh-FREE-nee-ah)
		(SKIT-soh-FREE-nee-ah)
		  schiz/o- *split*
		  phren/o- *diaphragm; mind*
		  -ia *condition; state; thing*
		Select the correct combining form meaning to get the definition of *schizophrenia: condition (of a) split mind.*
		
		hallucination
		(hah-LOO-sih-NAY-shun)
		  hallucin/o- *imagined perception*
		  -ation *being; having; process*
		
		neologism (nee-OH-loh-jizm)
		  ne/o- *new*
		  log/o- *study of; word*
		  -ism *disease from a specific*
		    cause; process
		
		catatonia (KAT-ah-TOH-nee-ah)
		  cata- *down*
		  ton/o- *pressure; tone*
		  -ia *condition; state; thing*
		
		catalepsy (KAT-ah-LEP-see)
		  cata- *down*
		  -lepsy *seizure*
		
		hebephrenia
		(HEE-bah-FREE-nee-ah)
		(HEB-eh-FREE-nee-ah)
		  hebe/o- *youth*
		  phren/o- *diaphragm; mind*
		  -ia *condition; state; thing*

DID YOU KNOW?

Insanity comes from two Latin words meaning *not sound.* Literature has long depicted an insane person as a lunatic who is influenced by the phases of the moon, with the most severe symptoms occurring during a full moon. *Lunatic* comes from the Latin word that means *moon.*

Childhood Disorders

Childhood disorders include any behavioral abnormality having to do with feeding, eating, elimination, learning, or motor skills—all major developmental areas during childhood. Treatment: Drug for ADHD, psychotherapy, group therapy, family therapy.

Word or Phrase	Description	Pronunciation/Word Parts
attention-deficit hyperactivity disorder (ADHD)	Distractability, short attention span, inability to follow directions, restlessness, hyperactivity, emotional lability, and impulsiveness. It may be caused by mild brain damage at birth, genetic factors, or other abnormalities. It is five times more common in boys than in girls. Most children outgrow the symptoms by late childhood. In the past, it was known as *minimal brain dysfunction* and *attention-deficit disorder.*	
autism spectrum disorder (ASD)	Inability to communicate, socialize, or form significant relationships with others, and a lack of interest in doing so. Patients may be of normal intelligence or mentally retarded. The patient may not speak or may have abnormal speech with **echolalia** (automatically repeating what someone else has said). The patient avoids physical contact and eye contact, but is fascinated by objects. There are ritualistic, repetitive behaviors. Asperger's syndrome is a less severe form within the range of the autism spectrum disorder.	**autism** (AW-tizm) **aut/o-** *self* **-ism** *disease from a specific cause; process* **echolalia** (EK-oh-LAY-lee-ah) **ech/o-** *echo of a sound wave* **-lalia** *condition of speech*
encopresis	Repeated passage of stool into the clothing in a child older than age 5 who does not have a gastrointestinal illness, mental retardation, or a physical disability	**encopresis** (EN-koh-PREE-sis) **en-** *in; inward; within* **copr/o-** *feces; stool* **-esis** *condition; process*
oppositional defiant disorder	Persistent, aggressive behavior (fighting, arguing, provoking, annoying), defiance of and refusal to obey rules, and disrespect for authority figures, with anger, stubbornness, and touchiness. **Conduct disorder** is a more severe form in which the patient physically and sexually assaults others, destroys property, steals, sets fires, or runs away from home.	**oppositional** (AW-poh-ZIH-shun-al) **oppos/o-** *forceful resistance* **-ition** *condition of having* **-al** *pertaining to*
reactive attachment disorder	Inability to emotionally bond and form intimate relationships with others because of severe abuse or neglect of the patient's basic needs before age 2 when trust is established. There is a lack of trust, watchful wariness, poor eye contact, lack of empathy, inability to show genuine affection, and a lack of a conscience. The patient is difficult to comfort and resists physical contact such as being held, but can show inappropriate friendliness to strangers.	**reactive** (ree-AK-tiv) **react/o-** *reverse movement* **-ive** *pertaining to*
Tourette's syndrome	Frequent, spontaneous, involuntary muscle tics (eye blinking, throat clearing, arm thrusting), vocal tics (grunts, barks), or spontaneous comments that are socially inappropriate, vulgar, obscene (**coprolalia**), or racist. The patient can only temporarily suppress these behaviors. The patient also can have echolalia, obsessive–compulsive disorder, and hyperactivity.	**Tourette's** (toor-ETZ) **coprolalia** (KAW-proh-LAY-lee-ah) **copr/o-** *feces; stool* **-lalia** *condition of speech*

Sexual Disorders

Sexual disorders are characterized by abnormalities of focusing sexual attention on an object or a person other than a consenting adult. Treatment: Aversion therapy, cognitive-behavioral therapy, group therapy, psychotherapy.

Word or Phrase	Description	Pronunciation/Word Parts
exhibitionism	Obtaining power, control, and **sexual** arousal by exposing the genital area in public places to strangers and seeing their reactions. The patient is an **exhibitionist.**	**exhibitionism** (EKS-hih-BIH-shun-izm) **exhibit/o-** *showing* **-ion** *action; condition* **-ism** *disease from a specific cause; process* **sexual** (SEK-shoo-al) **sex/o-** *sex* **-ual** *pertaining to*
fetishism	Obtaining sexual arousal from objects rather than a person. Patients devote a great deal of time to obtaining and using the object (a fetish), which, for men, often includes women's clothing.	**fetishism** (FET-ish-izm)
masochism	Obtaining sexual arousal for one's self through abuse, pain, humiliation, or bondage done deliberately by another person. The patient is a **masochist.**	**masochism** (MAS-oh-kizm)
pedophilia	Obtaining power, control, and sexual arousal through contact or sexual acts with preadolescent children. The patient is a **pedophile.**	**pedophilia** (PEE-doh-FIL-ee-ah) **ped/o-** *child* **phil/o-** *attraction to; fondness for* **-ia** *condition; state; thing* **pedophile** (PEE-doh-file) **ped/o-** *child* **-phile** *person who is attracted to; person who is fond of*
rape	Obtaining power, control, and sexual arousal through forced sexual intercourse with a nonconsenting adult. Statutory rape is sexual intercourse with a minor (defined by most states as a person under the age of 18). The patient is a **rapist. Incest** is rape of a child by a parent or relative.	**rape** (RAYP) **rapist** (RAY-pist) **rap/o-** *drag away; seize* **-ist** *person who specializes in; thing that specializes in* **incest** (IN-sest)
sadism	Obtaining power, control, and sexual arousal for one's self by deliberately causing abuse, pain, humiliation, or bondage to another person. The patient is a **sadist.**	**sadism** (SAY-dizm) (SAD-izm) **sadist** (SAY-dist)
voyeurism	Obtaining power, control, and sexual arousal by secretively viewing other people who are naked or having sexual relations. The elements of risk and danger as well as knowingly violating another's privacy are part of the experience. The patient is a **voyeur.**	**voyeurism** (VOY-er-izm)

Cognitive Disorders

Cognitive disorders are characterized by a temporary or permanent impairment of thinking and memory. Treatment: Supportive care, drugs to slow memory loss or improve cognitive function, or psychotherapy.	**cognitive** (KAWG-nih-tiv) **cognit/o-** *thinking* **-ive** *pertaining to*
amnesia Partial or total loss of long-term memory due to trauma or disease of the hippocampus. The patient is said to be **amnestic**. In **retrograde amnesia**, the patient cannot remember events that occurred before the onset of amnesia. In **anterograde amnesia**, the patient cannot remember events that occurred after the onset of amnesia. In **global amnesia**, all memories (past and present) are lost.	**amnesia** (am-NEE-zha) **amnes/o-** *forgetfulness* **-ia** *condition; state; thing* **amnestic** (am-NES-tik) **amnes/o-** *forgetfulness* **-tic** *pertaining to* **retrograde** (REH-troh-grayd) **retro-** *backward; behind* **-grade** *pertaining to going* **anterograde** (AN-ter-oh-GRAYD) **anter/o-** *before; front part* **-grade** *pertaining to going* **global** (GLOH-bal) **glob/o-** *comprehensive; shaped like a globe* **-al** *pertaining to*
delirium Acute confusion, disorientation, and agitation due to toxic levels of chemicals, drugs, or alcohol in the blood that affect the brain. These acute signs slowly subside as toxic levels of drugs or alcohol in the blood decrease. **Delirium tremens (DT)** is caused by withdrawal symptoms from alcoholic intoxication and includes restlessness, tremors of the hands, hallucinations, sweating, and increased heart rate.	**delirium** (deh-LEER-ee-um) (dee-LEER-ee-um) **delirium tremens** (dee-LEER-ee-um TREM-enz)
dementia Gradual but progressive deterioration of cognitive function due to old age or a neurologic disease. Alzheimer's disease is the most common type of dementia. There is a gradual decline in mental abilities, with forgetfulness, inability to learn new things, inability to perform daily activities, and difficulty making decisions. It can also include personality changes, anxiety, irritability, poor judgment, impulsiveness, hostility, combativeness, depression, and delusions.	**dementia** (deh-MEN-sha) **de-** *reversal of; without* **ment/o-** *chin; mind* **-ia** *condition; state; thing*

Impulse Control Disorders

Impulse control disorders are characterized by strong, persistent thoughts (impulses) that occupy the mind and cause tension as the patient decides whether or not to act on these often dangerous or illegal impulses. When the act is performed, the patient feels relief or even pleasure. Treatment: Psychotherapy, counseling with anger management, family therapy.

Word or Phrase	Description	Pronunciation/Word Parts
intermittent explosive disorder	Sudden, explosively violent, unprovoked attacks of rage that are out of proportion to the stress experienced. Patients always blame their anger on others or on circumstances. They commit assault and battery, which is often associated with domestic violence (spousal abuse, child abuse). During psychiatric interviews, patients are asked if they have any **homicidal ideation** about actually killing someone.	**homicidal** (HOH-mih-SY-dal) **hom/i-** *man* **cid/o-** *killing* **-al** *pertaining to* **ideation** (EYE-dee-AA-shun)
kleptomania	Overwhelming impulse to steal things that have little or no value. These things are not stolen out of anger or revenge, and the patient sometimes even secretly returns them. Unlike shoplifting, the patient does not steal in order to obtain something without paying for it. The patient is a **kleptomaniac**.	**kleptomania** (KLEP-toh-MAY-nee-ah) **klept/o-** *steal* **man/o-** *frenzy; thin* **-ia** *condition; state; thing*
pathological gambling	Constant gambling that interferes with normal life and work activities and creates severe financial problems. Patients lie about how much money they have lost and often place bigger bets to try to win back lost money.	**pathological** (PATH-oh-LAW-jih-kal)
pyromania	Deliberately setting fires for the pleasure of watching the fire and the people sent to fight the fire. Fires are not set to take revenge, conceal a crime, or collect insurance money. The patient is a **pyromaniac**.	**pyromania** (PY-roh-MAY-nee-ah) **pyr/o-** *burning; fire* **man/o-** *frenzy; thin* **-ia** *condition; state; thing*
trichotillomania	Repetitively pulling out hair from the head, eyebrows, or eyelashes. This is known as **hair-pulling disorder**. It is also related to excoriation disorder (skin-picking), both of which are a type of obsessive-compulsive behavior.	**trichotillomania** (TRIK-oh-TIL-oh-MAY-nee-ah) **trich/o-** *hair* **till/o-** *pull out* **man/o-** *frenzy; thin* **-ia** *condition; state; thing*

Personality Disorders

Personality disorders are characterized by a disturbance of one or more aspects of the personality (which is the combination of thoughts, beliefs, emotions, and behaviors that are unique to each person). Patients with personality disorders experience difficulty in interpersonal relationships (marriage, work, social). They are unable to adapt their rigid views, they fail to meet the needs of others, and they have a tendency to blame others for their own failures. Treatment: Psychotherapy, group therapy, family therapy.

Word or Phrase	Description	Pronunciation/Word Parts
antisocial personality	Disregard for the written and unwritten rules and standards of conduct (laws, morals, ethics) of society. Patients lie, steal, and manipulate, showing no empathy for others or guilt or remorse for their actions. There is also fighting, failure to attend school (truancy), vandalism, sexual promiscuity, excessive drinking, the use of illegal drugs, and criminal acts. These patients were previously known as *sociopaths* or *psychopaths*.	**antisocial** (AN-tee-SOH-shal) **anti-** *against* **soci/o-** *community; human beings* **-al** *pertaining to* **personality** (PER-son-AL-ih-tee) **person/o-** *person* **-al** *pertaining to* **-ity** *condition; state*
avoidant personality	Avoidance of social contact because of excessive shyness and extreme fear and sensitivity to criticism or rejection	

Word or Phrase	Description	Pronunciation/Word Parts
borderline personality	Inability to sustain a stable relationship. Patients fear abandonment and panic when they are alone, rushing into intense, but self-destructive relationships. They tend to see things in black and white—all good or all bad with no middle ground. They are hypersensitive, with strong emotions that can easily change. They have poor tolerance to stress and often overreact.	
dependent personality	Expects and wants to be told what to do and what to think. Patients are passive, have difficulty making decisions, and want others to take care of them and the details of their lives.	**dependent** (dee-PEN-dent) **depend/o-** *hang onto* **-ent** *pertaining to*
narcissistic personality	Exaggerated sense of self-worth and importance. Patients feel superior to others and believe they are entitled to be the center of attention and to receive compliments, admiration, and affection. They are angry, demanding, and manipulative if others receive more than they do. Their demand to be noticed can be emotional, dramatic, and done for its effect (**histrionic**). Also known as **narcissism**.	**narcissistic** (NAR-sih-SIS-tik) **narcissism** (NAR-sih-sizm) **histrionic** (HIS-tree-AW-nik)
obsessive–compulsive personality	Inflexible and perfectionistic. Patients feel that everything must be accounted for and in its place, nothing can be left to chance, and they are unwilling to compromise. Patients feel that there is always one best way to do everything and they expect others to agree with them. Patients keep lists and schedules and are concerned about productivity, but may be so consumed by minor details that they sometimes cannot get the job done. These patients do not have obsessive–compulsive disorder (which was discussed previously).	

Factitious Disorders

Factitious disorders are characterized by physical and/or psychological symptoms that are consciously made up (fabricated) by the patient, and that the patient knows are not true. Patients pretend to be sick (often with symptoms that are difficult to evaluate) or even make themselves sick because of a desire to be cared for. They are intelligent and knowledgeable about medicine, but they are experienced, expert liars who often fool physicians. Treatment: Psychotherapy, family therapy, cognitive-behavioral therapy.

Word or Phrase	Description	Pronunciation/Word Parts
malingering	Exhibiting **factitious** (false) medical or psychiatric symptoms in order to get a tangible reward, such as narcotic drugs or disability payments. Patients are aware that they are lying and know exactly what they want to achieve from their deceptions.	**malingering** (mah-LING-ger-ing) **factitious** (fak-TIH-shus) **factiti/o-** *artificial; made up* **-ous** *pertaining to*
Munchausen syndrome	Exhibiting factitious medical or psychiatric symptoms. Patients are aware that they are lying, but are unaware that their motivation is the desire for assistance, attention, compassion, pity, and being excused from the normal expectations of life. Patients are not concerned about the cost of multiple tests, treatments, or surgeries and, in fact, desire to have them.	**Munchausen** (moon-CHOW-zen)
Munchausen by proxy	A caregiver creates illness in another person (often a child or elderly person) in order to enjoy the attention that the sick person gets while simultaneously enjoying attention for being the sacrificing, loving caregiver. This is a form of child or elder abuse. The caregiver makes up a medical history, induces physical symptoms with drugs, or contaminates specimens for laboratory tests to prolong the sickness and the attention it brings.	**proxy** (PRAWK-see)

Dissociative Disorders

Dissociative disorders are characterized by a breakdown between the conscious mind and the person's identity, personality, and memory. This breakdown is precipitated by a traumatic event or by continuing trauma during childhood. Treatment: Psychotherapy.

Word or Phrase	Description	Pronunciation/Word Parts
depersonalization	Loss of connection (**dissociative process**) between personal thoughts and a sense of self and the environment. Patients feel as if they are in a dream or watching a movie of themselves, and events seem unreal and strange.	**depersonalization** (dee-PER-son-AL-ih-ZAY-shun) **dissociative** (dih-SOH-see-ah-TIV) **dis-** *away from* **soci/o-** *community; human beings* **-ative** *pertaining to*
fugue	Impulsive flight from one's life and familiar surroundings after a traumatic event. The patient begins a new life in a new location and functions normally but is unable to remember anything of the past.	**fugue** (FYOOG)
identity disorder	Loss of connection between the normally integrated functions of conscious thought, perception of the environment, identity, and memory, done in an effort to bury traumatic memories. Two or more distinct personalities are present, each with its own identity and history (made up of parts of the original personality). Each personality is capable of independent thoughts and actions and may be unaware of the other personalities. In the past, this was known as **multiple personality disorder** or **split personality.**	

Somatoform Disorders

Somatoform disorders are characterized by excessive physical complaints that are dramatic but do not fit any medical disease. Diagnostic tests are negative. There is pain in various places in the body with anxiety. Patients have poor insight into their problem and may have experienced trauma prior to the onset of symptoms. Treatment: Psychotherapy, antianxiety drug.

Word or Phrase	Description	Pronunciation/Word Parts
body dysmorphic disorder	The patient is continually concerned with minor defects in the appearance of the body, particularly of the face, and demands frequent plastic surgery	**dysmorphic** (dis-MOR-fik) **dys-** *abnormal; difficult; painful* **morph/o-** *shape* **-ic** *pertaining to*
conversion disorder	**Somatoform** (neurologic, sensory, or motor) deficits that occur without any physical basis. There may be sudden blindness, deafness, paralysis, or the inability to speak. This disorder begins with **repression** of overwhelming anxiety or internal conflict, which then undergoes a **conversion** to become physical symptoms.	**conversion** (con-VER-shun) **con-** *with* **vers/o-** *travel; turn* **-ion** *action; condition* **somatoform** (soh-MAT-oh-form) **somat/o-** *body* **-form** *having the form of* **repression** (ree-PREH-shun) **repress/o-** *press back* **-ion** *action; condition*
hypochondriasis	Preoccupation with, and misinterpretation of, minor body sensations with the fear that these indicate disease. Patients are convinced they have a serious illness and make frequent trips to the doctor despite medical evidence and reassurance to the contrary. The patient is known as a **hypochondriac**. Patients who do have significant physical symptoms but with excessive anxiety because of them are diagnosed as having **somatic symptom disorder**.	**hypochondriasis** (HY-poh-con-DRY-ah-sis) **hypo-** *below; deficient* **chondr/o-** *cartilage* **-iasis** *process; state* **somatic** (soh-MAT-ik) **somat/o-** *body* **-ic** *pertaining to*

Laboratory and Diagnostic Procedures

	Blood and Urine Tests	
Word or Phrase	**Description**	**Pronunciation/Word Parts**
drug level	Blood test to determine the level of an antipsychotic drug in patients who are noncompliant with taking their medicines.	
urine test for drugs	Urine test to detect illegal drugs	
	Radiologic Procedures	
CT scan or MRI scan	Procedure used to document loss of brain tissue or structural abnormalities of the brain that might be related to a psychiatric disorder	
PET scan	Procedure that shows areas of abnormal metabolism in the brain related to dementia and Alzheimer's disease	
	Psychiatric Procedures and Tests	
Beck Depression Inventory (BDI)	Screening tool that is filled out by the patient to assess the degree of depression. Each item offers four answers that show progressively more depressed emotions: I do not feel sad (0 points), I feel sad (1 point), I am sad all the time (2 points), and I am so sad I can't stand it (3 points). The patient selects the statement that most closely matches his/her feelings.	
Holmes Social Readjustment Rating Scale	Test that rates and assigns point values to various **stressors** (negative and positive life events) to measure the amount of stress in a patient's life: death of spouse (100 points), divorce (73 points), death of family member (63 points), personal illness (53 points), marriage (50 points), retirement (45 points), pregnancy (40 points), change in finances (38 points), change in jobs (36 points), change in schools (25 points), vacation (13 points), and Christmas (12 points)	**stressor** (STRES-or) **stress/o-** *disturbing stimulus* **-or** *person who does; person who produces; thing that does; thing that produces*
intelligence testing	Intelligence tests are administered if the patient is suspected of having any degree of mental impairment or retardation	
psychiatric diagnosis	Diagnosis of any mental or psychiatric illnesses. It is stated in a specific way, as required by the American Psychiatric Association's publication *Diagnostic and Statistical Manual of Mental Disorders,* fifth edition (DSM-5).	**psychiatric** (SY-kee-AT-rik) **psych/o-** *mind* **iatr/o-** *medical treatment; physician* **-ic** *pertaining to*
psychiatric interview	Technique that provides insights into the patient's mental illness. It can be done in a psychiatrist's office or clinic or during admission to an acute care hospital or psychiatric hospital. The patient (or other person if the patient is unable to answer) is asked why he/she came for care, who brought him/her for care, what stressors are going on in his/her life, and about any previous psychiatric illness. The psychiatrist notes the patient's general appearance and behavior and listens to the patient's answers to analyze speech, content of thoughts, abstract reasoning, insight, and judgment.	
Rorschach test	Test that uses a set of cards with black-and-white abstract shapes on them. Patients are asked to describe what the shape of the inkblot represents to them. It is also known as the **inkblot test**.	**Rorschach** (ROR-shak)
Thematic Apperception Test (TAT)	Test that assesses personality, emotions, attitudes, motivation, and conflicts. The patient is shown 31 different pictures of social or interpersonal situations. The patient describes what is happening in the picture or what the theme of the picture is.	**apperception** (AP-er-SEP-shun) **appercept/o-** *fully perceived* **-ion** *action; condition*

Psychiatric Therapies

Word or Phrase	Description	Pronunciation/Word Parts

art therapy	Therapy that uses drawing or creating other types of art while talking with an art therapist. Art therapy relieves stress, allows patients to express their thoughts and emotions safely, and helps them gain insight into their problems. Art therapy helps small children express something they saw or something that was done to them that they cannot describe in words.	**therapy** (THAIR-ah-pee)
		
		therapeutic (THAIR-ah-PYOO-tik)
		  therapeut/o- *therapy; treatment*
		  -ic *pertaining to*

aversion therapy	Therapy in which the patient thinks about a desired, but destructive, behavior and this is coupled with a mild electrical shock or a bad smell (such as ammonia). This is a form of conditioning that creates an aversion to doing that behavior. This therapy is used to treat drug and cigarette addiction.	**aversion** (ah-VER-shun)
		  a- *away from; without*
		  vers/o- *travel; turn*
		  -ion *action; condition*

cognitive-behavioral therapy (CBT)	Therapy based on the premise that cognitive beliefs and attitudes (not people or events) cause undesirable or destructive emotions, and that thought patterns and behaviors are learned and can be unlearned. Patients are taught to use guided imagery and self-counseling to produce desirable emotions and behavior. This therapy is used to treat anxiety, panic attacks, phobias, depression, eating disorders, and other behaviors.	**cognitive** (KAWG-nih-tiv)
		  cognit/o- *thinking*
		  -ive *pertaining to*
		
		behavioral (bee-HAY-vyoor-al)
		  behav/o- *activity; manner of acting*
		  -ior *pertaining to*
		  -al *pertaining to*

detoxication	Therapy that includes observation and medical treatment for a patient with alcoholism undergoing withdrawal. Drugs are given, as needed, to minimize withdrawal symptoms and prevent seizures. This therapy is also known as **detoxification**.	**detoxication** (dee-TAWK-sih-KAY-shun)
		  de- *reversal of; without*
		  toxic/o- *poison; toxin*
		  -ation *being; having; process*

electroconvulsive therapy (ECT)	Therapy that uses an electrical current and electrodes on the head to produce seizures (convulsions). Patients are given sedative and muscle relaxant drugs to make them unconscious and relaxed. The seizure lasts about 1 minute and the patient awakens within 1 hour. It is used to treat severe depression and schizophrenia. ECT relieves symptoms more quickly than antidepressant drugs (that can take up to a month to become effective). It is also known as **electroshock therapy**.	**electroconvulsive** (ee-LEK-troh-con-VUL-siv)
		  electr/o- *electricity*
		  convuls/o- *seizure*
		  -ive *pertaining to*

family therapy	Therapy that involves the entire family, not just the patient. The focus is on relationships and conflicts between family members (what they say to each other, how they say it, and how they act toward each other). The family often labels one family member as the troublemaker, while others can do no wrong. Unless corrected, these fixed roles keep the family members from adopting more appropriate behaviors.	

Word or Phrase	Description	Pronunciation/Word Parts
group therapy	Therapy that provides simultaneous therapy to several patients who have a similar mental illness (such as anxiety, depression, or being a victim of sexual abuse) (see Figure 17-10 ■). Group members share experiences and insights and provide feedback and emotional support to each other. **FIGURE 17-10 ■ Group therapy.** This psychologist is conducting a group psychotherapy session. Group members support or challenge each other while gaining insight into their own problems. *Source*: Photographee.eu/Shutterstock	

hypnosis	Therapy that places the patient in a sleeplike trance (the patient is still able to remember who they are and what is happening). The therapist makes suggestions that are incorporated in the patient's subconscious mind and later acted upon consciously to some degree. It is used to treat anxiety and phobias and to help patients stop smoking or lose weight. It is also known as **hypnotherapy**.	**hypnosis** (hip-NOH-sis)
		   hypn/o- *sleep*
		   -osis *condition; process*
		
		hypnotherapy
		(HIP-noh-THAIR-ah-pee)
		   hypn/o- *sleep*
		   -therapy *treatment*

play therapy	Therapy that uses toys and other objects (often dolls) to help young children express emotions and reenact traumatic or abusive events (on a small scale they can control). It is used to treat social withdrawal, anxiety, depression, aggression, and ADHD.	

psychoanalysis	Therapy based on the idea of a conscious and subconscious mind. It was developed by Sigmund Freud to analyze a patient's thoughts and behavior by using interpretation of dreams and hypnosis.	**psychoanalysis**
		(SY-koh-ah-NAL-ih-sis)
		   psych/o- *mind*
		   analy/o- *separate*
		   -sis *condition; process*

psychotherapy	Any therapy (except drug therapy and electroconvulsive therapy) that uses verbal or nonverbal communication between a patient or a group of patients and a psychologist or psychiatrist to treat a mental disorder	**psychotherapy**
		(SY-koh-THAIR-ah-pee)
		   psych/o- *mind*
		   -therapy *treatment*

systematic desensitization	Therapy technique in which a patient imagines 10 different scenarios involving a specific phobia (e.g., fear of spiders). Each scenario is associated with progressively greater anxiety. The patient practices relaxation techniques before and after visualizing the first scenario. When the first scenario no longer causes anxiety, the patient moves on to the second, and so forth, until that phobia no longer causes anxiety.	**desensitization**
		(dee-SEN-sih-tih-ZAY-shun)
		   de- *reversal of; without*
		   sensit/o- *affected by; sensitive to*
		   -ization *process of creating; process of inserting; process of making*

therapeutic milieu	Stable, structured, and safe emotional and physical environment that provides ongoing therapy of various types for a psychiatric patient	**milieu** (meel-YOO)

Drugs

These drug categories and drugs are used to treat psychiatric disorders. The most common generic and trade name drugs in each category are listed.

Category	Indication	Examples	Pronunciation/Word Parts
antianxiety drugs	Treat anxiety and neurosis. They are also known as **anxiolytic drugs** and **minor tranquilizers**.	alprazolam (Xanax), diazepam (Valium)	**antianxiety** (AN-tee-ang-ZY-eh-tee) **anti-** *against* **anxi/o-** *fear; worry* **-ety** *condition; state* **anxiolytic** (ANG-zee-oh-LIT-ik) **anxi/o-** *fear; worry* **lyt/o-** *break down; destroy* **-ic** *pertaining to* **tranquilizer** (TRANG-kwih-LY-zer) **tranquil/o-** *calm* **-izer** *thing that affects in a particular way*

> **DID YOU KNOW?**
> *Valium* comes from the Latin word *valere,* which means *to be healthy.* The plant valerian has been known since the time of Hippocrates to calm the nerves.

Category	Indication	Examples	Pronunciation/Word Parts
antidepressant drugs	Treat depression by prolonging the action of norepinephrine or serotonin. Categories include tricyclic, tetracyclic, monoamine oxidase inhibitors (MAOIs), selective serotonin reuptake inhibitors (SSRIs), and serotonin and norepinephrine reuptake inhibitors (SNRIs).	bupropion (Wellbutrin), doxepin (Sinequan), duloxetine (Cymbalta), fluoxetine (Prozac), paroxetine (Paxil), sertraline (Zoloft)	**antidepressant** (AN-tee-dee-PREH-sant) **anti-** *against* **depress/o-** *press down* **-ant** *pertaining to*
antipsychotic drugs	Treat psychosis, paranoia, and schizophrenia by blocking dopamine receptors in the limbic system. They are also known as **major tranquilizers**.	aripiprazole (Abilify), haloperidol (Haldol), risperidone (Risperdal)	**antipsychotic** (AN-tee-sy-KAW-tik) **anti-** *against* **psych/o-** *mind* **-tic** *pertaining to*

> **CLINICAL CONNECTIONS**
>
> **Pharmacology.** Many schizophrenic patients do not continue to take their prescribed antipsychotic drug because of **tardive dyskinesia**, a severe side effect that develops later in the treatment. It causes involuntary, repetitive movements of the face (grimacing, lip smacking, chewing, eye blinking, sticking out the tongue) and movements of the arms and legs (rocking back and forth, marching in place).
>
> **tardive** (TAR-dive) **tard/o-** *late; slow* **-ive** *pertaining to*
>
> **dyskinesia** (DIS-kih-NEE-zha) **dys-** *abnormal; difficult; painful* **kines/o-** *movement* **-ia** *condition; state; thing*

Category	Indication	Examples	Pronunciation/Word Parts
drugs for alcoholism	Inhibit an enzyme that metabolizes the breakdown products of alcohol. Patients on this drug who drink alcohol experience headache, dizziness, nausea, and even heart arrhythmias. This unpleasant reaction is a deterrent to drinking alcohol.	disulfiram (Antabuse)	

Category	Indication	Examples	Pronunciation/Word Parts
drugs for bipolar disorder	Lessen the severity of mood swings between the two emotional poles of mania and depression. These include antipsychotic drugs and anticonvulsant drugs.	lamotrigine (Lamictal), levetiracetam (Keppra), lithium (Lithobid)	
drugs for premenstrual dysphoric disorder (PMDD)	Treat the depression and anxiety associated with this psychiatric mood disorder	fluoxetine (Sarafem), paroxetine (Paxil), sertraline (Zoloft)	

Abbreviations

ADD	attention-deficit disorder	**OCD**	obsessive–compulsive disorder
ADHD	attention-deficit hyperactivity disorder	**OD**	overdose
ASD	autism spectrum disorder	**PCP**	phencyclidine ("angel dust," a street drug)
BDI	Beck Depression Inventory	**PMDD**	premenstrual dysphoric disorder
CBT	cognitive-behavioral therapy	**Psy**	psychiatry; psychology
CNS	central nervous system	**Psych**	psychiatry; psychology (pronounced "sike")
DT	delirium tremens	**PTSD**	posttraumatic stress disorder
ECT	electroconvulsive therapy	**SAD**	seasonal affective disorder
ETOH	ethanol (liquor); ethyl alcohol	**SSRI**	selective serotonin reuptake inhibitor (drug)
LSD	lysergic acid diethylamide	**TAT**	Thematic Apperception Test
MAO	monoamine oxidase		

WORD ALERT
Abbreviations

Abbreviations are commonly used in all types of medical documents; however, they can mean different things to different people and their meanings can be misinterpreted. Always verify the meaning of an abbreviation.

ASD means *autism spectrum disorder*, but it also means *atrial septal defect*.

OD means *overdose*, but *O.D.* means *right eye* or *Doctor of Optometry*.

PCP means *phencyclidine*, but it also means *primary care physician*.

IT'S GREEK TO ME!

Did you notice that some words have two different combining forms? Combining forms from both Greek and Latin remain a part of medical language today.

Word	Greek	Latin	Medical Word Examples
mind	phren/o-	ment/o-	schizophrenia, mental, dementia
	psych/o-		psychotherapy
self	aut/o-	su/i-	autism, suicide

CAREER FOCUS

Meet Patricia, a social worker

"There are all kinds of jobs you can do when you're a social worker. You can work in nursing homes. You can work in rehab centers. You can work on your own and do private counseling with people who've just gotten a terminal diagnosis. You can work with children. You can work in schools. One of the reasons why I love it is because you never know what you're going to be doing in a day. I'm assigned to a pulmonologist. Each day we go over his case list, and we prioritize who needs to be seen first, who needs home care, who needs nursing home placement, who needs help with prescriptions, who needs somebody to just go in and talk to them. I see my role as helping patients who are in an unfamiliar environment. It's not the best time of their lives. I use medical terminology all day long, especially when calling in the clinical information to the insurance companies."

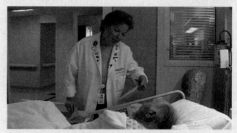

Source: Dan Frank/Ph College/Pearson Education

Social workers are allied health professionals who obtain medical, housing, financial, or other community services and support for patients or clients. Social workers work in the department of human services in government offices, clinics, nursing homes, hospitals, and in psychiatric hospitals.

    Psychologists are mental health practitioners who have a doctoral degree (Ph.D.) in **psychology**. They work in psychiatric hospitals, outpatient clinics, and school systems. They administer psychological and intelligence tests and act as therapists for various types of counseling and psychotherapy sessions (family, group, marriage). They are not physicians and cannot prescribe drug therapy.

    Psychiatrists are physicians who practice in the mental health specialty of psychiatry. They diagnose and treat patients with mental illness. Physicians can take additional training and become board certified in the subspecialties of child and adolescent psychiatry, geriatric psychiatry, psychosomatic medicine, addiction psychiatry, or forensic psychiatry.

social (SOH-shal)
   soci/o- *community; human beings*
   -al *pertaining to*

---

psychologist (sy-KAW-loh-jist)
   psych/o- *mind*
   log/o- *study of; word*
   -ist *person who specializes in; thing that specializes in*

---

psychology (sy-KAW-loh-jee)
   psych/o- *mind*
   -logy *study of*

---

psychiatrist (sy-KY-ah-trist)
   psych/o- *mind*
   iatr/o- *medical treatment; physician*
   -ist *person who specializes in; thing that specializes in*

MyMedicalTerminologyLab™   To see Patricia's complete video profile, log into MyMedicalTerminologyLab and navigate to the Multimedia Library for Chapter 17. Check the Video box, and then click the Career Focus - Social Worker link.

17.9 Analyze Medical Reports

ELECTRONIC PATIENT RECORD

This is a Consultation Report from a psychiatrist to the patient's primary care physician. Read the report and answer the questions.

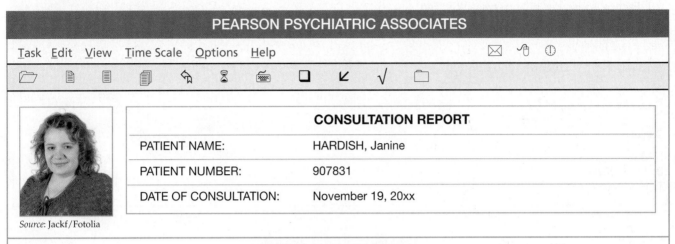

PEARSON PSYCHIATRIC ASSOCIATES

Task   Edit   View   Time Scale   Options   Help

CONSULTATION REPORT

PATIENT NAME:	HARDISH, Janine
PATIENT NUMBER:	907831
DATE OF CONSULTATION:	November 19, 20xx

Source: Jackf/Fotolia

DANIEL P. BENTLEY, M.D.
Pearson Psychiatric Associates
North Ridge Professional Building, Suite 702
Spring Garden, PA 17103
(717)-643-xxxx

Joseph Gildron, M.D., and Associates, Inc.

Centennial Medical Building, Suite 201
2859 Bonnie Brae Road
Ebensberg, PA 15890

Re: HARDISH, Janine

Dear Dr. Gildron:

Thank you for referring your patient, Mrs. Janine Hardish, to me for psychiatric evaluation.

The patient is a 39-year-old, divorced Caucasian female. She lives in a single-family dwelling with her two children. In the past, she has worked part time as a nurses' aide, but is not currently working because of feeling weak, dizzy, and tired. She states that she also feels depressed and hopeless. She claims that she has crying episodes every other day and difficulty sleeping at night.

She presents as a well-groomed lady whose clothes are neat, clean, and in good condition. Her hair is combed and her nails are clean and well manicured. Her affect is moderately bright, and she is alert and oriented to time, person, and place. She is able to answer questions easily, logically, and with a moderate amount of detail. Her thought content is well organized without evidence of flight of ideas or loose associations. Her fund of knowledge appears to be adequate. She is able to count backward from 100 and to do serial 7s. Her memory for recent and remote events is intact. She was able to name the last five presidents. She is able to think of 18 words that begin with the letter "f" in 45 seconds (an above-normal result). However, she states that she feels that her memory is impaired.

She denies delusions or hallucinations. She denies feelings of being persecuted or plotted against. She denies suicidal or homicidal ideation.

She has little contact with her ex-husband, even though they were just divorced. She is experiencing some difficulty with her finances at this time; her husband does send child support payments, but she is not currently working. Her oldest son is experiencing difficulties in his schoolwork and recently was pulled over by the police and given a ticket for speeding.

She has been taking Cymbalta 20 mg P.O. at bedtime, as prescribed by you; however, she has also obtained a prescription for a tricyclic antidepressant drug from another physician and is taking this as well as Ambien for sleep.

It is my opinion that this patient is able to care for her own personal needs, is mentally intact, and has little difficulty relating to others.

DIAGNOSIS

1. Normal mental status and psychiatric evaluation. A complete physical and neurologic examination was not performed. No known documented physical illness.
2. Moderate degree of psychosocial stressors.
3. Factitious disorder, not otherwise specified.

Thank you for your referral of this patient.

Sincerely,

Daniel P. Bentley, M.D.

Daniel P. Bentley, M.D.

DPB:jbt
D: 11/19/20xx
T: 11/19/20xx

---

1. Divide *psychosocial* into its three word parts and give the meaning of each word part.

   Word Part   **Meaning**

   _____   _____

   _____   _____

   _____   _____

2. Divide *factitious* into its two word parts and give the meaning of each word part.

   Word Part   **Meaning**

   _____   _____

   _____   _____

3. Divide *homicidal* into its three word parts and give the meaning of each word part.

   Word Part   **Meaning**

   _____   _____

   _____   _____

   _____   _____

4. A patient who has entertained ideas of suicide is said to be _____ (adjective).

5. Define *factitious disorder.* _____

6. Name three psychosocial stressors that the patient is currently experiencing.

   a. _____

   b. _____

   c. _____

7. What evidence of drug-seeking behavior is mentioned in this report? _____

8. Flight of ideas is associated with which of these disorders?   **bipolar disorder   impulse control disorder   suicide**

9. How are delusions different from hallucinations? _____

10. Feelings of being persecuted or plotted against can be labeled as what mental illness? _____

MyMedicalTerminologyLab™

MyMedicalTerminologyLab is a premium online homework management system that includes a host of features to help you study. Registered users will find:

- A multitude of quizzes and activities built within the MyLab platform

- Powerful tools that track and analyze your results—allowing you to create a personalized learning experience

- Videos and audio pronunciations to help enrich your progress

- Streaming lesson presentations (Guided Lectures) and self-paced learning modules

- A space where you and your instructor can check your progress and manage your assignments

Chapter 18
Oncology

Oncology (ong-KAW-loh-jee) is the medical specialty that studies the anatomy and physiology of a cancer cell and uses laboratory and diagnostic procedures, medical and surgical procedures, and drugs to treat cancerous diseases.

 ## Learning Outcomes

After you study this chapter, you should be able to

18.1 Identify structures of a cell.

18.2 Describe how a normal cell divides and how a normal cell becomes a cancerous cell.

18.3 List eight characteristics of cancerous cells and tumors.

18.4 Describe common types of cancer, laboratory and diagnostic procedures, medical and surgical procedures, radiation therapy, and drugs.

18.5 Give the meanings of word parts and abbreviations related to oncology.

18.6 Divide oncology words and build oncology words.

18.7 Spell and pronounce oncology words.

18.8 Analyze the medical content and meaning of oncology reports.

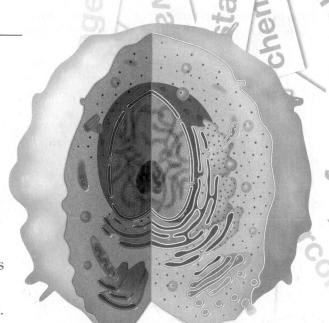

FIGURE 18-1 ■ A cell.
Each cell is a marvel of engineering, but a change in its structure or function can result in cancer.
Source: Pearson Education

Medical Language Key

To unlock the definition of a medical word, break it into word parts. Give the meaning of each word part. Put the meanings of the word parts in order, beginning with the meaning of the suffix, then the prefix (if present), then the combining form(s).

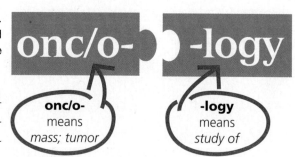

	Word Part	Word Part Meaning
Suffix	-logy	*study of*
Combining Form	onc/o-	*mass; tumor*

Oncology ▶ *Study of (a cancerous) mass or tumor.*

Anatomy and Physiology

Unlike other medical specialties, oncology is not based on a particular body system. Oncology encompasses all body systems because cancer can occur anywhere in the body. **Cancer** arises from various types of cells and tissues that often lend their names to the cancer.

Cancer begins as a single normal cell (see Figure 18-1 ■) that becomes an abnormal cell, and so we will begin our study of oncology by studying the structure and function of a normal cell.

Anatomy Related to Oncology

A **cell** is the smallest independently functioning structure in the body that can reproduce itself by division. All cells contain certain basic structures (see Figure 18-2 ■). The **cell membrane** around the cell is a permeable barrier that protects and supports the **intracellular contents**. It allows water and nutrients to enter the cell and cellular waste products to leave the cell. It also contains ion pumps that actively bring electrolytes (sodium, potassium, and so forth) in and out of the cell.

The **cytoplasm** is a gel-like substance that fills the cell. The cytoplasm contains dissolved substances as well as structures known as **organelles**.

- **Endoplasmic reticulum**. Network of channels throughout the cytoplasm that transports materials. It is also the site of protein, fat, and glycogen production.
- **Golgi apparatus**. Curved, stacked membranes that process and store proteins (such as hormones or enzymes) until they are released by the cell. It also makes lysosomes.
- **Lysosomes**. Small sacs that contain powerful digestive enzymes to destroy a bacterium or virus that invades the cell. When a cell dies, the lysosomes release their enzymes into the cytoplasm, and the cell is slowly dissolved.
- **Messenger RNA**. Messenger RNA (**ribonucleic acid**) duplicates the information contained in a gene and carries it to the ribosome where it is used to assemble amino acids to make a protein molecule.

Pronunciation/Word Parts

cancer (KAN-ser)

cancerous (KAN-ser-us)
   cancer/o- *cancer*
   -ous *pertaining to*
The combining form **carcin/o-** also means *cancer*.

cell (SEL)

cellular (SEL-yoo-lar)
   cellul/o- *cell*
   -ar *pertaining to*
The combining form **cyt/o-** also means *cell*.

intracellular (IN-trah-SEL-yoo-lar)
   intra- *within*
   cellul/o- *cell*
   -ar *pertaining to*

cytoplasm (SY-toh-plazm)
   cyt/o- *cell*
   -plasm *formed substance; growth*

organelle (OR-gah-NEL)
   organ/o- *organ*
   -elle *small thing*

endoplasmic (EN-doh-PLAS-mik)
   endo- *innermost; within*
   plasm/o- *plasma*
   -ic *pertaining to*

reticulum (reh-TIH-kyoo-lum)

Golgi (GOL-jee)

lysosome (LY-soh-sohm)
   lys/o- *break down; destroy*
   -some *body*
Add words to make a complete definition of *lysosome*: *body (that contains enzymes that) break down or destroy.*

ribonucleic acid
(RY-boh-noo-KLEE-ik AS-id)

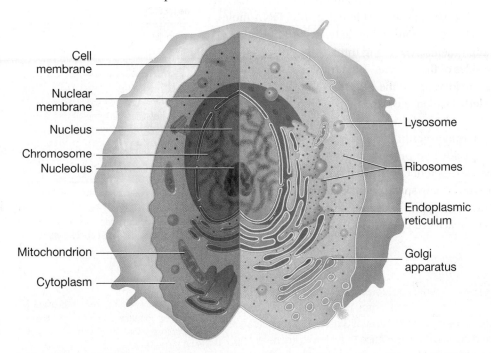

Cell membrane
Nuclear membrane
Nucleus
Chromosome
Nucleolus
Mitochondrion
Cytoplasm

Lysosome
Ribosomes
Endoplasmic reticulum
Golgi apparatus

FIGURE 18-2 ■ Structures of a cell.
A cell consists of many different structures, each of which plays a unique role in securing nutrients, producing energy, building proteins, and fighting invading pathogens. All of these functions are essential to the continuing health of the body.
Source: Pearson Education

- **Mitochondria**. Capsule-shaped structures with sectioned chambers that produce and store ATP, a high-energy molecule obtained from the metabolism of glucose. As needed, the mitochondria convert ATP to ADP to release energy for cellular activities.

- **Ribosomes**. Granular structures in the cytoplasm and on the endoplasmic reticulum. Ribosomes contain RNA and proteins and are the site where proteins are produced.

The **nucleus** is a large, round, centralized structure that is surrounded by a nuclear membrane. Through the action of DNA, it controls all of the activities that take place within the cell. The **nucleolus** is a round, central region within the nucleus. It produces RNA and ribosomes. **Chromosomes** are paired structures within the nucleus. Each cell nucleus contains 23 pairs of chromosomes for a total of 46 chromosomes. In each of the 23 pairs, one of the chromosomes was inherited from the mother and the other from the father. A single chromosome is made of one long DNA (**deoxyribonucleic acid**) molecule. A DNA molecule consists of repeating pairs of amino acids sequenced along two strands that form a double helix. A **gene** is one segment of a DNA molecule that contains enough amino acid pairs to provide the information to produce one protein molecule. In a cell that is not dividing, each long DNA molecule is loosely coiled, giving the nucleus a woven, grainy appearance under the microscope. As the cell prepares to divide, each DNA molecule coils tightly, making the chromosomes visible as rod-like structures in the nucleus.

> **DID YOU KNOW?**
> Most body cells contain one nucleus. However, a mature erythrocyte (red blood cell) does not contain any nucleus, and a skeletal muscle cell contains many nuclei.

Physiology of Cellular Division and Cancer

Mitosis is the process by which a cell divides. Mitosis begins in the cell's nucleus as each chromosome makes an exact copy of itself. (The double helix of its DNA molecule splits down its length and rebuilds to form another double helix.) All of the chromosomes and their identical copies align themselves along thread-like strands in the nucleus and then separate to opposite sides of the nucleus. Then the entire nucleus and cytoplasm split, forming two cells that are identical to the original cell.

Normal body cells divide in an orderly fashion and in response to a particular need. During childhood, growth hormone causes the body cells to divide rapidly as the child grows. During times of blood loss, the hormone erythropoietin from the kidneys stimulates stem cells in the bone marrow to divide and produce more mature erythrocytes (red blood cells). The rate of cell division is different for different types of cells. Skin cells have a high rate because they are constantly being shed from the surface of the body. In contrast, muscle cells divide less frequently. **Suppressor genes**, a group of genes in the DNA of each cell, inhibit mitosis and keep each cell from dividing excessively.

A CLOSER LOOK

The p53 gene is the most important suppressor gene. It is located on chromosome 17 in every cell. It is inactive until DNA in the cell's nucleus is damaged. Then, the p53 gene activates proteins to repair the DNA. While the DNA is being repaired, the p53 gene inhibits mitosis to decrease the chance of producing more defective cells. Because of their role in preventing the formation of cancer cells, suppressor genes are also known as *tumor suppressor genes*. If the damaged DNA cannot be repaired, the p53 gene directs the cell to shut down. This is **apoptosis** or programmed cell death.

Pronunciation/Word Parts

mitochondrion (MY-toh-CON-dree-on)

mitochondria (MY-toh-CON-dree-ah)
Mitochondrion is a Greek singular noun. Form the plural by changing *-on* to *-a*.

ribosome (RY-boh-sohm)
  rib/o- *ribonucleic acid*
  -some *body*

nucleus (NOO-klee-us)

nuclei (NOO-klee-eye)
Nucleus is a Latin singular noun. Form the plural by changing *-us* to *-i*. The combining form **kary/o-** means *nucleus of a cell*.

nuclear (NOO-klee-ar)
  nucle/o- *nucleus of an atom; nucleus of a cell*
  -ar *pertaining to*

nucleolus (noo-KLEE-oh-lus)

nucleoli (noo-KLEE-oh-lie)
Nucleolus is a Latin singular noun. Form the plural by changing *-us* to *-i*.

chromosome (KROH-moh-sohm)
  chrom/o- *color*
  -some *body*
Add words to make a complete definition of *chromosome*: (microscopic) body (that takes on) color (when stained).

deoxyribonucleic acid (dee-AWK-see-RY-boh-noo-KLEE-ik AS-id)

gene (JEEN)

genetic (jeh-NET-ik)
  gene/o- *gene*
  -tic *pertaining to*

mitosis (my-TOH-sis)
  mit/o- *thread-like strand*
  -osis *condition; process*
Add words to make a complete definition of *mitosis*: process (of cell division during which the chromosomes align along) thread-like strands (in the nucleus).

suppressor (soo-PRES-or)
  suppress/o- *press down*
  -or *person who does; person who produces; thing that does; thing that produces*

apoptosis (AP-awp-TOH-sis)
  apo- *away from*
  -ptosis *state of drooping; state of falling*
Add words to make a complete definition of *apoptosis*: state of falling away (of a cell) from (life to death).
The ending *-ptosis* contains a variation of the combining form *ptot/o-* (drooping; falling) and the suffix *-sis* (condition; process).

Types of damage to the DNA molecule of a chromosome include **genetic mutations** that delete genes, reverse their normal order, or break off segments of genes and insert those segments into other chromosomes (a process known as **translocation**).

Causes of DNA damage include carcinogens, pathogens, or heredity. These cause chronic tissue inflammation but do not immediately cause cancer. It is only after repeated exposure that the cellular DNA is damaged beyond repair.

Factors that Contribute to the Development of Cancer (see Figure 18-3 ■)

1. **Carcinogens** (environmental substances)

   radiation (sunlight, x-rays, radiation therapy, nuclear weapons)

   chemicals (insecticides, dyes)

   fumes (industrial pollution, radon gas from the soil, cigarette tar and smoke, automobile exhaust)

   foreign particles that cause chronic irritation (asbestos)

   some chemotherapy drugs

   some hormone drugs

2. **Pathogens** (bacteria and viruses)

   Chronic irritation and inflammation from a bacterial or viral infection can eventually damage DNA. Examples: The human papillomavirus causes genital warts and chronic inflammation that can lead to cervical cancer in women. Human

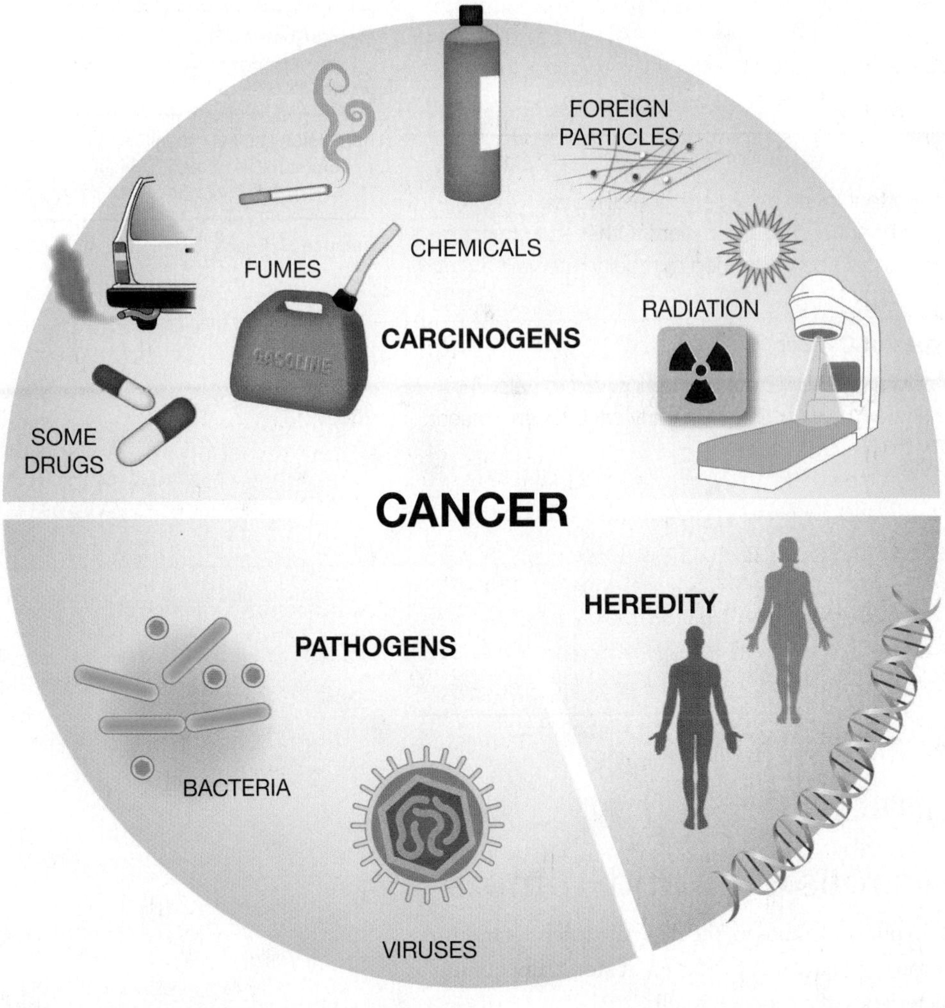

Pronunciation/Word Parts

mutation (myoo-TAY-shun)
   mutat/o- *change*
   -ion *action; condition*

translocation (TRANS-loh-KAY-shun)
   trans- *across; through*
   locat/o- *place*
   -ion *action; condition*

carcinogen (kar-SIN-oh-jen)
   carcin/o- *cancer*
   -gen *that which produces*

pathogen (PATH-oh-jen)
   path/o- *disease*
   -gen *that which produces*

FIGURE 18-3 ■ Causes of cancer.
Cancer is caused by carcinogens in the environment, heredity, pathogens (bacteria and viruses), and oncogenes (genes within a virus).
Source: Pearson Education

immunodeficiency virus (HIV) weakens the immune response until the body is unable to destroy newly formed cancerous cells. **Oncogenes** are mutated genes in the RNA of a virus. When the virus enters and infects a normal cell, its oncogene joins with the normal cell's DNA, changing it into a cancerous cell.

3. **Heredity**. Some persons inherit damaged DNA or an oncogene from one of their parents.

If the DNA in a chromosome is damaged, and the damaged area includes the p53 gene, then the cell loses its ability to repair itself. The damage remains, and the damaged cell cannot stop itself from dividing and producing more damaged cells. More than half of cancer cells have damage to the p53 gene.

A **neoplasm** is any new, growing tissue that is not part of the normal body structure. **Neoplasia** is the process by which a neoplasm develops. Neoplasms are also known as **tumors**. Neoplasms are either **malignant** (cancerous) or **benign** (not cancerous). Malignant neoplasms are known as **cancer**. The area where the cancerous cell first grew into a cancerous tumor is known as the **primary site**. When the tumor is still contained in that area it is said to be *in situ*. When the tumor spreads or a cancerous cell breaks away and metastasizes via the blood or lymphatic system to a distant part of the body, that is the **secondary site**. There is always just one primary site, but there may be several secondary sites. A **remission** is the period of time during which there are no symptoms or signs of cancer. A remission occurs after the successful treatment of cancer. A **relapse** is a return of the symptoms or signs of cancer after a period of improvement or even remission.

Pronunciation/Word Parts

oncogene (ONG-koh-jeen)
  onc/o- *mass; tumor*
  -gene *gene*

heredity (heh-RED-ih-tee)
  hered/o- *genetic inheritance*
  -ity *condition; state*

hereditary (heh-RED-ih-TAIR-ee)
  heredit/o- *genetic inheritance*
  -ary *pertaining to*

neoplasm (NEE-oh-plazm)
  ne/o- *new*
  -plasm *formed substance; growth*

neoplasia (NEE-oh-PLAY-zha)
  ne/o- *new*
  plas/o- *formation; growth*
  -ia *condition; state; thing*

tumor (TOO-mer)

malignant (mah-LIG-nant)
  malign/o- *cancer; intentionally causing harm*
  -ant *pertaining to*

benign (bee-NINE)

in situ (IN SY-too)

remission (ree-MIH-shun)
  remiss/o- *send back*
  -ion *action; condition*

relapse (REE-laps)

DID YOU KNOW?

Screening examinations are extremely important in the early detection of cancer. Self-examination of the breasts or testes is performed by the patient. Other examinations, such as mammography and colonoscopy, should be performed at regular intervals by healthcare professionals.

Warning Signs of Some Common Types of Cancer

The American Cancer Society uses the acronym CAUTION as a memory aid to help healthcare professionals and others remember the ways in which early cancer can present.

C   Change in bowel or bladder habits
A   A sore that does not heal
U   Unusual bleeding or discharge
T   Thickening or lump
I   Indigestion or trouble swallowing
O   Obvious changes in a wart or mole
N   Nagging cough or hoarseness

Characteristics of Cancerous Cells and Tumors

1. Cancerous cells are not part of, and do not contribute to, the normal structure and function of the body. Once a single cancerous cell has been produced, it stops functioning as a normal cell and takes on the characteristics of a cancerous cell.

2. Cancerous cells lack differentiation and cannot perform the specialized functions of normal cells.

3. Cancerous cells are not arranged in an orderly fashion (stacked on top of each other or all oriented in the same direction) like normal cells.

4. Cancerous cells often divide more rapidly than normal cells. Cancerous tumors often grow more quickly than normal tissue.

5. Cancerous cells can form a solid tumor. Cancerous tumors are irregular in shape and are not **encapsulated**. (Benign tumors do have a capsule.)

6. A cancerous tumor releases a substance that causes blood vessels in the surrounding tissues to grow into the tumor and provide it with nutrients. This is known as **angiogenesis**. The tumor grows rapidly but often has a central core of necrosis because the blood supply is inadequate.

7. Cancerous tumors are **invasive**. They penetrate (infiltrate) the normal tissues around them, interfere with tissue functions, and destroy normal cells (see Figure 18-4 ■).

8. Cancerous cells break off from a solid tumor and move through the blood vessels and lymphatic vessels to other sites in the body. This process is known as **metastasis**. The cancerous cells **metastasize** and are characterized as being **metastatic** (see Figure 18-5 ■).

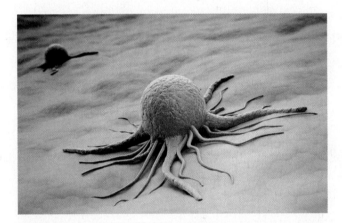

FIGURE 18-4 ■ Cancer cell.
A cancer cell has many projections of cytoplasm coming from it. These infiltrate into the surrounding tissues.
Source: Mopic/Fotolia

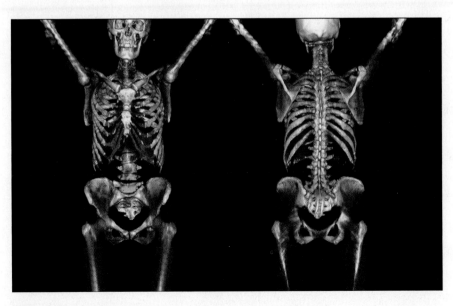

FIGURE 18-5 ■ Metastases.
This colorized bone scan shows green areas in the rib cage and spine that represent metastases from a breast carcinoma.
Source: Callista Images/Cultura/Corbis

Pronunciation/Word Parts

encapsulated (en-KAP-soo-LAY-ted)
  en- *in; inward; within*
  capsul/o- *capsule; enveloping structure*
  -ated *composed of; pertaining to a condition*

angiogenesis (AN-jee-oh-JEN-eh-sis)
  angi/o- *blood vessel; lymphatic vessel*
  gen/o- *arising from; produced by*
  -esis *condition; process*

invasive (in-VAY-siv)
  invas/o- *go into*
  -ive *pertaining to*

metastasis (meh-TAS-tah-sis)
  meta- *after; change; subsequent to; transition*
  -stasis *standing still; staying in one place*
The ending *-stasis* contains the combining form *stas/o-* and the suffix *-sis*.
Add words to make a complete definition of *metastasis: (a cell that is normally) staying in one place (but undergoes) change (and moves to another part of the body).*

metastases (meh-TAS-tah-seez)

metastasize (meh-TAS-tah-size)
  meta- *after; change; subsequent to; transition*
  stas/o- *standing still; staying in one place*
  -ize *affecting in a particular way*

metastatic (MET-ah-STAT-ik)
  meta- *after; change; subsequent to; transition*
  stat/o- *standing still; staying in one place*
  -ic *pertaining to*

The growth of cancerous cells and tumors cannot be easily controlled by the body. The body's defenses against cancerous cells and tumors include (1) the cell's p53 gene; (2) special lymphocytes known as *NK cells* (natural killer cells) that detect, engulf, and destroy cancerous cells; (3) lymph nodes that filter cancerous cells out of the lymph fluid; macrophages that engulf and destroy cancerous cells in the lymph nodes and tissues; and (4) **tumor necrosis factor** (TNF) released from lymph nodes that causes a cancerous tumor to become necrotic and die. However, the body's defenses are often overwhelmed by the cancer. Cancerous cells and tumors that are not destroyed by any of these means go on to multiply and metastasize.

Pronunciation/Word Parts

tumor (TOO-mor)

necrosis (neh-KROH-sis)
  necr/o- *dead body; dead cells; dead tissue*
  -osis *condition; process*

A CLOSER LOOK

A human being begins as a single cell that immediately begins to divide. By the end of the first week of life, those cells begin to differentiate, migrating to various parts of the body and producing specific tissues (such as muscle or bone) with different shapes and functions. This process is known as cellular **differentiation**. Cancer cells arise from a particular type of tissue, but then lose this differentiation and revert back to an immature, embryonal, **undifferentiated** state.

differentiation (DIF-er-EN-shee-AA-shun)
  differentiat/o- *distinct; specialized*
  -ion *action; condition*

undifferentiated
(un-DIF-er-EN-shee-AA-ted)
  un- *not*
  differentiat/o- *distinct; specialized*
  -ed *pertaining to*

DID YOU KNOW?

In his 1974 text *An Introduction to Drugs,* Michael C. Gerald wrote: "Cancerous cells are the anarchists of the body, for they know no law, pay no regard for the commonwealth, serve no useful function, and cause disharmony and death in their surrounds."

Vocabulary Review

Word or Phrase	Description	Combining Forms
angiogenesis	Process by which a cancerous tumor causes blood vessels in the surrounding tissues to grow into the tumor and provide it with nutrients	**angi/o-** *blood vessel; lymphatic vessel* **gen/o-** *arising from; produced by*
apoptosis	Programmed cell death in which the p53 gene directs the cell to shut down when its DNA is too damaged to be repaired	
cancer	Single abnormal cell that develops into a mass or tumor and is not encapsulated. Most grow rapidly and are invasive, growing into normal tissues around them.	**cancer/o-** *cancer* **carcin/o-** *cancer*
carcinogen	Environmental substance that can contribute to the development of cancer	**carcin/o-** *cancer*
cell	Smallest, independently functioning structure in the body that can reproduce itself by division	**cellul/o-** *cell* **cyt/o-** *cell*
cell membrane	Permeable barrier that surrounds a cell and holds in the cytoplasm. It allows water and nutrients to enter and waste products to leave the cell.	
chromosome	Paired, rodlike structures within the nucleus. Each cell contains 46 chromosomes (23 pairs).	**chrom/o-** *color*
cytoplasm	Gel-like intracellular substance. Organelles are embedded in it.	**cyt/o-** *cell*
differentiation	Process by which embryonic cells assume different shapes and functions in different parts of the body	**differentiat/o-** *distinct; specialized*
DNA	**Deoxyribonucleic acid.** Sequenced pairs of amino acids that form a double helix chain within a chromosome. One segment of DNA makes up a gene.	
encapsulated	Having a capsule or enveloping structure around it. Benign tumors have a capsule; cancerous tumors do not.	**capsul/o-** *capsule; enveloping structure*
endoplasmic reticulum	Organelle that is a network of channels that transport materials within the cell. It is also the site of protein, fat, and glycogen production.	**plasm/o-** *plasma*
gene	An area on a chromosome that contains all the DNA information needed to produce one type of protein molecule	**gene/o-** *gene*
genetic mutation	Damage to the DNA molecule that deletes genes, reverses the normal order of genes, or breaks off gene segments from one chromosome and inserts them in a place on another chromosome (**translocation**)	**gene/o-** *gene* **mutat/o-** *change* **locat/o-** *place*
Golgi apparatus	Organelle that consists of curved, stacked membranes that process and store hormones and enzymes. It also makes lysosomes.	
heredity	Genetic inheritance passed on from the DNA of the father and mother to the child. Genetic mutations that cause cancer can be inherited.	**hered/o-** *genetic inheritance*
in situ	The cancer is still contained to the area where it first appeared	
intracellular	Within a cell	**cellul/o-** *cell*
invasive	Characteristic of cancerous tumors. They penetrate and destroy the normal cells around them, compromising tissue function.	**invas/o-** *go into*
lysosome	Organelle that consists of a small sac with digestive enzymes in it. It destroys pathogens that invade the cell.	**lys/o-** *break down; destroy*

Word or Phrase	Description	Combining Forms
metastasis	Process by which cancerous cells break off from a tumor and move (**metastasize**) through the blood vessels or lymphatic vessels to other sites in the body. They are **metastatic**.	**stas/o-** *standing still; staying in one place* **stat/o-** *standing still; staying in one place*
mitochondria	Organelles that are capsule shaped and produce and store ATP and then convert it to ADP to release energy for cellular activities	
mitosis	Process of cellular division. The chromosomes duplicate, align along thread-like strands, and then migrate to either end of the nucleus as the cell divides.	**mit/o-** *thread-like strand*
neoplasm	Any new growing tissue that is not part of the normal body structure. **Neoplasia** is the process by which it develops. A neoplasm is a **tumor** that can be **malignant (cancer)** or **benign**.	**ne/o-** *new* **plas/o-** *formation; growth* **malign/o-** *cancer; intentionally causing harm* **cancer/o-** *cancer*
nucleolus	Round, central region within the nucleus. It makes RNA and ribosomes.	
nucleus	Large, round, centralized intracellular structure that contains chromosomes and their DNA. It controls all of the cell's activities. It is surrounded by a membrane.	**nucle/o-** *nucleus of an atom; nucleus of a cell* **kary/o-** *nucleus of a cell*
oncogenes	Damaged and mutated genes that cause a cell to become cancerous. A virus can carry an oncogene in its RNA. Then when it enters a normal cell, the oncogene becomes incorporated into the normal cell's DNA and it becomes a cancerous cell.	**onc/o-** *mass; tumor*
organelles	Small structures in the cytoplasm that have specialized functions. They include mitochondria, ribosomes, the endoplasmic reticulum, the Golgi apparatus, and lysosomes.	**organ/o-** *organ*
pathogen	Microorganism such as a bacterium or virus that causes infection	**path/o-** *disease*
primary site	Area where the cancer first appeared	
relapse	Return of the cancer after treatment	
remission	No symptoms of cancer after successful treatment	**remiss/o-** *send back*
ribosomes	Granular organelles in the cytoplasm and on the endoplasmic reticulum. Ribosomes contain RNA and proteins and are the site where proteins are produced.	**rib/o-** *ribonucleic acid*
RNA	**Ribonucleic acid**. It is created in the nucleolus and stored in ribosomes. Messenger RNA duplicates DNA information in the nucleus and carries it to the ribosome.	
secondary site	Area where the cancer has spread to	
suppressor genes	Group of genes in the DNA of each cell that inhibits mitosis. The p53 gene is the most important suppressor gene.	**suppress/o-** *press down*
tumor necrosis factor (TNF)	Substance released from lymph nodes that causes a cancerous tumor to become necrotic and die	**necr/o-** *dead body; dead cells; dead tissue*
undifferentiated	Cancerous cells that are immature and embryonal in appearance and behavior	**differentiat/o-** *distinct; specialized*

Give Word Part Meanings

Use the Answer Key at the end of the book to check your answers.

Combining Forms Exercise

Next to each combining form, write its meaning. The first one has been done for you.

Combining Form	Meaning	Combining Form	Meaning
1. **differentiat/o-**	distinct; specialized	17. malign/o-	_____
2. angi/o-	_____	18. mit/o-	_____
3. cancer/o-	_____	19. mutat/o-	_____
4. capsul/o-	_____	20. ne/o-	_____
5. carcin/o-	_____	21. necr/o-	_____
6. cellul/o-	_____	22. nucle/o-	_____
7. chrom/o-	_____	23. onc/o-	_____
8. cyt/o-	_____	24. organ/o-	_____
9. gene/o-	_____	25. path/o-	_____
10. gen/o-	_____	26. plasm/o-	_____
11. heredit/o-	_____	27. plas/o-	_____
12. hered/o-	_____	28. remiss/o-	_____
13. invas/o-	_____	29. rib/o-	_____
14. kary/o-	_____	30. stas/o-	_____
15. locat/o-	_____	31. stat/o-	_____
16. lys/o-	_____	32. suppress/o-	_____

Build Medical Words

Combining Form and Suffix Exercise

Read the definition of the medical word. Look at the combining form that is given. Select the correct suffix from the Suffix List and write it on the blank line. Then build the medical word and write it on the line. (Remember: You may need to remove the combining vowel. Always remove the hyphens and slash.) Be sure to check your spelling. The first one has been done for you.

SUFFIX LIST

-ant (pertaining to)
-ar (pertaining to)
-gen (that which produces)
-gene (gene)

-ion (action; condition)
-ity (condition; state)
-ive (pertaining to)
-osis (condition; process)
-ous (pertaining to)

-plasm (growth; formed substance)
-some (body)
-tic (pertaining to)

Definition of the Medical Word	Combining Form	Suffix	Build the Medical Word
	nucle/o-	-ar	nuclear
1. Pertaining to (the) nucleus of a cell			
(You think *pertaining to + nucleus of a cell* (nucle/o-). You change the order of the word parts to put the suffix last. You write *nuclear*.)			
2. Pertaining to cancer	cancer/o-	_____	_____
3. Condition (of) dead cells or dead tissue	necr/o-	_____	_____
4. Pertaining to go into	invas/o-	_____	_____
5. Pertaining to genes	gene/o-	_____	_____
6. Pertaining to intentionally causing harm	malign/o-	_____	_____
7. Pertaining to (a) cell	cellul/o-	_____	_____
8. That which produces cancer	carcin/o-	_____	_____
9. Gene (that causes a) mass or tumor	onc/o-	_____	_____
10. State (of) genetic inheritance	hered/o-	_____	_____
11. Formed substance (within a) cell	cyt/o-	_____	_____
12. (Microscopic) body (that takes on) color (when stained)	chrom/o-	_____	_____
13. Action (that causes to) change	mutat/o-	_____	_____
14. (Microscopic) body (that contains) ribonucleic acid	rib/o-	_____	_____
15. Process (of cell division during which the chromosomes align along) thread-like strands (in the nucleus)	mit/o-	_____	_____
16. Growth (that is) new	ne/o-	_____	_____

Cancer

	General	
Word or Phrase	**Description**	**Pronunciation/Word Parts**
anaplasia	Condition in which normal cells that are mature and differentiated become cancerous cells that are undifferentiated in appearance and behavior.	**anaplasia** (AN-ah-PLAY-zha) **ana-** *apart; excessive* **plas/o-** *formation; growth* **-ia** *condition; state; thing*
cancer	General word for any type of **cancerous** cell or tumor. There are four broad categories of cancer: carcinoma, sarcoma, leukemia, and embryonal cell carcinoma. Treatment: Chemotherapy drugs, radiation therapy, surgery, or a combination of these, depending on the type and extent of the cancer.	**cancer** (KAN-ser) **cancerous** (KAN-ser-us)
carcinoid tumor	Slow-growing cancerous tumor that occurs mainly in the digestive tract. It does not exhibit all of the characteristics of cancer, and it seldom metastasizes. **Carcinoid syndrome** is a set of symptoms caused by the release of the hormone serotonin from a carcinoid tumor.	**carcinoid** (KAR-sih-noyd) **carcin/o-** *cancer* **-oid** *resembling*
carcinomatosis	Condition in which cancerous tumors are present at multiple sites in the body.	**carcinomatosis** (KAR-sih-NOH-mah-TOH-sis) *Carcinomatosis* is a combination of *carcinomata* (the plural form of *carcinoma*) and the suffix *-osis* (condition; process).
dysplasia	Condition of atypical cells that are abnormal in size, shape, or organization, but have not yet become cancerous (see Figure 13-19). These cells are **dysplastic**. Dysplasia is the result of chronic irritation and inflammation.	**dysplasia** (dis-PLAY-zha) **dys-** *abnormal; difficult; painful* **plas/o-** *formation; growth* **-ia** *condition; state; thing* Select the correct prefix meaning to get the definition of *dysplasia*: *condition (of) abnormal formation or growth (of cells).* **dysplastic** (dis-PLAS-tik)
lymphadenopathy	Enlarged lymph nodes. The lymph nodes trap cancerous cells that break away from the site of the original tumor. The lymph node itself then becomes a site of cancer. Chains of lymph nodes in the neck, axillae, and groin regions are common sites of lymphadenopathy (see Figure 6-19).	**lymphadenopathy** (LIMF-ad-eh-NAW-pah-thee) **lymph/o-** *lymph; lymphatic system* **aden/o-** *gland* **-pathy** *disease*

Carcinomas

Word or Phrase	Description	Pronunciation/Word Parts
adenocarcinoma	An adenocarcinoma is cancer of a gland. Adenocarcinoma of the breast occurs in the epithelial cells lining the ducts of the milk glands of the breast (see Figures 18-6 ■ and 18-7 ■). An adenocarcinoma can also occur in the ducts of these glands: pancreas, prostate gland, or salivary glands. It is also known as **ductal cell carcinoma**. An adenocarcinoma of the ducts of the gallbladder is known as **cholangiocarcinoma**.	**adenocarcinoma** (AD-eh-noh-KAR-sih-NOH-mah) **aden/o-** *gland* **carcin/o-** *cancer* **-oma** *mass; tumor* **ductal** (DUK-tal) **duct/o-** *bring; duct; move* **-al** *pertaining to* **cholangiocarcinoma** (koh-LAN-jee-oh-KAR-sih-NOH-mah) **cholangi/o-** *bile duct* **carcin/o-** *cancer* **-oma** *mass; tumor*

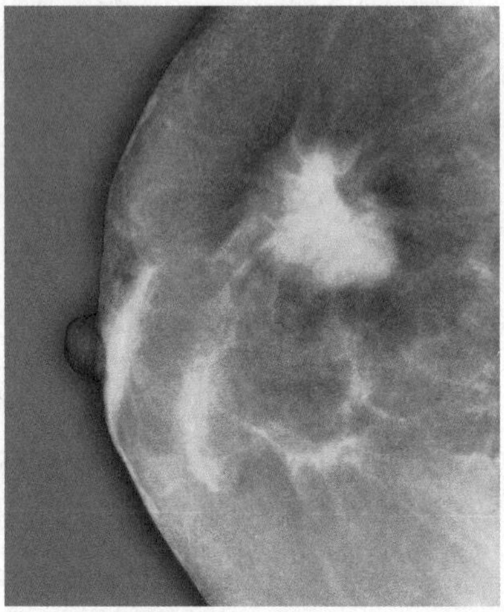

FIGURE 18-6 ■ Adenocarcinoma of the breast.
On a colorized mammogram, this patient has an adenocarcinoma of the breast, seen as a dense white mass in the center of the breast. Note the characteristic irregular edges of the tumor with infiltration into the surrounding breast tissue. Normal supporting fibers and lactiferous (milk-producing) ducts in the breast are visible as individual white streaks, and the fatty tissues of the breast appear as dark blue areas.
Source: Zephyr/Science Source

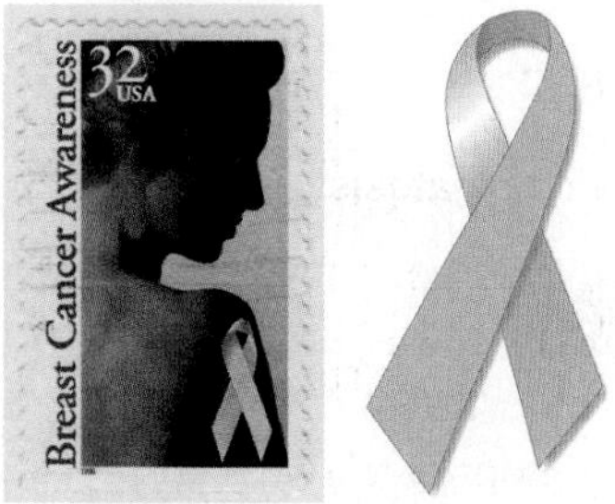

FIGURE 18-7 ■ The fight against breast cancer.
A pink ribbon is the universal symbol for the fight against breast cancer.
Source: Pearson Education

DID YOU KNOW?

Advanced adenocarcinoma of the breast can cause dimpling of the skin of the breast as the tumor pulls on supporting tissues around the ducts. This dimpling, known by the French phrase *peau d'orange* (peel of the orange), makes the breast skin look like the dimpled surface of an orange (see Figure 13-21).

Word or Phrase	Description	Pronunciation/Word Parts
carcinoma	Cancer of epithelial cells in the skin or mucous membranes. Carcinomas grow more slowly than sarcomas, but they occur more often. Carcinomas usually metastasize via the lymphatic system.	**carcinoma** (KAR-sih-NOH-mah) **carcin/o-** *cancer* **-oma** *mass; tumor* *Carcinoma* is a Greek singular noun. Form the plural by changing *-oma* to *-omata.* However, the English plural *carcinomas* is also used.

Word or Phrase	Description	Pronunciation/Word Parts
basal cell carcinoma	Cancer of the deepest layer (basal layer) of the epidermis of the skin (see Figure 18-8 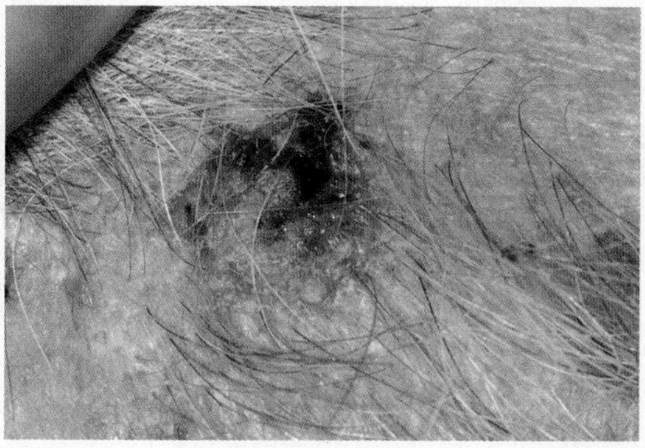 ■) **FIGURE 18-8 ■ Basal cell carcinoma.** This basal cell carcinoma of the skin shows a characteristic asymmetrical shape with an ulcerated area that has become necrotic. There is crusting from oozing tissue fluid and periodic bleeding that forms a scab. *Source*: Dr. P. Marazzi/Science Source	**basal** (BAY-sal) **bas/o-** *alkaline; base of a structure; basic* **-al** *pertaining to*
bronchogenic carcinoma	Cancer of the mucous membranes lining the bronchi of the lungs	**bronchogenic** (BRONG-koh-JEN-ik) **bronch/o-** *bronchus* **gen/o-** *arising from; produced by* **-ic** *pertaining to*
endometrial carcinoma	Cancer of the endometrium that lines the intrauterine cavity of the uterus	**endometrial** (EN-doh-MEE-tree-al) **endo-** *innermost; within* **metri/o-** *uterus; womb* **-al** *pertaining to*
hepatocellular carcinoma	Cancer of the liver cells (see Figure 18-9 ■). It is also known as a **hepatoma**. 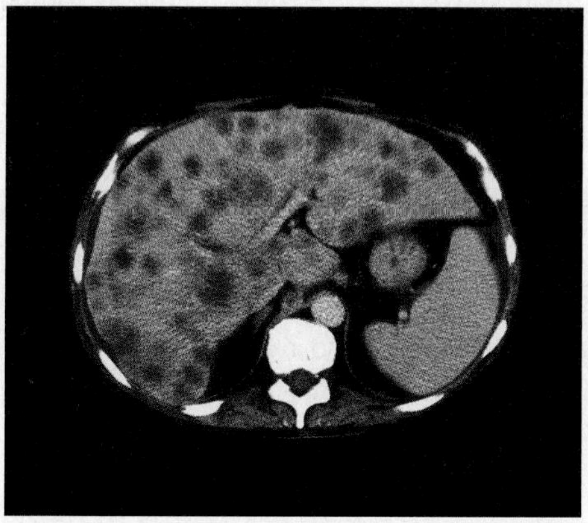 **FIGURE 18-9 ■ Hepatocellular carcinoma.** This colorized computerized tomography (CT) of the abdomen shows an enlarged (tan) liver nearly filling the abdominal cavity (on the left side), with many (red-brown) areas of cancer. An abdominal CT scan is read as if you were standing at the patient's feet, looking up, and so the (white) area in the center bottom of the scan is the vertebra of the spine. *Source*: Simon Fraser/Freeman Hospital, Newcastle upon Tyne/Science Source	**hepatocellular** (HEP-ah-to-SEL-yoo-lar) **hepat/o-** *liver* **cellul/o-** *cell* **-ar** *pertaining to* **hepatoma** (HEP-ah-TOH-mah) **hepat/o-** *liver* **-oma** *mass; tumor*
small cell carcinoma	Cancer of the epithelial cells of the lungs. These cancerous cells are small and round or oval (in contrast to large cell carcinoma, a less common type of lung cancer that has larger cancerous cells). It is also known as **oat cell carcinoma**.	
squamous cell carcinoma	Cancer of the squamous cells (top layer) of the epidermis of the skin	**squamous** (SKWAY-mus) **squam/o-** *scale-like cell* **-ous** *pertaining to*
transitional cell carcinoma	Cancer of the epithelial cells lining the urinary tract. Transitional cells are unique in that their shape transitions (changes) each time the bladder is filled with urine.	**transitional** (trans-ZIH-shun-al) **transit/o-** *change from one thing to another* **-ion** *action; condition* **-al** *pertaining to*

Word or Phrase	Description	Pronunciation/Word Parts
malignant melanoma	Cancer of melanocytes (melanin pigment cells) of the skin (see Figure 7-20)	**melanoma** (MEL-ah-NOH-mah) **melan/o-** *black* **-oma** *mass; tumor* Add words to make a complete definition of *melanoma: tumor (whose color is brown or) black.*

Sarcomas		
angiosarcoma	Cancer of a blood vessel or lymphatic vessel	**angiosarcoma** (AN-jee-OH-sar-KOH-mah) **angi/o-** *blood vessel; lymphatic vessel* **sarc/o-** *connective tissue* **-oma** *mass; tumor*
astrocytoma	Cancer of an astrocyte (star-shaped, branching cell that supports neurons) in the cerebrum of the brain. Cancer of an immature, embryonic astrocyte is known as **glioblastoma multiforme**.	**astrocytoma** (AS-troh-sy-TOH-mah) **astr/o-** *star-like structure* **cyt/o-** *cell* **-oma** *mass; tumor*
		glioblastoma multiforme (GLY-oh-blas-TOH-mah MUL-tee-FOR-may) **gli/o-** *supporting cells* **blast/o-** *embryonic; immature* **-oma** *mass; tumor*
chondrosarcoma	Cancer of the cartilage	**chondrosarcoma** (CON-droh-sar-KOH-mah) **chondr/o-** *cartilage* **sarc/o-** *connective tissue* **-oma** *mass; tumor*
Ewing's sarcoma	Cancer of the growth area (epiphysial plate) at the end of a long bone of an arm or leg	**Ewing** (YOO-ing)
Kaposi's sarcoma	Cancer of the skin and subcutaneous tissue. This previously rare cancer is commonly seen in AIDS patients because of their depressed immune response. These are irregularly shaped tumors on the skin and in the internal organs.	**Kaposi** (KAH-poh-see)
leiomyosarcoma	Cancer of the smooth muscle layer in the uterus, digestive tract, bladder, or prostate gland	**leiomyosarcoma** (LIE-oh-MY-oh-sar-KOH-mah) **lei/o-** *smooth* **my/o-** *muscle* **sarc/o-** *connective tissue* **-oma** *mass; tumor*
liposarcoma	Cancer of the fatty tissue	**liposarcoma** (LIP-oh-sar-KOH-mah) **lip/o-** *fat; lipid* **sarc/o-** *connective tissue* **-oma** *mass; tumor*
myosarcoma	Cancer of a muscle and connective tissue, such as a tendon or aponeurosis	**myosarcoma** (MY-oh-sar-KOH-mah) **my/o-** *muscle* **sarc/o-** *connective tissue* **-oma** *mass; tumor*

Word or Phrase	Description	Pronunciation/Word Parts
neurofibrosarcoma	Cancer of Schwann cells that produce myelin and surround the larger axons of neurons that make up the cranial nerves and spinal nerves	**neurofibrosarcoma** (NYOOR-oh-FY-broh-sar-KOH-mah) **neur/o-** *nerve* **fibr/o-** *fiber* **sarc/o-** *connective tissue* **-oma** *mass; tumor*
oligodendroglioma	Cancer of oligodendroglia, cells that surround the larger axons of neurons in the brain and spinal cord. They provide support and produce myelin. These cells have only a few branching structures.	**oligodendroglioma** (OH-lih-goh-DEN-droh-glee-OH-mah) **olig/o-** *few; scanty* **dendr/o-** *branching structure* **gli/o-** *supporting cells* **-oma** *mass; tumor*
osteosarcoma	Cancer of a bone (see Figure 18-10 ■). It is also known as **osteogenic sarcoma**. 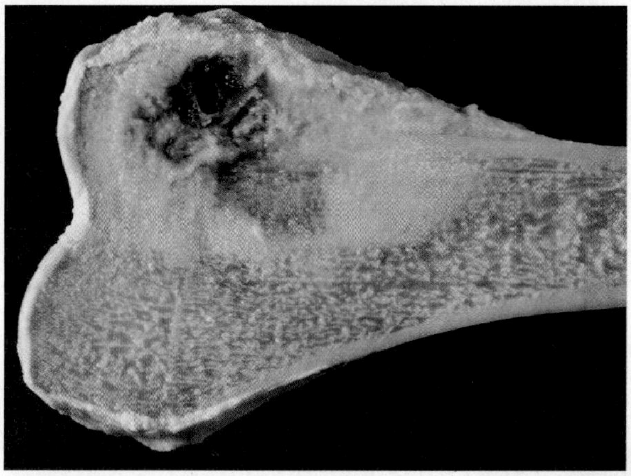 **FIGURE 18-10 ■ Osteosarcoma.** This patient, an 11-year-old girl, had an osteosarcoma of the distal end of her femur. The tumor also spread to the soft tissues around the bone. The tumor and part of the bone were removed during surgery. *Source*: CNRI/Science Source	**osteosarcoma** (AW-stee-OH-sar-KOH-mah) **oste/o-** *bone* **sarc/o-** *connective tissue* **-oma** *mass; tumor* **osteogenic** (AW-stee-oh-JEN-ik) **oste/o-** *bone* **gen/o-** *arising from; produced by* **-ic** *pertaining to*
rhabdomyo-sarcoma	Cancer of a skeletal (voluntary) muscle in the arms or legs	**rhabdomyosarcoma** (RAB-doh-MY-oh-sar-KOH-mah) **rhabd/o-** *rod shaped* **my/o-** *muscle* **sarc/o-** *connective tissue* **-oma** *mass; tumor* Each muscle cell in this tumor is shaped like a rod.
sarcoma	Cancer of connective tissues (cartilage, bone, tendon, ligament, aponeurosis, fascia, fat, subcutaneous tissue), muscles, or nerves. Sarcomas grow rapidly and most often show anaplasia of their cells. Sarcomas usually metastasize to other parts of the body via the circulatory system. A **fibrosarcoma** is a cancer composed entirely of immature fibroblasts (cells that, after they mature, produce cartilage and bone).	**sarcoma** (sar-KOH-mah) **sarc/o-** *connective tissue* **-oma** *mass; tumor* **fibrosarcoma** (FY-broh-sar-KOH-mah) **fibr/o-** *fiber* **sarc/o-** *connective tissue* **-oma** *mass; tumor*

Cancers of the Blood and Lymphatic System

Word or Phrase	Description	Pronunciation/Word Parts
leukemia	Cancer of leukocytes (white blood cells) (see Figure 6-17). Leukemia is named according to the type of leukocyte that is the most prevalent and whether the onset of symptoms is acute or chronic. Types of leukemia include acute **myelogenous leukemia** (AML), chronic myelogenous leukemia (CML), acute **lymphocytic leukemia** (ALL), and chronic lymphocytic leukemia (CLL).	**leukemia** (loo-KEE-mee-ah) **leuk/o-** *white* **-emia** *condition of the blood; substance in the blood* **myelogenous** (MY-eh-LAW-jeh-nus) **myel/o-** *bone marrow; myelin; spinal cord* **gen/o-** *arising from; produced by* **-ous** *pertaining to* **lymphocytic** (LIM-foh-SIT-ik) **lymph/o-** *lymph; lymphatic system* **cyt/o-** *cell* **-ic** *pertaining to*
lymphoma	Cancer of a lymph node, lymphoid tissue, or T or B lymphocytes. There are two types of lymphomas. **Hodgkin's lymphoma**, the most common type, shows characteristic Reed-Sternberg cells on biopsy (see Figure 18-11 ■). **Non-Hodgkin's lymphoma**, a group of more than 20 different lymphomas, does not have any Reed-Sternberg cells. A lymphoma that develops in a lymph node should not be confused with metastasis to a lymph node from a primary tumor located elsewhere in the body.	**lymphoma** (lim-FOH-mah) **lymph/o-** *lymph; lymphatic system* **-oma** *mass; tumor* **Hodgkin** (HAWJ-kin)
multiple myeloma	Cancer of the bone marrow. It contains malignant plasma cells. Normal plasma cells are B lymphocytes that produce antibodies (immunoglobulins) when activated by a pathogen. Malignant plasma cells produce abnormal antibodies known as Bence Jones proteins. Because the patient's immune response is abnormal with decreased levels of normal plasma cells and antibodies, the patient can develop serious infections.	**myeloma** (MY-eh-LOH-mah) **myel/o-** *bone marrow; myelin; spinal cord* **-oma** *mass; tumor* Select the correct combining form meaning to get the definition of *myeloma*: *tumor (of the) bone marrow.*

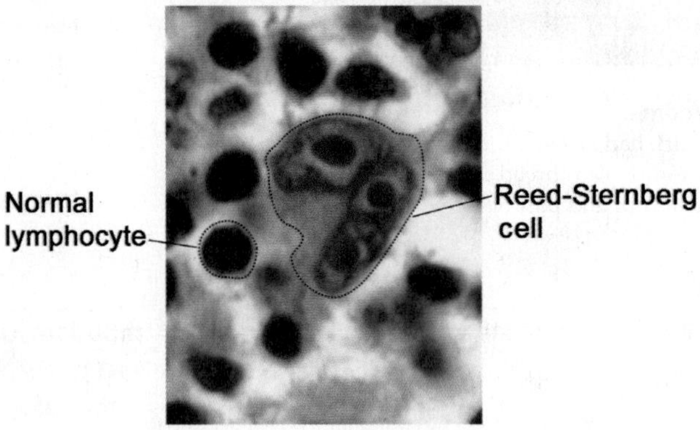

Normal lymphocyte — **Reed-Sternberg cell**

FIGURE 18-11 ■ Reed-Sternberg cell.
This Reed-Sternberg cell (circled) was in the biopsy of a lymph node from a patient who was then diagnosed with Hodgkin's lymphoma. It is a large, atypical, cancerous lymphocyte that often has two nuclei. It is shown here with smaller, normal lymphocytes.
Source: National Cancer Institutes

	Embryonal Cell Cancer	
Word or Phrase	**Description**	**Pronunciation/Word Parts**
choriocarcinoma	Cancer that develops during pregnancy. It involves the chorion, the membrane that surrounds the developing embryo and later becomes the placenta. This cancer only occurs when a woman is pregnant.	**choriocarcinoma** (KOR-ee-oh-KAR-sih-NOH-mah) **chori/o-** *chorion* **carcin/o-** *cancer* **-oma** *mass; tumor*
embryonal cell cancer	Cancer of an embryonal cell. It develops during childhood or adolescence. It includes choriocarcinoma, germ cell tumors, hepatoblastoma, neuroblastoma, retinoblastoma, teratoma, and Wilms' tumor.	**embryonal** (EM-bree-OH-nal) **embryon/o-** *embryo; immature form* **-al** *pertaining to*
germ cell tumor	Cancer of an embryonal cell (also known as a *germ cell*) in the ovary or testis. A **dysgerminoma** is cancer of an oocyte (immature cell that becomes an ovum) in the ovary. It occurs in young adult females. A **seminoma** is cancer of a spermatoblast (immature cell that becomes a spermatozoon) in the testis. It occurs in young adult males. **WORD ALERT** Germ cells have nothing to do with "germs" (bacteria, viruses). Germ cells are immature cells that "germinate" (grow or develop) into mature, specialized cells.	**dysgerminoma** (DIS-jer-mih-NOH-mah) **dys-** *abnormal; difficult; painful* **germin/o-** *embryonic tissue* **-oma** *mass; tumor* **seminoma** (SEM-ih-NOH-mah) **semin/o-** *sperm; spermatozoon* **-oma** *mass; tumor*
hepatoblastoma	Cancer of an embryonal cell in the liver. It occurs in young children.	**hepatoblastoma** (HEP-ah-TOH-blas-TOH-mah) **hepat/o-** *liver* **blast/o-** *embryonic; immature* **-oma** *mass; tumor*
neuroblastoma	Cancer of an embryonal nerve cell. It occurs in young children.	**neuroblastoma** (NYOOR-oh-blas-TOH-mah) **neur/o-** *nerve* **blast/o-** *embryonic; immature* **-oma** *mass; tumor*
retinoblastoma	Cancer of an embryonal cell in the retina of the eye. It occurs in young children.	**retinoblastoma** (RET-ih-NOH-blas-TOH-mah) **retin/o-** *retina* **blast/o-** *embryonic; immature* **-oma** *mass; tumor*
teratoma	Cancer of the ovary or testis that contains cells from other parts of the body. In the ovary, a teratoma can be malignant but usually is in the form of a benign dermoid cyst that contains hair and sometimes even teeth. However, a teratoma in the testis is almost always malignant.	**teratoma** (TAIR-ah-TOH-mah) **terat/o-** *bizarre form* **-oma** *mass; tumor*
Wilms' tumor	Cancer of an embryonal cell of the kidney. It occurs in young children. This is also known as **nephroblastoma**.	**Wilms' tumor** (WILMZ TOO-mor) **nephroblastoma** (NEH-froh-blas-TOH-mah) **nephr/o-** *kidney; nephron* **blast/o-** *embryonic; immature* **-oma** *mass; tumor*

Laboratory and Diagnostic Procedures

Cytology Tests		
Word or Phrase	**Description**	**Pronunciation/Word Parts**
bone marrow aspiration	Test that diagnoses leukemia or lymphoma and monitors its progression. A sample of bone marrow is taken from the posterior iliac crest. The stages of cell development (stem cell to mature cell) and the numbers of cells are examined under a microscope.	**aspiration** (AS-pih-RAY-shun) **aspir/o-** *breathe in; suck in* **-ation** *being; having; process*
exfoliative cytology	Test that examines cells found in secretions or cells that are scraped or washed off of tissue. The sample is examined under a microscope to look for abnormal or cancerous cells. Examples: Pap smear of the cervix (see Figures 13-25 and 13-26), bronchial or gastric washings, sputum.	**exfoliative** (eks-FOH-lee-ah-TIV) **cytology** (sy-TAW-loh-jee) **cyt/o-** *cell* **-logy** *study of*
frozen section	Test that involves freezing a tissue specimen obtained from a biopsy. Thin slices are stained and examined under a microscope. This is done in the laboratory during the surgery so that the surgeon knows immediately whether the tissue is cancerous or not. Freezing the tissue distorts some of the cell architecture, and so a permanent section is also done using a paraffin-like substance to make the tissue firm.	
HER2/neu	Test that detects a gene that affects the prognosis of, and treatment options for, breast cancer, ovarian cancer, and bladder cancer. A tumor that is HER2/neu positive is an aggressive tumor that is resistant to hormone therapy and some chemotherapy drugs.	**HER2/neu** (her-too-noo)
karyotype	Test that examines chromosomes under a microscope. A photograph of the karyotype (see Figure 18-12 ■) is studied to look for abnormal chromosomes with deletions or translocations. A translocation of chromosome 9 to chromosome 22 (known as the *Philadelphia chromosome*) is diagnostic of chronic myelogenous leukemia. A translocation between chromosomes 11 and 22 causes Ewing's sarcoma.	**karyotype** (KAIR-ee-oh-TYPE) **kary/o-** *nucleus of a cell* **-type** *model of*

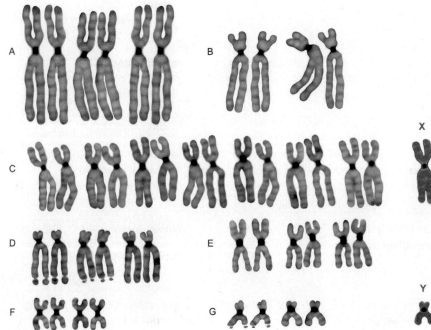

FIGURE 18-12 ■ Normal karyotype.
There are 23 pairs of chromosomes in a normal karyotype. Pairs 1–22 are shown here with pair 23 (the sex chromosomes) in the bottom right-hand corner. Two X sex chromosomes make this patient a female.
Source: BSIP/UIG/Universal Images Group/Getty Images

Word or Phrase	Description	Pronunciation/Word Parts
receptor assays	Cytology test that measures the number of **estrogen receptors (ER)** or **progesterone receptors (PR)** on the cell membrane of a cancer cell to determine the prognosis of, and treatment options for, breast cancer. A tumor with increased numbers of ER or PR receptors (known as *ER–positive* or *PR–positive*) is dependent on the estrogen (or progesterone) hormone, and so it is treated with a male hormone drug that creates the opposite hormonal environment.	**receptor** (ree-SEP-tor) **recept/o-** *receive* **-or** *person who does; person who produces; thing that does; thing that produces* **assay** (AS-say)

Blood Tests

Word or Phrase	Description	Pronunciation/Word Parts
alpha fetoprotein (AFP)	Test that detects a protein normally present in a fetus, but not in an adult. An elevated level of AFP is seen with cancer of the liver, ovaries, and testes. The higher the level, the more advanced the cancer. (An elevated level is also seen in noncancerous conditions, such as cirrhosis, hepatitis, neural tube defects, and Down syndrome.)	**alpha fetoprotein** (AL-fah FEE-toh-PRO-teen)
blood smear	Test in which a drop of blood is smeared on a glass slide and examined under a microscope. This test is done manually to examine the characteristics of leukocytes when an automated complete blood count (CBC) is abnormal and suggests leukemia.	
BRCA1 or BRCA2 gene	Test that detects the BRCA1 or BRCA2 gene, a genetic mutation that significantly increases the risk of breast cancer and ovarian cancer. This test is performed when there is a strong family history of breast or ovarian cancer. BRCA stands for **br**east **ca**ncer.	
carcinoembryonic antigen (CEA)	Test that detects a protein normally present in an embryo, but not in an adult. An elevated level of CEA is seen with several different cancers. The higher the level, the more advanced the cancer. (An elevated level is also seen in noncancerous conditions, such as diseases of the colon and liver or in patients who smoke.)	**carcinoembryonic** (KAR-sih-noh-EM-bree-AW-nik) **carcin/o-** *cancer* **embryon/o-** *embryo; immature form* **-ic** *pertaining to* **antigen** (AN-tih-jen)
human chorionic gonadotropin (HCG)	Test that detects a hormone normally present during pregnancy but not at other times. An elevated level of HCG is seen in choriocarcinoma in women and in cancer of the testes in men. (An elevated level is also seen in noncancerous conditions, such as cirrhosis, duodenal ulcer, and inflammatory bowel disease.)	**chorionic** (KOR-ee-AW-nik) **chorion/o-** *chorion* **-ic** *pertaining to* **gonadotropin** (GOH-nad-oh-TROH-pin) **gonad/o-** *gonad; ovary; testis* **trop/o-** *having an affinity for; stimulating; turning* **-in** *substance*
prostate-specific antigen (PSA)	Test that measures a protein in the prostate gland. An elevated level is seen in cancer of the prostate gland. The higher the level, the more advanced the cancer. Free PSA and total PSA levels are measured.	
tumor markers	Test that detects antigens on the surface of cancer cells. Tumor markers evaluate the extent of the cancer and the effectiveness of the treatment. Tumor markers include CA 15-3 and CA 27.29 (for breast cancer), CA 125 (for ovarian cancer), and CA 19-9 (for cancer of the pancreas and bile ducts). AFP, CEA, and HCG are also tumor markers.	

Urine Tests

urinalysis (UA)	Test that detects chemical compounds in the urine that indicate the presence of various cancers. These include Bence Jones protein (for multiple myeloma), vanillylmandelic acid (VMA) (for neuroblastoma), and 5-HIAA (for carcinoid syndrome).	**urinalysis** (YOOR-ih-NAL-ih-sis)

Radiology and Nuclear Medicine Procedures

Word or Phrase	Description	Pronunciation/Word Parts
computerized axial tomography (CAT, CT)	Procedure that uses x-rays to create many individual, closely spaced images or "slices" (see Figure 18-13 ■). The computer can combine these into a three-dimensional image to precisely locate a tumor or metastases. Radiopaque contrast dye can also be injected to provide more detail.	**tomography** (toh-MAW-grah-fee) **tom/o-** *cut; layer; slice* **-graphy** *process of recording*

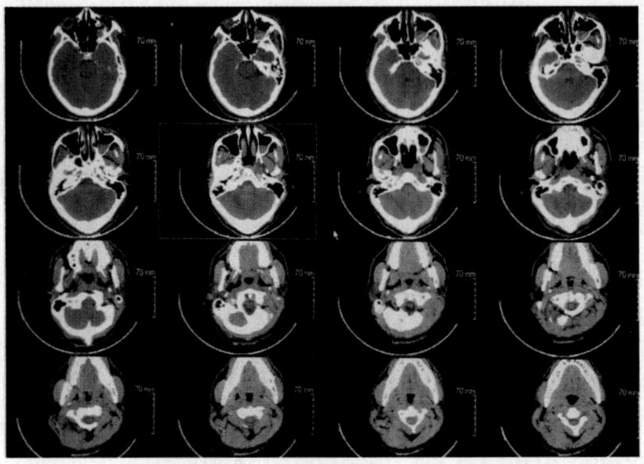

FIGURE 18-13 ■ CT scan.
These computerized tomography images of the head show multiple "slices" through different parts of the patient's head in order to pinpoint exactly where a tumor might be.
Source: Gca/Science Source

lymphangiography	Procedure in which a radiopaque contrast dye is injected into a lymphatic vessel. X-rays taken as the dye travels through the lymphatic vessels show enlarged lymph nodes, lymphomas, and areas of blocked lymph drainage. The x-ray image is a **lymphangiogram**.	**lymphangiography** (lim-FAN-jee-AW-grah-fee) **lymph/o-** *lymph; lymphatic system* **angi/o-** *blood vessel; lymphatic vessel* **-graphy** *process of recording* **lymphangiogram** (lim-FAN-jee-oh-GRAM) **lymph/o-** *lymph; lymphatic system* **angi/o-** *blood vessel; lymphatic vessel* **-gram** *picture; record*
magnetic resonance imaging (MRI)	Procedure that uses a magnetic field and radiowaves to align protons in the body and cause them to emit signals. MRI is a tomography that creates many individual "slice" images that the computer combines into a three-dimensional image to precisely locate a tumor or metastases. Radiopaque contrast dye can also be injected to provide more detail. An MRI scan does not use x-rays so the patient is not exposed to any radiation. Patients with extensive fibrocystic disease of the breast can be more accurately evaluated for breast cancer with an MRI scan instead of mammography.	**magnetic** (mag-NET-ik) **magnet/o-** *magnet* **-ic** *pertaining to*
mammography	Procedure that uses low-dose x-rays to produce an image of the breast to detect tumors. The breast is compressed between two flat surfaces to decrease its thickness and increase the quality of the image (see Figure 13-28). The x-ray image is a **mammogram** (see Figure 18-6).	**mammography** (mah-MAW-grah-fee) **mamm/o-** *breast* **-graphy** *process of recording* **mammogram** (MAM-oh-gram) **mamm/o-** *breast* **-gram** *picture; record*

Word or Phrase	Description	Pronunciation/Word Parts
scintigraphy	Nuclear medicine procedure that uses a radioactive tracer drug that collects in particular organs and tissues and emits gamma rays. A gamma camera counts the gamma rays and emits flashes of light to create a **scintigram**. Areas of increased uptake are abnormal and can be due to infection, cancer, or metastases.	**scintigraphy** (sin-TIH-grah-fee) 　**scint/i-** *point of light* 　**-graphy** *process of recording* **scintigram** (SIN-tih-gram) 　**scint/i-** *point of light* 　**-gram** *picture; record*
ultrasonography	Procedure that uses ultra high-frequency sound waves to produce an image. It is used to distinguish benign, fluid-filled tumors (cysts) from solid tumors that need to be biopsied. It is used to evaluate the breasts, abdominal organs, pelvic organs, and testes. It is also known as **sonography**, and the **ultrasound** image is a **sonogram**.	**ultrasonography** (UL-trah-soh-NAW-grah-fee) 　**ultra-** *beyond; higher* 　**son/o-** *sound* 　**-graphy** *process of recording* **ultrasound** (UL-trah-sound) **sonography** (soh-NAW-grah-fee) 　**son/o-** *sound* 　**-graphy** *process of recording* **sonogram** (SAW-noh-gram) 　**son/o-** *sound* 　**-gram** *picture; record*

Medical and Surgical Procedures and Radiation Therapy

Medical Procedures		
Word or Phrase	**Description**	**Pronunciation/Word Parts**
bone marrow transplantation (BMT)	Procedure for patients with leukemia and lymphoma. Bone marrow cells are harvested from the posterior iliac crest of a matched donor (see Figure 18-14 ■). The patient is treated with high-dose chemotherapy drugs or radiation to destroy all cancerous cells (this also destroys the patient's bone marrow cells). The donor bone marrow cells, which are administered through a central intravenous line, travel through the blood and implant in the patient's bone marrow. In 2–4 weeks, the donor cells begin to produce normal blood cells. In **stem cell transplantation**, stem cells from the patient or from a matched donor or from the umbilical cord blood of a matched donor can also be given. Also known as **bone marrow harvesting**.	**transplantation** (TRANS-plan-TAY-shun) 　**transplant/o-** *move something across and put in another place* 　**-ation** *being; having; process*

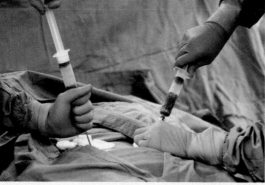

FIGURE 18-14 ■ Bone marrow harvest.
In this surgical procedure, a large needle attached to a syringe is inserted into the patient's (or a donor's) posterior iliac crest. The red marrow in the bone is aspirated into the syringe. After the patient's chemotherapy treatment is completed, this marrow is then given back to the patient through an intravenous line.
Source: Li Wa/Shutterstock

Word or Phrase	Description	Pronunciation/Word Parts
cryosurgery	Procedure in which cold liquid nitrogen is sprayed or painted onto a small malignant lesion. This freezes and destroys the cancerous cells.	**cryosurgery** (KRY-oh-SER-jer-ee) **cry/o-** *cold* **surg/o-** *operative procedure* **-ery** *process*
electrosurgery	Procedure in which an electrode and an electrical current are used to evaporate small, cancerous tumors on the skin. There are two types of electrosurgery. In **fulguration**, the electrode is held away from the skin and transmits the electrical current as a spark to the skin surface. In **electrodesiccation**, the electrode is touched to, or inserted into, the cancerous tumor.	**electrosurgery** (ee-LEK-troh-SER-jer-ee) **electr/o-** *electricity* **surg/o-** *operative procedure* **-ery** *process* **fulguration** (FUL-gyoor-AA-shun) **fulgur/o-** *spark of electricity* **-ation** *being; having; process* **electrodesiccation** (ee-LEK-troh-DES-ih-KAY-shun) **electr/o-** *electricity* **desicc/o-** *dry up* **-ation** *being; having; process*
grading	Procedure that classifies cancers by how differentiated their cells appear under a microscope. Normal cells appear well differentiated and characteristic of a particular tissue. Poorly differentiated or undifferentiated cancerous cells lack specialization and appear immature and embryonic. The greater the number of undifferentiated cells, the poorer the prognosis.	
insertion of a catheter to administer chemotherapy drugs	Procedure in which some chemotherapy drugs are given through an **intravenous line** in a vein. A **peripherally inserted central catheter** (PICC) is inserted in a vein in the arm and then threaded to the superior vena cava. An **intrathecal catheter** is inserted after a lumbar puncture is performed, so that the chemotherapy drug circulates through the cerebrospinal fluid. **Intravesical chemotherapy** is administered through a catheter inserted into the bladder. The chemotherapy drug is held in the bladder for several hours and then removed. This procedure is done weekly for several weeks.	**intravenous** (IN-trah-VEE-nus) **intra-** *within* **ven/o-** *vein* **-ous** *pertaining to* **peripheral** (peh-RIF-eh-ral) **peripher/o-** *outer aspects* **-al** *pertaining to* **intrathecal** (IN-trah-THEE-kal) **intra-** *within* **thec/o-** *dura mater; sheath* **-al** *pertaining to* **catheter** (KATH-eh-ter) **intravesical** (IN-trah-VES-ih-kal) **intra-** *within* **vesic/o-** *bladder; fluid-filled sac* **-al** *pertaining to*
staging	Procedure that classifies cancer by how far it has spread in the body. The TNM staging system is used to describe the size of the tumor and whether the tumor has spread to lymph nodes and other sites (see Table 18-1 ■).	

Table 18-1 Classification Systems for Cancer

TNM Staging System

T	Size of the primary **tumor** (on a scale of T1 through T4)
N	Number of regional lymph **nodes** affected (on a scale of N1 through N4)
M	Presence or absence of **metastases** to other sites in the body (on a scale of M0 or M1)

Other Staging Systems

Bethesda System	Cervical cancer
CIN Classification	Cervical cancer
Clark Level	Malignant melanoma
Dukes Classification	Cancer of the colon or rectum
FIGO Staging	Ovarian cancer
Gleason Score	Adenocarcinoma of the prostate gland
Jewett Classification	Bladder carcinoma

Surgical Procedures

Word or Phrase	Description	Pronunciation/Word Parts
biopsy (BX, Bx)	Procedure in which tissue is removed from a suspected cancerous tumor and sent to the pathology department for examination and diagnosis.	**biopsy** (BY-awp-see) **bi/o-** *life; living organism; living tissue* **-opsy** *process of viewing*
core needle biopsy	A large-gauge needle is inserted into the tumor to obtain several long cores of tissue (see Figure 18-15 ■).	

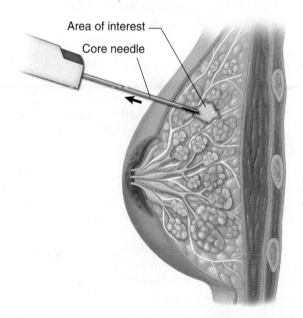

Area of interest
Core needle

FIGURE 18-15 ■ Core needle biopsy.
A core needle biopsy is performed on the breast after the area has been numbed with a local anesthetic drug. Three to six cores of tissue are obtained. An x-ray or an ultrasound may be used to pinpoint the exact location of the tumor to be biopsied.
Source: Pearson Education

excisional biopsy	An incision is made to expose the tumor, and the entire tumor is removed (excised) along with a surrounding margin of normal tissue.	**excisional** (ek-SIH-zhun-al) **excis/o-** *cut out* **-ion** *action; condition* **-al** *pertaining to*
fine-needle aspiration	A very fine needle is inserted into the tumor, and the fluid or tissue inside the tumor is aspirated into a syringe.	**aspiration** (AS-pih-RAY-shun) **aspir/o-** *breathe in; suck in* **-ation** *being; having; process*

Word or Phrase	Description	Pronunciation/Word Parts

incisional biopsy	An incision is made to expose the tumor, and part (but not all) of the tumor is removed.	**incisional** (in-SIH-zhun-al)
		  incis/o- *cut into*
		  -ion *action; condition*
		  -al *pertaining to*

optical biopsy	During an endoscopic procedure, a probe is inserted into the tumor. A laser from the probe creates a microscopic image of the cells of the tumor that can be used for diagnosis.	**optical** (AWP-tih-kal)
		  optic/o- *lenses; properties of light*
		  -al *pertaining to*

punch biopsy	Special forceps are used to grasp part of the tumor. As the forceps closes, it punches out a small, cylindrical tissue specimen. Multiple punch biopsies can be taken at one time.	
sentinel node biopsy	The sentinel lymph node, the first lymph node that receives drainage from the site of the primary tumor, is removed and examined.	**sentinel** (SEN-tih-nal)

stereotactic biopsy	Uses a CT scan to pinpoint the location of the tumor in three dimensions and guide the biopsy needle	**stereotactic** (STAIR-ee-oh-TAK-tik)
		  stere/o- *three dimensions*
		  tact/o- *touch*
		  -ic *pertaining to*

vacuum-assisted biopsy	A probe with a cutting device is inserted through the skin and rotated around to take multiple specimens. The specimens are then suctioned out.	
debulking	Procedure to excise (remove) part of a bulky, cancerous tumor. This reduces the size of the tumor and makes the patient more comfortable or leaves a smaller tumor that can be treated with chemotherapy or radiation therapy.	**debulk** (dee-BULK)

***en bloc* resection**	Procedure to excise (remove) a cancerous tumor and all surrounding tissues, which are removed as one block of tissue	***en bloc*** (en BLAWK)
		
		resection (ree-SEK-shun)
		  resect/o- *cut out; remove*
		  -ion *action; condition*

endoscopy	Procedure that uses a fiberoptic endoscope to examine a body cavity for signs of abnormal tissues or tumors. Grasping and cutting instruments are inserted through the endoscope to perform a biopsy. An optical biopsy can also be done at the same time.	**endoscopy** (en-DAW-skoh-pee)
		  endo- *innermost; within*
		  -scopy *process of using an instrument to examine*
		The ending -*scopy* contains the combining form *scop/o-* and the one-letter suffix -*y*.

excision of a tumor	Procedure to excise (remove) all or part of a cancerous tumor. In a wide excision, the tumor plus a wide margin of normal tissue around it is excised.	**excision** (ek-SIH-zhun)
		  excis/o- *cut out*
		  -ion *action; condition*

exenteration	Procedure to excise (remove) a cancerous tumor as well as all nearby organs. It is used to treat cancer that has metastasized throughout the abdominopelvic cavity.	**exenteration** (eks-EN-ter-AA-shun)
		  ex- *away from; out*
		  enter/o- *intestine*
		  -ation *being; having; process*

exploratory laparotomy	Procedure in which an abdominal incision is performed to widely open and explore the abdominopelvic cavity.	**exploratory** (eks-PLOR-ah-TOR-ee)
		  explorat/o- *search out*
		  -ory *having the function of*
		
		laparotomy (LAP-ar-AW-toh-mee)
		  lapar/o- *abdomen*
		  -tomy *process of cutting; process of making an incision*

Word or Phrase	Description	Pronunciation/Word Parts

insertion of a catheter or device to administer chemotherapy drugs	Procedure in which a **central venous catheter** (Broviac, Hickman, or Groshong catheter) is tunneled through the subcutaneous tissue in the upper chest. It is inserted into a large vein and advanced until its tip is positioned in the superior vena cava. The external end of the catheter is capped except when a chemotherapy drug is administered. An **intra-arterial catheter** is implanted in a main artery that brings blood to the organ where the cancerous tumor is located. A pump is also implanted under the skin or an externally worn portable infusion pump is used to administer regular doses of the chemotherapy drug. In **transarterial chemoembolization (TACE)**, a catheter is threaded through the femoral artery, aorta, and into the hepatic artery to deliver a one-time dose of chemotherapy to a cancerous tumor in the liver. After the drug is injected, a substance is added to block the flow of blood and keep the drug concentrated at the site of the cancerous tumor. An **intraperitoneal catheter** is inserted into the abdominopelvic cavity with a capped end on the surface of the body. The chemotherapy drug is injected into the peritoneal fluid and comes in contact with the surfaces of all the organs in the abdominopelvic cavity. An **implantable port** is a metal or plastic reservoir that is placed in a pocket in the subcutaneous tissue. The port is attached to a catheter in the superior vena cava. The chemotherapy drug is given by inserting a needle through the overlying skin and injecting the drug into the reservoir where it is released into the blood. An Ommaya reservoir is placed beneath the scalp with a connecting catheter placed in a ventricle in the brain, and the cerebrospinal fluid is used to circulate the chemotherapy drug. An **implantable wafer** is a dissolvable disk that contains a chemotherapy drug. It is surgically implanted in the area where a tumor has been excised.	**venous** (VEE-nus)
		  ven/o- *vein*
		  -ous *pertaining to*
		
		intra-arterial (IN-trah-ar-TEER-ee-al)
		  intra- *within*
		  arteri/o- *artery*
		  -al *pertaining to*
		
		transarterial (TRANS-ar-TEER-ee-al)
		  trans- *across; through*
		  arteri/o- *artery*
		  -al *pertaining to*
		
		chemoembolization
		(KEE-moh-EM-bol-ih-ZAY-shun)
		  chem/o- *chemical; drug*
		  embol/o- *embolus; occluding plug*
		  -ization *process of creating; process of inserting; process of making*
		
		intraperitoneal
		(IN-trah-PAIR-ih-toh-NEE-al)
		  intra- *within*
		  peritone/o- *peritoneum*
		  -al *pertaining to*
		
		implantable (im-PLANT-ah-bl)
		  implant/o- *placed within*
		  -able *able to be*
		
		port (PORT)

lumpectomy	Procedure to excise (remove) a small cancerous tumor without taking any surrounding tissue	**lumpectomy** (lump-EK-toh-mee) *Lumpectomy* is a combination of the English word *lump* and the suffix *-ectomy* (surgical removal).

lymph node dissection	Procedure to separate (dissect) lymph nodes from tissue and remove several or all of the lymph nodes in a lymph node chain during extensive cancer surgery. Involved lymph nodes represent metastases of the cancer from its original site.	**dissection** (dy-SEK-shun)
		  dissect/o- *cut apart*
		  -ion *action; condition*

percutaneous radiofrequency ablation	Procedure in which a needle electrode is placed through the skin into a small cancerous tumor (less than 2 inches in diameter). High-frequency radiowaves (similar to microwaves) heat and kill the cancerous cells.	**percutaneous**
		(PER-kyoo-TAY-nee-us)
		  per- *through; throughout*
		  cutane/o- *skin*
		  -ous *pertaining to*
		
		ablation (ah-BLAY-shun)
		  ablat/o- *destroy; take away*
		  -ion *action; condition*

radical resection	Procedure to excise (remove) a cancerous tumor, as well as all nearby lymph nodes, soft tissue, muscle, and even bone	**radical** (RAD-ih-kal)
		  radic/o- *root and all parts*
		  -al *pertaining to*

Radiation Therapy

Word or Phrase	Description	Pronunciation/Word Parts
brachytherapy	Category of radiation therapy that includes internal, interstitial, and intracavitary radiotherapy.	**brachytherapy** (BRAK-ee-THAIR-ah-pee) **brachy-** *short* **-therapy** *treatment* The ending -*therapy* contains the combining form *therap/o-* and the one-letter suffix -*y*.
internal radiotherapy	In **internal radiotherapy**, a radioactive substance (such as cesium, iridium, iodine, phosphorus, or palladium) that emits radiation is implanted near the cancerous tumor.	**internal** (in-TER-nal) **intern/o-** *inside* **-al** *pertaining to*
		radiotherapy (RAY-dee-oh-THAIR-ah-pee) **radi/o-** *forearm bone; radiation; x-rays* **-therapy** *treatment*
interstitial radiotherapy	In **interstitial radiotherapy**, radioactive implants (needles, wires, capsules, or pellets, which are known as *seeds*) are inserted into the tumor or into the tissue around the cancerous tumor.	**interstitial** (IN-ter-STIH-shal) **interstiti/o-** *spaces within tissue* **-al** *pertaining to*
intracavitary radiotherapy	In **intracavitary radiotherapy**, radioactive implants are inserted into a body cavity near the cancerous tumor.	**intracavitary** (IN-trah-KAV-ih-TAIR-ee) **intra-** *within* **cavit/o-** *hollow space* **-ary** *pertaining to*
fractionation	The total dose of external beam radiation is divided into smaller doses (fractions of the total dose) that are given each day to decrease the occurrence of side effects.	**fractionation** (FRAK-shun-AA-shun)
radiotherapy	Procedure that uses one of several types of **radiation** to disrupt the DNA in cancer cells. The radiation is in the form of waves (x-rays or gamma rays) or particles (electrons, neutrons, or protons). Radiotherapy is used to treat solid tumors, as well as leukemia and lymphoma, by radiating the bone marrow. Radiotherapy can be delivered from outside the body (conformal, external beam, or intravenous radiotherapy) or as implants inside the body (brachytherapy). Cancerous tumors that are readily destroyed by radiation therapy are said to be **radiosensitive**. Cancerous tumors that are not affected by radiation therapy are **radioresistant**.	**radiotherapy** (RAY-dee-oh-THAIR-ah-pee) **radi/o-** *forearm bone; radiation; x-rays* **-therapy** *treatment* Select the correct combining form meaning to get the definition of *radiotherapy*: treatment (using) radiation.
		radiation (RAY-dee-AA-shun) **radi/o-** *forearm bone; radiation; x-rays* **-ation** *being; having; process*
		radiosensitive (RAY-dee-oh-SEN-sih-tiv) **radi/o-** *forearm bone; radiation; x-rays* **sensit/o-** *affected by; sensitive to* **-ive** *pertaining to*
		radioresistant (RAY-dee-OH-ree-ZIS-tant) **radi/o-** *forearm bone; radiation; x-rays* **resist/o-** *withstand the effect of* **-ant** *pertaining to*

Word or Phrase	Description	Pronunciation/Word Parts
conformal radiotherapy	Uses a computer to map the location of the tumor and create a three-dimensional image of the tumor. The external beam radiation is then matched to conform to the exact shape of the tumor to protect nearby vital organs.	**conformal** (con-FOR-mal) **conform/o-** *having the same angle; having the same scale* **-al** *pertaining to*
external beam radiotherapy	Beams of radiation are generated by a machine outside the body and directed at the site of a cancerous tumor inside the body (see Figure 18-16 ■). Linear accelerators are used to increase the energy of the radiation so that it can penetrate more deeply into the body.	**external** (eks-TER-nal) **extern/o-** *outside* **-al** *pertaining to*

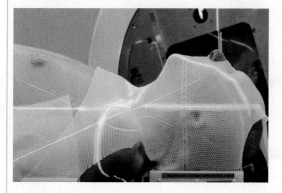

FIGURE 18-16 ■ External beam radiotherapy.
This patient is being prepared to receive external radiation therapy. The colored lines of light help the radiology technician correctly align the beam of radiation to treat this patient's throat cancer. The mesh mask helps keep the patient's head from moving from that position. Not all cancerous tumors can be treated with radiation therapy.
Source: Dr. P. Marazzi/Science Source

Word or Phrase	Description	Pronunciation/Word Parts
intravenous radiotherapy	Radioactive iodine is given intravenously. It concentrates in the thyroid gland and releases radiation to kill cancerous cells of the thyroid gland.	**intravenous** (IN-trah-VEE-nus) **intra-** *within* **ven/o-** *vein* **-ous** *pertaining to*

Drugs

These drug categories and drugs are used to treat cancer. The most common generic and trade name drugs in each category are listed.

Category	Indication	Examples	Pronunciation/Word Parts
alkylating chemotherapy drugs	Break DNA strands in the cancerous cell by substituting an alkyl group for a hydrogen molecule in the DNA	busulfan (Myleran), carmustine (Gliadel), chlorambucil (Leukeran), estramustine (Emcyt)	**alkylating** (AL-kih-LAY-ting)
antiemetic drugs	Not chemotherapy drugs. These drugs are used to treat the nausea and vomiting that are common side effects of chemotherapy.	dolasetron (Anzemet), dronabinol (Marinol), nabilone (Cesamet)	**antiemetic** (AN-tee-eh-MET-ik) **anti-** *against* **emet/o-** *vomiting* **-ic** *pertaining to*
antimetabolite chemotherapy drugs	Take the place of an important metabolite needed to build DNA, or they block an enzyme that produces an important metabolite. These drugs target cancerous cells that have a high rate of cell division.	capecitabine (Xeloda), fludarabine (Fludara), fluorouracil (5-FU, Adrucil), gemcitabine (Gemzar), methotrexate (Trexall)	**antimetabolite** (AN-tee-meh-TAB-oh-lite) **anti-** *against* **metabol/o-** *change; transformation* **-ite** *thing that pertains to*

Category	Indication	Examples	Pronunciation/Word Parts
chemotherapy antibiotic drugs	Inhibit the production of DNA and RNA, and this keeps the cancerous cell from dividing	bleomycin, doxorubicin (Adriamycin), epirubicin (Ellence)	**chemotherapy** (KEE-moh-THAIR-ah-pee) **chem/o-** *chemical; drug* **-therapy** *treatment*
			antibiotic (AN-tee-by-AW-tik) **anti-** *against* **bi/o-** *life; living organism; living tissue* **-tic** *pertaining to*

> **DID YOU KNOW?**
> Chemotherapy antibiotic drugs are not used to treat bacterial infections like regular antibiotic drugs are. Regular antibiotic drugs act on the cell wall of bacteria. Human cells have a cell membrane, not a cell wall. Chemotherapy antibiotic drugs affect rapidly dividing human cells, whether they are cancerous or normal.

Category	Indication	Examples	Pronunciation/Word Parts
chemotherapy enzyme drugs	Break down the amino acid asparagine. Normal body cells can synthesize their own supply of asparagine, but cancerous cells cannot.	asparaginase (Elspar), pegasparagase (Oncaspar)	

CLINICAL CONNECTIONS

Pharmacology. Chemotherapy protocols use a combination of several different chemotherapy drugs that are administered together. This increases their effectiveness against cancerous cells while minimizing the side effects caused by large doses of just one drug. A **protocol** is a standardized written plan of treatment for a particular type of cancer. A protocol details which chemotherapy drugs should be given, in what order they should be given, and at what doses. Protocols are named by combining the first letter of each drug name. For example, the ABVD chemotherapy protocol for treating Hodgkin's lymphoma consists of the chemotherapy drugs Adriamycin, bleomycin, vinblastine, and dacarbazine.

protocol (PROH-toh-kawl)

Adjuvant therapy is the use of chemotherapy drugs after another type of therapy (surgery, radiation therapy) has been used as the primary treatment.

adjuvant (AD-joo-vant) **adjuv/o-** *giving assistance; giving help* **-ant** *pertaining to*

Category	Indication	Examples	Pronunciation/Word Parts
hormonal chemotherapy drugs	Produce an opposite hormonal environment from the one that the cancer needs to reproduce. For example, estrogen (a female hormone drug) is given to men with prostate cancer.	anastrozole (Arimidex), goserelin (Zoladex), letrozole (Femara), leuprolide (Eligard, Lupron), megestrol (Megace), tamoxifen	**hormonal** (hor-MOH-nal) **hormon/o-** *hormone* **-al** *pertaining to*
mitosis inhibitor chemotherapy drugs	Cause DNA strands in the cancerous cell to break during the early stages of cell division (mitosis)	etoposide (Toposar), irinotecan (Camptosar), paclitaxel (Abraxane), topotecan (Hycamtin), vinblastine (Velban)	**inhibitor** (in-HIB-ih-tor) **inhibit/o-** *block; hold back* **-or** *person who does; person who produces; thing that does; thing that produces*

Category	Indication	Examples	Pronunciation/Word Parts
monoclonal antibody chemotherapy drugs	Bind to specific antigens on the surface of a cancerous cell and destroy the cell. Monoclonal antibodies are created using recombinant DNA technology. A human antibody is modified so that it will bind to a specific antigen on a cancerous cell.	alemtuzumab (Campath), trastuzumab (Herceptin)	**monoclonal** (MAW-noh-KLOH-nal) **mon/o-** *one; single* **clon/o-** *identical group derived from one; rapid contracting and relaxing* **-al** *pertaining to* **antibody** (AN-tih-BAW-dee) *Antibody* is a combination of the prefix *anti-* (against) and the English word *body* (structure or thing).
platinum chemotherapy drugs	Create crosslinks in the DNA strands that prevent the cancerous cell from dividing. These drugs actually contain the precious metal platinum.	carboplatin (Paraplatin), cisplatin	**platinum** (PLAT-ih-num)

Abbreviations

5-HIAA	5-hydroxyindoleacetic acid	**DNA**	deoxyribonucleic acid
AFP	alpha fetoprotein	**ER**	estrogen receptor
ALL	acute lymphocytic leukemia	**FIGO**	Federation Internationale de Gynécologie et Obstétrique scoring system
AML	acute myelogenous leukemia	**HCG, hCG**	human chorionic gonadotropin
BMT	bone marrow transplantation	**HER**	human epidermal (growth factor) receptor (2)
BRCA	breast cancer (gene)	**mets**	metastases (short form)
BX, Bx	biopsy	**MRI**	magnetic resonance imaging
Ca	cancer; carcinoma (pronounced "c-a")	**NK**	natural killer (cell)
CAT	computerized axial tomography	**PICC**	peripherally inserted central catheter
CEA	carcinoembryonic antigen	**PR**	progesterone receptor
chemo	chemotherapy (short form)	**PSA**	prostate-specific antigen
CIN	cervical intraepithelial neoplasia	**RNA**	ribonucleic acid
CIS	carcinoma *in situ*	**TACE**	transarterial chemoembolization
CLL	chronic lymphocytic leukemia	**TNF**	tumor necrosis factor
CML	chronic myelogenous leukemia	**TNM**	tumor, nodes, metastases
CRT	certified radiation therapist	**VMA**	vanillylmandelic acid
CT	computerized tomography		
CTR	certified tumor registrar		

WORD ALERT

Abbreviations

Abbreviations are commonly used in all types of medical documents; however, they can mean different things to different people and their meanings can be misinterpreted. Always verify the meaning of an abbreviation.

Ca means *cancer* or *carcinoma*, but it also means *calcium*.

ER means *estrogen receptor,* but it also means *emergency room*.

Mets is a short form for *metastases,* but it also is a unit of measurement that is used during cardiac treadmill stress tests to measure metabolic rate and oxygen consumption.

IT'S GREEK TO ME!

Did you notice that some words have two different combining forms? Combining forms from both Greek and Latin remain a part of medical language today.

Word	Greek	Latin	Medical Word Examples
cancer	carcin/o-	cancer/o-	carcinogen, cancerous
cell	cyt/o-	cellul/o-	lymphocytic, cellular
embryonic or immature	blast/o-	germin/o-	neuroblastoma, dysgerminoma
	embryon/o-		embryonal cell carcinoma
nucleus	kary/o-	nucle/o-	karyotype, nuclear

CAREER FOCUS

Meet Shah, a surgical assistant

"I'm a surgical assistant. I help the doctor from the beginnning to the end of the surgery. The very best part is assisting during cesarean sections. I like that part because sometimes there's a really sick baby or mom and, after the cesarean section, the baby is okay and the mom is okay. For a cesarean section, we have 50 different instruments. Each doctor uses different ways and different instruments. I keep track of the instruments and purchase new instruments."

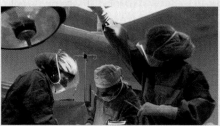

Source: Pearson Education

Surgical assistants are allied health professionals who assist surgeons in the operating room. They position and drape the patient and prepare the patient's surgical site by shaving and prepping the skin. Using sterile technique, they assist the surgeon during the operation by holding retractors, clamping or cutting tissues, and placing sutures.

Medical oncologists are physicians who specialize in treating patients with cancer. After the patient's cancer has been diagnosed, a medical oncologist assigns a grade and stage to the cancer and prescribes chemotherapy, radiation therapy, surgery, or a combination of all three, depending on the type of cancer and how advanced it is. Medical oncologists calculate the dose of the chemotherapy drugs based on the patient's body weight.

Radiation oncologists are physicians who have received additional training in using radiation therapy to treat cancer. They select the type of radiation and the most effective radiation technique for the type of cancer. They calculate the total dose of radiation to be given and then divide the dose into fractional amounts to be given each week.

surgical (SER-jih-kal)
  surg/o- *operative procedure*
  -ical *pertaining to*

medical (MED-ih-kal)
  medic/o- *medicine; physician*
  -al *pertaining to*

oncologist (ong-KAW-loh-jist)
  onc/o- *mass; tumor*
  log/o- *study of; word*
  -ist *person who specializes in; thing that specializes in*

radiation (RAY-dee-AA-shun)
  radi/o- *forearm bone; radiation; x-rays*
  -ation *being; having; process*

MyMedicalTerminologyLab™ To see Shah's complete video profile, log into MyMedicalTerminologyLab and navigate to the Multimedia Library for Chapter 18. Check the Video box, and then click the Career Focus - Surgical Technician link.

MULTIPLE COMBINING FORMS AND SUFFIX EXERCISE

Read the definition of the medical word. Select the correct suffix and combining forms. Then build the medical word and write it on the line. Be sure to check your spelling. The first one has been done for you.

SUFFIX LIST	COMBINING FORM LIST	
-ant (pertaining to)	aden/o- (gland)	onc/o- (mass; tumor)
-ery (process)	angi/o- (blood vessel; lymphatic vessel)	oste/o- (bone)
-graphy (process of recording)	blast/o- (embryonic; immature)	radi/o- (forearm bone; radiation; x-rays)
-ist (person who specializes in)	carcin/o- (cancer)	resist/o- (withstand the effect of)
-oma (mass; tumor)	chondr/o- (cartilage)	retin/o- (retina of the eye)
-pathy (disease)	cry/o- (cold)	sarc/o- (connective tissue)
	hepat/o- (liver)	surg/o- (operative procedure)
	lip/o- (fat; lipid)	
	log/o- (study of; word)	
	lymph/o- (lymph; lymphatic system)	
	my/o- (muscle)	
	nephr/o- (kidney; nephron)	

Definition of the Medical Word

Build the Medical Word

1. Tumor (of the) liver (with) immature (cells)   hepatoblastoma

2. Process of recording (the) lymph and lymphatic vessels

3. Tumor (of) fat (and) connective tissue

4. Tumor (of the) kidney (that has) embryonic, immature (cells)

5. Process (of using) cold (to kill cancer during an) operative procedure

6. Tumor (of the) muscle (and) connective tissue

7. Disease (of the) lymph gland

8. Tumor (of a) gland (that contains) cancer

9. Tumor (of the) retina of the eye (that has) embryonic, immature (cells)

10. Pertaining to (a cancer that is treated with) radiation (but) withstands the effect of (it)

11. Tumor (of the) cartilage (and) connective tissue

12. Tumor (of) bone (and) connective tissue

13. Person who specializes in tumors (and the) study of (them)

18.7A Spell Medical Words

HEARING MEDICAL WORDS EXERCISE

You hear someone speaking the medical words given below. Read each pronunciation and then write the medical word it represents. Be sure to check your spelling. The first one has been done for you.

1. AD-eh-noh-KAR-sih-NOH-mah   *adenocarcinoma*
2. KEE-moh-THAIR-ah-pee   _____
3. KRY-oh-SER-jer-ee   _____
4. HAWJ-kinz lim-FOH-mah   _____
5. LIM-fad-eh-NAW-pah-thee   _____

6. kar-SIN-oh-jen   _____
7. MET-ah-STAT-ik   _____
8. NEE-oh-plazm   _____
9. ong-KAW-loh-jist   _____
10. AW-stee-OH-sar-KOH-mah   _____

18.7B Pronounce Medical Words

PRONUNCIATION EXERCISE

Read the medical word and the syllables in its pronunciation. Circle the primary (main) accented syllable. The first one has been done for you.

1. cancer (ⓚⓐⓝ-ser)
2. angiosarcoma (an-jee-oh-sar-koh-mah)
3. benign (bee-nine)
4. biopsy (by-awp-see)
5. carcinogen (kar-sin-oh-jen)
6. carcinoma (kar-sih-noh-mah)
7. dysplasia (dis-play-zha)
8. genetic (jeh-net-ik)
9. lumpectomy (lump-ek-toh-mee)
10. metastatic (met-ah-stat-ik)

18.8 Analyze Medical Reports

ELECTRONIC PATIENT RECORD #1

This contains three related reports: an Operative Report and two Pathology Reports. Read all three reports and answer the questions.

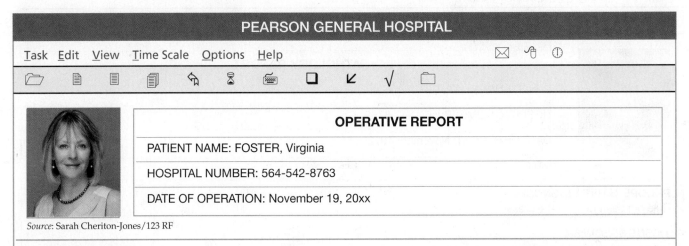

PEARSON GENERAL HOSPITAL

Task	Edit	View	Time Scale	Options	Help

OPERATIVE REPORT

PATIENT NAME: FOSTER, Virginia

HOSPITAL NUMBER: 564-542-8763

DATE OF OPERATION: November 19, 20xx

Source: Sarah Cheriton-Jones/123 RF

CLINICAL HISTORY

This is a 49-year-old white female with a right breast mass. She performs occasional self-examination of her breasts. While performing this procedure 2 days ago, she noted a lump in her right breast. She was seen by her primary care physician and referred for a mammogram. Mammography and subsequent ultrasound showed a solid rather than cystic mass. She was immediately scheduled for a biopsy. She has no family history of cancer.

PREOPERATIVE DIAGNOSIS

Rule out carcinoma of the breast.

OPERATION

Needle biopsy of right breast mass.

PLAN

This tissue specimen was sent to the Pathology Department for examination and diagnosis.

Alfredo P. Martinez, M.D.

Alfredo P. Martinez, M.D.

APM:rrg
D: 11/19/xx
T: 11/19/xx

ELECTRONIC PATIENT RECORD #2

PEARSON GENERAL HOSPITAL

Task   Edit   View   Time Scale   Options   Help

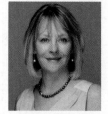

Source: Sarah Cheriton-Jones/123 RF

PATHOLOGY REPORT

PATIENT NAME: FOSTER, Virginia

HOSPITAL NUMBER: 564-542-8763

DATE OF REPORT: November 19, 20xx

PREOPERATIVE DIAGNOSIS
Rule out carcinoma of the breast.

TISSUE SPECIMEN
Needle biopsy, right breast mass.

GROSS DESCRIPTION
Specimen labeled "needle biopsy, right breast" is received in gauze. It consists of a single piece of tissue measuring 1.0 × 0.1 × 0.1 cm. It is cylindrical, tannish, soft, and pliable. It is submitted in its entirety for a frozen section.

MICROSCOPIC DESCRIPTION
Irregular nests of pleomorphic cells extend irregularly through the collagenous stroma. The margins of resection of the biopsy are not free of cancerous cells.

DIAGNOSIS
Infiltrating ductal carcinoma, poorly differentiated, grade 3.

Kevin V. Herzer, M.D.

Kevin V. Herzer, M.D.

KVH:smt
D: 11/19/xx
T: 11/19/xx

ELECTRONIC PATIENT RECORD #3

PEARSON GENERAL HOSPITAL

| Task | Edit | View | Time Scale | Options | Help | | ⊠ | ⌐⏚ | ① |

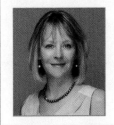

PATHOLOGY REPORT

PATIENT NAME:	FOSTER, Virginia
HOSPITAL NUMBER:	564-542-8763
DATE OF REPORT:	November 24, 20xx

CLINICAL HISTORY
This is a 49-year-old white female who presented to her primary care physician with a right breast mass. Subsequent needle biopsy on 11-19-xx revealed carcinoma of the breast. She was scheduled for a right mastectomy and axillary lymph node dissection.

PREOPERATIVE DIAGNOSIS
Carcinoma of the breast.

OPERATION
Right mastectomy and axillary lymph node dissection.

TISSUE SPECIMENS
Tumor and 28 axillary lymph nodes.

GROSS DESCRIPTION
The right breast tumor measures 3 cm at its greatest width and between 1.0 to 2.5 cm in length. A total of 28 right axillary lymph nodes of varying sizes are submitted.

MICROSCOPIC DESCRIPTION
Sections of the tumor reveal an invasive tumor composed of irregular nests of pleomorphic, anaplastic cells having prominent nucleoli. Some of the larger nests show central areas of necrosis. The tumor extends to an ulcerated skin surface. The margins of resection are free of tumor. A section of the nipple demonstrates tumor extending along the large lactiferous ducts. Ten axillary lymph nodes are positive for metastasis. The largest positive lymph node is 2.0 cm.

DIAGNOSIS
Infiltrating ductal carcinoma, poorly differentiated, grade 3. Metastatic carcinoma, involving 10 of 28 axillary lymph nodes.

Kevin V. Herzer, M.D.
_____
Kevin V. Herzer, M.D.

KVH:rrg
D: 11/24/xx
T: 11/24/xx

1. How did the patient discover her breast mass?

_____

2. What was the first test that the primary care physician ordered for her to have?

_____

3. A subsequent ultrasound showed what finding?

_____

4. What operative procedure was immediately scheduled and then performed?

_____

5. What was the preoperative diagnosis?

_____

6. Why is it important to know that the patient has no history of cancer in her family?

_____

7. What is a frozen section and how is it performed?

_____

8. What did the first pathology report say about the margins of resection of the biopsy?

_____

9. What was the Diagnosis on the first pathology report?

_____

10. Divide *carcinoma* into its two word parts and give the meaning of each word part.

    Word Part   **Meaning**

    _____   _____

    _____   _____

11. What second operation did the patient have done?

_____

12. Divide *dissection* into its two word parts and give the meaning of each word part.

    Word Part   **Meaning**

    _____   _____

    _____   _____

13. How many of the patient's axillary lymph nodes were positive for cancer?

_____

14. The patient had metastasis to the lymph nodes. If you wanted to use the adjective form of *metastasis,* you would say, "She had cancer that was _____."

15. What sentence in the second Pathology Report tells you that all of the tumor was removed?

_____

MyMedicalTerminologyLab™

MyMedicalTerminologyLab is a premium online homework management system that includes a host of features to help you study. Registered users will find:

- A multitude of quizzes and activities built within the MyLab platform

- Powerful tools that track and analyze your results—allowing you to create a personalized learning experience

- Videos and audio pronunciations to help enrich your progress

- Streaming lesson presentations (Guided Lectures) and self-paced learning modules

- A space where you and your instructor can check your progress and manage your assignments

Chapter 19
Radiology and Nuclear Medicine

Radiology (RAY-dee-AW-loh-jee) is the medical specialty that combines the study of anatomy and physiology, energy, and technology to create images of the internal structures and functions of the body for the purpose of diagnosis. Nuclear medicine (NOO-klee-ar MED-ih-sin) is the medical specialty that uses radioactive substances for this same purpose.

 ## Learning Outcomes

After you study this chapter, you should be able to

19.1 Describe radiology procedures that use x-rays.

19.2 Describe common x-ray projections (views) and patient positions.

19.3 Identify radiology procedures that use x-rays, x-rays with contrast, a magnetic field, sound waves, or an electron beam.

19.4 Identify nuclear medicine procedures that use gamma rays or positrons.

19.5 Give the meanings of word parts and abbreviations related to radiology and nuclear medicine.

19.6 Divide radiology and nuclear medicine words and build radiology and nuclear medicine words.

19.7 Spell and pronounce radiology and nuclear medicine words.

19.8 Analyze the medical content and meaning of radiology reports.

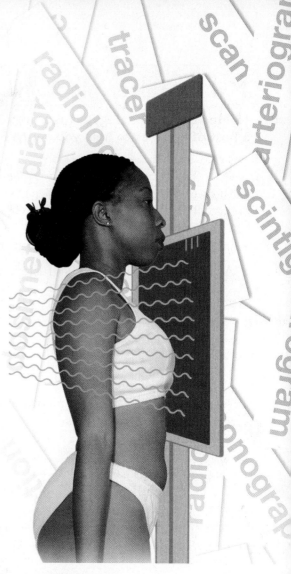

FIGURE 19-1 ■ Radiography.
Radiography is the most common subspecialty within the medical specialty of radiology.
Source: Pearson Education

Medical Language Key

To unlock the definition of a medical word, break it into word parts. Give the meaning of each word part. Put the meanings of the word parts in order, beginning with the meaning of the suffix, then the prefix (if present), then the combining form(s).

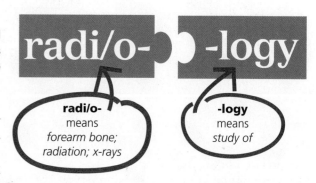

	Word Part	Word Part Meaning
Suffix	**-logy**	*study of*
Combining Form	**radi/o-**	*forearm bone; radiation; x-rays*

Radiology ▶ *Study of x-rays (and other imaging techniques).*

Anatomy and Physiology

The anatomy and physiology of the body can be seen in a whole new way in radiology and nuclear medicine, allowing us to view structures and functions within the body that are otherwise only accessible during surgery. Radiology is the medical specialty that uses x-rays, x-rays and contrast, a magnetic field, sound waves, or an electron beam to produce images (see Figure 19-1 ■). It includes the subspecialties of radiography, fluoroscopy, mammography, bone density testing, computerized axial tomography, magnetic resonance imaging, ultrasonography, and electron beam tomography. Nuclear medicine is the medical specialty that uses radioactive substances to produce images. All of these procedures are performed in the radiology and nuclear medicine department of a hospital or in an outpatient facility.

Diagnostic imaging (or medical imaging) includes radiology and nuclear medicine, but also includes medical photography, microscopic imaging of pathology tissue specimens, and other types of imaging.

Radiology

Radiography

Radiography is the most common subspecialty of radiology. Radiography uses x-rays to produce a diagnostic image. **X-rays** are a form of invisible **radiation**. They are produced when a positively charged metal plate inside a vacuum tube is bombarded with a stream of electrons. X-rays have a very short wavelength and contain so much energy that they are able to pass through the body.

During radiography (also known as **roentgenography**), the patient is placed between the x-ray machine and a large, flat, silver x-ray plate. X-ray beams travel through the patient's body to the x-ray plate (see Figure 19-2 ■). The image is in various shades of black, white, and gray that relate to the density of the various tissues. For example, air (in a body cavity or the lungs) has a low density, and x-rays pass through it, creating a nearly black area on the x-ray image; areas of low density are said to be **radiolucent**. Bone or a body organ has a high density that absorbs x-rays, creating a white area on the x-ray image (see Figure 19-2); areas of high density are said to be **radiopaque**. Areas of intermediate density create various shades of gray.

Pronunciation/Word Parts

diagnostic (DY-ag-NAW-stik)
  dia- *complete; completely through*
  gnos/o- *knowledge*
  -tic *pertaining to*

radiography (RAY-dee-AW-grah-fee)
  radi/o- *forearm bone; radiation; x-rays*
  -graphy *process of recording*

x-ray (EKS-ray)

radiation (RAY-dee-AA-shun)
  radi/o- *forearm bone; radiation; x-rays*
  -ation *being; having; process*
Select the correct combining form meaning to get the definition of *radiation*: *having radiation or x-rays.*

roentgenography (RENT-gen-AW-grah-fee)
  roentgen/o- *radiation; x-rays*
  -graphy *process of recording*

radiolucent (RAY-dee-oh-LOO-sent)
  radi/o- *forearm bone; radiation; x-rays*
  luc/o- *clear*
  -ent *pertaining to*

radiopaque (RAY-doo-oh-PAYK)

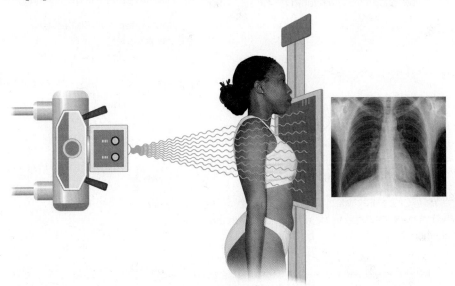

FIGURE 19-2 ■ PA chest x-ray.
This patient is having a PA (posteroanterior) chest x-ray. The x-ray machine projects a set of crossed lines onto the patient's back to help the technologist center the x-ray beam. The patient is asked to remain still so that the radiograph will not show motion artifact (a blurred image). The x-rays penetrate the patient's posterior chest. They exit through the patient's anterior chest, enter the x-ray plate, and create an image.
Source: Pearson Education; ksena32/Fotolia

The image on the x-ray plate is like the negative that is created when photographic film is exposed to light. The x-ray plate is then developed with chemicals, and the positive image is printed on flexible plastic film. The radiologist views or reads the x-ray film by placing it in front of a light box (see Figure 19-3 ■). The film image is a **radiograph**. See Table 19-1 ■ for other words and phrases related to radiography.

Obtaining radiographs of different parts of the body requires the patient to be placed in different positions. These positions are known as **projections** or **views**, and each position has a standardized, fixed orientation between the patient, the x-ray cassette, and the x-ray machine (see Table 19-2 ■).

Pronunciation/Word Parts

radiograph (RAY-dee-oh-GRAF)
  radi/o- *forearm bone; radiation; x-rays*
  -graph *instrument used to record*

projection (proh-JEK-shun)
  project/o- *orientation*
  -ion *action; condition*

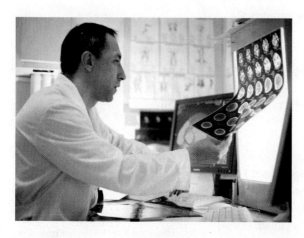

FIGURE 19-3 ■ Using a light box.
This radiologist is using a light box to view a series of images taken during a CT scan of the abdomen. The intense light of the light box illuminates fine details of the images.
Source: Moodboard Premium

Table 19-1 Radiography Words and Phrases		
Word or Phrase	**Description**	**Pronunciation/Word Parts**
film badge	A badge worn by all healthcare professionals who work in the radiology and nuclear medicine department. The badge contains a clear, unexposed piece of x-ray film that becomes progressively more opaque with cumulative exposure to radiation (x-rays, gamma rays from radioactive substances). Radiation exposure is measured in **rems**. **Dosimetry** is the process of measuring the amount of radiation exposure, as detected by a film badge and measured by a **dosimeter**.	**rem** (REM) *Rem* is an abbreviation for *roentgen-equivalent man.* **dosimetry** (doh-SIM-eh-tree) **dos/i-** *dose* **-metry** *process of measuring* **dosimeter** (doh-SIM-eh-ter) **dos/i-** *dose* **-meter** *instrument used to measure*
lead apron	Lead is an extremely dense substance that does not permit x-rays to pass through it. Lead aprons are used to shield parts of the patient's body that are not being x-rayed; they are also worn by the radiology department staff if they must be in the room with the patient while the procedure is being performed (see Figure 19-6). Otherwise, they stand behind a lead-lined shield that surrounds the x-ray control panel.	
plain film	Any radiograph that is taken without the use of a radiopaque contrast dye	
portable film	Radiograph taken at the patient's bedside on the nursing unit or in the emergency department when the patient cannot be transported to the radiology department	
scout film	Preliminary x-ray that is taken to provide an initial view of an area before a radiopaque contrast dye is administered	
x-ray cassette and bucky	A cassette is the case that holds the x-ray film. A bucky is an adjustable frame that is mounted on the wall, beneath the x-ray table, or is a mobile frame on wheels. It positions and holds the x-ray cassette.	

Table 19-2   Radiography Projections and Patient Positions

Projection	Description	Pronunciation/Word Parts
PA chest x-ray (posteroanterior)	The x-ray beam enters the patient's posterior upper back, exits through the anterior chest, and enters the x-ray plate. Position: The patient is in a standing position with the anterior chest next to the x-ray plate, and the x-ray machine by his/her back. This is the standard position and most common type of chest x-ray (see Figure 19-2).	**posteroanterior** (POHS-ter-OH-an-TEER-ee-or) **poster/o-** *back part* **anter/o-** *before; front part* **-ior** *pertaining to*
AP chest x-ray (anteroposterior)	The x-ray beam enters the patient's anterior chest, exits through the posterior upper back, and enters the x-ray plate. Position: The patient is in a lying position with the upper back next to the x-ray plate, and the x-ray machine is overhead. This position is most often used for portable chest x-rays taken at the patient's bedside.	**anteroposterior** (AN-ter-OH-pohs-TEER-ee-or) **anter/o-** *before; front part* **poster/o-** *back part* **-ior** *pertaining to*
lateral chest x-ray	The x-ray beam enters the patient's chest from the side and exits through the chest on the other side. Position: The patient is in a standing or lying position. In a left lateral x-ray, the left side of the chest is beside the x-ray plate, and the x-ray machine is on the other side. It is also known as a *lateral view* or *side view*.	**lateral** (LAT-er-al) **later/o-** *side* **-al** *pertaining to*
oblique x-ray	The x-ray beam enters the body from an oblique angle, midway between anterior and lateral. Position: The patient can be standing or lying.	**oblique** (oh-BLEEK)
cross-table lateral x-ray	The x-ray beam enters the patient's chest and abdomen from the side. Position: The patient is lying on his/her back on the x-ray table; the x-ray plate is on one side, and the x-ray machine is on the other. The x-ray beam travels across the x-ray table.	
lateral decubitus x-ray	The x-ray beam enters the patient's chest and abdomen from the side. Position: The patient is lying on his/her side on the x-ray table, the x-ray plate is beneath the x-ray table, and the x-ray machine is overhead. For a left lateral decubitus film, the patient is lying on the left side.	**decubitus** (dee-KYOO-bih-tus)
flat plate of the abdomen	The x-ray beam enters the patient's abdomen, exits through the lower back, and enters the x-ray plate. Position: The patient is lying on his/her back on the x-ray table, the x-ray plate is beneath the x-ray table, and the x-ray machine is overhead. *Flat plate* refers to the fact that the patient is lying down flat with the x-ray plate beneath.	
KUB	The x-ray beam enters the patient's chest and abdomen, exits through the back, and enters the x-ray plate. Position: The patient is lying on his/her back on the x-ray table, the x-ray plate is beneath the x-ray table, and the x-ray machine is overhead. *KUB* stands for *kidneys, ureters, and bladder,* the organs that are being x-rayed.	

Mammography

Mammography uses x-rays to create an image of the breast (see Figure 13-27). The breast is compressed to lessen its thickness and improve the quality of the image. Mammography is used to detect areas of microcalcifications, infection, cysts, and tumors, many of which cannot be felt on a breast examination. The image is a **mammogram** (see Figure 18-6). **Xeromammography** uses a special x-ray plate that is processed with dry chemicals, and the image, a **xeromammogram**, is printed on paper rather than on x-ray film.

Bone Density Testing

A bone density test uses x-rays to measure the bone mineral density (BMD) and determine if demineralization (from osteoporosis) has occurred. This is also known as **bone densitometry**. The heel or wrist bone can be tested, but the hip and spine bones give the most accurate results (see Figure 8-26).

There are two types of bone density tests: DEXA (or DXA) scan and quantitative computerized tomography (QCT). A **DEXA scan** (dual-energy x-ray absorptiometry) uses two (dual) x-ray beams with different energy levels to create a two-dimensional image. This scan can detect as little as a 1 percent loss of bone. **Quantitative computerized tomography (QCT)** uses x-rays and a CT scan (described in the next section) to create a three-dimensional image. QCT is able to take separate density measurements for the different areas within a bone.

Computerized Axial Tomography

Computerized axial tomography (CAT) or **computerized tomography (CT)** uses x-rays and a computer to create an image. Computerized tomography shows all types of tissues, but soft tissue structures are particularly clear (see Figures 11-12 and 16-13). The patient lies on a narrow bed inside the CT scanner. The x-ray emitter moves in a circle around the patient, while the x-ray detector moves along the opposite side of the circle. The paths of the x-ray emitter and detector are oriented along one of the imaginary planes of the body: coronal, sagittal, or transverse (see Figure 19-4 ■). The computer analyzes and creates a two-dimensional image or "slice" of that part of the body. Then the x-ray emitter and detector move a short distance (about 20 mm) proximally or distally and begin the process again to create another image or "slice." The radiologist views each of these individual images; together they make up a three-dimensional view of the area. Computerized

Pronunciation/Word Parts

mammography (mah-MAW-grah-fee)
    mamm/o- breast
    -graphy process of recording

mammogram (MAM-oh-gram)
    mamm/o- breast
    -gram picture; record

xeromammography
(ZEER-oh-mah-MAW-grah-fee)
The combining form xer/o- means dry.

densitometry (DEN-sih-TAW-meh-tree)
    densit/o- density
    -metry process of measuring

DEXA (DEK-sah)

quantitative (KWAN-tih-TAY-tiv)
    quantitat/o- amount; quantity
    -ive pertaining to

tomography (toh-MAW-grah-fee)
    tom/o- cut; layer; slice
    -graphy process of recording

axial (AK-see-al)
    axi/o- axis
    -al pertaining to

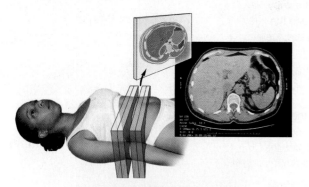

VENTRAL

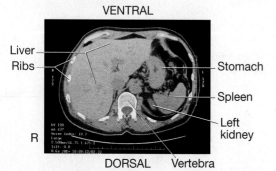

Liver
Ribs
Stomach
Spleen
Left kidney
R
DORSAL   Vertebra

FIGURE 19-4 ■ Computerized axial tomography (CAT) of the abdomen taken in the transverse plane.
The radiologist reads a CAT scan image as if he/she were standing at the feet of the patient who is lying in the scanner. This CAT scan image shows the liver on the left side, which is actually the patient's right side when viewed from his/her feet.
Source: Geoff Tompkinson/Science Source

tomography is also known as a scan because the machine scans (moves across) the body. A multidetector-row CT scanner (MDCT) has an area of x-ray detectors (not just a row), and it can quickly scan multiple "slices" simultaneously. A spiral CT scan moves the patient's bed through the scanner as the x-ray emitter rotates around the patient. This produces a spiral image; this procedure is 10 times faster than a regular CT scan.

An iodinated contrast dye can be injected intravenously or into a body cavity to produce an enhanced CT image. A CT scan that uses no contrast dye is said to be unenhanced. Often two sets of images are obtained, one set before contrast dye is given and another set after contrast dye is given. These are known as precontrast and postcontrast images.

When a CT scan is used to guide the insertion of a needle (for a biopsy), this is known as **interventional radiology**.

interventional (IN-ter-VEN-shun-al)
  inter- *between*
  vent/o- *coming*
  -ion *action; condition*
  -al *pertaining to*

CLINICAL CONNECTIONS

Obstetrics (Chapter 13). Pregnant women are generally advised to avoid x-rays. However, sometimes x-rays are necessary. Although an exposure of 5000 mrems has been shown to cause a risk of fetal deformity, most x-rays involve significantly less radiation, as shown below. The abbreviation *mrem* stands for *microrem* (one-thousandth of a rem).

dental x-ray	1 mrem	chest x-ray (two views)	8 mrems
mammography	2 mrems	CT scan	1,000 mrems

Radiography with Contrast

The details on an x-ray image can be enhanced by using barium contrast medium or an **iodinated contrast dye** to outline anatomical structures.

iodinated (EYE-oh-dih-NAY-ted)
  iodin/o- *iodine*
  -ated *composed of; pertaining to a condition*

Word or Phrase	Description	Pronunciation/Word Parts
angiography	Iodinated contrast dye is injected to outline a blood vessel. The x-ray image is an **angiogram**. In **digital subtraction angiography (DSA)**, two x-ray images are obtained, without contrast dye and then with contrast dye. A computer compares the two images and digitally "subtracts" the image of the soft tissues, bones, and muscles, leaving just the image of the blood vessels. In **rotational angiography**, the x-ray machine moves around the area to be examined, taking multiple x-rays after contrast dye has been injected. The computer creates a three-dimensional image that can be rotated and viewed from all angles. This is useful when arteries have a twisted path or when normal anatomy is distorted. In **arteriography**, contrast dye is injected into an artery to show blockage, narrowed areas, or aneurysms (see Figures 19-5 ■ and 5-17). The x-ray image is an **arteriogram**. **Aortography** uses contrast dye injected into the aorta, the largest artery. In **venography**, contrast dye is injected into a vein to show weakened valves and dilated walls. The x-ray image is a **venogram**.	**angiography** (AN-jee-AW-grah-fee) **angi/o-** *blood vessel; lymphatic vessel* **-graphy** *process of recording* **angiogram** (AN-jee-oh-GRAM) **angi/o-** *blood vessel; lymphatic vessel* **-gram** *picture; record* **arteriography** (ar-TEER-ee-AW-grah-fee) **arteri/o-** *artery* **-graphy** *process of recording* **arteriogram** (ar-TEER-ee-oh-GRAM) **arteri/o-** *artery* **-gram** *picture; record* **aortography** (AA-or-TAW-grah-fee) **aort/o-** *aorta* **-graphy** *process of recording* **venography** (vee-NAW-grah-fee) **ven/o-** *vein* **-graphy** *process of recording* **venogram** (VEE-noh-gram) **ven/o-** *vein* **-gram** *picture; record*

Word or Phrase	Description	Pronunciation/Word Parts

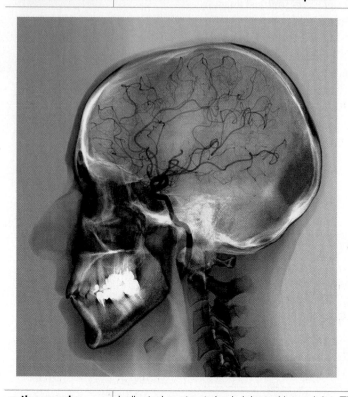

FIGURE 19-5 ■ Arteriogram of the cerebral arteries.
This procedure is also known as *cerebral angiography* or *carotid arteriography*. The injected dye outlines the carotid artery (coming up from the neck) and the many smaller branches of cerebral arteries within the cranial cavity.
Source: Zephyr/Science Source

Word or Phrase	Description	Pronunciation/Word Parts

arthrography	Iodinated contrast dye is injected into a joint. The dye outlines the bones, joint capsule, and soft tissue structures. The image is an **arthrogram**.	**arthrography** (ar-THRAW-grah-fee)
		  arthr/o- *joint*
		  -graphy *process of recording*
		
		arthrogram (AR-throh-gram)
		  arthr/o- *joint*
		  -gram *picture; record*

barium enema	Barium contrast medium is inserted into the rectum. The barium outlines the colon and rectum and shows tumors, polyps, or diverticula in the bowel wall (see Figure 3-24). For a **double contrast (air contrast) enema**, the barium is removed and air is instilled as a second contrast. Fluoroscopy and individual radiographs are done to document the procedure.	**barium** (BAIR-ee-um) **enema** (EN-eh-mah)

cholangiography, intravenous (IVC)	Iodinated contrast dye is injected intravenously. The dye travels through the blood to the liver and is then excreted with bile into the gallbladder. It outlines the gallbladder and bile ducts and shows thickening of the gallbladder wall and gallstones. The x-ray image is a **cholangiogram**. In **endoscopic retrograde cholangiopancreatography**, an endoscope is passed through the mouth and into the duodenum. A catheter is passed through the endoscope, and contrast dye is injected to visualize the pancreatic duct and the common bile duct (see Figure 3-25).	**cholangiography**
		(KOH-lan-jee-AW-grah-fee)
		  cholangi/o- *bile duct*
		  -graphy *process of recording*
		
		intravenous (IN-trah-VEE-nus)
		  intra- *within*
		  ven/o- *vein*
		  -ous *pertaining to*
		
		cholangiogram
		(koh-LAN-jee-oh-GRAM)
		  cholangi/o- *bile duct*
		  -gram *picture; record*
		
		cholangiopancreatography (koh-LAN-jee-oh-PAN-kree-ah-TAW-grah-fee)
		  cholangi/o- *bile duct*
		  pancreat/o- *pancreas*
		  -graphy *process of recording*

Word or Phrase	Description	Pronunciation/Word Parts
cholecystography, oral (OCG)	Iodinated contrast dye in a tablet form is taken orally. After the tablet dissolves in the small intestine, the dye enters the blood, is processed by the liver, and then excreted with bile into the gallbladder. It outlines the gallbladder and shows thickening of the gallbladder wall and gallstones. The x-ray image is a **cholecystogram**.	**cholecystography** (KOH-lee-sis-TAW-grah-fee) **cholecyst/o-** *gallbladder* **-graphy** *process of recording* **cholecystogram** (KOH-lee-SIS-toh-gram) **cholecyst/o-** *gallbladder* **-gram** *picture; record*
hysterosalpingography	Iodinated contrast dye is inserted through a catheter that was passed through the vagina and into the uterus. The dye outlines the cavity of the uterus and the uterine tubes and shows narrowing, scarring, and blockage of the tubes. The x-ray image is a **hysterosalpingogram**.	**hysterosalpingography** (HIS-ter-oh-SAL-ping-GAW-grah-fee) **hyster/o-** *uterus; womb* **salping/o-** *uterine tube* **-graphy** *process of recording* **hysterosalpingogram** (HIS-ter-OH-sal-PING-goh-GRAM) **hyster/o-** *uterus; womb* **salping/o-** *uterine tube* **-gram** *picture; record*
lymphangiography	Iodinated contrast dye is injected into a lymphatic vessel. The dye outlines the vessel and shows enlarged lymph nodes, lymphomas (tumors), and blockages of lymphatic drainage. The x-ray image is a **lymphangiogram**.	**lymphangiography** (lim-FAN-jee-AW-grah-fee) **lymph/o-** *lymph; lymphatic system* **angi/o-** *blood vessel; lymphatic vessel* **-graphy** *process of recording* **lymphangiogram** (lim-FAN-jee-oh-GRAM) **lymph/o-** *lymph; lymphatic system* **angi/o-** *blood vessel; lymphatic vessel* **-gram** *picture; record*
myelography	Iodinated contrast dye is injected into the subarachnoid space between the L3 and L4 vertebrae. The dye outlines the spinal cavity, spinal nerves, nerve roots, intervertebral disks, and shows tumors and herniated disks. The x-ray image is a **myelogram**. Because a myelogram can have the side effect of a severe headache, a CT scan or MRI scan of the spine is often performed instead.	**myelography** (MY-eh-LAW-grah-fee) **myel/o-** *bone marrow; myelin; spinal cord* **-graphy** *process of recording* **myelogram** (MY-eh-loh-GRAM) **myel/o-** *bone marrow; myelin; spinal cord* **-gram** *picture; record*

Word or Phrase	Description	Pronunciation/Word Parts
pyelography	In **intravenous pyelography**, iodinated contrast dye is injected into a vein, circulates through the blood, and is excreted in the urine by the kidneys. It outlines the urinary tract and shows narrowing, blockage, and stones (see Figure 11-18). It is also known as **excretory urography**. In **retrograde pyelography**, a cystoscopy is performed, and iodinated contrast dye is injected through a catheter inserted through the urethra, bladder, and then into each ureter. The x-ray image is a **pyelogram** or **urogram**.	**pyelography** (PY-eh-LAW-grah-fee) **pyel/o-** *renal pelvis* **-graphy** *process of recording* **excretory** (EKS-kreh-TOR-ee) **excret/o-** *removing from the body* **-ory** *having the function of* **urography** (yoor-AW-grah-fee) **ur/o-** *urinary system; urine* **-graphy** *process of recording* **pyelogram** (PY-eh-loh-GRAM) **pyel/o-** *renal pelvis* **-gram** *picture; record* **urogram** (YOOR-oh-gram) **ur/o-** *urinary system; urine* **-gram** *picture; record*
upper gastrointestinal series (UGI)	Barium contrast medium as a liquid is swallowed. The barium outlines the esophagus and stomach to show ulcers and blockage. This is also known as a **barium swallow**. A **small-bowel follow-through** follows the barium as it outlines the small intestine. To evaluate a patient's ability to swallow, liquid barium is mixed with crackers and swallowed (a barium meal).	**gastrointestinal** (GAS-troh-in-TES-tih-nal) **gastr/o-** *stomach* **intestin/o-** *intestine* **-al** *pertaining to*

Radiography with Contrast and Fluoroscopy

Fluoroscopy uses continuous x-rays to capture the moving images of the internal organs as they occur. The x-rays pass through the patient's body to a fluorescent screen that transforms the x-rays into long wavelengths of light that the eye can see as they are displayed on a computer monitor. Fluoroscopy is used to follow the movement of iodinated contrast dye during a cardiac catheterization or angiography, and to follow barium contrast medium during an upper GI series (barium swallow) (see Figure 19-6 ■), a small-bowel follow-through, and other procedures. Individual x-ray images are taken

fluoroscopy (floor-AW-skoh-pee)
  fluor/o- *fluorescence*
  -scopy *process of using an instrument to examine*

cineradiography
(SIN-eh-RAY-dee-AW-grah-fee)
  cin/e- *movement*
  radi/o- *forearm bone; radiation; x-rays*
  -graphy *process of recording*

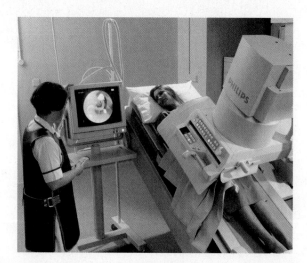

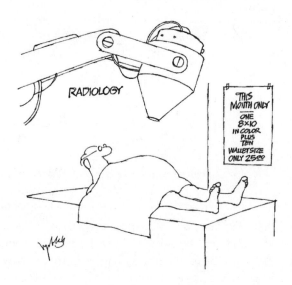

FIGURE 19-6 ■ Fluoroscopy.
This patient swallowed the contrast medium barium, and the tilted table allows the barium to flow through the stomach and intestine, coating and outlining them to make them visible during fluoroscopy. The radiologist has a hand-held device that allows her to create individual x-ray images from the continuously moving images on the computer screen. The radiologist is wearing a lead apron to protect her from exposure to x-rays.
Source: Hank Frentz/Shutterstock

to capture the most important aspects of the procedure. The entire fluoroscopy can be recorded digitally, a procedure known as **cineradiography**.

Magnetic Resonance Imaging

Magnetic resonance imaging (MRI) uses a scanner and a strong magnetic field (see Figure 19-7 ■) to align protons in the atoms of the patient's body. Then high-frequency radio-waves are sent through the patient's body. The protons absorb the radiowaves and emit signals. The signals, which vary according to the type of tissue, create an image. An MRI scan does not use x-rays so the patient is not exposed to any radiation. Like a CT scan, magnetic resonance imaging is a type of tomography that creates many individual "slice" images (see Figure 19-8 ■). Magnetic resonance imaging is the best procedure for showing soft tissues, blood vessels, intervertebral disks, muscles, nerves, organs, tumors, and areas of infection. **Gadolinium**, a metallic element that responds to a magnetic field, can be injected intravenously during magnetic resonance angiography (MRA) or into a body cavity to produce an enhanced MRI image. An unenhanced MRI uses no gadolinium. An open MRI is performed on a modified MRI scanner that is not enclosed on all sides. Open MRI is ideal for pediatric, older adult, claustrophobic, anxious, or extremely obese patients.

Pronunciation/Word Parts

magnetic (mag-NET-ik)
  magnet/o- *magnet*
  -ic *pertaining to*

gadolinium (GAD-oh-LIN-ee-um)

ultrasonography
(UL-trah-soh-NAW-grah-fee)
  ultra- *beyond; higher*
  son/o- *sound*
  -graphy *process of recording*

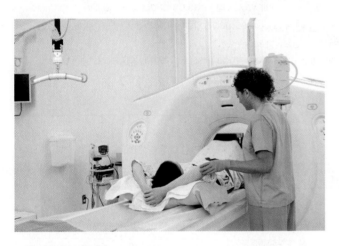

FIGURE 19-7 ■ MRI scan.
This radiologic technologist is positioning and reassuring the patient before the bed slides into the MRI scanner. During the scan, the technologist is in contact with the patient via an intercom inside the scanner.
Source: Trish23/Fotolia

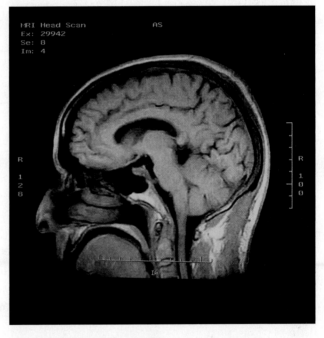

FIGURE 19-8 ■ MRI of the head.
This MRI image was created along the midsagittal plane that divides the right half from the left half of the head. This is just one of many thin "slices" that were individually imaged. The computer then merges the individual images into a three-dimensional image.
Source: CGinspiration/Shutterstock

Ultrasonography

Ultrasonography or **sonography** uses pulses of inaudible, ultra high-frequency sound waves to create an image. A handheld **ultrasound transducer** that emits sound waves is held against the skin over the organ or structure to be imaged (see Figure 5-25). A conducting gel on the skin optimizes transmission of the sound waves. The transducer is moved back and forth to view the organ or structure from different angles. Alternately, an **ultrasound probe** can be placed inside a body cavity. Sound waves from either a transducer or probe are reflected as echoes from the internal structures. The echoes are changed into electrical signals and analyzed by a computer. The strongest echoes produce the brightest areas on the ultrasound image. The ultrasound image is a **sonogram**. Ultrasonography can produce several different types of images (see Table 19-3 ■). Ultrasonography can also be used to guide the insertion of a needle for a biopsy or for amniocentesis (see Figure 13-26).

sonography (soh-NAW-grah-fee)
  son/o- *sound*
  -graphy *process of recording*

ultrasound (UL-trah-sound)

transducer (trans-DOO-ser)
  trans- *across; through*
  duc/o- *bring; move*
  -er *person who does; person who produces; thing that does; thing that produces*

sonogram (SAW-noh-gram)
  son/o- *sound*
  -gram *picture; record*

DID YOU KNOW?

Patients who undergo an MRI scan must sign a consent form that describes what types of metal items can or cannot be subjected to the magnetic field. You might be surprised to see which items are allowed and which are not.

Allowed Items

- Permanent metal dental work such as crowns are allowed because they will not detach, although they may produce artifact (an unwanted image) on the MRI image.
- Artificial metal or ceramic prostheses in joints and orthopedic hardware (screws, nails, plates, and rods).

Items Not Allowed

- All metal objects that are not permanently attached to the body. These include glasses, watches, jewelry, hairpins, metal false teeth, artificial limbs, and clothing with metal zippers, buttons, or snaps. These objects respond to the magnetic field and can be forcefully pulled into the scanner, causing damage to the scanner.
- Nose rings, lip rings, tongue studs, pierced earrings, and other piercings must be removed or they could be moved by the magnetic field, causing damage to the patient's tissues.
- Implanted devices such as pacemakers, pacing wires, some heart valves, aneurysm clips, cochlear implants, some penile implants, artificial eyes, and some intrauterine devices may be moved by the magnetic field, causing internal tissue damage.
- Hearing aids, some pacemakers, TENS units, and insulin pumps can have their working parts damaged by the magnetic field.
- Metal workers, gunshot victims, or military personnel with shrapnel injuries are presumed to have metal fragments in their tissues and should not undergo MRI scans.
- Transdermal patches that deliver heart, pain, contraceptive, or smoking cessation drugs must be removed because some contain a small metal wire that can cause burns to the skin.
- Metallic eye shadow may cause the eyelids to flutter as they are moved by the magnetic field.

Table 19-3 Types of Ultrasonography

Type	Description
Two-dimensional	Creates an image in various shades of gray. It is also known as **grayscale ultrasonography** or a **B scan**.
Three-dimensional	In addition to signals sent by the transducer or probe, a position sensor relays information that the computer uses to create an image in three dimensions. The computer also colorizes the image in shades of brown.
Four-dimensional	Creates a computer-colorized image that is continuously moving. The computer updates the ultrasound image on the screen as it receives new signals from the transducer or probe and position sensor. It is also known as **real-time ultrasonography**.

Ultrasonography is used to differentiate solid tumors and stones from fluid-filled cysts of the breast, gallbladder, kidney, ovary, or uterus (see Figure 11-19). It can be used to assess the internal structures of the eye. It can provide images of a fetus in the uterus (see Figure 13-28), and the fetal parts can be measured to estimate the gestational age and the mother's due date. Unlike many types of radiologic procedures, ultrasonography does not expose the patient to harmful radiation (see Table 19-4 ■).

ECHOCARDIOGRAPHY **Echocardiography** uses ultra high-frequency sound waves to show real-time, moving images of the heart during contraction and relaxation (see Figure 19-9 ■). The ultrasound image, which is viewed on a computer screen or as individual still images, is an **echocardiogram**. **Transesophageal echocardiography (TEE)** may be ordered when a standard echocardiogram cannot produce a good-quality image. During a TEE, the patient swallows an endoscope that contains a tiny sound wave–emitting transducer at its tip. The tip is positioned in the esophagus directly behind the heart.

Pronunciation/Word Parts

echocardiography
(EK-oh-KAR-dee-AW-grah-fee)
  ech/o- *echo of a sound wave*
  cardi/o- *heart*
  -graphy *process of recording*

echocardiogram
(EK-oh-KAR-dee-oh-GRAM)
  ech/o- *echo of a sound wave*
  cardi/o- *heart*
  -gram *picture; record*

transesophageal
(TRANS-eh-SAW-fah-JEE-al)
  trans- *across; through*
  esophag/o- *esophagus*
  -eal *pertaining to*

Table 19-4   Radiologic Procedures and Exposure to Radiation

Source	Radiologic Procedure	Exposure to Radiation
X-rays	Radiography (plain films or with contrast)	Yes
	Fluoroscopy	Yes
	Mammography, xeromammography	Yes
	Bone density testing	Yes
	Computerized tomography (CT scan)	Yes
Electron beam	Electron beam tomography (usually combined with CT scan)	Yes
Radiowaves and magnetic field	Magnetic resonance imaging (MRI scan)	No
Ultra high-frequency sound waves	Ultrasonography	No
	Echocardiography	No
	Doppler ultrasonography	No

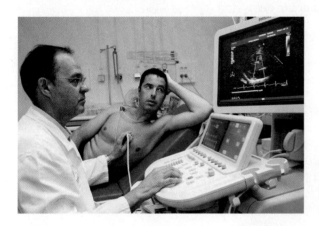

FIGURE 19-9 ■ Echocardiography.
This patient is having an echocardiography. The ultrasound technician is holding a transducer that produces sound waves. These bounce off the structures of the heart as echoes that the computer displays on the monitor screen.
Source: Philippe Garo/AP-HP Groupe hospitalier Pitié-Salpêtrière/Science Source

DOPPLER ULTRASONOGRAPHY   Doppler ultrasonography uses ultra high-frequency sound waves and Doppler technology to produce the audible sound of blood flowing through an artery. The transducer emits and then collects reflected sound waves. If the artery is patent, a loud "swish . . . swish . . . swish" will be heard as the blood is pumped through the artery. If the artery is blocked, little or no sound will be heard. Doppler technology is also used in automatic blood pressure machines that give a digital readout of the blood pressure and in fetal monitors that, when placed on the mother's abdomen, make the heartbeat of the fetus audible.

Color flow duplex ultrasonography combines a two-dimensional ultrasound with Doppler technology to create an image that shows anatomy as well as colors that correlate to the velocity, direction, and turbulence of the blood flow in that area. It is used to image the coronary arteries, carotid arteries, or arteries of the legs.

Electron Beam Tomography

Electron beam tomography (EBT) uses a beam of electrons and a computer to create an image. EBT is also known as a full body scan, although only the area from the shoulders to the upper legs is actually scanned. These scans are being marketed directly to consumers and do not need to be ordered by a physician. They are considered screening tests, not diagnostic tests. The Virtual Physical and the Virtual Colonoscopy use a spiral CT scan combined with an EBT scan to produce a detailed three-dimensional image. The Virtual Physical is able to reveal small areas of plaque in the coronary arteries, early signs of emphysema in the lungs, and early stages of cancer. The Virtual Colonoscopy produces results that are as reliable as those of a colonoscopy, but it costs only about one-third as much.

Pronunciation/Word Parts

Doppler (DAW-pler)

duplex (DOO-pleks)

electron (ee-LEK-tron)
 electr/o- *electricity*
 -on *structure; substance*

tomography (toh-MAW-grah-fee)
 tom/o- *cut; layer; slice*
 -graphy *process of recording*

Nuclear Medicine

Nuclear medicine is the medical specialty that uses **radioactive** substances (radionuclides) to create an image of the internal structures and function of the body. When a radioactive substance decays, it produces alpha particles, beta particles, gamma rays, positrons, or other subatomic particles that are a form of radiation. Radioactive substances that produce gamma rays or positrons are used for nuclear medicine imaging. *Note:* Radioactive substances that produce alpha and beta particles are used in radiation therapy (in the medical specialty of oncology) to destroy cancerous cells (see "Oncology," Chapter 18).

Radiopharmaceuticals are man-made or naturally occurring radioactive substances (radionuclides) that have been processed and measured so that they can be given as a drug dose. They are administered intravenously, except for radioactive gases, which are administered by inhalation. Radiopharmaceuticals are also known as **tracers** because their presence in the body can be traced by the gamma rays they produce. The radiopharmaceuticals used in nuclear medicine have short half-lives of a few hours to a few days. This means that the patient is exposed to a minimal amount of radiation. The length of time it takes for half of the atoms in a radioactive substance to decay and become stable (non-radioactive) is the **half-life**.

> **DID YOU KNOW?**
>
> In 1898, while working with uranium, Polish physicist Marie Curie and her husband, French physicist Pierre Curie, discovered the radioactive chemical element radium and coined the word *radioactivity*. They were awarded the Nobel Prize in physics, the first time a woman had won the Nobel Prize. Marie Curie's subsequent work with radium also earned her a Nobel Prize in chemistry, making her the first person to ever receive a Nobel Prize in two disciplines. The Curies often had severe radiation burns from handling radium or carrying it in their pockets. Marie Curie died in 1934, from leukemia or aplastic anemia, most likely from long-term exposure to radiation. Her oldest daughter, Irene Joliot-Curie, discovered how to produce radioactive elements artificially. She was awarded the Nobel Prize in chemistry 1 year after her mother's death.

Nuclear Medicine Procedures That Use Gamma Rays

Radiopharmaceutical drugs that emit gamma rays are listed in Table 19-5 ■.

After a radiopharmaceutical drug is administered, a gamma scintillation camera scans the area. When a gamma ray from the radioactive radiopharmaceutical drug enters the scintillation camera, it strikes a crystal structure, the crystal emits a flash of visible light (a photon), and a computer compiles the flashes of light into a two-dimensional image. This is known as **scintigraphy**. It is also known as a **scintiscan** because the scintillation camera moves back and forth (scanning) across the body. The image is a **scintigram**.

Areas of increased uptake on a scintigram are known as "hot spots," and areas of decreased uptake are known as "cold spots." When the blood flow (perfusion) to an organ is being studied, areas of decreased uptake are known as filling defects.

Bone scintigraphy is used to detect areas of increased uptake related to arthritis, fracture, osteomyelitis, cancerous tumors of the bone, or areas of bony metastasis.

Cholescintigraphy or a **HIDA scan** is used to detect areas of decreased uptake in the gallbladder that are related to cystic duct obstruction and acute cholecystitis. HIDA stands for hydroxyiminodiacetic acid, a molecule that carries the radiopharmaceutical drug to the liver.

Table 19-5 Radiopharmaceutical Drugs That Emit Gamma Rays		
Radiopharmaceutical	**Description**	**Pronunciation/Word Parts**
gallium-67	Intravenous drug used to detect inflammation, infection, and benign and cancerous tumors. Gallium is a soft, silvery metal that is a liquid at room temperature.	**gallium** (GAL-ee-um)
indium-111	Intravenous drug used to detect cancerous tumors. Indium-111 is combined with a hormone that is attracted to cancerous cells of the endocrine system, or it is combined with a monoclonal antibody that is attracted to cancerous cells of the ovary or colon. Indium is a soft, silvery metal.	**indium** (IN-dee-um)
iodine-123 and iodine-131	Intravenous drug used to image the thyroid gland. Iodine is a purple-black, shiny crystalline solid that is a trace element in the soil.	**iodine** (EYE-oh-dine)
krypton-81m	Inhaled gas used to image the lung. It is also used in krypton lasers in surgery. Krypton is a colorless, odorless gas that is present in trace amounts in the atmosphere.	**krypton** (KRIP-tawn)
technetium-99m	Intravenous drug used to image many different areas of the body. It is the most common radiopharmaceutical used in nuclear imaging. Technetium is a silvery gray metal.	**technetium** (tek-NEE-shee-um)
thallium-201	Intravenous drug used to image the heart. Thallium is a gray metal that is so soft it can be cut with a knife.	**thallium** (THAL-ee-um)
xenon-133	Inhaled gas used to image the lungs. Xenon is a colorless, odorless gas that is present in trace amounts in the atmosphere.	**xenon** (ZEE-nawn)

A liver-spleen scan is used to detect areas of decreased uptake that indicate non-functioning tissue due to inflammation, infection, benign tumors, or cancer in the liver or spleen.

A **MUGA (multiple-gated acquisition) scan** is used to detect how well the heart walls move as they contract. It also calculates the ejection fraction (how much blood the ventricle can pump out in one contraction). The ejection fraction is the most accurate predictor of overall heart function. The gamma camera is coordinated (gated) with the patient's EKG. This procedure is also known as a **radionuclide ventriculography (RNV)** or a **gated blood pool scan**, and the image is a **nuclear ventriculogram**. A **SPECT (single-photon emission computed tomography) scan** is a MUGA scan of the heart in which the gamma camera moves in a circle around the patient to create individual images as "slices" of the heart (tomography).

An **OncoScint scan** is used to detect areas of increased activity that are metastases from a cancerous tumor's primary site in the colon or ovary. OncoScint is the trade name for the combination of indium-111 and a monoclonal antibody that binds to receptors on those cancerous cells. A **ProstaScint scan** does the same thing for metastases from prostate cancer.

A thyroid scan is used to detect areas of increased activity that indicate a hyperfunctioning, benign thyroid nodule or goiter or decreased activity that indicate a cyst or cancerous tumor of the thyroid (see Figure 19-10 ■). It is also known as a radioactive iodine uptake (RAIU) and thyroid scan.

A **ventilation-perfusion scan (V/Q)** is a two-part test that uses two radio-active substances, one that is inhaled (to evaluate air flow and ventilation) and one that is given intravenously (to evaluate blood flow and perfusion of tissues). It is used to detect areas of decreased uptake that indicate poor air flow, pneumonia, atelectasis, or a pleural effusion. Areas of decreased uptake on the perfusion scan indicate poor blood flow to the lung tissues. It is also known as a **lung scan**. The *Q* stands for quotient.

Pronunciation/Word Parts

MUGA (MUG-ah)

ventriculography (ven-TRIH-kyoo-LAW-grah-fee)
   venticul/o- *chamber that is filled; ventricle*
   -graphy *process of recording*

ventriculogram (ven-TRIH-kyoo-loh-GRAM)
   ventricul/o- *chamber that is filled; ventricle*
   -gram *picture; record*

SPECT (SPEKT)

OncoScint (AWN-koh-sint)

ProstaScint (PRAW-stah-sint)

ventilation (VEN-tih-LAY-shun)
   ventilat/o- *movement of air*
   -ion *action; condition*

perfusion (per-FYOO-zhun)
   per- *through; throughout*
   fus/o- *pouring*
   -ion *action; condition*

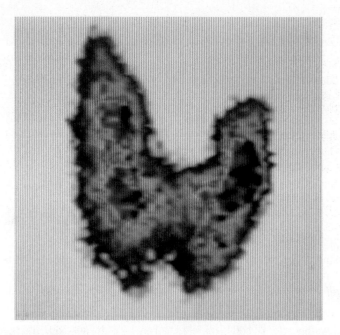

FIGURE 19-10 ▪ Thyroid scan.
The radiopharmaceutical drug technetium-99m outlines the size and shape of the thyroid gland. At the same time, the radiopharmaceutical drug iodine-123 is taken up by the thyroid gland cells and shows their rate of metabolism. This scan shows two dark blue "cold spots" in the right lobe of the thyroid gland and one large dark blue "cold spot" in the left lobe, where the cells are not taking up iodine. These areas could be benign cysts or cancerous tumors. (Remember, when you view the image, your right side corresponds to the patient's left side.)
Source: SIU/Encyclopedia/Corbis

Nuclear Medicine Procedures That Use Positrons

A positron is a positively charged particle that has the same mass as an electron, but the opposite charge. Radioactive substances that emit positrons are used in **positron emission tomography (PET)**. Like a CT scan or an MRI scan, a PET scan is a tomography that produces individual images of the body in "slices." However, unlike CT and MRI scans that produce images of the anatomy of an organ, a PET scan produces images of the physiology and metabolism of an organ. PET scans are of particular value in identifying areas of cancer (because cancerous cells have a higher metabolic rate than normal cells). They also show areas of ischemia in the heart (because ischemic cells have poor blood flow and a lower metabolic rate than normal cells). PET scans also show areas of abnormally increased or decreased metabolism in the brains of patients with Alzheimer's disease (see Figure 10-15), Parkinson's disease, epilepsy, and schizophrenia.

Pronunciation/Word Parts

positron (PAW-zih-trawn)

tomography (toh-MAW-grah-fee)
  tom/o- *cut; layer; slice*
  -graphy *process of recording*

A CLOSER LOOK

A cyclotron (subatomic particle accelerator) is needed to produce a radioactive substance that emits positrons. The half-life of radioactive substances that emit positrons is very brief (a few minutes in length). Therefore the cyclotron must be at the hospital where the PET scan is performed. A cyclotron, however, is a large, expensive piece of equipment, so PET scans are only available in the largest hospitals. For a PET scan, a positron-emitting radioactive substance is combined with glucose molecules and injected intravenously. The higher the rate of metabolism in a cell, the more glucose is consumed and the more radioactive substance that is carried into the cell. As the radioactive substance decays, it releases a positron. Almost immediately the positron collides with a nearby electron. The collision simultaneously produces two gamma rays that move in opposite directions from each other. A special circular gamma camera is set so that it only records simultaneously produced gamma rays. A computer traces the rays back to identify where they originated in an organ. This then becomes a point on the PET scan image.

Abbreviations

AP	anteroposterior		**MRI**	magnetic resonance imaging
Ba	barium		**MUGA**	multiple-gated acquisition (scan) (pronounced "MUG-ah")
BE	barium enema		**PA**	posteroanterior
CAT	computerized axial tomography		**PET**	positron emission tomography
CT	computerized tomography		**QCT**	quantitative computerized tomography
CXR	chest x-ray		**R, r**	roentgen (unit of exposure to x-rays or gamma rays)
DEXA	dual-energy x-ray absorptiometry		**rad**	radiation absorbed dose
DSA	digital subtraction angiography		**RAIU**	radioactive iodine uptake
DXA	dual-energy x-ray absorptiometry		**rem**	roentgen-equivalent man
EBT	electron beam tomography		**RRT**	registered radiologic technologist
ERCP	endoscopic retrograde cholangiopancreatography		**SPECT**	single-photon emission computerized tomography
HIDA	hydroxyiminodiacetic acid		**TEE**	transesophageal echocardiogram; transesophageal echocardiography
IVC	intravenous cholangiogram; intravenous cholangiography		**UGI**	upper gastrointestinal (series)
IVP	intravenous pyelogram; intravenous pyelography		**US**	ultrasonography; ultrasound
KUB	kidneys, ureters, bladder		**V/Q**	ventilation-perfusion (scan)
Lat	lateral			
MRA	magnetic resonance angiography			

CAREER FOCUS

Meet Jennifer, a radiologic technologist

"I became an x-ray technologist because I wanted to work in a profession where I worked with all different patients. You get to work in the emergency room; you get to work doing procedures alongside a physician, dealing with acutely ill patients. You also get to go to the operating room. We also deal with outpatients. We not only do routine x-rays, but we're also involved in minor procedures, along with assisting the radiologists during upper GIs, barium enemas, etc. You're not in any single area all the time, and it's just very nice to see every aspect of the hospital. We use medical terminology every day in our profession. When reading the requisitions that are sent over from the doctors' offices or notifying nurses if we have questions about a patient's exam, we need to use appropriate medical terminology."

Radiologic technologists are allied health professionals who perform and document a variety of radiologic procedures and assist the physician during radiologic procedures in the radiology and nuclear medicine department in a hospital or in a diagnostic imaging outpatient facility.

Radiologists are physicians who practice in the medical specialty of radiology. They view and interpret the results of radiologic procedures to diagnose conditions of all body systems. Nuclear medicine physicians practice in the medical specialty of nuclear medicine. They view and interpret the results of nuclear medicine procedures. Radiation oncologists use radiation to treat patients who have cancer.

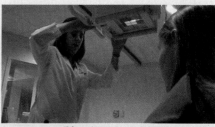

Source: Pearson Education

radiologic (RAY-dee-oh-LAW-jik)
  radi/o- *forearm bone; radiation; x-rays*
  log/o- *study of; word*
  -ic *pertaining to*

technologist (tek-NAW-loh-jist)
  techn/o- *technical skill*
  log/o- *study of; word*
  -ist *person who specializes in; thing that specializes in*

radiologist (RAY-dee-AW-loh-jist)
  radi/o- *forearm bone; radiation; x-rays*
  log/o- *study of; word*
  -ist *person who specializes in; thing that specializes in*

MyMedicalTerminologyLab™ To see Jennifer's complete video profile, log into MyMedicalTerminologyLab and navigate to the Multimedia Library for Chapter 19. Check the Video box, and then click the Career Focus - Radiologic Technician link.

CHAPTER REVIEW EXERCISES

Test your knowledge of the chapter by completing these review exercises. Use the Answer Key at the end of the book to check your answers. Note: Each of the numbered exercise headers corresponds to a numbered learning outcome on the first page of the chapter. Headers that include a number with an A or with a B after it show that there are two different parts to that learning outcome.

19.1 Describe X-ray Procedures

19.2 Describe X-ray Projections and Positions

19.3 Identify Radiology Procedures That Use X-rays, X-rays and Contrast, a Magnetic Field, Sound Waves, or an Electron Beam

19.4 Identify Nuclear Medicine Procedures That Use Gamma Rays or Positrons

MATCHING EXERCISE

Match each word or phrase to its description.

1. arthrography
2. fluoroscopy
3. gamma scintillation camera
4. krypton-81m
5. portable film
6. OncoScint scan
7. radiolucent
8. radiopharmaceutical
9. MRI
10. V/Q scan

_____ Pertaining to an area of low density on a radiograph

_____ Uses a continuous x-ray and a monitor

_____ Uses a magnetic field and radiowaves

_____ Contrast dye is injected into a joint

_____ Radioactive substance measured to be given as a drug dose

_____ Radiopharmaceutical drug that is inhaled as a gas and used in nuclear medicine

_____ Detects gamma rays from radioactive substances

_____ Used to detect metastases from colon or ovary cancer

_____ Ventilation-perfusion scan of the lungs

_____ Radiograph performed somewhere other than the radiology department

CIRCLE EXERCISE

Circle the correct word from the choices given.

1. A (**plain**, **portable**, **scout**) film is a preliminary radiograph taken before contrast dye is given.
2. A spiral scan is one type of a/an (**CT**, **MRI**, **PET**) scan.
3. The Virtual Physical uses what technology? (**arteriography**, **EBT**, **MRI**)
4. During all of these procedures, the patient is exposed to radiation, *except* during a/an (**CT scan**, **mammography**, **MRI scan**).
5. During a (**MUGA**, **PET**, **SPECT**) scan, the ejection fraction of the heart can be calculated.
6. In a (**cross-table lateral**, **KUB**, **oblique**) x-ray, the patient is lying on his/her back with the x-ray plate on one side and the x-ray machine on the other side.

RECALL AND LIST EXERCISE

List 10 metal items that might be on or inside a patient that should not be subjected to an MRI scan.

1. _____   2. _____   3. _____

4. _____   5. _____   6. _____

7. _____   8. _____   9. _____

10. _____

FILL IN THE BLANK EXERCISE

Fill in the blank with the correct word from the word list.

Doppler	film badge	gadolinium	half-life	light box	PA (posteroanterior)

1. The radiologist uses a _____ to view radiographs.

2. A _____ chest x-ray is the most common type of chest x-ray.

3. Every healthcare professional working in radiology must wear a _____ to detect exposure to radiation.

4. _____ is a metallic element that is used in MRI scans because it responds to a magnetic field.

5. _____ technology produces the audible sound of blood flowing through an artery.

6. The _____ is the length of time it takes for half of the atoms in an amount of a radioactive substance to decay and become stable.

TRUE OR FALSE EXERCISE

Indicate whether each statement is true or false by writing T or F on the line.

1. _____ Postcontrast images are taken after the injection of contrast dye.

2. _____ Both radiology and nuclear medicine use radioactive substances to create images of the internal structures of the body.

3. _____ The process of measuring the amount of radiation exposure is known as *densitometry*.

4. _____ Using a CT scan to guide the placement of a needle for biopsy is known as *interventional radiology*.

5. _____ Fluoroscopy is used during a bone densitometry test.

6. _____ IVC and OCG are both types of radiologic procedures that use contrast dye to view the gallbladder.

7. _____ Ultrasonography uses ultra high-frequency sound waves generated by a transducer or a probe.

8. _____ A PET scan detects positrons and shows areas of cellular metabolism.

9. _____ Iodinated contrast dye contains iodine.

10. _____ The contrast medium barium is used during SPECT scans.

MULTIPLE CHOICE EXERCISE

Circle the correct answer from the choices given.

1. Roentgenography is the same thing as _____.
   a. IVP
   b. radiography
   c. KUB
   d. tomography

2. All of the following procedures use x-rays *except* _____.
   a. mammography
   b. cross-table lateral
   c. KUB
   d. ultrasonography

3. When standard echocardiography cannot produce a good-quality image, the physician may order a _____.
   a. KUB
   b. TEE
   c. MRI
   d. DSA

4. PET scans are useful in detecting or studying _____.
   a. epilepsy
   b. Alzheimer's disease
   c. schizophrenia
   d. all of the above

MATCHING EXERCISE

Match each word or phrase to its description.

1. barium swallow
2. B scan
3. bone densitometry
4. cineradiography
5. enhanced
6. filling defect
7. HIDA scan
8. pyelography
9. radiopharmaceutical
10. ultrasonography
11. xeromammogram

_____ Fluoroscopy captured digitally
_____ Breast image from x-rays captured on paper rather than on film
_____ DEXA scan and QCT
_____ Any procedure that uses a contrast dye
_____ Another name for *urography*
_____ Upper GI series
_____ Another name for *sonography*
_____ Two-dimensional, gray-scale ultrasound
_____ Drug that acts as a tracer in the body
_____ Area of decreased uptake in an organ on a perfusion scan
_____ Another name for *cholescintigraphy*

19.5A Give Word Part Meanings

WORD PARTS EXERCISE

Next to each word part, write its meaning. The first one has been done for you.

Word Part	Meaning	Word Part	Meaning
1. act/o-	*action*	10. cardi/o-	
2. angi/o-		11. cholangi/o-	
3. anter/o-		12. cholecyst/o-	
4. aort/o-		13. cin/e-	
5. arteri/o-		14. cyst/o-	
6. arthr/o-		15. densit/o-	
7. -ated		16. dos/i-	
8. -ation		17. duc/o-	
9. axi/o-		18. ech/o-	

Word Part	Meaning	Word Part	Meaning
19. electr/o-	_____	42. nucle/o-	_____
20. esophag/o-	_____	43. -ory	_____
21. excret/o-	_____	44. pancreat/o-	_____
22. fluor/o-	_____	45. pharmaceutic/o-	_____
23. fus/o-	_____	46. poster/o-	_____
24. gastr/o-	_____	47. project/o-	_____
25. gnos/o-	_____	48. pyel/o-	_____
26. -gram	_____	49. quantitat/o-	_____
27. -graph	_____	50. rad/io-	_____
28. -graphy	_____	51. roentgen/o-	_____
29. hyster/o-	_____	52. salping/o-	_____
30. intestin/o-	_____	53. scint/i-	_____
31. iodin/o-	_____	54. -scopy	_____
32. -ion	_____	55. son/o-	_____
33. later/o-	_____	56. techn/o-	_____
34. log/o-	_____	57. tom/o-	_____
35. luc/o-	_____	58. trac/o-	_____
36. lymph/o-	_____	59. ur/o-	_____
37. magnet/o-	_____	60. ven/o-	_____
38. mamm/o-	_____	61. ventilat/o-	_____
39. -meter	_____	62. vent/o-	_____
40. -metry	_____	63. ventricul/o-	_____
41. myel/o-	_____	64. xer/o-	_____

19.5B Define Abbreviations

ABBREVIATION EXERCISE

Write the meaning of each abbreviation. The first one has been done for you.

1. MUGA *multiple-gated acquisition (scan)* _____
2. PET _____
3. BE _____
4. CXR _____
5. US _____
6. CAT _____
7. IVP _____
8. AP _____
9. KUB _____
10. MRI _____

19.6A Divide Medical Words

DIVIDING WORDS EXERCISE

Separate these words into their component parts (prefix, combining form, suffix). Note: Some words do not contain all three word parts. The first one has been done for you.

Medical Word	Prefix	Combining Form	Suffix	Medical Word	Prefix	Combining Form	Suffix
1. radiology	___	radi/o-	-logy	5. tomography	___	___	___
2. fluoroscopy	___	___	___	6. angiogram	___	___	___
3. intravenous	___	___	___	7. dosimeter	___	___	___
4. ultrasonography	___	___	___	8. diagnostic	___	___	___

19.6B Build Medical Words

COMBINING FORM AND SUFFIX EXERCISE

Read the definition of the medical word. Select the correct suffix from the Suffix List. Select the correct combining form from the Combining Form List. Build the medical word and write it on the line. Be sure to check your spelling. The first one has been done for you.

SUFFIX LIST	COMBINING FORM LIST	
-al (pertaining to)	angi/o- (blood vessel; lymphatic vessel)	nucle/o- (nucleus of an atom; nucleus of a cell)
-ar (pertaining to)	arteri/o- (artery)	
-ated (composed of; pertaining to a condition)	arthr/o- (joint)	pyel/o- (renal pelvis)
-er (person who produces; thing that produces)	axi/o- (axis)	radi/o- (forearm bone; radiation; x-rays)
	cholangi/o- (bile duct)	
-gram (picture; record)	densit/o- (density)	scint/i- (point of light)
-graphy (process of recording)	dos/i- (dose)	son/o- (sound)
-meter (instrument used to measure)	fluor/o- (fluorescence)	tom/o- (cut; layer; slice)
-metry (process of measuring)	iodin/o- (iodine)	trac/o- (visible path)
-scopy (process of using an instrument to examine)	mamm/o- (breast)	ur/o- (urinary system; urine)
		ven/o- (vein)

Definition of the Medical Word	Build the Medical Word
1. Pertaining to (the) nucleus of an atom	nuclear
2. Process of recording (an image of a) blood vessel	___
3. (Contrast dye that is) composed of iodine	___
4. Process of recording x-rays	___
5. Picture or record (of the) breast	___
6. Process of recording (an image of a) cut, layer, or slice	___
7. Process of using an instrument to examine fluorescence	___
8. Picture or record (of an) artery	___
9. Pertaining to (an) axis	___
10. Process of recording sound	___
11. Process of recording (the image of a) joint	___
12. Process of measuring (a) dose (of radiation)	___
13. Process of recording (the image of a) vein	___
14. Process of recording (a) point of light	___
15. Thing that produces (a) visible path	___

Definition of the Medical Word

16. Picture or record (of) sound
17. Picture or record (of structures of the) urinary system
18. Process of recording (an image of a) breast
19. Process of measuring (the) density (of bone)
20. Instrument used to measure (a) dose (of radiation)
21. Picture or record (of the) renal pelvis
22. Process of recording (the) bile duct

Build the Medical Word

_____

_____

_____

_____

_____

_____

_____

MULTIPLE COMBINING FORMS AND SUFFIX EXERCISE

Read the definition of the medical word. Select the correct suffix and combining forms. Then build the medical word and write it on the line. Be sure to check your spelling. The first one has been done for you.

SUFFIX LIST	COMBINING FORM LIST	
-al (pertaining to)	angi/o- (blood vessel; lymphatic vessel)	lymph/o- (lymph; lymphatic system)
-gram (picture; record)	anter/o- (before; front part)	mamm/o- (breast)
-graphy (process of recording)	cardi/o- (heart)	pharmaceutic/o- (drug; medicine)
-ior (pertaining to)	cin/e- (movement)	poster/o- (back part)
-ist (person who specializes in; thing that specializes in)	ech/o- (echo of a sound wave)	radi/o- (forearm bone; radiation; x-rays)
	hyster/o- (uterus; womb)	salping/o- (uterine tube)
	log/o- (study of; word)	techn/o- (technical skill)
		xer/o- (dry)

Definition of the Medical Word

1. Pertaining to (the) back part (and the) front part
2. A picture or record (of the) uterus (and) uterine tubes
3. Process of recording movement (during an) x-ray
4. A picture or record (of) lymph (and a) lymphatic vessel
5. A picture or record (processed with) dry (chemicals of the) breast
6. Process of recording (the) echo of a sound wave (reflected from the) heart
7. Pertaining to radiation (from a) drug or medicine
8. Person who specializes in technical skill (in the) study of (radiology)

Build the Medical Word

posteroanterior _____

_____

_____

_____

_____

_____

_____

_____

19.7A Spell Medical Words

HEARING MEDICAL WORDS EXERCISE

You hear someone speaking the medical words given below. Read each pronunciation and then write the medical word it represents. Be sure to check your spelling. The first one has been done for you.

1. BAIR-ee-um   _barium_
2. ar-TEER-ee-oh-GRAM   _____
3. KOH-lee-SIS-toh-gram   _____
4. DEN-sih-TAW-meh-tree   _____
5. EK-oh-KAR-dee-oh-GRAM   _____

6. HIS-ter-OH-sal-PING-goh-GRAM   _____
7. lim-FAN-jee-oh-GRAM   _____
8. SAW-noh-gram   _____
9. toh-MAW-grah-fee   _____
10. ZEER-oh-mah-MAW-grah-fee   _____

19.7B Pronounce Medical Words

PRONUNCIATION EXERCISE

Read the medical word and the syllables in its pronunciation. Circle the primary (main) accented syllable. The first one has been done for you.

1. angiography (an-jee-(aw)-grah-fee)
2. arthrogram (ar-throh-gram)
3. arthrography (ar-thraw-grah-fee)
4. dosimeter (doh-sim-eh-ter)
5. fluoroscopy (floor-aw-skoh-pee)
6. lymphangiogram (lim-fan-jee-oh-gram)
7. mammogram (mam-oh-gram)
8. mammography (mah-maw-grah-fee)
9. tomography (toh-maw-grah-fee)
10. venogram (vee-noh-gram)

19.8 Analyze Medical Reports

This is a Radiology Report. Read the report and answer the questions.

ELECTRONIC PATIENT RECORD #1

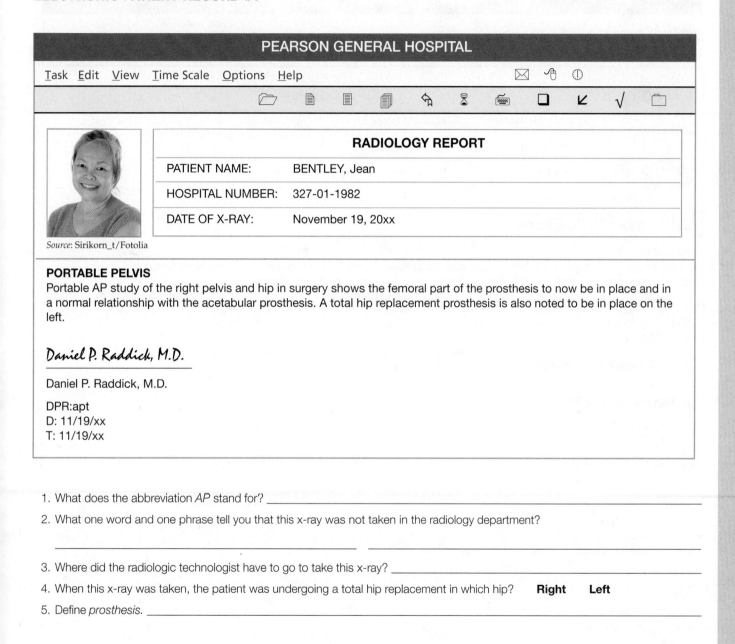

PEARSON GENERAL HOSPITAL

Task   Edit   View   Time Scale   Options   Help

RADIOLOGY REPORT

PATIENT NAME:	BENTLEY, Jean
HOSPITAL NUMBER:	327-01-1982
DATE OF X-RAY:	November 19, 20xx

Source: Sirikorn_t/Fotolia

PORTABLE PELVIS
Portable AP study of the right pelvis and hip in surgery shows the femoral part of the prosthesis to now be in place and in a normal relationship with the acetabular prosthesis. A total hip replacement prosthesis is also noted to be in place on the left.

Daniel P. Raddick, M.D.

Daniel P. Raddick, M.D.

DPR:apt
D: 11/19/xx
T: 11/19/xx

1. What does the abbreviation *AP* stand for? _____

2. What one word and one phrase tell you that this x-ray was not taken in the radiology department?

   _____   _____

3. Where did the radiologic technologist have to go to take this x-ray? _____

4. When this x-ray was taken, the patient was undergoing a total hip replacement in which hip?   **Right**   **Left**

5. Define *prosthesis.* _____

ELECTRONIC PATIENT RECORD #2

This is a Radiology Report. Read the report and answer the questions.

PEARSON GENERAL HOSPITAL

Task   Edit   View   Time Scale   Options   Help

RADIOLOGY REPORT

PATIENT NAME:	ADAMS, Bryce
HOSPITAL NUMBER:	11-98-64370
DATE OF X-RAY:	November 19, 20xx

Source: Leungchopan/Fotolia

AIR CONTRAST BARIUM ENEMA

PROCEDURE
Under fluoroscopic control, the barium was allowed to flow in a retrograde manner to fill the cecum. Using a double-contrast technique, multiple films were obtained. Several small diverticula are noted. There is also some displacement of the small bowel. A soft tissue density is seen within the lower abdomen. No mucosal ulcerations or polypoid lesions are identified.

IMPRESSION
Barium and air contrast study shows displacement of the small bowel with a tissue density. This is suggestive of a pelvic mass. No evidence of polypoid lesions is seen in the colon.

Robert C. Johnson, M.D.

Robert C. Johnson, M.D.

RCJ:smt
D: 11/19/xx
T: 11/19/xx

---

1. What type of radiologic procedure was done?

   a. KUB

   b. flat plate of the abdomen

   c. fluoroscopy

2. Name the two types of contrast that were used for this procedure.

   _____

   _____

3. In addition to watching the procedure on a monitor, how many radiographs (films) were taken?

   _____

4. Divide *fluoroscopic* into its three word parts and give the meaning of each word part.

Word Part	**Meaning**
_____	_____
_____	_____
_____	_____

ELECTRONIC PATIENT RECORD #3

This is a Nuclear Medicine Report. Read the report and answer the questions.

PEARSON GENERAL HOSPITAL

Task Edit View Time Scale Options Help

NUCLEAR MEDICINE REPORT

PATIENT NAME:	MATHESON, Latrise
HOSPITAL NUMBER:	901156-48376
DATE OF X-RAY:	November 19, 20xx

Source: Jaimie Duplass/Fotolia

RADIOACTIVE IODINE UPTAKE

The patient was given an oral capsule containing 100 microcuries of I-123, and uptake by the thyroid gland was measured at 6 hours and 24 hours. The 6-hour uptake was 5.5% (normal 4–12%). The 24-hour uptake was 14.0% (normal 7–24%).

THYROID SCAN

Fifteen minutes after the intravenous injection of 10 millicuries of technetium-99m, views of the -thyroid gland were performed. The thyroid gland was in a normal position in the neck. The overall size of the gland was within normal limits, and there was uniform uptake throughout both the right and left lobes.

IMPRESSION

1. Normal thyroid radioiodine uptake.

2. Normal thyroid scan.

Victoria J. Evans, M.D.

Victoria J. Evans, M.D.

VJE:mja
D: 11/19/xx
T: 11/19/xx

---

1. What are the names and atomic numbers of the two radiopharmaceuticals given in this procedure?

   _____

   _____

2. What are the two units of measurement for the doses of these radiopharmaceuticals?

   _____

   _____

3. What is the range of normal values for the 24-hour uptake? _____

4. How was the radioactive iodine administered? _____

5. How was the radioactive technetium-99m administered? _____

6. Divide *radioactive* into its three word parts and give the meaning of each word part.

Word Part	**Meaning**
_____	_____
_____	_____
_____	_____

7. What phrase tells you that there was an equal amount of radioactive tracer present in all parts of the thyroid gland?

   _____

MyMedicalTerminologyLab™

MyMedicalTerminologyLab is a premium online homework management system that includes a host of features to help you study. Registered users will find:

- A multitude of quizzes and activities built within the MyLab platform
- Powerful tools that track and analyze your results—allowing you to create a personalized learning experience
- Videos and audio pronunciations to help enrich your progress
- Streaming lesson presentations (Guided Lectures) and self-paced learning modules
- A space where you and your instructor can check your progress and manage your assignments

Appendix A

Glossary of Medical Word Parts: Prefixes, Suffixes, and Combining Forms

Prefixes

A

a-	away from; without
ab-	away from
ad-	toward
an-	not; without
ana-	apart; excessive
ant-	against
ante-	before; forward
anti-	against
apo-	away from

B

bi-	two
brachy-	short
brady-	slow

C

cata-	down
circa-	about
circum-	around
con-	with
contra-	against

D

de-	reversal of; without
di-	two
dia-	complete; completely through
dis-	away from
dys-	abnormal; difficult; painful

E

e-	out; without
ec-	out; outward
ecto-	outermost; outside
em-	in
en-	in; inward; within
endo-	innermost; within
epi-	above; upon
eu-	good; normal
ex-	away from; out
extra-	outside

H

hemi-	one half
hyper-	above; more than normal
hypo-	below; deficient

I

im-	not
in-	in; not; within
infra-	below; beneath
inter-	between
intra-	within

K

kilo-	one thousand

M

mal-	bad; inadequate
mega-	large
meso-	middle
meta-	after; change; subsequent to; transition
mid-	middle

N

non-	not

P

pan-	all
par-	beside
para-	abnormal; apart from; beside; two parts of a pair
per-	through; throughout
peri-	around
poly-	many; much
post-	after; behind
pre-	before; in front of
pro-	before

Q

quadri-	four

R

re-	again and again; backward; unable to
retro-	backward; behind

S

semi-	half; partly
sub-	below; underneath
super-	above; beyond
supra-	above
sym-	together; with
syn-	together

T

tachy-	fast
trans-	across; through
tri-	three

U

ultra-	beyond; higher
un-	not
uni-	not paired; single

Suffixes

A

-able	able to be
-ac	pertaining to
-ad	in the direction of; toward
-ade	action; process
-al	pertaining to
-alis	pertaining to
-amnios	amniotic fluid
-an	pertaining to
-ance	state
-ancy	state
-ant	pertaining to
-ar	pertaining to
-arche	beginning
-arian	pertaining to a person
-aris	pertaining to

-ary	pertaining to
-ase	enzyme
-ate	composed of; pertaining to
-ated	composed of; pertaining to a condition
-atic	pertaining to
-ation	being; having; process
-ative	pertaining to
-ator	person who does; person who produces; thing that does; thing that produces
-atory	pertaining to
-ature	system composed of

B

-blast	immature cell
-body	structure; thing

C

-cele	hernia
-centesis	procedure to puncture
-cephalus	head
-cere	waxy substance
-clast	cell that breaks down substances
-cle	small thing
-clonus	rapid contracting and relaxing
-cnemius	leg
-coccus	spherical bacterium
-collis	condition of the neck
-crasia	condition of a mixing
-crine	thing that secretes
-crit	separation of
-cyte	cell

D

-dactyly	condition of fingers; condition of toes
-derma	skin
-desis	procedure to fuse together
-didymis	testicle; testis
-dose	measured quantity
-drome	running
-duct	duct; tube

E

-eal	pertaining to
-ectasis	condition of dilation
-ectomy	surgical removal
-ed	pertaining to
-edema	swelling
-ee	person who is the object of an action; person who receives; thing that is the object of an action; thing that receives
-elasma	plate-like structure
-elle	small thing
-ema	condition
-emia	condition of the blood; substance in the blood
-emic	pertaining to a condition of the blood; pertaining to a substance in the blood
-ence	state
-encephaly	condition of the brain
-ency	condition of being; condition of having
-ent	pertaining to
-entery	condition of the intestine
-eon	person who performs

-er	person who does; person who produces; thing that does; thing that produces
-ergy	activity; process of working
-ery	process
-esis	condition; process
-etic	pertaining to
-ety	condition; state

F

-flux	flow
-form	having the form of
-frice	cleaning agent

G

-gen	that which produces
-gene	gene
-glia	cells that provide support
-grade	pertaining to going
-graft	tissue for implant; tissue for transplant
-gram	picture; record
-graph	instrument used to record
-graphy	process of recording
-gravida	pregnancy

I

-ia	condition; state; thing
-iac	pertaining to
-ial	pertaining to
-ian	pertaining to
-ias	condition
-iasis	process; state
-iatic	pertaining to a process; pertaining to a state
-iatry	medical treatment
-ic	pertaining to
-ical	pertaining to
-ice	quality; state
-ician	skilled expert; skilled professional
-ics	knowledge; practice
-id	origin; resembling; source
-ide	chemically modified structure
-ie	thing
-il	thing
-ile	pertaining to
-immune	immune response
-in	substance

-ine	pertaining to; thing pertaining to
-ing	doing
-ion	action; condition
-ior	pertaining to
-ious	pertaining to
-ism	disease from a specific cause; process
-ist	person who specializes in; thing that specializes in
-istry	process related to a specialty
-isy	condition of infection; condition of inflammation
-ite	thing that pertains to
-itian	skilled expert; skilled professional
-itic	pertaining to
-ition	condition of having
-itis	infection of; inflammation of
-ity	condition; state
-ium	chemical element; structure
-ive	pertaining to
-ix	thing
-ization	process of creating; process of inserting; process of making
-ize	affecting in a particular way
-izer	thing that affects in a particular way

K

-kine	movement

L

-lalia	condition of speech
-lepsy	seizure
-lith	stone
-logy	study of
-ly	going toward
-lysis	process to break down; process to destroy
-lyte	dissolved substance

M

-megaly	enlargement
-ment	action; state
-meter	instrument used to measure
-metry	process of measuring
-mileusis	process of carving

N

-nate	thing that is born
-nine	pertaining to a single chemical substance

O

-oid	resembling
-ol	chemical substance
-ole	small thing
-oma	mass; tumor
-omatosis	condition of masses; condition of tumors
-on	structure; substance
-one	chemical substance
-opsy	process of viewing
-or	person who does; person who produces; thing that does; thing that produces
-ory	having the function of
-ose	full of; thing full of
-osing	condition of making
-osis	condition; process
-ous	pertaining to

P

-path	person involved with disease
-pathy	disease
-pause	cessation
-penia	condition of deficiency
-pexy	process of surgically fixing in place
-phage	thing that eats; thing that swallows
-pharynx	pharynx; throat
-phil	attraction to; fondness for
-phile	person who is attracted to; person who is fond of
-phylaxis	condition of guarding; condition of protecting
-phyma	growth; tumor
-physis	state of growing
-phyte	growth
-plant	procedure to graft; procedure to transfer
-plasm	formed substance; growth
-plasty	process of reshaping by surgery
-plex	parts
-pnea	breathing
-poiesis	process of formation
-poietin	substance that forms
-probe	rod-like instrument
-ptosis	state of drooping; state of falling
-ptysis	condition of coughing up

R

-rrhage	excessive discharge; excessive flow
-rrhaphy	procedure of suturing
-rrhea	discharge; flow
-rubin	red substance

S

-salpinx	uterine tube
-scope	instrument used to examine
-scopy	process of using an instrument to examine
-sin	substance
-sis	condition; process
-some	body
-spasm	sudden, involuntary muscle contraction
-sphere	ball; sphere
-stasis	standing still; staying in one place
-steroid	steroid
-sterol	lipid-containing compound
-stomy	surgically created opening
-systole	contraction

T

-therapy	treatment
-thorax	chest; thorax
-tic	pertaining to
-tion	being; having; process
-tome	area with distinct edges; instrument used to cut
-tomy	process of cutting; process of making an incision
-tope	place; position

-tor	person who does; person who produces; thing that does; thing that produces
-tous	pertaining to
-tresia	hole; opening
-tripsy	process of crushing
-triptor	thing that crushes
-tron	instrument
-trophy	process of development
-ty	quality; state
-type	model of

U

-ual	pertaining to
-ula	small thing
-ule	small thing
-um	period of time; structure
-ure	result of; system
-us	condition; thing

V

-verse	travel; turn

Z

-zoon	animal; living thing

Combining Forms

A

abdomin/o-	abdomen
ablat/o-	destroy; take away
abort/o-	stop prematurely
abras/o-	scrape off
absorpt/o-	absorb; take in
access/o-	contributing part; supplemental part
accommod/o-	adapt
acetabul/o-	hip socket
acid/o-	acid; low pH
acous/o-	hearing; sound
acr/o-	extremity; highest point
actin/o-	rays of the sun
act/o-	action
acu/o-	needle; sharpness

addict/o-	controlled by; surrender to
aden/o-	gland
adenoid/o-	structure resembling a gland
adhes/o-	stick to
adip/o-	fat
adjuv/o-	giving assistance; giving help
adnex/o-	accessory connecting parts
adolesc/o-	beginning of being an adult
adrenal/o-	adrenal gland
adren/o-	adrenal gland
affect/o-	have an influence on; mood; state of mind
affer/o-	toward the center
agglutin/o-	clumping; sticking
aggreg/o-	crowding together
ag/o-	lead to

agon/o-	causing action
agor/a-	open area; open space
albin/o-	white
albumin/o-	albumin
alges/o-	sensation of pain
alg/o-	pain
align/o-	arranged in a straight line
aliment/o-	food; nourishment
alkal/o-	base; high pH
allerg/o-	allergy
all/o-	other; strange
alopec/o-	bald
alveol/o-	air sac
ambly/o-	dimness
ambulat/o-	walking
amnes/o-	forgetfulness
amni/o-	amnion; membrane around the fetus
amputat/o-	cut off
amput/o-	cut off
amygdal/o-	almond shape
amyl/o-	carbohydrate; starch
anabol/o-	building up
analy/o-	separate
anastom/o-	create an opening between two structures
ancill/o-	accessory; servant
andr/o-	male
aneurysm/o-	aneurysm; dilation
angin/o-	angina
angi/o-	blood vessel; lymphatic vessel
anis/o-	unequal
ankyl/o-	fused together; stiff
an/o-	anus
antagon/o-	oppose; work against
anter/o-	before; front part
anthrac/o-	coal
anxi/o-	fear; worry
aort/o-	aorta
apher/o-	withdrawal
aphth/o-	ulcer
apic/o-	apex; tip
appendic/o-	appendix
appendicul/o-	limb; small attached part
append/o-	appendix; small structure hanging from a larger structure
appercept/o-	fully perceived
aque/o-	watery substance
arachn/o-	spider; spider web
areol/o-	small, circular area
arteri/o-	artery

arteriol/o-	arteriole
arter/o-	artery
arthr/o-	joint
articul/o-	joint
asbest/o-	asbestos
ascit/o-	ascites
aspir/o-	breathe in; suck in
asthen/o-	lack of strength
asthm/o-	asthma
astr/o-	star-like structure
atel/o-	incomplete
ather/o-	soft, fatty substance
atheromat/o-	fatty deposit; fatty mass
athet/o-	without place; without position
atri/o-	atrium; chamber that is open at the top
attenu/o-	weakened
audi/o-	hearing
audit/o-	sense of hearing
augment/o-	increase in degree; increase in size
aur/i-	ear
auricul/o-	ear
auscult/o-	listening
aut/o-	self
autonom/o-	independent; self-governing
axill/o-	armpit
axi/o-	axis

B

bacteri/o-	bacterium
balan/o-	glans penis
bar/o-	weight
basil/o-	base of an organ
bas/o-	alkaline; base of a structure; basic
behav/o-	activity; manner of acting
bili/o-	bile; gall
bilirubin/o-	bilirubin
bi/o-	life; living organism; living tissue
blast/o-	embryonic; immature
blephar/o-	eyelid
botul/o-	sausage
brachi/o-	arm
bronchi/o-	bronchus
bronchiol/o-	bronchiole
bronch/o-	bronchus
brux/o-	grind the teeth
buccinat/o-	cheek
bucc/o-	cheek
bulb/o-	bulb-like structure

bunion/o-	bunion
burs/o-	bursa

C

cac/o-	bad; poor
calcane/o-	calcaneus; heel bone
calc/i-	calcium
calcific/o-	hard from calcium
calci/o-	calcium
calc/o-	calcium
calcul/o-	stone
calic/o-	calyx
cali/o-	calyx
calor/o-	heat
cancell/o-	lattice structure
cancer/o-	cancer
candid/o-	*Candida*; yeast
can/o-	dog like
capill/o-	capillary; hair-like structure
capn/o-	carbon dioxide
capsul/o-	capsule; enveloping structure
carb/o-	carbon
carbox/y-	carbon monoxide
carcin/o-	cancer
card/i-	heart
cardi/o-	heart
cari/o-	caries; tooth decay
carot/o-	sleep; stupor
carp/o-	wrist
cartilagin/o-	cartilage
catabol/o-	breaking down
catheter/o-	catheter
caud/o-	tail bone
caus/o-	burning
cavit/o-	hollow space
cav/o-	hollow space
cec/o-	cecum
celi/o-	abdomen
cellul/o-	cell
centr/o-	center; dominant part
cephal/o-	head
cerebell/o-	cerebellum
cerebr/o-	cerebrum
cervic/o-	cervix; neck
cheil/o-	lip
chem/o-	chemical; drug
chez/o-	pass feces
chir/o-	hand
chlor/o-	chloride

cholangi/o-	bile duct
chol/e-	bile; gall
cholecyst/o-	gallbladder
choledoch/o-	common bile duct
cholesterol/o-	cholesterol
chol/o-	bile; gall
chondr/o-	cartilage
chori/o-	chorion
chorion/o-	chorion
choroid/o-	choroid of the eye
chrom/o-	color
chron/o-	time
cid/o-	killing
cili/o-	hair-like structure
cin/e-	movement
cingul/o-	structure that surrounds
circulat/o-	movement in a circular route
circul/o-	circle
cirrh/o-	yellow
cis/o-	cut
claudicat/o-	limping pain
claustr/o-	enclosed space
clavicul/o-	clavicle, collar bone
clav/o-	clavicle, collar bone
cleid/o-	clavicle, collar bone
clinic/o-	medicine
clon/o-	identical group derived from one; rapid contracting and relaxing
coagul/o-	clotting
coarct/o-	pressed together
cocc/o-	spherical bacterium
coccyg/o-	coccyx; tail bone
cochle/o-	cochlea; spiral-shaped structure
cognit/o-	thinking
coit/o-	sexual intercourse
coll/a-	fibers that hold together
col/o-	colon
colon/o-	colon
colp/o-	vagina
comat/o-	unconsciousness
comminut/o-	break into small pieces
communicat/o-	impart; transmit
communic/o-	impart; transmit
compens/o-	compensate; counterbalance
compress/o-	press together
compromis/o-	exposed to danger
compuls/o-	compel; drive
concept/o-	conceive; form
concuss/o-	violent impact

conduct/o-	carrying; conveying
conform/o-	having the same angle; having the same scale
congenit/o-	present at birth
congest/o-	accumulation of fluid
coni/o-	dust
conjug/o-	joined together
conjunctiv/o-	conjunctiva of the eye
con/o-	cone
constip/o-	compacted feces
constrict/o-	drawn together; narrowed
construct/o-	build
contin/o-	hold together
contract/o-	pull together
contus/o-	bruising
converg/o-	coming together
convuls/o-	seizure
copr/o-	feces; stool
corne/o-	cornea of the eye
cor/o-	pupil of the eye
coron/o-	structure that encircles like a crown
corpor/o-	body
cortic/o-	cortex; outer region
cosmet/o-	adorned; attractive
cost/o-	rib
crani/o-	cranium; skull
crin/o-	secrete
cry/o-	cold
crypt/o-	hidden
cubit/o-	elbow
culd/o-	cul-de-sac
cusp/o-	point; projection
cutane/o-	skin
cut/i-	skin
cyan/o-	blue
cycl/o-	ciliary body of the eye; circle; cycle
cyst/o-	bladder; fluid-filled sac; semisolid cyst
cyt/o-	cell

D

dacry/o-	lacrimal sac; tears
dactyl/o-	digit; finger; toe
dec/i-	one tenth
decidu/o-	falling off
defici/o-	inadequate; lacking
degluti/o-	swallowing
delt/o-	triangle
delus/o-	false belief
dem/o-	people; population
dendr/o-	branching structure

densit/o-	density
dent/i-	tooth
dentit/o-	eruption of teeth
dent/o-	tooth
depend/o-	hang onto
depress/o-	press down
derm/a-	skin
dermat/o-	skin
derm/o-	skin
desicc/o-	dry up
dextr/o-	right; sugar
diabet/o-	diabetes
diaphor/o-	sweating
diaphragmat/o-	diaphragm
diaphys/o-	shaft of a bone
diastol/o-	dilating
didym/o-	testicle; testis
dietet/o-	diet; foods
diet/o-	diet; foods
differentiat/o-	distinct; specialized
different/o-	different; distinct
digest/o-	break down food; digest
digit/o-	digit; finger; toe
dilat/o-	dilate; widen
dipl/o-	double
dips/o-	thirst
disk/o-	disk
dissect/o-	cut apart
dissemin/o-	scattered throughout the body
distent/o-	distended; stretched
dist/o-	away from the center; away from the point of origin
diverticul/o-	diverticulum
donat/o-	gift; giving
dors/o-	back; dorsum
dos/i-	dose
drom/o-	running
duc/o-	bring; move
duct/o-	bring; duct; move
du/o-	two
duoden/o-	duodenum
dur/o-	dura mater
dynam/o-	movement; power
dyn/o-	pain

E

ecchym/o-	blood in the tissue
ech/o-	echo of a sound wave
eclamps/o-	seizure

ectat/o-	dilation
ectop/o-	outside
edentul/o-	without teeth
efface/o-	do away with; obliterate
effer/o-	away from the center
effus/o-	pouring out
ejaculat/o-	expel suddenly
elast/o-	flexing; stretching
electr/o-	electricity
emaci/o-	make thin
embol/o-	embolus; occluding plug
embryon/o-	embryo; immature form
eme/o-	vomiting
emet/o-	vomiting
emiss/o-	send out
emot/o-	moving; stirring up
emulsific/o-	liquid with suspended particles
encephal/o-	brain
enter/o-	intestine
enucle/o-	remove the main part
enur/o-	urinate
eosin/o-	eosin; red, acidic dye
ependym/o-	cellular lining
epilept/o-	seizure
epiphys/o-	enlarged area at the end of a long bone
episi/o-	vulva
erect/o-	stand up
erg/o-	activity; work
erupt/o-	breaking out
erythemat/o-	redness
erythr/o-	red
es/o-	inward
esophag/o-	esophagus
esthes/o-	feeling; sensation
esthet/o-	feeling; sensation
estr/a-	female
estr/o-	female
ethm/o-	sieve
eti/o-	cause of disease
etym/o-	word origin
exacerb/o-	increase; provoke
excis/o-	cut out
excori/o-	take out skin
excret/o-	removing from the body
exhibit/o-	showing
ex/o-	away from; external; outward
explorat/o-	search out
express/o-	communicate
extens/o-	straightening

extern/o-	outside
extrins/o-	outside
exud/o-	oozing fluid

F

faci/o-	face
factiti/o-	artificial; made up
fallopi/o-	uterine tube
fasci/o-	fascia
fec/a-	feces; stool
fec/o-	feces; stool
femor/o-	femur; thigh bone
fer/o-	bear
ferrit/o-	iron
ferr/o-	iron
fertil/o-	conceive; form
fet/o-	fetus
fibrill/o-	muscle fiber; nerve fiber
fibrin/o-	fibrin
fibr/o-	fiber
fibul/o-	fibula; lower leg bone
filtrat/o-	filtering; straining
filtr/o-	filter
fiss/o-	splitting
fixat/o-	make stable; make still
flatul/o-	flatus; gas
flex/o-	bending
fluor/o-	fluorescence
foc/o-	point of activity
foli/o-	leaf
follicul/o-	follicle; small sac
foramin/o-	foramen; opening into a cavity; opening into a channel
forens/o-	court proceedings in criminal law
format/o-	arrangement; structure
fove/o-	small, depressed area
fract/o-	bend; break up
fratern/o-	close association; close relationship
front/o-	front
fruct/o-	fruit
fulgur/o-	spark of electricity
fund/o-	fundus; part farthest from the opening
fundu/o-	fundus; part farthest from the opening
fung/o-	fungus
fus/o-	pouring

G

galact/o-	milk
ganglion/o-	ganglion

gangren/o-	gangrene
gastr/o-	stomach
gemin/o-	group; set
gene/o-	gene
gener/o-	creation; production
genit/o-	genitalia
gen/o-	arising from; produced by
germin/o-	embryonic tissue
ger/o-	old age
gestat/o-	conception to birth
gest/o-	conception to birth
gigant/o-	giant
gingiv/o-	gums
glandul/o-	gland
glauc/o-	silver gray
glen/o-	socket of a joint
gli/o-	supporting cells
glob/o-	comprehensive; shaped like a globe
globul/o-	shaped like a globe
glomerul/o-	glomerulus
gloss/o-	tongue
glott/o-	glottis of the larynx
gluc/o-	glucose; sugar
glycer/o-	glycerol; sugar alcohol
glyc/o-	glucose; sugar
glycos/o-	glucose; sugar
gnos/o-	knowledge
gonad/o-	gonad; ovary; testis
goni/o-	angle
gon/o-	ovum; seed; spermatozoon
grad/o-	going
granul/o-	granule
graph/o-	record
gustat/o-	sense of taste
gynec/o-	female; woman

H

habilitat/o-	give ability
halit/o-	breath
hallucin/o-	imagined perception
hal/o-	breathe
hebe/o-	youth
hec/o-	habitual condition of the body
hedon/o-	pleasure
helic/o-	coil
hemat/o-	blood
hem/o-	blood

hemoglobin/o-	hemoglobin
hemorrh/o-	flowing of blood
hemorrhoid/o-	hemorrhoid
hepat/o-	liver
heredit/o-	genetic inheritance
hered/o-	genetic inheritance
herni/o-	hernia
heter/o-	other
hex/o-	habitual condition of the body
hiat/o-	gap; opening
hidr/o-	sweat
hil/o-	indentation
hirsut/o-	hairy
histi/o-	tissue
home/o-	same
hom/i-	man
hormon/o-	hormone
humer/o-	humerus; upper arm bone
hyal/o-	clear, glass-like substance
hydatidi/o-	fluid-filled sacs
hydr/o-	fluid; water
hygien/o-	health
hy/o-	U–shaped structure
hypn/o-	sleep
hypophys/o-	pituitary gland
hyster/o-	uterus; womb

I

iatr/o-	medical treatment; physician
icter/o-	jaundice
ict/o-	seizure
idi/o-	individual; unknown
ile/o-	ileum
ili/o-	hip bone; ilium
illus/o-	false perception
immun/o-	immune response
impact/o-	wedged in
implant/o-	placed within
incarcer/o-	imprison
incis/o-	cut into
incud/o-	anvil-shaped bone; incus
induct/o-	leading in
infarct/o-	small area of dead tissue
infect/o-	disease within
infer/o-	below
inflammat/o-	redness and warmth
inguin/o-	groin
inhibit/o-	block; hold back

inject/o-	insert; put in
insemin/o-	sow a seed
insert/o-	introduce; put in
inspect/o-	looking at
insulin/o-	insulin
insul/o-	island
integument/o-	skin
integu/o-	cover
intern/o-	inside
interstiti/o-	spaces within tissue
intestin/o-	intestine
intrins/o-	inside
intussuscept/o-	receive within
invas/o-	go into
involut/o-	enlarged organ returns to normal size
iodin/o-	iodine
iod/o-	iodine
irid/o-	iris of the eye
ir/o-	iris of the eye
ischi/o-	hip bone; ischium
isch/o-	block; keep back

J

jaund/o-	yellow
jejun/o-	jejunum
jugul/o-	jugular; throat

K

kal/i-	potassium
kary/o-	nucleus of a cell
kel/o-	tumor
kerat/o-	cornea of the eye; hard, fibrous protein
ket/o-	ketones
keton/o-	ketones
kines/o-	movement
kin/o-	movement
klept/o-	steal
kyph/o-	bent; humpbacked

L

labi/o-	labium; lip
laborat/o-	testing place; workplace
labyrinth/o-	labyrinth of the inner ear
lacer/o-	tearing
lacrim/o-	tears
lact/i-	milk
lact/o-	milk

lamin/o-	flat area on a vertebra; lamina
lapar/o-	abdomen
laryng/o-	larynx; voice box
later/o-	side
lei/o-	smooth
lenticul/o-	lens of the eye
lent/o-	lens of the eye
leuk/o-	white
lev/o-	left
lex/o-	word
ligament/o-	ligament
ligat/o-	bind; tie up
limb/o-	border; edge
lingu/o-	tongue
lipid/o-	fat; lipid
lip/o-	fat; lipid
lith/o-	stone
lob/o-	lobe of an organ
locat/o-	place
loc/o-	one place
log/o-	study of; word
lord/o-	swayback
luc/o-	clear
lumb/o-	area between the ribs and pelvis; lower back
lumin/o-	lumen; opening
lun/o-	moon
lymph/o-	lymph; lymphatic system
ly/o-	break down; destroy
lys/o-	break down; destroy
lyt/o-	break down; destroy

M

macr/o-	large
macul/o-	small area; spot
magnet/o-	magnet
malac/o-	softening
malign/o-	cancer; intentionally causing harm
malle/o-	hammer-shaped bone; malleus
malleol/o-	malleolus
mamm/a-	breast
mamm/o-	breast
mandibul/o-	lower jaw; mandible
man/o-	frenzy; thin
manu/o-	hand
masset/o-	chewing
mastic/o-	chewing
mast/o-	breast; mastoid process

mastoid/o-	mastoid process
matur/o-	mature
maxill/o-	maxilla; upper jaw
mediastin/o-	mediastinum
medic/o-	medicine; physician
medi/o-	middle
medull/o-	inner region; medulla
megal/o-	large
melan/o-	black
melen/o-	black
meningi/o-	meninges
mening/o-	meninges
menisc/o-	crescent-shaped cartilage; meniscus
men/o-	month
menstru/o-	monthly discharge of blood
ment/o-	chin; mind
mesenter/o-	mesentery
mesi/o-	middle
metabol/o-	change; transformation
metri/o-	uterus; womb
metr/o-	measurement; uterus; womb
micr/o-	one millionth; small
micturi/o-	making urine
mineral/o-	electrolyte; mineral
mi/o-	narrowing
mit/o-	thread-like strand
mitr/o-	structure like a tall hat with two points
mitt/o-	send
mobil/o-	movement
mon/o-	one; single
morbid/o-	disease
morb/o-	disease
morph/o-	shape
mort/o-	death
motil/o-	movement
mot/o-	movement
muc/o-	mucus
mucos/o-	mucous membrane
mult/i-	many
muscul/o-	muscle
mutat/o-	change
myc/o-	fungus
mydr/o-	widening
myelin/o-	myelin
myel/o-	bone marrow; myelin; spinal cord
my/o-	muscle
myop/o-	near vision
myos/o-	muscle
myring/o-	eardrum; tympanic membrane

myx/o-	mucus-like substance

N

narc/o-	sleep; stupor
nas/o-	nose
nat/o-	birth
necr/o-	dead body; dead cells; dead tissue
ne/o-	new
nephr/o-	kidney; nephron
nerv/o-	nerve
neur/o-	nerve
neutr/o-	not taking part
nid/o-	focus; nest
noct/o-	night
nocturn/o-	night
nod/o-	knob of tissue; node
nodul/o-	small, knobby mass
norm/o-	normal; usual
nosocomi/o-	hospital
nuch/o-	neck
nucle/o-	nucleus of an atom; nucleus of a cell
null/i-	none
nutri/o-	nourishment
nutrit/o-	nourishment

O

obes/o-	fat
obsess/o-	besieged by thoughts
obstetr/o-	pregnancy and childbirth
obstip/o-	severe constipation
obstruct/o-	blocked by a barrier
occipit/o-	back of the head; occiput
occlus/o-	close against
ocul/o-	eye
odont/o-	tooth
odyn/o-	pain
olfact/o-	sense of smell
olig/o-	few; scanty
olisthe/o-	slipping
oment/o-	omentum
om/o-	mass; tumor
omphal/o-	navel; umbilicus
onc/o-	mass; tumor
onych/o-	fingernail; toenail
o/o-	egg; ovum
oophor/o-	ovary
operat/o-	perform a procedure; surgery
ophidi/o-	snake

ophthalm/o-	eye
op/o-	vision
opportun/o-	taking advantage of an opportunity; well timed
oppos/o-	forceful resistance
optic/o-	lenses; properties of light
opt/o-	eye; vision
orbicul/o-	small circle
orbit/o-	eye socket
orchid/o-	testicle; testis
orchi/o-	testicle; testis
orch/o-	testicle; testis
orex/o-	appetite
organ/o-	organ
or/o-	mouth
orth/o-	straight
osm/o-	sense of smell
osse/o-	bone
ossic/o-	bone
ossicul/o-	ossicle; small bone
ossificat/o-	changing into bone
oste/o-	bone
ot/o-	ear
ovari/o-	ovary
ov/i-	egg; ovum
ov/o-	egg; ovum
ovul/o-	egg; ovum
ox/i-	oxygen
ox/o-	oxygen
ox/y-	oxygen; quick

P

palat/o-	palate
palliat/o-	reduce the severity
palpat/o-	feeling; touching
palpit/o-	throb
pancreat/o-	pancreas
papill/o-	elevated structure
parenchym/o-	functional cells of an organ
pareun/o-	sexual intercourse
pariet/o-	wall of a cavity
par/o-	giving birth
paroxysm/o-	sudden, sharp attack
part/o-	childbirth; labor
parturit/o-	childbirth; labor
patell/o-	kneecap; patella
pathet/o-	suffering
path/o-	disease
pat/o-	open

paus/o-	cessation
pect/o-	stiff
pector/o-	chest
pedicul/o-	lice
ped/o-	child
pelv/i-	hip bone; pelvis; renal pelvis
pelv/o-	hip bone; pelvis; renal pelvis
pendul/o-	hanging down
pen/o-	penis
pepsin/o-	pepsin
peps/o-	digestion
pept/o-	digestion
percuss/o-	tapping
perfor/o-	opening
perine/o-	perineum
peripher/o-	outer aspects
peritone/o-	peritoneum
periton/o-	peritoneum
perone/o-	fibula; lower leg bone
person/o-	person
petechi/o-	petechiae
phac/o-	lens of the eye
phag/o-	eating; swallowing
phak/o-	lens of the eye
phalang/o-	digit; finger; toe
pharmaceutic/o-	drug; medicine
pharmac/o-	drug; medicine
pharyng/o-	pharynx; throat
phas/o-	speech
phe/o-	gray
phil/o-	attraction to; fondness for
phim/o-	closed tight
phleb/o-	vein
phob/o-	avoidance; fear
phor/o-	bear; carry; range
phosph/o-	phosphorus
phot/o-	light
phren/o-	diaphragm; mind
phylact/o-	guarding; protecting
physic/o-	body
physi/o-	physical function
phys/o-	distend; grow; inflate
pigment/o-	pigment
pil/o-	hair
pituitar/o-	pituitary gland
pituit/o-	pituitary gland
placent/o-	placenta
plak/o-	plaque
plasm/o-	plasma

plas/o-	formation; growth
plast/o-	formation; growth
pleg/o-	paralysis
pleur/o-	lung membrane
pne/o-	breathing
pneum/o-	air; lung
pneumon/o-	air; lung
pod/o-	foot
poikil/o-	irregular
polar/o-	negative state; positive state
pol/o-	pole
polyp/o-	polyp
poplite/o-	back of the knee
por/o-	pores; small openings
port/o-	point of entry
poster/o-	back part
potent/o-	capable of doing
pract/o-	medical practice
pregn/o-	being with child
presby/o-	old age
press/o-	pressure
preventat/o-	prevent
prevent/o-	prevent
priap/o-	persistent erection
prim/i-	first
proct/o-	rectum and anus
product/o-	produce
project/o-	orientation
pronat/o-	face down
propri/o-	one's own self
prostat/o-	prostate gland
prosthet/o-	artificial part
protein/o-	protein
prote/o-	protein
proxim/o-	near the center; near the point of origin
prurit/o-	itching
psor/o-	itching
psych/o-	mind
puber/o-	growing up
pub/o-	hip bone; pubis
pulmon/o-	lung
pulsat/o-	rhythmic throbbing
punct/o-	hole; perforation
pupill/o-	pupil of the eye
purul/o-	pus
pyel/o-	renal pelvis
pylor/o-	pylorus
py/o-	pus

pyret/o-	fever
pyr/o-	burning; fire

Q

quadr/o-	four
quantitat/o-	amount; quantity

R

radic/o-	root and all parts
radicul/o-	spinal nerve root
radi/o-	forearm bone; radiation; x-rays
rap/o-	drag away; seize
react/o-	reverse movement
recept/o-	receive
recess/o-	move back
rect/o-	rectum
recuper/o-	recover
reduct/o-	bring back; decrease
refract/o-	bend; deflect
regurgitat/o-	backward flow
relax/o-	relax
remiss/o-	send back
ren/o-	kidney
repress/o-	press back
resect/o-	cut out; remove
resist/o-	withstand the effect of
resuscit/o-	raise up again; revive
retard/o-	delay; slow down
retent/o-	hold back; keep
reticul/o-	small network
retin/o-	retina of the eye
rex/o-	see *orex/o-*
rhabd/o-	rod shaped
rheumat/o-	watery discharge
rhin/o-	nose
rhiz/o-	spinal nerve root
rhythm/o-	rhythm
rhytid/o-	wrinkle
rib/o-	ribonucleic acid
roentgen/o-	radiation; x-rays
rotat/o-	rotate
rrhag/o-	excessive discharge; excessive flow
rrhe/o-	discharge; flow
rrhythm/o-	rhythm
rub/o-	red
rug/o-	fold

S

sacchar/o-	sugar
sacr/o-	sacrum
sagitt/o-	front to back
saliv/o-	saliva
salping/o-	uterine tube
saphen/o-	clearly visible
sarc/o-	connective tissue
satur/o-	filled up
scal/o-	series of graduated steps
scaph/o-	boat shaped
scapul/o-	scapula; shoulder blade
schiz/o-	split
scient/o-	knowledge; science
scint/i-	point of light
scintill/o-	point of light
scler/o-	hard; sclera of the eye
scoli/o-	crooked; curved
scop/o-	examine with an instrument
scot/o-	darkness
script/o-	write
scrot/o-	bag; scrotum
sebace/o-	oil; sebum
seb/o-	oil; sebum
secret/o-	produce; secrete
sect/o-	cut
sedat/o-	calm an agitation
semin/i-	sperm; spermatozoon
semin/o-	sperm; spermatozoon
sen/o-	old age
sensitiv/o-	affected by; sensitive to
sensit/o-	affected by; sensitive to
sens/o-	sensation
sensor/i-	sensory
septic/o-	infection
sept/o-	dividing wall; septum
ser/o-	serum-like fluid; serum of the blood
sex/o-	sex
sial/o-	saliva; salivary gland
sigmoid/o-	sigmoid colon
sin/o-	channel; hollow cavity
sinus/o-	sinus
skelet/o-	skeleton
soci/o-	community; human beings
somat/o-	body
somn/o-	sleep
som/o-	body
son/o-	sound

sorb/o-	suck up
spad/o-	opening; tear
spasm/o-	spasm
spasmod/o-	spasm
spast/o-	spasm
spermat/o-	sperm; spermatozoon
sperm/o-	sperm; spermatozoon
sphen/o-	wedge shape
sphenoid/o-	sphenoid bone; sphenoid sinus
spher/o-	ball; sphere
sphincter/o-	sphincter
sphygm/o-	pulse
spin/o-	backbone; spine
spir/o-	breathe; coil
splen/o-	spleen
spondyl/o-	vertebra
squam/o-	scale-like cell
stal/o-	contraction
staped/o-	stapes; stirrup-shaped bone
stas/o-	standing still; staying in one place
stat/o-	standing still; staying in one place
steat/o-	fat
sten/o-	constriction; narrowness
stere/o-	three dimensions
stern/o-	breastbone; sternum
steroid/o-	steroid
steth/o-	chest
sthen/o-	strength
stigmat/o-	mark; point
stimul/o-	exciting; strengthening
stomat/o-	mouth
stom/o-	mouth; surgically created opening
strangul/o-	constrict
strept/o-	curved
stress/o-	disturbing stimulus
styl/o-	stake
sucr/o-	cane sugar; sugar
suct/o-	suck
sudor/i-	sweat
su/i-	self
superfici/o-	near the surface; on the surface
super/o-	above
supinat/o-	lying on the back
supposit/o-	placed beneath
suppress/o-	press down
suppur/o-	pus formation
surg/o-	operative procedure
suspens/o-	hanging

symptomat/o-	collection of symptoms
syncop/o-	fainting
synovi/o-	joint membrane; synovium
synov/o-	joint membrane; synovium
system/o-	body as a whole
systol/o-	contracting

T

tact/o-	touch
tampon/o-	stop up
tard/o-	late; slow
tars/o-	ankle
tax/o-	coordination
techn/o-	technical skill
tele/o-	distance
tempor/o-	side of the head; temple
tendin/o-	tendon
ten/o-	tendon
tens/o-	pressure; tension
terat/o-	bizarre form
termin/o-	boundary; end; word
testicul/o-	testicle; testis
test/o-	testicle; testis
tetr/a-	four
thalam/o-	thalamus
thanat/o-	death
thec/o-	dura mater; sheath
theli/o-	cellular layer
then/o-	thumb
therapeut/o-	therapy; treatment
therap/o-	treatment
therm/o-	heat
thorac/o-	chest; thorax
thromb/o-	blood clot
thym/o-	rage; thymus
thyr/o-	shield-shaped structure; thyroid gland
thyroid/o-	thyroid gland
tibi/o-	shin bone; tibia
till/o-	pull out
toc/o-	childbirth; labor
toler/o-	become accustomed to
tom/o-	cut; layer; slice
ton/o-	pressure; tone
tonsill/o-	tonsil
topic/o-	specific area
tort/i-	twisted position
toxic/o-	poison; toxin

tox/o-	poison
trabecul/o-	mesh
trache/o-	trachea; windpipe
trac/o-	visible path
tract/o-	pulling
tranquil/o-	calm
transit/o-	change from one thing to another
transmitt/o-	send across; send through
transplant/o-	move something across and put in another place
traumat/o-	injury
tremul/o-	shaking
trich/o-	hair
triglycerid/o-	triglyceride
trochanter/o-	trochanter
trochle/o-	structure shaped like a pulley
troph/o-	development
trop/o-	having an affinity for; stimulating; turning
tubercul/o-	nodule; tuberculosis
tuber/o-	nodule
tuberos/o-	knob-like projection
tub/o-	tube
tubul/o-	small tube
turbin/o-	scroll-like structure; turbinate
tuss/o-	cough
tympan/o-	eardrum; tympanic membrane

U

ulcerat/o-	ulcer
uln/o-	forearm bone; ulna
umbilic/o-	navel; umbilicus
ungu/o-	fingernail; toenail
ureter/o-	ureter
urethr/o-	urethra
urin/o-	urinary system; urine
ur/o-	urinary system; urine
uter/o-	uterus; womb
uve/o-	uvea of the eye

V

vaccin/o-	vaccine
vagin/o-	vagina
vag/o-	vagus nerve; wandering
valv/o-	valve
valvul/o-	valve
varic/o-	varicose vein; varix

vas/o-	blood vessel; vas deferens
vascul/o-	blood vessel
vegetat/o-	growth
veget/o-	vegetable
venere/o-	sexual intercourse
ven/i-	vein
ven/o-	vein
ventilat/o-	movement of air
ventil/o-	movement of air
vent/o-	coming
ventricul/o-	chamber that is filled; ventricle
ventr/o-	abdomen; front
verd/o-	green
vers/o-	travel; turn
vertebr/o-	vertebra
vert/o-	travel; turn
vesic/o-	bladder; fluid-filled sac
vesicul/o-	fluid-filled sac
vestibul/o-	entrance; vestibule
vest/o-	dress

viril/o-	masculine
vir/o-	virus
viscer/o-	large internal organs
viscos/o-	thickness
vis/o-	sight; vision
vitre/o-	transparent substance; vitreous humor
voc/o-	voice
volunt/o-	person's own free will
vuls/o-	tear
vulv/o-	vulva

X

xanth/o-	yellow
xen/o-	foreign
xer/o-	dry
xiph/o-	sword

Z

zygomat/o-	cheekbone; zygoma

Appendix B

Glossary of Medical Abbreviations, Acronyms, and Short Forms

*An asterisk beside an abbreviation means it is included (or may be included in the future) on a list compiled by The Joint Commission. The list contains abbreviations that have been the cause of errors. These abbreviations should not be used, and they also must appear on a healthcare facility's "Do Not Use" list. That is a short list because it is the minimum required by The Joint Commission to obtain facility accreditation. However, because these abbreviations are still used by some healthcare providers, they are included here.

**Many hospitals have removed this abbreviation from their official list of abbreviations because it has an undesirable meaning that is unrelated to the respiratory system.

■A square beside an abbreviation means it is from a more comprehensive list of abbreviations that should not be used, as compiled by the Institute for Safe Medication Practices (ISMP).

5-HIAA	5-hydroxyindoleacetic acid

A

A&O	alert and oriented
A&P	anatomy and physiology; auscultation and percussion
A	blood type A in the ABO blood group
AAA	abdominal aortic aneurysm
AB	blood type AB in the ABO blood group
AB, Ab	abortion
ABD, abd	abdomen
ABG	arterial blood gases
ABR	auditory brainstem response
AC, a.c.	before meals (Latin, *ante cibum*)
ACE	angiotensin-converting enzyme
Ach	acetylcholine
ACS	acute coronary syndrome
ACT	activated clotting time
ACTH	adrenocorticotropic hormone
AD, A.D.*■	right ear (Latin, *auris dextra*)
ADA	American Dental Association; American Diabetes Association; American Dietetic Association; Americans with Disabilities Act
ADD	attention-deficit disorder

ADH	antidiuretic hormone
ADHD	attention-deficit hyperactivity disorder
ADLs	activities of daily living
AED	automatic external defibrillator
AFB	acid-fast bacillus
A fib	atrial fibrillation
AFP	alpha fetoprotein
AGA	appropriate for gestational age
AI	aortic insufficiency; apical impulse; artificial insemination; artificial intelligence
AICD	automatic implantable cardiac defibrillator; automatic implantable cardioverter-defibrillator
AIDS	acquired immunodeficiency syndrome
AKA	above-the-knee amputation
alk phos	alkaline phosphatase
ALL	acute lymphocytic leukemia
ALP	alkaline phosphatase
ALS	amyotrophic lateral sclerosis
ALT	alanine aminotransferase; alanine transaminase
AMD	age-related macular degeneration
AMI	acute myocardial infarction
AML	acute myelogenous leukemia
ANS	autonomic nervous system
anti-CCP	anti-cyclic citrullinated peptide
AODM	adult-onset diabetes mellitus

AP	anteroposterior
aPTT	activated partial thromboplastin time
ARDS	acute respiratory distress syndrome; adult respiratory distress syndrome
ARF	acute renal failure; acute respiratory failure; acute rheumatic fever
ARM	artificial rupture of membranes
ARMD	age-related macular degeneration
ART	assisted reproductive technology
AS	aortic stenosis
AS, A.S.*■	left ear (Latin, *auris sinister*)
ASC	ambulatory surgery center
ASC-H	atypical squamous cells, cannot exclude HSIL
ASC-US	atypical squamous cells of undetermined significance
ASCVD	arteriosclerotic cardiovascular disease
ASD	atrial septal defect; autism spectrum disorder
ASHD	arteriosclerotic heart disease
ASIS	anterior-superior iliac spine
AST	aspartate aminotransferase; aspartate transaminase
ATN	acute tubular necrosis
AU, A.U.*■	both ears (Latin, *auris unitas*); each ear (Latin, *auris uterque*)
AV	atrioventricular
AVM	arteriovenous malformation

B

B	blood type B in the ABO blood group
Ba	barium
BAEP	brainstem auditory evoked potential
BAER	brainstem auditory evoked response
bagged	manually ventilated with an Ambu bag (short form)
basos	basophils (short form)
BBT	basal body temperature
BDI	Beck Depression Inventory
BE	barium enema; base excess (in the blood)
BKA	below-the-knee amputation
BM	bowel movement
BMD	bone mineral density
BMT	bone marrow transplantation
BOM	bilateral otitis media
BP	blood pressure
BPD	biparietal diameter (of the fetal head)
BPH	benign prostatic hypertrophy
BPM, bpm	beats per minute
BPP	biophysical profile
BRBPR	bright red blood per rectum
BRCA	breast cancer (gene)
BS	bowel sounds; breath sounds

BSE	breast self-examination
BSO	bilateral salpingo-oophorectomy
BUN	blood urea nitrogen
BX, Bx	biopsy

C

C&S	culture and sensitivity
C1–C7	cervical vertebrae 1–7
Ca	cancer; carcinoma (pronounced "c-a")
Ca, Ca++	calcium
CABG	coronary artery bypass graft (pronounced "cabbage")
CAD	coronary artery disease
CAPD	continuous ambulatory peritoneal dialysis
CAT	computerized axial tomography
cath	catheterization; catheterize (short form)
CBC	complete blood count
CBD	common bile duct
CBT	cognitive-behavioral therapy
CC	chief complaint
cc*■	cubic centimeter (measure of volume)
CCPD	continuous cycling peritoneal dialysis
CCU	coronary care unit
CD4	helper T cell
CD8	suppressor T cell
CDC	Centers for Disease Control
CDCP	Centers for Disease Control and Prevention
CDE	certified diabetes educator
CDH	congenital dislocation of the hip
CEA	carcinoembryonic antigen
CF	cystic fibrosis
chemo	chemotherapy (short form)
CHF	congestive heart failure
CIN	cervical intraepithelial neoplasia
CIS	carcinoma *in situ*
CK	conductive keratoplasty; creatine kinase
CKD	chronic kidney disease
CK-MB	creatine kinase-MB (band)
Cl, Cl−	chloride
CLL	chronic lymphocytic leukemia
CLO	*Campylobacter*-like organism
CMG	cystometrogram
CML	chronic myelogenous leukemia
cmm	cubic millimeter
CN1–CN12	cranial nerves 1–12
CNM	certified nurse midwife
CNS	central nervous system
CO	carbon monoxide

CO₂	carbon dioxide
COMT	catechol-*O*-methyltransferase
COPD	chronic obstructive pulmonary disease
COTA	certified occupational therapy assistant
CP	cardiopulmonary; cerebral palsy
CPAP	continuous positive airway pressure (pronounced "SEE-pap")
CPD	cephalopelvic disproportion
CPK-MB	creatine phosphokinase-MB (band)
CPK-MM	creatine phosphokinase-MM (band)
CPR	cardiopulmonary resuscitation
CRF	cardiac risk factors; chronic renal failure
CRNA	certified registered nurse anesthetist
CRP	C-reactive protein
CRPS	chronic regional pain syndrome; complex regional pain syndrome
CRT	certified radiation therapist
CS	cesarean section ("C-section", short form)
CSF	cerebrospinal fluid
CT	computerized tomography
CTD	cumulative trauma disorder
CTR	certified tumor registrar
CTS	carpal tunnel syndrome
CV	cardiovascular
CVA	cerebrovascular accident
CVS	chorionic villus sampling
CXR	chest x-ray
cysto	cystoscopy (short form)

D

D/C*■	discharge; discontinue
D&C	dilation and curettage
dB, db	decibel
D.C.	Doctor of Chiropracty or Chiropractic Medicine
D.D.S.	Doctor of Dental Surgery
Derm	dermatology (short form)
DEXA	dual-energy x-ray absorptiometry
DI	diabetes insipidus
DIC	disseminated intravascular coagulation
diff	differential count of WBCs (short form)
DIP	distal interphalangeal (joint)
DJD	degenerative joint disease
DKA	diabetic ketoacidosis
DM	diabetes mellitus
DNA	deoxyribonucleic acid
D.O.	Doctor of Osteopathy or Osteopathic Medicine
DOE	dyspnea on exertion
D.P.M.	Doctor of Podiatry or Podiatric Medicine
Dr.	doctor

DRE	digital rectal examination
DS	discharge summary
DSA	digital subtraction angiography
DSM-5	*Diagnostic and Statistical Manual of Mental -Disorders,* 5th edition
DT	delirium tremens
DTR	deep tendon reflex
DUB	dysfunctional uterine bleeding
DVT	deep venous thrombosis
DX, Dx	diagnosis
DXA	dual-energy x-ray absorptiometry

E

EAC	external auditory canal
EBT	electron beam tomography
EBV	Epstein-Barr virus
ECCE	extracapsular cataract extraction
ECG	electrocardiogram; electrocardiography
echo	echocardiogram; echocardiography (short form)
ECT	electroconvulsive therapy
ECV	external cephalic version
ED	emergency department; erectile dysfunction
EDB	estimated date of birth
EDC	estimated date of confinement; extensor digitorum communis
EDD	estimated date of delivery
EEG	electroencephalogram; electroencephalography
EGA	estimated gestational age
EGD	esophagogastroduodenoscopy
EHR	electronic health record
EKG	electrocardiogram; electrocardiography
ELISA	enzyme-linked immunosorbent assay
EMB	endometrial biopsy
EMG	electromyogram; electromyography
EMR	electronic medical record
END	electroneurodiagnostic (technician)
ENT	ears, nose, and throat
eos	eosinophils (short form)
EOM	extraocular movements; extraocular muscles
EOMI	extraocular muscles intact
epi	epinephrine (short form)
epis	epithelial cells (in a urine specimen) (short form)
EPO	erythropoietin
EPR	electronic patient record
EPS	electrophysiologic study
ER	emergency room; estrogen receptor
ERCP	endoscopic retrograde cholangiopancreatography
ESRD	end-stage renal disease
ESWL	extracorporeal shock wave lithotripsy

ESWT	extracorporeal shock wave therapy
ET	endotracheal
ETOH	ethanol (liquor); ethyl alcohol
ETT	endotracheal tube

F

FBG	fasting blood glucose
FBS	fasting blood sugar
Fe	ferritin (iron)
FEV$_1$	forced expiratory volume (in one second)
FH	family history
FHR	fetal heart rate
fib	fibula (short form)
FIGO	Federation Internationale de Gynécologie et Obstétrique (scoring system)
FiO$_2$	fraction (percentage) of inhaled oxygen
FOBT	fecal occult blood test
FSH	follicle-stimulating hormone
FTI	free thyroxine index
FVC	forced vital capacity
FX, Fx	fracture

G

G	gravida; gauge (of a needle)
G/TPAL	see G and *TPAL*
GC	gonococcus (*Neisseria gonorrhoeae*)
GCS	Glasgow Coma Scale (or Score)
G-CSF	granulocyte colony-stimulating factor
GDM	gestational diabetes mellitus
GERD	gastroesophageal reflux disease
GGPT, GGT	gamma-glutamyl transpeptidase
GH	growth hormone
GI	gastrointestinal
GIFT	gamete intrafallopian transfer
GM-CSF	granulocyte-macrophage colony-stimulating factor
GTT	glucose tolerance test
gtt.	drops
GU	genitourinary; gonococcal urethritis
GVHD	graft-versus-host disease
GYN	gynecology

H

H&H	hemoglobin and hematocrit
H&P	history and physical (examination)
HAV	hepatitis A virus
Hb	hemoglobin
HbA$_{1C}$	hemoglobin A$_{1C}$

HbCO	carboxyhemoglobin
HBV	hepatitis B virus
HCG, hCG	human chorionic gonadotropin
HCl	hydrochloric acid
HCO$_3^-$	bicarbonate
HCT	hematocrit
HCTZ	hydrochlorothiazide (drug)
HCV	hepatitis C virus
HDL	high-density lipoprotein
HEENT	head, eyes, ears, nose, and throat
HER	human epidermal (growth factor) receptor (2)
Hg	mercury
HGB, Hgb	hemoglobin
HIDA	hydroxyiminodiacetic acid
HIPAA	Health Insurance Portability and Accountability Act (pronounced "HIP-ah")
HIV	human immunodeficiency virus
HLA	human leukocyte antigen
HMD	hyaline membrane disease
HNP	herniated nucleus pulposus
HoLAP	holmium laser ablation of the prostate
hpf	high-power field
HPI	history of present illness
HPV	human papillomavirus
HRT	hormone replacement therapy
HSG	hysterosalpingogram; hysterosalpingography
HSIL	high-grade squamous intraepithelial lesion
HSV	herpes simplex virus
HTN	hypertension
HX, Hx	history
Hz	hertz

I

I&D	incision and drainage
I&O	intake and output
IBD	inflammatory bowel disease
IBS	irritable bowel syndrome
ICCE	intracapsular cataract extraction
ICD-10	*International Classification of Diseases,* 10th edition
ICP	intracranial pressure
ICSI	intracytoplasmic sperm injection
ICU	intensive care unit
IDDM	insulin-dependent diabetes mellitus
IgA	immunoglobulin A
IgD	immunoglobulin D
IgE	immunoglobulin E
IgG	immunoglobulin G
IgM	immunoglobulin M

IM	intramuscular
INR	international normalized ratio
IOL	intraocular lens
IOP	intraocular pressure
IRS	insulin resistance syndrome
ISMP	Institute for Safe Medication Practices
IUGR	intrauterine growth retardation
IVC	intravenous cholangiogram; intravenous cholangiography
IVF	*in vitro* fertilization
IVP	intravenous pyelogram; intravenous pyelography

J

JOD	juvenile-onset diabetes (mellitus)
JVD	jugular venous distention

K

K, K⁺	potassium
KS	Kaposi's sarcoma
KUB	kidneys, ureters, bladder

L

L&D	labor and delivery
L/S	lecithin/sphingomyelin (ratio)
L1–L5	lumbar vertebrae 1–5
LA	left atrium
LADA	latent autoimmune diabetes in adults
LASIK	laser-assisted *in situ* keratomileusis (pronounced "LAY-sik")
Lat	lateral
LBBB	left bundle branch block
LDH	lactic dehydrogenase
LDL	low-density lipoprotein
LEEP	loop electrocautery excision procedure
LES	lower esophageal sphincter
LFTs	liver function tests
LGA	large for gestational age
LH	luteinizing hormone
LLE	left lower extremity
LLL	left lower lobe (of the lung)
LLQ	left lower quadrant (of the abdomen)
LMP	last menstrual period
LOC	loss of consciousness
LP	lumbar puncture
LPN	licensed practical nurse
LSD	lysergic acid diethylamide (a street drug)
LSIL	low-grade squamous intraepithelial lesion
LTK	laser thermal keratoplasty

LUE	left upper extremity
LUL	left upper lobe (of the lung)
LUQ	left upper quadrant (of the abdomen)
LV	left ventricle
LVAD	left ventricular assist device
LVH	left ventricular hypertrophy
LVN	licensed vocational nurse
lymphs	lymphocytes (short form)

M

MAO	monoamine oxidase
MCH	mean cell hemoglobin
MCHC	mean cell hemoglobin concentration
MCP	metacarpophalangeal (joint)
MCV	mean cell volume
M.D.	Doctor of Medicine
MD	macular degeneration; muscular dystrophy
MDCT	multidetector-row computerized tomography
MDI	metered-dose inhaler
mets	metastases (short form); unit of measurement during cardiac treadmill stress test
MI	myocardial infarction
mL	milliliter (measure of volume)
mm Hg	millimeters of mercury
mm³	cubic millimeter
MMSE	mini mental status examination
mono	mononucleosis (short form)
monos	monocytes (short form)
MR	mitral regurgitation
MRA	magnetic resonance angiography
mrem	one thousandth of a rem
MRI	magnetic resonance imaging
MS*■	magnesium sulfate; morphine sulfate; multiple sclerosis
MSH	melanocyte-stimulating hormone
MUGA	multiple-gated acquisition (scan) (pronounced "MUG-ah")
MVP	mitral valve prolapse

N

N&V	nausea and vomiting
Na, Na⁺	sodium
NB	newborn
NCS	nerve conduction study
NG	nasogastric
NICU	neonatal intensive care unit (pronounced "NIK-yoo"); neurologic intensive care unit (pronounced "NIK-yoo")
NIDDM	non-insulin-dependent diabetes mellitus

NK	natural killer (cell)
NP	nurse practitioner
NPH	neutral protamine Hagedorn (insulin); normal pressure hydrocephalus
NPO, n.p.o.	nothing by mouth (Latin, *nil per os*)
NSAID	nonsteroidal anti-inflammatory drug
NSR	normal sinus rhythm
NST	nonstress test
NSVD	normal spontaneous vaginal delivery

O

O	blood type O in the ABO blood group
O&P	ova and parasites
O_2	oxygen
OA	osteoarthritis; Overeaters Anonymous
OB	obstetrics
OB/GYN	obstetrics and gynecology
OCD	obsessive–compulsive disorder
OCG	oral cholecystogram; oral cholecystography
OCP	oral contraceptive pill
OD, O.D.*■	right eye (Latin, *oculus dexter*); overdose
O.D.	Doctor of Optometry
OGTT	oral glucose tolerance test
OOB	out of bed
ORIF	open reduction and internal fixation
ortho	orthopedics (short form)
OS, O.S.*■	left eye (Latin, *oculus sinister*)
OSHA	Occupational Safety and Health Administration
OT	occupational therapist; occupational therapy
OU, O.U.*■	both eyes (Latin, *oculus unitas*); each eye (Latin, *oculus uterque*)

P

P	para; phosphorus; pulse (rate)
PA	physician's assistant; posteroanterior
PAC	premature atrial contraction
PACU	postanesthesia recovery room (pronounced "PAK-yoo")
PAD	peripheral artery disease
Pap	Papanicolaou (smear or test) (short form)
PAP	prostatic acid phosphatase
PC, p.c.	after meals (Latin, *post cibum*)
PCI	percutaneous coronary intervention
PCO_2, pCO_2	partial pressure of carbon dioxide
PCP	phencyclidine ("angel dust," a street drug); primary care physician
PD	prism diopter
PDA	patent ductus arteriosus

PDT	photodynamic therapy
PE	physical examination; pressure-equalizing (tube); pulmonary embolus
PEG	percutaneous endoscopic gastrostomy
PEJ	percutaneous endoscopic jejunostomy
PERRL	pupils equal, round, and reactive to light
PERRLA	pupils equal, round, reactive to light and accommodation
PET	positron emission tomography
PFT	pulmonary function test
pH	potential of hydrogen (acid or alkaline)
Pharm.D.	Doctor of Pharmacy
PICC	peripherally inserted central catheter
PICU	pediatric intensive care unit (pronounced "PIK-yoo")
PID	pelvic inflammatory disease
PIP	proximal interphalangeal (joint)
PM&R	physical medicine and rehabilitation
PMDD	premenstrual dysphoric disorder
PMH	past medical (and surgical) history
PMI	point of maximum impulse
PMN	polymorphonuclear (leukocyte)
PMS	premenstrual syndrome
PND	paroxysmal nocturnal dyspnea; postnasal drainage; postnasal drip
PO, p.o.	by mouth (Latin, *per os*)
PO_2, pO_2	partial pressure of oxygen
polys	polymorphonuclear leukocytes (short form)
PPD	packs per day (of cigarettes); purified protein derivative (TB test)
PR	progesterone receptor
PRBCs	packed red blood cells
primip	primiparous (short form)
PRK	photorefractive keratectomy
PRN, p.r.n.	as needed (Latin, *pro re nata*)
pro time	prothrombin time (short form)
PROM	passive range of motion; premature rupture of membranes
PSA	prostate-specific antigen
Psy	psychiatry; psychology
Psych	psychiatry; psychology (pronounced "sike")
PT	physical therapist; physical therapy; prothrombin time
PTC	percutaneous transhepatic cholangiography
PTCA	percutaneous transluminal coronary angioplasty
PTSD	posttraumatic stress disorder
PTT	partial thromboplastin time
PUD	peptic ulcer disease
PUVA	psoralen (drug and) ultraviolet A (light therapy)
PVC	premature ventricular contraction
PVD	peripheral vascular disease

PVP	photoselective vaporization of the prostate

Q

QCT	quantitative computerized tomography

R

R, r	roentgen (unit of exposure to x-rays or gamma rays)
RA	rheumatoid arthritis; right atrium; room air (no supplemental oxygen)
rad	radiation absorbed dose (short form)
RAIU	radioactive iodine uptake
RAST	radioallergosorbent test
RBBB	right bundle branch block
RBC	red blood cell
RDS	respiratory distress syndrome
rehab	rehabilitation (short form)
rem	roentgen-equivalent man
REM	rapid eye movement
RF	rheumatoid factor
RFA	radiofrequency ablation
RIA	radioimmunoassay
RICE	rest, ice, compression, and elevation
RIND	reversible ischemic neurologic deficit
RLE	right lower extremity
RLL	right lower lobe (of the lung)
RLQ	right lower quadrant (of the abdomen)
RML	right middle lobe (of the lung)
RN	registered nurse
RNA	ribonucleic acid
RNV	radionuclide ventriculography
R/O, r/o	rule out
ROM	range of motion; rupture of membranes
ROP	retinopathy of prematurity
ROS	review of systems
RP	retinitis pigmentosa
RPR	rapid plasma reagin (test)
RRT	registered radiologic technologist; registered respiratory therapist
RSI	repetitive strain injury
RUE	right upper extremity
RUL	right upper lobe (of the lung)
RUQ	right upper quadrant (of the abdomen)
RV	right ventricle

S

S1	first sacral vertebra
S₁	first heart sound
S₂	second heart sound
S₃	third heart sound
S₄	fourth heart sound
SA	sinoatrial
SAB	spontaneous abortion
SAD	seasonal affective disorder
SARS	severe acute respiratory syndrome
SBE	subacute bacterial endocarditis
SCC	squamous cell carcinoma
SCI	spinal cord injury
segs	segmented neutrophils (short form)
SG	specific gravity
SGA	small for gestational age
SGOT	serum glutamic-oxaloacetic transaminase
SGPT	serum glutamic-pyruvic transaminase
SH	social history
SIADH	syndrome of inappropriate ADH
SICU	surgical intensive care unit (pronounced "SIK-yoo")
SIDS	sudden infant death syndrome
SLE	systemic lupus erythematosus
SMA	sequential multichannel analysis
SMAC	sequential multichannel analysis with computer (pronounced "smack")
SNF	skilled nursing facility (pronounced "sniff")
SOB**	shortness of breath
SOM	serous otitis media
SPECT	single-photon emission computerized tomography
SPEP	serum protein electrophoresis (pronounced "S-pep")
sp gr	specific gravity
SQ*■	subcutaneous
SSEP	somatosensory evoked potential
SSER	somatosensory evoked response
SSRI	selective serotonin reuptake inhibitor (drug)
STD	sexually transmitted disease
STI	sexually transmitted infection
subcu	subcutaneous (short form)
subQ■	subcutaneous (short form)
SVT	supraventricular tachycardia
SX, Sx	symptoms

T

T&A	tonsillectomy and adenoidectomy
T1–T12	thoracic vertebrae 1–12
T₃, T3■	triiodothyronine
T₄	thyroxine
T₇	free thyroxine index (FTI)
TAB	therapeutic abortion
TACE	transarterial chemoembolization

TAH-BSO	total abdominal hysterectomy and bilateral salpingo-oophorectomy
TAT	Thematic Apperception Test
TB	tuberculosis
TEE	transesophageal echocardiogram; transesophageal echocardiography
TENS	transcutaneous electrical nerve stimulation (unit)
TFTs	thyroid function tests
THR	total hip replacement
TIA	transient ischemic attack
tib	tibia (short form)
TIBC	total iron-binding capacity
tib-fib	tibia and fibula (short form)
TM	tympanic membrane
TMJ	temporomandibular joint
TNF	tumor necrosis factor
TNM	tumor, nodes, metastases
TnT	troponin T
TNTC	too numerous to count
TPA	tissue plasminogen activator (drug)
TPAL	term newborns, premature newborns, abortions, living children
TPR	temperature, pulse, and respiration
trach	tracheostomy (short form)
TRAM	transverse rectus abdominis muscle (flap) (pronounced "tram")
TRUS	transrectal ultrasound
TSE	testicular self-examination
TSH	thyroid-stimulating hormone
TUMT	transurethral microwave therapy
TUNA	transurethral needle ablation
TURBT	transurethral resection of bladder tumor
TURP	transurethral resection of the prostate
TVH	total vaginal hysterectomy
TX, Tx	treatment
TXM	type and crossmatch (short form)

U

UA	urinalysis
UGI	upper gastrointestinal (series)
UPEP	urine protein electrophoresis (pronounced "U-pep")
URI	upper respiratory infection
US	ultrasonography; ultrasound
UTI	urinary tract infection
UVB	ultraviolet light B

V

V fib	ventricular fibrillation (short form)
V tach	ventricular tachycardia (short form)
V/Q	ventilation-perfusion (scan)
VBAC	vaginal birth after ceserean section (pronounced "V-back")
VCUG	voiding cystourethrogram; voiding cystourethrography
VD	venereal disease
VDRL	Venereal Disease Research Laboratory (test)
VEP	visual evoked potential
VER	visual evoked response
VF	visual field
VLDL	very low-density lipoprotein
VMA	vanillylmandelic acid
VS	vital signs
VSD	ventricular septal defect

W

WBC	white blood cell

Z

ZIFT	zygote intrafallopian transfer

Answer Key

Chapter 1: The Structure of Medical Language

1.1 Identify Medical Language Skills

Fill in the Blank Exercise (p. 24)

1. **a.** reading
   b. listening
   c. thinking, analyzing, and understanding
   d. writing (or typing) and spelling
   e. speaking and pronouncing

1.2 Describe Medical Language Origins

True or False Exercise (p. 24)

1. T
3. F
5. T

1.3 Form Plural Nouns

Latin and Greek Plural Nouns Exercise (p. 24)

Latin Singular	Latin Plural
1. vertebra	vertebrae
3. alveolus	alveoli
5. nucleus	nuclei
7. diverticulum	diverticula
9. ovum	ova
11. diagnosis	diagnoses

Greek Singular	Greek Plural
13. epididymis	epididymides
15. carcinoma	carcinomata
17. ganglion	ganglia

Circle Exercise (p. 25)

1. phalanx
3. vertebrae
5. alveoli

1.4 Identify and Describe Word Parts

Matching Exercise (p. 25)

2, __, 1, __, 3, __

True or False Exercise (p. 25)

1. F
3. F
5. T

Fill in the Blank Exercise (pp. 25–26)

1. **a.** combining form
   b. suffix
   c. prefix
   b. sub-
   c. post-
3. **a.** hyper-

1.5 Give Word Part Meanings

Word Parts Exercise #1 (pp. 26–27)

1.	P	away from; without
3.	S	pertaining to
5.	P	not; without
7.	CF	appendix; small structure hanging from a larger structure
9.	CF	artery
11.	S	pertaining to
13.	P	two
15.	P	slow
17.	CF	heart
19.	CF	colon
21.	CF	impart; transmit
23.	CF	skin
25.	CF	skin
27.	CF	break down food; digest
29.	S	surgical removal
31.	CF	intestine
33.	CF	feeling; sensation
35.	P	good; normal
37.	CF	group; set
39.	S	process of recording
41.	CF	liver
43.	P	below; deficient
45.	S	condition; state; thing
47.	S	pertaining to
49.	P	between
51.	P	within
53.	S	disease from a specific cause; process
55.	S	infection of; inflammation of
57.	CF	abdomen
59.	CF	side
61.	P	bad; inadequate
63.	CF	medicine; physician
65.	CF	monthly discharge of blood
67.	S	process of measuring
69.	CF	nose
71.	CF	nourishment
73.	S	condition; process
75.	S	disease
77.	P	around
79.	CF	paralysis
81.	P	many; much
83.	P	before; in front of
85.	P	four
87.	S	instrument used to examine
89.	CF	sperm; spermatozoon
91.	S	surgically created opening
93.	P	fast

95. CF   treatment
97. CF   thyroid gland
99. CF   tonsil
101. P   across; through
103. CF   urinary system; urine
105. CF   vagina

Word Parts Exercise #2 (p. 27)

1. poly-   polyneuritis; polyneuropathy
3. -logy   cardiology; etymology; neurology, psychology; technology; terminology
5. brady-   bradycardia
7. muscul/o-   muscular
9. -ism   euthyroidism; hypothyroidism; organism
11. -itis   appendicitis; arthritis; hepatitis; laryngitis; neuritis; polyneuritis; tonsillitis
13. -megaly   cardiomegaly
15. gastr/o-   gastric; gastrointestinal; gastroscopy
17. -scopy   gastroscopy

Matching Exercise (p. 28)

4, __, 12, __, 5, __, 2, __, 1, __, 3, __

1.6A Divide Medical Words

Dividing Words Exercise #1 (pp. 28–30)

1. -ac   cardi/o-
pertaining to   heart
pertaining to the heart
3. -itis   laryng/o-
infection of; inflammation of   larynx
infection of or inflammation of the larynx
5. -logy   neur/o-
study of; word   nerve
study of the nerves
7. -ia   pneumon/o-
condition; state; thing   air; lung
condition of the lung
9. -scopy   gastr/o-
process of using an instrument to examine   stomach
process of using an instrument to examine the stomach
11. -ia   an-   esthes/o-
condition; state; thing   not; without   feeling; sensation
condition of (being) without feeling or sensation
13. -ia   tachy-   cardi/o-
condition; state; thing   fast   heart
condition of a fast heart
15. -al   intra-   nas/o-
pertaining to   within   nose
pertaining to within the nose

Dividing Long Words Exercise #2 (p. 31)

1. -scopy   process of using an instrument to examine
esophag/o-   esophagus
gastr/o-   stomach
duoden/o-   duodenum
process of using an instrument to examine the esophagus, stomach and duodenum

1.6B Build Medical Words

Combining Form and Suffix Exercise (p. 31)

1. cardiac
3. intestinal
5. neuroma
7. therapist
9. urinary
11. arthropathy
13. cardiomegaly

Prefix Exercise (p. 32)

1. hyper-   hyperthyroidism
3. epi-   epigastric
5. intra-   intramuscular
7. post-   postnasal

1.7A Spell Medical Words

Spelling Exercise (p. 32)

1. cardiac
3. subcutaneous
5. mammography
7. tachycardia
9. urination

Circle Exercise (p. 33)

1. gastric
3. cardiac
5. urinary

Hearing Medical Words Exercise (p. 33)

1. cardiac
3. urination
5. intravenous
7. tonsillitis
9. subcutaneous

1.7B Pronounce Medical Words

Pronunciation Exercise (p. 33)

1. kar
3. tray
5. kar
7. meg
9. koh

1.8 Describe the Medical Record

True or False Exercise (p. 33)

1. T
3. T
5. F

Fill in the Blank Exercise (p. 34)

1. a. Several healthcare professionals can access the same record at the same time.
    b. The record cannot be lost or damaged because there is always a back-up electronic copy.
    c. It only takes seconds to retrieve a patient's past medical records.
3. a. electronic medical record (EMR)
    b. electronic patient record (EPR)
    c. electronic health record (EHR)

1.9 Define Abbreviations

Fill in the Blank Exercise (p. 34)

1. electronic patient record
3. chief complaint
5. diagnosis

Chapter 2: The Body in Health and Disease

Labeling Exercise (pp. 57–60)

FIRST EXERCISE

1. posterior (dorsal)
3. medial
5. proximal

SECOND EXERCISE

1. cranial cavity
3. thoracic cavity
5. abdominal cavity

THIRD EXERCISE

1. right hypochondriac region
3. right lumbar region
5. right inguinal region
7. left lumbar region
9. hypogastric region

FOURTH EXERCISE

1. cell membrane
3. nucleolus
5. mitochondrion
7. lysosome
9. endoplasmic reticulum

FIFTH EXERCISE

1. cardiovascular system
3. integumentary system
5. urinary system
7. gastrointestinal system

GIVE WORD PART MEANINGS

COMBINING FORMS EXERCISE (pp. 61–62)

1. back; dorsum
3. before; front part
5. tail bone
7. cell
9. cartilage
11. cranium; skull
13. cell
15. skin
17. away from the center; away from the point of origin
19. intestine
21. front
23. genitalia
25. female; woman
27. medical treatment; physician
29. below
31. skin
33. intestine
35. larynx; voice box
37. area between the ribs and pelvis; lower back
39. break down; destroy
41. medicine; physician
43. one millionth; small
45. birth
47. nerve
49. nucleus of an atom; nucleus of a cell
51. mass; tumor
53. organ
55. ear
57. hip bone; pelvis; renal pelvis
59. physical function
61. produce
63. mind
65. four
67. ribonucleic acid
69. examine with an instrument
71. backbone; spine
73. above
75. cut; layer; slice
77. urinary system; urine
79. blood vessel
81. travel; turn

BUILD MEDICAL WORDS

COMBINING FORM AND SUFFIX EXERCISE (pp. 62–63)

1. -al   abdominal
3. -ar   lumbar
5. -al   distal
7. -al   cranial
9. -logy   dermatology
11. -al   lateral
13. -logy   cardiology
15. -logy   urology
17. -logy   ophthalmology
19. -logy   gynecology
21. -ous   nervous
23. -logy   oncology
25. -al   inguinal
27. -logy   hematology
29. -logy   neurology
31. -al   medial
33. -logy   cardiology
35. -ics   dietetics
37. -al   visceral

PREFIX EXERCISE (p. 63)

1. endo-   endocrine
3. mid-   midsagittal
5. re-   respiratory
7. re-   reproductive

GIVE WORD PART MEANINGS

COMBINING FORMS EXERCISE (p. 74)

1. boundary; end; word
3. accessory; servant
5. time
7. present at birth
9. increase; provoke
11. creation; production
13. genitalia
15. give ability
17. medical treatment; physician
19. disease within
21. study of; word
23. new
25. nourishment
27. feeling; touching
29. tapping
31. formation; growth
33. recover
35. operative procedure
37. technical skill
39. treatment

BUILD MEDICAL WORDS

COMBINING FORM AND SUFFIX EXERCISE (p. 75)

1. -ion   inspection
3. -ist   therapist
5. -ive   palliative
7. -ary   hereditary
9. -logy   symptomatology
11. -ation auscultation
13. -ic   therapeutic
15. -ion   percussion
17. -al   congenital

PREFIX EXERCISE (p. 76)

1. dia-   diagnosis
3. a-   asymptomatic
5. re-   refractory

2.1 Describe Approaches to Organize the Body

2.2 Identify Planes, Directions, Quadrants, Regions, Cavities, Systems, Medical Specialties, and Cell Structures

Matching Exercise (p. 78)

7, __, 1, __, 4, __, 6, __, 3

Circle Exercise (p. 78)

1. blood   7. thoracic
3. cells   9. distal
5. anatomical

True or False Exercise (pp. 78–79)

1. T   7. F
3. F   9. T
5. F   11. F

2.3 Categorize Diseases

2.4 Describe a Physical Examination

2.5 Describe Healthcare Professionals and Settings of Care

Circle Exercise (p. 79)

1. physician's office   5. hereditary
3. refractory

Fill in the Blank Exercise (p. 79)

1. subacute   5. idiopathic
3. auscultation   7. clinic

True or False Exercise (p. 79)

1. F   5. T
3. T   7. F

2.6A Give Word Part Meanings

Word Parts Matching Exercise (p. 80)

13, __, 7, __, 6, __, 16, __, 17, __, 15, __, 14, __, 5, __, 3

2.6B Define Abbreviations

Matching Exercise (p. 80)

4, __, 6, __, 1, __, 2, __, 10, __, 7

2.7A Divide Medical Words

Dividing Words Exercise (p. 81)

1. ana-   tom/o-   -ical
3. ____   cephal/o-   -ad
5. ____   gynec/o-   -logy
7. ____   ophthalm/o- -logy
9. ____   poster/o-   -ior
11. ____   thorac/o-   -ic

2.7B Build Medical Words

Combining Form and Suffix Exercise (p. 81)

1. neurology   9. congenital
3. microscope   11. dermatology
5. cardiology   13. symptomatology
7. superior

2.8A Spell Medical Words

You Write the Medical Report (p. 82)

1. gynecology   7. neonatology
3. otolaryngology   9. orthopedics
5. dermatology

Proofreading and Spelling Exercise (p. 82)

1. anatomical   7. otolaryngology
3. thoracic   9. gynecology
5. cardiovascular

English and Medical Word Equivalents Exercise (p. 83)

1. anterior or ventral   7. superior
3. lateral   9. cephalad
5. supine

Hearing Medical Words Exercise (p. 83)

1. disease   9. integumentary
3. cardiovascular   11. palliative
5. epigastric   13. prognosis
7. hereditary

2.8B Pronounce Medical Words

Pronunciation Exercise (p. 83)

1. teer   7. path
3. tay   9. pel
5. naw

Chapter 3: Gastroenterology

Labeling Exercise (pp. 98–99)

FIRST EXERCISE

1. oral cavity   5. submandibular gland
3. teeth   7. pharynx

SECOND EXERCISE

1. esophagus   7. rugae
3. pancreas   9. cardia
5. pylorus   11. omentum

THIRD EXERCISE

1. liver   9. appendix
3. pancreas   11. anal sphincter
5. ascending colon   13. jejunum
7. descending colon   15. sigmoid colon

GIVE WORD PART MEANINGS
COMBINING FORMS EXERCISE (p. 100)

1. fluid; water
3. absorb; take in
5. carbohydrate; starch
7. appendix
9. bile; gall
11. abdomen
13. chloride
15. bile; gall
17. common bile duct
19. colon
21. break down food; digest
23. liquid with suspended particles
25. esophagus
27. feces; stool
29. tongue
31. liver
33. intestine
35. movement
37. abdomen
39. fat; lipid
41. chewing
43. ear
45. hip bone; pelvis; renal pelvis
47. digestion
49. peritoneum
51. rectum and anus
53. rectum
55. saliva
57. sigmoid colon
59. mouth

BUILD MEDICAL WORDS
COMBINING FORM AND SUFFIX EXERCISE (p. 101)

1. -al   intestinal
3. -cyte   hepatocyte
5. -ary   salivary
7. -ation   mastication
9. -ase   lipase
11. -ary   alimentary
13. -ive   digestive
15. -gen   pepsinogen
17. -ary   biliary
19. -ory   gustatory
21. -in   gastrin
23. -al   jejunal
25. -al   fecal
27. -ase   lactase
29. -al   peritoneal

PREFIX EXERCISE (p. 102)

1. sub-   submandibular
3. meso-   mesenteric
5. sub-   sublingual

MULTIPLE COMBINING FORMS AND SUFFIX
EXERCISE (p. 102)

1. hydr/o-   chlor/o-   -ic   hydrochloric
3. abdomin/o-   pelv/o-   -ic   abdominopelvic
5. gastr/o-   enter/o-   -logy   gastroenterology

3.1 Identify Anatomical Structures
3.2 Describe Physiology

Matching Exercise (p. 131)
7, __, 12, __, 11, __, 10, __, 4, __, 3, __, 2

Circle Exercise (p. 131)

1. duodenum   5. hydrochloric acid
3. cardia   7. bile

True or False Exercise (pp. 131–132)

1. T   7. F
3. F   9. F
5. F

Sequencing Exercise (p. 132)

1. oral cavity   7. ileum
3. esophagus   9. colon
5. duodenum   11. anus

3.3A Describe Diseases

Matching Exercise (p. 132)
13, __, 2, __, 7, __, 12, __, 11, __, 3, __, 10

True or False Exercise (p. 133)

1. T   5. F
3. T   7. T

3.3B Describe Laboratory, Radiology, Surgery, and Drugs

Fill in the Blank Exercise (p. 133)

1. stoma   7. barium swallow
3. albumin   9. herniorrhaphy
5. cholangiography

Circle Exercise (p. 133)

1. liver transplantation   7. CLO
3. cholecystectomy   9. gastrectomy
5. obesity

3.4 Form Plurals and Adjectives

Plural Noun and Adjective Exercise (p. 134)

1. ____   abdominal
3. ____   appendiceal
5. ____   cecal
7. diverticula diverticular
9. ____   esophageal
11. ____   hepatic
13. ____   pancreatic
15. ____   pharyngeal
17. ____   rectal

3.5A Give Word Part Meanings

Word Parts Exercise (pp. 134–135)
1. create an opening between two structures
3. being; having; process
5. procedure to puncture
7. yellow
9. hold together
11. diverticulum
13. surgical removal
15. that which produces
17. process of recording
19. hemorrhoid
21. gap; opening
23. process; state
25. groin
27. action; condition
29. thing
31. stone
33. study of; word
35. enlargement
37. blocked by a barrier
39. navel; umbilicus
41. appetite
43. disease
45. opening
47. process of reshaping by surgery
49. polyp
51. backward flow
53. procedure of suturing
55. instrument used to examine
57. spleen
59. surgically created opening
61. process of cutting; process of making an incision
63. navel; umbilicus

Related Combining Forms Exercise (p. 135)
1. steat/o-, lip/o-
3. gloss/o-, lingu/o-

3.5 Define Abbreviations

Matching Exercise (p. 135)
13, __, 3, __, 8, __, 6, __, 11, __, 12, __, 10,

3.6A Divide Medical Words

Dividing Words Exercise (p. 136)
1.	an-	orex/o-	-ia
3.	meso-	enter/o-	-ic
5.	____	sial/o-	-lith
7.	____	herni/o-	-rrhaphy
9.	____	cirrh/o-	-osis
11.	de-	fec/o-	-ation
13.	____	append/o-	-ix
15.	____	rect/o-	-cele

3.6B Build Medical Words

Combining Form and Suffix Exercise (pp. 136–137)
1. constipation
3. nasogastric
5. appendicitis
7. cholecystectomy
9. laparotomy
11. polypectomy
13. appendectomy
15. sigmoidoscopy
17. anastomosis
19. colostomy
21. hemorrhoidectomy
23. sialolith
25. cholangiogram

Prefix Exercise (p. 137)
1.	in-	indigestion
3.	dys-	dyspepsia
5.	sub-	sublingual
7.	anti-	antiemetic
9.	im-	imperforate
11.	hyper-	hyperemesis

Multiple Combining Forms and Suffix Exercise (p. 138)
1.	bilirubin	7.	colorectal
3.	gastroenteritis	9.	choledocholithotomy
5.	nasogastric	11.	hematemesis

3.7A Spell Medical Words

Proofreading and Spelling Exercise (p. 138)
1.	gastroenterology	7.	lumen
3.	esophagus	9.	rectocele
5.	hemorrhoids		

English and Medical Word Equivalents Exercise (p. 139)
1.	abdomen	9.	oral cavity
3.	intestine	11.	deglutition
5.	mastication	13.	emesis
7.	pyrosis		

You Write the Medical Report (pp. 139–140)
1. anorexia
3. gastroenteritis
5. colonoscopy
7. esophageal, hematemesis, cirrhosis, ascites
9. cholelithiasis, cholecystectomy

Hearing Medical Words Exercise (p. 140)
1.	anorexia	9.	gastroenteritis
3.	duodenum	11.	herniorrhaphy
5.	cholecystitis	13.	lipase
7.	colostomy	15.	sigmoidoscopy

3.7B Pronounce Medical Words

Pronunciation Exercise (p. 140)
1.	gas	9.	pat
3.	sy	11.	ty
5.	nee	13.	ling
7.	aw	15.	loh

3.8 Research Medical Words

On the Job Challenge Exercise (p. 141)

1. aerophagia   condition (caused by) air (that is) swallowed (while eating)
3. tenesmus   painful straining to have a stool
5. borborygmus   a rumbling sound due to gas in the intestines

Sound-Alike Words (p. 141)

1. celiac trunk: an arterial branch of the abdominal aorta. It supplies blood to the stomach, small intestine, liver, gallbladder, and pancreas.

   celiac disease: an autoimmune disorder and toxic reaction to the gluten found in certain grains (wheat, barley, rye, oats). It is also known as gluten sensitivity enteropathy.

3. stoma: a surgically created opening like a mouth; it is formed when the edges of the colon are brought out through the abdominal wall and rolled to make a mouth-like opening and then sutured to the abdominal wall. A stoma is created when part of the ileum and colon are removed during a colostomy surgical procedure.

   stomatitis: an inflammation of the oral mucosa; it can be caused by poorly fitted dentures or infection.

3.9 Analyze Medical Reports

Electronic Patient Record #2 and #3 (pp. 142–145)

1. anorexic   an-   not; without   orex/o-   appetite
   -ic   pertaining to
   dyspepsia   dys-   abnormal; difficult; painful
   peps/o-   digestion
   -ia   condition; state; thing
   gastroenteritis   gastr/o- stomach
   enter/o-   intestine
   -itis infection of; inflammation of
3. eating food from a food truck at the county fair

Electronic Patient Records #2 and #3 (p. 143–145)

1. gastric
3. fec/a-   feces; stool
   -lith   stone
5. N&V
7. emesis
9. worm-like
11. acute appendicitis
13. gastroenteritis
15. peritonitis
17. liver
19. Peritonitis is infection and inflammation of the peritoneum that occurs when an ulcer, diverticulum, or cancerous tumor eats through the wall of the stomach or intestines or when an inflamed appendix ruptures; drainage and bacteria spill into the abdominopelvic cavity.

Chapter 4: Pulmonology

Labeling Exercise (p. 156)

FIRST EXERCISE

1. larynx
3. cluster of alveoli
5. diaphragm
7. pharynx
9. apex of lung
11. sternum

SECOND EXERCISE

1. bronchiole
3. carbon dioxide
5. capillary wall

GIVE WORD PART MEANINGS

COMBINING FORMS EXERCISE (p.157)

1. air sac
3. bronchiole
5. carbon dioxide
7. cell
9. diaphragm
11. comprehensive; shaped like a globe
13. breathe
15. indentation
17. change; transformation
19. mucous membrane
21. mouth
23. oxygen
25. wall of a cavity
27. pharynx; throat
29. lung membrane
31. air; lung
33. lung
35. breathe; coil
37. chest; thorax
39. scroll-like structure; turbinate
41. large internal organs

BUILD MEDICAL WORDS

COMBINING FORM AND SUFFIX EXERCISE (p. 158)

1. -ar   alveolar
3. -al   tracheal
5. -ic   phrenic
7. -ic   thoracic
9. -ation   ventilation
11. -al   bronchial
13. -eal   laryngeal
15. -ic   diaphragmatic

PREFIX EXERCISE (p. 159)

1. in-   inspiration
3. re-   respiration
5. ex-   exhalation

MULTIPLE COMBINING FORMS AND SUFFIX
EXERCISE (p. 159)

1. -ary cardi/o- pulmon/o- cardiopulmonary
3. -ary bronch/o- pulmon/o- bronchopulmonary

4.1 Identify Anatomical Structures

Matching Exercise (p. 184)

6, __, 2, __, 5, __, 8, __, 1, __, 4

Circle Exercise (p. 184)

1. lobe
3. hilum

True or False Exercise (p. 184)

1. F
3. F

4.2 Describe Physiology

Circle Exercise (p. 184)

1. epiglottis
3. phrenic nerve

True or False Exercise (p.185)

1. T
3. T

4.3A Describe Diseases

Matching Exercise (p. 185)

3, __, 4, __, 2, __, 8, __

True or False Exercise (p. 185)

1. I
3. F
5. T
7. T
9. F

Fill in the Blank Exercise (p. 185)

1. bronchopneumonia
3. wheezing
5. tachypnea
7. carcinoma
9. tuberculosis

4.3B Describe Laboratory, Radiology, Surgery, and Drugs

Matching Exercise (p. 186)

6, __, 8, __, 3, __, 4, __, 5, __

Circle Exercise (p. 186)

1. lung
3. carboxyhemoglobin

4.4 Form Plurals and Adjectives

Plural Noun and Adjective Exercise (p. 186)

1. ____ nasal
3. ____ anoxic
5. ____ apneic
7. bronchi bronchial
9. ____ diaphragmatic
11. ____ laryngeal
13. ____ mucosal
15. ____ pleural
17. ____ thoracic

4.5A Give Word Part Meanings

Word Parts Exercise (p. 187)

1. gland
3. breathe in; suck in
5. incomplete
7. pertaining to
9. slow
11. cancer
13. spherical bacterium
15. blue
17. abnormal; difficult; painful
19. condition of dilation
21. condition
23. picture; record
25. above; more than normal
27. condition; state; thing
29. disease from a specific cause; process
31. infection of; inflammation of
33. instrument used to measure
35. blocked by a barrier
37. condition; process
39. tapping
41. breathing
43. pus
45. cut out; remove
47. instrument used to examine
49. sudden, involuntary muscle contraction
51. fast
53. chest; thorax
55. nodule; tuberculosis
57. cough

Related Combining Forms Exercise (p. 187)

1. spir/o-, hal/o-
3. pneum/o-, pulmon/o-, pneumon/o-

4.5B Define Abbreviations

Matching Exercise (p. 188)

7, __, 5, __, 1, __, 6, __

4.6A Divide Medical Words

Dividing Words Exercise (p. 188)

1. in- hal/o- -ation
3. re- spir/o- -atory
5. circum- or/o- -al
7. pan- lob/o- -ar
9. inter- cost/o- -al
11. epi- glott/o- -ic
13. auscult/o- -ation
15. thorac/o- -tomy
17. pneumon/o- -ia
19. ex- pector/o- -ant
21. cyan/o- -tic
23. a- pne/o- -ic

4.6B Build Medical Words

Combining Form and Suffix Exercise (pp. 189–190)
1. asthmatic
3. pyothorax
5. cyanosis
7. hemoptysis
9. stethoscope
11. bronchiectasis
13. ventilator
15. pleurisy
17. anthracosis
19. bronchoscopy
21. therapist
23. hemothorax
25. resuscitation
27. thoracocentesis

Prefix Exercise (p. 190)
1. in-   intubation
3. pan-   panlobar
5. anti-   antitussive
7. an-   anoxia
9. endo-   endotracheal

Multiple Combining Forms and Suffix Exercise (pp. 190–191)
1. cardiothoracic
3. bronchodilator
5. pneumococcal
7. pulmonologist

4.7A Spell Medical Words

Hearing Medical Words (p. 190)
1. anoxia
3. auscultation
9. pneumothorax
5. emphysema
7. laryngeal

English and Medical Word Equivalents Exercise (p. 191)
1. pharynx
3. thorax
5. sudden infant death syndrome
7. dyspnea
9. larynx

4.7B Pronounce Medical Words

Pronunciation Exercise (p. 191)
1. ky
3. noh
5. ray
7. tray

4.8 Research Medical Words

On the Job Challenge Exercise (p. 191)
1. second word of the phrase;   fibrosis
3. Word search by looking under the noun, not the adjectives in a phrase.

Sound-Alike Words (p. 192)
1. mucosa: the mucous membrane that lines the entire respiratory system.
   mucous: adjective that describes a mucous membrane
   mucus: substance produced by the mucous membranes
3. emphysema: a disease in which the alveoli become hyperinflated and often rupture, creating large air pockets in the lungs
   empyema: a disease of a localized collection of purulent material (pus) in the thoracic cavity from an infection in the lungs; it is also known as *pyothorax*.

4.9 Analyze Medical Reports

Electronic Patient Record #1 (p. 192)
1. asthma
3. stethoscope
5. a. ox/i-   -meter
      oxygen   instrument used to measure
   b. auscult/o-   -ation
      listening   process
7. metered-dose inhaler

Electronic Patient Record #2 (pp. 193–194)
1. shortness of breath;   (SOB)
3. bronch/o- bronchus
   -scopy   process of using an instrument to examine
5. a. culture and sensitivity
   b. chronic obstructive pulmonary disease
   c. left lower lobe
7. bronchoscopy and a biopsy
9. consolidative changes; density in LLL, patchy infiltrates; atelectasis
11. barrel chest
13. right-sided pneumonia

Chapter 5: Cardiology

Labeling Exercise (pp. 213–214)
FIRST EXERCISE
1. right pulmonary artery
3. superior vena cava
5. pulmonary trunk
7. tricuspid valve
9. chordae tendineae
11. aortic arch
13. pulmonary valve
15. left atrium
17. left ventricle
19. apex of heart

SECOND EXERCISE
1. atrioventricular node
3. right atrium
5. bundle branches
7. left atrium
9. Purkinje fibers

THIRD EXERCISE
1. ascending aorta
3. abdominal aorta
5. subclavian artery
7. brachial artery
9. renal artery
11. radial artery
13. femoral artery
15. tibial artery

GIVE WORD PART MEANINGS
COMBINING FORMS EXERCISE (p. 215)
1. armpit
3. blood vessel; lymphatic vessel
5. apex; tip
7. arteriole
9. atrium; chamber that is open at the top
11. capillary; hair-like structure
13. heart
15. movement in a circular route
17. carrying; conveying

19. structure that encircles like a crown
21. dilating
23. outside
25. bend; break up
27. jugular; throat
29. structure like a tall hat with two points
31. wall of a cavity
33. vein
35. back of the knee
37. lung
39. kidney
41. dividing wall; septum
43. body as a whole
45. cellular layer
47. shin bone; tibia
49. valve
51. blood vessel
53. vein
55. large internal organs

BUILD MEDICAL WORDS

COMBINING FORM AND SUFFIX EXERCISE (p. 216)

1.	-ic	thoracic
3.	-ar	valvular
5.	-ac	cardiac
7.	-ous	venous
9.	-al	atrial
11.	-ole	arteriole
13.	-ic	aortic
15.	-ic	systolic
17.	-ar	ventricular

MULTIPLE COMBINING FORMS AND SUFFIX EXERCISE (p. 217)

1.	vas/o-	dilat/o-	vasodilation
3.	cardi/o-	vascul/o-	cardiovascular
5.	vas/o-	constrict/o-	vasoconstriction
7.	atri/o-	ventricul/o-	atrioventricular

5.1 Identify Anatomical Structures

5.2 Describe Physiology

Matching Exercise (p. 246)

9, __, 6, __, 4, __, 5, __, 7, __

True or False Exercise (p. 246)

1.	F	9.	F
3.	F	11.	T
5.	F	13.	T
7.	T		

Sequencing Exercise (p. 247)

1.	right atrium	9.	left ventricle
3.	right ventricle	11.	arteries and arterioles
5.	lungs	13.	venules and veins
7.	left atrium		

Circle Exercise (p. 247)

1.	aorta	5.	jugular
3.	auscultation	7.	calcium

5.3A Describe Diseases

Fill in the Blank Exercise (p. 248)

1.	claudication	7.	thrombus
3.	arrhythmia	9.	cardiomegaly
5.	necrosis		

Circle Exercise (p. 248)

1.	bradycardia	3.	aneurysm

True or False Exercise (p. 248)

1.	F	7.	T
3.	T	9.	T
5.	F		

5.3B Describe Laboratory, Radiology, Surgery, and Drugs

Laboratory Test Exercise (pp. 248–249)

80061	✓	Lipid Panel
80162	✓	Digoxin Drug Level
82465	✓	Cholesterol
82553	✓	Creatine Kinase, MB
83718	✓	HDL Lipoprotein
83719	✓	VLDL Lipoprotein
83721	✓	LDL Lipoprotein
84478	✓	Triglycerides
84484	✓	Troponin
86140	✓	C-Reactive Protein
36415	✓	Venipuncture

True or False Exercise (p. 249)

1.	F	5.	F
3.	T	7.	T

5.4 Form Plurals and Adjectives

Plural Noun and Adjective Exercise (p. 249)

1.		pericardial
3.	atria	atrial
5.		septal
7.	valves	valvular
9.	veins	venous
11.	arterioles	arteriolar

5.5A Give Word Part Meanings

Word Parts Exercise (pp. 250–252)

1. angina
3. abdomen
5. pertaining to
7. pertaining to
9. aneurysm; dilation
11. against
13. apex; tip

15. artery

17. artery

19. enzyme

21. soft, fatty substance

23. being; having; process

25. atrium; chamber that is open at the top

27. listening

29. two

31. slow

33. heart

35. sleep; stupor

37. procedure to puncture

39. movement in a circular route

41. clavicle; collar bone

43. pressed together

45. carrying; conveying

47. drawn together; narrowed

49. structure that encircles like a crown

51. skin

53. complete; completely through

55. dilate; widen

57. abnormal; difficult; painful

59. echo of a sound wave

61. outside

63. condition of the blood; substance in the blood

65. pertaining to

67. pertaining to

69. femur; thigh bone

71. bend; break up

73. tissue for implant; tissue for transplant

75. process of recording

77. below; deficient

79. pertaining to

81. origin; resembling; source

83. hip bone; ilium

85. small area of dead tissue

87. block; keep back

89. infection of; inflammation of

91. process of creating; process of inserting; process of making

93. fat; lipid

95. study of; word

97. lumen; opening

99. frenzy; thin

101. enlargement

103. process of measuring

105. muscle

107. close against

109. mass; tumor

111. full of; thing full of

113. pertaining to

115. wall of a cavity

117. disease

119. chest

121. around

123. fibula; lower leg bone

125. vein

127. process of reshaping by surgery

129. back of the knee

131. before; in front of

133. lung

135. again and again; backward; unable to

137. kidney

139. rhythm

141. hard; sclera of the eye

143. dividing wall; septum

145. sound

147. constriction; narrowness

149. above

151. contraction

153. fast

155. technical skill

157. pressure; tension

159. cellular layer

161. chest; thorax

163. shin bone; tibia

165. area with distinct edges; instrument used to cut

167. across; through

169. three

171. process of development

173. forearm bone; ulna

175. period of time; structure

177. valve

179. varicose vein; varix

181. blood vessel

183. vein

185. travel; turn

187. foreign

Related Combining Forms Exercise (p. 252)

    1. angi/o-, vas/o-, vascul/o-

    3. phleb/o-, ven/o

5.5B Define Abbreviations

Matching Exercise (p. 252)

10, __, 3, __, 4, __, 7, __, 8, __

5.6A Divide Medical Words

Dividing Words Exercise (p. 252)

1.		circulat/o-	-ion
3.		ischm/o-	-emia
5.	a-	rrhythm/o-	-ia
7.		aneurysm/o-	-al
9.		angi/o-	-plasty

5.6B Build Medical Words

Combining Form and Suffix Exercise (p. 253)

    1. necrotic

    3. atheroma

    5. aneurysmectomy

    7. infarction

    9. auscultation

    11. telemetry

    13. patent

    15. angiography

    17. palpitation

    19. valvuloplasty

Prefix Exercise (p. 254)

1. hyper-   hypercholesterolemia
3. hyper-   hypertension
5. peri-   pericardiocentesis
7. brady-   bradycardia
9. supra-   supraventricular
11. peri-   pericarditis
13. hypo-   hypotensive

Multiple Combining Forms and Suffix Exercise (pp. 254–255)

1. arteriosclerosis
3. echocardiography
5. atherosclerosis
7. thrombophlebitis
9. sphygmomanometer
11. cardioversion

5.7A Spell Medical Words

Proofreading and Spelling Exercise (p. 255)

1. sphygmomanometer
3. atheromatous
5. tachycardia
7. angioplasty
9. infarction

You Write the Medical Report (p. 255)

1. angina pectoris, diaphoresis
3. atherosclerosis, claudication, necrotic

Hearing Medical Words (p. 256)

1. cardiac
3. cardiothoracic
5. coronary artery
7. cardiomegaly
9. atherosclerosis
11. angioplasty

5.7B Pronounce Medical Words

Pronunciation Exercise (p. 256)

1. kar
3. lay
5. dy
7. lay
9. tay

5.8 Research Medical Words

Sound-Alike Words (p. 256)

1. cardiac: The adjective for the word *heart*.
   cardia: The first part of the stomach, just after the esophagus.
3. palpation: Using the fingers to press on a body part to detect a mass, an enlarged organ, tenderness, or pain.
   palpitation: An uncomfortable sensation felt in the chest during a contraction of the heart.

5.9 Analyze Medical Reports

Electronic Patient Record #1 (pp. 257–258)

1. HTN
3. **a.** congestive heart failure
   b. creatine kinase, MB
   c. cardiopulmonary resuscitation
   d. left ventricular hypertrophy

5. cardi/o-   heart
   -megaly   enlargement
7. 70–80 beats per minute
9. cardiac arrest
11. asystole
13. left
15. fluid retention from congestive heart failure

Electronic Patient Records #2 (p. 259)

1. Atrial fibrillation is a very fast, uncoordinated quivering of the myocardium, specifically the atria.
3. Asystole is the complete absence of a heart rate. It is treated with cardiopulmonary resuscitation.

Chapter 6: Hematology and Immunology

Labeling Exercise (pp. 279–280)

FIRST EXERCISE

1. eosinophil
3. lymphocyte
5. monocyte

SECOND EXERCISE

1. tonsils and adenoids
3. mediastinal lymph nodes
5. appendix and Peyer's patches
7. cervical lymph nodes
9. spleen
11. red bone marrow

GIVE WORD PART MEANINGS
COMBINING FORMS EXERCISE (p. 281)

1. crowding together
3. alkaline; base of a structure; basic
5. cell
7. eosin; red, acidic dye
9. fibrin
11. comprehensive; shaped like a globe
13. granule
15. blood
17. nucleus of a cell
19. lymph; lymphatic system
21. one; single
23. bone marrow; myelin; spinal cord
25. normal; usual
27. oxygen; quick
29. eating; swallowing
31. formation; growth
33. spleen
35. blood clot
37. poison

BUILD MEDICAL WORDS

COMBINING FORM AND SUFFIX EXERCISE (p. 282)

1. -poiesis   hematopoiesis
3. -ation   coagulation
5. -cyte   phagocyte
7. -logy   hematology
9. -phil   eosinophil
11. -cyte   thrombocyte
13. -lyte   electrolyte
15. -ation   aggregation
17. -cyte   granulocyte
19. -phil   basophil

PREFIX EXERCISE (p. 283)

1. endo-   endotoxin
3. poly-   polymorphonuclear
5. mega-   megakaryocyte

MULTIPLE COMBINING FORMS AND SUFFIX EXERCISE (p. 283)

1. cyt/o-   tox/o-   -ic   cytotoxic
3. immun/o-   globul/o-   -in   immunoglobulin

6.1 Identify Anatomical Structures
6.2 Describe Physiology

Matching Exercise (p. 303)

6, __, 16, __, 9, __, 13, __, 5, __, 11, __, 3, __, 10, __

True or False Exercise (p. 303)

1. T   7. T
3. T   9. T
5. F

Circle Exercise (p. 304)

1. blood
3. fibrin
5. electrolytes
7. heme

Multiple Choice Exercise (p. 304)

1. d   3. d

Fill in the Blank Exercise (p. 304)

1. A, B, AB, O
3. (Pick any three): segmented neutrophil, segmenter, seg, polymorphonuclear leukocyte, PMN, poly

Matching Exercise (p. 305)

7, __, 3, __, 8, __, 6, __, 2, __

6.3A Describe Diseases

Matching Exercise (p. 305)

5, __, 8, __, 13, __, 7, __, 12, __, 2, __, 3, __, 9

True or False Exercise (p. 305)

1. F   7. F
3. F   9. T
5. T

Multiple Choice Exercise (p. 306)

1. a   3. d

6.3B Describe Laboratory, Radiology, Surgery, and Drugs

Circle Exercise (p. 306)

1. ferritin level
3. MCV
5. electrophoresis
7. thrombolytic

Matching Exercise (p. 306)

4, __, 7, __, 10, __, 8, __, 2, __

6.4 Form Plurals and Adjectives

Plural Noun and Adjective Exercise (p. 307)

1. indices   ____
3. ____   anemic
5. ____   hemolytic
7. thrombi   ____

6.5A Give Word Part Meanings

Word Parts Exercise (pp. 307–308)

1. gland
3. other; strange
5. unequal
7. weakened
9. life; living organism; living tissue
11. calcium
13. clotting
15. separation of
17. cell
19. cut apart
21. embolus; occluding plug
23. cut out
25. pouring
27. picture; record
29. blood
31. other
33. below; deficient
35. immune response
37. disease from a specific cause; process
39. study of; word
41. break down; destroy
43. large
45. one millionth; small
47. shape
49. mass; tumor
51. all
53. disease

55. attraction to; fondness for
57. vein
59. formation; growth
61. substance that forms
63. many; much
65. excessive discharge; excessive flow
67. spleen
69. rage; thymus
71. vaccine

Related Combining Forms Exercise (p. 308)

1. cyt/o-, cellul/o-
3. phleb/o-, ven/o-

6.5B Define Abbreviations

Matching Exercise (p. 308)

5, __, 11, __, 1, __, 3, __, 7, __, 10

6.6A Divide Medical Words

Dividing Words Exercise (p. 308)

1. ____	eosin/o-	-phil
3. trans-	fus/o-	-ion
5. ____	immun/o-	-ization
7. ____	bi/o-	-opsy

6.6B Build Medical Words

Combining Form and Suffix Exercise (p. 309)

1. microcyte	11. phlebotomy
3. leukemia	13. splenectomy
5. embolism	15. autoimmune
7. septicemia	17. splenomegaly
9. thrombosis	19. attenuated

Prefix Exercise (p. 310)

1. a-	aplastic
3. pan-	pancytopenia
5. anti-	anticoagulant
7. intra-	intravascular

Multiple Combining Forms and Suffix Exercise (pp. 310–311)

1. poikilocytosis	9. thrombolytic
3. lymphadenopathy	11. anisocytosis
5. normocytic	13. hematologist
7. immunodeficiency	

6.7A Spell Medical Words

Hearing Medical Words Exercise (p. 311)

1. anemia
3. embolism
5. hemorrhage
7. leukemia
9. mononucleosis

6.7B Pronounce Medical Words

Pronunciation Exercise (p. 311)

1. loo	7. see
3. sin	9. baw
5. lay	

6.8 Research Medical Words

Sound-Alike Words (p. 311)

1. albumen: the white of an egg
   albumin: the most abundant protein in the plasma
3. mono: short form for *mononucleosis*, an infectious disease caused by the Epstein-Barr virus. Often called the "kissing disease."
   monos: short form for *monocytes*, the largest of the leukocytes

6.9 Analyze Medical Reports

Electronic Patient Record #1 (p. 312)

1. complete blood count
3. millions per milliliter
5. one thousand

Electronic Patient Records #2 (pp. 313–314)

1. b
3. 500, 100, 500
5. CD4 count
7. intravenous heroin use
9. Because he had an opportunistic infection (*Pneumocystis jiroveci* pneumonia) and a CD4 count below 200 (his was 100, and that qualifies for a change from HIV positive to a diagnosis of AIDS.

Chapter 7: Dermatology

Labeling Exercise (p. 323)

FIRST EXERCISE

1. hair shaft	7. artery
3. sebaceous gland	9. sweat gland
5. duct of sweat gland	11. dermis

SECOND EXERCISE

| 1. nail root | 5. nail bed |
| 3. lunula | |

GIVE WORD PART MEANINGS

COMBINING FORMS EXERCISE (p. 324)

1. follicle; small sac
3. other; strange
5. fibers that hold together
7. skin
9. skin
11. sweating
13. stand up

15. away from; external; outward
17. leaf
19. skin
21. cornea of the eye; hard, fibrous protein
23. one place
25. black
27. guarding; protecting
29. oil; sebum
31. affected by; sensitive to
33. sweat
35. cellular layer
37. fingernail; toenail

BUILD MEDICAL WORDS

COMBINING FORM AND SUFFIX EXERCISE (p. 325)

1. -in   elastin
3. -tome   dermatome
5. -gen   collagen
7. -cyte   melanocyte
9. -ous   sebaceous
11. -ary   integumentary
13. -ment   integument

PREFIX EXERCISE (p. 325)

1. ex-   exfoliation
3. sub-   subcutaneous

7.1 Identify Anatomical Structures
7.2 Describe Physiology

Matching Exercise (p. 351)

6, __, 8, __, 4, __, 1, __, 9

Circle Exercise (p. 351)

1. nail bed
3. hair
5. dermatome

True or False Exercise (p. 351)

1. T
3. T
5. T

7.3A Describe Diseases

Circle Exercise (p. 352)

1. fissure
3. macule

Matching Exercise (p. 352)

5, __, 1, __, 12, __, 11, __, 4, __, 8, __

True or False Exercise (p. 352)

1. F
3. T
5. F
7. T

Circle Exercise (p. 353)

1. flat
3. excoriation
5. feet
7. xanthoma

Fill in the Blank Exercise (p. 353)

1. herpes whitlow
3. scabies
5. shingles
7. verruca
9. furuncle

7.3B Describe Laboratory, Radiology, Surgery, and Drugs

Matching Exercise (p. 353)

4, __, 2, __, 1, __, 6

Circle Exercise (p. 354)

1. debridement
3. intradermal
5. incisional biopsy
7. antifungal drugs

7.4 Form Plurals and Adjectives

Plural Noun and Adjective Exercise (p. 354)

1. follicles   follicular
3. ____   epidermal
5. nails   ungual
7. vesicles   vesicular
9. ____   cyanotic
11. ____   icteric
13. ____   gangrenous
15. malignancies   malignant
17. ____   psoriatic
19. comedoes   ____

7.5A Give Word Part Meanings

Word Parts Exercise (pp. 354–355)

1. scrape off
3. white
5. not; without
7. being; having; process
9. life; living organism; living tissue
11. cell
13. bruising
15. blue
17. skin
19. abnormal; difficult; painful
21. surgical removal
23. redness
25. cut out
27. outside
29. splitting
31. fungus
33. tissue for implant; tissue for transplant
35. blood
37. hairy
39. process; state
41. cut into
43. action; condition
45. infection of; inflammation of
47. tearing
49. cancer; intentionally causing harm

51. new
53. resembling
55. fingernail; toenail
57. condition; process
59. pigment
61. formation; growth
63. before; in front of
65. itching
67. excessive discharge; excessive flow
69. connective tissue
71. old age
73. area with distinct edges; instrument used to cut
75. blood vessel; vas deferens
77. yellow
79. dry

Related Combining Forms Exercise (p. 355)

1. lip/o-, adip/o-
3. trich/o-, hirsut/o-, pil/o-
5. derm/a-, derm/o-, dermat/o-, cutane/o-, cut/i-, integument/o-

7.5B Define Abbreviations

Matching Exercise (p. 355)

4, __, 1, __, 5, __, 2

7.6A Divide Medical Words

Dividing Words Exercise (p. 356)

1. an-   esthes/o-   -ia
3. epi-   derm/o-   -al
5. ana-   phylact/o-   -ic
7. ____   hemat/o-   -oma

7.6B Build Medical Words

Combining Form and Suffix Exercise (pp. 356–357)

1. dermatoplasty
3. xeroderma
5. abrasion
7. cyanosis
9. pruritic
11. neoplasm
13. necrotic
15. keloid
17. exudate
19. biopsy
21. dermatome
23. rhytidectomy

Prefix Exercise (p. 357)

1. anti-   antifungal
3. an-   anesthesia
5. an-   anhidrosis
7. pre-   premalignant

7.7A Spell Medical Words

English and Medical Word Equivalents Exercise (p. 358)

1. eczema
3. alopecia
5. furuncle (or abscess)
7. urticaria
9. scabies
11. tinea
13. verruca

Hearing Medical Words Exercise (p. 358)

1. acne vulgaris
3. blepharoplasty
5. cyanosis
7. dermatologist
9. pruritus

7.7B Pronounce Medical Words

Pronunciation Exercise (p. 358)

1. bray
3. pee
5. ly
7. lip
9. eye

7.8 Research Medical Words

On the Job Challenge Exercise (p. 359)

1. Condition of fingernail and/or toenail eating and swallowing.
3. Condition of hair (being) pulled out (in a) frenzy

Sound-Alike Words (p.359)

1. dermatome: a specific area of the skin that sends sensory information through a nerve to the spinal cord
   dermatome: a surgical instrument used to make a shallow, continuous cut to form a skin graft
3. excoriation: superficial injury with a sharp object such as a fingernail, animal claw, or thorn that creates a linear scratch in the skin
   exfoliation: normal process of the constant shedding of dead skin cells from the most superficial part of the epidermis

7.9 Analyze Medical Reports

Electronic Patient Record (pp. 360–361)

1. cellul/o-   cell
   -itis   infection of; inflammation of
3. pruritus
5. welts
7. drug reaction
9. erythema nodosum

Chapter 8: Orthopedics (Skeletal)

Labeling Exercise (pp. 382–383)

FIRST EXERCISE

1. temporal bone
3. sphenoid bone
5. nasal bone
7. zygoma
9. mandible
11. parietal bone

SECOND EXERCISE

1. tarsal bones
3. phalanges
5. talus

THIRD EXERCISE

1. clavicle
3. humerus
5. costal cartilage
7. ulna
9. phalanges
11. patella
13. tibia
15. manubrium
17. sternum
19. ilium
21. coccyx
23. pubis or pubic bone

GIVE WORD PART MEANINGS

COMBINING FORMS EXERCISE (p. 384)

1. hip socket
3. joint
5. calcaneus; heel bone
7. wrist
9. cervix; neck
11. clavicle; collar bone
13. cortex; outer region
15. cranium; skull
17. shaft of a bone
19. sieve
21. fibula; lower leg bone
23. socket of a joint
25. U-shaped structure
27. hip bone; ischium
29. ligament
31. lower jaw; mandible
33. maxilla; upper jaw
35. nose
37. bone
39. bone
41. wall of a cavity
43. hip bone; pelvis; renal pelvis
45. digit; finger; toe
47. forearm bone; radiation; x-rays
49. scapula; shoulder blade
51. wedge shape
53. vertebra
55. stake
57. joint membrane; synovium
59. side of the head; temple
61. shin bone; tibia
63. vertebra

BUILD MEDICAL WORDS

COMBINING FORM AND SUFFIX EXERCISE (p. 385)

1. -al cranial
3. -al costal
5. -ous ligamentous
7. -eal phalangeal
9. -ation articulation
11. -al vertebral
13. -ar ulnar
15. -ion ossification
17. -al sternal
19. -ar clavicular
21. -ic pubic
23. -ar patellar

8.1 Identify Anatomical Structures
8.2 Describe Physiology

Matching Exercise (p. 404)

12, __, 11, __, 18, __, 15, __, 6, __, 3, __, 1, __, 2, __, 5, __

Circle Exercise (p. 404)

1. humerus
3. ilium
5. ankle
7. elbow
9. clavicle

True or False Exercise (p. 405)

1. T
3. F
5. T

8.3A Describe Diseases

True or False Exercise (p. 405)

1. T
3. F
5. F
7. F

Fill in the Blank Exercise (p. 405)

1. osteoarthritis
3. arthralgia
5. osteosarcoma
7. compound
9. arthropathy

Circle Exercise (pp. 405–406)

1. osteomyelitis
3. demineralization
5. pectus excavatum
7. hairline

8.3B Describe Laboratory, Radiology, Surgery, and Drugs

Circle Exercise (p. 406)

1. goniometer
3. arthrodesis
5. a blood test
7. arthrography
9. allograft

True or False Exercise (p. 406)

1. T
3. T
5. F
7. F

8.4 Form Plurals and Adjectives

Plural Noun and Adjective Exercise (p. 406)

1. ____ cranial
3. ____ thoracic
5. vertebrae vertebral
7. ____ iliac
9. patellae patellar

8.5A Give Word Part Meanings

Word Parts Exercise (p. 407)

1. away from; without
3. pain
5. cut off
7. fused together; stiff
9. procedure to puncture
11. break into small pieces
13. reversal of; without
15. right; sugar
17. disk
19. person who is the object of an action; person who receives; thing that is the object of an action; thing that receives

21. creation; production
23. picture; record
25. blood
27. action; condition
29. bent; humpbacked
31. place
33. bad; inadequate
35. action; state
37. process of measuring
39. bone marrow; myelin; spinal cord
41. mass; tumor
43. condition; process
45. disease
47. child
49. growth
51. pores; small openings
53. connective tissue
55. instrument used to examine
57. area with distinct edges; instrument used to cut
59. blood vessel

Related Combining Forms Exercise (p. 407)

1. oste/o-, osse/o-
3. arthr/o-, articul/o-
5. perone/o-, fibul/o-

8.5B Define Abbreviations

Abbreviation Exercise (p. 408)

3, __, 5, __, 7, __, 4

8.6A Divide Medical Words

Dividing Words Exercise (p. 408)

1. ____   oste/o-   -cyte
3. meta-   tars/o-   -al
5. ____   densit/o- -metry
7. ____   scoli/o-   -osis
9. ____   arthr/o-   -graphy

8.6B Build Medical Words

Combining Form and Suffix Exercise (pp. 408–409)

1. arthropathy   9. goniometer
3. kyphosis   11. arthrodesis
5. congenital   13. amputee
7. osteoma   15. lordosis

Prefix Exercise (p. 409)

1. a-   avascular
3. intra-   intra-articular
5. mal-   malalignment
7. an-   analgesic

Multiple Combining Forms and Suffix Exercise (pp. 409–410)

1. levoscoliosis   7. arthralgia
3. osteoporosis   9. osteosarcoma
5. hemarthrosis

8.7A Spell Medical Words

English and Medical Word Equivalents Exercise (p. 410)

1. cranium   13. patella
3. fontanel   15. calcaneus
5. mandible   17. lordosis
7. sternum   19. genu valgum
9. olecranon   21. osteophyte
11. coccyx

Hearing Medical Words Exercise (p. 410)

1. arthritis   7. orthopedist
3. chondroma   9. phalanx
5. dextroscoliosis

8.7B Pronounce Medical Words

Pronunciation Exercise (p. 411)

1. tay   7. foh
3. thraw   9. kar
5. troh

8.8 Research Medical Words

Test Yourself (p. 411)

1. osteoblast: bone cell that deposits new bone
3. osteocyte: bone cell that maintains and monitors the mineral content (calcium, phosphorus) of bone
5. The first three are all cells, but an osteophyte is not a cell; it is a bone spur.

Sound-Alike Words (p. 411)

1. ileum: the third part of the small intestine
   ilium: most superior hip bone
3. humerus: long bone of the upper arm
   humorous: an English adjective that means *funny*

On the Job Challenge Exercise (p. 411)

1. A fracture whose pieces do not break through the overlying skin
3. A fracture whose pieces do break through the overlying skin

8.9 Analyze Medical Reports

Electronic Patient Record (pp. 412–413)

1. dextr/o-   right
   scoli/o-   curved; crooked
   -osis   condition; process
3. orth/o-   straight
   ped/o-   child
   -ist   person who specializes in; thing that specializes in
5. tibia
7. vertebrae
9. to the right
11. the number of degrees of curvature of the dextroscoliosis

Chapter 9: Orthopedics (Muscular)

Labeling Exercise (pp. 432–433)

FIRST EXERCISE

1. temporalis muscle
3. trapezius muscle
5. triceps brachii muscle
7. brachioradialis muscle
9. gastrocnemius muscle
11. frontalis muscle
13. pectoralis major muscle
15. rectus abdominis muscle
17. tibialis anterior muscle

SECOND EXERCISE

1. rotation
3. slight flexion
5. plantar flexion

GIVE WORD PART MEANINGS
COMBINING FORMS EXERCISE (p. 434)

1. person's own free will
3. before; front part
5. cheek
7. clavicle; collar bone
9. rib
11. bring; duct; move
13. outside
15. fiber
17. front
19. introduce; put in
21. chewing
23. muscle
25. muscle
27. small circle
29. fibula; lower leg bone
31. forearm bone; radiation; x-rays
33. breastbone; sternum
35. side of the head; temple
37. tendon
39. shin bone; tibia
41. development
43. travel; turn

BUILD MEDICAL WORDS
COMBINING FORM AND SUFFIX EXERCISE (p. 435)

1. -or   rotator
3. -ar   muscular
5. -al   fascial
7. -oid   deltoid
9. -er   masseter
11. -alis   pectoral
13. -ion   contraction

9.1 Identify Anatomical Structures
9.2 Describe Physiology

Fill in the Blank Exercise (p. 449)

1. gastrocnemius muscle
3. deltoid muscle
5. rectus femoris muscle
7. biceps brachii muscle
9. rectus abdominis muscle
11. masseter muscle
13. biceps femoris muscle

Circle Exercise (p. 449)

1. origin   5. deltoid
3. musculature

Matching Exercise (p. 450)

11, __, 1, __, 4, __, 6, __, 2, __, 3, __

Recall and Describe Exercise (p. 450)

1. Moving the arm away from the midline of the body
3. Turning the palm of the hand posteriorly or downward
5. Bending the knee joint to decrease the angle between the upper and lower leg

9.3A Describe Diseases

Matching Exercise (p. 450)

8, __, 4, __, 9, __, 5, __, 3

True or False Exercise (p. 451)

1. F   7. T
3. F   9. T
5. F

Circle Exercise (p. 451)

1. ataxia   5. Dupuytren's
3. athetoid

9.3B Describe Laboratory, Surgery, and Drugs

Multiple Choice Exercise (p. 451)

1. a   5. d
3. a

Circle Exercise (p. 452)

1. fibromyalgia   3. thymectomy

9.4 Form Plurals and Adjectives

Plural Noun and Adjective Exercise (p. 452)

1. muscles   muscular
3. bursae   bursal
5. ____   fascial

9.5A Give Word Part Meanings

Word Parts Exercise (pp. 452–453)

1. away from; without
3. pain

5. lack of strength

7. life; living organism; living tissue

9. bursa

11. rapid contracting and relaxing

13. pull together

15. skin

17. surgical removal

19. condition; process

21. picture; record

23. give ability

25. condition; state; thing

27. medical treatment

29. redness and warmth

31. person who specializes in; thing that specializes in

33. condition; state

35. movement

37. movement

39. mass; tumor

41. straight

43. condition; process

45. physical function

47. many; much

49. rod shaped

51. connective tissue

53. joint membrane; synovium

55. treatment

57. process of cutting; process of making an incision

59. development

61. tear

Related Combining Forms Exercise (p. 453)

1. kin/o-, kines/o-, mobil/o-, mot/o-

3. ten/o-, tendin/o-

9.5B   Define Abbreviations

Define And Match Exercise (p. 453)

1. electromyography

3. nonsteroidal anti-inflammatory drug

5. occupation therapy or occupational therapist

7. intramuscular

1, __, 5, __, 2, __, 3

9.6A   Divide Medical Words

Dividing Words Exercise (p. 453)

1.	ab-	duct/o-	-ion
3.	brady-	kines/o-	-ia
5.	____	fasci/o-	-al
7.	____	myos/o-	-itis
9.	re-	habilitat/o-	-ion

9.6B   Build Medical Words

Combining Form and Suffix Exercise (p. 454)

1. fasciectomy

3. inflammation

5. fasciitis

7. fasciotomy

9. myoclonus

11. tenorrhaphy

13. ganglionectomy

15. bursitis

Prefix Exercise (p. 455)

1.	re-	rehabilitation
3.	brady-	bradykinesia
5.	hyper-	hyperextension
7.	a-	atrophic
9.	a-	avulsion
11.	poly-	polymyositis

Multiple Combining Forms and Suffix Exercise (pp. 455–456)

1. musculoskeletal

3. neuromuscular

5. fibromyalgia

7. rhabdomyoma

9. podiatrist

9.7A   Spell Medical Words

Proofreading and Spelling Exercise (p. 456)

1. orthopedics

3. fascia

5. fibromyalgia

7. ganglion

9. dystrophy

English and Medical Word Equivalents Exercise (p. 456)

1. bursitis

3. torticollis

5. hyperextension-hyperflexion injury (or acceleration-deceleration injury)

7. medial epicondylitis

Hearing Medical Words Exercise (p. 456)

1. bursa

3. bradykinesia

5. fascia

7. myalgia

9. rehabilitation

9.7B   Pronounce Medical Words

Pronunciation Exercise (p. 457)

1. duk

3. prak

5. per

7. skel

9.8   Research Medical Words

On the Job Challenge Exercise (p. 457)

1. musculus

3. muscles (muscle or musculus)

Sound-Alike Words (p. 457)

1. rectum: short straight segment that is the last part of the large intestine after the sigmoid colon. It connects to the outside of the body.
   rectus: Latin word for *straight*

3. contraction: shortening of the length of all of the muscle fibers and of the muscle itself.
   contracture: progressive flexion of an arm or leg muscle in which it is progressively drawn into a position where it becomes nearly immovable because of inactivity or because of paralysis

9.9   Analyze Medical Reports

Electronic Patient Records #1 and #2 (pp. 458–460)

1.	my/o-	muscle
	-pathy	disease
3.	bi/o-	life; living organism; living tissue
	-opsy	process of viewing

5. muscle biopsy x 3
7. anterior and lateral upper leg
9. climbing stairs, getting up from a chair or from a bed
11. myopathy of undetermined etiology
13. b
15. When the report comes back from the Armed Forces Institute of Pathology

Chapter 10: Neurology

Labeling Exercise (pp. 480–481)

FIRST EXERCISE

1. frontal lobe
3. parietal lobe
5. cerebellum

SECOND EXERCISE

1. cranium
3. arachnoid
5. pia mater
7. white matter of the cerebrum

THIRD EXERCISE

1. cerebrum
3. gyrus
5. hypothalamus
7. pons
9. corpus callosum
11. cerebellum

GIVE WORD PART MEANINGS

COMBINING FORMS EXERCISE (p. 482)

1. group; set
3. toward the center
5. star-like structure
7. independent; self-governing
9. cerebellum
11. cochlea; spiral-shaped structure
13. cranium; skull
15. branching structure
17. dura mater
19. brain
21. feeling; sensation
23. face
25. front
27. sense of taste
29. meninges
31. movement
33. bone marrow; myelin; spinal cord
35. nerve
37. eye
39. few; scanty
41. wall of a cavity
43. outer aspects
45. spinal nerve root
47. spinal nerve root
49. body
51. side of the head; temple
53. send across; send through
55. vagus nerve; wandering
57. abdomen; front
59. sight; vision

BUILD MEDICAL WORDS

COMBINING FORM AND SUFFIX EXERCISE (p. 483)

1. -ic   somatic
3. -al   cranial
5. -ory   auditory
7. -oid   arachnoid
9. -cyte   astrocyte
11. -ite   dendrite
13. -ure   fissure
15. -ic   thalamic
17. -or   receptor
19. -ic   autonomic
21. -al   temporal
23. -ar   cerebellar
25. -al   dural

PREFIX EXERCISE (p. 484)

1. sym-   sympathetic
3. epi-   epidural
5. sub-   subarachnoid
7. hypo-   hypoglossal

10.1 Identify Anatomical Structures
10.2 Describe Physiology

Matching Exercise (p. 512)

7, __, 9, __, 11, __, 2, __, 14, __, 8, __, 5, __, 3

Circle Exercise (p. 512)

1. cerebrum
3. pia mater
5. left hemisphere of the cerebrum
7. oculomotor

True or False Exercise (p. 513)

1. F
3. F
5. T
7. T

Fill in the Blank Exercise (p. 513)

1. dura mater, arachnoid, pia mater
3. hemisphere
5. hypothalamus

Multiple Choice Exercise (p. 513)

1. c
3. d

10.3A Describe Diseases

True or False Exercise (p. 514)

1. T
3. F
5. T
7. T

Circle Exercise (p. 514)

1. shingles
3. subdural hematoma
5. paresthesias

Fill in the Blank Exercise (p. 514)

1. multiple sclerosis
3. narcolepsy
5. status epilepticus

7. sciatica
9. nuchal rigidity
11. syncope

Multiple Choice Exercise (p. 515)

1. b

3. d

10.3B Describe Laboratory, Radiology, Surgery, and Drugs

True or False Exercise (p. 515)

1. T
3. F

5. T
7. F

Matching Exercise (p. 515)

9, __, 7, __, 3, __, 5, __, 6

Fill in the Blank Exercise (p. 516)

1. corticosteroid drug
3. alpha fetoprotein
5. EEG
7. polysomnography

10.4 Form Plurals and Adjectives

Plural Noun and Adjective Exercise (p. 516)

1. ____   cerebral
3. ____   comatose
5. gyri   ____
7. ____   meningeal
9. ____   spinal

10.5A Give Word Part Meanings

Word Parts Exercise (pp. 516–517)

1. away from; without
3. pain
5. not; without
7. artery
9. composed of; pertaining to a condition
11. embryonic; immature
13. hernia
15. head
17. unconsciousness
19. bruising
21. cranium; skull
23. reversal of; without
25. disk
27. abnormal; difficult; painful
29. away from the center
31. brain
33. cellular lining
35. feeling; sensation
37. communicate
39. arrangement; structure
41. supporting cells
43. picture; record
45. process of recording
47. one half

49. fluid; water
51. condition; state; thing
53. pertaining to
55. within
57. block; keep back
59. flat area on a vertebra; lamina
61. word
63. lymph; lymphatic system
65. bad; inadequate
67. meninges
69. chin; mind
71. movement
73. myelin
75. sleep; stupor
77. neck
79. mass; tumor
81. having the function of
83. abnormal; apart from; beside; two parts of a pair
85. speech
87. light
89. many; much
91. before; in front of
93. mind
95. four
97. receive
99. spinal nerve root
101. sensation
103. body
105. below; underneath
107. fainting
109. process of cutting; process of making an incision
111. pulling
113. development
115. blood vessel

Related Combining Forms Exercise (p. 518)

1. psych/o-, ment/o-
3. rhiz/o-, radicul/o-
5. epilept/o-, convuls/o-, ict/o-

10.5B Define Abbreviations

Matching Exercise (p. 518)

6, __, 1, __, 7, __, 5, __

10.6A Divide Medical Words

Dividing Words Exercise (p. 518)

1. a-   phas/o-   -ia
3. epi-   dur/o-   -al
5. intra-   crani/o-   -al
7. ____   narc/o-   -lepsy
9. post-   ict/o-   -al

10.6B Build Medical Words

Combining Form and Suffix Exercise (p. 519)

1. mental
3. hematoma

5. biopsy
7. meningitis

9. hydrocephalus
11. concussion
13. infarction
15. neuropathy
17. convulsion
19. comatose
21. syncopal
23. radiculopathy
25. diskectomy

Prefix Exercise (p. 520)

1. intra-   intraventricular
3. post-   postictal
5. poly-   polyneuritis
7. dys-   dyslexic
9. a-   aphasia
11. sub-   subdural
13. poly-   polysomnography
15. dys-   dysphagia

Multiple Combining Forms and Suffix Exercise (p. 520)

1. neurologic
3. myelomeningocele
5. neurofibromatosis
7. neuralgia
9. cerebrovascular
11. cephalalgia

10.7A Spell Medical Words

Proofreading and Spelling Exercise (p. 521)

1. neurosurgery
3. meningioma
5. infarct
7. paralyzed
9. epilepsy

Hearing Medical Words Exercise (p. 521)

1. seizure
3. craniotomy
5. migraine
7. occipital
9. meningitis

10.7B Pronounce Medical Words

Pronunciation Exercise (p. 552)

1. ner
3. fay
5. sef
7. nin
9. at

10.8 Research Medical Words

Sound-Alike Words (p. 522)

1. convulsion: Another name for a seizure
   seizure: Another name for a convulsion
   epilepsy: The condition of having convulsions or seizures. A recurring condition in which a group of neurons in the brain spontaneously sends out electrical impulses in an abnormal, uncoordinated way.
3. The ventricles in the brain contain cerebrospinal fluid. The ventricles in the heart contain blood.

10.9 Analyze Medical Reports

Electronic Patient Record #1 (p. 523)

1. epilepsy
3. *EEG* stands for *electroencephalography*. Multiple electrodes are placed on the scalp overlying specific lobes of the brain. The electrodes are attached by wire leads to an electroencephalograph, a machine that records brain waves.

Electronic Patient Record #2 (pp. 524–525)

1. neur/o-   nerve
   log/o-   study of; word
   -ic   pertaining to
3. VER
5. paresthesias
7. a. light touch
   b. pinprick
   c. vibration
   d. position
   e. 2-point discrimination
9. Romberg
11. blockage of an artery
13. c
15. coordination
17. multiple sclerosis

Chapter 11: Urology

Labeling Exercise (pp. 538–539)

FIRST EXERCISE

1. renal pyramid
3. major calyx
5. cortex
7. hilum

SECOND EXERCISE

1. ureter
3. penis
5. urethral meatus
7. prostatic urethra

THIRD EXERCISE

1. glomerular capsule
3. renal arteriole
5. renal venule
7. distal convoluted tubule

GIVE WORD PART MEANINGS

COMBINING FORMS EXERCISE (pp. 539–540)

1. absorb; take in
3. calyx
5. bladder; fluid-filled sac; semisolid cyst
7. electricity
9. red
11. filtering; straining
13. genitalia

15. indentation
17. kidney; nephron
19. penis
21. prostate gland
23. renal pelvis
25. contraction
27. small tube
29. urethra
31. urinary system; urine

BUILD MEDICAL WORDS

COMBINING FORMS AND SUFFIX EXERCISE (p. 540)

1. -al   mucosal
3. -eal   caliceal
5. -al   vesical
7. -ar   glomerular
9. -ory   excretory
11. -ary   urinary
13. -al   ureteral
15. -al   urethral
17. -tion   micturition

11.1 Identify Anatomical Structures

11.2 Describe Physiology

Unscramble and Match Exercise (p. 563)

1. bladder   9. prostate
3. hilum   11. calices
5. sphincter   13. urethra
7. glomerulus
10, __, 8, __, 7, __, 5, __, 1, __, 11, __, 6

Sequencing Exercise (p. 563)

1. renal artery
3. proximal convoluted tubule
5. distal convoluted tubule
7. calyx
9. ureter
11. urethra

True or False Exercise (p. 563)

1. F   5. T
3. F

11.3A Describe Diseases

Matching Exercise (p. 564)

3, __, 2, __, 9, __, 4, __, 7, __

Antonyms Exercise (p. 564)

1. chronic
3. hypospadias
5. urinary incontinence or enuresis

Synonyms Exercise (p. 564)

1. proteinuria
3. childhood bedwetting
5. Wilms' tumor

True or False Exercise (p. 564)

1. T   7. F
3. F   9. T
5. F   11. T

11.3B Describe Laboratory, Radiology, Surgery, and Drugs

Laboratory Test Exercise (p. 565)

82040	✓	Albumin
82565	✓	Creatinine, Blood
82575	✓	Creatinine Clearance
84520	✓	Blood Urea Nitrogen (BUN)
84550	✓	Uric Acid
81001	✓	Urinalysis, Automated
87086	✓	Urine Culture

Circle Exercise (p. 566)

1. sound waves
3. nephrectomy
5. UA
7. contrast dye

Multiple Choice Exercise (p. 566)

1. c   3. a

11.4 Form Plurals and Adjectives

Plural Noun and Adjective Exercise (p. 566)

1. cortices   cortical
3. glomeruli   glomerular
5. kidneys   renal
7. tubules   tubular
9.   urethral

11.5A Give Word Part Meanings

Word Parts Exercise (pp. 566–567)

1. albumin
3. walking
5. blood vessel; lymphatic vessel
7. composed of; pertaining to
9. bacterium
11. embryonic; immature
13. cancer
15. catheter
17. time
19. hold together
21. cell
23. abnormal; difficult; painful
25. surgical removal
27. state
29. above; upon
31. bend; break up
33. glucose; sugar

35. process of recording
37. blood
39. fluid; water
41. condition; state; thing
43. in; not; within
45. spaces within tissue
47. action; condition
49. condition; state
51. potassium
53. white
55. break down; destroy
57. instrument used to measure
59. dead body; dead cells; dead tissue
61. night
63. mass; tumor
65. condition; process
67. process of surgically fixing in place
69. many; much
71. state of drooping; state of falling
73. pus
75. hold back; keep
77. instrument used to measure
79. affected by; sensitive to
81. sound
83. spasm
85. cut; layer; slice
87. poison
89. move something across and put in another place
91. thing that crushes
93. vagina

Related Combining Forms Exercise (p. 568)

1. cyst/o-; vesic/o-
3. lith/o-; calcul/o-
5. enur/o-; micturi/o-; urin/o-; ur/o-

11.5B Define Abbreviations

Define and Match Exercise (p. 568)

1. blood urea nitrogen
3. chronic renal failure
5. extracorporeal shock wave lithotripsy
7. intravenous pyelography (or pyelogram)
9. kidneys, ureters, bladder
11. urinalysis
7, __, 3, __, 9, __, 10, __, 6, __, 8, __

11.6A Divide Medical Words

Dividing Words Exercise (p. 568)

1.	retro-	peritone/o-	-al
3.	____	electr/o-	-lyte
5.	____	nephr/o-	-pathy
7.	____	vesic/o-	-cele
9.	dys-	ur/o-	-ia
11.	____	catheter/o-	-ization

11.6B Build Medical Words

Combining Form and Suffix Exercise (p. 570)

1. urethritis
3. pyelography
5. cystitis
7. nephropathy
9. cystoscopy
11. urogram
13. lithotripsy
15. nephropexy

Prefix Exercise (p. 570)

1.	hypo-	hypokalemia
3.	poly-	polycystic
5.	an-	anuria
7.	poly-	polyuria
9.	epi-	epispadias

Multiple Combining Forms and Suffix Exercise (pp. 570–571)

1. lithogenesis
3. glomerulosclerosis
5. nephroblastoma
7. nephrolithiasis
9. hematuria
11. glycosuria
13. oliguria
15. ketonuria
17. nocturia

11.7A Spell Medical Words

Hearing Medical Words Exercise (p. 571)

1.	catheter	7.	hemodialysis
3.	cystitis	9.	nocturia
5.	dysuria		

11.7B Pronounce Medical Words

Pronunciation Exercise (p. 571)

1.	nay	7.	frek
3.	taw	9.	fry
5.	mair		

11.8 Research Medical Words

On the Job Challenge Exercise (p. 572)

1. Strangury is a slow and painful discharge of urine because of spasms of the bladder and urethra.

Sound-Alike Words (p. 572)

1. A calculus is a kidney stone.
   The calcaneus is the largest of the ankle bones. It is also known as the *heel bone*.
3. The cortex of the kidney is the outer layer of the kidney, just below the fibrous capsule that surrounds it.
   The cerebral cortex or gray matter is the outermost layer of tissue that follows the curves of the gyri and sulci on the surface of the brain.

The cortex of the adrenal cortex is the outer layer of the adrenal gland; it secretes three groups of hormones: mineralocorticoids, glucocorticoids, and androgens.

11.9 Analyze Medical Reports

Electronic Patient Record (pp. 573–574)

1. ur/o-   urinary system; urine
   log/o-   study of; word
   -ist   person who specializes in; thing that specializes in
3. hemat/o- blood
   ur/o-   urinary system; urine
   -ia   condition; state; thing
5. kidneys, ureters, bladder
   Intravenous
7. clean-catch urine
9. Renal colic is a spasm of the smooth muscle of the ureter or bladder as a kidney stone's jagged edges scrape the mucosa. This causes severe pain, nausea and vomiting, and hematuria.
   Suprapubic pain is pain that is located above the pubis, one of the hip bones.
11. She was given a strainer to strain her urine to catch a kidney stone so that it could be sent to a laboratory for analysis.
13. Because the patient could not be pregnant and the pain was from another source.
15. Because the blood in the urine could not have been from menstruation and was from another source.

Chapter 12: Male Reproductive Medicine

Labeling Exercise (p. 585)

1. vas deferens
3. corpus cavernosum of the penis
5. glans penis
7. ejaculatory duct
9. epididymis
11. scrotum

GIVE WORD PART MEANINGS

COMBINING FORMS EXERCISE (p. 586)

1. beginning of being an adult
3. bulb-like structure
5. testicle; testis
7. stand up
9. genitalia
11. ovum; seed; spermatozoon
13. spaces within tissue
15. testicle; testis
17. testicle; testis
19. penis
21. produce
23. growing up
25. sperm; spermatozoon

27. sperm; spermatozoon
29. testicle; testis
31. tube
33. urinary system; urine
35. blood vessel; vas deferens

BUILD MEDICAL WORDS

COMBINING FORM AND SUFFIX EXERCISE (p. 587)

1. -al   perineal
3. -ty   puberty
5. -ule   tubule
7. -ence   adolescence
9. -ar   testicular
11. -ic   prostatic
13. -al   inguinal

12.1 Identify Anatomical Structures

12.2 Describe Physiology

Fill in the Blank Exerise (p. 601)

1. spermatogenesis
3. testes
5. lumen
7. epididymis
9. spermatic cord
11. flagellum
13. ductus deferens
15. prostate gland

True or False Exercise (p. 601)

1. F   7. T
3. T   9. F
5. F

Circle Exercise (p. 602)

1. scrotum   5. meiosis
3. seminiferous tubules 7. FSH

Sequencing Exercise (p. 602)

1. seminiferous tubules 5. prostatic urethra
3. vas deferens   7. urethral meatus

12.3A Describe Diseases

Matching Exercise (p. 602)

12, __, 7, __, 11, __, 1, __, 5, __, 8, __

Circle Exercise (pp. 602–603)

1. breasts   7. phimosis
3. oligospermia   9. phimosis
5. syphilis

12.3B Describe Laboratory, Radiology, Surgery, and Drugs

Circle Exercise (p. 603)

1. sperm count   5. erectile dysfunction
3. orchiopexy

Fill in the Blank Exercise (p. 603)
1. prosthesis
3. acid phosphatase
5. digital rectal examination
7. vasovasostomy

12.4 Form Plurals and Adjectives

Plural Noun and Adjective Exercise (p. 603)

1.	tubules	tubular
3.	____	perineal
5.	epididymides	____
7.	____	penile

12.5A Give Word Part Meanings

Related Combining Forms Exercise (p. 604)
1. balan/o-, pen/o-
3. didym/o-, test/o-, testicul/o-, orchid/o-, orchi/o-, orch/o-

Word Parts Exercise (p. 604)
1. away from; without
3. state
5. against
7. being; having; process
9. cancer
11. around
13. hidden
15. abnormal; difficult; painful
17. condition of being; condition of having
19. conceive; form
21. picture; record
23. female; woman
25. pertaining to
27. cut into
29. disease from a specific cause; process
31. condition; state
33. study of
35. breast; mastoid process
37. movement
39. mass; tumor
41. condition; process
43. closed tight
45. persistent erection
47. discharge; flow
49. sound
51. development
53. urethra
55. sexual intercourse

12.5B Define Abbreviations

Definition Exercise (p. 605)
1. benign prostatic hypertrophy
3. gonococcus
5. prostate-specific antigen
7. transurethral resection of the prostate

12.6A Divide Medical Words

Dividing Words Exercise (p. 605)

1.	dys-	pareun/o-	-ia
3.	circum-	cis/o-	-ion
5.	a-	sperm/o-	-ia
7.	re-	product/o-	-ive

12.6B Build Medical Words

Prefix Exercise (p. 606)

1.	trans-	transurethral
3.	ultra-	ultrasonography
5.	circum-	circumcision
7.	post-	postcoital
9.	in-	infertility

Combining Form and Suffix Exercise (pp. 606–607)
1. motility
3. cancerous
5. seminoma
7. morphology
9. orchiopexy
11. balanitis
13. biopsy
15. venereal
17. prostatitis
19. phimosis

Multiple Combining Forms and Suffix Exercise (p. 607)
1. immunodeficiency
3. vasovasostomy
5. spermatogenesis
7. oligospermia

12.7A Spell Medical Words

Proofreading and Spelling Exercise (p. 608)

1.	glans	7.	gametes
3.	scrotum	9.	seminal
5.	inguinal		

English and Medical Word Equivalents Exercise (p. 608)
1. seminoma
3. erectile dysfunction
5. cryptorchidism (or cryptorchism)
7. benign prostatic hypertrophy

Hearing Medical Words Exercise (p. 608)

1.	perineum	7.	orchitis
3.	chancre	9.	seminoma
5.	epididymis		

12.7B Pronounce Medical Words

Pronunciation Exercise (p. 609)

1.	pyoo	7.	til
3.	lay	9.	tih
5.	tay		

12.8 Research Medical Words

Sound-Alike Words (p. 609)

1. glans penis: the tip of the penis is known as the *glans penis*
   glands: structures in the endocrine system that produce and secrete hormones directly into the blood and not through ducts

12.9 Analyze Medical Reports

Electronic Patient Record #1 (p. 610)

1. Phimosis is a congenital condition in which the opening of the foreskin is too small to allow the foreskin to pull back over the glans penis.
3. The bladder is full on physical examination because of the patient's inability to initiate a urinary stream, which results in retaining urine in the bladder.
5. Proscar is an androgen inhibitor drug.
7. That procedure reduces the size of the prostate gland. A resectoscope is inserted through the urethra and is used to cut pieces of the prostate gland and cauterize bleeding blood vessels. Chips of prostatic tissue are then irrigated out.

Electronic Patient Record #2 (pp. 611–612)

1. orchi/o-   testicle; testis
   -pexy   process of surgically fixing in place
3. back
5. suprapubic skin on the left side; scrotum (scrotal incision)
7. under the skin
9. before

Chapter 13: Gynecology and Obstetrics

Labeling Exercise (p. 634)

FIRST EXERCISE

1. mons pubis
3. clitoris
5. vaginal introitus
7. vulva
9. anus

SECOND EXERCISE

1. uterine tube
3. intrauterine cavity
5. myometrium
7. cervical canal
9. lumen of uterine tube
11. follicle at time of ovulation
13. fimbriae
15. uterine cervix

GIVE WORD PART MEANINGS

COMBINING FORMS EXERCISE (p. 635)

1. ovum; seed; spermatozoon
3. accessory connecting parts

5. small, circular area
7. cervix; neck
9. vagina
11. pull together
13. blue
15. do away with; obliterate
17. vulva
19. female
21. bear
23. fetus
25. close association; close relationship
27. milk
29. arising from; produced by
31. gonad; ovary; testis
33. uterus; womb
35. block; keep back
37. milk
39. lobe of an organ
41. breast
43. month
45. uterus; womb
47. muscle
49. new
51. ovary
53. egg; ovum
55. egg; ovum
57. giving birth
59. childbirth; labor
61. placenta
63. produce
65. produce; secrete
67. childbirth; labor
69. navel; umbilicus
71. urinary system; urine
73. uterus; womb
75. vulva

BUILD MEDICAL WORDS

COMBINING FORM AND SUFFIX EXERCISE (pp. 636–637)

1. -al   fundal
3. -ine   uterine
5. -an   ovarian
7. -ation   ovulation
9. -al   cervical
11. -tic   amniotic
13. -al   adnexal
15. -ion   conception
17. -ic   embryonic
19. -al   vaginal
21. -ancy   pregnancy
23. -al   perineal
25. -al   placental
27. -ar   vulvar
29. -ion   gestation

PREFIX EXERCISE (p. 637)

1. pre- prenatal
3. re- reproductive
5. peri perimetrium
7. endo- endometrium

MULTIPLE COMBINING FORMS AND SUFFIX
EXERCISE (p. 638)

1. lact/i- fer/o- -ous lactiferous
3. o/o- gen/o- -esis oogenesis
5. ox/y- toc/o- -in oxytocin
7. genit/o- urin/o- -ary genitourinary

13.1 Identify Anatomical Structures
13.2 Describe Physiology
13.3 Describe the Neonate

Matching Exercise (p. 670)
3, __, 3, __, 4, __, 6, __, 7, __, 3, __, 1, __, 6

True or False Exercise (p. 670)

1. T   9. F
3. T   11. F
5. F   13. F
7. T

Fill in the Blank Exercise (p. 671)

1. zygote   9. fetus
3. presenting part 11. trimester
5. gamete   13. false labor
7. umbilical cord

Sequencing Exercise (p. 671)

1. engagement   5. placenta delivered
3. crowning

Matching Exercise (p. 671)
7, __, 9, __, 5, __, 6, __, 2

13.4A Describe Diseases

Matching Exercise (p. 672)
7, __, 1, __, 5, __, 6, __, 8

Circle Exercise (p. 672)

1. breasts
3. ovarian
5. candidiasis
7. hemosalpinx
9. prolapsed cord
11. dyspareunia

Matching Exercise (p. 672)
1, __, 5, __, 4, __, 6, __

13.4B Describe Laboratory, Radiology, Surgery, and Drugs

True or False Exercise (p. 673)

1. F   7. F
3. F   9. T
5. F

Matching Exercise (p. 673)
8, __, 6, __, 2, __, 10, __, 7, __

Multiple Choice Exercise (p. 673)

1. d   3. b

13.5 Form Plurals and Adjectives

Plural Noun and Adjective Exercise (p. 674)

1. areolaè   areolar
3. breasts   mammary
5. fetuses   fetal
7. ova   ____
9. ____   placental
11. ____   uterine

13.6A Give Word Part Meanings

Word Parts Exercise (pp. 674–675)

1. away from; without
3. stop prematurely
5. not; without
7. life; living organism; living tissue
9. *Candida*; yeast
11. procedure to puncture
13. cone
15. bladder; fluid-filled sac; semisolid cyst
17. dura mater
19. seizure
21. outside
23. picture; record
25. pregnancy
27. fluid-filled sacs
29. condition; state; thing
31. sow a seed
33. infection of; inflammation of
35. smooth
37. study of
39. many
41. none
43. few; scanty
45. process of viewing
47. child
49. hanging down
51. process of surgically fixing in place
53. process of reshaping by surgery
55. before; in front of
57. pus
59. backward; behind
61. excessive discharge; excessive flow

63. uterine tube

65. instrument used to examine

67. operative procedure

69. process of cutting; process of making an incision

71. dry

Related Combining Forms Exercise (p. 675)

1. oophor/o-, ovari/o-

3. episi/o-, vulv/o-

5. toc/o-, part/o-, parturit/o-

7. gynec/o-, estr/a-, estr/o-

9. hyster/o-, uter/o-, metri/o-, metr/o-

13.6B Define Abbreviations

Matching Exercise (p. 675)

5, __, 8, __, 11, __, 3, __, 9, __, 6, __, 14, __

13.7A Divide Medical Words

Dividing Words Exercise (p. 676)

1. ____	menstru/o-	-ation
3. ____	ne/o-	-nate
5. poly-	cyst/o-	-ic
7. ____	lact/o-	-ation
9. retro-	vers/o-	-ion

13.7B Build Medical Words

Combining Form and Suffix Exercise (pp. 676–677)

1. nuchal

3. salpingitis

5. cystocele

7. vaginitis

9. cryoprobe

11. laparoscope

13. episiotomy

15. mastitis

17. rectocele

19. colposcopy

21. conization

23. culdoscopy

25. colporrhaphy

27. hysterectomy

29. mammoplasty

Prefix Exercise (pp. 677–678)

1. dys-	dysplasia
3. poly-	polycystic
5. endo-	endometriosis
7. bi-	bimanual
9. pre-	preeclampsia
11. an-	anovulation
13. epi-	epidural

Multiple Combining Forms and Suffix Exercise (p. 678)

1. pyometritis

3. cephalopelvic

5. multiparous

7. cryosurgery

9. oligomenorrhea

13.8A Spell Medical Words

Proofreading and Spelling Exercise (p. 679)

1. gynecologic

3. uterus

5. obstetrical

7. amniocentesis

9. hysterectomy

English and Medical Word Equivalents Exercise (p. 679)

1. mammary glands

3. neonate

5. Braxton Hicks contractions

7. fontanel

9. hyperemesis gravidarum

You Write the Medical Report (pp. 679–680)

1. failure of lactation

3. leukorrhea, *Candida albicans* (or *Candida*), antifungal

5. infertility, salpingitis, polycystic, dyspareunia, laparoscopy, endometriosis

Hearing Medical Words Exercise (p. 680)

1. biopsy

3. mammography

5. amniocentesis

7. dyspareunia

13.8B Pronounce Medical Words

Pronunciation Exercise (p. 680)

1. men

3. mam

5. yoo

7. jy

9. tek

11. aw

13. aw

13.9 Research Medical Words

Sound-Alike Words (p. 680)

1. perineum: area of skin between the vulva and the anus.
peritoneum: double-layer serous membrane that lines the abdominopelvic cavity and surrounds each gastrointestinal organ. It secretes peritoneal fluid to fill the spaces between the organs.

3. colposcopy: procedure that uses a magnifying, lighted scope to visually examine the vagina and cervix.
colonoscopy: procedure that uses a colonoscope inserted through the rectum to visualize and examine the colon.

13.10 Analyze Medical Reports

Electronic Patient Record #1 (p. 681)

1. Menorrhagia: A menstrual period with excessively heavy flow or a menstrual period that lasts longer than 7. days. It is caused by a hormone imbalance, uterine fibroids, or endometriosis.
Oligomenorrhea: A menstrual period with very light flow or intermittent menstrual cycles (longer than 35 days before the next cycle begins) in a woman who previously had normal menstruation. It is caused by a hormone imbalance.
Dysmenorrhea: Painful menstruation. It is caused by pelvic inflammatory disease, endometriosis, or uterine fibroids.
Dyspareunia: Painful or difficult sexual intercourse. It is caused by a hymen across the vaginal introitus or because of infection (of the vagina, cervix, or uterus), pelvic inflammatory disease, endometriosis, or retroflexion of the uterus.

3. No, because during a tubal ligation, a section of the uterine tubes is removed and there is no path for a fertilized ovum to take to get to the uterus.

5. A colposcopy is a medical procedure that uses a magnifying, lighted scope to visually examine the vagina and cervix

7. FSH: follicle-stimulating hormone. LH: luteinizing hormone.

Electronic Patient Record #2 (pp. 682–683)

1. a. appropriate for gestation age

    b. estimated date of confinement

    c. estimated gestational age

    d. neonatal intensive care unit

3. gestat/o- conception to birth

    -ion   action; condition

    -al   pertaining to

5. NSVD

7. version

9. molding

11. The anterior fontanel or soft spot is a soft area on the top of the head. There is also a small posterior fontanel at the back of the head.

13. Mother's temperature was 103.2. degrees, and she was started on an antibiotic drug. The newborn's temperature was 101.2. degrees, and a chest x-ray was taken to rule out pneumonia.

Chapter 14: Endocrinology

Labeling Exercise (pp. 698–699)

FIRST EXERCISE

1. thyroid gland

3. pancreas

5. ovary

7. hypothalamus

9. thymus

SECOND EXERCISE

1. thyroid cartilage of the larynx

3. trachea

5. parathyroid glands

GIVE WORD PART MEANINGS

COMBINING FORMS EXERCISE (p. 700)

1. ovary

3. adrenal gland

5. lead to

7. oppose; work against

9. calcium

11. secrete

13. female

15. milk

17. glucose; sugar

19. glucose; sugar

21. same

23. pituitary gland

25. insulin

27. iodine

29. black

31. nerve

33. pancreas

35. pituitary gland

37. kidney

39. standing still; staying in one place

41. testicle; testis

43. thalamus

45. shield-shaped structure; thyroid gland

47. childbirth; labor

49. having an affinity for; stimulating; turning

51. masculine

BUILD MEDICAL WORDS

COMBINING FORM AND SUFFIX EXERCISE (p. 701)

1. -ic   thymic

3. -gen   androgen

5. -stasis homeostasis

7. -oid   thyroid

9. -ar   testicular

11. -ism   antagonism

PREFIX EXERCISE (p. 701)

1. ad-   adrenal

3. para- parathyroid

5. pro-   prolactin

14.1 Identify Anatomical Structures

14.2 Describe Physiology

Location Exercise (p. 723)

1. in the center of the brain, on top of the brainstem, below the thalamus

3. between the two lobes of the thalamus

5. on the posterior surface of the thyroid gland

7. posterior to the stomach within the abdominal cavity

9. in the pelvic cavity, near the end of each uterine tube

Matching Exercise (p. 723)

anterior pituitary gland 3, 5, 10

pineal gland 11

pancreas 1, 6

adrenal medulla 8

ovaries 9, 12

Circle Exercise (pp. 723–724)

1. adrenal medulla

3. parathyroid glands

5. thymus

7. melatonin

9. antagonism

14.3A Describe Diseases

Matching Exercise (p. 724)

4, __, 2, __, 9, __, 5, __, 6

True or False Exercise (p. 724)

1. T

3. F

5. F

7. F

14.3B Describe Laboratory, Radiology, Surgery, and Drugs

Circle Exercise (p. 724)
1. virilism
3. diabetes insipidus
5. thyroid gland
7. estradiol

Matching Exercise (p. 725)
6, __, 1, __, 3, __

Laboratory Test Exercise (p. 725)

80051	✓	Electrolyte Panel
80053	✓	Metabolic Panel, Comprehensive
82310	✓	Calcium, Total Blood
82670	✓	Estradiol
82947	✓	Glucose, Fasting
82951	✓	Glucose Tolerance Test (GTT)
83036	✓	Hemoglobin A$_{1c}$
84132	✓	Potassium
84144	✓	Progesterone
84146	✓	Prolactin
84295	✓	Sodium
84403	✓	Testosterone, Total
84443	✓	Thyroid-stimulating Hormone (TSH)
84436	✓	Thyroxine (T$_4$), Total
84480	✓	Triiodothyronine (T$_3$), Total

14.4 Form Plurals and Adjectives

Plural Noun and Adjective Exercise (p. 726)
1. ____   pituitary
3. cortices   cortical
5. hormones   hormonal
7. ovaries   ovarian
9. testes   testicular

14.5A Give Word Part Meanings

Word Parts Exercise (p. 726)
1. acid; low pH
3. against
5. life; living organism; living tissue
7. cell
9. right; sugar
11. thirst
13. swelling
15. conceive; form
17. conception to birth
19. female; woman
21. above; more than normal
23. condition; state; thing
25. disease from a specific cause; process
27. ketones
29. breast; mastoid process
31. month
33. mucus-like substance
35. nerve

37. not
39. process of viewing
41. childbirth; labor
43. cessation
45. gray
47. retina of the eye
49. sphenoid bone; sphenoid sinus
51. poison; toxin
53. urinary system; urine

14.5B Define Abbreviations

Abbreviation Exercise (p. 727)
1. IDDM
3. FBG or FBS
5. ADA
7. SAD
9. IRS

14.6A Divide Medical Words

Dividing Words Exercise (p. 727)
1. syn-   erg/o-   -ism
3. ____   home/o-   -stasis
5. ____   galact/o-   -rrhea
7. hypo-   glyc/o-   -emia
9. ____   thyroid/o-   -ectomy

14.6B Build Medical Words

Combining Form and Suffix Exercise (pp. 727–728)
1. toxic
3. hypophysectomy
5. adenoma
7. diabetic
9. hirsutism
11. myxedema
13. gigantism
15. virilism

Prefix Exercise (p. 728)
1. hyper-   hypercalcemia
3. in-   infertility
5. en-   endemic
7. para-   parathyroidectomy
9. hyper-   hyperglycemia

Multiple Combining Forms and Suffix Exercise (p. 729)
1. multinodular
3. adrenogenital
5. gynecomastia

14.7A Spell Medical Words

Proofreading and Spelling Exercise (p. 729)
1. endocrinology
3. mellitus
5. medulla
7. thyroidectomy
9. thyromegaly

Hearing Medical Words Exercise (p. 729)
1. diabetes
3. glandular
5. infertility
7. thyroidectomy

14.7B Pronounce Medical Words

Pronunciation Exercise (p. 730)
1. hor
3. kor
5. naw
7. too

14.8 Research Medical Words

Sound-Alike Words (p. 730)

1. endocrine gland: gland of the endocrine system that produces and secretes one or more hormones into the blood
   exocrine gland: gland that secretes substances through a duct.
3. diabetes insipidus: hyposecretion of antidiuretic hormone by the posterior pituitary gland.
   diabetes mellitus: hyposecretion of insulin by the beta cells of the pancreas.

14.9 Analyze Medical Reports

Electronic Patient Record (pp. 731–732)

1. endo-   innermost; within
   crin/o-   secrete
   log/o-   study of; word
   -ist   person who specializes in; thing that specializes in
3. TSH
5. testosterone (transdermal patches), thyroid replacement hormone (Synthroid)
7. hypothyroidism
9. pituitary gland (surgical removal of an adenoma)

Chapter 15: Ophthalmology

Labeling Exercise (p. 746)

FIRST EXERCISE

1. lacrimal gland
3. iris
5. pupil
7. lacrimal sac
9. nasolacrimal duct

SECOND EXERCISE

1. sclera
3. conjunctiva
5. cornea
7. iris
9. choroid
11. optic disk
13. fovea
15. posterior cavity

GIVE WORD PART MEANINGS

COMBINING FORMS EXERCISE (p. 747)

1. adapt
3. watery substance
5. capsule; enveloping structure
7. choroid of the eye
9. conjunctiva of the eye
11. pupil of the eye
13. lacrimal sac; tears
15. bend; break up
17. fundus; part farthest from the opening
19. iris of the eye
21. cornea of the eye; hard, fibrous protein
23. side

25. lens of the eye
27. middle
29. movement
31. nose
33. eye
35. eye; vision
37. lens of the eye
39. pupil of the eye
41. hard; sclera of the eye
43. three dimensions
45. mesh
47. sight; vision

BUILD MEDICAL WORDS

COMBINING FORM AND SUFFIX EXERCISE (p. 748)

1. -al   corneal
3. -ual   visual
5. -al   scleral
7. -ic   optic
9. -ar   macular
11. -ion   vision
13. -al   conjunctival

15.1 Identify Anatomical Structures

15.2 Describe Physiology

Matching Exercise (p. 767)

8, __, 9, __, 5, __, 10, __, 12, __, 2, __

Circle Exercise (p. 767)

1. iris
3. sclera
5. cones

True or False Exercise (p. 767)

1. F
3. T
5. T
7. T

Sequencing Exercise (p. 768)

1. light rays from an object
3. cornea
5. lens
7. fovea of the retina

15.3A Describe Diseases

Circle Exercise (p. 768)

1. nystagmus
3. glaucoma
5. hyperopia

Matching Exercise (p. 768)

7, __, 3, __, 6, __, 2, __

15.3B Describe Laboratory, Radiology, Surgery, and Drugs

True or False Exercise (p. 768)

1. T
3. T

Fill in the Blank Exercise (p. 769)
1. peripheral vision
3. accommodation
5. penlight
7. tonometry
9. retinopexy
11. angiogram
13. trabeculoplasty
15. phacoemulsification

15.4 Form Plurals and Adjectives

Plural Noun and Adjective Exercise (p. 769)
1. pupils   pupillary
3. irides   iridal
5. fundi   fundal

15.5A Give Word Part Meanings

Word Parts Exercise (p. 770)
1. away from; without
3. not; without
5. unequal
7. embryonic; immature
9. joined together
11. cold
13. double
15. surgical removal
17. liquid with suspended particles
19. inward
21. angle
23. process of recording
25. above; more than normal
27. jaundice
29. action; condition
31. infection of; inflammation of
33. instrument used to measure
35. process of measuring
37. process of carving
39. new
41. elevated structure
43. process of surgically fixing in place
45. bear; carry; range
47. process of reshaping by surgery
49. before; in front of
51. state of drooping; state of falling
53. process of using an instrument to examine
55. sound
57. process of cutting; process of making an incision
59. having an affinity for; stimulating; turning
61. blood vessel

Related Combining Forms Exercise (p. 770)
1. kerat/o-, corne/o-
3. cor/o-, pupill/o-
5. phac/o-, phak/o-, lent/o-, lenticul/o-

15.5B Define Abbreviations

Matching Exercise (p. 771)
7, __, 1, __, 3, __, 4, __

15.6A Divide Medical Words

Dividing Words Exercise (p. 771)
1. intra-   capsul/o-   -ar
3. extra-   ocul/o-   -ar
5. a-   phak/o-   -ia
7. a-   stigmat/o-   -ism

15.6B Build Medical Words

Combining Form and Suffix Exercise (pp. 771–772)
1. conjunctivitis
3. blepharitis
5. gonioscopy
7. blepharoptosis
9. convergence
11. cryotherapy
13. funduscopy
15. blepharoplasty

Prefix Exercise (p. 772)
1. en-   entropion
3. extra-   extracapsular
5. an-   anicteric
7. retro-   retrolental

Multiple Combining Forms and Suffix Exercise (p. 773)
1. esotropia
3. microkeratome
5. retinoblastoma
7. cycloplegia
9. phacoemulsification
11. optometrist
13. presbyopia

15.7A Spell Medical Words

Proofreading and Spelling Exercise (p. 774)
1. visual
3. conjunctiva
5. macula
7. cataract
9. funduscopic

Hearing Medical Words Exercise (p. 774)
1. amblyopia
3. cycloplegia
5. ophthalmologist
7. presbyopia
9. tonometer

15.7B Pronounce Medical Words

Pronunciation Exercise (p. 774)
1. ty
3. vy
5. koh
7. taw
9. pek

15.8 Research Medical Words

Sound-Alike Words (p. 774)
1. fundus of the eye: general word for the retina because it is the area farthest from the opening (pupil)
   fundus of the stomach: rounded, top part of the stomach
   fundus of the uterus: rounded top part of the uterus
3. macula: Dark yellow-orange area with indistinct edges on the retina. It contains the fovea.
   macule: A skin lesion that is a flat circle and is pigmented brown or black, such as a freckle or age spot.

15.9 Analyze Medical Reports

Electronic Patient Record (p. 775)

1. fundal or funduscopic
3. an-not; without

   icter/o-   jaundice

   -ic   pertaining to
5. myopia
7. False. It is just scar tissue.
9. O.D.
11. sclerae were nonicteric
13. because of her mild exophthalmos bilaterally

Chapter 16: Otolaryngology

Labeling Exercise (pp. 789–790)

FIRST EXERCISE

1. temporal bone
3. incus
5. tympanic membrane
7. mastoid bone
9. eustachian tube
11. oval window
13. cochlear branch of the vestibulocochlear nerve
15. vestibule

SECOND EXERCISE

1. sphenoid sinus	13. frontal sinus
3. adenoids	15. nasal cavity
5. nasopharynx	17. oral cavity
7. palatine tonsil	19. mandible
9. lingual tonsil	21. trachea
11. laryngopharynx	

GIVE WORD PART MEANINGS

COMBINING FORMS EXERCISE (p. 791)

1. hearing; sound
3. structure resembling a gland
5. sense of hearing
7. ear
9. hollow space
11. circle
13. back; dorsum
15. outside
17. tongue
19. anvil-shaped bone; incus
21. labium; lip
23. larynx; voice box
25. hammer-shaped bone; malleus
27. breast; mastoid process
29. maxilla; upper jaw
31. mucous membrane
33. nose
35. bone
37. ear
39. pharynx; throat
41. dividing wall; septum
43. wedge shape
45. above
47. tonsil
49. eardrum; tympanic membrane
51. voice

BUILD MEDICAL WORDS

COMBINING FORM AND SUFFIX EXERCISE (p. 792)

1.	-al	palatal
3.	-ory	auditory
5.	-al	septal
7.	-ar	tonsillar
9.	-ial	stapedial
11.	-eal	pharyngeal
13.	-pharynx	nasopharynx
15.	-al	mucosal
17.	-al	oral
19.	-cle	auricle
21.	-eal	laryngeal

16.1 Identify Anatomical Structures

16.2 Describe Physiology

Matching Exercise (p. 810)

External ear	5, 12, 16
Inner ear	3, 13, 18
Nasal cavity	4, 9, 17

True or False Exercise (p. 810)

1.	T	5.	T
3.	T	7.	F

Sequencing Exercise (p. 810)

1.	external auditory canal	7.	vestibule
3.	malleus	9.	vestibulocochlear nerve
5.	stapes		

16.3A Describe Diseases

True or False Exercise (p. 811)

1.	F	5.	F
3.	T	7.	F

Matching Exercise (p. 811)

1, __, 8, __, 4, __, 5, __, 10, __

16.3B Describe Laboratory, Radiology, Surgery, and Drugs

Fill in the Blank Exercise (p. 811)

1.	Rinne test	7.	antihistamine
3.	CT scan	9.	cochlear implant
5.	culture		

16.4 Form Plurals and Adjectives

Plural Noun and Adjective Exercise (p. 812)
1. incudes   incudal
3. stapedes   stapedial
5. ____   pharyngeal

16.5A Give Word Part Meanings

Word Parts Exercise (p. 812)
1. pain
3. not; without
5. two
7. accumulation of fluid
9. pouring out
11. blood
13. action; condition
15. side
17. study of; word
19. instrument used to measure
21. nerve
23. condition; process
25. all
27. growth; tumor
29. process of reshaping by surgery
31. after; behind
33. discharge; flow
35. examine with an instrument
37. process of using an instrument to examine
39. serum-like fluid; serum of the blood
41. surgically created opening
43. area with distinct edges; instrument used to cut
45. cough

Related Combining Forms Exercise (p. 813)
1. tympan/o-, myring/o-
3. rhin/o-, nas/o-
5. acous/o-, audi/o-, audit/o-

16.5B Define Abbreviations

Matching Exercise (p. 813)
6, __, 5, __, 4, __, 3

16.6A Divide Medical Words

Dividing Words Exercise (p. 813)
1. ____   tympan/o-   -ic
3. semi-   circul/o-   -ar
5. sub-   lingu/o-   -al
7. ____   rhin/o-   -plasty

16.6B Build Medical Words

Combining Form and Suffix Exercise (pp. 814–815)
1. acoustic
3. labyrinthitis
5. rhinorrhea
7. tonsillitis
9. rhinophyma
11. suppurative
13. septoplasty
15. myringotome
17. otorrhea
19. cheiloplasty
21. glossectomy
23. laryngitis
25. rhinoplasty
27. rhinitis
29. allergic

Prefix Exercise (p. 815)
1. bi-   bilateral
3. post-   postnasal
5. de-   decongestant
7. pan-   pansinusitis

Multiple Combining Forms and Suffix Exercise (p. 816)
1. sensorineural
3. lymphadenopathy
5. otosclerosis
7. otorhinolaryngologist

16.7A Spell Medical Words

English and Medical Word Equivalents Exercise (p. 816)
1. external auditory canal
3. cerumen
5. incus
7. naris
9. larynx
11. upper respiratory infection
13. epistaxis
15. pharyngitis

Hearing Medical Words Exercise (p. 817)
1. adenoids
3. cheiloplasty
5. epistaxis
7. laryngitis
9. sinusitis

16.7B Pronounce Medical Words

Pronunciation Exercise (p. 817)
1. koh
3. rih
5. tim
7. tal
9. dih

16.8 Research Medical Words

Sound-Alike Words (p. 817)
1. epistaxis: sudden, sometimes severe bleeding from the nose. It is due to irritation or dryness of the nasal mucous membranes and the rupture of a small artery, or it can be caused by trauma to the nose.
   rhinorrhea: clear mucus discharge from the nose.
3. mastoiditis: infection or inflammation of the bony projection of the temporal bone that is behind the ear.
   mastitis: infection or inflammation of the breast.

16.9 Analyze Medical Reports

Electronic Patient Record #1 (p. 818)
1. rhinitis medicamentosa: inflammation of the nose (mucous membranes) due to the excessive use of topical nasal decongestant drugs.
3. Because of allergies

Electronic Patient Record #2 (pp. 819–820)

1. sinus/o-   sinus
   -itis   infection of; inflammation of
3. tympanic membranes
5. palpation of the forehead and cheekbone areas bilaterally
7. amoxicillin
9. frontal sinuses and maxillary sinuses
11. increased fever, severe pain and pressure in the sinuses, increasing fatigue, dizziness, pain in the ears

Chapter 17: Psychiatry

GIVE WORD PART MEANINGS
COMBINING FORMS EXERCISE (p. 827)

1. almond shape
3. structure that surrounds
5. border; edge
7. send across; send through

BUILD MEDICAL WORDS
COMBINING FORM AND SUFFIX EXERCISE (p. 827)

1. -oid   amygdaloid
3. -ion   emotion

17.1 Identify Anatomical Structures
17.2 Describe Physiology

Matching Exercise (p. 847)

6, __, 1, __, 1, __, 3, __

True or False Exercise (p. 847)

1. F
3. F
5. F
7. T

Matching Exercise (p. 847)

1, 4, 5; __; 2; __; 2; __

17.3A Describe Mental Disorders

Circle Exercise (p. 848)

1. panic
3. delirium tremens
5. echolalia
7. depression
9. Munchausen by proxy

Matching Exercise (p. 848)

6, __, 1, __, 5, __, 13, __, 4, __, 3, __, 9, __

True or False Exercise (p. 848)

1. T
3. F
5. F
7. T

Matching Exercise (p. 849)

4, __, 5, __, 3, __, 1, __

17.3B Describe Laboratory and Diagnostic Procedures, Therapies, and Drugs

True or False Exercise (p. 849)

1. T
3. T
5. F
7. F
9. T

Matching Exercise (p. 849)

7, __, 2, __, 4, __, 6

17.4 Form Plurals and Adjectives

Plural Noun and Adjective Exercise (p. 849)

1. emotions   emotional
3. ____   manic
5. delusions   delusional
7. ____   affective

17.5A Give Word Part Meanings

Word Parts Exercise (p. 850)

1. extremity; highest point
3. open area; open space
5. not; without
7. fear; worry
9. being; having; process
11. two
13. enclosed space
15. compel; drive
17. ciliary body of the eye; circle; cycle
19. press down
21. echo of a sound wave
23. condition; process
25. artificial; made up
27. imagined perception
29. pleasure
31. sleep
33. medical treatment; physician
35. disease from a specific cause; process
37. condition of speech
39. frenzy; thin
41. one millionth; small
43. new
45. snake
47. attraction to; fondness for
49. avoidance; fear
51. diaphragm; mind
53. after; behind
55. burning; fire
57. split
59. community; human beings
61. disturbing stimulus
63. death
65. treatment
67. pull out
69. injury
71. foreign

17.5B Define Abbreviations

Matching Exercise (p. 851)

5, __, 3, __, 9, __, 6, __, 2

17.6A Divide Medical Words

Dividing Words Exercise (p. 851)

1. an-   orex/o-   -ia
3. dys- thym/o-   -ia
5. bi-   pol/o-   -ar
7. de-   ment/o-   -ia

17.6B Build Medical Words

Combining Form and Suffix Exercise (pp. 851–852)

1. compulsion
3. hypnosis
5. cognitive
7. hallucinogen
9. psychotherapy
11. factitious
13. autism
15. obsession
17. rapist

Prefix Exercise (p. 852)

1. dys-   dysmorphic
3. post-   posttraumatic
5. an-   anhedonia

Multiple Combining Forms and Suffix Exercise (p. 853)

1. microphobia
3. claustrophobia
5. suicidal
7. arachnophobia
9. psychiatric
11. ophidiophobia
13. homicidal
15. pyromania

17.7A Spell Medical Words

Proofreading and Spelling Exercise (p. 854)

1. psychiatry
3. dopamine
5. dysthymia
7. homicidal
9. personality
11. narcissistic
13. therapeutic

Hearing Medical Words Exercise (p. 854)

1. addiction
3. delusion
5. euphoria
7. milieu
9. psychiatrist

17.7B Pronounce Medical Words

Pronunciation Exercise (p. 854)

1. pan
3. leer
5. noh
7. ky

17.8 Research Medical Words

Sound-Alike Words (p. 854)

1. anorexia nervosa: extreme, chronic fear of being fat and an obsession to become thinner. The patient decreases food intake to the point of starvation.

   anorexia: decreased appetite because of disease or the gastrointestinal side effects of a drug.

17.9 Analyze Medical Reports

Electronic Patient Record (pp. 855–856)

1. psych/o-   mind
   soci/o-   community; human beings
   -al   pertaining to
3. hom/i-   man
   cid/o-   killing
   -al   pertaining to
5. A factitious disorder is a mental illness characterized by physical or psychological symptoms that are consciously made up (fabricated) by the patient and that the patient knows are not true.
7. She has been taking Cymbalta 20 P.O. at bedtime, as prescribed; however, she has also obtained another prescription for a tricyclic antidepressant drug from another physician and is taking this as well as Ambien for sleep.
9. A delusion is a continued false belief concerning events of everyday life. A hallucination is also a false belief, but it is a false impression of the senses.

Chapter 18: Oncology

GIVE WORD PART MEANINGS

COMBINING FORMS EXERCISE (p. 867)

1. distinct; specialized
3. cancer
5. cancer
7. color
9. gene
11. genetic inheritance
13. go into
15. place
17. cancer; intentionally causing harm
19. change
21. dead body; dead cells; dead tissue
23. mass; tumor
25. disease
27. formation; growth
29. ribonucleic acid
31. standing still; staying in one place

BUILD MEDICAL WORDS

COMBINING FORM AND SUFFIX EXERCISE (p. 868)

1. -ar   nuclear
3. -osis   necrosis
5. -tic   genetic
7. -ar   cellular
9. -gene   oncogene
11. -plasm   cytoplasm
13. -ion   mutation
15. -osis   mitosis

18.1 Identify Cellular Structures
18.2A Describe Normal Cell Division

Matching Exercise (p. 889)

2, __, 6, __, 7, __, 8, __, 9, __

True or False Exercise (p. 889)

1. F
3. F

5. F
7. F

18.2B Describe How a Normal Cell Becomes Cancerous

Circle Exercise (p. 889)

1. Translocation
3. carcinogen

5. benign

18.3 Describe Characteristics of Cancerous Cells

True or False Exercise (p. 890)

1. F
3. T

5. F
7. T

18.4A Describe Types of Cancer

True or False Exercise (p. 890)

1. F
3. F
5. F

7. T
9. T

Matching Exercise (p. 890)

9, __, 6, __, 4, __, 3, __, 1, __, 8

Fill in the Blank Exercise (p. 891)

C: Change in bowel or bladder habits.
U: Unusual bleeding or discharge.
I: Indigestion or trouble swallowing.
N: Nagging cough or hoarseness.

18.4B Describe Laboratory, Surgery, Radiation Therapy, and Drugs

Matching Exercise (p. 891)

8, __, 6, __, 5, __, 1, __

True or False Exercise (p. 891)

1. F
3. T

5. F
7. F

Matching Exercise (p. 891)

8, __, 4, __, 3, __, 5, __

Circle Exercise (p. 892)

1. Adjuvant therapy
3. excising the tumor and surrounding structures as one block of tissue

18.5A Give Word Part Meanings

Word Parts Exercise (pp. 892–893)

1. gland
3. star-like structure
5. embryonic; immature
7. cancer
9. bile duct
11. chorion
13. cell
15. cut apart
17. embolus; occluding plug
19. condition of the blood; substance in the blood
21. cut out
23. arising from; produced by
25. picture; record
27. liver
29. within
31. process of creating; process of inserting; process of making
33. white
35. study of; word
37. cancer; intentionally causing harm
39. black
41. muscle
43. new
45. nerve
47. mass; tumor
49. process of viewing
51. bone
53. formed substance; growth
55. forearm bone; radiation; x-rays
57. send back
59. withstand the effect of
61. rod shaped
63. process of using an instrument to examine
65. sound
67. operative procedure
69. treatment
71. beyond; higher

Related Combining Forms Exercise (p. 893)

1. carcin/o-, cancer/o-
3. kary/o-, nucle/o-

18.5B Define Abbreviations

Matching Exercise #1 (p. 893)

2, __, 1, __, 6, __

Matching Exercise #2 (p. 893)

7, __, 2, __, 6, __, 1

18.6A Divide Medical Words

Dividing Words Exercise (p. 894)

1. ____	carcin/o-	-gen
3. ____	kary/o-	-type
5. en-	capsul/o-	-ated
7. meta-	stat/o-	-ic
9. ____	leuk/o-	-emia

18.6B Build Medical Words

Combining Form and Suffix Exercise (p. 894)

1. carcinoid		**9.** leukemia
3. seminoma		**11.** biopsy
5. neoplasm		**13.** cytology
7. carcinoma		**15.** karyotype

Multiple Combining Forms and Suffix Exercise (p. 895)

1. hepatoblastoma		**9.** retinoblastoma
3. liposarcoma		**11.** chondrosarcoma
5. cryosurgery		**13.** oncologist
7. lymphadenopathy		

18.7A Spell Medical Words

Hearing Medical Words Exercise (p. 896)

1. adenocarcinoma		**7.** metastatic
3. cryosurgery		**9.** oncologist
5. lymphadenopathy		

18.7B Pronounce Medical Words

Pronunciation Exercise (p. 896)

1. kan		**7.** play
3. nine		**9.** ek
5. sin		

18.8 Analyze Medical Reports

Electronic Patient Records #1, #2, and #3 (pp. 897–900)

1. She performs occasional self-examination of her breasts. While doing this 2 days ago, she noted a lump in her right breast.
3. A solid rather than cystic mass
5. Rule out carcinoma of the breast
7. A frozen section involves freezing a tissue specimen obtained from a biopsy. Thin slices of the specimen are stained and then examined under a microscope.
9. Infiltrating ductal carcinoma, poorly differentiated, grade 3.
11. Right mastectomy and axillary lymph node dissection.
13. 10 of the 28 axillary lymph nodes were positive for metastasis
15. The margins of resection are free of tumor.

Chapter 19: Radiology and Nuclear Medicine

19.1 Describe X-ray Procedures

19.2 Describe X-ray Projections and Positions

19.3 Identify Radiology Procedures That Use X-rays, X-rays and Contrast, a Magnetic Field, Sound Waves, or an Electron Beam

19.4 Identify Nuclear Medicine Procedures That Use Gamma Rays or Positrons

Matching Exercise (p. 918)

7, __, 9, __, 8, __, 3, __, 10, __

Circle Exercise (p. 918)

1. scout		**5.** MUGA
3. EBT		

Recall and List Exercise (p. 919)

Any 10 of these items are correct answers: glasses, watches, jewelry, hairpins, metal false teeth, artificial limbs, clothing with metal zippers, metal buttons or snaps, nose rings, lip rings, tongue studs, pierced earrings, implanted pacemakers or pacing wires, some heart valves, aneurysm clips, cochlear implants, some penile implants, artificial eyes, some intrauterine devices, hearing aids, TENS units, insulin pumps, persons who are metal workers, persons who are gunshot victims, persons who are military personnel, transdermal patches, metallic eye shadow.

Fill in the Blank Exercise (p. 919)

1. light box		**5.** Doppler
3. film badge		

True or False Exercise (p. 919)

1. T		**7.** T
3. F		**9.** T
5. F		

Multiple Choice Exercise (p. 920)

1. b		**3.** b

Matching Exercise (p. 920)

4, __, 3, __, 8, __, 10, __, 9, __, 7

19.5A Give Word Part Meanings

Word Parts Exercise (pp. 920–921)

1. action
3. before; front part
5. artery
7. composed of; pertaining to a condition
9. axis
11. bile duct

13. movement

15. density

17. bring; move

19. electricity

21. removing from the body

23. pouring

25. knowledge

27. instrument used to record

29. uterus; womb

31. iodine

33. side

35. clear

37. magnet

39. instrument used to measure

41. bone marrow; myelin; spinal cord

43. having the function of

45. drug; medicine

47. orientation

49. amount; quantity

51. radiation; x-rays

53. point of light

55. sound

57. cut; layer; slice

59. urinary system; urine

61. movement of air

63. chamber that is filled; ventricle

19.5B Define Abbreviations

Abbreviation Exercise (p. 921)

1. multiple-gated acquisition (scan)

3. barium enema

5. ultrasound

7. intravenous pyelography

9. kidneys, ureters, bladder

19.6A Divide Medical Words

Dividing Words Exercise (p. 922)

1. ____ radi/o- -logy

3. intra- ven/o- -ous

5. ____ tom/o- -graphy

7. ____ dos/i- -meter

19.6B Build Medical Words

Combining Form and Suffix Exercise (pp. 922–923)

1. nuclear

3. iodinated

5. mammogram

7. fluoroscopy

9. axial

11. arthrography

13. venography

15. tracer

17. urogram

19. densitometry

21. pyelogram

Multiple Combining Forms and Suffix Exercise (p. 923)

1. posteroanterior

3. cineradiography

5. xeromammogram

7. radiopharmaceutical

19.7A Spell Medical Words

Hearing Medical Words Exercise (p. 924)

1. barium

3. cholecystogram

5. echocardiogram

7. lymphangiogram

9. tomography

19.7B Pronounce Medical Words

Pronunciation Exercise (p. 924)

1. aw

3. thraw

5. aw

7. mam

9. maw

19.8 Analyze Medical Reports

Electronic Patient Record #1 (p. 925)

1. anteroposterior

3. operating room

5. an orthopedic device, such as an artificial joint

Electronic Patient Record #2 (p. 926)

1. c

3. multiple

Electronic Patient Record #3 (p. 927)

1. iodine-123 (I-123), technetium-99m

3. 7–24%

5. intravenous injection

7. uniform uptake throughout both the right and left lobes

Index